ANTE BILIĆ D.M.D.
41000 ZAGREB — NAZOROVA 2
Telefon: (041) 437 - 012
YUGOSLAVIA

Ante Bilić
09. 08. 1987.

HANDBOOK OF EXPERIMENTAL IMMUNOLOGY
VOLUME 2: CELLULAR IMMUNOLOGY

HANDBOOK OF EXPERIMENTAL IMMUNOLOGY
IN FOUR VOLUMES

Volume 2: Cellular Immunology

EDITED BY

D. M. WEIR MD, FRCP

Professor of Microbial Immunology,
University of Edinburgh, Scotland

CO-EDITORS

L. A. Herzenberg PhD

Professor of Genetics,
Stanford University, USA

Caroline Blackwell PhD

Lecturer, Department of Bacteriology,
University of Edinburgh, Scotland

Leonore A. Herzenberg DSc

Senior Research Associate, Department of Genetics,
Stanford University, USA

FOURTH EDITION

BLACKWELL SCIENTIFIC PUBLICATIONS

OXFORD   LONDON   EDINBURGH

BOSTON   PALO ALTO   MELBOURNE

First published 1967
Second edition 1973
Third edition 1978
Reprinted 1979
Fourth Edition 1986

Printed in Great Britain
at the Alden Press, Oxford

DISTRIBUTORS
USA
    Blackwell Scientific Publications Inc
    PO Box 50009, Palo Alto
    California 94303

    Blackwell Mosby Book Distributors
    11830 Westline Industrial Drive
    St Louis, Missouri 63141

Canada
    The C. V. Mosby Company
    5240 Finch Avenue East
    Scarborough, Ontario

Australia
    Blackwell Scientific Publications
        (Australia) Pty Ltd
    107 Barry Street
    Carlton, Victoria 3053

British Library
Cataloguing in Publication Data

Handbook of experimental immunology.—4th ed. 1.
    Immunology—Laboratory manuals I. Weir,
    D.M. II. Herzenberg, L.A. III. Blackwell,
    C. IV. Herzenberg, Leonore A. 599.02′9′028
    QR183

ISBN 0-632-01499-7
ISBN 0-632-00975-6 v. 1
ISBN 0-632-01378-8 v. 2
ISBN 0-632-01379-6 v. 3
ISBN 0-632-01381-8 v. 4

Contents

List of contributors   xi

Preface   xvii

VOLUME 2
CELLULAR IMMUNOLOGY

Phagocytes

41 Overview: The function of receptors in phagocytosis
S. D. WRIGHT AND S. C. SILVERSTEIN

42 Overview: The mononuclear phagocyte system
R. VAN FURTH

43 Plasma membrane markers to study differentiation, activation and localization of murine macrophages. Ag F4/80 and the mannosyl, fucosyl
receptor
S. GORDON, PHYLLIS M. STARKEY, D. HUME,
R. A. B. EZEKOWITZ, S. HIRSCH AND J.
AUSTYN

44 Methods for studying the ontogeny of
mononuclear phagocytes
C. C. STEWART

45 Macrophage cell lines
P. RALPH

46 *In vitro* determination of phagocytosis and
intracellular killing by polymorphonuclear and
mononuclear phagocytes
P. C. J. LEIJH, R. VAN FURTH AND THEDA L.
VAN ZWET

47 Secreted proteins of resting and activated mac-
rophages
ZENA WERB, M. J. BANDA, R. TAKEMURA
AND S. GORDON

48 Macrophage membrane receptors
J. STEWART, ELIZABETH J. GLASS, D. M.
WEIR AND M. R. DAHA

49 Dendritic cells
R. M. STEINMAN, W. C. VAN VOORHIS AND
D. M. SPALDING

50 Reduction and excitation of oxygen by phagocytic leukocytes: biochemical and cytochemical
techniques
J. A. BADWEY, J. M. ROBINSON, M. J. KAR-
NOVSKY AND M. L. KARNOVSKY

51 Locomotion and chemotaxis of leukocytes
P. C. WILKINSON

52 Assays for phagocyte ecto-enzymes
P. J. EDELSON

The lymphoid system

53 Overview: Lymphocytes and their relations
H. S. MICKLEM

54 Physical methods for separation of lymphocyte
subpopulations
R. G. MILLER

55 Preparative immunoselection of lymphocyte
populations
S. V. HUNT

56 Genetic markers for following cell populations
J. D. ANSELL AND H. S. MICKLEM

57 Following cellular traffic: methods of labelling
lymphocytes and other cells to trace their migration *in vivo*
E. C. BUTCHER AND W. L. FORD

58 Human leukocyte subpopulations
P. BEVERLEY

59 Lymphokines
J. KAPPLER AND PHILLIPA MARRACK

60 Natural killer cells
H. WIGZELL AND U. RAMSTEDT

61 Genetics and cell distributions of mouse cell
surface alloantigens
LORRAINE FLAHERTY AND J. FORMAN

Lymphocyte responses

62 Overview: Lymphocyte responses
G. J. V. NOSSAL

63 Lymphocyte responses to polyclonal B and T cell activators
EVA SEVERINSON AND EVA-LOTTA LARSSON

64 Assays for immunoglobulin-secreting cells
D. W. DRESSER

65 Limiting dilution analysis of effector cells and their precursors *in vitro*
M. ZAUDERER

66 *In vitro* evaluation of human lymphocyte function
H. C. LANE, GAIL WHALEN AND A. S. FAUCI

67 Assay for *in vivo* adoptive immune response
G. M. IVERSON

68 Analysis of cytotoxic T cell responses
ELIZABETH SIMPSON AND P. CHANDLER

69 T cell lines and hybrids in mouse and man
C. G. FATHMAN AND E. G. ENGLEMAN

70 B cell growth factors
MAUREEN HOWARD

Immunoregulation

71 Overview: Helper and suppressor T cells
K. OKUMARA AND T. TADA

72 Overview: Ir genes
B. BENACERRAF

73 Overview: Idiotypic regulation
K. RAJEWSKY

74 Overview: Epitope-specific regulation
LEONORE A. HERZENBERG

75 Overview: T cell clones
H. CANTOR

76 Subtractive cDNA hybridization and the T-cell receptor genes
M. M. DAVIS

77 Detection of suppressor cells and suppressor factors for delayed-type hypersensitivity responses
S. D. MILLER AND M. K. JENKINS

78 Detection of suppressor cells and suppressor factors for antibody responses
C. WALTENBAUGH AND B. S. KIM

79 Contrasuppressor T cells: a practical guide to the identification of contrasuppressive effects in immunoregulatory systems
D. R. GREEN

80 Antigen-specific suppressor molecules produced by T cells
M. TANIGUCHI AND T. TOKUHISA

81 Immunosuppressive agents
D. J. G. WHITE AND J. F. L. SHAW

82 Studies of autoimmune diseases
ELIZABETH S. RAVECHE AND A. D. STEINBERG

83 Primary immunodeficiencies: definitions and diagnosis
F. S. ROSEN

84 Studying immune regulation with protein and peptide antigens
N. SHASTRI AND E. E. SERCARZ

**VOLUME 1
IMMUNOCHEMISTRY**

Antigens

1 Overview: Antigens
M. SELA

2 Preparation of synthetic antigens
M. SELA AND SARA FUCHS

3 Haptens and carriers
O. MÄKELÄ AND I. J. T. SEPPÄLÄ

4 Isolation and identification of bacterial antigens
I. R. POXTON AND C. CAROLINE BLACKWELL

5 Preparation of viral antigens
C. J. BURRELL

6 Antigens of parasites
T. W. PEARSON AND M. W. CLARK

7 Fungal antigens
JOAN L. LONGBOTTOM AND P. K. C. AUSTWICK

8   Immunization of experimental animals
    D. W. DRESSER

9   Carbohydrate antigens in higher animals
    S. HAKOMORI AND R. KANNAGI

10 The chemistry and standardization of allergens
    S. DREBORG, R. EINARSSON, JOAN L. LONG-BOTTOM

Immunoglobulins:
Purification and characterization

11 Overview: The quest for antibody homogeneity: the *sine qua non* for structural and genetic insights into antibody complementarity
    E. A. KABAT

12 Immunochemical analysis of human and rabbit immunoglobulins and their subunits
    D. R. STANWORTH AND M. W. TURNER

13 Purification and characterization of monoclonal antibodies
    R. R. HARDY

14 Preparation and purification of active fragments from mouse monoclonal antibodies
    P. PARHAM

15 Determination of the three-dimensional structures of immunoglobulins
    A. B. EDMUNDSON AND KATHERYN R. ELY

16 Immunoadsorbants
    SARA FUCHS AND M. SELA

17 Two-dimensional crystals of immunoglobulins
    J. REIDLER, E. E. UZGIRIS AND R. D. KORNBERG

18 Sources of myeloma proteins, and M-components
    M. POTTER

Mammalian cell membrane antigens

19 Overview: Mammalian cell surface antigens
    R. D. KORNBERG

20 Membrane and secretory immunoglobulins: structure, biosynthesis and assembly
    J. W. GODING

21 Class I MHC antigens of mouse and humans
    J. E. COLIGAN AND T. J. KINDT

22 Glycoprotein antigens of the lymphocyte surface and their purification by antibody affinity chromatography
    A. F. WILLIAMS AND A. N. BARCLAY

23 Immunofluorescence methods to study cell surface and cytoplasic proteins, and their dynamics
    E. R. UNANUE AND J. BRAUN

24 Measurement of lateral diffusion by fluorescence photobleaching recovery
    N. O. PETERSEN, S. FELDER AND E. L. ELSON

Antibody interaction with soluble and cellular antigens

25 Overview: Introduction to methods used to study the affinity and kinetics of antibody-antigen reactions
    M. W. STEWARD

26 Radioimmunoassays and related methods
    A. E. BOLTON AND W. M. HUNTER

27 Enzyme immunoassays: heterogenous and homogeneous systems
    R. M. NAKAMURA, A. VOLLER AND D. E. BIDWELL

28 Preparation and use of fluorochrome conjugates
    G. D. JOHNSON AND E. J. HOLBOROW

29 Flow cytometry and fluorescence activated cell sorting (FACS)
    D. R. PARKS, L. L. LANIER AND L. A. HERZENBERG

30 Data analysis in flow cytometry
    W. A. MOORE AND R. A. KAUTZ

31 Purification and coupling of fluorescent proteins for use in flow cytometry
    R. R. HARDY

32 Immunodiffusion and immunoelectrophoresis
    Ö. OUCHTERLONY AND L.-Å. NILSSON

33 Passive cutaneous anaphylaxis
    Z. OVARY

34 Solid-phase radioimmune assays
    C. J. NEWBY, K. HAYAKAWA AND LEONORE
    A. HERZENBERG

35 Immunological techniques for the identification
    of antigens and antibodies by electron micros-
    copy
    G. A. ANDRES, K. C. HSU AND BEATRICE C.
    SEGAL

36 Affinity targeting and fusion of vesicles to cells
    W. GODFREY, J. GUYDEN AND L. WOFSY

37 Immunotoxins
    OLIVIA MARTINEZ AND L. WOFSY

38 Kinetics of antibody reaction and the analysis of
    cell surface antigens
    D. W. MASON AND A. F. WILLIAMS

Complement

39 Complement technology
    R. A. HARRISON AND P. J. LACHMANN

40 Complement fixation by monoclonal antigen-
    antibody complexes
    R. R. HARDY

VOLUME 3
GENETICS AND
MOLECULAR IMMUNOLOGY

Molecular approaches to immunology

85. Overview: Introductory comments on molecu-
     lar immunology
     D. BALTIMORE

86 Construction and screening of recombinant
    DNA libraries in bacteriophage lambda
    P. W. TUCKER

87 The major histocompatibility complex of the
    mouse
    L. SMITH, M. STEINMETZ AND L. HOOD

88 The murine immunoglobulin heavy chain con-
    stant region gene locus
    N. M. GOUGH AND SUZANNE CORY

89 The Igh-V genes of the mouse
    R. RIBLET AND P. H. BRODEUR

90 Classification of mouse V_H sequences
    RENATE DILDROP

91 Transfection for lymphocyte cell surface
    antigens
    PAULA KAVATHAS AND L. A. HERZENBERG

92 Lymphoid cell gene transfer
    SHERIE L. MORRISON AND V. T. OI

Immunoglobulin genetics

93 Overview: Allotypes
    H. H. FUDENBERG

94 Human immunoglobulin allotypes
    M. S. SCHANFIELD AND ERNA VAN LOGHEN

95 New methods for human allotyping
    D. ZELASCHI, M. J. JOHNSTON, C. J. NEWBY
    AND LEONORE A. HERZENBERG

96 Gm and disease
    Y. NAKAO AND T. SASAZUKI

97 Mouse immunoglobulin allotypes
    MARILYN PARSON, LEONORE A. HERZEN-
    BERG, A. M. STALL AND L. A. HERZENBERG

98 Rat immunoglobulin allotypes
    G. A. GUTMAN

99 Rabbit immunoglobulin allotypes
    ROSE G. MAGE

Genetics of the major histocompatibility complex

100 Overview: The murine MHC
     D. B. MURPHY

101 The MHC of the laboratory rat, *Rattus norve-
     gicus*
     G. W. BUTCHER AND J. C. HOWARD

102 Human HLA genetics and disease associations
     GLENYS THOMSON

103 Common assays for identifying immune re-
     sponse genes
     C. WALTENBAUGH AND S. D. MILLER

Resources

104 The mouse linkage map
     MARGARET C. GREEN

105 Sonatic cell genetics and the human gene map
     M. E. KAMARCK AND F. H. RUDDLE

106 Inbred, congenic, recombinant-inbred and
     mutant mouse strains
     R. W. MELVOLD

VOLUME 4
APPLICATIONS OF IMMUNOLOGICAL
METHODS IN BIOMEDICAL
SCIENCES

Monoclonal antibodies

107 Overview: Monoclonal antibodies
     C. MILSTEIN

108 Schemata for the production of monoclonal
     antibody-producing hybridomas
     T. J. KIPPS AND L. A. HERZENBERG

109 Hybridoma immunoglobulin isotype switch
     variant selection with the fluorescence activated
     cell sorter
     T. J. KIPPS AND L. A. HERZENBERG

110 Isotype switch variants
     A. RADBRUCH

111 Growing hybridoma and producing monoclon-
     al antibodies *in vivo*
     K. OKUMURA AND S. HABU

Applications:
Monoclonal Antibodies

112 Neurobiology
     JANET WINTER, KAREN L. VALENTINO AND
     L. F. REICHARDT

113 Monoclonal antibodies in the study of parasites
     and host-parasite relationships
     E. HANDMAN AND G. F. MITCHELL

114 Application of monoclonal antibodies in bacter-
     iology
     C. CAROLINE BLACKWELL AND F. P. WIN-
     STANLEY

115 Applications of monoclonal antibodies in viro-
     logy
     W. GERHARDT AND T. BACHI

116 Special applications of tissue section immunolo-
     gic staining in the characterization of monoclon-
     al antibodies and in the study of normal and
     neoplastic tissues
     R. V. ROUSE AND R. A. WARNKE

117 Monoclonal antibodies directed to carbo-
     hydrate antigens
     R. KANNAGI AND S. HAKOMORI

118 Macrophages
     J. C. UNKELESS AND T. A. SPRINGER

Applications:
Immunological methods

119 Application of immunological techniques in
     bacteriology
     F. P. WINSTANLEY AND C. CAROLINE
     BLACKWELL

120 Application of immunological methods in viro-
     logy
     E. J. STOTT AND D. A. J. TYRRELL

121 Applications of immunological methods in
     mycology
     JOAN L. LONGBOTTOM

122 Applications of immunological methods in pro-
     tozoology
     E. H. R. LUMSDEN

123 Applications of immunological methods in hel-
     minthology
     W. J. L. SOULSBY AND SHEELAGH LLOYD

124 Immunological aspects of human pregnancy
     J. A. MACINTYRE AND W. PAGE FAULK

125 Applications of immunological techniques to
     the study of the tumour-host relationship
     G. J. DOUGHERTY, C. A. ALLEN AND NANCY
     M. HOGG

Additional clinical applications of
immunological methods

126 Tests of immune function
     S. J. URBANIAK, M. C. MCCANN, A. G.
     WHITE, G. R. BARCLAY AND A. B. KAY

x   *Contents*

127 Provocation tests and measurements of media-
     tors from mast cells and basophils in asthma and
     allergic rhinitis
     O. CROMWELL, S. R. DURHAM, R. J. SHAW,
     JUDITH A. MACKAY AND A. B. KAY

128 Methods for detecting immune complexes in
     biological fluids
     M. H. KLEIN AND K. SIMINOVITCH

129 Immunohistochemistry in pathology
     EADIE HEYDERMAN, I. STRUDLEY AND T. C.
     RICHARDSON

130 Quantification of IgE and IgG4 both as total
     immunoglobulins and as allerge-specific anti-
     bodies
     T. G. MERRETT

General methods for immunologic studies

131 Statistical aspects of planning and design of
     immunological experiments
     R. A. ELTON AND W. H. MCBRIDE

132 Guidelines to statistical analysis
     W. LUTZ

133 Laboratory animal techniques for immunology
     W. J. HERBERT, F. KRISTENSEN, with RUTH
     M. AITKEN, M. B. ESLAMI, ANNE FERGUSON,
     KATHLEEN G. GRAY, W. J. PENHALE

Index to Volume 2   xix

Contributors

C. A. Allen, *Imperial Cancer Research Fund, London, UK*

G. A. Andres, *Department of Pathology, State University of New York at Buffalo, NY, USA*

J. D. Ansell, *Department of Zoology, University of Edinburgh, Edinburgh, UK*

P. K. C. Austwick, *Department of Allergy and Clinical Immunology, Cardiothoracic Institute, London, UK*

J. Austyn, *Sir William Dunn School of Pathology, University of Oxford, Oxford, UK*

T. Bachi, *Institute for Immunology and Virology, University of Zurich, Zurich, Switzerland*

J. A. Badwey, *Department of Biological Chemistry, Harvard Medical School, Boston, Mass, USA*

D. Baltimore, *Whitehead Institute for Biomedical Research, Cambridge, Mass, USA*

M. J. Banda, *Laboratory of Radiobiology and Environmental Health, University of California, San Francisco, Ca, USA*

A. N. Barclay, *MRC Cellular Immunology Unit, Sir William Dunn School of Pathology, University of Oxford, Oxford, UK*

G. R. Barclay, *Blood Transfusion Centre, Royal Infirmary, Edinburgh, UK*

B. Benacerraf, *Department of Pathology, Harvard Medical School, Boston, Mass, USA*

P. Beverley, *ICRF Human Tumour Immunology Group, School of Medicine, University College London, London, UK*

D. E. Bidwell, *Nuffield Laboratories of Comparative Medicine, Zoological Society of London, London, UK*

C. Caroline Blackwell, *Department of Bacteriology, University of Edinburgh, Edinburgh, UK*

A. E. Bolton, *Department of Biological Science. Sheffield City Polytechnic, Sheffield, UK*

J. Braun, *Department of Pathology, University of California, Los Angeles, Ca, USA*

P. H. Brodeur, *Department of Pathology, Tufts University, Boston, Mass, USA*

C. J. Burrell, *Division of Virology, Institute of Medical and Veterinary Science, Adelaide, Australia*

E. C. Butcher, *Department of Pathology, Stanford University Medical School, Stanford, Ca, USA*

G. C. Butcher, *Institute of Animal Physiology, Agricultural Research Council, Babraham, Cambridge, UK*

H. Cantor, *Department of Pathology, Harvard Medical School, Boston, Mass, USA*

P. Chandler, *Transplantation Biology Section, Clinical Research Centre, Harrow, UK*

M. W. Clark, *Department of Biochemistry and Microbiology, University of Victoria, BC, Canada*

J. E. Coligan, *National Institute of Allergy and Infectious Diseases, Bethesda, Md, USA*

Suzanne Cory, *The Walter and Eliza Hall Institute of Medical Research, Royal Melbourne Hospital, Victoria, Australia*

O. Cromwell, *Department of Allergy and Clinical Immunology, Cardiothoracic Institute, London, UK*

M. R. Daha, *Department of Nephrology, University Hospital, Leiden, The Netherlands*

M. M. Davis, *Department of Medical Microbiology, Stanford University Medical School, Stanford, Ca, USA*

R. Dildrop, *Institute of Genetics, University of Cologne, Cologne, Federal Republic of Germany*

G. J. Dougherty, *Imperial Cancer Research Fund, London, UK*

S. Dreborg, *Allergy and Diagnostics Division, Pharmacia AB, Uppsala, Sweden*

D. W. Dresser, *Division of Immunology, National Institute for Medical Research, Mill Hill, London, UK*

S. R. Durham, *Department of Allergy and Clinical Immunology, Cardiothoracic Institute, London, UK*

P. J. Edelson, *Department of Pediatrics, New York Hospital, Cornell Medical Centre, New York, NY, USA*

A. B. Edmundson, *Department of Biology, University of Utah, Salt Lake City, Utah, USA*

R. Einarsson, *Biochemistry Division, Pharmacia AB, University of Uppsala, Uppsala, Sweden*

E. L. Elson, *Department of Biological Chemistry, Washington University Medical Centre, St. Louis, Mo, USA*

R. A. Elton, *Medical Computing and Statistics Group, University of Edinburgh, Edinburgh, UK*

Katherine R. Ely, *Department of Biology, University of Utah, Salt Lake City, Utah, USA*

E. G. Engleman, *Department of Medicine, Stanford University, School of Medicine, Stanford, Ca, USA*

R. A. B. Ezekowitz, *Sir William Dunn School of Pathology, University of Oxford, Oxford, UK*

C. G. Fathman, *Department of Medicine, Stanford University School of Medicine, Stanford, Ca, USA*

A. S. Fauci, *Laboratory of Immunoregulation, National Institute of Health, Bethesda, Md, USA*

S. Felder, *Department of Biological Chemistry, Washington University School of Medicine, St. Louis, Mo, USA*

Lorraine Flaherty, *Centre for Laboratories and Research, New York State Department of Health, Albany, NY, USA*

The late W. L. Ford, *Department of Immunology, University of Manchester, Manchester, UK*

J. Forman, *Department of Microbiology, University of Texas Southwestern Medical School, Dallas, Texas, USA*

Sara Fuchs, *Department of Clinical Immunology, The Weizmann Institute of Science, Rehovot, Israel*

H. H. Fudenberg, *Department of Basic and Clinical Immunology and Microbiology, Medical University of South Carolina, Charleston, SC, USA*

W. Gerhard, *Wistar Institute of Anatomy and Biology, Philadelphia, Pa, USA*

Elizabeth J. Glass, *Animal Breeding Research Organisation, Edinburgh, UK*

W. Godfrey, *Department of Microbiology, University of California, San Francisco, Ca, USA*

J. W. Goding, *Department of Pathology and Immunology, Monash Medical School, Victoria, Australia*

S. Gordon, *Sir William Dunn School of Pathology, University of Oxford, Oxford, UK*

D. R. Green, *Department of Immunology, University of Alberta, Edmonton, Canada*

Margaret C. Green, *The Jackson Laboratory, Bar Harbor, Maine, USA*

N. M. Gough, *Ludwig Institute for Cancer Reseach, Royal Melbourne Hospital, Victoria, Australia*

G. A. Gutman, *Department of Microbiology and Molecular Genetics, University of California, Irvine, Ca, USA*

J. Guyden, *Department of Microbiology and Immunology, University of California, San Francisco, Ca, USA*

S. Habu, *Department of Cell Biology, Tokai University, Japan*

S. Hakomori, *Division of Biochemical Oncology, Fred Hutchinson Cancer Research Center, Seattle, Wash, USA*

E. Handman, *Laboratory of Immunoparasitology, The Walter and Eliza Hall Institute of Medical Research, Royal Melbourne Hospital, Victoria, Australia*

R. R. Hardy, *Institute for Molecular and Cellular Biology, Osaka University, Osaka, Japan*

R. A. Harrison, *Mechanisms in Tumour Immunity Unit, MRC Centre, Cambridge, UK*

K. Hayakawa, *Department of Genetics, Stanford University School of Medicine, Stanford, Ca, USA*

W. J. Herbert, *Animal Services Unit, University of Dundee, Dundee, UK*

L. A. Herzenberg, *Department of Genetics, Stanford University School of Medicine, Stanford, Ca, USA*

Leonore A. Herzenberg, *Department of Genetics, Stanford University School of Medicine, Stanford, Ca, USA*

Eadie Heyderman, *Department of Histopathology, St. Thomas's Hospital Medical School, London, UK*

S. Hirsch, *Sir William Dunn School of Pathology, University of Oxford, Oxford, UK*

Nancy M. Hogg, *Imperial Cancer Research Fund, London, UK*

E. J. Holborow, *Bone and Joint Research Unit, London Hospital Medical College, London, UK*

L. Hood, *Division of Biology, California Institute of Technology, Pasadena, Ca, USA*

J. C. Howard, *Institute of Animal Physiology, Agricultural Research Council, Babraham, Cambridge, UK*

Maureen Howard, *National Institute of Allergy and Infectious Diseases, Bethesda, Md, USA*

K. C. Hsu, *Department of Microbiology, College of Physicians and Surgeons of New York, NY, USA*

D. A. Hume, *Sir William Dunn School of Pathology, University of Oxford, Oxford, UK*

S. V. Hunt, *MRC Cellular Immunology Unit, Sir William Dunn School of Pathology, University of Oxford, Oxford, UK*

W. M. Hunter, *Celltec Ltd, Slough, Berkshire, UK*

G. M. Iverson, *Dept of Pathology, Howard Hughes Medical Institute, Yale University, New Haven, Conn, USA*

M. K. Jenkins, *Department of Microbiology-Immunology, Northwestern University, Chicago, Ill, USA*

G. D. Johnson, *Department of Immunology, University of Birmingham, Birmingham, UK*

M. J. Johnston, *Department of Genetics, Stanford University Medical School, Stanford, Ca, USA*

E. A. Kabat, *Department of Microbiology, College of Physicians and Surgeons of Columbia University, New York, NY, USA*

M. E. Kamarck, *Department of Biology, Yale University, New Haven, Conn, USA*

R. Kannagi, *Division of Biochemical Oncology, Fred Hutchinson Cancer, Seattle, Wash, USA*

J. Kappler, *Department of Medicine, National Jewish Hospital and Research Center, Denver, Co, USA*

M. J. Karnovsky, *Department of Biological Chemistry, Harvard Medical School, Boston, Mass, USA*

M. L. Karnovsky, *Department of Pathology, Harvard Medical School, Boston, Mass, USA*

R. A. Kautz, *Department of Genetics, Stanford University School of Medicine, Stanford, Ca, USA*

Paula Kavathas, *Department of Genetics, Stanford University School of Medicine, Stanford, Ca, USA*

A. B. Kay, *Department of Allergy and Clinical Immunology, Cardiothoracic Institute, London, UK*

B. S. Kim, *Department of Microbiology-Immunology, Northwestern University, Chicago, Ill, USA*

T. J. Kindt, *National Institute of Allergy and Infectious Disease, Bethesda, Md, USA*

T. J. Kipps, *Scripps Clinic and Research Foundation, La Jolla, Ca, USA*

M. Klein, *Department of Immunology, Toronto Western Hospital, Ontario, Canada*

R. D. Kornberg, *Department of Cell Biology, Stanford University Medical School, Stanford, Ca, USA*

P. J. Lachmann, *Mechanisms in Tumour Immunity Unit, MRC Centre, Cambridge, UK*

H. C. Lane, *Laboratory of Immunoregulation, National Institute of Health, Bethesda, Maryland, USA*

L. L. Lanier, *Becton Dickinson Monoclonal Center Inc, Mountain View, Ca, USA*

P. C. J. Leijh, *Department of Infectious Diseases, University Hospital, Leiden, The Netherlands*

Sheelagh Lloyd, *Department of Clinical Veterinary Medicine, University of Cambridge, Cambridge, UK*

Joan L. Longbottom, *Department of Clinical Immunology, Cardiothoracic Institute, London, UK*

Eva Lotta Larsen, *Department of Immunobiology, Karolinska Institute, Stockholm, Sweden*

W. H. R. Lumsden, *19a Merchiston Crescent, Edinburgh, UK*

W. Lutz, *Medical Computing and Statistics Group, University of Edinburgh, Edinburgh, UK*

W. H. McBride, *Department of Radiation Oncology, University of California, Los Angeles, USA*

M. C. McCann, *Blood Transfusion Centre, Royal Infirmary, Edinburgh, UK*

J. A. McIntyre, *Department of Obstetrics and Gynaecology, Southern Illinois School of Medicine, Springfield, Ill, USA*

Judith A. MacKay, *Department of Allergy and Clinical Immunology, Cardiothoracic Institute, London, UK*

Rose A. Mage, *Laboratory of Immunology, National Institute of Allergy and Infectious Diseases, Bethesda, Md, USA*

O. Mäkelä, *Department of Bacteriology and Immunology, University of Helsinki, Helsinki, Finland*

Phillipa Marrack, *Department of Medicine, National Jewish Hospital and Research Center, Denver, Co, USA*

Olivia Martinez, *Department of Microbiology and Immunology, University of California, Berkeley, Ca, USA*

D. W. Mason, *MRC Cellular Immunology Unit, Sir William Dunn School of Pathology, University of Oxford, Oxford, UK*

R. Melvold, *Dept of Microbiology and Immunology, Northwestern University Medical School, Chicago, Ill, USA*

T. G. Merrett, *RAST Allergy Unit, Benenden Chest Hospital, Cranbrook, Kent, UK*

H. S. Micklem, *Department of Zoology, University of Edinburgh, Edinburgh, UK*

R. G. Miller, *Ontario Cancer Institute, University of Toronto, Toronto, Ontario, Canada*

S. D. Miller, *Department of Microbiology Immunology, The Medical and Dental Schools, Ill, Northwestern University, Chicago, USA*

C. Milstein, *Laboratory of Molecular Biology, Medical Research Council The Medical School, Cambridge, UK*

G. F. Mitchell, *Laboratory of Immunoparasitology, The Walter and Eliza Hall Institute of Medical Research, Royal Melbourne Hospital, Victoria, Australia*

W. A. Moore, *Department of Genetics, Stanford University School of Medicine, Stanford, Ca, USA*

Sherie L. Morrison, *Department of Microbiology, Columbia University College of Physicians and Surgeons, New York, NY, USA*

D. B. Murphy, *Department of Pathology, Yale University, New Haven, Conn, USA*

R. M. Nakamura, *Department of Pathology, Scripps Clinic and Research Foundation, La Jolla, Ca, USA*

Y. Nakao, *Department of Medicine, University of Kobe, Japan*

C. J. Newby, *Department of Genetics, Stanford University Medical School, Stanford, Ca, USA*

L. A. Nilsson, *Department of Medical Microbiology, University of Gothenburg, Gothenburg, Sweden*

G. J. V. Nossal, *Walter and Eliza Hall Institute of Medical Research, Royal Melbourne Hospital, Victoria, Australia*

V. Oi, *Becton Dickinson Monoclonal Center, Mountain View, Ca, USA*

K. Okumura, *Department of Immunology, Juntendo University, Tokyo, Japan*

Ö. Ouchterlony, *Department of Medical Microbiology, University of Gothenborg, Gothenburg, Sweden*

Z. Ovary, *Department of Pathology, New York University Medical Center, New York, NY, USA*

W. Page Faulk, *Medi-Search AG, Meiringen, Switzerland*

P. Parham, *Department of Cell Biology, Stanford University School of Medicine, Stanford, Ca, USA*

D. R. Parks, *Department of Genetics, Stanford University School of Medicine, Stanford, Ca, USA*

M. Parson, *Department of Genetics, Stanford University School of Medicine, Stanford, Ca, USA*

T. W. Pearson, *Department of Biochemistry and Microbiology, University of Victoria, BC, Canada*

N. O. Petersen, *Department of Chemistry, University of Western Ontario, London, Ontario, Canada*

M. Potter, *Laboratory of Genetics, National Cancer Institute, Bethesda, Md, USA*

I. R. Poxton, *Department of Bacteriology, University Medical School, Edinburgh, UK*

A. Radbruch, *Institute of Genetics, University of Cologne, Cologne, Federal Republic of Germany*

P. Ralph, *Department of Cell Biology, Cetus Corporation, Emeryville, Ca, USA*

K. Rajewsky, *Institute of Genetics, University of Cologne, Cologne, Federal Republic of Germany*

U. Ramstedt, *Department of Immunology, Karolinska Institute, Stockholm, Sweden*

Elizabeth Raveche, *National Institute of Health, Bethesda, Md, USA*

L. F. Reichardt, *Department of Neurology, University of California, San Francisco, Ca, USA*

J. Reidler, *Department of Cell Biology, Stanford University School of Medicine, Stanford, Ca, USA*

R. Riblet, *Department of Immunology, Medical Biology Institute, La Jolla, Ca, USA*

J. M. Robinson, *Department of Pathology, Harvard Medical School, Boston, Mass., USA*

F. S. Rosen, *Division of Immunology, Children's Hospital Medical Center, Boston, Mass, USA*

R. V. Rouse, *Department of Pathology, Stanford University School of Medicine, Stanford, Ca, USA*

F. A. Ruddle, *Department of Biology, Yale University, New Haven, Conn, USA*

T. Sasazuki, *Department of Genetics, Medical Institute of Bioregulation, Kyushu University, Fukuoka, Japan*

M. S. Schanfield, *Genetic Testing Institute, Atlanta, Georgia, USA*

Beatrice C. Seegal, *Department of Microbiology, College of Physicians and Surgeons of Columbia University, New York, NY, USA*

M. Sela, *Department of Chemical Immunology, The Weizmann Institute of Science, Rehovot, Israel*

I. J. T. Seppälä, *Department of Bacteriology and Immunology, University of Helsinki, Helsinki, Finland*

E. E. Sercarz, *Department of Microbiology, University of California, Los Angeles, Ca, USA*

Eva Severinson, *Department of Immunobiology, Karolinska Institute, Stockholm, Sweden*

N. Shastri, *Department of Microbiology, University of California, Los Angeles, Ca, USA*

J. F. L. Shaw, *Department of Surgery, University of Cambridge, Cambridge, UK*

S. C. Silverstein, *Laboratory of Cellular Physiology and Immunology, The Rockefeller University, New York, NY, USA*

R. J. Shaw, *Department of Allergy and Clinical Immunology, Cardiothoracic Institute, London, UK*

K. Simonovitch, *Department of Immunology, Toronto Western Hospital, Ontario, Canada*

Elizabeth Simpson, *Transplantation Biology Section, Clinical Research Centre, Harrow, UK*

L. Smith, *Division of Biology, California Institute of Technology, Pasadena, Ca, USA*

E. J. L. Soulsby, *Department of Clinical Veterinary Medicine, University of Cambridge, UK*

D. M. Spalding, *Division of Clinical Immunology and Rheumatology, University of Alabama in Birmingham, Birmingham, Alabama, USA*

T. A. Springer, *Dana Farber Cancer Institute, Harvard Medical School, Boston, Mass, USA*

D. R. Stanworth, *Department of Immunology, University of Birmingham, Birmingham, UK*

Phyllis M. Starkey, *Sir William Dunn School of Pathology, University of Oxford, Oxford, UK*

A. D. Steinberg, *National Institute of Health, Bethesda, Md, USA*

R. M. Steinman, *Laboratory of Cellular Physiology, and Immunology, The Rockefeller University, New York, NY, USA*

M. Steinmetz, *Basel Institute for Immunology, Basel, Switzerland*

M. W. Steward, *Department of Medical Microbiology, London School of Hygiene and Tropical Medicine, London, UK*

C. C. Stewart, *Experimental Pathology Group, Los*

Alamos National Laboratory, Los Alamos, New Mexico, USA

J. Stewart, *Department of Bacteriology, University of Edinburgh, Edinburgh, UK*

E. J. Stott, *Institute for Research on Animal Diseases, Newbury, Berkshire, UK*

T. Tada, *Department of Immunology, University of Tokyo, Tokyo, Japan*

N. Takemura, *Medical Research Institute, Tokyo Medical and Dental University, Tokyo, Japan*

R. Takemura, *Laboratory of Radiobiology and Environmental Health, University of California, San Francisco, Ca, USA*

M. Taniguchi, *Department of Immunology, Chiba University, Chiba, Japan*

Glenys Thomson, *Department of Genetics, University of California, Berkeley, Ca, USA*

P. W. Tucker, *Department of Microbiology, University of Texas, Southwestern Medical School, Dallas, Texas, USA*

T. Tokuhisa, *Department of Immunology, Chiba University, Chiba, Japan*

M. W. Turner, *Department of Immunology, Institute of Child Health, London, UK*

D. A. J. Tyrrell, *MRC Common Cold Unit, Harvard Hospital, Salisbury, Wiltshire, UK*

E. R. Unanue, *Department of Pathology, Harvard Medical School, Boston, Mass, USA*

J. Unkeless, *The Rockefeller University, New York, NY, USA*

R. J. Urbaniak, *Aberdeen and North East of Scotland Blood Transfusion Service, Aberdeen, UK*

E. E. Uzgiris, *Department of Cell Biology, Stanford University School of Medicine, Stanford, Ca, USA*

Karen L. Valentino, *Department of Physiology, University of California School of Medicine, San Francisco, Ca, USA*

R. van Furth, *Department of Infectious Diseases, University Hospital, Leiden, The Netherlands*

E. van Loghem, *The Netherlands Red Cross Blood Transfusion Service, Amsterdam, The Netherlands*

W. C. van Voorhis, *Laboratory of Cellular Physiology, The Rockefeller University, New York, NY, USA*

Theda L. van Zwet, *Department of Infectious Diseases, University Hospital, Leiden, The Netherlands*

A. Voller, *Nuffield Laboratories of Comparative Medicine, Zoological Society of London, London, UK*

C. Waltenbaugh, *Department of Microbiology-Immunology, Northwestern University, Chicago, Ill, USA*

R. A. Warnke, *Department of Pathology, Stanford University Medical School, Stanford, Ca, USA*

D. M. Weir, *Department of Bacteriology, University of Edinburgh, Edinburgh, UK*

Zena Werb, *Laboratory of Radiobiology and Environmental Health, University of California, San Francisco, Ca, USA*

G. Whalen, *Laboratory of Immunoregulation, National Institute of Health, Md, USA*

A. G. White, *Department of Surgery, Faculty of Medicine, Kuwait University, Kuwait*

D. J. G. White, *Department of Surgery, University of Cambridge, Cambridge, UK*

H. Wigzell, *Department of Immunology, Karolinska Institute, Stockholm, Sweden*

P. C. Wilkinson, *Department of Bacteriology and Immunology, University of Glasgow, Glasgow, UK*

A. F. Williams, *MRC Cellular Immunology Unit, Sir William Dunn School of Pathology, University of Oxford, Oxford, UK*

F. P. Winstanley, *Armed Services University, Washington, DC, USA*

Janet Winter, *Department of Physiology, University of California, San Francisco, Ca, USA*

L. Wofsy, *Department of Microbiology and Immunology, University of California, Berkeley, Ca, USA*

S. D. Wright, *Laboratory of Cellular Physiology and Immunology, The Rockefeller University, New York, NY, USA*

M. Zauderer, *Department of Microbiology and Oncology, University of Rochester, Rochester, NY, USA.*

D. Zelaschi, *Department of Genetics, Stanford University School of Medicine, Stanford, Ca, USA*

Preface

The pace of progress in immunology has not slackened since the last edition of this handbook. The subject now draws heavily on molecular biology and genetics and this has necessitated the inclusion of an additional volume on **Genetics and Molecular Immunology**. The explosion in the development of hybridoma technology and cell culture, since the last edition, can be seen from the many chapters in each volume that employ monoclonal reagents and cell lines. Some idea of the expansion of the field can be gained from the **Cellular Immunology** volume where contributions on phagocytes and lymphocytes now occupy 30 chapters compared to 12 in the previous edition. A new section on immunoregulation contains 14 chapters and there are now 6 chapters devoted to mammalian cell membrane antigens in the **Immunochemistry** volume.

It is now no longer possible for one editor to keep in touch with the enormous expansion in this field, and I am much indebted to my co-editors Len and Leonore Herzenberg who have joined me in the task of co-opting research workers in the wide range of disciplines now contributing to the field of immu-nology. I am particularly grateful to my wife Dr Caroline Blackwell for her help with the massive editing task.

Amongst the many new features of this edition is the provision of overviews for many of the sections. I am most grateful to our contributors in the methodology sections for their efforts to achieve a consistent style of presentation of the procedures, and I hope that this will help in the accessibility of the descriptive material. A work of this size inevitably takes a number of years to put together but considerable effort has gone into introducing up to date material into the chapters. This has been achieved by enabling and encouraging contributors to introduce new material and references during the proof stages of their chapters.

I wish to thank Hilary Flenley for her careful and thorough index, and Nigel Palmer and his staff at Blackwell Scientific Publications Edinburgh office without whom production of the new edition would have been impossible. Per Saugman has as always, maintained a benevolent paternal interest in the project.

D.M.W.

Chapter 41
Overview: the function of receptors in phagocytosis

S. D. WRIGHT & S. C. SILVERSTEIN

The attachment step, 41.1
Receptors function independently of one another, 41.3
Engulfment, 41.3

Cytoskeletal proteins, cell motility, and the energetics of phagocytosis, 41.5
Transmembrane signals, 41.6

Fc receptors are constitutively active, 41.6
Some problems and strategies in the study of the roles of receptors in phagocytosis, 41.9

Mononuclear phagocytes together with polymorphonuclear leucocytes comprise the most numerous classes of phagocytic cells in higher organisms. Rabinovitch has termed these cells 'professional' phagocytes because they have made a full-time occupation out of eating. Leucocytes are not the only 'professional' phagocytes in the body. The pigmented epithelial cells of the retina phagocytose the fragments of rod outer segments that are shed daily by the rod cells [1]. Thus being a professional phagocyte is not a unique property of motile cells of haematopoietic (mesenchymal) origin.

A role for phagocytosis in antimicrobial defence has been recognized since the time of Metchnikoff [2]. Less widely appreciated is the role phagocytosis plays in homoeostatic functions such as the turnover of surfactant in the lung [3], and the removal of senescent erythrocytes [4]. In each of these instances, the material to be removed is specifically and selectively phagocytosed without apparent injury to neighbouring cells and tissues. The authors believe that this specificity is a consequence of receptor–ligand interactions that govern the ingestion process.

Macrophages have on their plasma membranes binding sites for more than forty ligands (Table 41.1). Receptors of defined molecular weight and subunit composition have been identified for a few of these ligands (e.g. IgG [5], complement [6,7]). The presence of specific receptor proteins for the remaining ligands is inferred by their specific and saturable binding to leucocytes and by the inability of other ligands to compete for binding.

At present, only a few of these receptors (i.e. those for IgG, complement, oligosaccharides) are known to promote ingestion of particles. It seems unlikely that the remaining receptors play a major role in phagocytosis since their ligands are soluble and bind poorly to micro-organisms or other particulate matter. (Fibronectin is a special case and will be discussed later in this chapter.) For this reason, the authors have focussed on mechanisms by which IgG, complement, and oligosaccharides promote phagocytosis. Implicit in their discussion is the assumption that uptake of all particulate materials by phagocytic leucocytes, be they latex beads or IgG-coated bacteria, is governed by receptor–ligand interactions; and that the general principles established in studies of the uptake of IgG-, complement-, or oligosaccharide-coated particles will be broadly applicable to other receptor–ligand systems.

The attachment step

Phagocytosis can be divided both conceptually and experimentally into a series of processes that culminate in the total engulfment of a particle. The first step in this series is the attachment of the particle to the phagocyte's surface [8]. In general, attachment occurs over a broad temperature range and independently of the expenditure of metabolic energy by the phagocyte. Engulfment, on the other hand, is strictly dependent on cellular metabolism and is entirely halted at temperatures below 18–20 °C [9,10]. Particles coated with some ligands (e.g. complement) bind more efficiently to their corresponding receptors at 37 °C than at 4 °C; particles coated with other ligands, such as IgG, bind with roughly equal efficiency at both temperatures.

Attachment per se does not predestine the particle for ingestion. Erythrocytes or smooth encapsulated bacteria can be bound to the surfaces of phagocytic leucocytes with concanavalin A [11], F(ab)₂ antibody fragments [12], fibronectin [13], or complement [14,15], and will remain on the phagocyte's surface for

Table 41.1. Receptors on the surface of macrophages[1]

Ligand	Name of receptor (if different from ligand)	Comments	Reference
Receptors that constitutively promote phagocytosis			
IgG_{2a}	FcRI	Murine	[5]
$IgG_{1/2b}$	FcRII	Murine	[5]
IgG_3		Murine	[5]
IgG_1	$Fc_\gamma R_{hi}$	Human	[86]
Immune complexes	$Fc_\gamma R_{lo}$	Human	[86]
IgE			[87]
Mannose/G1cNAc-containing oligosaccharides			[88]
Galactose-containing oligosaccharides			[4]
Receptors that promote phagocytosis in a regulated fashion			
C3b and C4b	CR1	Also inhibits complement enzymes	[6]
C3bi	CR3		[7]
C3d and C3dg	CR2		[57]
Receptors for fast-acting regulators			
Fibronectin			[13]
Serum amyloid P component			[60]
'lymphokine'		Secreted by lymphocytes in response to a factor from phagocytosing macrophages	[58]
Insulin			[89]
Adrenalin			[90]
Histamine			[91]
Somatomedin			[92]
Calcitonin			[93]
Parathormone			[93]
Receptors for long-term regulators			
γ-Interferon (macrophage activating factor)			[94]
Colony stimulating factor			[95]
Receptors that mediate pinocytic uptake of ligands			
α_2Macroglobulin–protease complex			[96]
LDL			[97]
Acetyl-LDL			[97]
VLDL			[98]
Transferrin			[99]
(Receptors for Fc, C3, and oligosaccharides also mediate pinocytosis)			
Receptors for chemoattractants			
Formyl-methionyl-leucyl-phenylalanine			[100]
C5a			[100]
Thrombin			[101]
Miscellaneous receptors			
Elastase			[102]
Lactoferrin			[103]
Fibrin			[104]
Tumour cell		Presumed to exist because 'activated' macrophages bind tumour cells	[105]
C1q			[106]

[1] It should be noted that for each ligand there may be multiple distinct receptors. Additional surface proteins that may be receptors are described in Table 118.1 in the chapter by Unkeless & Springer.

several hours at 37 °C. That these particles can be ingested is evident when IgG directed against the surface of the particle is added to the cultures. Under these conditions the particles are ingested [16,17]. These results indicate that signals generated by the ligation of specific membrane receptors are required to promote internalization.

Receptors function independently of one another

Phagocytosis-promoting receptors diffuse freely in the plane of the plasma membrane [18,19] and function independently of one another in mediating particle ingestion. For example, macrophages that are functionally depleted of Fc receptors after spreading on IgG-coated surfaces still phagocytose via their receptors for C3 and for oligosaccharides; conversely, macrophages whose complement receptors have been depleted by spreading on a complement-coated surface or inactivated by treatment with proteolytic enzymes still phagocytose via their Fc receptors [18]. Moreover, signals generated via one class of phagocytosis-promoting receptors are not transmitted to other classes of phagocytosis-promoting receptors on the same cell. For example, ligation of macrophage Fc receptors does not stimulate complement receptor function [18]. Nevertheless, two receptors may complement one another if ligands for each are present on a single particle. Ehlenberger & Nussenzweig [20] reported that erythrocytes bearing complement and a limiting number of IgG molecules are phagocytosed to a greater extent than erythrocytes bearing the same number of IgG molecules alone. Under the conditions of their experiment, complement receptors were unable to promote ingestion. However, attachment is the rate limiting step in Fc-receptor mediated phagocytosis [21]. Thus ligands that enhance attachment such as complement thereby enhance the efficiency of interaction of ingestion-promoting ligands, such as IgG with their corresponding receptors.

Engulfment

Generation of a signal that promotes membrane internalization, as occurs when Fc receptors are ligated, produces a membrane response that is restricted to the segments of membrane in contact with the particle initiating the signal [16]. The advancing pseudopods adhere closely to the surface of the particle (Fig. 41.1), even to the point of enveloping each particle in a separate vacuole. These and other observations led Griffin *et al.* [16,22] to propose a general hypothesis (the 'zipper' mechanism) to explain these findings. Essentially, the 'zipper' concept predicts that movement of a phagocyte's plasma membrane along the surface of a ligand-coated particle is governed by the availability of receptors on the surface of the phagocyte and is guided by the distribution of ligands on the surface of the particle. Several lines of evidence support this hypothesis, the most compelling of which is an experiment in which B lymphocytes were coated circumferentially or hemispherically with IgG antibodies to membrane IgM and then incubated with macrophages. Lymphocytes coated circumferentially with IgG were engulfed. Lymphocytes coated on one hemisphere with IgG were bound to the macrophages via this IgG cap, but they were not engulfed. Ultrastructural histochemistry confirmed that the macrophage membrane extends over the surface of the IgG-coated capped lymphocyte only in the areas of the IgG cap [22]. Thus, engulfment requires the sequential and circumferential interaction of receptors on the surface of the phagocyte with corresponding ligands on the surface of the particle.

Scanning electron micrographs of the engulfment of IgG-coated erythrocytes by macrophages show that these phagocytes extend several broad, relatively flat pseudopods over the particle. As these pseudopods advance they form a smooth cup-like structure whose rim ultimately covers the entire particle. There is no evidence that these advancing pseudopods fuse with one another; rather, formation of the phagocytic cup involves considerable membrane flow and remodelling such that the final event in closure of the phagocytic vacuole is the fusion of membranes over a small hole (punctum) at the point where the advancing pseudopods meet [23]. Thus the extent of membrane fusion required to close a phagocytic vacuole may be no greater than that required to close a pinocytic vesicle.

Within a span of 15–30 min macrophages can ingest sufficient particles to cause the interiorization of 30–40% of their total surface area. These cells have large internal stores of plasma membrane (perhaps as much as two-fold the amount of the surface [24,25]) and the authors presume that these internal membrane stores are inserted into the cell surface to replace plasma membrane interiorized with the ingested particles. Such redistribution of membrane from internal stores to the cell surface has been shown to accompany phagocytosis in amoebae [26,27] and in leucocytes [28], and may explain the constancy of plasma membrane composition in phagocytosing leucocytes suggested by the experiments of Tsan & Berlin [29] over a decade ago.

Cohn, Hubbard, Steinman and their associates [10,30,31] have made imaginative use of lactoperoxidase (LPO) catalysed surface iodination to examine the surface proteins incorporated into the membrane of the phagosome. These investigators labelled the surface membranes of fibroblasts [31,32] and macro-

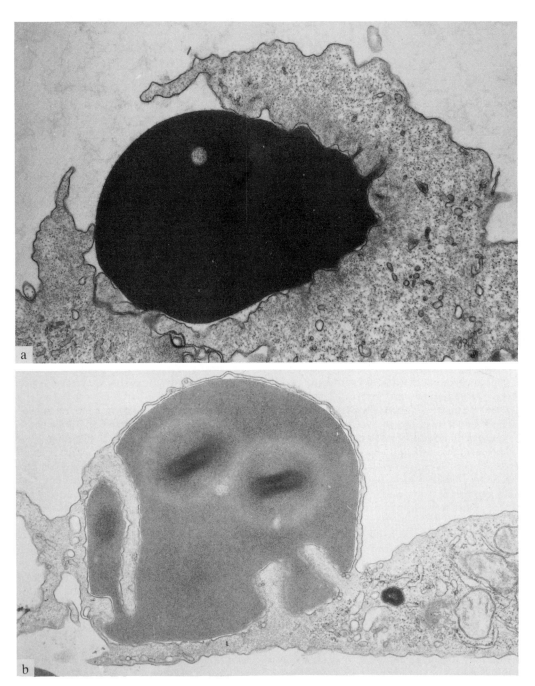

Fig. 41.1. Phagocytosis of IgG-coated erythrocytes. (a) The dense filamentous mesh seen at the base of the forming phagosome in this cultured human monocyte is a hallmark of receptor-mediated phagocytosis. (b) This murine peritoneal phagocyte illustrates the close, circumferential adhesion that forms between the macrophage plasma membrane and the surface of the IgG-coated erythrocyte during phagocytosis.

phages [33] with ^{125}I and then allowed these cells to ingest latex beads. The latex-containing phagolysosomes were then isolated and their ^{125}I-labelled membrane proteins were analysed by SDS–PAGE and compared with the ^{125}I-labelled proteins originally present on the cell surface. No significant differences were noted, leading them to conclude that latex particles are enveloped within vacuoles whose membranes contain a random and representative sample of plasma membrane proteins. This conclusion was reinforced by the experiments of Muller *et al.* [34] who iodinated the inner surface of the phagolysosome membrane with LPO coupled to latex. SDS–PAGE analysis of the membrane proteins labelled in this way confirmed that the protein composition of phagolysosome membrane is remarkably similar to that of the plasma membrane.

The authors have no information regarding the identity of the 'receptors' that mediate uptake of latex beads or their fate after phagocytosis of latex. However, in the case of phagocytosis of IgG-coated particles mediated by Fc receptors, Mellman *et al.* [35] found that phagocytosis of these particles enhanced the internalization and degradation of Fc receptors. Such phagocytosis also caused a marked reduction in the number of Fc receptors remaining at the cell's surface, indicating that phagocytosis of IgG-coated particles promotes concentration of a subset of plasma membrane proteins into the membrane of the phagocytic vacuole. Further work is needed to determine whether, in addition to the ligated receptors, a specific subset of membrane proteins other than the ligated receptor is internalized when a ligand-coated particle is ingested.

Cytoskeletal proteins, cell motility, and the energetics of phagocytosis

Macrophages contain 10% by weight actin and about 1% by weight myosin and actin binding proteins. Common sense and analogy to other known motile systems dictate that these cytoplasmic contractile proteins, together with their regulatory elements (e.g. actin-binding proteins [36], gelsolin [37]), promote the extension of membrane pseudopods during phagocytosis. Nevertheless, this common sense view is buttressed by only three types of evidence, all of which are indirect. First, polymorphonuclear leucocytes from a child with the 'lazy leucocyte syndrome' exhibited defective chemotaxis and phagocytosis. An abnormality in actin filament assembly was identified in extracts of these leucocytes [38]. Second, cytoplasmic contractile proteins, especially actin, are found at the tips of advancing pseudopods and are especially enriched in the zone of cytoplasm directly beneath the

nascent phagocytic vacuole [39,40]. Third, cytochalasins halt assembly of g-actin into f-actin, and inhibit phagocytosis [40].

Two groups of investigators have suggested a role for clathrin in phagocytosis. Montesano *et al.* [41] used tannic acid to visualize clathrin on the cytoplasmic face of the plasma membranes of macrophages ingesting IgG-coated erythrocytes. The clathrin was prominent at foci of tight contact between the macrophage and the IgG-coated erythrocyte. Aggeler & Werb [42], on the other hand, observed large sheets of assembled clathrin on the inner surface of the plasma membrane of macrophages ingesting 0.8 μm diameter latex beads. Since cytochalasin B is relatively inefficient as an inhibitor of the uptake of small (< 1 μm) latex beads compared with its effect on the uptake of large particles, it is possible that these small beads, like animal viruses [43], are internalized within coated vesicles. However, the identification of clathrin on the nascent phagosome of macrophages ingesting IgG-coated particles suggests an additional role for this protein in phagocytosis of large particles.

Several lines of evidence indicate that microtubules and 10 nm filaments are not essential participants in the ingestion process. The most compelling of these is the observation that isolated fragments of neutrophil cytoplasm (cytoplasts), which appear to lack these cytoskeletal elements, retain the capacity to phagocytose particulate materials [44].

A role for myosin in phagocytosis remains to be established. We do not know whether actomyosin contraction, as occurs in skeletal muscle, is required for pseudopod extension, or whether actin filament assembly, as occurs in Thyone sperm [45], is sufficient. Since phagocytosis can only be observed in intact cells, novel methods, such as the selection of mutant cell lines with phagocytic defects [46,47,48], or the microinjection of antibodies that inhibit the function of specific cytoskeletal proteins [49,50,107] will be needed to gain further insight into these issues.

That phagocytosis reflects muscle-like activity at the single cell level is emphasized by the similarities in the metabolic processes of phagocytosing macrophages and contracting skeletal muscle cells. Both cell types exhibit increased rates of glycolysis and lactate production [51]; both contain creatine kinase and large stores of creatine phosphate (three- to fivefold molar excess of ATP); and both utilize their creatine phosphate stores to rephosphorylate ADP during periods of high metabolic demand [52]. Thus it is evident that particle internalization imposes a large demand for ATP. In muscle, where actin filaments are relatively stable structures and the ratio of actin to myosin is roughly 4:1, a significant proportion of the ATP required is consumed by actomyosin ATPase. In phagocytic leucocytes, where actin rapidly interconverts between g- and f-actin and the ratio of actin to myosin is about 100:1, we do not know the relative importance of myosin ATPase and the conversion of g- to f-actin in ATP utilization.

As noted above, it is conventional wisdom that cytoskeletal proteins provide the motile force for membrane extension. However, it is possible that in phagocytic leucocytes membrane extension is powered by a local influx of salt and water, that this extension is facilitated by *dis*assembly of the adjacent cytoskeleton, and that the dense actin lattice observed beneath the nascent phagosome acts only to stabilize and direct the movement caused by hydrostatic pressure.

Transmembrane signals

Implicit in the zipper concept [16,17,22] is the notion that receptor ligation *per se* is insufficient to produce particle engulfment. Rather, ligated receptors must generate transmembrane signals that regulate subsequent structural changes and activate metabolic processes in the underlying cytoplasm. This view is supported by the findings that uniformly opsonized particles bind to metabolically poisoned [53] or cytochalasin-treated [40] phagocytes but are not ingested by them. Recent studies of isolated Fc receptors provide insight into the nature of the transmembrane signals they generate.

Fc receptors are constitutively active

Several distinct types of Fc receptors have been identified on phagocytic leucocytes and on mast cells [reviewed in 5]. In all cases studied, ligation of these receptors with particle-bound immunoglobulins simultaneously initiates the entire known panoply of responses (i.e. phagocytosis, secretion of peroxide and arachidonate metabolites, release of histamine, etc.). Because ligation of these receptors constitutively, immediately and maximally signals the several cellular responses listed above, we think of Fc receptors as 'unregulated' receptors.

The Fc receptor on mouse macrophages that binds antibodies of subclasses $\gamma 1$ and $\gamma 2b$ (termed FcRII) has been characterized, largely through the work of Unkeless and his associates. In its unligated form the M_r 55 000 receptor diffuses rapidly ($D = 2-3 \times 10^{-9}$ cm^2/s [19]) in the plane of the macrophage membrane and therefore does not appear to be linked to the cytoskeleton. Young *et al.* have presented evidence that this receptor is a ligand-dependent ion channel [54]. When purified and incorporated into artificial lipid bilayers, the Fc receptor generates discrete channels that are selective for monovalent cations.

The channels open only upon binding of ligand and thereafter decay with a time constant of approximately 250 ms. In living macrophages, the ion flux caused by ligation of Fc receptors causes a transient depolarization of the plasma membrane which is inhibited when choline is substituted for Na$^+$ in the medium [55]. These findings suggest that the initial event occurring upon ligation of FcRII is the influx of Na$^+$ into the cytoplasm. Is Na$^+$ influx sufficient to elicit the spectrum of secretory and endocytic activities that accompany ligation of FcRII? We do not know. However, comparative studies of the effects of ligation of complement receptors provide some insight into the complexity of the problem.

The function of complement receptors is regulated

Human macrophages express two distinct receptors for the cleavage products of the third component of complement (C3) [6,7,56]. One receptor (CR1) recognizes C3b, and the other receptor (CR3) recognizes a cleavage product of C3b, termed C3bi.

Separate receptors for C3b and C3bi have not been demonstrated on murine macrophages because purified murine complement proteins from which to form these ligands are not available. While murine macrophages probably do have separate CR1 and CR3 proteins, the methods commonly used to generate particles coated with mouse complement yield particles coated predominantly with C3bi. Thus most studies of C3 receptors in the murine system have, of necessity, focussed on CR3.

Under some conditions, polymorphonuclear leucocytes and macrophages also express a receptor that recognizes a further degradation product of C3 termed C3d [57]. This receptor appears to be distinct from CR1 and CR3, yet limited experimental evidence suggests that it functions in a manner similar to that of CR1 and CR3.

CR1 and CR3 exist in one of two states; an inactive state in which the receptors bind ligand but do not signal phagocytosis, and an active state in which ligation immediately initiates ingestion. For example, resident peritoneal macrophages of mice have inactive C3 receptors, but after a brief incubation (10 min) of these cells with a specific T cell derived lymphokine, their C3 receptors promote phagocytosis [58]. Similarly, in human macrophages, CR1 and CR3 bind their respective ligands, but neither receptor signals the cell to initiate phagocytosis. Both receptors, however, promote phagocytosis of erythrocytes coated with the corresponding ligands after brief incubation of the macrophages with tumour-promoting phorbol esters [15].

The activity of C3 receptors on human macrophages is regulated in a similar fashion by the plasma protein, fibronectin [59,60]. C3 receptors are activated when macrophages attach to fibronectin-coated surfaces though, interestingly, C3 receptors are not activated by soluble fibronectin [60]. Interaction of surface-bound fibronectin with fibronectin receptors on the basal portion of the macrophage activates C3 receptors on the apical portion of the cell [60]. This observation indicates that C3 receptors throughout the surface of the macrophage can be activated by signals initiated within a small segment of the macrophage's plasma membrane.

Activation enables C3 receptors to generate transmembrane signals. This point is confirmed by studies on the nature of the interaction of macrophages with ligand-coated surfaces [61]. When macrophages with active (i.e. phagocytosis-competent) complement receptors contact a complement-coated surface, the cells spread enormously as though attempting to phagocytose the coverslip, and the zone between macrophage and substrate becomes inaccessible to soluble proteins in the medium. In contrast, when macrophages with inactive complement receptors contact a complement-coated surface, they attach and spread, but the zone between the macrophage and the surface remains accessible to soluble proteins in the medium [61]. Thus the seal between macrophage and ligand-coated substrate is not a consequence of receptor ligation *per se*. Rather, its formation requires cytoskeletal functions that can be inhibited by cytochalasins (unpublished observations) and that are initiated only when active phagocytosis-promoting receptors are ligated. The authors interpret this as evidence that activated receptors generate transmembrane signals.

The ability of C3 receptors to promote phagocytosis has been correlated with their mobility in the plane of the membrane. Griffin *et al.* [62] plated macrophages on C3-coated surfaces and then assayed receptor activity on the non-adherent surface of the macrophage. In this type of experiment, loss of C3 receptor activity from the non-adherent portion of the cell appears to be due to diffusion of mobile receptors to the adherent surface of the cell where they are 'trapped' by interaction with ligand [19]. Resident peritoneal macrophages that have inactive C3 receptors did not show loss of C3 receptors when plated on C3-coated surfaces, indicating that the C3 receptors of these cells are relatively immobile in the plasma membrane. In contrast, when these macrophages were plated on C3-coated surfaces and treated with a lymphokine, their C3 receptors rapidly disappeared from the cells' apical surfaces indicating that they had become mobile in the plasma membrane. This change in receptor mobility correlated temporally with activation of C3 receptors for phagocytosis. Studies employing similar methods have shown that receptors that are constitutively active in phagocytosis (Fc and oligosaccharide receptors) are constitutively mobile [18,63], suggesting that receptor mobility is a necessary condition for receptors to promote phagocytosis. That induction of C3 receptor mobility *per se* is not sufficient to activate C3 receptor function is shown in studies of CR1 and CR3 of human monocytes and macrophages. These receptors are mobile in the membranes of unstimulated human phagocytes, even though they do not mediate phagocytosis [15]. Thus mobility appears to be a necessary but not a sufficient condition for receptors to generate a phagocytic response.

Little is known of the structural basis for the regulated function of CR1 and CR3. In both mouse and man, activation of the receptors occurs rapidly (within 10 min), does not require protein synthesis, and is halted by agents that depolymerize microtubules [15,58]. Activation of C3 receptors requires the continuous presence of lymphokines [58], fibronectin, or phorbol esters [64] and is rapidly reversed when these substances are removed, thus ruling out irreversible modifications such as proteolysis as the basis for activation. Activation is not caused by enhanced expression or altered distribution of C3 receptors since treatment with fibronectin or phorbol esters does not change the number or distribution of C3 receptors on the surface of the macrophage [64]. Thus it appears that the capacity for signal transduction by CR1 and CR3 is regulated by reversible reactions (such as phosphorylation or methylation) and that these reactions can be initiated by ligation of a different class of receptors (e.g. fibronectin receptors) on the surface of the same cell. Similar activation of one receptor by signals generated by ligation of another type of receptor on the same cell may represent a common strategy employed by many different types of cells to regulate their behaviour on a short time scale. Viewed in this context, fibronectin-mediated activation of C3 receptors reflects information processing at the unicellular level.

Diversity of signals generated by one receptor

As mentioned above, macrophages release large quantities of reactive oxygen intermediates (hydrogen peroxide and superoxide) [65] and arachidonic acid metabolites [66] during Fc-mediated phagocytosis. Secretion of these substances does not require engulfment and closure of the phagosome since IgG-coated beads or substrates that are too large to be ingested readily promote release of peroxide [67] and arachidonate [68]. Nonetheless, this secretory activity has been viewed as a consequence of phagocytosis, perhaps triggered by the same transmembrane signals that initiate engulfment (Fig. 41.2a). Recent experiments, however, suggest that the problem is more complex than was recognized previously. Receptors for C3 promote phagocytosis without signalling the release of peroxide [69,70] or arachidonic acid [109]. Thus, if Fc receptors transmit a single message that initiates both secretion and phagocytosis, this signal must be different from the signal employed by C3 receptors to initiate phagocytosis (Fig. 41.2b). The hypothesis that Fc and C3 receptors initiate phagocytosis via different messages is consistent with the observations of Kaplan [71] who noted morphological differences in macrophages phagocytosing IgG- and C3-coated erythrocytes: IgG-coated particles are engulfed by pseudopods thrown up from the body of the macrophage while C3-coated erythrocytes sink into the cytoplasm of the macrophage.

An alternative view of Fc and C3 receptor signalling is shown in Fig. 41.2c. C3 and Fc receptors may employ a common signal to initiate phagocytosis, but the Fc receptors may send additional signals to promote secretion of peroxide and arachidonic acid. Admittedly, the authors know of no examples of receptors that generate two or more distinct transmembrane signals, but we would like to suggest a plausible mechanism for such a phenomenon. A number of receptors possess the ability to phosphorylate specific intracellular substrates in a ligand-dependent fashion [72]. Each phosphorylation may alter an enzyme or ion-channel activity that could constitute an intracellular message. The specificity of phosphorylation is presumably governed by enzyme–substrate interactions so that each kinase could phosphorylate one or several substrates and a given substrate could be phosphorylated by one of several kinases. Thus a receptor could send several signals by phosphorylating different substrates, and several receptors could send

identical signals by phosphorylating the same substrate.

The response to a given ligand depends on the differentiation state of the macrophage

Macrophages at different stages of differentiation exhibit different responses to ligation of the same receptors. For example, mouse macrophages elicited by BCG immunization secrete large amounts of peroxide upon ligation of their Fc receptors, while resident peritoneal macrophages secrete very small amounts of peroxide in response to the same ligand [73]. Conversely, oligosaccharide receptors of resident macrophages promote release of large amounts of arachidonic acid metabolites (both lipoxygenase and cyclo-oxygenase products) while ligation of these same receptors on BCG-elicited macrophages causes a much smaller response, and the arachidonate metabolites released are exclusively derived from the cyclo-oxygenase pathway [74]. The authors do not know which of these differences in macrophage responsiveness reflect reversible, short-term responses to modulatory ligands (such as the effect of fibronectin on C3 receptors) and which are relatively stable changes resulting from altered patterns of gene expression.

Are phagocytosis and spreading identical processes?

Spreading of cells on a surface has been likened to phagocytosis of a particle of infinite diameter. There are, however, several reasons to question this view. First, some receptors promote spreading but not phagocytosis: receptors for fibronectin show this behaviour [13,60,75]. Second, spreading and phagocytosis exhibit dissimilar morphological features. Macrophages spread on glass or plastic contact the substrate at punctate adhesion plaques, leaving the remainder of the undersurface of the cell freely accessible to soluble proteins in the extracellular

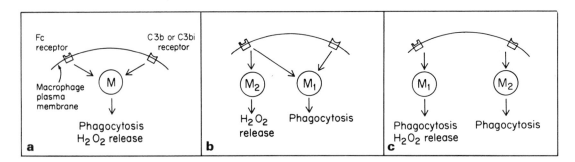

Fig. 41.2. Three models for signal generation by C3 and Fc receptors. See text for details.

medium. On the other hand, macrophages that have spread on a surface coated with ligands that promote phagocytosis (i.e. IgG or C3) exhibit a band of tight attachment to the surface that extends continuously around the periphery of the cell [61, 108]. This band of attachment forms a seal that renders the undersurface of the macrophage inaccessible to soluble proteins in the medium. Third, the rates of spreading and phagocytosis are different. Spreading of human macrophages at 37 °C requires over an hour to complete while ligand-induced 'frustrated phagocytosis' induces maximal cellular extension in 10–15 min [108].

Some problems and strategies in the study of the roles of receptors in phagocytosis

Problems

Many of the particles commonly used to assay phagocytosis (e.g. yeast cell walls, oil emulsions, laboratory strains of bacteria) contain on their surfaces ligands that promote their ingestion. For instance, yeast cell walls bind weakly to macrophages and thus are ingested inefficiently. When these particles are coated with complement they are ingested efficiently even when the macrophage complement receptors are inactive in promoting phagocytosis. This occurs because complement receptors on macrophages enhance binding of the complement-coated yeast particle to the phagocyte, thereby promoting contact between oligosaccharides on the surface of the yeast and their corresponding receptors on the surface of the macrophage. In this instance, the signal to engulf the yeast is initiated by the ligated oligosaccharide receptors.

An investigator who is unaware of the presence of these endogenous ligands on the yeast might conclude that the complement receptors signalled engulfment of these particles. For this reason the authors feel it is difficult to interpret experiments that employ particles bearing multiple ligands. Native erythrocytes and some encapsulated bacteria do not suffer from this defect. Since their surfaces are not recognized by any of the known receptor systems on phagocytes, they provide convenient surfaces to which antibodies and complement bind.

Even homogeneous ligands on erythrocytes can, at times, elicit the participation of more than one class of receptor on phagocytic leucocytes. For example, rabbit IgG* ligates at least two distinct receptors (FcRI and FcRII) on murine phagocytes [5]. In this case the reaction of two receptors with a single ligand results from using ligands from one species (rabbit) with phagocytes from another species (mouse). Such pro-

* There are no subclasses of IgG in the rabbit.

miscuity in receptor behaviour is encountered to a much smaller degree when immunoglobulins of homogeneous isotype are used in conjunction with phagocytes from the homologous species [76].

The observations of Nose & Wigzell [77] on the ligands recognized by murine Fc receptor may further complicate our view of Fc receptor specificity. These investigators prepared murine anti-erythrocyte IgG_{2b} monoclonal antibodies from hybridoma cells treated with tunicamycin (a drug which prevents glycosylation). The resulting unglycosylated IgG2b antibodies bind to antigens on erythrocytes but do not promote binding or ingestion of these erythrocytes by macrophages. These results led Nose & Wigzell to conclude that oligosaccharide residues on the Fc domain of IgG may be the ligands for Fc receptors. The authors have observed co-modulation of FcRII when mouse macrophages are plated for 4 h on substrates coated with mannose-containing oligosaccharide [110]. These findings raise the possibility that some classes of murine Fc receptor recognize oligosaccharides and have a much broader specificity than previously suspected.

A further complication in interpretation of some phagocytosis experiments arises from the findings that macrophages secrete opsonins and regulatory ligands. Two examples illustrate this point. First, macrophages incubated with yeast cell walls secrete and deposit C3 on those particles such that this macrophage-derived C3 may function as an opsonin [78]. Second, macrophages secrete fibronectin [79], and this fibronectin may alter the behaviour of their C3 receptors.

Strategies

Of the variety of experimental approaches available to dissect receptor function in macrophages and other cells, there are two that the authors think are especially worthy of comment here. The first is the use of monoclonal anti-receptor antibodies to block a single species of receptor. This approach has confirmed the presence of multiple receptors for IgG [80] and C3 [7] on macrophages, and also has been useful in functional studies of these receptors. However, three caveats must be observed in the use of monoclonal antibodies.

1 Monoclonal antibodies are not always specific for a single receptor. For example, the monoclonal antibodies IB4 [7] and TS1/18 [81] bind not only the C3bi receptor, but two additional (and homologous) receptors on human macrophages.

2 Monoclonal antibodies often block not only their target antigen but also Fc receptors on macrophages [82]. For example, monoclonal IgGs directed against

CR3 of human macrophages also block the Fc receptors of these cells (S.D. Wright & S.C. Silverstein, unpublished observations). It appears that binding of IgGs to surface antigens brings their Fc domain into close proximity with Fc receptors, thereby blocking these receptors. Fab or F(ab)₂ fragments of anti-receptor antibodies must, therefore, be used to achieve selectivity.

3 Monoclonal antibodies that bind to a receptor may not block its ligand-binding activity and may even enhance it [7,83].

A second approach to dissection of receptor function utilizes substrates that are covalently derivatized with ligands or anti-receptor antibodies. When macrophages are plated on these substrates, receptors that are mobile in the plane of the membrane move to the adherent portion of the phagocyte and can be trapped in this location by ligands or anti-receptor antibodies bound to the substrate. The cell's apical surface (the surface exposed to the medium and therefore to ligand-coated particles) thus becomes depleted of a specific class of receptor. With this technique, antibodies that bind but do not block the ligand-binding site of a receptor can be used to remove that receptor from the cells' apical surface, thereby facilitating the identification of its ligand specificity and/or function.

Ligand-coated surfaces offer a potential solution to another problem that is inherent in the study of phagocytosis. Ligand-coated particles are multivalent (10^3–10^4 ligands per particle) and thus they attach to macrophages with an enormous net affinity†. So tight is their binding that monovalent ligands are ineffective competitive inhibitors. For example, soluble IgG monomers are inefficient as inhibitors of the binding and ingestion of IgG-coated erythrocytes by macrophages [76].

The efficiency of soluble ligands can be enhanced enormously by attaching them to a culture surface. The high local concentration of ligand that can be achieved on a surface (10^{-3}–10^{-4} M [19]) can cause complete down-modulation of receptors and thereby abolish the binding of ligand-coated particles to macrophages. Employed in this way, ligand- and antibody-coated surfaces are powerful tools for investigating the complexities of a variety of processes regulated by surface receptors.

Summary and speculations

Phagocytosis is a dynamic process that requires co-ordinated interactions of cytoskeletal elements and plasma membrane. To direct the motile force for

† Given a monovalent ligand with a binding affinity of K, the net affinity for the interaction of dimers of the ligand with two receptors is roughly K^2, for trimers it is K^3, and so on.

pseudopod extension and membrane movement, cytoskeletal proteins must be assembled into structures of higher order. To allow continued membrane movements, remodelling of the adjacent cytoplasm, and passage of the ingested particle through the cortical cytoplasm into the cytocentre, these same cytoskeletal elements must be *dis*assembled. Assembly and disassembly processses must be co-ordinated spatially and temporally to achieve engulfment of the particle, much as agonist and antagonist muscles must work co-ordinately to allow limb movement.

The authors believe that plasma membrane receptors and their associated proteins are the principal molecules that regulate and co-ordinate the phagocytic process. Thus they presume that the signals generated by phagocytosis-promoting receptors must be transient or biphasic to accommodate sequential assembly and disassembly of the phagocytic machinery. Interestingly, FcRII displays exactly this property. Ligation of FcRII opens a monovalent cation channel that then closes with a pre-programmed time constant of 250 ms [54]. The ion flux initiated by FcRII ligation is brief and, due to its short duration, probably local. The authors do not know whether these ion fluxes are sufficient or even necessary signals to induce changes in the cytoplasm, but their transient nature satisfies one requirement for phagocytosis-promoting signals. Thus the authors consider receptor-mediated ion fluxes likely candidates for one class of intracellular signals that initiates phagocytosis.

Engulfment is initiated by the interaction of particle-bound ligands with their corresponding membrane receptors. Once ligated, these receptors must orchestrate a series of reactions that lead to pseudopod extension and the apposition of additional membrane with the surface of the particle. Since unligated receptors have high diffusion rates (2–3×10^{-9} cm²/s for Fc receptors [19]), they soon encounter a ligand on the surface of the particle and are themselves bound to it. This leads to the vectorial propagation of engulfment signals.

An increase in cytosolic Ca^{2+} accompanies Fc receptor ligation [84]. Hoffstein's work [85] suggests that this Ca^{2+} may be derived from storage depots associated with the segments of plasma membrane in which receptor–ligand interactions have occurred. This released Ca^{2+} may be used in concert with gelsolin to disassemble the actin network. Immunofluorescence analyses of the locations of cytoskeletal proteins during phagocytosis show gelsolin to be concentrated at the base of the nascent phagocytic vacuole and relatively scarce at the tips of the advancing pseudopods [39]. The authors presume that cellular homeostatic processes are responsible for removal of the monovalent cations that enter the cytoplasm as a result of receptor ligation, and for the return of free Ca^{2+} concentrations to their resting levels. Reduction in local Ca^{2+} concentrations should stop the action of gelsolin.

The authors believe that the entire sequence of events described above is repeated many times during phagocytosis. Ultimately, engulfment is completed, no more receptors are ligated, no more signals are generated, and the phagocyte is free to digest the fruits of its labours.

Many problems remain to be solved. Listed below are a number of questions that the authors believe are central to further progress. Motivating their choice of questions is the belief that structural information will be essential to understanding receptor function.

1 What is the structure of phagocytosis-promoting receptors, especially in their cytoplasmic domains? Do these receptors interact with other membrane or cytosolic proteins? What is the nature of these interactions?

2 Do all phagocytosis-promoting receptors generate ionic signals? How many different signals can be generated by a single type of receptor? Which of these mediate phagocytosis?

3 How are regulated receptors (such as CR1 and CR3) switched on and off by receptors for other ligands?

4 What receptors and mechanisms are involved in the 'non-specific' uptake of particles such as latex?

5 Do receptors co-ordinate the phagocytic process as postulated, or is control vested in other membrane or cytosolic molecules?

6 How are the forces that move pseudopods around particles generated and directed? What roles, if any, do myosin and clathrin play in phagocytosis?

Acknowledgement

The research described in this review was supported by grant CA30198, AI08697, AI22003 and NS18793 from the USPHS, by JFRA-103 from the ACS and by a grant from the Muscular Dystrophy Association.

References

1 BESHARSE J.C. (1982) The daily light–dark cycle and rhythmic metabolism in the photoreceptor-pigment epithelial complex. In *Progress in Retinal Research*, (eds. Osborne N. & Chader G.). Pergamon Press, Oxford.

2 METCHNIKOFF E. (1887) Sur la lutta des cellules de l'organismes centre l'invasion des microbes. *Anals Inst. Pasteur, Paris*, **1**, 321.

3 NICHOLS B.A. (1976) Normal rabbit alveolar macro-phages. (I) The phagocytosis of tubular myelin. *J. exp. Med.* **144**, 906.

4 SCHLEPPER-SCHAFER J., KOLB-BACHOFEN V. & KOLB H. (1983) Identification of a receptor for senescent erythro-cytes on liver macrophages. *Biochem. biophys. Res. Commun.* **112**, 551.

5 UNKELESS J.C., FLEIT H. & MELLMAN I.S. (1981) Structural aspects and heterogeneity of immunoglobulin Fc receptors. *Adv. Immunol.* **32**, 247.

6 FEARON D.T. (1980) Identification of the membrane glycoprotein that is the C3b receptor of the human erythrocyte, polymorphonuclear leukocyte, B lympho-cyte, and monocytes. *J. exp. Med.* **152**, 20.

7 WRIGHT S.D., RAO P.E., VAN VOORHIS W.C., CRAIG-MYLE L.S., IIDA K., TALLE M.A., WESTBERG E.F., GOLDSTEIN G. & SILVERSTEIN S.C. (1980) Identification of the C3bi receptor of human monocytes and macro-phages by using monoclonal antibodies. *Proc. natn. Acad. Sci. U.S.A.* **80**, 5699.

8 RABINOVITCH M. (1967) The dissociation of the attach-ment and ingestion phases of phagocytosis by macro-phages. *Exptl Cell Res.* **46**, 19.

9 MAHONEY E.M., HAMILL A.L., SCOTT W.A. & COHN Z.A. (1977) Response of endocytosis to altered fatty acyl composition of macrophage phospholipids. *Proc. natn. Acad. Sci. U.S.A.* **74**, 4895.

10 SILVERSTEIN S.C., STEINMAN R.M. & COHN Z.A. (1977) · Endocytosis. *Ann. Rev. Biochem.* **46**, 669.

11 HORWITZ M.A. & SILVERSTEIN S.C. (1980) Influence of the *Escherichia coli* capsule on complement fixation and on phagocytosis and killing by human phagocytes. *J. clin. Invest.* **65**, 82.

12 GRIFFIN F.M. JUN. & SILVERSTEIN S.C. (1974) Segmental response of the macrophage plasma membrane to a phagocytic stimulus. *J. exp. Med.* **139**, 323.

13 BEVILACQUA M.P., AMRANI D., MOSESSON M.W. & BIANCO C. (1981) Receptors for cold-insoluble globulin (plasma fibronectin) on human monocytes. *J. exp. Med.* **153**, 42.

14 BIANCO C., GRIFFIN F.M. JUN. & SILVERSTEIN S.C. (1975) Studies of the macrophage complement receptor. Alteration of receptor function upon macrophage acti-vation. *J. exp. Med.* **141**, 1278.

15 WRIGHT S.D. & SILVERSTEIN S.C. (1982) Tumor-pro-moting phorbol esters stimulate C3b and C3b′ receptor-mediated phagocytosis in cultured human monocytes. *J. exp. Med.* **156**, 1149.

16 GRIFFIN F.M., GRIFFIN J.A., LEIDER J.E. & SILVERSTEIN S.C. (1975) Studies on the mechanism of phagocytosis. (I) Requirements for circumferential attachment of particle-bound ligands to specific receptors on the macrophage plasma membrane. *J. exp. Med.* **142**, 1263.

17 SHAW P.R. & GRIFFIN F.M. JUN. (1981) Phagocytosis requires repeated triggering of macrophage phagocytic receptors during particle ingestion. *Nature*, **289**, 409.

18 MICHL J., PIECZONKA M.M., UNKELESS J.C. & SILVER-STEIN S.C. (1979) Effects of immobilized immune com-plexes on Fc- and complement-receptor function in resident and thioglycollate-elicited mouse peritoneal macrophages. *J. exp. Med.* **150**, 607.

19 MICHL J., PIECZONKA M.M., UNKELESS J.C., BELL G.I.

& SILVERSTEIN S.C. (1983) Fc receptor modulation in mononuclear phagocytes maintained on immobilized immune complexes occurs by diffusion of the receptor molecule. *J. exp. Med.* **157**, 2121.

20 EHLENBERGER A.G. & NUSSENZWEIG V. (1977) The role of membrane receptors for C3b and C3d in phagocytosis. *J. exp. Med.* **145**, 357.

21 MICHL J., UNKELESS J.C., PIECZONKA M.M. & SILVERSTEIN S.C. (1983) Modulation of Fc receptors of mononuclear phagocytes by immobilized antigen–antibody complexes. Quantitative analysis of the relationship between ligand concentration and Fc receptor response. *J. exp. Med.* **157**, 1746.

22 GRIFFIN F.M. JUN., GRIFFIN J.A. & SILVERSTEIN S.C. (1977) Studies on the mechanism of phagocytosis. (II) The interaction of macrophages with anti-immunoglobulin IgG-coated bone marrow-derived lymphocytes. *J. exp. Med.* **144**, 788.

23 ORENSTEIN J.M. & SHELTON E. (1977) Membrane phenomena accompanying erythrophagocytosis. *Lab. Invest.* **36**, 363.

24 PHAIRE-WASHINGTON L., WANG E. & SILVERSTEIN S.C. (1980) Phorbol myristate acetate stimulates pinocytosis and membrane spreading in mouse peritoneal macrophages. *J. Cell Biol.* **86**, 634.

25 UNKELESS J.C. & HEALEY G.A. (1983) Quantitation of proteins and internal antigen pools by a monoclonal sandwich radioimmune assay. *J. immunol. Meth.* **56**, 1.

26 BOWERS B., OLSZEWSKI T.E. & HYDE J. (1983) Morphometric analysis of volumes and surface area in membrane compartments during endocytosis in *Acanthamoeba*. *J. Cell Biol.* **88**, 509.

27 RYTER A. & DE CHASTELLIER C. (1977) Morphometric and cytochemical studies of *Dictyostelium discoideum* in vegetative phase. Digestive system and membrane turnover. *J. Cell Biol.* **75**, 200.

28 MULLER W.A., STEINMAN R.M. & COHN Z.A. (1982) The membrane proteins of the vacuolar system. (III) Further studies on the composition and recycling of endocytic vacuole membrane in cultured macrophages. *J. Cell. Biol.* **96**, 29.

29 TSAN M.F. & BERLIN R.D. (1971) Effect of phagocytosis on membrane transport of nonelectrolytes. *J. exp. Med.* **134**, 1016.

30 STEINMAN R.M., MELLMAN I.S., MULLER W.A. & COHN Z.A. (1983) Endocytosis and the recycling of plasma membrane. *J. Cell Biol.* **96**, 1.

31 HUBBARD A.L. & COHN Z.A. (1975) Externally disposed plasma membrane proteins. (I) Enzymatic iodination of mouse L cells. *J. Cell Biol.* **64**, 438.

32 HUBBARD A.L. & COHN Z.A. (1975) Externally disposed plasma membrane proteins. (II) Metabolic fate of iodinated polypeptides of mouse L cells. *J. Cell Biol.* **64**, 461.

33 MULLER W.A., STEINMAN R.M. & COHN Z.A. (1980) The membrane proteins of the vacuolar system. (II) Bidirectional flow between secondary lysosomes and plasma membrane. *J. Cell Biol.* **86**, 305.

34 MULLER W.A., STEINMAN R.M. & COHN Z.A. (1980) The membrane proteins of the vacuolar system. (I)

35 MELLMAN I.S., PLUTNER H., STEINMAN R.M., UNKELESS J.C. & COHN Z.A. (1983) Internalization and degradation of macrophage Fc receptors during receptor mediated phagocytosis. *J. Cell Biol.* **96**, 887.

36 HARTWIG J.H. & STOSSEL T.P. The structure of actin-binding protein molecules in solution and interacting with actin filaments. *J. Mol. Biol.* **145**, 563.

37 YIN H.L. & STOSSEL T.P. (1980) Purification and structural properties of gelsolin, a Ca^{++}-activated regulatory protein of macrophages. *J. Biol. Chem.* **255**, 9490.

38 BOXER L.A., HEDLEY-WHITE E.T. & STOSSEL T.P. (1974) Neutrophil actin dysfunction and abnormal neutrophil behaviour. *New Engl. J. Med.* **291**, 1093.

39 STENDAHL O.I., HARTWIG J.H. & BROTSCHI E.A. (1980) Distribution of actin-binding protein and myosin in macrophages during spreading and phagocytosis. *J. Cell Biol.* **84**, 215.

40 AXLINE S.G. & REAVEN E.P. (1974) Inhibition of phagocytosis and plasma membrane mobility of the cultivated macrophage by cytochalasin B. Role of subplasmalemmal microfilaments. *J. Cell Biol.* **62**, 647.

41 MONTESANO R., MOSSAZ A., VASSALLI P. & ORCI L. (1983) Specialization of the macrophage plasma membrane at sites of interaction with opsonized erythrocytes. *J. Cell Biol.* **96**, 1227.

42 AGGELER J. & WERB Z. (1982) Initial events during phagocytosis by macrophages viewed from the outside and the inside of the cell: membrane–particle interaction and clathrin. *J. Cell Biol.* **94**, 613.

43 HELENIUS A., MARSH M. & WHITE J. (1980) Virus entry into animal cells. *Trends biochem. Sci.* **6**, 104.

44 ROOS D., VOETMAN A.A. & MEERHOF L.J. (1983) Functional activity of enucleated human polymorphonuclear leukocytes. *J. Cell Biol.* **97**, 368.

45 TILNEY L.G., HATANO S., ISHIKAWA H. & MOOSEKER M. (1973) The polymerization of actin: Its role in the generation of the acrosomal process of certain echinoderm sperm. *J. Cell Biol.* **81**, 608.

46 MUSCHEL R.L., ROSEN N. & BLOOM B.R. (1977) Isolation of variants in phagocytosis of a macrophage-like continuous cell line. *J. exp. Med.* **145**, 175.

47 UNKELESS J.C., KAPLAN G., PLUTNER H. & COHN Z.A. (1979) Fc-receptor variants of a mouse macrophage cell line. *Proc. natn. Acad. Sci. U.S.A.* **76**, 1400.

48 TAKASAKI S., EMLING F. & LEIVE L. (1984) Variants deficient in phagocytosis of latex beads isolated from the murine macrophage-like cell line. *J. Cell Biol.* **98**, 2198.

49 KIEHART D.P., MABUCHI I. & INOUE S. (1982) Evidence that myosin does not contribute the force production in chromosome movement. *J. Cell Biol.* **94**, 165.

50 SANDOVAL I.V., BONIFACINO J.S., KLAUSNER R.D., HENKART M. & WEHLAND J. (1984) Role of microtubules in the organization and localization of the Golgi apparatus. *J. Cell Biol.* **99**, 113s.

51 COHN Z.A. & MORSE S.I. (1960) Functional and metabolic properties of polymorphonuclear leukocytes. (I) Observations on the requirements and consequences of particle ingestion. *J. exp. Med.* **111**, 667.

52 LOIKE J.D., KOZLER V.F. & SILVERSTEIN S.C. (1979) Increased ATP and creatine phosphate turnover in phagocytosing mouse peritoneal macrophages. *J. Biol. Chem.* **154**, 9558.

53 MICHL J., OHLBAUM D.J. & SILVERSTEIN S.C. (1976) 2-Deoxyglucose selectively inhibits Fc and complement receptor-mediated phagocytosis in mouse peritoneal macrophages. (I) Description of the inhibitory effect. *J. exp. Med.* **144**, 1465.

54 YOUNG J.D.-E., UNKELESS J.C., YOUNG T.M., MAURO A. & COHN Z.A. (1983) Role for mouse macrophage IgG Fc receptor as ligand-dependent ion channel. *Nature*, **306**, 186.

55 YOUNG J.D.-E., UNKELESS J.C., KABACK H.R. & COHN Z.A. (1983) Macrophage membrane potential changes associated with the $\gamma 2b/\gamma 1$ Fc receptor–ligand binding. *Proc. natn. Acad. Sci. U.S.A.* **80**, 1357.

56 CARLO J.R., RUDDY S., STUDER E.J. & CONRAD D.H. (1979) Complement receptor binding of C3b-coated cells treated with C3b inactivator, $\beta 1$H globulin and trypsin. *J. Immunol.* **123**, 523.

57 INADA S., BROWN E.J., GAITHER T.A., HAMMER C.H., TAKAHASHIJ T. & FRANK M.M. (1983) C3d receptors are expressed on human monocytes after *in vitro* cultivation. *Proc. natn. Acad. Sci. U.S.A.* **80**, 2351.

58 GRIFFIN J.A. & GRIFFIN F.M. JUN. (1979) Augmentation of macrophage complement receptor function *in vitro*. (I) Characterization of the cellular interactions required for the generation of a T-lymphocyte product that enhances macrophage complement receptor function. *J. exp. Med.* **150**, 653.

59 POMMIER C.G., INADA S., FRIES L.F., TAKAHASHI T., FRANK M.M. & BROWN E.J. (1983) Plasma fibronectin enhances phagocytosis of opsonized particles by human peripheral blood monocytes. *J. exp. Med.* **157**, 1844.

60 WRIGHT S.D., CRAIGMYLE L.S. & SILVERSTEIN S.C. (1983) Fibronectin and serum amyloid P component stimulate C3b- and C3bi-mediated phagocytosis in cultured human monocytes. *J. exp. Med.* **158**, 1338.

61 WRIGHT S.D. & SILVERSTEIN S.C. (1982) Phagocytosing macrophages exclude soluble macromolecules from the zone of contact with ligand-coated targets. *Nature*, **309**, 359.

62 GRIFFIN F.M. JUN. & MULLINAX P.J. (1981) Augmentation of macrophage complement receptor function *in vitro*. (III) C3b receptors that promote phagocytosis migrate within the plane of the macrophage membrane. *J. exp. Med.* **154**, 291.

63 SUNG S.J., NELSON R.S. & SILVERSTEIN S.C. (1983) Yeast mannans inhibit binding and phagocytosis of zymosan by mouse peritoneal macrophages. *J. Cell Biol.* **96**, 160.

64 WRIGHT S.D., LICHT M.R., CRAIGMYLE L.S. & SILVERSTEIN S.C. (1984) Communication between receptors for different ligands on a single cell; ligation of fibronectin receptors induces a reversible alteration of the function of complement receptors on cultured human monocytes. *J. Cell Biol.* **99**, 336.

65 NATHAN C.F. & ROOT R.K. (1977) Hydrogen peroxide release from mouse peritoneal macrophages. *J. exp. Med.* **146**, 1648.

66 SCOTT W.A., ZRIKE J.M., HAMMILL A.L., KEMPE J. & COHN Z.A. (1980) Regulation of arachidonic acid metabolites in macrophages. *J. exp. Med.* **152**, 324.

67 JOHNSTON R.B. JUN., LEHMEYER J.E. & GUTHRIE L.A. (1976) Generation of superoxide anion and chemiluminescence by human monocytes during phagocytosis and on contact with surface-bound immunoglobulin G. *J. exp. Med.* **143**, 1551.

68 ROUZER C.A., SCOTT W.A., KEMPE J. & COHN Z.A. (1980) Prostaglandin synthesis by macrophages requires a specific receptor–ligand interaction. *Proc. natn. Acad. Sci. U.S.A.* **77**, 4279.

69 WRIGHT S.D. & SILVERSTEIN S.C. (1983) Receptors for C3b and C3bi promote phagocytosis but not the release of toxic oxygen from human phagocytes. *J. exp. Med.* **158**, 2016.

70 YAMAMOTO K. & JOHNSTON R.B. JUN. (1984) Dissociation of phagocytosis from stimulation of the oxidative metabolic burst in macrophages. *J. exp. Med.* **159**, 405.

71 KAPLAN G. (1977) Differences in the mode of phagocytosis with Fc and C3 receptors in macrophages. *Scand. J. Immunol.* **6**, 797.

72 COBB M.H. & ROSEN O.M. (1983) The insulin receptor and tyrosine protein kinase activity. *Biochim. biophys. Acta*, **738**, 1.

73 EZEKOWITZ R.A.B., BAMPTON M. & GORDON S. (1983) Macrophage activation selectively enhances expression of Fc receptors for IgG2a. *J. exp. Med.* **157**, 807.

74 SCOTT W.A., PALOWSKI N.A., MURRAY H.W., ANDREACH M., ZRIKE J. & COHN Z.A. (1982) Regulation of arachidonic acid metabolism by macrophage activation. *J. exp. Med.* **155**, 1148.

75 VAN DE WATER L., DESTREE A.T. & HYNES R.O. (1983) Fibronectin binds to some bacteria but does not promote their uptake by phagocytic cells. *Science*, **220**, 201.

76 DIAMOND B., BLOOM B.R. & SCHARFF M.D. (1978) The Fc receptors of primary and cultured phagocytic cells studied with homogeneous antibodies. *J. Immunol.* **121**, 1329.

77 NOSE M. & WIGZELL H. (1983) Biological significance of carbohydrate chains on monoclonal antibodies. *Proc. natn. Acad. Sci. U.S.A.* **80**, 6632.

78 EZEKOWITZ R.A.B., SIM R.B., HILL M. & GORDON S. (1984) Local opsonization by secreted macrophage complement components. Role of receptors for complement in uptake of zymosan. *J. exp. Med.* **159**, 244.

79 ALITALO K., HOVI T. & VAHERI A. (1980) Fibronectin is produced by human macrophages. *J. exp. Med.* **151**, 602.

80 UNKELESS J.C. (1979) Characterization of a monoclonal antibody against mouse macrophage and lymphocyte Fc receptors. *J. exp. Med.* **150**, 580.

81 SANCHEZ-MADRID F., NAGY J.A., ROBBINS E., SIMON P. & SPRINGER T.A. (1983) Characterization of a human leukocyte differentiation antigen family with distinct α subunits and a common β subunit: The lymphocyte-function associated antigen (LFA-1), the C3bi complement receptor (OKM1/Mac-1), and the p150,95 molecule. *J. exp. Med.* **158**, 1785.

82 KURLANDER R.J. (1983) Blockade of Fc receptor-mediated binding to U-937 cells by murine monoclonal

antibodies directed against a variety of surface antigens. *J. Immunol.* **131**, 140.

83 SIMON P., SANCHEZ-MADRID F. & SPRINGER T.A. (1983) Enhancement of complement receptor type 3 with monoclonal antibody to the MAC-1 β subunit. *Fedn Proc.* **41**, 841.

84 YOUNG J.D.-E. (1983) Rise of free intracellular Ca^{2+} in mouse macrophage associated with γ2b/γ1 Fc receptor–ligand and interaction. *Biol. Bull.* **165**, 498.

85 HOFFSTEIN S.T. (1979) Ultrastructural demonstration of calcium loss from local regions of the plasma membrane of surface-stimulated human granulocytes. *J. Immunol.* **123**, 1395.

86 FLEIT H.B., WRIGHT S.D. & UNKELESS J.C. (1982) Human neutrophil Fcγ receptor distribution and structure. *Proc. natn. Acad. Sci. U.S.A.* **79**, 3275.

87 SPIEGELBERG H.L., BOLTZ-NITULESCU G., PLUMMER J.M. & MELEWICZ F.M. (1983) Characterization of the IgE Fc receptors on monocytes and macrophages. *Fedn Proc.* **42**, 124.

88 STAHL P.D., RODMAN J.S., MILLER M.J. & SCHLESINGER P.H. (1978) Evidence for receptor-mediated binding of glycoproteins, glycoconjugates and lysosomal glycosidases by alveolar macrophages. *Proc. natn. Acad. Sci. U.S.A.* **75**, 1399.

89 BLECHER M. & GOLDSTEIN S. (1977) Hormone receptors: VI. On the nature of binding of glucagon and insulin to human circulating mononuclear leukocytes. *Mol. cell. Endocr.* **8**, 301.

90 KALISKER A., NELSON H.E. & MIDDLETON E. JUN. (1977) Drug-induced changes of adenylate cyclase activity in cells from asthmatic and nonasthmatic subjects. *J. Allergy clin. Immunol.* **60**, 259.

91 SELIGMANN B.E., FLETCHER M.P. & GALLIN J.I. (1983) Histamine modulation of human neutrophil oxidative metabolism, locomotion, degranulation, and membrane potential changes. *J. Immunol.* **130**, 1902.

92 ROSENFELD R., THORSSON A.V. & HINTZ R.L. (1979) Increased somatomedin receptor sites in newborn circulating mononuclear cells. *J. clin. Endocr. Metab.* **48**, 456.

93 LUBEN R.A., WONG G. & COHN D.V. (1976) Biochemical characterization with parathormone and calcitonin of isolated bone cells: Provisional identification of osteoclasts and osteoblasts. *Endocrinology*, **99**, 526.

94 SCHREIBER R.D., PACE J.L., RUSSEL S.W., ALTMAN A. & KATZ D.H. (1983) Macrophage-activating factor produced by a T cell hybridoma: Physiochemical and biosynthetic resemblance to α-interferon. *J. Immunol.* **131**, 826.

95 GUILBERT L.J. & STANLEY E.R. (1980) Specific interaction at murine colony-stimulating factors with mononuclear phagocytic cells. *J. Cell Biol.* **85**, 153.

96 KAPLAN J. & NEILSEN M.L. (1979) Analysis of macrophage surface receptors. (I) Binding of α2-macroglobulin–protease complexes to rabbit alveolar macrophages. *J. Biol. Chem.* **254**, 7323.

97 GOLDSTEIN J.L., HO K.Y., BASU S.K. & BROWN M.S. (1979) A binding site on macrophages that mediates the uptake and degradation of acetylated low density lipoproteins, producing massive cholesterol deposition. *Proc. natn. Acad. Sci. U.S.A.* **76**, 333.

98 KRAEMER F.B., CHEN Y.D., LOPEZ R.D. & REAVEN G.M. (1983) Characterization of the binding site on thioglycolate-stimulated mouse peritoneal macrophages that mediates the uptake of very low density lipoproteins. *J. Biol. Chem.* **158**, 12190.

99 WYLLIE J.C. (1977) Transferrin uptake by rabbit alveolar macrophages *in vitro*. *Br. J. Haematol.* **37**, 17.

100 SYNDERMAN R. & PIKE M.C. (1984) Chemoattractant receptors on phagocytic cells. *Ann. Rev. Immunol.* **2**, 257.

101 BAR-SHAVIT R., KAHN A., FENTON J.W. & WILNER G.D. (1983) Chemotactic response of monocytes to thrombin. *J. Cell Biol.* **96**, 282.

102 CAMPBELL E.J., WHITE R.R., SENIOR R.M., RODRIGUEZ R.J. & KUHN C. (1979) Receptor-mediated binding and internalization of leukocyte elastase by alveolar macrophages *in vitro*. *J. clin. Invest.* **64**, 824.

103 VAN SNICK J.L. & MASSON P.L. (1976) The binding of human lactoferrin to mouse peritoneal cells. *J. exp. Med.* **144**, 1568.

104 SHERMAN L.A. & LEE J. (1977) Specific binding of soluble fibrin to macrophages. *J. exp. Med.* **145**, 76.

105 ADAMS D.O. & HAMILTON T.A. (1984) The cell biology of macrophage activation. *Ann. Rev. Immunol.* **2**, 283.

106 TENNER A.S. & COOPER N.R. (1980) Analysis of receptor mediated C1q binding to human peripheral blood mononuclear cells. *J. Immunol.* **125**, 1658.

107 MCNEIL P.L., MURPHY R.F., LANNI F. & TAYLOR D.L. (1984) A method for incorporating macromolecules into adherent cells. *J. Cell Biol.* **98**, 1565.

108 HEIPLE J.M., ALLEN N.S., WRIGHT S.D. & SILVERSTEIN S.C. (1984) Cell–substrate interactions during frustrated phagocytosis: reflection-interference microscopic analysis. *J. Cell Biol.* **99**, 326a (abstract).

109 ADEREM A.A., WRIGHT S.D., SILVERSTEIN S.C. & COHN Z.A. (1985) Ligated complement receptors do not activate the arachidonic acid cascade in resident peritoneal macrophages. *J. exp. Med.* **161**, 617.

110 SUNG S.S.J., NELSON R. & SILVERSTEIN S.C. (1985) Mouse peritoneal macrophages plated on mannan- and horseradish peroxidase-Fc receptors. J. Immunol. (in press).

Chapter 42
Overview: the mononuclear phagocyte system

R. VAN FURTH

General aspects of the
mononuclear phagocyte
system, 42.1

'Mononuclear phagocytes' is the name given to a cell line comprising macrophages, monocytes, pro-monocytes, and monoblasts. The monoblast and the pro-monocyte, which are localized in the bone marrow, are dividing cells that give rise to monocytes [1–4]. Monocytes leave the bone marrow and are transported via the peripheral blood to the tissues, where they become macrophages [1–4, 17].

General aspects of the mononuclear phagocyte system

Characterization

For the study of the physiological functions of mononuclear phagocytes, as well as their role in pathophysiology, adequate characterization of the cells under study is necessary. Until recently, use was mainly made of morphological criteria. This is not sufficient, because the group of mononuclear phagocytes includes many different forms. Therefore more advanced techniques must be used to characterize a cell as a mononuclear phagocyte and to distinguish it from other cells with similar morphology. Methods to characterize mononuclear phagocytes are:

(1) light, phase-contrast, and electron microscopy;
(2) cytochemical determination of cytoplasmic, lysosomal, and ecto-enzymes;
(3) determination of membrane antigens and receptors with (monoclonal) antibodies;
(4) determination of the presence and function of receptors (e.g. Fc and C receptors, immune phagocytosis).

Because neither the specificity of the available markers nor the sensitivity of the techniques used is optimal yet, classification must be based on more than one property. One of the most reliable markers for the identification of mononuclear phagocytes of human or animal origin is non-specific esterase with α-naphthyl butyrate or acetate as substrate [5,6]. In these cells the non-specific esterase is localized diffusely in the cytoplasm; in T lymphocytes, which show two or more positive dots, the enzyme occurs in granules. Lyso-

zyme is another good marker and can be demonstrated with an immunofluorescent and immune peroxidase method using a species-specific, anti-lysozyme antibody [6]. Unlike these two enzymes, peroxidase is a useful marker to distinguish various developmental stages of mononuclear phagocytes (Fig. 42.1). At the light- and electron-microscopical levels, the localization of peroxidase is different in monoblasts, pro-monocytes, monocytes, and macrophages. Granules are only positive in monoblasts, pro-monocytes, monocytes, and exudate macrophages; resident macrophages are negative, which means that with light microscopy no peroxidatic activity is seen in resident macrophages. The demonstration of peroxidatic activity in the rough endoplasmic reticulum, nuclear envelope, and Golgi apparatus of mononuclear phagocytes is only possible with electron microscopy (Fig. 42.1).

Other enzymes suitable for the characterization of mononuclear phagocytes are the ecto-enzymes 5'-nucleotidase, leucine aminopeptidase, and alkaline phosphodiesterase I, which occur in the plasma membrane of these cells and can be determined cytochemically. 5'-Nucleotidase is helpful for distinguishing normal (resident) macrophages from activated macrophages, since its activity is high in the former and extremely low in the latter, whereas that of the other two ecto-enzymes increases upon activation.

The availability of monoclonal antibodies has greatly facilitated the characterization of cells. These antibodies react specifically with antigens or receptors on the cell membrane or with cytoplasmic structures or enzymes. However, cross-reactivity of a given kind of monoclonal antibody with antigens, receptors, or other structures of completely unrelated cells sometimes causes problems. Furthermore, the antigenic structure to which the monoclonal antibody is directed is usually species specific.

Receptors for the Fc part of IgG and for C3 on the cell surface, along with a number of functional characteristics including endocytosis, are intrinsic properties of mononuclear phagocytes. These cells

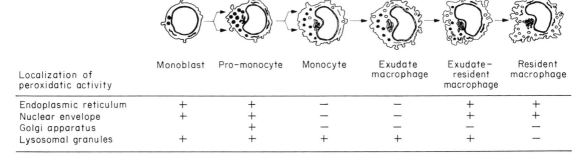

Localization of peroxidatic activity	Monoblast	Pro-monocyte	Monocyte	Exudate macrophage	Exudate-resident macrophage	Resident macrophage
Endoplasmic reticulum	+	+	−	−	+	+
Nuclear envelope	+	+	−	−	+	+
Golgi apparatus		+	−	−	−	−
Lysosomal granules	+	+	+	+	+	−

Fig. 42.1. Peroxidase activity patterns and sequence of development of monoblasts, pro-monocytes, monocytes, and macrophages.

carry Fc and C receptors in all stages of their development, but in immature stages (monoblasts and pro-monocytes) the percentage of cells with receptors may be lower than in the monocytes and macrophages [7]. Ingestion of opsonized bacteria or IgG-coated red cells (immune phagocytosis) is a very important criterion that must be fulfilled before a cell can be called a mononuclear phagocyte. However, ingestion of complement-coated red cells (EIgMC) does not occur unless mononuclear phagocytes have been activated; this does not hold for bacteria, which are readily ingested by monocytes and non-activated macrophages when coated with complement or IgM plus complement.

All mononuclear phagocytes pinocytose avidly but pinocytosis is also performed by other kinds of cell (e.g. fibroblasts), although to a much smaller degree. Non-toxic vital dyes and colloidal carbon are not suitable for the characterization of endocytic activity in mononuclear phagocytes because other kinds of cell also ingest these substances to some extent.

The minimum requirements to be satisfied before a cell can be called a mononuclear phagocyte are difficult to define. It is generally accepted that mononuclear phagocytes must be at least esterase-positive, contain Fc receptors in their membranes, and ingest IgG-coated particles. Often, because of differences in developmental stage and state of activation, not all of the cell types are positive for a given criterion. However, it is generally accepted that positivity of 90% or more of the cells in a population is sufficient to call a population positive for the criterion in question.

Origin and kinetics

Mononuclear phagocytes form a cell line that originates from the pluripotent stem cell in the bone marrow. The most immature cell of this line is the monoblast (Figs 42.1 and 42.2). In the mouse, the cell cycle of the monoblast is about 12 h, and after division one cell gives rise to two pro-monocytes. The pro-monocyte too divides only once (cell-cycle time about 16 h) and gives rise to two monocytes (Fig. 42.2). Thus from monoblast to monocyte there is a fourfold amplification. Monocytes do not divide further, and leave the bone marrow randomly within 24 h after they are formed. These cells remain in the circulation for a relatively long time (mouse: half-time about 17 h; man: half-time about 71 h) compared with granulocytes (half-time about 7 h), and they leave this compartment randomly.

During the last twenty years, considerable attention has been given to the origin of the macrophages. The bone marrow origin of macrophages in the peritoneal cavity, liver, spleen, and lung, as well as that of synovial type-A cells and osteoclasts, has been proven by a large number of chimera studies [8]. In addition, *in vitro* labelling studies with the DNA precursor ^{3}H-thymidine showed a labelling index of less than 5% for macrophages at various sites; these mononuclear phagocytes are not resident macrophages but have very recently (less than 24–48 h before harvesting) arrived in the tissues from the bone marrow. Kinetic studies with *in vivo*-labelled monocytes done in normal and monocytopenic mice and in irradiated mice with partial bone marrow shielding, have provided proof that the monocytes migrate from the blood into the tissues, where they become macrophages (Figs 42.1 and 42.2) [1–4]. The current view is that in the normal steady state the maintenance of the population of macrophages in a tissue compartment depends on the influx of monocytes from the circulation and on local division of mononuclear phagocytes that also derive from the bone marrow and divide once in the tissues. Quantitative kinetic studies in normal mice have shown that of the monocytes leaving the circulation about 56% become Kupffer cells, about 30% become

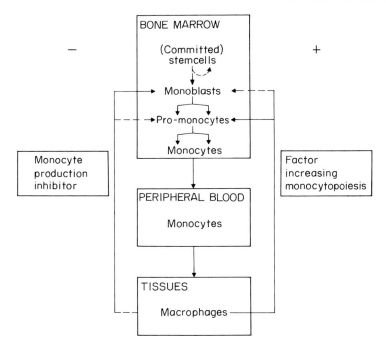

Fig. 42.2. Schematic representation of the origin and kinetics of mononuclear phagocytes, and the humoral control (positive and negative feedback mechanisms) of the production of monocytes.

spleen macrophages, about 15% become pulmonary macrophages, and about 8% become peritoneal macrophages. Calculations have further shown that on average, 75% or more of the macrophage population is supplied by the influx of monocytes and 25% or less by local division of (immature) mononuclear phagocytes. Based on these data, the calculated mean turn-over time of macrophages in the tissues would be about 6–7 days, which is much shorter than the turnover time previously reported.

In the normal steady state the combination of a constant influx of monocytes into tissues (where they become macrophages) and a constant local production, implies a constant cell death in the tissues and/or a constant efflux of cells from the tissue compartments. Almost nothing is known about this point, except that the latter cells in all probability migrate to the local lymph nodes and that lung macrophages leave the body via air spaces.

Another important point which should be considered in the study of experimental or pathological lesions in which mononuclear phagocytes are involved is whether these cells accumulate or proliferate in the tissues. These terms are often used erroneously: proliferation should be reserved for cases in which the increase in the number of cells is known to be due to the division of cells already present at, or recruited to, a site and the term accumulation for increases due to the migration of (non-dividing) cells from other sites (e.g. the circulation).

Regulation of monocyte production

As soon as tissue injury occurs, the mechanisms by which injurious agents are eliminated start to operate. In general, granulocytes appear first at the site of the lesion, and after a short delay the number of exudate macrophages in the inflammatory exudate begins to increase. During various kinds of inflammation the number of circulating monocytes increases as well. When a large number of macrophages is required at the site of inflammation, a regulatory mechanism acting at the level of the dividing mononuclear phagocytes in the bone marrow is needed to form more monocytes. Since increased production of monocytes occurs by augmentation of the rate of division of the monoblasts and of the pro-monocytes, chemical signals influencing the rate of division of these monocyte precursors in the bone marrow should be demonstrable in the circulation during certain periods of the inflammatory reaction.

Recent investigations have shown that plasma and sera collected during the onset of an inflammatory reaction contain a factor that stimulates monocytopoiesis [9–12]. This factor, called 'factor increasing monocytopoiesis' (FIM), is synthesized and secreted by macrophages at the site of inflammation and then transported via the circulation to the bone marrow where it exerts its stimulatory action (Fig. 42.2).

In mice and rabbits this factor has been fairly well characterized. FIM is a small protein with a relative molecular mass of about 20 000 Da, has no carbohydrate moieties essential for its function, is cell line specific (i.e. has no effect on the formation of granulocytes and lymphocytes), is not species specific (i.e. rabbit FIM is active in mice and vice versa), is not related to complement factors or clotting factors, has no chemotactic activity towards macrophages and is not identical with CSF.

Indications were obtained that in the second phase of an inflammatory response the increased monocyte production is decreased by a serum factor that inhibits monocytopoiesis (Fig. 42.2). This factor, 'monocyte production inhibitor' (MPI), has a molecular mass of approximately 50 000 Da; the site of its production has not yet been established [13]. Although FIM and MPI are not detectable under steady-state conditions with the available assay methods, it is conceivable that they

regulate monocytopoiesis under steady-state conditions as well.

Mononuclear phagocyte system

On the basis of the data then available, the concept of the Mononuclear Phagocyte System (MPS) [14] was put forward in 1969. Later research confirmed the assumptions underlying this concept, and supplementary evidence was also obtained. The cells assigned to the mononuclear phagocyte system at present are shown in Fig. 42.3.

Several types of cell (i.e. dendritic cells, interdigitating cells in lymphoid tissues, follicular and germinal-centre dendritic cells, epidermal Langerhans' cells, and veiled cells in lymph) all differ from monocytes and macrophages in a number of morphologic and func-

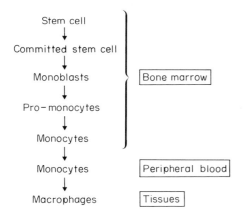

Stem cell
↓
Committed stem cell
↓
Monoblasts
↓   } Bone marrow
Pro-monocytes
↓
Monocytes
↓
Monocytes   Peripheral blood
↓
Macrophages   Tissues

Normal state
  Connective tissue (histiocyte)
  Liver (Kupffer cell)
  Lung (alveolar macrophage)
  Lymph nodes (free and fixed
    macrophages, interdigitating cell?)
  Spleen (free and fixed macrophages)
  Bone marrow (fixed macrophages)
  Serous cavities (pleural and
    peritoneal macrophages)
  Bone (osteoclasts)
  Central nervous system (CSF macrophages;
    brain macrophages)
  Skin (histiocyte; Langerhans' cell?)
  Synovia (type A cell)
  Other organs (tissue macrophage)

Inflammation
  Exudate macrophage
  Exudate-resident macrophage
  Epithelioid cell
  Multinucleated giant cell (Langerhans'
    type and foreign-body type)

Fig. 42.3. Cells included in the Mononuclear phagocyte system (MPS) in normal and inflamed tissues.

tional characteristics and, furthermore, their origin has not yet been definitely established [15,16]. Consequently, these cells have not yet been assigned definitely to the MPS, even though some of them (e.g. the interdigitating cell, the Langerhans' cell, and the veiled cells) are good candidates.

References

1 VAN FURTH R. (1970) The origin and turnover of promonocytes, monocytes and macrophages in normal mice. In *Mononuclear phagocytes*, (ed. van Furth R.), p. 151. Blackwell Scientific Publications, Oxford.

2 VAN FURTH R. (1975) Mononuclear phagocytes in human pathology. Proposal for an approach to improved classification. In *Mononuclear phagocytes in immunity, infection and pathology*, (ed. van Furth R.), p. 1. Blackwell Scientific Publications, Oxford.

3 VAN FURTH R. (1980) Cells of the mononuclear phagocyte system. Nomenclature in terms of sites and conditions. In *Mononuclear phagocytes. Functional aspects*, (ed. van Furth R.), p. 1. Martinus Nijhoff Publishers, Boston, Dordecht, Lancaster.

4 VAN FURTH R., DIESSELHOF-DEN DULK M.M.C., RAEBURN J.A., VAN ZWET TH.L., CROFTON R. & BLUSSÉ VAN OUD ALBLAS A. (1980) Characteristics, origin and kinetics of human and murine mononuclear phagocytes. In *Mononuclear phagocytes. Functional aspects*, (ed. van Furth R.), p. 297. Martinus Nijhoff Publishers, Boston, Dordecht, Lancaster.

5 VAN FURTH R. (1981) Identification of mononuclear phagocytes. Introduction and definitions. In *Methods for studying mononuclear phagocytes*, (ed. Edelson P.J., Koren H. & Adams D.O.), p. 243. Academic Press, London, New York, San Francisco.

6 DIESSELHOFF-DEN DULK M.M.C. & VAN FURTH R. (1981) Characteristics of mononuclear phagocytes from different tissues. In *Methods for studying mononuclear phagocytes*, (eds. Edelson P.J., Koren H. & Adams D.O.), p. 253. Academic Press, London, New York, San Francisco.

7 VAN FURTH R. & DIESSELHOFF-DEN DULK M.M.C. (1982) Characterization of mononuclear phagocytes from the mouse, guinea pig, rat, and man. *Inflammation*, **39**, 53.

8 VAN FURTH R., VAN DER MEER J.W.M., BLUSSÉ VAN OUD ALBLAS A. & SLUITER W. (1982) Development of mononuclear phagocytes. In *Self-defense mechanisms— Role of macrophages*, (eds. Mizuno D., Cohn Z.A., Takeya K. & Ishida N.), p. 25. University of Tokyo Press–Elsevier Biomedial Press, New York, Amsterdam.

9 VAN WAARDE D., HULSING-HESSELINK E. & VAN FURTH R. (1977) Humoral regulation of monocytopoiesis during the early phase of an inflammatory reaction caused by particulate substances. *Blood*, **50**, 141.

10 VAN WAARDE D., HULSING-HESSELINK E. & VAN FURTH R. (1977) Properties of factor increasing monocytopoiesis (FIM) occurring in the serum during the early phase of an inflammatory reaction. *Blood*, **50**, 727.

11 SLUITER W., VAN WAARDE D., HULSING-HESSELINK E., ELZENGA-CLAASEN I. & VAN FURTH R. (1980) Humoral control of monocyte production during inflammation. In *Mononuclear phagocytes. Functional aspects*, (ed. van Furth R.), p. 325. Martinus Nijhoff Publishers, Boston, Dordecht, Lancaster.

12 SLUITER W., ELZENGA-CLAASEN I., VAN DER VOORT VAN DER KLEY-VAN ANDEL A.E. & VAN FURTH R. (1983) Presence of the factor increasing monocytopoiesis (FIM) in rabbit peripheral blood during an acute inflammation. *J. Reticuloendothel. Soc.* **34**, 235.

13 VAN WAARDE E., HULSING-HESSELINK E. & VAN FURTH R. (1978) Humoral control of monocytopoiesis by an activator and an inhibitor. *Agents Actions*, **8**, 432.

14 VAN FURTH R., COHN Z.A., HIRSCH J.G., HUMPHREY SPECTOR W.G. & LANGEVOORT H.L. (1972) The mononuclear phagocyte system. A new classification of macrophages, monocytes and their precursor cells. *Bull. Wld Hlth Org.* **46**, 651.

15 VAN VOORHIS W.C., WITMER M.D. & STEINMAN R.M. (1983) The phenotype of dendritic cells and macrophages. *Fedn Proc.* **42**, 3114.

16 THORBECKE G.J., SILBERBERG-SINAKIN J. & FLOTTE, T.J. (1980) Langerhans cell as macrophages in skin and lymphoid organs. *J. invest. Dermatol.* **75**, 32.

17 VAN FURTH R., DIESSELHOFF-DEN DULK M.M.C., SLUITER W. & VAN DISSEL J.T. (1985) New perspectives on the kinetics of mononuclear phagocytes. In *Mononuclear phagocytes. Characteristics, physiology and function*, (ed. van Furth R.), Chapter 21. Martinus Nijhoff Publishers, Boston, Dordrecht, Lancaster.

Chapter 43
Plasma membrane markers to study differentiation, activation and localization of murine macrophages. Ag F4/80 and the mannosyl, fucosyl receptor

S. GORDON, PHYLLIS M. STARKEY, D. HUME,
R. A. B. EZEKOWITZ, S. HIRSCH & J. AUSTYN

General considerations, 43.1
Methods for radioimmunoassay
  of Ag F4/80 and other Mϕ
  antigens, 43.4

Methods for immunofluorescence
  assays of Mϕ antigens, 43.8
Methods for
  immunocytochemical assay of
  Ag F4/80 and other Mϕ Ag,
  43.9

Method for MFR assay, 43.11
Conclusion, 43.13

Cells of the mononuclear phagocyte system are found in different compartments (bone marrow, blood, tissues) and vary considerably in maturity and function. Tissue macrophages (Mϕ) can be classified as resident (unstimulated), elicited (stimulation by an inflammatory agent such as thioglycollate broth) or activated (enhanced antimicrobial or cytocidal activity after exposure to lymphokines, e.g. during infection by bacillus Calmette-Guerin, BCG). Differentiation antigens and specific plasma membrane receptors provide markers to study Mϕ heterogeneity, to localize Mϕ in tissues, and to isolate and selectively ablate cells. A differentiation antigen (Ag) defined by the rat monoclonal antibody (Ab), F4/80, is restricted to mature mouse Mϕ and has been used to identify Mϕ in situ by a sensitive immunocytochemical method (Tables 43.1 and 43.2). The lectin-like mannosyl, fucosyl receptor (MFR) expressed by mature Mϕ of all species studied (man, rat, mouse), mediates endocytosis and secretory responses (Table 43.3). Its expression is selectively down-regulated by immunologic stimuli which activate Mϕ. Table 43.4 compares changes in MFR and other plasma membrane constituents upon Mϕ activation. In this chapter the authors describe methods to measure expression of Ag F4/80 and MFR activity by various Mϕ populations. These assays can be readily applied to other markers of cell differentiation and activation. The immunochemical characterization of other Mϕ plasma membrane molecules is dealt with by Unkeless & Springer (Chapter 118).

General considerations

Cell isolation and cultivation

All assays described employ defined ligands to study Ag and receptor activity in Mϕ populations isolated from various sources. Cells are assayed in situ or in culture, intact (live or fixed) or after lysis, adherent or non-adherent. Results reflect the activity of a population or of individual cells. The origin, purity and handling of cells markedly influence the choice of assay, expression of Ag and interpretation of results and will be considered first. Detailed protocols of cell isolation and cultivation are described elsewhere [35] and the authors limit their comments to murine cells.

Primary Mϕ and Mϕ-like cell lines differ in homogeneity, maturity, growth properties and adherence. Suspensions of mouse peritoneal Mϕ can be readily obtained as resident, elicited or activated populations from inbred strains. 'Resident' Mϕ are a sensitive indicator of animal house care, subclinical infection and exposure to endotoxin. Inflammatory Mϕ are obtained from mice 4–5 days after intraperitoneal injection of Brewer's complete thioglycollate broth [36] and activated Mϕ 10–21 days after infection with BCG ($\sim 1 \times 10^7$ live organisms/mouse) or 4–14 days after injection of Corynebacterium parvum [9]. These populations vary in Mϕ yield and purity and contain lymphocytes and neutrophils as major contaminants. Adherence to tissue culture plastic or glass is often used as a relatively simple way to purify Mϕ. Adher-

Table 43.1. Properties of Ag F4/80

1 Determinant defined by rat IgG2b non-cytotoxic Ab.
2 Molecule is a 160 kDa glycoprotein which is synthesized by Mϕ.
3 Expressed on plasma membrane and inside phagolysosomes.
4 Mouse-restricted, although a similar Ag has been found on rat Mϕ. No strain or sex differences.
5 Stable to trypsin and elastase, which cleave molecule.
6 Stable to glutaraldehyde, methanol and acetone.
7 Expressed by nearly all Mϕ in culture, including cells derived from blood, peritoneum, lung, bone marrow and Mϕ-like cell lines.
8 Maturity marker for all Mϕ in independent colonies derived from bone marrow in culture.
9 Pan-Mϕ marker in tissues, as defined by immunocytochemistry.
10 Not expressed by any cell type, *in vitro* or *in vivo*, which is clearly not a Mϕ, including neutrophils, lymphocytes, dendritic cells and fibroblasts.
11 Expression influenced by cell stimulation *in vivo* and adherence in culture.

[References 1–11 and unpublished observations.]

Table 43.2. Expression of Ag F4/80 by cells of the mononuclear phagocyte system

Bone marrow	Blood	Tissues	Note
CFU-S ?– * CFU-C– CFC– Promonocyte± Monocyte± Macrophage+	Monocyte±	Resident+ Serous cavities Haemopoietic Lymphoid Liver Gastro-intestinal tract Respiratory tract Genito-urinary tract Skin Bone, connective tissue Endocrine organs Nervous system Inflammatory elicited+ Immunologically activated+	 T cell areas– Interdigitating cells– Langerhans' cells+ Osteoclast– Microglia+ Choroid plexus+

* –, F4/80 negative; +, F4/80 positive.
[References 1–9]

ence may influence expression of plasma membrane Ag and receptors [1,2], depending on the nature of the substratum [37]. Subsequent detachment of viable cells can prove difficult—most Mϕ can be removed from gelatin-coated vessels by trypsin or local anaesthetics such as lignocaine [19], agents which influence surface markers. Use of heterologous sera during cultivation introduces further artefacts. Prolonged adherence and spreading of Mϕ also alter their properties profoundly. Less adhesive substrata (e.g. Teflon, poly-2-hydroxyethyl methacrylate (poly-

HEMA) or gelatin-coated plastic vessels provide a useful alternative [38]).

Isolation of Mϕ from organs such as liver and spleen depends on proteolytic digestion, e.g. with collagenase, and introduces another possible source of surface marker variation. Bone marrow cultures can be used to generate mass or clonal populations of Mϕ in liquid or semi-solid media. Growth and differentiation of Mϕ *in vitro* depends on specific colony-stimulating factors, e.g. CSF-1, found in conditioned medium from L cell fibroblasts. The analysis of

Table 43.3. Properties of MFR

---

1   Lectin-like receptor for mannosyl- or fucosyl-terminal glycoconjugates. Ligands include neoglycoproteins (Man-BSA ~ Fuc-BSA > Glc NAc-BSA), core oligosaccharides, ribonuclease B, β-glucuronidase and other lysosomal hydrolases, and horseradish peroxidase.
2   Found on Mϕ from rat, mouse and man.
3   Expressed by nearly all mature Mϕ from lung, peritoneum and bone marrow in culture. Many Mϕ like cell lines lack MFR, which can be restored by Mϕ × Mϕ somatic cell hybridization.
4   Human blood monocytes lack MFR which appears during maturation to Mϕ in culture.
5   Expressed by Kupffer cells and possibly liver endothelial cells *in vivo*.
6   Low levels may be found on neutrophils and undetectable on lymphocytes, fibroblasts and dendritic-like cells.
7   Mediates pinocytosis and phagocytosis and triggers respiratory burst.
8   Binding of ligand depends on calcium, receptor is sensitive to trypsin and recycles from an intracellular compartment.
9   Modulated by adherence of Mϕ to mannan-coated substratum or immobilized zymosan.
10   Down-regulated by Mϕ activating stimuli including lymphokines and interferon-γ.
11   Variable enhancement by glucocorticoids which counteract effect of lymphokine and interferon-γ on human monocytes or Mϕ.

[References 12–23 and unpublished observations.]

Table 43.4. Plasma membrane changes associated with immune activation of macrophages

Marker	Decreased	No change	Increased	References
Antigens				
Ia			+	[21,24–26]
F4/80	+			[9,21]
7/4			+	[27]
Receptors				
FcR IgG2a			+	[28]
FcR IgG1/2b	+			[9,28]
CR3 (Mac-1 Ag expression)		+		[9,21]
MFR	+			[9,21]
Ecto-enzymes				
5′ Nucleotidase	+			[29]
Alkaline phosphodiesterase			+	[30]
Product release				
Reactive O$_2$ metabolites			+	[31]
Platelet activating factor	+/0			[33]
Prostaglandins	+			[32]
Apolipoprotein E	+			[34]

marker expression by independent colonies provides a powerful tool to study Mϕ heterogeneity [2]. Effects of growth on Mϕ surface properties have received little study. Clonal populations of continuous cell lines, e.g. J774, can be cultivated in bulk, an advantage for purification. These lines vary in development and can be induced to differentiate by agents such as PMA and lymphokines. Cell lines which express markers of Mϕ maturation such as Ag F4/80 lack other markers such as the MFR [15].

Fixation

Live target cells are required to assay many cell functions and binding of a ligand to intact cells indicates expression on the external surface of the plasmalemma. However, prior fixation is often employed for convenience of washing and storage of target cells for immunoassays. Many determinants are stable to glutaraldehyde in the range 0.125–1.25%, although mobility of molecules within the plane of the plasma membrane is destroyed. It is important to titrate the effects of fixation on stability of each Ag. Glutaraldehyde-fixed cells are impermeable to ligands. To detect an intracellular or cytoskeletal Ag, cells can be permeabilized with ice-cold methanol or acetone and some cytoplasmic components can be extracted at the same time by a non-ionic detergent, e.g. Triton X-100.

Binding of ligands

Binding of Ab or other ligands can be measured directly or by an indirect method, using a radio-labelled, fluorescent or enzymatic detection system. Theoretical aspects of immunoassays of cell Ag are dealt with by Mason & Williams in Chapter 38. In trace indirect binding assays (IBA) only the first Ab is present at saturation. When saturating amounts of a second detecting Ab are also used ('saturation IBA') binding of the second Ab is proportional to the amount of first Ab bound. The number of second-stage Ab molecules bound per cell can be calculated from the formula

$$\frac{\text{c.p.m.} \times (\text{ng cold second Ab}) \times 6.2 \times 10^9 \text{ molecules}}{\text{Input c.p.m.} \times \text{no. of cells}}$$

Direct binding assays at saturation give a more precise measure of the number of Ag sites. Specific binding of ligands to cells is derived by including cell-free controls and by competition with excess unlabelled ligand or inhibitors, e.g. mannose-rich yeast mannan in the MFR assay. Macrophages pose unique problems in their ability to bind immunoglobulins, glycoproteins and other ligands by specific mechanisms involving other than the supposed binding sites. Best-defined is Fc-dependent binding of certain classes of immuno-globulins to one of several Fc receptors expressed on $M\phi$ [39]. These receptors vary in their affinity for monomeric or aggregated/complexed immunoglobu-lins from the same or different species and FcR expression is selectively modulated during $M\phi$ differ-entiation and activation [28]. Ideally, only rigorously purified $F(ab')_2$ or Fab fragments can exclude binding of an Ab to a $M\phi$ FcR. In practice, hybridomas can be screened on $M\phi$ of the same species as that im-munized, to exclude cytophilic binding. Specific monoclonal Ab directed against an FcR can be included in screening assays, e.g. the rat anti-FcR Ab 2.4G2 blocks the mouse FcR for IgG1/2b but not a distinct FcR for IgG2a [39]. Aggregated non-specific immunoglobulins are not efficient inhibitors of FcR; ligands directed against the Fc region of Ab molecules can also be considered.

Carbohydrate residues on immunoglobulins and other glycoproteins may bind to MFR or other lectin-like receptors on $M\phi$. Inhibitors such as man-nan can be incorporated in assays. It is possible for immunoglobulins to interact with components of the alternative pathway of complement secreted by living $M\phi$ and bind to receptors for complement under certain conditions [22]. Finally, $M\phi$ could express ill-defined 'receptors' for denatured or aggregated proteins generated during labelling or storage of ligands. Clearing by high-speed centrifugation may not suffice to eliminate such 'non-specific' labelling.

Methods for radioimmunoassay of Ag F4/80 and other $M\phi$ antigens

Equipment

Gamma counter.
Swing-out bench centrifuge, e.g. MSE 'Super' Minor.
Microtitre tissue culture plates from Sterilin, Tedding-ton, Middlesex TW11 8QZ, UK.
Terasaki tissue culture plates from Falcon, 1950 Williams Drive, Oxnard, CA 93030, USA.
LP3 plastic round-bottom tubes, 64×11 mm from LIP (Equipment A Services) Ltd., 111, Dockfield Road, Shipley, West Yorkshire BD17 7AS, UK.

Materials

Glutaraldehyde, 0.125% solution in PBS made up freshly from 25% stock solution (EM grade) from Agar Aids, 66a Cambridge Road, Stansted, Essex CM24 8DA, UK.
PBS—(Dulbecco 'A') 137 mM-NaCl, 3 mM-KCl, 10 mM-Na_2HPO_4, pH 7.3.
PBA—PBS containing 0.1% bovine serum albumin (Cohn fraction V) and 10 mM-sodium azide.
Fetal calf serum (FCS).
First antibody solution—either conditioned medium from hybridoma cells or ascites fluid. Alternatively, the Ab can be purified partially or totally by Na_2SO_4 precipitation alone or followed by affinity chromato-graphy on DEAE-cellulose (for details, see Chapter 13). Ab F4/80 is available from the authors.
Second antibody solution—$F(ab')_2$ fragment is pre-pared and isolated from the chosen polyclonal or monoclonal Ab preparation (see Chapter 13) stored lyophilized at $-20\,°C$ in aliquots. MRC OX-12 is available from Serotec, Bicester, Oxon, UK. As required, 50 μg of $F(ab')_2$ is iodinated by the chlora-mine T method, the iodinated protein is separated from free iodine by chromatography on Sephadex G-10 and stored in PBS containing 10 mM-azide as 4 °C.

Procedure for intact cells

Plate assay with immobilized cells

This is the most convenient method for adherent target cells, though it can also be used for non-adherent cells if they are first immobilized on poly-L-lysine coated plastic plates.

Preparation of target cells

1 For adherent target cells, distribute cells in plastic microtitre plates under sterile conditions ($0.5–1 \times 10^6$ cells/ml in 200 μl of appropriate medium). Incubate 1–2 h or longer, as desired.
2 Wash cells three times with PBS to remove non-adherent cells and medium. If fixed target cells are required add glutaraldehyde (0.125% v/v in PBS) for 10 min at room temperature.
3 Wash cells three times with PBS. Incubate with fetal calf serum (10% in PBS) for 30 min at room temperature to block remaining cross-linking sites.
4 Wash cells three times with PBS and store at 4 °C in PBA.
5 For non-adherent target cells, microtitre plates are incubated with 0.1 mg/ml poly-L-lysine in PBS for 1 h at 37 °C (200 μl per well) then washed well with PBS twice. One hundred microlitres of cell suspension (2×10^6/ml) are added per well.
6 The plates are centrifuged at 200 *g* (e.g. MSE Mistral 2L centrifuge) for 4 min at room temperature.
7 One hundred microlitres of 0.25% glutaraldehyde is then added to each microtitre well. After 10 min, plates are washed twice with PBS and stored in PBA. Before use, pre-soak with medium containing 2% fetal calf serum for 1 h at 37 °C, to block non-specific binding.

Notes and recommendations

The choice of target cells and duration of cultivation depends on the level of Ag expression and the availability of a reasonably homogeneous population in adequate amounts. For F4/80, thioglycollate-elicited mouse peritoneal Mϕ are cultured for at least 24 h before fixation as F4/80 Ag is modulated on adherence.

Assays with unfixed cells avoid loss of Ag activity due to fixation and give lower backgrounds, but cells must be prepared freshly, assays done at 4 °C to prevent uptake, and care taken during washes to avoid losses. Only fixed target cells can be used with samples containing detergents.

For each Ag, fixation conditions must be optimized empirically to retain maximal specific binding with minimal non-specific binding.

Fixed targets can be stored at 4 °C in the presence of azide for months without loss of Ag. Pre-incubate with fresh PBA and wash before use.

Indirect radioimmune binding assay

1 Pour off liquid and to each well add 30–50 μl of first Ab, diluted in PBA. Leave at 4 °C for 1 h.
2 Wash cells three times with PBA. The most convenient washing procedure is to hold the plate at an angle and fill each well with PBA from a wash bottle held so that the stream of liquid hits the side of each well. The plate can then be inverted to flick out the liquid and the procedure repeated. To each well add 30 μl of ^{125}I-labelled second Ab diluted in PBA. Leave at 4 °C for 1 h.
3 Wash cells three times with PBA. Solubilize bound radioactivity with 200 μl 0.5 M-NaOH per well, remove 180 μl and assay in gamma counter.
4 As controls, include cell-free blank wells and cell blanks without first Ab. If using fixed cells, then the cell-free blank wells should be incubated with medium alone and then fixed and washed as for the cells.

Notes and recommendations

The concentration of first Ab should be just sufficient to saturate all the Ag. This is determined empirically by titrating serial dilutions of Ab against the target cells. Unpurified Ab, e.g. conditioned medium or ascites fluid, often gives the lowest background. Some monoclonal Ab bind to cell-free tissue culture plastic blanks, especially after treatment with fixatives.

Second antibody: use of F(ab′)$_2$ is critical to prevent Fc binding. Polyclonal rabbit anti-rat Ab allows the assay of several different rat monoclonal Ab, but will cross-react with mouse Ig on B lymphocytes or Mϕ unless cross-reacting Ab are removed by immunoadsorption. Monoclonal second Ab may be useful, e.g. MRC OX-12 (mouse anti-rat^k) gives lower backgrounds but reacts with fewer determinants and does not react with IgG from all rat strains [40].

In trace assays, where the relative levels of Ag on different cells are being measured, the concentration of second Ab should be about 5 μCi/ml (8×10^6 c.p.m./ml). In saturation assays, to determine the number of bound first Ab molecules, labelled F(ab′)$_2$ is diluted with non-radioactive F(ab′)$_2$ which should compete with its binding and the concentration required to saturate is determined empirically (usually 20 μg/ml).

Incubation times: optimal times should be determined empirically for each Ab. In practice, most Ab/Ag interactions reach equilibrium in 30–60 min at

4 °C. If the 'off rate' of the first Ab is relatively high, the second incubation should be kept short.

Microassays: if the supply of target cells or Ab is limiting, Terasaki plates can be used instead of microtitre plates. The methods are the same, but 8 μl of cell suspension (0.5–1.0 × 10^6 cells/ml) are plated per well, and if fixation is required, the plates are flooded with 0.125% glutaraldehyde. In the assay itself, 8 μl of first and second Ab solutions are used, with the second Ab at 15 μCi/ml. Cells are solubilized with 8 μl of NaOH.

Tube assay

This method is best suited for use with non-adherent target cells. An advantage over the plate assay is that large cell numbers can be used facilitating detection of low levels of Ag/cell, disadvantages are that it is more time consuming and fewer samples can be assayed at once.

Cells are washed three times in PBS by centrifugation, and assayed live or fixed in suspension. Cells are fixed by incubation for 10 min at room temperature in glutaraldehyde 0.125% in PBS, then washed three times in PBS, resuspended in PBS + 10% FCS for 30 min at room temperature, and finally washed three times in PBS and stored at 4 °C in PBA.

For assay, 50 μl of cell suspension (0.5–2 × 10^6 cells/ml) in PBA are dispensed to each LP3 tube and centrifuged at 380 **g** for 5 min. The liquid is aspirated and 50 μl of first Ab diluted in PBA, is added and the cells incubated at 4 °C for 1 h. The cells are washed twice by centrifugation with 2 ml cold PBA. Fifty microlitres of ^{125}I-labelled second Ab (2.5 μCi/ml in PBS) is added and the cells are incubated for 1 h at 4 °C. The cells are washed as above three times with cold PBA and the pellets assayed in the gamma counter. 'No cell' blanks should be included to measure binding of Ab to the plastic tube, as well as blanks without first Ab.

Autoradiography

Coverslips with adherent Mϕ are incubated with first and second Ab as above. If live targets are used, the cells are subsequently washed and fixed for 10 min with methanol. Bound radioactivity is determined directly by counting the coverslips, which are then mounted, cell side uppermost, on glass slides and processed for autoradiography by standard methods. Non-adherent cells are assayed in suspension and processed as cytocentrifuge preparations.

Procedure for soluble antigen

Competition assay for Ag F4/80 or other Mϕ Ag

A solution of Ab F4/80 is pre-incubated with samples containing Ag, and the remaining free Ab is measured as above by the plate assay against glutaraldehyde-fixed target cells, e.g. J774 cells or 2-day cultured TPM. Tube assays of detergent lysates are difficult as cells do not pellet well in detergent solutions and losses occur on washing, giving poor replication.

Procedure

1 The Ab F4/80 solution diluted with PBA is titrated against the target cells and a dilution chosen which is just sub-saturating (see Fig. 43.1, top panel). The concentration of the Ab solution used at (c) is then fixed at twice this level.

2 Cells are suspended in lysis buffer (1% Triton X-100 in PBS, pH 7.4, containing 3 mM-Pms-F, 3 mM-iodoacetic acid and 10 mM-EDTA) and disrupted by homogenization with a Dounce type homogenizer. Insoluble material is removed by centrifugation. All procedures are at 4 °C.

3 A series of doubling dilutions is made for each sample to be tested, the diluent containing the same detergent concentration as the lysis buffer. Diluted Ag samples are each incubated at 4 °C for 1 h with an equal volume of diluted Ab F4/80. Controls include diluent in place of Ag to measure maximal Ab binding (100%) and PBA in place of F4/80 to measure the non-specific binding of second Ab (0%). If the units of antigen are to be calculated with reference to a standard Ag solution (e.g. J774 lysate) then dilutions of this standard Ag solution must be assayed each time.

4 Aliquots of the Ag–Ab mixtures are assayed for binding of free Ab by the plate assay described above (see 'Plate assay with immobilized cells', p. 43.5).

5 *Calculation of Ag concentrations*: for each sample, the results obtained in the plate assay are plotted as in Fig. 43.1 lower panel, with Ag dilution as the x-axis and specific bound radioactivity (active control) as the y-axis. The Ag dilution which inhibits Ab binding by 50% is then read off the graph (1/8 for sample A and 1/16 for sample B). If no standard Ag solution is available as a reference, then arbitrary units of Ag can be defined such that a sample of 1 u/ml would give 50% inhibition. The concentration of Ag in each sample is then the reciprocal of the dilution required to give 50% inhibition (8 Ag u/ml sample A, 16 Ag u/ml for sample B). If a standard Ag solution is used, where the concentration of Ag is known or has been arbitrarily set, then samples are related to this standard. Thus in

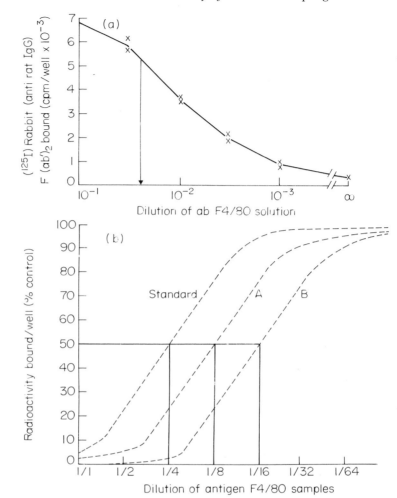

Fig. 43.1. (a) Titration curve for Ab F4/80 solution in the plate assay against glutaraldehyde-fixed mouse TPM as target cells. The arrow indicates the dilution used in the competition assay for soluble Ag F4/80. (b) Theoretical titration curves of Ag F4/80 samples in the competition assay. Curves are shown for two unknowns, A and B and for a standard Ag solution. The amount of radiolabelled second Ab bound, for each dilution of Ag pre-incubated with Ab F4/80, has been corrected for nonspecific binding due to the Ag alone and is then expressed as a percentage of the binding measured with Ab F4/80 alone.

Fig. 43.1, if the standard contained 10 Ag u/ml, sample A would be 20 Ag u/ml and sample B 40 Ag u/ml.

Notes and recommendations

Solubilization of Ag: the choice of detergent varies with the Ag and with the goal, e.g. purification. Triton X-100 or NP40 have a high E_{280} and cannot be removed by dialysis and would therefore need to be removed at an early stage in any purification by displacement with another detergent. Brij 96 is relatively poor as a solubilizing agent, but some Ag are stable in Brij 96 whilst being unstable in other detergents. Sodium deoxycholate can be removed by dialysis and has a low E_{280}, but disrupts nuclei so that a two-step lysis schedule is advocated, e.g. lyse cells in 3% Brij 96, centrifuge at 2000 *g* for 10 min to remove nuclei and debris and make 1% in DOC [41].

Apart from its effectiveness in solubilizing a particular Ag, the stability of Ag and/or Ab to the chosen detergent should be checked. In a competition assay, Ag levels should be measured on (1) intact cells, (2) cells + detergent, (3) supernatant from cells + detergent, (4) pellet from cells + detergent. Fig. 43.2 illustrates the results expected when (A) both Ag and Ab are stable, (B) Ag is unstable, and (C) the Ab is unstable.

Typically, Ab binding to target cells is increased by the presence of detergents, as is non-specific binding of second Ab. Dilutions of Ag should therefore always be made so as to keep a concentration of the detergent constant throughout, and control samples should contain the same detergent concentration.

Incubation times: for Ag F4/80 all incubations are for 30–60 min at 4 °C. Equilibrium is usually reached by 60 min, but incubations of Ag–Ab mixtures and the

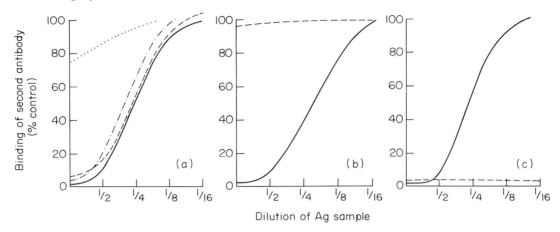

Fig. 43.2. Testing the stability of Ag and/or Ab to detergent. Theoretical curves obtained in the competition assay for Ag are shown (A) where both Ag and Ab are stable to the detergent, (B) where only the Ab is stable, and (C) where only the Ag is stable. Samples pre-incubated with first Ab are intact cells suspended in PBS (---), cells suspended in PBS containing detergent (- -), the soluble fraction from cells lysed in PBS containing detergent (----) and the insoluble pellet from cells lysed in PBS containing detergent (...).

second Ab with the target cells should be kept short, as an appreciable off rate for the Ag–Ab complexes will lead to underestimates of Ag concentration. Long incubations favour dissociation of the soluble Ag–Ab complexes and, because of the high concentration of Ag on target cells, free Ab would be most likely to bind to the target cells rather than rebinding to soluble Ag. Optimal incubation times are determined empirically for each Ag–Ab system.

Controls include lysates from cells or tissues which lack the Ag. Beware of carry-over of IgG from tissue into final assay.

The indirect competition assay is relatively insensitive. Unkeless & Healey (1983) describe direct binding assays for soluble Ag which use ^{125}I-Fab fragments of monoclonal Ab with polyvalent antibodies to precipitate Ag–Ab complexes [42]. Dot immunobinding assays may also be applicable [55].

Methods for immunofluorescence assays of Mϕ antigens

Immunofluorescence assays are described in detail elsewhere in this volume. The authors only comment on aspects which relate to FACS analysis of Mϕ populations. Equipment and reagents are as described elsewhere or above.

Procedure

1 For FACS analysis, live cell suspensions (1×10^7/ml in PBA) are incubated with first and second Ab as described above. To diminish losses through adherence all steps are at 4 °C, in the presence of azide, and in siliconized tubes. Cells are obtained in suspension by direct harvesting, cultivation in non-adherent vessels, or by scraping gently from a substratum at 4 °C with a rubber policeman. The second Ab is a FITC-conjugated rabbit F(ab')$_2$ anti-rat Fab or FITC-OX-12 which should be cleared by centrifugation before use. Both first and second Ab are used at saturation. Incubation with FITC–Ab should be in the dark. Include control cells without first Ab and without either first or second Ab (autofluorescence). If desired, lyse erythrocytes in Tris-buffered NH$_4$Cl [43] before labelling. Analyse low-angle forward scatter and fluorescence. Macrophages tend to be larger than lymphocytes or neutrophils.

For cell sorting higher cell numbers are needed (e.g. 3×10^8 nucleated bone marrow to sort Mϕ progenitors) and cells are collected into tubes containing 2 ml Leibovitz medium, which is not bicarbonate-based.

Mϕ are readily lost through adherence to tubes during prolonged processing, especially if the cells are activated.

Mϕ resuspended after prior adherence may be damaged by the detachment procedure, especially if the cells are activated. These cells are lost during processing.

Cultivated Mϕ show high levels of autofluorescence (see Chapter 44).

Labelling by second Ab in the absence of first Ab can be due to (1) mouse IgG cytophilically bound to Mϕ, (2) aggregates, or (3) carbohydrate. Cross-reaction of RAR with mouse Ig can be avoided by immunoabsorption of the RAR by passage over Sepharose–mouse IgG or by adding 2–5% mouse serum during the second incubation. The use of monoclonal second Ab, e.g. OX-12, eliminates this problem, provided that the rat first Ab is detected by this allotype-restricted reagent. Aggregates can be removed by centrifugation, sugar-specific binding eliminated by inhibitors, e.g. mannan. Even when all these precautions are taken, there are unexplained instances of binding of FITC-labelled second Ab to particular Mφ populations, e.g. cultured non-adherent populations of bone marrow.

Sorting of Mφ precursors combined with growth in the presence of defined colony stimulating activities provides a powerful method to analyse heterogeneity among independent clones of Mφ [2].

Method for immunocytochemical assay of Ag F4/80 and other Mφ Ag

The authors describe an immunoperoxidase method based on the avidin–biotin-complex (ABC) procedure of Hsu *et al.* [44] to detect Ag F4/80 and other glutaraldehyde-stable mouse Mφ antigens in tissue sections or isolated cells.

Equipment

Perfusion apparatus [45]: a cannula (pp50, end very slightly bevelled) is connected to two vessels with a two-way tap system. Both vessels are connected to a pressure chamber (e.g. a large flask) in which a pressure of 120 mmHg is generated by a sphygmomanometer attached to a separate inlet.
Dissecting board and instruments.
Staining tray.

Reagents

Perfusion fixation

Sodium cacodylate (Agar Aids, Stanstead, Essex, UK: R1104).
Sucrose (BDH, Poole, Dorset, UK: 10274).
PBS tablets (Oxoid, Basingstoke, Hampshire, UK: BR14a).
Glutaraldehyde, 8% aqueous, EM1 grade (Polysciences, Pennsylvania 0216, USA).

Embedding

Polywax (MP 57 °C) (Difco, West Molesey, Sussex, UK).

Immunocytochemistry

Vectastain kit (rabbit anti-rat Ig, Seralab PK 4004).
Avidin (Sigma, A 9275).
Biotin (Sigma, B 4501).
Diaminobenzidine tetra-HCl (DAB) (Polysciences 04008).
Analar ethanol (BDH 10107).
Rabbit anti-mouse IgG serum. Cross-reacting Ab against rat IgG is removed by passage over rat IgG–Sepharose.
Glucose oxidase, type V (Sigma).
H_2O_2 (30%) (BDH 28519).
Other materials standard.

Procedure

Perfusion fixation of mouse tissues

Perfusion through aorta

1 Anaesthetize with ether. Carefully open abdominal cavity.
2 Open thoracic cavity by carefully snipping diaphragm without cutting liver.
3 Cut ribs upwards on both sides, clamp flap of ribs with artery forceps and use this to pull the flap over the animal's head (the clamp also serves to reduce bleeding).
4 Grip the heart with straight forceps and push the cannula into the base of the left ventricle (*c.* half-way up the ventricle). Tape the tubing to the operation board and it will stay in place in the heart, provided it is not violently disturbed.

Other perfusions

To clear particular tissues other modes of perfusion may be desirable.
1 To perfuse the pulmonary circulation: first, cannulate the trachea with a pp 50 tube attached to a 5 ml syringe filled with air; tie in place. Insert perfusion tube into the right instead of the left ventricle and perfuse at 30–40 mmHg.
2 To perfuse the lower body: first, tie off the portal vein, thereby excluding the mesenteric and hepatic circulations. Further restriction of alternative blood flow can be achieved by clamping the neck with artery forceps. Cannulate the left ventricle as usual and perfusate is directed to the gonads and hind quarters.

Perfusion sequence

Ensure that there are no air bubbles in the perfusion system. When the cannula is in place, cut the inferior vena cava immediately below the liver (take care not to cut the adjacent descending aorta) and open the tap to the first vessel. This should contain *warm* heparinized PBS (37 °C) to clear the animal of blood. When the animal is exsanguinated (the liver should turn a light brown colour) after 2–5 min, switch the perfusion over to the fixative (0.5% E.M. grade glutaraldehyde, 1% sucrose, 0.1 M-cacodylate buffer, pH 7.4). The animal will begin to twitch if the perfusion is successful. Continue fixation for 20 min. The gastro-intestinal tract, skeletal muscle, etc. should be quite yellow. During this time exchange the other perfusion vessel's contents, replace with sucrose-cacodylate without fixative. Perfuse the animal for 10 min with the buffer to remove the excess fixative. Excise the desired tissue and store in sucrose-cacodylate.

Tissue section preparations

The tissue is dehydrated and embedded in polywax as follows: 70% ethanol, 1 h; 90% ethanol, 2 h; 100% ethanol, 3 h; isopropanol overnight; ligroin, 1 h; embed in polywax (melting point 57 °C). Sections (6 μm) are cut and placed on microscope slides. Multiwell slides (4 spots) have the advantage of being easily labelled with pencil so that one can tell which side the sample is on and of allowing multiple sections on one slide to conserve reagents.

Alternative embedding in polyethylene glycol 4000-distearate following dehydration in ethanol or in low-temperature (42 °C) paraffin RAL wax may improve antigen preservation. Prolonged clearing in xylene, toluene or chloroform instead of ligroin may be undesirable.

Cell preparations

Fix the cells adherent or in suspension with glutaraldehyde in sucrose-cacodylate buffer. For cytocentrifuge preparations coat slides with poly-L-lysine by smearing with a 1% solution in water prior to using them in the cytocentrifuge.

Staining

The method is essentially as described in the Vectastain kit with a few modifications.

1 Rehydration: remove the paraffin wax with xylene (do not leave in xylene for more than *c.* 1 min). Place sequentially for *c.* 30 s in ethanol baths: 100%, 100%, 99.8% (analar grade); 90%, 70%, 50% (laboratory grade) and finally H_2O for 5 min.

2 Transfer to 0.3% H_2O_2 in methanol (1 ml of stock H_2O_2/100 ml methanol) to kill endogenous peroxidase. Incubate for 30 min.

3 H_2O—5 min.

4 Remove excess water from the slide by running a tissue down the edge on both sides of the specimens. Place on flat surface (e.g. staining tray). Add 1/50–1/100 of rabbit mouse IgG serum with no cross-reaction against rat IgG and 2 drops of Vectastain rabbit serum/10 ml in PBS.

5 Incubate for 45–60 min. Leave controls without specific Ab. For tests remove the excess blocking antibody and add diluted first Ab. Dilution is made in PBS-rabbit serum (1 drop/10 ml). It is critical that the Ab is titrated and used at just saturating concentrations, or the background can be too high.

6 Incubate *c.* 2 h (not critical).

7 Remove excess Ab and place slides in PBS bath, wash for 20 min, not less, as washing diminishes background.

8 Remove excess PBS, place in tray and add biotinylated second Ab (e.g. rabbit anti-rat IgG), incubate for 1 h (Vectastain blue reagent: 1 drop/10 ml in PBS).

9 Wash as above for 10 min.

10 Add ABC (avidin–biotin–peroxidase) as detailed in kit: incubate for 1 h (2 drops avidin in 10 ml PBS, 2 drops biotin peroxidase: mix for 15 min before use).

11 Wash for 10 min in PBS.

12 Add substrate: 10 mg DAB in 20 ml PBS + 10 mM-imidazole, pH 7.4. Pass through 0.45 μm filter; add 15 μl of stock (30%) H_2O_2.

13 Incubate until brown colour develops, usually 10–15 min (view under microscope if necessary).

14 Wash off DAB and dip slide for 30–40 s (no longer: for some purposes lighter counterstain may be desirable) in Mayer's haematoxylin blue in tap-water.

15 Dehydrate through the ethanol series as above. Use two separate 100% ethanol baths for the ascending series to avoid contamination with wax.

16 Take through two xylene baths (not the xylene used for dewaxing) and finally mount under DPX.

Microscopy and photography

It is often difficult to obtain convincing black and white pictures of sections in which the peroxidase stain is readily visible in colour. Alternative approaches: (1) omit the counterstain; (2) photograph using a blue filter (e.g. Ilford 303); (3) use $CoCl_2$ in developing the DAB reaction (see below) to yield a darker reaction product; (4) photograph under dark field; the DAB reaction product scatters light and glows against the dark background.

Notes and recommendations

Antigen stability should be checked for fixation, embedding and all processing steps. A useful alternative to glutaraldehyde that is less damaging to many antigens is periodate-lysine-paraformaldehyde (PLP) [46]. Frozen sections may be necessary if a particular Ag is labile during processing, but do not preserve detailed morphology as well as the above protocol. Waxes which melt at lower temperature (e.g. 42 °C) help to preserve Ag with an acceptable loss of morphology, but may require sectioning in the cold.

Clearance of blood cells from the vasculature is more efficient under controlled pressure. Small veins will appear distended.

Adequate perfusion fixation may be difficult to achieve for organs such as testis or embryonic tissues. Direct injection of fixative into an organ may be feasible (e.g. into uterus) but could also distort structures. Tissue fragments can be fixed as blocks but penetration by glutaraldehyde is poor; PLP may be better in this regard. If fixation is inadequate F4/80 (and most other antigens) will not withstand embedding procedures. This can lead to false-negative results.

Ag F4/80 is stable after decalcification of adult bone by 10 mM-EDTA in Ca^{2+}, Mg^{2+} free PBS or 10% citrate-formate buffer (pH 5.7).

Unlike its efficacy in perfusion-fixed material, the methanol-peroxide treatment does not eliminate all endogenous peroxidase activity in mouse bone marrow leucocytes fixed *in vitro*. An alternative method proposed by Klebanoff (personal communication) is based on studies by Locksley *et al.* [47]. After fixation, preparations are washed and incubated at 37 °C for 15 min with 10^{-3} M-sodium azide, 10^{-2} M-glucose, 2 units glucose oxidase in PBS.

Staining in the absence of first Ab could be due to binding of peroxidase, a glycoprotein, to the Mφ MFR. Straus showed that such staining could be prevented by mannan or chelators [48]. The perfusion fixation method destroys this type of staining.

Cross-reaction of RAR with mouse Ig contributes to non-specific staining especially in lymphoid tissue, but may be less of a problem in cultivated Mφ. Monoclonal second Ab such as OX-12 gives more specific but weaker staining.

Optimal dilutions of first Ab must be titrated for each Ab.

The imidazole buffer is optimal for peroxidase activity. It is possible to include $CoCl_2$ (3 ml 1% $CoCl_2$ per 100 ml substrate before addition of H_2O_2) to enhance sensitivity.

Some tissues contain endogenous avidin-binding constituents [49]. These can be blocked by incubation in 0.01% avidin followed by 0.01% biotin, after killing endogenous peroxidase.

Method for MFR assay

These are adapted from procedures developed by Stahl *et al.* [9,12,13,15].

Equipment

Gamma counter.
24-well tissue culture trays (Linbro Chemical Co., Flow, Irvine, England).
LP3 plastic round-bottom tubes, 64 × 11 mm.
Microfuge (Beckman B, Beckman Dickinson).
Microfuge tubes—0.4 ml.

Materials

Ligands

A glycoconjugate of mannose-bovine serum albumin (mannose BSA) with 33–37 mol of sugar per mole of protein can be obtained from E-Y Laboratories, 127 N Amphlett Blvd, San Mateo, CA94401, U.S.A.
β-glucuronidase, a glycoprotein with terminal mannose can be purified from rat preputial glands [50].
Inhibitors: mannan from baker's yeast (obtained from Sigma Chemical Co., St. Louis, MO: catalogue M-7304) is made up to a 50 mg/ml stock in DMEM and used at 1 mg/ml final concentration. An alternative inhibitor is ribonuclease B (Sigma) used at 7.5 mg/ml final concentration.

Other materials

PBS—(Dulbecco's A) 137 mM-NaCl, 3 mM-KCl, 10 mM-Na_2HPO_4, pH 7.3—for washing cell monolayers.
Dulbecco's modification of Eagle's minimal essential medium (DMEM) from Gibco-Biocult Ltd., Paisley, Scotland.
Fetal bovine serum.
Four parts silicone oil: one part mineral oil (Dextrex Chem. Industries Inc., Elizabethtown, Kentucky 42701, USA).
Alternative solution for cell washing after suspension assay: one part bovine serum albumin (ρ 1.088): one part Versilube F50 oil (Alfa Chemicals Ltd., P.O. Box 9, Staines, Middlesex TW18 4OS, UK).

Procedure

Iodination of ligands

Neoglycoconjugates and β-glucuronidase are trace labelled with $Na^{125}I$ by a modified chloramine T method [50]. Forty microlitres of mannose BSA (100 μg/ml) or β-glucuronidase (360 μg/ml) in 0.1 M-sodium phosphate buffer, pH 7.6, are incubated with 1 mCi Na^{125}I and 300 μg (30 μl) chloramine T on ice for 10 min. The reaction is terminated by the addition of 436 μg sodium metabisulphite (190 μl) and 1.9 mg potassium iodide (190 μl). All reagents are suspended in 0.1 M-sodium phosphate buffer, pH 7.6. The reaction products are passed down a Sephadex G-10 column (Pharmacia Fine Chemicals), pre-washed with 0.1 M-phosphate buffer, pH 7.6. Aliquots of 300 μl are collected and the first labelled peak is pooled, diluted in 5 ml of DMEM + 5% FBS and filtered through a 0.22 μm Micropore filter which has been washed with 1% bovine serum albumin and DMEM + 5% FBS.

The ligand is tested for trichloroacetic acid (TCA) precipitability (10% v/v) and screened by uptake or degradation assay using Mϕ which express MFR activity (e.g. TPM).

Binding and uptake of mannose-specific ligands

Binding and uptake are assayed at saturating concentrations of ligand using trace labelled mannose-BSA (saturation 120 ng/ml ligand/5 $\times$ 10^5 Mϕ) or β-glucuronidase (saturation 300 μg/ml/5 $\times$ 10^5 Mϕ) in the presence or absence of mannan. Binding is assayed at 4 °C, uptake at 37 °C. The reaction mixture contains Ca^{2+} and Mg^{2+}, which are required for binding, and FCS, which does not inhibit mannose-specific binding, unlike many other sera.

Adherent macrophage populations

Macrophages/monocytes (5 $\times$ 10^5) are adhered for at least 1 h in 24-well Linbro trays, washed in PBS and incubated in 300 μl DMEM + 5% FBS, with HEPES buffer, pH 7.0, and 0.1–0.5 μg/well ^{125}I-mannose-BSA (3 $\times$ 10^6 c.p.m./μg), with or without 1.25–2.5 mg mannan. Cells are incubated in duplicate for 60 min at 4 °C or for 20–30 min at 37 °C and washed three times in ice-cold PBS with 10 mM-sodium azide. Then 200 μl/well of 1 N-NaOH are added to dissolve the cells and the cell-associated radioactivity is measured in a Packard gamma spectrometer (Packard Instrument Co. Inc., Downes Grove, IL, USA). Cell protein is assayed by the Lowry method [52]. Results are expressed as nanograms of mannose-BSA specifically bound or taken up per 5 $\times$ 10^5 Mϕ plated or per μg cell protein.

Non-adherent cells

Cells in suspension are assayed in microfuge tubes over a layer of oil. The media and cells (100 μl) are placed in a 0.4 ml microfuge tube over 0.15 ml oil (Silicone/mineral oil or versilube/BSA) with an air bubble separating oil from the media. During incubation cells tend to sediment towards the water–oil interface. Following incubation for 60 min at 4 °C or 20–30 min at 37 °C the tubes are spun in a microfuge for 30 s and the tips of the tubes, containing the cell pellet, are cut off with a scalpel. The cells and the media are measured separately for radioactivity.

Degradation assays

Degradation of ^{125}I-mannose-BSA by Mϕ can be measured by the appearance of TCA-soluble labelled material in the medium. Degradation of ^{125}I-mannose-BSA is detectable after ~40 min incubation at 37 °C and continues at a linear rate for several days if Mϕ are maintained in the continuous presence of ligand. Trace amounts of sterile ligand (*c.* 1 $\times$ 10^6 c.p.m. in 5–20 μl) are added to monolayers of adherent Mϕ populations (5 $\times$ 10^5–1 $\times$ 10^6 Mϕ/well) in 96- or 24-well multiwell trays, in culture media (0.2–1.0 ml) supplemented with fetal calf serum, in the absence or presence of mannan (1–2 mg/ml). Cell-free blanks are included, with and without mannan. After 1–2 days incubation an aliquot of medium is removed and the TCA-soluble radioactivity determined. Cell-dependent, mannan-inhibitable degradation per unit time is calculated as a function of Mϕ number or protein.

Single cell assays

Uptake of ^{125}I-mannose BSA or ^{125}I β-glucuronidase by Mϕ can be detected at the single cell level by autoradiography. To increase the cell-associated radioactivity a higher specific activity ligand should be used (5 $\times$ 10^6 c.p.m./μg) at saturation. Coverslips with adherent Mϕ are incubated as above for 20–30 min at 37 °C, washed well and fixed. Radioactivity associated with the coverslips can be determined directly before processing.

Notes and recommendations

Kinetic parameters of specific binding and uptake of ligand can be determined [15]. The degradation assay is not saturable, but is sensitive and linear for prolonged periods of incubation. Specificity can be established by using other neoglycoprotein inhibitors. Other glycoprotein ligands, including horseradish-peroxidase, can be taken up by the MFR [14].

In prolonged degradation assays, cell viability should be monitored by phase-contrast microscopy. Lysozyme secretion is a useful measure of cellular biosynthetic activity. Optimal culture conditions are essential, pH variations in crowded cultures may perturb MFR activity [54]. Sera of some species contain inhibitors, presumably mannosyl-, fucosyl-terminal glycoproteins.

Mannan is non-toxic at relatively high concentrations, but, if used in other assays, e.g. of respiratory burst activity, scavenge O_2^- [19], unlike ribonuclease B [27].

Conclusion

As summarized in Tables 43.1–4, Ag F4/80 and MFR expression are profoundly altered by Mϕ maturation and activation, by culture conditions and by extrinsic regulators such as lymphokines. Different assays vary markedly in sensitivity, e.g. the immunocytochemical method readily detects Ag F4/80 on BCG-activated peritoneal Mϕ, unlike FACS analysis. The interpretation of results obtained with these, as with other assays of cell antigens and receptors, requires an appreciation of the value and limits of each analysis.

Acknowledgements

Work in the authors' laboratory was supported in part by the Medical Research Council, UK. The authors thank the following for helpful discussions: N. Barclay, S.H. Lee, D. Mason, T. Miokoena, V.H. Perry, S. Rabinowitz, P. Stahl, P. Tree and A.F. Williams.

Note added in proof

The absorption immunoassay for Ag F4/80 has been used to estimate total macrophage content in murine tissues [56]. Biochemical and immunocytochemical results obtained with Ab F4/80 have been extended and summarized [57–60].

References

1 AUSTYN J.M. & GORDON S. (1981) F4/80: a monoclonal antibody directed specifically against the mouse macrophage. *Eur. J. Immunol.* **11**, 805–815.

2 HIRSCH S., AUSTYN J.M. & GORDON S. (1981) Expression of the macrophage-specific antigen F4/80 during differentiation of mouse bone marrow cells in culture. *J. exp. Med.* **154**, 713–725.

3 HUME D.A. & GORDON S. (1983) The mononuclear phagocyte system of the mouse defined by immunohistochemical localisation of antigen F4/80. Identification of resident macrophages in renal medullary and cortical interstitium and the juxtaglomerular complex. *J. exp. Med.* **157**, 1704–1709.

4 HUME D.A., ROBINSON A.P., MacPHERSON G.G. & GORDON S. (1983a) The mononuclear phagocyte system of the mouse defined by immunohistochemical localisation of antigen F4/80. The relationship between macrophages, Langerhans cells, reticular cells and dendritic cells in lymphoid and hematopoietic organs. *J. exp. Med.* **158**, 1522–1536.

5 HUME D.A., PERRY V.H. & GORDON S. (1983b) Immunohistochemical localisation of a macrophage-specific antigen in developing mouse retina. Phagocytosis of dying neurons and differentiation of microglial cells to form a regular array in the plexiform layers. *J. Cell Biol.* **97**, 253–257.

6 HUME D.A., LOUTIT J.F. & GORDON S. (1984a) The mononuclear phagocyte system of the mouse defined by immunohistochemical localisation of antigen F4/80. Macrophages of bone and associated connective tissue. *J. Cell Sci.* **66**, 189–194.

7 HUME D.A., HALPIN D., CHARLTON H. & GORDON S. (1984b) The mononuclear phagocyte system of the mouse defined by immunohistochemical localisation of antigen F4/80. Macrophages of endocrine organs. *Proc. natn. Acad. Sci. U.S.A.* **81**, 4174–4177.

8 HUME D.A., PERRY V.H. & GORDON S. (1984) The mononuclear phagocyte system of the mouse defined by immunohistochemical localisation of antigen F4/80. Macrophages associated with epithelia. *Anat. Rec.* **210**, 503.

9 EZEKOWITZ R.A.B., AUSTYN J., STAHL P.D. & GORDON S. (1981) Surface properties of bacillus Calmette-Guerin-activated mouse macrophages. Reduced expression of mannose-specific endocytosis, Fc receptors and antigen F4/80 accompanies induction of Ia. *J. exp. Med.* **154**, 60–76.

10 MULLER W.A., STEINMAN R.M. & COHN Z.A. (1983) Membrane proteins of the vacuolar system. (III) Further studies on the composition and recycling of endocytic vacuole membrane in cultured macrophages. *J. Cell Biol.* **96**, 29–36.

11 NUSSENZWEIG M.C., STEINMAN R.M., UNKELESS J.C., WITMER M.D., GUTCHINOV B. & COHN Z.A. (1981) Studies of the cell surface of mouse dendritic cells and other leukocytes. *J. exp. Med.* **154**, 168.

12 STAHL P., RODMAN J., MILLER J. & SCHLESINGER P. (1978) Evidence for receptor-mediated binding of glycoproteins, glycoconjugates and lysosomal glycosidases by alveolar macrophages. *Proc. natn. Acad. Sci. U.S.A.* **75**, 1399.

13 STAHL P., SCHLESINGER P., SIGARDSON E., RODMAN J.S. & LEE Y.C. (1980) Receptor mediated pinocytosis of mannose glycoconjugates by macrophages, characterisation and evidence for receptor recycling. *Cell*, **19**, 207.

14 SUNG S.S.J., NELSON R.S. & SILVERSTEIN S.C. (1983) Yeast mannose inhibits binding and phagocytosis of zymosan by mouse peritoneal macrophages. *J. Cell Biol.* **96**, 160.

15 STAHL P. & GORDON S. (1982) Expression of a mannose-fucosyl receptor for endocytosis on cultured primary macrophages and their hybrids. *J. Cell Biol.* **93**, 49.

16 SHEPHERD V.L., CAMPBELL E.J., SENIOR R.M. & STAHL P.D. (1982) Characterization of the mannose/fucosyl receptor on human mononuclear phagocytes. *J. Res.* **32**, 423–432.

17 HUBBARD A.L. & STUBENBROK H. (1979) An electron microscopic autoradiographic study of the carbohydrate recognition systems in rat liver. *J. Cell Biol.* **83**, 65.

18 WARR J.A. (1980) A macrophage receptor for mannose/glycosamine glycoproteins of potential importance in

phagocytic activity. *Biochem. biophys. Res. Commun.* **93**, 737.

19 BERTON G. & GORDON S. (1983) Modulation of macrophage mannosyl-specific receptors by cultivation on immobilised zymosan. Effects on phagocytosis and superoxide anion release. *Immunology*, **49**, 705–715.

20 PUGH C.W., MACPHERSON G.G. & STEER H.W. (1983) Characterization of nonlymphoid cells derived from rat peripheral lymph. *J. exp. Med.* **157**, 1758–1779.

21 EZEKOWITZ R.A.B. & GORDON S. (1982) Down regulation of mannosyl-receptor mediated endocytosis and antigen F4/80 on BCG activated mouse macrophages. Role of T lymphocytes and lymphokines. *J. exp. Med.* **155**, 1623.

22 EZEKOWITZ R.A.B., SIM R., HILL M. & GORDON S. (1984) Local opsonisation by secreted macrophage complement components. Role of receptors for complement in uptake of zymosan. *J. exp. Med.* **159**, 244.

23 MOKOENA T. & GORDON S. (1985) Activation of human macrophages. Modulation of mannosyl, fucosyl receptors for endocytosis by lymphokine, interferon and dexamethasone. *J. clin. Invest.* **75**, 624.

24 STEEG P.S., MOORE R.N. & OPPENHEIM J.J. (1980) Regulation of murine macrophage Ia antigen expression by products of activated spleen cells. *J. exp. Med.* **152**, 1734.

25 STEINMAN R.M., NOGUEIRA N., WITMER M.D., TYDINGS J.P. & MELLMAN I.S. (1980) Lymphokine enhances the expression and synthesis of Ia antigens on cultured mouse peritoneal macrophages. *J. exp. Med.* **152**, 1248.

26 SCHER M., BELLER D.I. & UNANUE E.R. (1980) Demonstration of a soluble mediator that induces exudates rich in Ia positive macrophages. *J. exp. Med.* **152**, 1684.

27 HIRSCH S. & GORDON S. (1983) Polymorphic expression of a neutrophil differentiation antigen revealed by monoclonal antibody 7/4. *Immunogenetics*, **18**, 229–339.

28 EZEKOWITZ R.A.B., BAMPTON M. & GORDON S. (1983) Macrophage activation selectively enhances expression of Fc receptors for IgG2a. *J. exp. Med.* **157**, 807.

29 EDELSON P.J. (1980) Macrophage ectoenzymes. Their identification, metabolism, and control. In *Mononuclear Phagocytes: Functional Aspects*, (ed. van Furth R.). Nijhoff (Martinus) Publishers B.V.

30 MORAHAN P.S., EDELSON P.J. & GASS K. (1980) Changes in macrophage ectoenzymes upon *in vivo* or *in vitro* activation for antitumour activity. *J. Immunol.* **125**, 1313.

31 NATHAN C.F. & ROOT R.K. (1977) Hydrogen peroxide release from mouse peritoneal macrophages. Dependence on sequential activation and triggering. *J. exp. Med.* **146**, 1648.

32 SCOTT W.A., PAWLOWSKI N.A., MURRAY H.W., ANDREACH M., ZRIKE J. & COHN Z.A. (1982) The regulation of arachidonic acid metabolism by macrophage activation. *J. exp. Med.* **155**, 1148.

33 ROUBIN R., MENCIA-HUERTA J.M. & BENVENISTE J. (1982) Release of platelet-activating factor (PAF-acether) and leukotrienes C and D from inflammatory macrophages. *Eur. J. Immunol.* **12**, 141–146.

34 WERB Z. & CHIN J.R. (1983) Apoprotein E is synthesised and secreted by resident and thioglycollate-elicited Mϕ

35 KOREN H., EDELSON P. & ADAMS D. (1981) *Methods for Studying Mononuclear Phagocytes*. Academic Press, London.

36 UNKELESS J.C., GORDON S. & REICH E. (1974) Secretion of plasminogen activator by stimulated macrophages. *J. exp. Med.* **139**, 834–850.

37 KAPLAN G. & GAUDERNACK G. (1982) *In vitro* differentiation of human monocytes. Differences in monocyte phenotype induced by cultivation on glass or on collagen. *J. exp. Med.* **156**, 1101.

38 BERTON G. & GORDON S. (1983) Superoxide release by peritoneal and bone marrow-derived mouse macrophages. Modulation by adherence and cell activation. *Immunology*, **49**, 693–704.

39 UNKELESS J., FLEIT H. & MELLMAN I.S. (1981) Structural aspects and heterogeneity of immunoglobulin Fc receptors. *Adv. Immunol.* **31**, 247–270.

40 HUNT S.V. & FOWLER M.H. (1981) A repopulation assay for B and T lymphocyte stem cells employing radiation chimaeras. *Cell Tissue Kinet.* **14**, 445–464.

41 BROWN W.R.A., BARCLAY A.N., SUNDERLAND C.A. & WILLIAMS A.F. (1981) Identification of a glycophorin-like molecule at the cell surface of rat thymocytes. *Nature*, **289**, 456–460.

42 UNKELESS J.C. & HEALEY G.A. (1983) Quantitation of proteins and internal antigen pools by a monoclonal sandwich radioimmune assay. *J. immunol. Meth.* **56**, 1–11.

43 BOYLE W. (1968) An extension of the 51-Cr rlease assay for the estimation of mouse cytotoxins. *Transplantation*, **6**, 761–764.

44 HSU S.M., RAINE L. & FANGER H. (1981) The use of avidin–biotin-peroxidase (ABC) complex in immunoperoxidase techniques. A comparison between ABC and unlabelled antibody (PAP) procedures. *J. Histochem. Cytochem.* **29**, 577–580.

45 GLAUERT A.M. (1975) *Fixation, dehydration and embedding of biological specimens*, p. 82. North–Holland Publishing Co., Oxford.

46 McLEAN I.W. & NAKANE P.K. (1974) Periodate-lysine-paraformaldehyde fixative. A new fixative for immunoelectron microscopy. *J. Histochem. Cytochem.* **22**, 1077–1083.

47 LOCKSLEY R.M., WILSON C.B. & KLEBANOFF S.J. (1983) Increased respiratory burst in myeloperoxidase-deficient monocytes. *Blood*, **62**, 902–909.

48 STRAUS W. (1981) Cytochemical detection of mannose-specific receptors for glycoproteins with horseradish/peroxidase as a ligand. *Histochemistry*, **73**, 39–47.

49 WOOD G.S. & WARNKE R. (1981) Suppression of endogenous avidin-binding activity in tissues and its relevance to biotin–avidin detection systems. *J. Histochem. Cytochem.* **29**, 1196–1204.

50 KELLER R.K. & TOUSTER O. (1975) Physical and chemical properties of B glucuronidase from preputial glands of the female rat. *J. Biol. Chem.* **250**, 4765.

51 GREENWOOD F., HUNTER W. & GLOVER J. (1975) The preparation of I-labelled human growth hormone of high specific activity. *J. Biochem.* **89**, 114.

52 LOWRY D.H., ROSEBOROUGH N.J., FARR A.L. & RAN-DALL R.J. (1951) Protein measurement with folin phenol reagent. *J. Biol. Chem.* **193,** 265.

53 GORDON S., TODD J. & COHN Z.A. (1974) *In vitro* synthesis and secretion of lysozyme by mononuclear phagocytes. *J. exp. Med.* **139,** 1228–1248.

54 STAHL P., SCHLESINGER P.H., SIGARDSON E., RODMAN J.S. & LEE Y.C. (1980) Receptor mediated pinocytosis of mannose glucoconjugates by macrophages. Characterisation and evidence for receptor recycling. *Cell,* **19,** 207.

55 TOWBIN H., STAEHELIN T. & GORDON J. (1979) Electrophoretic transfer of proteins from polyacrylamide gels to nitrocellulose sheets: procedure and some applications. *Proc. natn. Acad. Sci. U.S.A.* **76,** 4350–4354.

56 LEE S-H., STARKEY P.M. & GORDON S. (1985) Quantitative analysis of total macrophage content in adult mouse tissues. Immunochemical studies with monoclonal antibody F4/80. *J. exp. Med.* **161,** 475.

57 PERRY V.H., HUME D.A. & GORDON S. (1985) Immunohistochemical localization of macrophages and microglia in the adult and developing mouse brain. *Neuroscience,* (in press).

58 HUME D.A. & GORDON S. (1985) The mononuclear phagocyte system of the mouse defined by immunohistochemical localization of antigen F4/80. In Mononuclear phagocytes. Characterisitcs, physiology and function, (ed. van Furth R.), (in press). Martinus Nijhoff Publishers, Boston, Dordrecht, Lancaster.

59 GORDON S., HIRSCH S. & STARKEY P.M. (1985) Differentiation antigens of mouse macrophages and polymorphonuclear leukocytes. In Mononuclear phagocytes. Characteristics, physiology and function, (ed. van Furth R.), (in press). Martinus Nijhoff Publishers, Boston, Dordrecht, Lancaster.

60 GORDON S., CROCKER P., MORRIS L., LEE S-H., PERRY V.H. & HUME D.A. (1985) Localization and function of tissue macrophages. Ciba Foundation Symposium 118, (in press).

Chapter 44
Methods for studying the ontogeny of mononuclear phagocytes

C. C. STEWART

Method for obtaining cells from mice, 44.2

Method for counting cells, 44.4

Method for culturing cells, 44.5

Removal of adherent cells, 44.6

Method for labelling murine

macrophages with MAbs, 44.6

Analysis of positive cells, 44.10

Solutions, 44.16

Mononuclear phagocytes represent one of the most primitive host defence systems retained by higher organisms. These cells, while preserving characteristics (like phagocytosis) of the most primitive cells, have also acquired many specialized functions such as: (1) antigen presentation; (2) microbicidal and tumoricidal activity; (3) secretion of mediators that regulate the proliferation, differentiation and function of other cells; and (4) secretion of enzymes important in the host defence [for review see refs. 1 and 2].

These cells also represent an important system with which to study the regulation of normal cell proliferation and differentiation. Mononuclear phagocytes will not proliferate unless macrophage growth factor (also called colony stimulating factor-1) is present in adequate concentrations. This growth factor, constitutively produced by fibroblasts, has been purified by Stanley et al. [3]. It interacts with distinct receptors found only on mononuclear phagocytes. When the factor is present in adequate concentrations, the cells will proliferate; when it is removed, the cells will stop proliferating after completing the DNA synthetic phase and mitosis [4]. Thus this cell system offers a unique model system for studying the molecular biology of cell proliferation resulting from a single ligand–receptor interaction.

Not all mononuclear phagocytes are capable of proliferation. Monoblasts, promonocytes and monocytes all appear to be able to proliferate but as monocytes differentiate into tissue macrophages, some of these cells retain proliferative capacity while others senesce and lose their proliferative ability. Thus the system also offers a unique model to study the biology of cellular senescence.

As mentioned above, macrophages arise from an orderly differentiation process through morphologically identifiable cell types. In the bone marrow, the first recognizable cell type is the monoblast; these differentiate into promonocytes, then into monocytes, which are released into the blood [5]. From the blood, the monocytes go to the tissues where they become macrophages. During an inflammatory reaction, large numbers of monocytes are recruited into the lesion. The functionally diverse subpopulations of these cells, however, are not revealed by their morphology. Thus new methodologies must be developed to identify and isolate functionally different monocytes similar to the way in which lymphocyte subpopulations have been resolved.

Although all mononuclear phagocytes pass through the morphological stages described above, their heterogeneous functional expression may not be so simple to resolve. Two different modes of functional heterogeneity, illustrated in Fig. 44.1, have been postulated: the single lineage hypothesis (maturational heterogeneity), and the multilineage hypothesis (clonal heterogeneity). In maturational heterogeneity it is assumed that a single lineage of cells expresses different functions at different stages of differentiation and maturity. A subpopulation of cells expressing a particular function represents a window in the life of the maturing cell. A particular function, therefore, is expressed only during a unique stage(s) of maturation. Some functions may be expressed for only a short period while other functions, such as phagocytic activity, may be retained throughout the maturational sequence. Alternatively, mononuclear phagocyte lineages exhibiting a particular function may be derived from progenitor cells whose progeny express unique functions. In this case, the functional future of the lineage is determined at the level of the most primitive precursor cells found in the bone marrow. Thus all progeny, even though maturing through the classical morphological stages, retain the specialized function so that only cells within that lineage are capable of expressing that function. This kind of

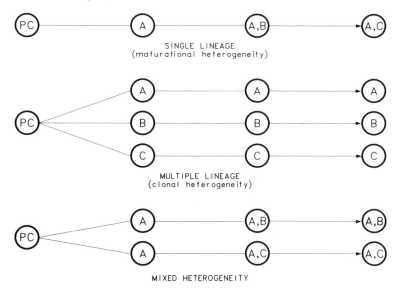

Fig. 44.1. Mononuclear phagocyte heterogeneity. In the single lineage hypothesis, all functional cells are derived from a single precursor cell. As they differentiate, progeny may express some function (A) throughout their lifetime while other functions (B and C) are expressed only at a particular stage of differentiation. In the multiple lineage hypothesis, a precursor cell (PC) gives rise to functionally distinct lineages A, B, and C. It is most likely that mononuclear phagocytes are a mixture of the two extremes in which both maturational and clonal heterogeneity is expressed. Thus both lineages are capable of expressing a common function (A), but one lineage expresses B, while the other expresses C.

differentiation would be analogous to that for T or B cell subpopulations. Neither of the two hypotheses are mutually exclusive, however, and cells within the series may share common functions that depend on the level of maturation while other functions may be clonally distributed (Fig. 44.1). The mononuclear phagocyte system offers a unique model for studying the mechanism of cellular differentiation.

In this chapter, the techniques for isolating and growing mononuclear phagocyte subpopulations will be described. Flow cytometry and monoclonal antibodies have provided a powerful means to identify and study unique subsets of lymphocytes. The author's work has been directed toward applying these same principles to identify specific differentiation stages and to study the heterogeneity of mononuclear phagocytes. Unlike lymphocytes, mononuclear phagocytes are very difficult to study using monoclonal antibodies; the pitfalls that the author has experienced, along with the possible solutions to them, will also be described.

Abbreviations used in this chapter

αMOPS: alpha morpholinopropane sulphonic acid.
PAB: phosphate-buffered saline with 0.1% sodium azide and 0.5% BSA.
BSA: bovine serum albumin.
PI: propidium iodide.
MEM: minimum essential medium.

Method for obtaining cells from mice

Materials

Three millilitre syringes with 25-gauge needles.
Ten millilitre syringes with 22-gauge needles.
Fifteen millilitre centrifuge tubes.
Fifty millilitre centrifuge tubes.
Dissecting board, pins.
Scissors—$3\frac{3}{4}$ in. curved blunt pointed dissecting (Roboz No. RS-521).
70% Ethanol in a squeeze bottle.
Sterile $5\frac{3}{4}$ in. cotton plugged Pasteur pipettes with 1 ml bulb.
One, five and ten millilitre pipettes.
Fifty millilitre beaker with ether-saturated sponge.
Intravenous saline drip pack and administration set.
Ring stand.
Three-way stopcock.
Eighteen-gauge catheter start kit (Becton-Dickinson #6707).
5% CO_2 in air.

Procedure

Bone marrow cells

1 Fill 3 ml syringe (25-gauge needle) with alpha morpholinopropane sulphonic acid (αMOPS).
2 Sacrifice the animal by cervical dislocation and pin supinely to a board; wash legs and lower part of animal with 70% ethanol.

3 Make an incision in the skin of the leg and retract it, exposing the femur.

4 Pin the skin to the board.

5 Using the forceps, hold the tendons at the posterior femur joint, clip with scissors, and pull muscle and tissue back to the anterior end of the femur; the entire femur is now exposed.

6 With scissors, scrape underside clean of tissue and muscle.

7 Hold the femur with forceps and cut both the anterior and posterior ends at the joints with scissors.

8 While holding the femur with forceps, insert the 25-gauge needle through the entire length, making a channel; pull the needle back to within 1 mm of the end and syringe 1.5 ml of the αMOPS through the femur and into the 15 ml centrifuge tube.

9 Remove the needle, turn the femur around, and repeat, flushing the remaining αMOPS through this end and into the centrifuge tube.

10 Repeat to obtain the required number of cells. All cells may be pooled and placed on ice. The usual cell yield per femur is between 6 and 9×10^6 cells, depending on the age and strain of the mice.

Peritoneal exudate cells

1 Inject mice i.p. with 1.5 ml Brewer's thioglycollate medium (or other phlogogenic agent) 3 days prior to harvesting cells (for resident peritoneal cells omit this step).

2 Sacrifice mouse by cervical dislocation and pin supinely to board.

3 Soak abdominal cavity with 70% ethanol.

4 Make a vertical incision in the abdominal midline through the skin without puncturing the peritoneal membrane.

5 Pull the skin up. This exposes the lower rib cage and a 'window' for aspirating the peritoneal fluid.

6 Inject 10 ml αMOPS containing 5 units/ml heparin into this 'window' with a 10 ml syringe and a 22-gauge needle.

7 Do not remove the needle but turn bevel side down. Lift up with the needle, making a 'tent' and aspirate slowly; use little pressure and be careful not to aspirate part of the intestine.

8 Average recovery volume is 9 ml.

9 Inspect each suspension microscopically for bacterial contamination which can occur if the intestine is punctured.

10 Pool acceptable suspensions in a 50 ml conical centrifuge tube and replace the cap; place on ice.

Peripheral blood mononuclear cells

1 Place the animal in a container with an ether sponge to anaesthetize; maintain anaesthesia by secur-ing a 50 ml beaker with an ether-saturated pad over the animal's nose.

2 Pin animal supinely to the board and soak with 70% ethanol.

3 Make a midline incision into the chest wall; do not cut into the peritoneal membranes but expose the rib cage by retracting the skin and cut through the sternum, exposing the heart.

4 Cut the atrium and aspirate the blood as it fills the chest cavity using a Pasteur pipette; transfer it to a centrifuge tube containing 5 ml αMOPS with 20 units/ml heparin.

5 Rinse the chest cavity by transferring 2 ml medium into the chest and very gently aspirating it with the pipette; this rinse with heparin prevents clotting.

6 For each collection tube, put in a maximum of 5 ml of blood; the average yield per mouse is about 1 ml blood.

7 Centrifuge cells at 150 *g* for 10 min.

8 Resuspend cells in 10 ml αMOPS, pooling samples as desired with a maximum of 3 ml packed cells; adjust to 10 ml αMOPS.

9 Overlay cell suspension (10 ml) on 5 ml Ficoll–Hypaque in a 15 ml centrifuge tube by holding the tube at a 45° angle and pipetting suspension carefully down the side of the tube.

10 Centrifuge at 1200 *g* and 15 °C for 10 min.

11 Aspirate and discard the top layer of medium to within 0.5 ml above the band.

12 Use a sterile cotton plugged Pasteur pipette with a bulb to collect the middle layer of mononuclear cells; move the tip of the pipette around the outside edge of the tube because the cells have a tendency to adhere to the side of the tube; collect all cells to within 0.5 ml above the bottom erythrocyte layer.

13 Transfer the cells to a 50 ml centrifuge tube.

14 Wash by adjusting each 15 ml of cell suspension to 50 ml with αMOPS to dilute the Ficoll–Hypaque.

15 Centrifuge at 200 *g* for 10 min at 4 °C.

16 Aspirate and discard the supernatant fluid to just above the cell pellet; add 10 ml αMOPS with a 10 ml pipette; resuspend the cells in it.

17 Repeat three times to disperse the cells; if still clumped, aspirate more vigorously; pool when all cells are dispersed and place on ice.

Alveolar cells

1 Attach a saline i.v. drip pack to a ring stand with the top of the solution 25 cm above the working surface.

2 Insert the i.v. administration set into the saline pack; attach a three-way stopcock to the free end.

3 Attach a 10 ml syringe to the stopcock and fill all tubing with saline to eliminate air bubbles.

4 Anaesthetize the animal by placing it in an atmosphere of 5% CO_2.
5 Cut open the abdomen exposing the inferior vena cava and diaphragm.
6 Sever the inferior vena cava and exsanguinate the animal before lung lavage to reduce blood contamination in lavage fluid.
7 Cut away lower half of rib cage to expose collapsed lungs.
8 Expose trachea and pin neck back by inserting a rubber band around the pinboard and through the mouth.
9 Place suture silk under the trachea; insert an 18-gauge catheter placement unit about 5 mm deep into the trachea and secure it with a suture thread; remove the stylet and attach the unit to the three-way stopcock.
10 Allow the lungs to fill with saline by gravity; change the stopcock position to the syringe and slowly aspirate the saline from the lungs. Repeat for ten cycles.
11 Transfer the lavage to a centrifuge tube containing diluting fluid with an equal volume of αMOPS. The usual yield is about 5×10^5 cells in a total lavage fluid of 10 ml; pool suspension and place on ice.

Notes and recommendations

In the above procedures, each cell suspension has been obtained in αMOPS, a buffer the pH of which does not depend on CO_2. Mononuclear phagocytes are exquisitely sensitive to pH values greater than 7.4, and they will die if left very long in medium above this pH. The author has used this buffered medium for manipulations. While there are many short-term viability assays which may indicate good viability of cells over a few hours, cell growth reveals the true long-term viability of the cells.

It is best to obtain the cells after the entire experiment has been set up. This includes labelling all culture tubes and dishes, preparing the medium, and arranging the materials for easy access. The last procedure is to obtain the cells, dilute, and plate them. In this way, the time for which the cells will be manipulated is minimized. This is most important if good growth is to be achieved.

Method for counting cells

Equipment

Electronic particle counter.

Materials

Pasteur pipettes with 1 ml bulb.
Twenty dram vials.

Procedure

Counting cells in suspension

1 Add an appropriate amount of cells (usually 100 μl) to an equal volume of pronase and incubate for 10 min at 37 °C.
2 Add the entire sample to 10 ml of cetrimide counting solution.
3 Count the sample using an electronic particle counter (the same settings that would be used to count erythrocytes.)
4 Calculate the cells per ml of the cell suspension.

Counting adherent cells

1 Resuspend the non-adherent cells completely in medium contained in the culture and remove it.
2 Add 1.5 ml, 3 ml, or 5 ml cetrimide counting solution to 35 mm, 60 mm, or 100 mm culture dish, respectively.
3 Using a Pasteur pipette with 1 ml bulb, resuspend the adherent cells in the counting solution by systematically aspirating and flushing the solution over the dish's surface. Do not allow air into the pipette as this will produce bubbles.
4 Transfer the solution to 10 ml cetrimide counting solution and rinse the dish once.
5 Count the sample and calculate the number of adherent cells per dish.

Notes and recommendations

The advantage of the above procedure is that nuclei are counted and adherent cells are quickly removed from the dish. Pronase is used to digest the dead cells in the non-adherent cell suspension so that the count obtained on suspensions is for viable cells only [6]. The author does not treat the adherent cells with pronase because his experience has been that dead cells are not adherent. When an adherent cell dies it detaches from the plate. The procedure described, however, is not conducive to haemocytometer counting because the cells are too dilute. If a haemocytometer is used, cells in suspension can be counted directly using standard techniques, and the adherent cells can be removed using only 1.5 ml of the cetrimide counting solution.

Method for culturing cells

Equipment

CO_2 incubator.
Centrifuge.
Laminar air flow hood (optional).
Pipette aid.

Materials

Culture dishes (35 and 100 ml).
Culture flasks (75 cm^2).
One, five and ten millilitre pipettes.
L-929 cells (ATCC).

Procedure

Preparation of conditioned medium (LCM)

1　Adjust L cells in culture medium to 5000 cells per ml.
2　Put 20 ml in each 75 cm^2 culture flask.
3　Incubate for 7 days in CO_2 incubator with 7–10% CO_2 in humidified air.
4　Remove medium and centrifuge.
5　Freeze LCM until needed; just prior to use filter through a 0.22 μm Micropore filter after thawing.

Preparation of macrophage cell suspensions

1　Determine the cell concentration of each cell suspension obtained in the section named 'Method for obtaining cells; note the volume. Calculate the total number of cells.
2　Centrifuge cells at 150 g for 10 min and discard supernatant fluid.
3　Referring to Table 44.1, determine the appropriate cell concentration and resuspend the cell pellet in growth medium.
4　Make the appropriate dilutions in growth medium and plate the cells in 35 or 100 ml dishes.
5　Incubate the dishes of flasks in a CO_2 incubator.

Notes and recommendations

Murine mononuclear phagocytes will proliferate in medium containing colony stimulating factor-1 (CSF-1 [7]). The author has found that the best source of CSF-1 is L-929 cell conditioned medium. He recommends using an automatic pipetter when manipulating the cell suspension. Mouth pipetting is almost certain to result in mycoplasma contamination of the cells or the possibility that the operator might be contaminated by the cells.

When growing macrophages in 35 mm culture dishes, the author puts two dishes inside a 100×20 mm Petri dish along with a third dish containing distilled H_2O. The larger plate is covered and put in the incubator. This produces a chamber which improves humidification of the culture.

The single most important variable affecting macrophage growth is pH. Cells should be cultured at 7–10% CO_2 (pH 7–7.2). A pH variation, which occurs with frequent opening of the incubator door, will definitely cause poor growth. If an incubator must be used which

Table 44.1. Optimal cell concentrations for culturing mononuclear phagocytes

	Percentage colony forming cells	Initial cell concentration*		Lag period	Doubling time
		Colonies	Bulk		
Bone marrow					
Day 7	0.8	10^4	10^5	1 day	24 h
Day 14	3.0	10^3	10^4	5–7 days	40 h
Blood		10^3	10^4	5–7 days	40 h
Alveolar cell	5.0	10^3	10^4	5–7 days	40 h
Spleen cells	1.0	10^4	10^5	5–7 days	40 h
Resident peritoneal cells	0.1	10^4	10^5	5–7 days	40 h
Peritoneal exudate cells	15.0	10^2	10^4	5–7 days	40 h

* If colonies are desired, plate 3 ml of cells at the concentration indicated in 35 mm culture dishes. If confluent monolayers of macrophages are desired, plate cells at the higher concentration. The author uses 3 ml for 35 mm dishes, 5 ml for 60 mm dishes, and 15 ml for 100 ml dishes.

is frequently opened, the author suggests putting the cultures in a lucite box or desiccator which has been pre-gassed. Make sure the growth medium is pre-gassed with 10% CO_2 prior to obtaining the cells. This will ensure the proper medium pH of 7–7.3. When gassing, do not bubble the gas through the medium because this will cause bubbles to form; instead, use a cotton plugged transfer pipette and allow the gas to flow in the void volume above the medium; stopper the bottle and invert it several times. Repeat as necessary to obtain the appropriate pH as determined by the colour of the medium.

The second most important variable which affects macrophage growth is the quality of the batch of fetal bovine serum used. It is most important to screen each batch of fetal serum for its ability to support maximum growth. Peritoneal exudate cells are the most sensitive target cell to use in the screening assay. A good batch of serum will yield 100 to 150 colonies per 1000 cells and the cells with colonies will be nicely spread out. If a bad batch is used, it will yield only a few colonies and round or dendritic looking cells will be obtained. The author has found that batches of serum that support good macrophage growth are universally excellent for both lymphocyte cultures and for carrying all other cell lines.

For the peritoneal exudate cells, do not pool the suspensions until each has been inspected for bacterial contamination, which can occur if the intestine has been accidently punctured. Pool acceptable suspensions in 15 ml conical centrifuge tubes, and replace the cap; place on ice.

Table 44.1 lists the best initial concentrations to use for growing macrophages derived from various sources. Cells will proliferate as long as an adequate concentration of CSF-1 is present. Once the cells have consumed the CSF-1 (0.017 units/cell/day), they will stop growing. The author has found that 1 ml of growth medium will support the growth of macrophages to a maximum concentration of 1.0×10^5 cells/ml regardless of the initial concentration. Thus, if 50 000 colony-forming macrophages are cultured in 1 ml medium, they will undergo only one doubling. If 10 000 cells are cultured, these cells will undergo four doublings. Table 44.1 also indicates the lag period and generation times for the different populations from which the length of time to obtain the desired number of cells can be determined, e.g. if one desires 10^6 cells, one would need to use 10 ml of growth medium. These growth kinetics have been completely described in other reports [4,6–10].

Removal of adherent cells

Materials

2.5 mM-Sodium pyrophosphate (Sigma, S-390).
Rubber policeman.

Procedure

1   Remove medium from culture and flood the culture dish with 2 mM-sodium pyrophosphate solution.
2   Incubate for 10 min at room temperature.
3   Carefully remove the sodium pyrophosphate, discard, and add an appropriate amount of medium.
4   Gently scrape off cells with a rubber policeman.

Notes and recommendations

The author has not found a technique for the successful removal of adherent macrophages in which the majority of cells are not severely damaged. The best recovery of viable cells he has found is only 30–50%. The advantage of the procedure described above over scraping alone is that a higher viable cell recovery is obtained than when cells are scraped off and aggregation is less severe. This system does not work for human cells and the author has been unsuccessful in finding a good method for removing them.

Method for labelling murine macrophages with MAbs

Materials

Desired monoclonal antibodies (MAbs), preferably directly labelled with a fluorochrome or biotin.
Note: if the antibody is biotinated, add the appropriate amount of labelled avidin; incubate cells for 15 min; centrifuge; pour off supernatant fluid and blot.
Appropriate second reagent labelled with a fluorochrome or conjugated to a fluorochrome (preferably the F(ab')$_2$ fragment which has been affinity purified).
Test tubes (10 × 75 mm).
Microlitre pipetting device.

Procedures

Using directly labelled MAbs (LMAb) on macrophages

1   Adjust cells in phosphate-buffered saline with 0.1% sodium azide and 0.5% BSA (PAB) to 2×10^7 cells/ml.
2   Distribute 50 μl of cells into each 10 × 75 mm glass tube on ice.
3   Add a tenfold excess of myeloma protein mixture; incubate for 10 min.

4 Add appropriate amount of LMAb; incubate for 15 min on ice.
5 Add 4 ml PAB and centrifuge for 10 min at 200 *g*.
6 Pour off supernatant fluid and blot well.
7 Resuspend cells in 2 ml PAB, filter and analyse.

Using MAbs on macrophages with labelled second reagent

1 Adjust cells in PAB to 2×10^7 cells/ml.
2 Distribute 50 μl of cells into each 10×75 mm glass test tube on ice.
3 When the MAb is from a different species than the macrophages (e.g. murine macrophages and rat MAbs), add a tenfold excess of myeloma protein mixture; incubate for 10 min.
4 Add MAb to the tubes.
5 When the MAb is from the same species as the macrophages (e.g. murine macrophages and murine MAbs), separate control tubes must be prepared using a myeloma protein of the same isotype and subclass as the MAb. Add the same weight of myeloma protein to the control tubes as that of MAb added to experimental tubes.
6 Incubate samples for 15 min on ice.
7 Add 4 ml PAB and centrifuge for 10 min at 200 *g*.
8 Pour off supernatant fluid and blot well.
9 Add appropriate amount of labelled second reagent and resuspend cells in it.
10 Incubate cells on ice for 15 min.
11 Add 4 ml PAB and centrifuge for 10 min at 200 *g*.
12 Pour off supernatant fluid and blot well.
13 Repeat **11** and **12.**
14 Add 2 ml PAB, filter and analyse.

Determining viability

Materials

200 μg/ml solution of propidium iodide (PI).

Procedure

1 To each millilitre of cell sample, add 10 μl of PI solution per millilitre of sample (2 μg/ml final).
2 Incubate for at least 5 min.
3 Analyse cells.

Testing second reagents

1 Obtain peritoneal cells or peritoneal exudate cells.
2 Prepare five serial 1:2 dilutions of the second reagent, starting with no dilution at all.
3 Prepare two groups of cells, one group with five tubes containing a first reagent MAb of known titre

and a second group of five tubes with PAB only (no first reagent).
4 Process as described above (label with second reagents); however, no myeloma blocking protein should be added. For each dilution add 10 μl of labelled second reagent.
5 Complete labelling procedure and analyse.

Fixation of cells

1 After the last wash in the first or second procedure above, resuspend the cell pellet in 0.5 ml saline instead of PAB.
2 Add 1.5 ml of 1% buffered paraformaldehyde.
3 Analyse samples within 2 weeks of fixation.
4 Do not use PI with this procedure.

Notes and recommendations

The following conditions are likely to be encountered when macrophages are stained with MAbs:
   (1) the MAb can bind via Fc receptors if it is of the appropriate subclass;
   (2) the MAb can bind to the specific epitope;
   (3) the second reagent can bind to cytophilic antibody;
   (4) the second reagent can bind to the Fc receptors;
   (5) the second reagent can bind to the MAb.
   Obviously, the ideal situation would be conditions (2) and (5) only. One approach would be to use the F(ab')$_2$ fragment of both the MAb and the second reagent. This would eliminate problems (1) and (4), but not (3) if the second reagent is an anti-Ig against the same species as the target cells since the second reagent can, therefore, bind to the cytophilic antibody on the cells. For example, a goat anti-mouse Ig will have heavy and light chain activity for mouse Ig and label B cells (κ) as well as macrophages with cytophilic antibody on their surface. This will cause a high background fluorescence and considerably reduce the sensitivity with which the specific MAb bound to the macrophage can be resolved.
   All MAbs should be centrifuged at 80 000 *g* for 5 min prior to their use to remove aggregated Ig. The accumulation of a significant precipitate indicates aggregation, and the antibody may need to be periodically retired as it is coming out of solution. Store MAbs at $-20\,^\circ$C or $-70\,^\circ$C for long-term storage and at 4 $^\circ$C for short-term use. Do not freeze-thaw MAbs more than once. The author generally aliquots a month's supply into microtitre vials and freezes them.
   The author highly recommends using F(ab')$_2$ fragments of the second reagent. There are several problems, however, using F(ab')$_2$ fragments of rodent

MAbs which make this solution far from satisfactory for the first reagent:

(1) the preparation of F(ab')$_2$ fragments is time consuming;

(2) F(ab')$_2$ fragments of sufficient purity are technically difficult to make from mice and rats;

(3) the yield of F(ab')$_2$ fragments from mice and rats can be very low and may be prohibitively expensive when purchased MAbs are used.

The author has described a general procedure for labelling macrophages with either directly labelled MAbs or unlabelled MAbs which are stained using a labelled second reagent. When the MAb is labelled with a fluorochrome such as fluorescein or with biotin, the Fc binding can be blocked by pre-incubation of the macrophages with a tenfold excess of the appropriate myeloma protein prior to the addition of the labelled MAb. An example of the effectiveness of this blocking is shown in Fig. 44.2.

Using a second reagent to stain the bound MAb, however, is somewhat more complex and depends on the species from which the reagents and target cells are derived. For example, suppose murine MAbs are to be used on murine cells. It is not possible to block Fc binding by pre-incubating with a blocking murine myeloma protein because it too will be labelled by the second reagent. Thus, for each isotype and subclass of murine MAb used, it is necessary to incubate a separate tube of control cells with a myeloma protein of the same isotype and subclass before addition of the second reagent. This will provide a background level above which the MAb specific staining can be compared. The extent to which positive cells can be resolved will determine the sensitivity of the system. When, however, MAbs are not the same as the target macrophages (e.g. rat MAb against mouse macrophages) it is possible to pre-block using murine myeloma proteins since the anti-rat Ig presumably will not stain bound mouse Ig. Some commercially available anti-rat Ig, however, will cross-react with mouse Ig (predominantly κ) and unless the antibody has been affinity purified for rat Ig, it must be exhaustively absorbed with murine spleen cells.

To illustrate this problem, consider a goat antiserum (that has not been affinity purified or absorbed) against rat immunoglobulin. This reagent is a heterogeneous antiserum and contains a varying amount of each goat isotype with antibody activity against each rat immunoglobulin isotype. The antiserum can also cross-react with mouse immunoglobulins. This situation is shown in Fig. 44.3, where three goat anti-rat Ig preparations have been tested against mouse spleen cells.

If the major antibody subclass is a goat γ2a and the contaminating cross-reactivity is against mouse κ light

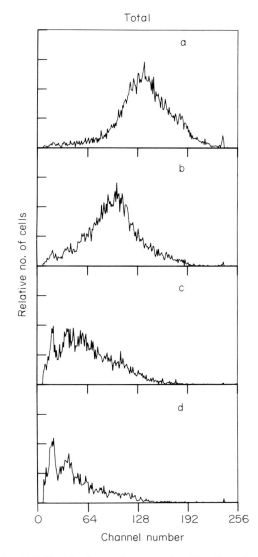

Fig. 44.2. Blocking by myeloma proteins. The effect of adding a γ2a myeloma protein to block the non-specific binding of a fluoresceinated MAb of the γ2a subclass is shown. Note that the binding of the MAb to the macrophages is extremely strong in (a). As cells are pre-incubated for 10 min with increasing amounts of the γ2a myeloma protein, the binding of the MAb decreases. At a ninefold excess of myeloma protein (w/w), the distribution (c) is closest to the autofluorescent control (d).

chains, this antibody will bind to γ2a Fc receptors on macrophages as well as to the light chains on cytophilic antibodies bound to the macrophages. In addition, all the B lymphocytes will be labelled because of the mouse light chain activity. This situation is illustrated in Fig. 44.4 for Brand B.

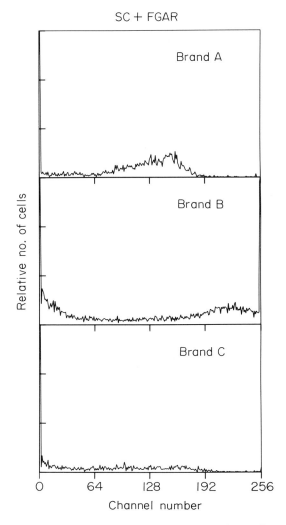

SC + FGAR

Brand A

Brand B

Brand C

Relative no. of cells

0   64   128   192   256

Channel number

Fig. 44.3. Goat anti-rat Ig binding to murine spleen cells. The fluoresceinated Ig fractions of goat antisera to rat immunoglobulins (FGAR) were obtained from three different suppliers. The recommended amount was added to murine spleen cells. Both Brand A and B stained the B cells due to cross-reactivity of the antibody with murine Ig. Brand C, which was the only one that was affinity purified for rat immunoglobulins, did not significantly stain the spleen cells.

If the antibody is absorbed exhaustively with spleen cells (or affinity purified on rat Ig column) to remove the contaminating light chain activity, B lymphocytes will no longer be labelled as illustrated in Fig. 44.4. The macrophages, however, can still bind the antibody due to their FcR activity. Exhaustive absorption with macrophages can result in the removal of virtually all of the anti-rat Ig activity. If none of these measures are

taken, however, the sensitivity for detecting bound first reagents using this antibody will be very poor. To minimize these problems, the author recommends using reagents that have been affinity purified for the species desired. The author also recommends the use of F(ab')$_2$ fragments to reduce Fc binding. The only problem with the latter is that they are not always commercially available. Each batch of second reagent should be tested as it is the author's unfortunate experience that many of the affinity purified F(ab')$_2$ reagents that are commercially available are of poor quality. They are often only partial digests, contaminated with significant amounts of the Fc portion of the molecule, over-fluoresceinated so antibody activity is low, or are contaminated by unknown products that bind to macrophages.

In titring second reagents, the dilution that produces the least binding while still retaining activity for the MAb should be chosen (see Fig. 44.5). We are seeking the dilution that resolves positive cells but has the least amount of staining by itself. When rat MAbs are used with mouse macrophages, the pre-treatment of the cells with the myeloma protein mixture will reduce the non-specific binding of the second labelled anti-rat Ig second reagent. This procedure cannot be used for mouse MAbs because the labelled anti-mouse Ig reagent will also bind to the myeloma proteins bound to the cells. The author has found that it is necessary to wash the cells twice after adding avidin because it tends to bind loosely to some mononuclear phagocyte populations.

The author finds it advisable to add PI to a final concentration of 2 μg/ml for 5 min prior to running so that dead cells are not analysed. This is because dead cells will bind antibodies non-specifically even with the blocking protocols. Thus positive subpopulations for a particular MAb may represent dead cells rather than a true subpopulation. The PI-stained nuclei of the dead cells are brightly fluorescent while viable cells are unstained as they exclude the dye [12]. Since the dead cells are so brightly stained with PI there is no interference with the resolution of viable cells which have been stained with a fluorochrome of either fluorescein or one of the rhodamines. The author recommends adding PI to five samples and waiting 5 min. After sample 1 has been analysed, add PI to sample 6, etc. In this way, each sample will have had PI for at least 5 min and analysis can proceed without further interruptions. It is, however, inadvisable to incubate samples longer than 1 h with PI prior to running because PI may be toxic with prolonged incubation. Although it is often believed that dead cells can be distinguished from live cells based on their physical parameters (Coulter volume or low-angle light scatter), this is only possible when a very

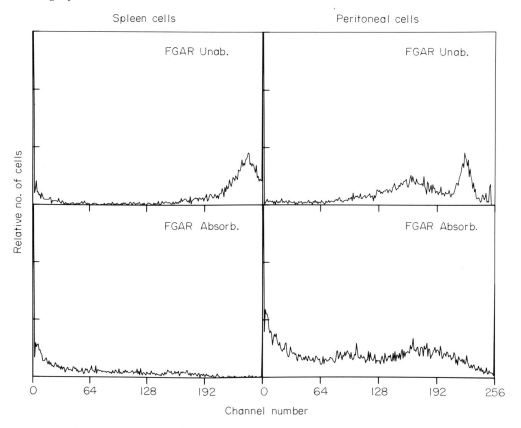

Fig. 44.4. Binding of goat anti-rat Ig to murine lymphocytes and macrophages. The Ig fraction of goat antiserum to rat Ig (FGAR) was fluoresceinated and sold by a commercial supplier to be used as a second reagent. When used at the recommended amount, the unabsorbed reagent, which had not been affinity purified, labelled all spleen B cells as well as macrophages from the peritoneal cavity because of the cross-reactivity with mouse Ig on the membranes of these cells. When the reagent was absorbed using the equivalent of ten spleens per millilitre, the reactivity of the FGAR for B cells was reduced considerably, but the reagent strongly bound to peritoneal macrophages through their Fc receptors. This latter binding could be blocked using a mixture of murine myeloma proteins, as illustrated in Fig. 44.2.

homogeneous population of cells are being labelled. For macrophages, it has been the author's experience that reprocessing data based on this assumption may be risky. As shown in Fig. 44.5, dead cells have been labelled with PI. When the data is reprocessed on the cells which have taken up PI, it can be clearly seen that the electronic volume and autofluorescence distributions are virtually identical to that of the viable cells.

It may not always be possible to run freshly isolated cells on the same day. The paraformaldehyde fixed cells retain both physical and fluorescent characteristics remarkably well [13]. Cell viability data, however, will be lost, and care must be taken to ensure that most of the cells are viable at the time of staining; if they are not, procedures for live cells should be used. It is inadvisable to fix cells prior to staining with MAbs

because epitopes can be altered or reduced in number by denaturation. This was dramatically shown to be the case recently by Walker *et al.* [14] for the expression of Ia by mononuclear phagocytes.

Analysis of positive cells

Equipment

Flow cytometer.
Fluorescence microscope.

Materials

Appropriate labelled samples as described above.

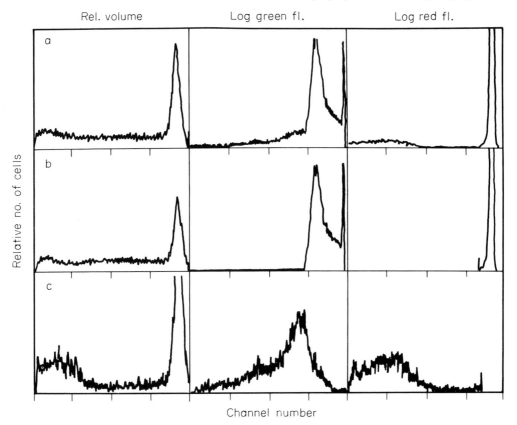

Fig. 44.5. Viability assessment using propidium iodide. Bone marrow cells from C3H murine femors were cultured for five days in growth medium. The cells were then removed using sodium pyrophosphate. The volume, autofluorescence and propidium iodide distributions, respectively, are shown for these cells in the top row. The corresponding distributions of the dead cells are shown in the next row after reprocessing the data on the PI-labelled cells. The last row shows the distribution of viable cells after reprocessing the data on the cells which had excluded the dye.

Procedure

Microscopic method

1 Prepare coverslips with vaseline around each edge. This is easily done by putting a film of vaseline on the palm of the hand and scraping the edge of the coverslip along it.
2 Place 20 μl of stained cells (to which 2 μl stock PI (1 mg/ml) has been added) on a microscope slide and cover it with the coverslip.
3 Match fluorescence excitation and emission to the fluorochrome using the appropriate filtration.
4 Determine the proportion of stained viable cells. Exclude the cells that have been stained with PI (red nuclei). (It may be necessary to alternate filters if PI and fluorochrome are widely separated.)

Use of a flow cytometer

1 A typical experiment is shown in Table 44.2. It illustrates the appropriate control and experimental samples.
2 Set the gain for the physical parameters (e.g. low-angle light scatter) to include all the cells.
3 Using the control sample for the group, set the fluorescence gain so that half of the cells appear above channel zero and the PI stained cells are off scale (last channel).
4 Collect 10 000 or more events.

    Depending on the flow cytometer configuration, it may not be possible to get half the viable cells in channel zero and the dead cells in the last channel. There are ways of doing this for four possible configurations.

Autofluorescence

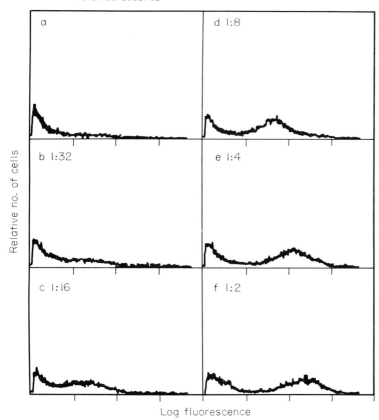

Fig. 44.6. Titration of a second reagent. Murine peritoneal cells were
incubated with a previously determined optimal concentration of the
MAb MAC-1. After washing the cells,
a constant amount (10 μl) of various
dilutions of a fluoresceinated goat
anti-rat Ig (FGAR) was added and
the samples were incubated for an
additional 15 min. After washing, the
cells were analysed. As the dilution is
decreased from (a) 1/32 to (d) 1/8, an
increasing proportion of cells are
resolved as positive. However, with
dilutions less than 1/8 there is no improvement in the proportion of cells
resolved although the mean channel
continues to shift slightly to the right.
The author selects a 1/4 dilution of
this reagent because it is the highest
dilution producing the greatest shift in
fluorescence to the right, indicating
complete saturation but not a significant excess of the second reagent.
Note that the unstained cells are
beginning to shift to the right when a
1/2 dilution of the FGAR is used
(compare fluorescence distributions in
the left quarter of e and f).

Table 44.2. Staining murine macrophages with MAbs

Sample		Myeloma protein	First reagent	Second reagent
Directly labelled MAbs				
Autofluorescence				
labelled MAbs				
	Control	None	None	None
	MAbs	Yes	Yes	None
MAbs with labelled second reagent				
Murine MAb				
	Control	Yes[3]	None	Yes[1]
	MAbs	Yes[3]	Yes	Yes
Rat MAb				
	Control	Yes	None	Yes[2]
	MAbs	Yes	Yes	Yes

[1] The author recommends using affinity purified goat anti-mouse Ig F(ab′)$_2$ labelled with
the appropriate fluorochrome.
[2] The author recommends using affinity purified goat anti-rat Ig F(ab′)$_2$ labelled with the
appropriate fluorochrome.
[3] Myeloma proteins should be of the same isotype and subclass as the MAb.

(1) Single fluorescence detector with linear amplifier

Set gain so that PI-stained cells are in the last channel but no viable cells are in the last channel. This is accomplished by increasing the gain until PI-stained cells are in the last channel but no viable cells are in the last channel even though they may be spread out in the region of display (see Fig. 44.7a). (A comparison to a control sample that has not been stained with PI may facilitate this.)

(2) Dual fluorescence detector with linear amplifier (list mode data acquisition only)

1 Using one fluorescence channel to measure the fluorescence of the fluorochrome bound to the antibody, set the gain so that one-half of the cells are above channel zero when the cells are not labelled with a MAb. Use appropriate filters.
2 Using the second fluorescence detector, set the gain so the peak of the PI-stained cells are in channel 100 (Fig. 44.7b). Use appropriate filters. (For example, if the MAb is labelled with FITC, collect PI emission > 580 nm.)
3 After analysis, reprocess the data on the viable cells which are in channels 0–10 of the PI channel.

(3) Single fluorescence detector with logarithmic amplifier

The same procedure as described in (1) above is used. The advantage of the log amp is the extended range it affords. When the log amp is used, it is nearly always possible to get half of the cells above channel zero and all dead cells in the last channel.

(4) Dual fluorescence detector with log amplifier

The same procedure as described in (2) above is used. A log amp can be used for the channel which measures PI fluorescence but it is not necessary.

Notes and recommendations

One of the most powerful methods to resolve cell populations is to combine flow cytometry with the use of specific antibodies against cell membrane determinants. This methodology allows for a finer and more objective discrimination of subpopulations than do classical histological procedures with the advantage that viable cells can be obtained using cell sorting procedures. Even though the function of the epitope labelled by the antibody may not always be known, the labelling pattern may be unique to a particular subpopulation.

Table 44.3 lists the various wavelengths for the argon and krypton lasers as well as the relative power

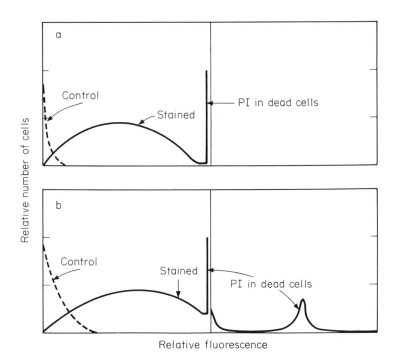

Fig. 44.7. Setting up the flow cytometer. Cells were stained with the fluoresceinated second reagent only (negative cells) or with a MAb and fluoresceinated second reagent. Propidium iodide (PI) was added 5 min prior to analysis. (a) When using a linear amplifier with a single fluorescence detector, it is possible that the range of the region of display will not be great enough to include negative cells if the positive cells are prevented from going into the last channel. (b) When using one channel to measure green fluorescence and a second channel to measure the red fluorescence from PI, it is possible to increase the range of detection by allowing positively stained cells to accumulate in the last channel. Since no FITC (green) labelled cells will appear in the red channel, the data can be reprocessed on viable cells only, thereby eliminating them from the green channel distribution.

Table 44.3. Available wavelengths and power for typical argon and krypton lasers

Wavelength (nm)	Laser power (mW)	
	5 W Argon	800 mW Krypton
Ultraviolet		
351,363	200	—
337,350,356	—	100
Violet		
406,413,415	—	100
454	120	—
457	350	—
Blue		
465	150	—
472	200	—
476	600	50
482	—	300
488	1500	—
496	600	—
Green		
501	400	—
514	2000	—
520	—	700
Yellow		
528	350	—
530	—	200
568	—	150
Red		
647	—	500
676	—	120
Infra-red		
752	—	100
793,799	—	30

for each line. It is also possible to obtain other wavelengths that might be even more useful by using dye lasers. There will undoubtedly be more use of dye lasers on flow cytometers in the future. In Table 44.4, the current popular fluorochromes are listed, with their excitation and emission maxima, the recommended laser line for excitation, and the appropriate filters to use.

Mononuclear phagocytes represent one of the most difficult cell populations on which to measure cell diversity using membrane markers and flow cytometry because of the high degree of autofluorescence, which increases even more when they are cultured. This problem is illustrated in Fig. 44.8 where the log fluorescence spectrum of normal mouse spleen lymphocytes is compared to bone marrow derived mononuclear phagocytes obtained after 6 days of culture in growth medium. The higher fluorescence of the macrophages is readily apparent. Using an antibody labelled with an average of three fluorescein molecules, it would be possible to resolve a lymphocyte subpopulation having bound only 5000 antibody molecules. In contrast, the cultured macrophages would need to have bound over 70 000 antibody molecules to be detected as positive, and for peritoneal macrophages over 50 000 antibody molecules would have to be bound (data not shown). Thus cells having epitopes for a particular antibody may not be resolved even though they have specific epitopes for that antibody. The level of sensitivity with which positive cells can be detected is much lower for macrophages than it is for lymphocytes. It is not possible, therefore, to be sure that a macrophage is negative for a particular marker when it cannot be explicitly resolved as positive.

Thus the autofluorescence of cells determines the sensitivity with which a particular epitope can be

Table 44.4. Common fluorochromes used to label monoclonal antibodies

Fluorochrome*	Wavelength (nm)				
			Laser		
	Excitation	Emission	Argon	Krypton	Filtration
Fluorescein	490	520	488	—	515–580
R-Phyco-erythrin	565	575	528	530	570–610
X-Rhodamine isothiocyanate	580	600	—	568	>610
Tetramethyl rhodamine	550	575	528	530	570–610
Sulpharhodamine 101 (Texas red)	585	605	—	568	>610

* Excitation and emission spectra of fluorochromes bound to immunoglobulins.

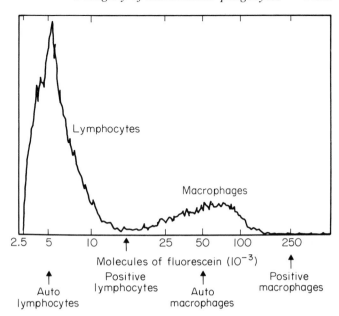

Fig. 44.8. Relative autofluorescence of lymphocytes and cultured macrophages. Spleen lymphocytes and macrophages obtained 6 days after culturing mouse bone marrow with MFG, were analysed for autofluorescence intensity at 488 nm using a flow cytometer. Cells were analysed after resuspension in phosphate-buffered saline containing 0.1% bovine serum albumin and 0.1% sodium azide. The mean autofluorescence of spleen cells and macrophages is shown. For spleen cells to be positive, they would need to have a mean fluorescence of at least 15 000 fluorescein molecules while macrophages would need to have a mean fluorescence of 200 000 molecules.

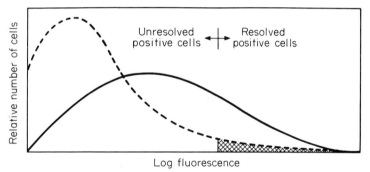

Fig. 44.9. Resolution of positive cells. One major problem illustrated in this figure is the overlap between positively stained cells and control cells. In this example, the entire population has shifted to the right after addition of the MAb but the shift is not sufficient to cause complete resolution. Most of the cells still overlap the negative control sample and cannot be resolved as explicitly positive. A lower limit is selected, above which 5% of the control cells are found (cross-hatched area) as a means of determining a region above which positive cells will most likely be resolved. This situation is often encountered when macrophages are stained with monoclonal antibodies due to the high degree of autofluorescence exhibited by them.

resolved. Using a flow cytometer, there is no spatial resolution, such as bright areas (patching) on the membrane that might be resolved microscopically, because the total fluorescence of the cell is integrated. When the number of bound molecules is less than the number required for resolution, there may only be a slight shift in the distribution to the right, and this overlaps the autofluorescence distribution. Under these conditions, it is not possible to determine whether there are a few cells that are positive or whether all the cells are faintly positive (Fig. 44.9).

This assumes that there is no binding of the second reagent other than to the epitope of interest. If the second reagent binds to the cells either by Fc or by specific binding to cytophilic antibodies on the cells as described above, the sensitivity is even further decreased.

In determining the percentage of positive cells, the appropriate control sample is used as a baseline and the channel above which 5% of the cells are found becomes the lower limit. Cells found above this lower limit are considered positive. Using the following formula, the author determines the percentage of cells that have been bound by a specific monoclonal antibody:

$$\% \text{ Positive cells} = \frac{P - fT}{T - fT} \times 100$$

where P is the number of cells in the experimental sample above the selected channel; T is the total number of cells evaluated in the experimental sample; f is the fraction of cells in the control sample which are above the selected channel; and fT represents the number of cells which appear positive in both the control and experimental sample. Since the cells cannot be evaluated, they are subtracted from both the numerator and the denominator.

Solutions

Preparation medium (α-MOPS)

10 g α-Minimum essential medium (αMEM) without sodium bicarbonate (Gibco, Cat. No. 410.2000).
4 g 2 N-Morpholinopropane sulphonic acid (MOPS) (Sigma, Cat. No. M-1254).
0.4 g NaCl.
2.7 ml 5 M-NaOH.
20 ml 100 Penicillin–streptomycin solution.
Adjust to one litre with distilled water, pH 7.2–7.4.
Filter through a 0.22 μm Micropore filter.

Preparation medium with serum (α-10 MOPS)

Add 10 ml fetal bovine serum to 90 ml αMOPS.
Filter through 0.22 μm Micropore filter.

Preparation medium with heparin

For peritoneal cells

Add 500 units heparin* per 100 ml αMOPS.

For peripheral blood

Add 2000 units of heparin* per 100 ml αMOPS.
1 ml = 1000 USP units.

Culture medium

10 g αMEM in powder form with l-glutamine *without* sodium bicarbonate and *without* nucleosides.
Add 2.2 g sodium bicarbonate.
Adjust to one litre with distilled water.
Add 100 ml fetal bovine serum to 900 ml of αMEM.
Filter through 0.22 μm Micropore filter.

Growth medium

800 ml αMEM with bicarbonate.
100 ml Fetal bovine serum.
100 ml L cell conditioned medium.
Filter through a 0.22 μm Micropore filter.

* Liquaemin sodium (Organon Inc.).

Phosphate-buffered saline (without calcium or magnesium)

4 g NaCl.
0.1 g KCl.
0.1 g KH_2PO_4.
0.575 g Na_2HPO_4.
Adjust to one litre with distilled water.

Sodium pyrophosphate

500 ml Phosphate-buffered saline without calcium and magnesium.
0.56 g $Na_4P_2O_7.10H_2O$ (Fisher Scientific Company S-390).
pH to 7.2 using 1 M-HCl.

Pronase (10 × stock solution)

2.5 g Pronase Grade B (Calbiochem #537088).
0.85 g Sodium chloride.
Dissolve in 100 ml distilled H_2O.
Aliquot and freeze. Prior to use, thaw, dilute 1/10 saline, and filter through 0.45 μm Micropore filter.

Cetrimide counting solution

90 g Hexadecyltrimethylammonium bromide (Sigma, H-5882).
25.5 g NaCl.
1.11 g EDTA (disodium salt).
Adjust to 3 litres with distilled water (35–40 °C).
Filter through 0.45 μm Micropore filter.

Thioglycollate

10.1 g Brewer's thioglycollate (DIFCO).
Add 250 ml distilled water.
Boil for 1 min to dissolve.
Autoclave to sterilize.

PBS azide BSA (PAB)

500 ml Phosphate-buffered saline with Ca^{2+} or Mg^{2+}.
2.5 g Bovine albumin Fraction V (Sigma, Cat. No. A-9647).
5.0 ml 10% Sodium azide (Sigma, Cat. No. S-2002).
Filter through 0.22 μm Micropore filter.

10% Sodium azide

10 g Sodium azide.
Add 100 ml saline (0.15 M-sodium chloride).

Ficoll

90 g Ficoll (Sigma, Cat. No. F-4375).
One litre distilled water.
Stir, heat to 40 °C.
Filter through 0.22 μm Micropore filter.

Ficoll–Hypaque solution

7 ml Ficoll solution.
2 ml Hypaque (sodium hypaque 50%, Winthrop).
1 ml sterile water.

Myeloma protein mixture

Obtain murine myeloma proteins (μ, $\gamma1$, $\gamma2a$, $\gamma3$) in lyophilized form.
Resuspend each protein in distilled H_2O to 40 mg/ml, and then mix equal amounts of each together.
Dialyse against one litre PBS containing 0.1% sodium azide.
For solutions of individual myeloma proteins, do not mix together but dilute in PAB to working solutions of either 10 or 1 mg/ml.

Buffered paraformaldehyde

Dissolve 10.7 g sodium cacodylate (Sigma C-0250) in one litre deionized water.
Adjust pH to 7.2 with 1N HCl (about 2 ml).
Dissolve 10 g paraformaldehyde in above solution (bring to boil to dissolve).
Add 7.5 g sodium chloride.
Conductivity should read between 14000 and 17000 μmho/cm.
Filter through 0.2 μm Micropore filter.

Propidium iodide solution (200 μg/ml)

10 ml Propidium iodide (Calbiochem #537059).
Dissolve in 50 ml PBS without calcium and magnesium.

Acknowledgements

This investigation was performed under the auspices of the DOE and the Los Alamos National Flow Cytometry and Sorting Research Resource and was supported by grant numbers CA27908, AI19490 and P41-RR01315-02 awarded by the National Institutes of Health, Department of Health and Human Services.

References

1 VAN FURTH R. (ed.) (1980) *Mononuclear Phagocytes, Functional Aspects.* Nijhoff (Martinus) Publishers, Boston.
2 FORSTER O. & LANDY M. (1981) *Heterogeneity of Mononuclear Phagocytes.* Academic Press, New York.
3 STANLEY E.R., GUILBERT L.J., TUSHINSKI R.J. & BARTELMEZ S.H. (1983) CSF-1-A mononuclear phagocyte lineage-specific hemopoietic growth factor. *J. cell. Biochem.* **21**, 151.
4 VAN DER ZEIJST B.A.M., STEWART C.C. & SCHLESINGER S. (1978) Proliferative capacity of mouse peritoneal macrophages *in vitro. J. exp. Med.* **147**, 1253.
5 VAN FURTH R. (1980) Origin and kinetics of mononuclear phagocytes. In *Mononuclear Phagocytes, Functional Aspects*, (ed. van Furth R.), p. 1. Nijhoff (Martinus) Publishers, Boston.
6 STEWART C.C., YEN S. & SENIOR R.M. (1981) Colony-forming ability of mononuclear phagocytes. In *Manual of Macrophage Methodology*, (eds. Herscowitz H.B., Holden H.T., Bellanti J.A. & Ghaffar A.), p. 171. Marcel Dekkar, New York.
7 STEWART C.C. & LIN H. (1978) Macrophage growth factor and its relationship to colony stimulating factor. *J. Reticuloendothel. Soc.* **23**, 269.
8 STEWART C.C. (1980) Formation of colonies by mononuclear phagocytes outside the bone marrow. In *Mononuclear Phagocytes, Functional Aspects*, (ed. van Furth R.), p. 377. Nijhoff (Martinus) Publishers, Boston.
9 STEWART C.C. (1984) Regulation of mononuclear proliferation. In *The Reticuloendothelial System: A Comprehensive Treatise*, (eds. Reichard S. & Filkins J.P.), Vol. 7A, p. 37. Plenum Press, New York.
10 WALKER E.B., WARNER N.L. & STEWART C.C. (1985) Characterization of subsets of bone marrow-derived macrophages by flow cytometry analysis. *J. Reticuloendothel. Soc.* **37**, 121.
11 STEWART C.C. (1981) Murine mononuclear phagocytes from bone marrow. In *Methods for Studying Mononuclear Phagocytes*, (eds. Adams D.O., Koren H. & Edelson P.), p. 5. Academic Press, New York.
12 VISSER J.W.M. & VAN DEN ENGH G.J. (1982) Immunofluorescence measurements by flow cytometry. In *Immunofluorescence Technology, Selected Theoretical and Clinical Aspects*, (eds. Wick G., Traill K.N. & Schauenstein K.), p. 95. Elsevier, Biomedical Press.
13 LANIER L.L. & WARNER N.L. (1981) Paraformaldehyde fixation of hemapoietic cells for quantitative flow cytometry (FACS) analysis. *J. immunol. Meth.* **47**, 25.
14 WALKER W.S., HESTER R.B. & BEELEN R.H.J. (1983) Persistent expression of Ia-antigen on a subpopulation of murine resident peritoneal macrophages. *Cell. Immunol.* **79**, 125.

Chapter 45
Macrophage cell lines

P. RALPH

Advantages of cell lines, 45.1
Derivation and availability of
   macrophage cell lines, 45.1

Method for the culture of
   macrophage cell lines, 45.3
Applications, 45.5

Advantages of cell lines

Macrophage cell lines are a resource which has been introduced into most areas of mononuclear phagocyte research. The cell lines can be easily maintained by laboratory personnel familiar with tissue culture methods. The lines differ in degree of maturity and functional properties, but almost all macrophage characteristics have been found in one or more of the lines.

Macrophage-related cell lines offer many advantages for the study of macrophage function. These advantages range from *convenience*, in obtaining large numbers of relatively homogeneous cells by growth in culture, to *purity* of the cell population, ensuring that experimental results obtained are due only to macrophages. A variety of cell lines and *variants* exist which stably differ in degree of maturation, sensitivity to inducing agents, and extent of mature macrophage characteristics. Examples of special uses of macrophage cell lines are given in Table 45.1.

Derivation and availability of macrophage cell lines

Species of macrophage-related cell lines

Most macrophage lines were derived from murine macrophage tumours. However, a number of murine lines have been obtained by spontaneous outgrowth from long-term cultures of normal macrophages (Table 45.2). One or a few lines has been described from chicken, rabbit, hamster, pig, goat, sheep, guinea-pig, dog, cat [19] and rat [161]. Immature human macrophage-related lines which were derived from leukaemia or lymphoma patients and immature murine lines are listed in Table 45.6.

Adaptation of macrophage tumours to culture

Murine tumours

The first step for adapting murine tumours to growth in culture has often been to obtain passage of the tumour as ascites cells upon intraperitoneal (i.p.) injection. This is favourable to culture growth for haemic tumour lines in general; it simplifies handling and allows facile comparison with peritoneal macrophages [20]. Ascites cells collected sterilely are washed twice with a balanced salt solution (BSS) and cultured at $1-2 \times 10^6$/ml in a rich medium (see next section). Five to ten vessels, e.g. Petri dishes, are preferable to a single large one in case some become contaminated. Large numbers of RBC in the ascites can be removed by several low-speed centrifugations that leave most of the RBC in the supernatant. Alternatively, the cells can be separated by Ficoll-Hypaque centrifugation or the cell pellet can be suspended in $1-2$ ml H_2O and then 10 ml BSS added after 30 s. This lyses the RBC, leaving the macrophage cells viable. Up to ten RBC per tumour cell can be tolerated. Usually 90% of tumour cells will die during the next few days in culture. Half the culture supernate should be replaced with fresh medium twice a week, or more often if there is extensive metabolism seen by change in the phenol red indicator to acid yellow. If considerable death occurs, cells should be harvested, centrifuged, and recultured at higher cell densities between 3 and 10×10^5/ml.

If cells appear to be dying rapidly, or if a microbial contamination occurs that cannot be eliminated with antibiotics, the cells can be transplanted back into a mouse of original strain. Priming mice with 1 ml mineral oil or pristane i.p. on, or up to one month before, the day of tumour cell inoculation appears to aid macrophage growth, as described for myeloma and Abelson lymphomas [21]. Several cycles of cell culture or *in vivo* growth may be necessary before obtaining growth *in vitro*. As lines adapt to culture, viable cells will increase in number with population doubling times of $1-7$ days. This will allow periodic splitting, making two cultures from one. Culturing on a sparse feeder layer of normal fibroblasts may be beneficial. Ascitic forms of cell lines already adapted to culture will begin rapid growth within several days of *in vitro* culture.

Table 45.1. Special uses of macrophage cell lines

Property	Examples[a]	References
Convenience	Production of IL-1	[1]
	Production of CSF	[2]
Homogeneity		
Biochemical	Corticosteroid receptors	[3]
	Insulin receptors	[4]
	Intracellular signals and gene activation	[5,6]
	Oxygen metabolite variants	[7]
Immunochemical	Hybridoma antibody to MØ subsets	[8]
Functional	Cytotoxic activity in MØ subsets	[9]
	Receptor differences in response to modulators	[10]
Exclusion of other cell types	Direct effect of agents on macrophages	[9–14]
Variant sublines	(Table 45.12)	
Cell cycle		
functions	Cessation of endocytosis at mitosis	[15]
	High latex uptake and FcR in G_2	[16]
Rapid growth	Cell type-specific growth inhibitors	[10,12,14,17]
Malignancy	Cancer type-specific chemotherapy	[18]

[a] CSF, myeloid colony-stimulating factors; MØ, macrophage; FcR, immunoglobulin Fc receptor.

Human tumours

Human lines have been derived from pleural effusion, bone marrow or blood of patients with diffuse histiocytic lymphoma, monocytic and myelomonocytic leukaemia. They were adapted to autonomous growth in culture by the use of feeder-layers of normal human glial cells [22], and growth in low oxygen (5%) and human embryo conditioned media [23].

In vitro *derivation of macrophage cell lines*

Viral transformation and cell fusion techniques

The first macrophage lines to be described were obtained by SV40 virus transformation *in vitro*. The key to this method is the use of a growth factor to induce cell division prior to viral infection [24]. Other murine lines produced by SV40 have been described [25–28], suggesting that this may be a general method. In principle, macrophage lines could be obtained from any species using similar methods and suitable transforming viruses. A number of human lines have been derived using nonlytic SV40 DNA as a transforming agent [160]. The introduction of conditions for maintaining pluripotent bone marrow stem cell replication and differentiation into myeloid and monocyte lineages [29] has led to a number of macrophage lines as spontaneous outgrowths or during RNA viral infections [30,31].

Another murine line is FC-1 developed during an experimental fusion of a myeloma with spleen cells, which has many of the properties of macrophages [27,32,33]. Hybridoma lines derived from fusing peritoneal exudate macrophages with a myeloma [162] or P388D1 with adherent spleen cells [163] present antigen and induce IL-2 production in T cells and can stimulate or inhibit mixed lymphocyte reactions.

Outgrowth of macrophage cell lines from normal cultures of mononuclear phagocytes

Long-term cultures of murine peritoneal or spleen cells have occasionally yielded permanent macrophage lines [30]. Long-term bone marrow ('Dexter') cultures from mice have also provided outgrowth of macrophage lines without introducing a transforming agent. These cultures use horse serum, or fetal bovine serum plus hydrocortisone, and continually produce myeloid progenitors and differentiated granulocytes and macrophages [29]. After some time, about 4–6 months, only macrophages remain in the cultures, apparently non-proliferating. By weekly feeding with ordinary fetal bovine serum medium, macrophage lines from several strains of mice have been obtained [8,30,31]. A method for deriving cell lines from long-term culture of blood monocytes of rabbit, hamster, pig, goat, sheep, guinea-pig, dog, and cat emphasizes daily feedings with complete removal of the spent medium which appears to contain inhibitors of proliferation [34]. Long-term culture of CSF-dependent macrophage lines from 17 mouse strains has been described [164].

The presumably general methods of SV40 transformation and long-term bone marrow culture are difficult to perfect and should be used to obtain macrophage lines only with full-time dedication, or with help of a 'next door' expert in these techniques.

Repositories of macrophage cell lines

Commonly studied murine lines, WEHI-3, J774, P388D1, RAW264, PU5-1.8, RAW309Cr, WR19M.1, immature lines M1, and human U937, are available from American Type Culture Collection (ATCC), 12301 Parklawn Avenue, Rockville, MD 20852 (telephone: 800-638-6597; 301-881-2600). Some lines are also maintained at Meloy Laboratories, 6715 Electronic Drive, Springfield, VA 22151 (telephone: 703-354-2600).

Originators of important lines are encouraged to deposit them at the ATCC, which will oversee their distribution to the scientific community but preserve the commercial interests of the originator.

Method for the culture of macrophage cell lines

Lines have been maintained in culture in a variety of ways, depending on the preference of the investigator and beliefs about how to maintain strong expression of the macrophage property being studied. The author will describe methods used in his laboratory that allow cell doubling times from 16 to 24 h (20–30 h for human U937), maximum cell numbers of $1–2 \times 10^6$/ml, and relatively constant expression of lysozyme production, Fc and C receptors, phagocytosis of latex beads and RBC, and non-specific and antibody-dependent tumour killing.

Reagents

Fetal bovine serum

Fetal bovine sera from a variety of commercial sources have been suitable, but each serum lot has to be tested for good cell growth. Sera screened for low endotoxin contamination (e.g. < 0.1 ng/ml from Sterile Systems, Logan, UT) is necessary due to the extreme sensitivity of some cell lines to growth inhibition and functional stimulation by ng/ml concentrations of lipopolysaccharide [9,10]. Screening for mycoplasma and viruses is prudent. Heat inactivation (30 min at 56 °C) is unnecessary but can be utilized to further prevent microbial contamination.

Media

Media used are MEM alpha (GIBCO, without nucleosides), RPMI 1640, or McCoy's 5A (available from several vendors, also as powdered formulations). The lines will grow in other media, such as Dulbecco's MEM with high glucose, but some lines grow faster in a richer medium.

Procedure

Mature macrophage lines, in contrast to lymphoid cell lines, will remain viable for a week or more at saturating densities ($1–2 \times 10^6$/ml). However, for most studies cultures should be kept at lower concentrations, allowing logarithmic growth, or else fed three times a week. Lines can be subcultured by diluting the cells 1:10 or 1:100 into fresh media. Population doubling times should be 16–24 h. At dilution to low cell concentrations, there may be a lag before initiation of rapid growth. The all-purpose medium is RPMI 1640, 10% fetal calf serum, with 20 mg L-glutamine per 100 ml added within 2 weeks of use. Penicillin (50 u/ml) and streptomycin (50 µg/ml) are useful in preventing microbial contaminations; 50 µg/ml Gentamicin (Schering Corp.) may be substituted as a more stable antibiotic with a broader spectrum of activity. In cases of fungal contamination, Fungizone (E. R. Squibb & Sons) at 2–5 µg/ml is suitable. Cells are grown in plastic Petri dishes in volumes of 2 ml (e.g. Falcon Plastics No. 1008), 5 ml (No. 1007), 20 ml (No. 1005), or 100 ml (No. 1013). Petri dishes must be kept in a humidified 37 °C incubator with 5–10% CO_2-air. Closed flasks with cells maintained above 5×10^5/ml will generate enough CO_2 to maintain proper pH conditions without external CO_2. If cultured in glass, or plastic tissue culture dishes (Falcon 3000 series) or flasks, cells of some lines will bind tightly to the substrate, spread out, grow slowly, and yield less than 30% of Petri dish saturation densities. This may be an advantage for certain studies on macrophage physiology [35]. Large volume spinner cultures have been used with macrophage cell lines [36].

Harvesting macrophage cell lines

With plastic Petri dishes, or flasks in most cases, the majority of cells can be harvested by vigorous pipetting. For complete single cell recovery without compromising viability or other functions, the Petri dishes or flasks are scraped with a rubber policeman. Other methods of harvesting which may be necessary in special situations include the use of 0·125% trypsin [11] or 12 mM-lignocaine [37].

Storage of macrophage cell lines in liquid nitrogen

It is necessary to maintain cell lines in liquid nitrogen (1) as a source if growing cultures are lost, (2) as a source if a line changes properties, and (3) as a convenience. Cells are frozen at about 10^7/ml growth medium containing 10% (v/v) DMSO (dimethyl sulphoxide). Slow cooling between 0 and $-60\ ^\circ$C, at a rate of about 1 °C per minute, is important to preserve viability. An inexpensive method suspends freezing vials containing cells above the liquid phase of a liquid nitrogen container (BF-5 Linde Cryogenic Freezer, Union Carbide, Inc.). After 3 h in the polystyrene plug, the vials can be placed directly in liquid nitrogen.

For recovery of cells, put a vial in water at 20–37 °C. When the contents have thawed, wipe the vial with 70% ethanol and dilute the contents at least 1:20 with growth medium. DMSO at 10% is toxic to cells at warm temperature; therefore cells should be initiated into freezing as soon as they are put into the freezing solution, and they should be diluted into growth medium as soon as they are thawed. Washing out the DMSO by centrifugation sometimes lyses the cells in their fragile condition.

Critical comments

Mycoplasma contamination

This contaminant may coexist with cell lines for years and be a scientific problem only in certain kinds of experiments. However, since this represents an unknown variable, it is important to assay cultures for mycoplasma and replace contaminated cultures with axenic ones whenever possible (see [38] for further details).

Table 45.2. Murine macrophage cell lines

Name	Strain	Aetiology[a]	Special properties[b]	References
WEHI-3	BALB/c	S	Requires own growth factor	[39]
			Monocyte-like migration	[40]
J774	BALB/c	Oil	Phosphokinase studies	[5,6]
PU5-1.8	BALB/c	S?	Strongly cytotoxic	[9]
			Tumoricidal factor (TNF)	[42]
Fc-1	BALB/c	Fusion[c]	Migration sensitive to MIF	[33]
SKW2	BALB/c	A-MuLV		[9]
RAW264	BAB/14	A-MuLV	Strongly cytotoxic	[9]
			Sensitive to ng/ml LPS	[10]
RAW309Cr	CX BALB.B	A-MuLV		[41]
ABLS23	CAL-20	A-MuLV		[9]
IC-21	C57BL/6	SV40	Unresponsive to stimulators	[11,24]
M5076	C57BL/6	S	Ovarian origin	[43]
P388D1	DBA/2	S?	Purification of calmodulin	[44]
			Many defects	Table 45.11
426C	DBA/2	OS virus[c]		[31]
SK2.2	CBA/J	S[c]		[31]
A	A/J	S[c]		[8]
NCTC1469	C3H/HeAnf	S	Liver origin	[45]
Mm1	SL	S		[46]
BJ-1	C3H/HeJ	SV40	Pulmonary origin	[25]
427E	B6D2F1	F-MuLV[c]		[29]
Several	NZBxB,NZW	SV40		[26]
28-2	ICR	SV40[c]	Reversible phagocytosis	[28]
Several	Several	c	CSF-dependent	[164]

These cell lines manifest general macrophage properties of Fc and C receptors, latex bead phagocytosis, and lysozyme production.
[a] Tumours except as noted; S = spontaneous; A-MuLV = Abelson murine leukaemia virus; SV40 virus; OS = osteosarcoma virus; F-MuLV = Friend virus.
[b] A number of lines exhibit chemotaxis [40,47], receptors for CSF-1 [48], and cytotoxic capacity (see below).
[c] Experimental cell fusion or virus transformation *in vitro* or spontaneous outgrowth in culture.

Table 45.3. Secretions of macrophage lines

Product	Cell line	References
Haemopoietic factors		
Granulocyte-macrophage CSF	Many	[10]
Separate granulocyte and macrophage CSFs	WEHI-3	[2]
Granulocyte precursor renewal	WEHI-3	[52]
Megakaryocyte CSF and potentiation factor	Several	[53]
Platelet-stimulating factor	WEHI-3	[54]
Erythroid burst-promoting factor (BPA)	WEHI-3	[55]
Erythroid-potentiating factor	U937	[56]
Mast cell CSF	WEHI-3	[57–59]
Acidic isoferritin inhibitor	Many	[60]
Pluripotent stem cell factor	WEHI-3	[59]
Eosinophil CSF	WEHI-3	[61]
Lymphocyte regulators		
IL-1[a]	U937	[62,63]
IL-1[a]	P388D1	[1,64,65]
IL-1	Several	[50]
B cell differentiation factor (IL-1?)	Several	[66]
Prostaglandin E	Several	[13]
55K suppressor factor	RAW264	[67]
Cytotoxic T cell inducer ($\neq$IL-1)	WEHI-3,J774	[68]
H_2O_2 and O_2^-	J774	[7]
	Several	[69]
Tumoricidal factors	P388D1	[70]
	RAW264	[71]
	PU5-1.8	[42]
	THP-1	[165]
Fibroblast growth factor	4 lines	[72]
	THP-1	[166]
Interferon	PU5-1.8	[73]
	J774,IC-21	[74]
	BJ-1	[25]
Arachidonic acid metabolites	3 lines	[75]
Endogenous pyrogen	Many	[76,77]
Procoagulant[b]	PU5-1.8	[78]
FcR inducer	WR19M	[79]
Fibronectin	RAW309Cr.1	[80]
Cachectin	RAW264	[164]
Complement component D	U937	[168]
Apolipoprotein E	THP-1	[169]

[a] Stimulated by human C5a, human LK, phorbol ester, etc.
[b] Stimulated by lymphokine and LPS.

Stability of cell line characteristics and cross-contamination

Cell line characteristics are generally stable over periods of a year. However, the possibility of contamination of a culture with a different cell line, or overgrowth of the parent line by variant clones, requires continual quality control and occasionally recloning to maintain or select the desired macrophage properties. It cannot be assumed that a cell line obtained from laboratory A will be identical in all properties to that described in publications from laboratory B.

Applications

Mature macrophage cell lines

Table 45.2 lists a number of well-characterized murine lines. All these lines have strong expression of surface receptors for immunoglobulin Fc and complement, produce lysozyme, and are highly active in phagocytosis of latex or zymosan beads [e.g. 12]. Most of these lines also exhibit immune or antibody-dependent phagocytosis of red blood cells [9,41,49] and varying degrees of cytolytic activity toward RBC and tumour targets induced by lymphokine, lipopolysaccharide

Table 45.4. Enzymes of macrophage lines

Enzyme	Cell line	References
Lysozyme	Many	[81]
Neutral proteases		
Plasminogen activator	J774	[74]
	P388D1	[82]
	RAW264	[83]
Elastase, collagenase	P388D1	[3]
Lysosomal enzymes	J774	[84]
	U937	[85]
	Several	[47,86]
Ecto-enzymes	J774	[87]
Lipogenic enzymes	M1	[88]
Peroxidase	M1	[89]
	Several	[86]
	U937	[22]
Adenosine deaminase	J774,P388D1	[47]
Thymidine kinase	P388D1	[90]
Transglutaminase	IC-21,J774,P388D1	[91]
Lipoprotein lipase	THP-1	[169]
Phospholipases	P388D1	[170]

(LPS), phorbol myristic acetate (PMA), antitarget antibody, lymphokine and other agents [9,31].

WEHI-3 is perhaps the most immature in this group with lysozyme, production of endogenous pyrogen, interleukin-1 (IL-1), myeloid colony-stimulating activities (CSA) and prostaglandin E (PGE), zymosan and latex bead phagocytosis but little immune phagocytosis or cytotoxicity [9,12,13,50] and very low pinocytosis [51]. Other lines have most of the functions of peritoneal macrophages.

None of the lines is as adherent as their normal counterparts, but adherence can be increased by transferring from suspension culture to glass or plastic tissue culture substrate in assays [35]. Cells also adhere more strongly when incubated without serum, with activating agents such as LPS, or with PGE or cholera toxin.

Constitutive and induced production of enzymes and secreted products

Monokines produced by cell lines include colony-stimulating and related factors for megakaryocyte, erythrocyte, mast cell or basophil, neutrophil, eosinophil, and macrophage progenitors and their precursors (Table 45.3). Factors that stimulate induction of cytotoxic T cells and immunoglobulin secretion by B lymphocytes have been described; some are probably the same as IL-1 or LAF. The cell lines require LPS, BCG, PMA, or other stimulation to produce most of these factors. The dose response for induction is closely associated with growth inhibition of the macrophage lines, suggesting induction of terminal maturation or differentiation [10].

For CSF production by PU5–1.8, induction represents a gene activation requiring new RNA and protein synthesis [14]. Under certain growth conditions, perhaps due to stimulation by fetal calf serum, PGE and CSF are secreted continuously [13]. LPS, zymosan, concanavalin A, poly I:C, PPD, and even CSF induce or enhance PGE production.

Oxygen metabolites, peroxide, and superoxide anion are secreted by some macrophage lines upon stimulation with PMA, zymosan, or antigen–antibody

Table 45.5. Properties of immature murine macrophage-lineage lines

Name	Strain	Aetiology[a]	Macrophage properties	Induced properties	References
M1	SL	S		Enzymes, PGE, CSF Fc receptors	[92]
				Mac-1 and 3 antigens	[8]
R453	C57BL/6	R-MuLV		Peroxidase, phagocytosis	[89]
RAW8	BALB/c	A-MuLV	Endogenous pyrogen	Fc receptors	[76,93]
WEHI-3D⁺	BALB/c	Oil(S?)		Morphology, lysozyme	[94]
WEHI-265	BALB/c	K-MuLV			[78,95]
WEHI-274	BALB/c				[78]

[a] S = spontaneous; R-MuLV = Rauscher murine leukaemia virus; A-MuLV = Abelson murine leukaemia virus.

Table 45.6. Human (immature) macrophage lines

Name	Aetiology[a]	Properties	Induced properties	References
U937	DHL	Lysozyme		[81]
		Peroxidase, esterase[b]		[22,85]
		Pyrogen		[77]
		PGE$_2$		[96]
		FGF[c]		[97]
		Elastase		[98]
		EZ sites[d]		[99]
			Fc and C receptors	[17,100,101]
			ADCC[e], phagocytosis	[17,100]
			Non-specific cytotoxicity	[17,102]
			Chemotactic receptor	[103]
			Surface antigens	[101,104–106]
			Resistance to parasite growth	[107]
			O$_2^-$	[108]
			NBT reduction	[109]
			C2	[110]
			IL-1	[62,63]
			T suppressor	[111]
HL-60	APML		Several[b]	[86,89]
DHL-2	DHL	Several[b]		[112]
CM-S	DBS	IL-1	Several[b]	[113]
RC-2A	AMML	Several[b]		[17,23]
THP-1	AMoL	Several[b]		[114]
			IL-1	[115]
CTV-1				[171]
P39	CMML		Transplantable ascites	[172]

[a] APML = acute promyelocytic leukaemia; DHL, diffuse histiocytic lymphoma; DBS = Diamond-Blackfan syndrome; AMML = acute myelomonocytic leukaemia; AMoL = acute monocytic leukaemia; CMML = chronic myelomonocytic leukaemia.
[b] Fc receptors, C receptors and latex bead phagocytosis weakly expressed.
[c] Fibroblast growth factor.
[d] Surface receptors for several enzymes.
[e] ADCC = antibody-dependent cellular cytotoxicity to RBC and tumour targets.

complexes [7], although this activity is difficult to maintain [69]. Spontaneous release of tumoricidal factors and poly I:C-induced interferon production have been reported as well as a number of enzymes (Table 45.4).

Immature murine and human cell lines

Some cell lines express a plurality of macrophage characteristics only after culture with inducing agents (Tables 45.5 and 45.6). These immature lines can be induced with endogenous mediators resembling CSF, with activating agents like LPS and PMA, and with unphysiological agents such as polar solvents and nucleotide analogues [8,17,92]. Even inhibitors of normal macrophage growth or function such as corticosteroids [3,116] and PGE [117,118] can induce some maturation in immature cell lines [8,92,119].

Macrophage characteristics induced in these cells include receptors for complement and Fc region of IgG immunoglobulin; production of CSF, lysozyme, and prostaglandin; mobility in agar; adherence; peroxidase and lysosomal enzymes; and non-specific phagocytosis. There appears to be a limit to the degree of maturation possible in the immature murine cell lines since induction of antibody-dependent phagocytosis and lysis of RBC and tumour targets have not been detected [9]. Human line U937 shows greater capacity for differentiation in response to lymphokine, non-lymphoid sources of CSF, and tumour promoter PMA

Table 45.8. Fc and C receptors expressed on macrophage lines

| Line | Receptors for murine proteins: | | | | | |
	IgG$_1$	IgG$_{2a}$	IgG$_{2b}$	IgG$_3$	Other	References
J774	+	+	+	+		[129]
J774.2.1	+	+	+	−		[129]
J774-ICR		+	−			[37]
FC1,P388D1	+	+	+	+		[129]
RAW264	+	+	+	+		[130,131]
IC-21		+	+			[132]
6 lines					IgE	[133]
P388D1,IC-21					C3b,C3d	[134]
P388D1					C5a	[135]
U937	Human IgG$_1$ = IgG$_3$ >					
	IgG$_4$ > IgG$_2$					[136]
U937					Human IgE	[137]

Table 45.7. Growth of microbial parasites in cell lines

Species	References
Reovirus	[120]
Flavivirus, Bunyavirus	[121]
Avian leukaemia virus	[30]
Yellow fever virus	[122]
Abelson murine leukaemia virus	[41]
Herpesvirus	[123]
Rickettsia akari	[124]
Leishmania donovani amastigotes	[125]
Leishmania donovani promastigotes	[126,127]
Leishmania tropica amastigotes	[124]
Leishmania tropica promastigotes	[127]
Candida	[69]
Toxoplasma gondii	[107]
Chlamydia psittaci	[51]
Trypanosoma cruzi	[128]

[17]. Two other lymphoid human monoblast-like lines, RC-2A and THP-1, have weak expression of macrophage characteristics.

In addition to these lines, several human myeloid leukaemia lines have surface antigens and other properties in common with macrophages, or can be induced to express these characteristics [17,86,104]. The HL-60 promyelocytic line HL-60 has been widely studied for differentiation into the macrophage pathway [e.g. 86,104]. The induction of high levels of tumor necrosis factor prodction in HL-60 has led to the cloning of this gene and its expression in bacterial and mammalian cells [173,174].

Parasite–host interactions

Macrophage cell lines support the growth of a variety of viruses, bacteria, and protozoal parasites (Table 45.7). Lymphokine and/or LPS stimulate murine macrophage cell line cytotoxicity to *Leishmania tro-*

Table 45.9. Fc-mediated effects in macrophage lines

Effect	Line	References
Phagocytosis and lysis of erythrocytes	Many	[9]
DMSO induction of EA phagocytosis	P388D1	[138]
IgG$_{2a}$ stimulates adenyl cyclase, IgG$_{2b}$ stimulates PGE	P388D1	[139]
Fc but not C receptor loss during IgG-vesicle ingestion	RAW264	[140]
αIFN stimulates G$_{2a}$- and G$_{2b}$-mediated phagocytosis	J774	[141]
Antibody stimulation of viral infectivity	P388D1	[120–122]
Antibody-dependent killing (ADCC) of tumours	Many	Table 47.11
ADCC of Coxiella virus	J774	[176]

Table 45.10. Expression of Ia and macrophage-restricted antigens on cell lines

Antigen	Line	Comment	References
Murine lines			
Mac-1	10 lines	170+95K[a], induced on M1	[8,142,143]
Mac-2	10 lines	32K[a], not induced on M1	[8]
Mac-3	10 lines	100-170K[a], induced on M1	[8]
F4/80	4 lines	160K	[144]
Pgp-1	5 lines	100K	[143]
Ia	3 lines	Induced by lymphokine[b]	[145]
Ia	WEHI-3	Induced by lymphokine	[146]
Ia	P388D1	Induced by lymphokine[b]	[147]
Ia	P388D1	Induced by γ-interferon	[148]
Ia	M1 clone		[46]
Ia	P388AD2	Presents tolerogen	[177]
Ia	Hybrids		[162,163]
Human lines			
Mac-1	U937	Induced by PMA, γ-interferon	[101]
Mac-3	U937	Induced by PMA	[101]
M206	U937	180K, constitutive	[106]
DR	U937	Induced by γ-interferon	[112,149]
DR	DHL-2		[112]
DR	U937	Induced by azacytidine	[178]

[a] Size in kilodaltons.
[b] Ia-positive cells present antigen to H-2-restricted T-cell lines.

Table 45.11. Tumour cytotoxicity

Induction	Line	References
Spontaneous	Many	[11,70[a],71[a]]
LPS, PMA, MDP	Many	[9,11,42[a],71]
	U937	[17]
Lymphokine	Many	[11,31,71,150,151,152]
Antibody (ADCC)	Many	[9]
Stimulation of ADCC by LPS, PMA, LK (lymphokine)	RAW264	[9]
Stimulation of ADCC by microtubule inhibitors	RAW264	[153]
Induction of ADCC by LK, PMA	U937	[8,100]

[a] Soluble toxic factor.

pica [127], *Toxoplasma gondii*, and *Chlamydia psittaci* [51] and human U937 line toxicity to *Toxoplasma gondii* [107].

Fc and C receptors and Fc-mediated events

Macrophage cell lines have played a key role in identification of at least three different receptors for mouse IgG isotypes: IgG$_3$, IgG$_{2b}$ or 'immune complex', and monomer IgG$_{2a}$. Cell lines selectively lacking one type of receptor have aided this research (Table 45.8). A receptor for IgM has not been identified. Most macrophage lines studied have IgE receptors, and receptors for complement components C3b, C3d, C5a have been described.

Specific classes of IgG immunoglobulins induce physiological events in the cell lines (Table 45.9), including phagocytosis and lysis of erythrocyte [130] and killing of tumour targets by monoclonal antibodies of all four murine IgG isotypes [131]. IgE

Table 45.12. Singular absence of function or defect in macrophage lines

Trait	Comment	Line	References
EA phagocytosis	Induced by cAMP, insulin	J774 variants	[33,141]
EA phagocytosis	Induced by DMSO	P388D1	[138]
EA phagocytosis		NCTC1469	[154]
E-IgG$_{2b}$ phagocytosis		P388D1	[16]
E-IgG$_{2a}$ phagocytosis		FC1 variants	[129]
C-mediated phagocytosis		J774 variants	[155]
C-mediated phagocytosis		NCTC1469	[154]
EA phagocytosis, PGE		28-12 variant	[28]
CHO (M,NAG,G) receptors		J774	[156]
Procoagulant activity	Induced by LPS or LK	P388D1, J774	[78]
Plasminogen activator		IC-21	[74]
Plasminogen activator		NCTC1469	[157]
Interferon induced by LPS		P388D1	[74]
Fibronectin		P388D1	[80]
Fc receptor for IgG$_3$		J774 variant	[129]
Fc receptor for IgG$_{2b}$		J774 variants	[37]
H$_2$O and O$_2{}^-$		J774 variants	[7]
Killing *T. cruzi*	Restored by H$_2$O$_2$ generator	J774 variant	[158]
Pinocytosis		J774 variants	[159]
Ia	Not inducible	PU5, WEHI-274	[145]

antibody also mediates phagocytosis of erythrocytes [137].

Ia and macrophage-restricted antigens on lines

Macrophage-specific antigens and other antigens found mainly on mononuclear phagocytes which are defined by monoclonal antibodies have been studied in cell lines (Table 45.10). Ia or human DR antigens are present or inducible on a few lines, and in some cases these lines can present antigen to antigen-specific T cells in an Ia-restricted manner to stimulate DNA synthesis (Table 45.10).

Cytotoxicity towards tumour targets

Spontaneous cytotoxicity; non-specific killing induced by lymphokine, LPS, tumour promoter PMA and other agents; ADCC to tumour targets mediated by macrophage cell lines; all of these have been described. In some cases a soluble toxic factor has been identified (Table 45.11).

Macrophage cell line: defects and maturation sequences studied in cell lines

Cell lines which differ in their properties are useful to simplify scientific study of the bewildering number of reactions in macrophages. A variant line selected for (the absence of) a particular trait is even more valuable

since it is likely to be similar to its parent in markers other than those selected. Variant lines or lines missing typical macrophage properties are listed in Table 45.12.

Attempts have been made to put macrophage cell lines into a single maturation sequence, based on cytotoxic capacity [9,11,49], production of neutral proteases and interferon [74,82,83], CSF and prostaglandin [10,13], phagocytosis and lysozyme production [9,12,49,81], or surface antigens [143]. However, these schemes are mutually contradictory. The diversity of macrophage lines may be due to the existence of sublineages of normal macrophages, physiological regulation of functions, laboratory differences in maintaining cell lines, and idiosyncratic effects of malignancy and long-term culture.

Acknowledgment

The author thanks Mrs Rose Vecchiolla for her patience and excellent editorial help.

References

1 FARRAR J.J., MIZEL S.B., FULLER-FARRAR J., FARRAR W.L. & HILFIKER M.L. (1980) Macrophage-independent activation of helper T cells. (I) Production of interleukin 2. *J. Immunol.* **125**, 793.
2 WILLIAMS N., EGER R.R., MOORE M.A.S. & MENDELSOHN N. (1978) Differentiation of mouse bone marrow

precursor cells into neutrophil granulocytes by an activity separation from WEHI-3 cell-conditioned medium. *Differentiation*, **11**, 59.

3 WERB Z., FOLEY R. & MUNCK A. (1978) Glucocorticoid receptors and glucocorticoid-sensitive secretion of neutral proteinases in a macrophage cell line. *J. Immunol.* **121**, 115.

4 BAR R.S., KAHN C.R. & KOREN H.S. (1977) Insulin inhibition of antibody-dependent cytotoxicity and insulin receptors in macrophages. *Nature*, **265**, 632.

5 KIKUTANI H., KISHIMOTO T., SAKAGUCHI N., NISHIZAWA Y., RALPH P. & YAMAMURA Y. (1981) Activation of cyclic AMP-dependent protein kinase activity during LPS stimulation of macrophage tumor cell line, J774.1. *Int. J. Immunopharmac.* **3**, 57.

6 ROSEN N., PISCITELLO J., SCHNECK J., MUSCHEL R., BLOOM B.R. & ROSEN O. (1979) Properties of protein kinase and adenylate cyclase-deficient variants of a macrophage-like cell line. *J. cell. Physiol.* **98**, 125.

7 DAMIANI G., KIYOTAKI C., SOELLER W., SASADA M., PEISACH J. & BLOOM B.R. (1980) Macrophage variants in oxygen metabolism. *J. exp. Med.* **152**, 808.

8 RALPH P., HO M.-K., LITCOFSKY P.B. & SPRINGER T.A. (1983) Expression and induction *in vitro* of macrophage-restricted antigens on murine cell lines. *J. Immunol.* **130**, 108.

9 RALPH P. & NAKOINZ I. (1981) Differences in antibody-dependent cellular cytotoxicity and activated killing of tumor cells by macrophage cell lines. *Cancer Res.* **41**, 3546.

10 RALPH P., BROXMEYER H., NAKOINZ I. & MOORE M.A.S. (1978). Induction of myeloid colony-stimulating activity (CSA) in murine monocyte tumor cell lines by macrophage activators and in a T cell line by Con A. *Cancer Res.* **38**, 1414.

11 TANIYAMA T. & HOLDEN H.T. (1980) Cytolytic activity against tumor cells by macrophage cell lines and augmentation by macrophage stimulants. *Int. J. Cancer*, **26**, 61.

12 RALPH P. & NAKOINZ I. (1977). Direct toxic effects of immunopotentiators on monocytic, myelomonocytic, and histiocytic tumor cells in culture. *Cancer Res.* **37**, 546.

13 KURLAND J.I., PELUS L., RALPH P., BOCKMAN R.S. & MOORE M.A.S. (1979) Synthesis of prostaglandin E by normal and neoplastic macrophages is dependent upon colony-stimulating factors (CSF). *Proc. natn. Acad. Sci. U.S.A.* **76**, 2326.

14 RALPH P., BROXMEYER H. & NAKOINZ I. (1977) Immunostimulators induce granulocyte/macrophage colony-stimulating activity and block proliferation in a monocyte tumor cell line. *J. exp. Med.* **146**, 611.

15 BERLIN R.D., OLIVER J.M. & WALTER R.J. (1978) Surface functions during mitosis: phagocytosis, pinocytosis and mobility of surface-bound Con A. *Cell*, **15**, 327.

16 GANDOUR D.M. & WALKER W.S. (1983) Macrophage cell cycling: influence on Fc receptors and antibody-dependent phagocytosis. *J. Immunol.* **130**, 1108.

17 RALPH P., WILLIAMS N., MOORE M.A.S. & LITCOFSKY P.B. (1982) Induction of antibody-dependent and nonspecific tumor killing in human monocytic leukemia cells by nonlymphocyte factors and phorbol ester. *Cell. Immunol.* **71**, 215.

18 TARNOWSKI G.S., RALPH P. & STOCK C.C. (1979) Sensitivity to chemotherapeutic and immunomodulating agents of two mouse lymphomas and of a macrophage tumor. *Cancer Res.* **39**, 3964.

19 RALPH P. (1984) Diversity and regulatory events in human and murine macrophage-related cell lines. In *Mononuclear Phagocyte Biology*, (ed. Volkman A.), p. 333. Marcel Dekker, Inc., New York.

20 RALPH P., PRICHARD J. & COHN M. (1975) Reticulum cell sarcoma: *in vitro* model for mediator of cellular immunity. *J. Immunol.* **114**, 898.

21 SKLAR M.D., SHEVACH E.M., GREEN I. & POTTER M. (1975) Transplantation and preliminary characteristics of lymphocyte surface markers of Abelson virus-induced lymphomas. *Nature*, **253**, 550.

22 SÜNDSTROM C. & NILSSON K. (1976) Establishment and characterization of a human histiocytic lymphoma cell line (U-937). *Int. J. Cancer*, **17**, 565.

23 BRADLEY T.R., PILKINGTON G., GARSON M., HODGSON G.S. & KRAFT N. (1982) Cell lines derived from a human myelomonocytic leukaemia. *Br. J. Haematol.* **51**, 595.

24 DEFENDI V. (1976) Macrophage cell lines and their uses in immunobiology. In *Immunobiology of the Macrophage*, (ed. Nelson D.S.) p. 275. Academic Press, New York.

25 CAHOON B.E. & MILLS J. (1981) Development and characterization of a continuous line of alveolar macrophages from C3H/HeJ mice. *J. Reticuloendothel. Soc.* **29**, 357.

26 LEVY J.A., BARRETT S.G., LEONG J.C. & DIRKSEN E.R. (1981) Transformation of macrophages from NZB hybrid mice by Simian Virus 40. *J. Reticuloendothel. Soc.* **29**, 35.

27 BLOOM B.R., DIAMOND B., MUSCHEL R., ROSEN N., SCHNECK J., DAMIANI G., ROSEN O. & SCHARFF M. (1978) Genetic approaches to the mechanisms of macrophage function. *Fedn Proc.* **37**, 2765.

28 TANIGAWA T., SUZUKI T., TAKAYAMA H. & TAKAGI A. (1982) Changes in prostaglandin levels in cultures of SV40-transformed macrophage cell lines in relation to their phenotypic expression. *Microbiol. Immunol.* **26**, 59.

29 TESTA N.G., DEXTER T.M., SCOTT D. & TEICH N.M. (1980) Malignant myelomonocytic, cells after *in vitro* infection of marrow cells with Friend leukaemia virus. *Br. J. Cancer*, **41**, 37.

30 RALPH P., WILLIAMS N., SHERIDAN A., NAKOINZ I., JACKSON H. & MOORE M. (1980) Effector cell functions in long-term culture of murine, prosimian and human bone marrow. In *Mononuclear Phagocytes—Functional Aspects*, (ed. van Furth R.), p. 363. Nijhoff (Martinus) Publishers B.V.

31 RALPH P., NAKOINZ I., POTTER J.E.R. & MOORE M.A.S. (1980) Activity of macrophage cell lines in tumor cytotoxicity. In *Genetic Control of Natural Resistance to Malignancy and Infection*, (eds. Skamene E., Kongshavn P.A.S. & Landy M.), p. 519. Academic Press, New York.

32 DIAMOND B., BLOOM B.R. & SCHARFF M.D. (1978) The Fc receptors of primary and cultured phagocytic cells

studied with homogeneous antibodies. *J. Immunol.* **121**, 1329.

33 NEWMAN W., DIAMOND B., FLOMENBERG P., SCHARFF M.D. & BLOOM B.R. (1979) Response of a continuous macrophage-like cell line to MIF. *J. Immunol.* **123**, 2292.

34 WARDLEY R.C., LAWMAN M.J. & HAMILTON F. (1980) The establishment of continuous macrophage cell lines from peripheral blood monocytes. *Immunology*, **39**, 67.

35 MUSCHEL R.J., ROSEN N., ROSEN O.M. & BLOOM B.R. (1977) Modulation of Fc-mediated phagocytosis by cyclic AMP and insulin in a macrophage-like cell line. *J. Immunol.* **119**, 1813.

36 KAPLAN A.M., BEAR H.D., KIRK L., CUMMINS C. & MOHANAKUMAR T. (1978) Relationship of expression of a cell-surface antigen on activated murine macrophages to tumor cell cytotoxicity. *J. Immunol.* **120**, 2080.

37 UNKELESS J.C. (1979) Characterization of a monoclonal antibody directed against mouse macrophage and lymphocyte Fc receptors. *J. exp. Med.* **150**, 580.

38 McGARRITY G.J. & NICHOLS W.W. (eds.) (1978) *Mycoplasma Infection of Cell Cultures.* Plenum Press, New York.

39 BROXMEYER H.E. & RALPH P. (1977) *In vitro* regulation of a mouse myelomonocytic leukemia line in culture. *Cancer Res.* **37**, 3578.

40 AKSAMIT R.R., FALK W. & LEONARD E.J. (1981) Chemotaxis by mouse macrophage cell lines. *J. Immunol.* **126**, 2194.

41 RASCHKE W.C., BAIRD S., NAKOINZ I. & RALPH P. (1978) Functional macrophage cell lines transformed by Abelson leukemia virus. *Cell*, **15**, 261.

42 MÄNNEL D.N., MOORE R.N. & MERGENHAGEN S.E. (1980) Macrophages as a source of tumoricidal activity (TNF). *Infect. Immun.* **30**, 523.

43 TALMADGE J.E., KEY M.E. & HART I.R. (1981) Characterization of a murine ovarian reticulum cell sarcoma of histiocytic origin. *Cancer Res.* **41**, 1271.

44 JAMIESON G.A. & VANAMAN T.C. (1980) Isolation and characterization of calmodulin from a murine macrophage-like cell line. *J. Immunol.* **125**, 1171.

45 VAN LOVEREN H., VAN DER ZEIJST B.A.M., DEWEGER R.A., VAN BASTEN C., PIJPERS H. & DEN OTTER W. (1981) Identification of the neonatal liver cell line NCTC 1469 as a macrophage-like cell line. *J. Reticuloendothel. Soc.* **29**, 433.

46 KYOIZUMI S., NORO N., TESHIGAWARA K., SAKAGUCHI S. & MASUDA T. (1981) A cloned cell line, Mk1, possessing Ia antigens and accessory cell activity. *J. Immunol.* **128**, 2586.

47 SNYDERMAN R.M., PIKE M.C., FISCHER D.G. & KOREN H.S. (1977) Biologic and biochemical activities of continuous macrophage cell lines P388D1 and J774.1. *J. Immunol.* **119**, 2060.

48 GUILBERT J.L. & STANLEY E.R. (1980) Specific interaction of murine colony-stimulating factor with mononuclear phagocytic cells. *J. Cell Biol.* **85**, 153.

49 RALPH P. & NAKOINZ I. (1980) Environmental and chemical dissociation of antibody-dependent phagocytosis from lysis mediated by macrophages: stimulation of lysis by sulfhydryl-blocking and esterase-inhibiting

agents and depression by trypan blue and trypsin. *Cell. Immunol.* **50**, 94.

50 LACHMAN L.B. & METZGAR R.S. (1980) Characterization of high and low ML lymphocyte-activating factor (interleukin I) from P388D1 and J774.1 mouse macrophage cell lines. *J. Reticuloendothel. Soc.* **27**, 621.

51 JONES T.C. & BYRNE G.I. (1980) Interactions of macrophages with intravacuolar bacteria and protozoa. In *Mononuclear Phagocytes Functional Aspects*, (ed. van Furth R.), p. 1611. Nijhoff (Martinus) Publishers B.V.

52 DEXTER T.M., GARLAND J., SCOTT D., SCOLNICK E. & METCALF D. (1980) Growth of factor-dependent hemopoietic precursor cell lines. *J. exp. Med.* **152**, 1036.

53 WILLIAMS N., JACKSON H., RALPH P. & NAKOINZ I. (1981) Cell interactions influencing murine marrow megakaryocytes: nature of the potentiator cell in bone marrow. *Blood*, **57**, 157.

54 KRIZSA K. & DEXTER T.M. (1978) Cell interactions in long term murine bone marrow culture. *Biomedicine Express*, **29**, 162.

55 ISCOVE N., unpublished observations.

56 ASCENSAO J.L., KAY N.E., EARENFIGHT-ENGLER T., KOREN H.S. & ZANJANI E.D. (1981) Production of erythroid potentiating factor(s) by a human monocytic cell line. *Blood*, **57**, 170.

57 NAGAO K., YOKORO K. & AARONSON S.A. (1981) Continuous lines of basophil-mast cells derived from normal mouse bone marrow. *Science*, **212**, 333.

58 YUNG Y.-P., EGER R., TERTIAN G. & MOORE M.A.S. (1981) Purification of a mast cell growth factor and its dissociation from TCGF. *J. Immunol.* **127**, 794.

59 GREENBERGER J.S., SAKAKEENY M.A., HUMPHRIES R.K., EAVES C.J. & ECKNER R.J. (1983) Demonstration of permanent factor-dependent multipotential (erythroid/ neutrophil/basophil) hematopoetic progenitor cell lines. *Proc. natn. Acad. Sci. U.S.A.* **80**, 2931.

60 BROXMEYER H.E., BOGNACKI J., RALPH P., DORNER M.H., LI L. & CASTRO-MALASPINA H. (1982) Monocyte-macrophage derived acidic isoferritins: normal feedback regulators of granulocyte-macrophage progenitor cells. *Blood*, **60**, 595.

61 METCALF D., PARKER J., CHESTER H.M. & KINCADE P.W. (1974) Growth of eosinophil-like granulocytic colonies by mouse bone marrow cells *in vitro*. *J. cell. Physiol.* **84**, 275.

62 PALACIOS R., IVHED I., SIDERAS P., NILSSON K., SUGAWARA I. & FERNANDEZ C. (1982) Accessory function of human tumor cell lines: production of interleukin 1 by the human histiocytic lymphoma cell line U-937. *Eur. J. Immunol.* **12**, 895.

63 AMENTO E.P., KURNICK J.T., EPSTEIN A. & KRANE S.M. (1982) Modulation of synovial cell products by a factor from a human cell line: T lymphocyte induction of a mononuclear cell factor. *Proc. natn. Acad. Sci. U.S.A.* **79**, 5307.

64 GOODMAN M.G., CHENOWETH D.E. & WEIGLE W.O. (1982) Induction of Interleukin 1 secretion and enhancement of humoral immunity by binding of human C5A to macrophage surface C5A receptors. *J. exp. Med.* **156**, 912.

65 PALACIOS R. (1982) Cloned lines of Interleukin 2 producer human T lymphocytes. *J. Immunol.* **129**, 2586.

66 HOFFMANN M.K., KOENIG S., MITTLER R.S., OETTGEN H.F., RALPH P., GALANOS C. & HÄMMERLING U. (1979) Macrophage factor controlling differentiation of B cells. *J. Immunol.* **122**, 497.

67 ARENE T. & PIERCE C. (1980) Properties of a nonspecific suppressor factor produced by SIRS-treated macrophages. *Fedn Proc.* **39**, 1156.

68 IGARASHI T., IKEDA Y., SAITO H., TAKANO S., KISHIMOTO Y. & SHIDA L. (1982) Induction of the differentiation of memory T killer cells with factors released from macrophage-like cell lines. *Cell. Immunol.* **70**, 11.

69 SASADA M. & JOHNSTON R.B. (1980) Macrophage microbicidal activity. Correlation between phagocytosis-associated oxidative metabolism and the killing of *Candida* by macrophages. *J. exp. Med.* **152**, 85.

70 AKSAMIT R.R. & KIM K.J. (1979) Macrophage cell lines produce a cytotoxin. *J. Immunol.* **122**, 1785.

71 RUSSELL S.W., GILLESPIE G.Y. & PACE J.L. (1980) Comparison of responses made to activating agents by mouse peritoneal macrophages and cells of the macrophage line RAW264. *J. Reticuloendothel. Soc.* **27**, 607.

72 WHARTON W., GILLESPIE G.Y., RUSSELL S.W. & PLEDGER W.J. (1982) Mitogenic activity elaborated by macrophage-like cell lines acts as competence factor(s) for BALB/c 3T3 cells. *J. cell. Physiol.* **110**, 93.

73 DJEU J.Y., HEINBAUGH J.A., HOLDEN H.T. & HERBERMAN R.B. (1979) Role of macrophages in the augmentation of mouse natural killer cell activity by poly I:C and interferon. *J. Immunol.* **122**, 182.

74 NEUMANN C. & SORG C. (1981) Independent induction of plasminogen activator and interferon in murine macrophages. *J. Reticuloendothel. Soc.* **30**, 79.

75 STENSON W.F., NICKELLS M.W. & ATKINSON J.P. (1981) Metabolism of exogenous arachidonic acid by murine macrophage-like tumor cell lines. *Prostaglandin*, **21**, 675.

76 BODEL P. (1978) Spontaneous pyrogen production by mouse histiocytic and myelomonocytic tumor cell lines *in vitro. J. exp. Med.* **147**, 1503.

77 BODEL P., RALPH P., WENC K. & LONG J.C. (1980) Endogenous purogen production by Hodgkin's disease and human histiocytic lymphoma cell lines *in vitro. J. clin. Invest.* **65**, 514.

78 FARRAM E., GECZY C.L., MOON D.K. & HOPPER K. (1983) The ability of lymphokine and lipopolysaccharide to induce procoagulant activity in mouse macrophage cell lines. *J. Immunol.* **130**, 2750.

79 CALCAGNO M., PEREZ J.R., WALDO M.G., CABRERA G. & WEISS-STEIDER B. (1982) Evidence of the existence of a factor that induces Fc receptors on bone marrow cells. *Blood*, **59**, 756.

80 VAN DE WATER L., DESTREE A.T. & HYNES R.O. (1983) Fibronectin binds to some bacteria but does not promote their uptake by phagocytic cells. *Science*, **220**, 201.

81 RALPH P., MOORE M.A.S. & NILSSON K. (1976) Lysozyme synthesis by established human and murine histiocytic lymphoma cell lines. *J. exp. Med.* **143**, 1528.

82 WERB Z., BANDA M.J. & JONES P.A. (1980) Degradation of connective tissue matrices by macrophages. *J. exp. Med.* **152**, 1340.

83 HAMILTON J.A. & MOORE M.A.S. (1980) Regulation of the plasminogen activator activity of macrophage tumor cell lines. *Int. J. Immunopharmac.* **2**, 353.

84 KAPLAN G. & MØRLAND B. (1978) Properties of a murine monocytic tumor cell line J-774 *in vitro.* (I) Morphology and endocytosis. *Expl Cell Res.* **115**, 53.

85 SÜNDSTROM C. & NILSSON K. (1977) Cytochemical profile of human hematopoietic biopsy cells and derived cell lines. *Br. J. Haematol.* **25**, 601.

86 GREENBERGER J.S., NEWBERGER P.C., KARPAS A. & MOLONEY W.C. (1978) Constitutive and inducible granulocyte-macrophage functions in mouse, rat and human myeloid leukemia-derived culture lines. *Cancer Res.* **38**, 3340.

87 EDELSON P.J. (1981) Plasma membrane ectoenzymes: macrophage differentiation antigens. In *Heterogeneity of Mononuclear Phagocytes*, (eds. Forster O. & Landy M.), p. 143. Academic Press, New York.

88 OKUMA M., ICHIKAWA Y., YAMASHITO S., KITAJIMA K. & NUMA S. (1976) Studies on some lipogenic enzymes of cultured myeloid leukemic cells. *Blood*, **47**, 439.

89 ICHIKAWA Y., MAEDA M. & HORIUCHI M. (1976) *In vitro* differentiation of Rauscher virus-induced myeloid leukemia cells. *Int. J. Cancer*, **17**, 789.

90 STADECKER M.J. (1981) Comparison of pyrimidine and purine nucleoside secretion and nucleoside kinase expression in resident and elicited peritoneal macrophages. *J. Immunol.* **126**, 1724.

91 SCHROFF G., NEUMANN C. & SORG C. (1981) Transglutaminase as a marker for subsets of murine macrophages. *Eur. J. Immunol.* **11**, 637.

92 SACHS L. (1978) Control of normal cell differentiation and the phenotypic reversion of malignancy in the myeloid leukemia. *Nature*, **274**, 535.

93 RALPH P., NAKOINZ I. & RASCHKE W.C. (1982) Induction of differentiated functions coupled with growth inhibition in lymphocyte and macrophage tumor cell lines. In *Maturation Factors in Cancer*, (ed. Moore M.A.S.), p. 245. Raven Press, New York.

94 COOPER P.C., METCALF D. & BURGESS A.W. (1982) Biochemical and functional characterization of mature progeny purified from a myelomonocytic leukemia cell line. *Leuk. Res.* **6**, 313.

95 WALKER E.B., LANIER L.L. & WALKER N.L. (1982) Characterization and functional properties of tumor cell lines in accessory cell replacement assays. *J. Immunol.* **128**, 852.

96 COBB M.A., HSUEH W., PACHMAN L.M. & BARNES W.T. (1983) Prostaglandin biosynthesis by a human macrophage-like cell line, U937. *J. Reticuloendothel. Soc.* **33**, 197.

97 WHARTON W. (1983) Human macrophage-like cell line U937-1 elaborates mitogenic activity for fibroblasts. *J. Reticuloendothel. Soc.* **33**, 151.

98 SENIOR R.M., CAMPBELL E.J., LANDIS J., COX F.R., KUHN C. & KOREN H.S. (1982) Elastase of U937 monocyte-like cells: comparisons with elastases derived from human monocytes and neutrophils and murine macrophage-like cells. *J. clin. Invest.* **69**, 384.

99 CAMPBELL E.J. (1982) Human leukocyte elastase, cathepsin G, and lactoferrin: family of neutrophil granule

glycoproteins that bind to an alveolar macrophage receptor. *Proc. Natn. Acad. Sci. U.S.A.* **79**, 6941.

100 LARRICK J.W., FISCHER D.G., ANDERSON S.J. & KOREN H. (1980) Characterization of a human macrophage-like cell line stimulated *in vitro*: a model of macrophage functions. *J. Immunol.* **125**, 6.

101 RALPH P., HARRIS P.E., PUNJABI C.J., WELTE K., LITCOFSKY P.B., RUBIN B.Y., MOORE M.A.S., HO M.-K. & SPRINGER T.A. (1983) Lymphokine inducing 'terminal differentiation' of the human monoblast leukemia line U937: a role for γ interferon. *Blood*, **62**, 1169.

102 GIDLUNG M., ORN A., PATTENGALE P.K., JANNSON M., WIGZELL H. & NILSSON K. (1981) Natural killer cells kill tumor cells at a given stage of differentiation. *Nature*, **292**, 848.

103 PIKE M.C., FISHER D.G., KOREN H.S. & SYNDERMAN R. (1980) Development of specific receptors for *N*-formylated chemotactic peptides in a human monocyte cell line stimulated with lymphokines. *J. exp. Med.* **152**, 31.

104 GRIFFIN J.D., RITZ J., NADLER L.M. & SCHLOSSMAN S.F. (1981) Expression of myeloid differentiation antigens on normal and malignant myeloid cells. *J. clin. Invest.* **68**, 912.

105 WALDREP J.C., MOHANAKUMAR T. & KAPLAN A.M. (1981) Human mononuclear phagocyte-associated antigens. (II) Lymphokine-inducible antigens on the macrophage cell line U937. *Cell. Immunol.* **62**, 140.

106 MARUYAMA S., NAITO T., KAKITA H., KISHIMOTO S., YAMAMURA Y. & KISHIMOTO T. (1983) Preparation of a monoclonal antibody against human monocyte lineage. *J. clin. Immunol.* **3**, 57.

107 WING E.J., KOREN H.S., FISCHER D.G. & KELLEY V. (1981) Stimulation of a human macrophage-like cell line (U937) to inhibit multiplication of an intracellular pathogen. *J. Reticuloendothel. Soc.* **29**, 321.

108 CLEMENT L.T. & LEHMEYER J.E. (1983) Regulation of the growth and differentiation of a human monocytic cell line by lymphokines; induction of superoxide anion production and chemiluminescence. *J. Immunol.* **130**, 2763.

109 OLSSON I. & BREITMAN T.R. (1982) Induction of differentiation of the human histiocytic lymphoma cell line U-937 by retinoic acid and cyclic adenosine 3′:5′-monophosphate-inducing agents. *Cancer Res.* **42**, 3924.

110 LITTMAN B.H., HALL R.E. & MUCHMORE A.V. (1983) Lymphokine and phorbol (PMA) regulation of complement (C2) synthesis using U937. *Cell. Immunol.* **76**, 189.

111 WILKINS J.A., SIGURDSON L., JORDON Y., RUTHERFORD W.J. & WARRINGTON R.J. (1983) Immunoregulatory factors from a human macrophage-like cell line: a human T-cell lymphokine-induced suppressor factor for lymphocyte proliferation. *Cell. Immunol.* **77**, 329.

112 NILSSON K., KIMURA A., KLARESKOG L., ANDERSON L.C., GAHMBERG C.G. & WIGZELL H. (1981) Cell surface characteristics of human histiocytic lymphoma cell lines: expression of *Helix pomatia* A hemagglutinin binding surface glycoproteins, HLA-DR and common acute lymphocytic leukemia (cALL) antigen. *Leuk. Res.* **5**, 185.

113 BUTLER R.H., REVOLTELLA R.P., MUSIANI P. & PIANTELLI M. (1983) Constitutive production of interleukin-1

by the human continuous cell line, CM-S. *Cell. Immunol.* **78**, 368.

114 TSUCHIYA S., YAMABE M., YAMAGUCHI Y., KOBAYASHI Y. & KONNO T. (1980) Establishment and characterization of a human acute monocytic leukemia cell line (THP-1). *Int. J. Cancer*, **26**, 171.

115 MAIZEL S.B. & ANDERSON B.J. (1982) Interleukin 1 production by a human monocytic leukemia cell line (THP-1). *Cell. Immunol.* **70**, 396.

116 RALPH P., ITO M., BROXMEYER H.E. & NAKOINZ I. (1978) Corticosteroids block newly induced but not constitutive functions of macrophage cell lines: CSA production, latex phagocytosis, antibody-dependent lysis of RBC and tumor targets. *J. Immunol.* **121**, 300.

117 WILLIAMS N. (1979) Preferential inhibition of murine macrophage colony formation by prostaglandin E. *Blood*, **53**, 1089.

118 PELLUS L.M., BROXMEYER H.E., KURLAND J.I. & MOORE M.A.S. (1979) Regulation of macrophage and granulocyte proliferation. Specificities of prostaglandin E and lactoferrin. *J. exp. Med.* **150**, 277.

119 HONMA Y., KASUKABE T. & HOZUMI M. (1978) Production of differentiation-stimulating factor in cultured mouse myeloid leukemia cells treated with glucocorticoids. *Expl Cell Res.* **111**, 261.

120 BURSTIN S.J., BRANDRISS M.W. & SCHLESINGER J.J. (1983) Infection of a macrophage-like cell line, P388D1, with reovirus. *J. Immunol.* **130**, 2915.

121 PEIRIS J.S.M., GORDON S., UNKELESS J.C. & PORTERFIELD J.S. (1981) Monoclonal anti-Fc receptor IgG blocks antibody enhancement of viral replication in macrophages. *Nature*, **289**, 189.

122 SCHLESINGER J.J. & BRANDRISS M.W. (1981) Growth of 17D yellow fever virus in a macrophage-like cell line, U937: role of Fc and viral receptors in antibody-mediated infection. *J. Immunol.* **127**, 659.

123 LOPEZ C., unpublished observations.

124 NACY C. & RALPH P., unpublished observations.

125 BERENS R.L. & MARR J.J. (1979) Growth of *Leishmania donovani* amastigotes in a continuous macrophage-like cell culture. *J. Protozool.* **26**, 453.

126 CHANG K.-P. (1980) Human cutaneous *Leishmania* in a mouse macrophage line: propagation and isolation of intracellular parasites. *Science*, **209**, 1240.

127 MURRAY H.W. (1981) Interaction of *Leishmania* with a macrophage cell line. Correlation between intracellular killing and the generation of oxygen intermediates. *J. exp. Med.* **153**, 1690.

128 TANAKA Y., KIYOTAKI C., TANOWITZ H. & BLOOM B.R. (1982) Reconstitution of a variant macrophage cell line defective in oxygen metabolism with an H_2O_2 generating system. *Proc. natn. Acad. Sci. U.S.A.* **79**, 2584.

129 DIAMOND B. & YELTON D.E. (1981) A new Fc receptor on mouse macrophages binding IgG_3. *J. exp. Med.* **153**, 514.

130 RALPH P., NAKOINZ I., DIAMOND B. & YELTON D. (1980) All classes of murine IgG antibody mediate macrophage phagocytosis and lysis of erythrocytes. *J. Immunol.* **125**, 1885.

131 RALPH P. & NAKOINZ I. (1983) Monoclonal antibodies of all murine IgG classes, but not IgM, mediate

macrophage ADCC to tumor targets. *J. Immunol.* **131**, 1028.

132 WALKER W.S. (1976) Separate Fc-receptors for immunoglobulins IgG$_{2a}$ and IgG$_{2b}$ on an established cell line of mouse macrophages. *J. Immunol.* **116**, 911.

133 BOLTZ-NITULESCU G., PLUMMER J.M. & SPIEGELBERG H.L. (1982) Fc receptors for IgE on mouse macrophages and macrophage-like cell lines. *J. Immunol.* **128**, 2265.

134 WALKER W.S. & GANDOUR D.M. (1980) Detection and functional assessment of complement receptors on two macrophage-like cell lines. *Exptl Cell Res.* **129**, 15.

135 CHENOWITH D.E., GOODMAN M.G. & WEIGLE W.O. (1982) Demonstration of a specific receptor for human C5A anaphylatoxin on murine macrophages. *J. exp. Med.* **156**, 68.

136 ANDERSON C.L. (1982) Isolation of the receptor for IgG from a human monocyte cell line (U937) and from human peripheral blood monocytes. *J. exp. Med.* **156**, 1794.

137 MELEWICZ F.M., PLUMMER J.M. & SPIEGELBERG H.L. (1982) Comparison of the Fc receptors for IgE on human lymphocytes and monocytes. *J. Immunol.* **129**, 563.

138 TAKASAKI S. & LEWE L. (1982) Induction by dimethylsulfoxide of Fc fragment-mediated phagocytosis in the mouse macrophage-like cell line P388D1. *Proc. natn. Acad. Sci. U.S.A.* **79**, 4980.

139 NITIA T. & SUZUKI T. (1982) Biochemical signals transmitted by Fcγ receptors triggering mechanisms of the increased synthesis of adenosine-3-5-cyclic monophosphate mediated by Fcγ2b receptors of a murine macrophage-like cell line (P388D). *J. Immunol.* **129**, 2708.

140 PETTY H.R., HAFEMAN D.G. & McCONNELL H.M. (1980) Specific antibody-dependent phagocytosis of lipid vesicles by RAW264 macrophages results in the loss of cell surface Fc but not C3b receptor activity. *J. Immunol.* **125**, 2391.

141 SCHNECK J., RAGER-ZISMAN B., ROSEN O.M. & BLOOM B.R. (1982) Genetic analysis of the role of cAMP in mediating effects of interferon. *Proc. natn. Acad. Sci. U.S.A.* **79**, 1879.

142 TROWBRIDGE I.S. & OMARY M.B. (1981) Molecular complexity of leukocyte surface glycoproteins related to the macrophage differentiation antigen Mac-1. *J. exp. Med.* **154**, 1517.

143 VAN LOVEREN H., HILGERS J., DEBAKKER J.M., DE-WEGER P.A., BREDEROO P. & DEN OTTER W. (1983) Macrophage-like cell lines: endogenous peroxidatic activity, cell surface antigens, and colony-stimulating factor production. *J. Reticuloendothel. Soc.* **33**, 221.

144 AUSTYN J.M. & GORDON S. (1981) F4/80, a monoclonal antibody directed specifically against the mouse macrophage. *Eur. J. Immunol.* **11**, 805.

145 WALKER E.B., LANIER L.L. & WARNER N.L. (1982) Concomitant induction of the cell surface expression of Ia determinants and accessory cell function by a murine macrophage tumor cell line. *J. exp. Med.* **155**, 629.

146 McNICHOLAS J.M., KING D.P. & JONES, P.P. (1983) Biosynthesis and expression of Ia and H-2 antigens on a macrophage cell line are stimulated by products of activated spleen cells. *J. Immunol.* **130**, 449.

147 BIRMINGHAM J.R., CHESNUT R.W., KAPPLER J.W., MARRACK P., KUBO R. & GREY H.M. (1982) Antigen presentation to T cell hybridomas by a macrophage cell line: an inducible function. *J. Immunol.* **128**, 1491.

148 STEEG P.S., JOHNSON H.M. & OPPENHEIM J.J. (1982) Regulation of murine macrophage Ia antigen expression by an immune interferon-like lymphokine: inhibitory effect of endotoxin. *J. Immunol.* **129**, 2402.

149 BROXMEYER H.E., unpublished observations.

150 VAN LOVEREN H., SNOEK M. & DEN OTTER W. (1977) Effects of silica on macrophages and lymphocytes. *J. Reticuloendothel. Soc.* **22**, 523.

151 KELSO A., GLASEBROOK A.L., KANAGAWA O. & BRUNNER K.T. (1982) Production of macrophage-activating factor by T lymphocyte clones and correlation with other lymphokine activities. *J. Immunol.* **129**, 550.

152 RALPH P., WILLIAMS N., NAKOINZ I., JACKSON H. & WATSON J.D. (1982) Distinct signals for antibody-dependent and nonspecific killing of tumor targets mediated by macrophages. *J. Immunol.* **129**, 427.

153 RALPH P. & NAKOINZ I. (1982) Augmentation of macrophage antibody-dependent killing of tumor targets by microtubule inhibitors. *Cell. Immunol.* **70**, 321.

154 VAN BASTEN C.D.H., DEWEGER R.A. & VAN LOVEREN H. (1983) NCTC 1469 CB, a subline of the macrophage-like cell line NCTC 1469 with reduced phagocytic activity. *J. Reticuloendothel. Soc.* **33**, 47.

155 LIANG-TAKASAKI C.-J., MÄKELÄ P.H. & LIEVE L. (1982) Phagocytosis of bacteria by macrophages: changing the carbohydrate of lipopolysaccharide alters interaction with complement and macrophages. *J. Immunol.* **128**, 1229.

156 STAHL P.D. & GORDON S. (1981) Expression of the mannose/fucose pinocytosis receptor by primary macrophages and macrophage hybrids. *J. supramol. Struct. cell. Biochem.* **5**, 870.

157 DEWEGER R.A., VAN LOVEREN H., VAN BASTEN C.D.H., OSKAM R., VAN DER ZEIJST, B.A.M. & DEN OTTER W. (1983) Functional activities of the NCTC 1469 macrophage-like cell line: comparison of the NCTC 1469 cell line with various other macrophage-like cell lines. *J. Reticuloendothel. Soc.* **33**, 55.

158 TANAKA Y., KIYOTAKI C., TANOWITZ H. & BLOOM B.R. (1982) Reconstitution of a variant macrophage cell line defective in oxidative metabolism with a H$_2$O$_2$-generating system. *Proc. natn. Acad. Sci. U.S.A.* **79**, 2584.

159 NORIN A.J. (1980) Macrophage cell line mutants deficient in phagocytosis have reduced pinocytic activity. In *Genetic Control of Natural Resistance to Infection and Malignancy*, (eds. Skamene E., Kungshavn P.A.L. & Landy M.), p. 531. Academic Press, New York.

160 NAGATA Y., DIAMOND B. & BLOOM B.R. (1983) The generation of human monocyte/macrophage cell lines. *Nature*, **306**, 597.

161 FUJII T., TAKEICHI N., KASAI M., MORIUCHI T. & KOBAYASHI H. (1983) Establishment and characterization of a differentiating myeloid cell line obtained from a rat myelomonocytic leukemia. *Cancer Res.* **43**, 1875.

162 TAKEDA Y., WOO H.J. & OSAWA T. (1985) Mouse

macrophage hybridomas secreting a cytotoxic factor and interleukin 1. *Cell. Immunol.* **90**, 493.

163 JU S. & DORF M.E. (1985) Functional analysis of cloned macrophage hybridomas. IV. Induction and inhibition of mixed lymphocyte responses. *J. Immunol.* **134**, 3722.

164 JOHNSON C.R., KITZ, D. & LITTLE J.R. (1983) A method for the derivation and continuous propagation of cloned murine bone marrow macrophages. *J. Immunol. Meth.* **65**, 319.

165 ARMSTRONG C.A., KLOSTERGAARD J. & GRANGER G.A. (1985) Isolation and initial characterization of tumoricidal monokine(s) from the human monocytic leukemia cell line THP-1. *J. Nat. Cancer Inst.* **74**, 1.

166 GAFFNEY E.V., TSAI S., LINGENFELTER S.E., DELL' AQUILA M.L. & GONDA J.E. (1984) Stimulation of diploid fibroblast growth with serum-free medium conditioned by mezerein-treated monocytic leukemia cells. *J. Leukocyte Biol.* **35**, 489.

167 MAHONEY J.R. JUN., BEUTLER B.A., TRANG N.L. VINE W., IKEDA Y., KAWAKAMI M. & CERAMI A. (1985) Lipopolysaccharide-treated RAW 264.7 cells produce a mediator that inhibits lipoprotein lipase in 3T3-L1 cells. *J. Immunol.* **134**, 1673.

168 BARNUM S.R. & VOLANAKIS J.E. (1985) *In vitro* biosynthesis of complement protein D by U937 cells. *J. Immunol.* **134**, 1799.

169 TAJIMA S., HAYASHI R., TSUCHIYA S., MIYAKE Y. & YAMAMOTO A. (1985) Cells of a human monocytic leukemia cell line (THP-1) synthesize and secrete apolipoprotein E and lipoprotein lipase. *Biochem. biophys. Res. Commun.* **126**, 526.

170 ROSS M.I., DEEMS R.A., JESIATIS A.J., DENNIS E.A. & ULEVITCH R.J. (1985) Phospholipase activities of the P388D1 macrophage-like cell line. *Archs Biochem. Biophys.* **238**, 247.

171 CHEN P., CHIU C., CHIOU T., MAEDA S., CHIANG H., TZENG C., SUGIYAMA T. & CHIANG B.N. (1984) Establishment and characterization of a human monocytoid leukemia cell line, CTV-1. *Gann,* **75**, 660.

172 NAGAI M., SEKI S., KITAHARA T., ABE T., MINATO K., WATANABE S. & SHIMOYAMA M. (1984) A novel human myelomonocytoid cell line, P39/Tsugane, derived from overt leukemia following myelodysplastic syndrome. *Gann,* **75**, 1100.

173 PENNICA D., NEDWIN G.E., HAYFLICK J.S., SEEBURG P.H., DERYNCK R., PALLADINO M.A., KOHR W.J., AGGARWAL B.B. & GOEDDEL D.V. (1984) Human tumour necrosis factor: precursor structure, expression and homology to lymphotoxin. *Nature,* **312**, 724.

174 WANG A.M., CREASEY A.A., LADNER M.B., LIN L.S., STRICKLER J., VAN ARSDELL J.N., YAMAMOTO R. & MARK D.F. (1985) Molecular cloning of the complementary DNA for human tumor necrosis factor. *Science,* **228**, 149.

175 KING A.A., SANDS J.J. & PORTERFIELD J.S. (1984) Antibody-mediated enhancement of rabies virus infection in a mouse macrophage cell line (P388D1). *J. gen. Virol.* **65**, 1091.

176 KOSTER F.T., KIRKPATRICK T.L., ROWATT J.D. & BACA O.G. (1984) Antibody-dependent cellular cytotoxicity of *Coxiella burnetii*-infected J774 macrophage target cells. *Infect. Immun.* **43**, 253.

177 PHIPPS R.P., PILLAI P.S. & SCOTT D.W. (1984) Conversion of a tolerogenic to an immunogenic signal by P388AD.2 cells, a lymphoid dendritic cell-like tumour line. *J. Immunol.* **132**, 2273.

178 PETERLIN B.M., GONWA T.A. & STOBO J.D. (1984) Expression of HLA-DR by a human monocyte cell line is under transcriptional control. *J. Mol. cell. Immunol.* **1**, 191.

Chapter 46
In vitro determination of phagocytosis and intracellular killing by polymorphonuclear and mononuclear phagocytes

P. C. J. LEIJH, R. VAN FURTH & T. L. VAN ZWET

Methods to measure phagocytosis and intracellular killing, 46.3

Materials, 46.5
Methods, 46.7

Notes, recommendations and results, 46.9

One of the most important host-defence mechanisms against invading micro-organisms is the phagocytosis, followed by intracellular killing and digestion, of micro-organisms by phagocytic cells.

The two lines of professional phagocytes are the polymorphonuclear leucocytes and the mononuclear phagocytes. Cells of both lines originate in the bone marrow and, after circulating in the blood, migrate to the tissues where they carry out their functions (Fig. 46.1) [1–4]. Tissue macrophages are divided into free macrophages, which are present in connective tissues and serous cavities, and fixed macrophages of organs, for instance the liver (Kupffer cells), spleen, and lymph nodes.

One of the requirements for the initiation of phagocytosis is the establishment of contact between particulate matter and phagocytic cells. This contact can be brought about by transport of particles via the blood or lymph to the sites of fixed phagocytic cells (i.e. tissue macrophages) or by migration of mobile phagocytic cells (i.e. granulocytes and monocytes) to the site of the particles. The former process is exemplified by the macrophages of the liver, spleen, and lymph nodes, which by endocytosis clear the blood and lymph of particulate matter (micro-organisms, effete cells, or antigen–antibody complexes); the latter by the accumulation of granulocytes and monocytes at sites of injury, where they participate in the inflammatory reaction by ingesting micro-organisms, non-microbial foreign matter, pathological cells, and antigen–antibody complexes.

The process of phagocytosis can be separated into several stages (Fig. 46.2): opsonization of the particles by serum factors, recognition and attachment of the opsonized particles to the cell surface, engulfment of such particles, intracellular killing of micro-organisms, and digestion of micro-organisms and other ingested matter.

Recognition and attachment of particles by phagocytes

Although phagocytosis of particles was shown as early as 1862 by Haeckel [5], and Metchnikoff [6] described macrophages and microphages as early as 1892, the role of serum factors in this process first became clear in 1904, when Wright & Douglas [7] showed that such substances are obligatory for optimal ingestion. Opsonization is achieved by the covering of particles with specific antibodies of the IgG class, with or without complement. IgG antibodies bind to particles at their $(Fab^1)_2$ sites, thus exposing their Fc part on the surface of the particles. Since phagocytes have membrane receptors for the Fc part of IgG [8–11], they recognize these IgG-coated particles. IgM has no opsonic capacity, but binding of IgM antibodies to particles induces activation of the complement system. This leads to deposition of C3b on the particles, which may result in the recognition of these particles by the phagocytes via C3b receptors [10,12–14].

Although the recognition of particles coated with IgG and/or C3b via their Fcγ and C3b receptors, is the main mechanism underlying the ingestion of foreign material, called 'immune phagocytosis' [15–17], there are other factors which influence or mediate this process [18–22].

Ingestion

When micro-organisms have been recognized and are attached to the phagocytes, ingestion can occur. The mechanism underlying the ingestion of particles by macrophages was studied in detail by Silverstein &

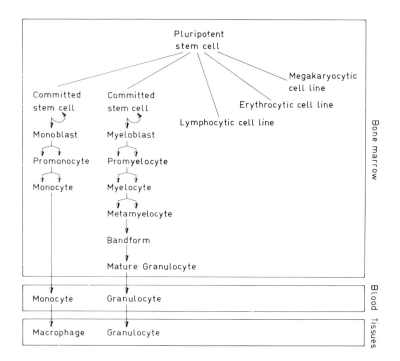

Fig. 46.1. Schematic representation of the differentiation and localization of cells derived from the haemopoietic stem cell.

Griffin [15,16,23]. Their experiments showed that one single-point receptor–ligand interaction is not enough to trigger complete ingestion of the particle, but that the phagocyte membrane surrounds the particle in a zipper-like way due to receptor–opsonin interactions. When the tips of the pseudopodia of a phagocyte that surround a particle fuse together, the micro-organism is lodged in a phagosome, whose wall is formed by the inverted cell membrane (Fig. 46.3). During and after formation of the phagosome, adjacent lysosomes fuse with the phagocytic vacuole, and the contents of the lysosome discharge into the phagocytic vacuole after rupture of the common membrane, giving a phago-lysosome.

Killing of micro-organisms by phagocytes

The interaction between opsonized micro-organisms and the phagocyte membrane does not only result in the ingestion of the organisms but also evokes a metabolic burst, which is characterized, for example, by an increased oxygen (O_2) consumption, and the production of superoxide anion (O_2^-) and hydrogen peroxide (H_2O_2) [24–27] Both O_2^- and H_2O_2 have microbicidal activity. H_2O_2 forms an even more powerful microbicidal system in concert with halide ions and myeloperoxidase of the phagocytes [28,29]. The importance of this microbicidal system is best illustrated by the defects in microbicidal activity of

granulocytes and monocytes of patients suffering from chronic granulomatous disease (CGD). This rare disease has an incidence of 1–2 in 10^6 members of the population. Phagocytes of these patients are unable to convert O_2 into H_2O_2 and cannot kill catalase-positive micro-organisms [30,31]. Deficiency of myeloperoxidase in the phagocytes, a more common disorder than CGD (incidence 2 in 10^4), is associated with a normal O_2 consumption, and a normal or slightly diminished intracellular killing capacity of the phagocytes.

Besides this oxygen-dependent microbicidal system there are also oxygen-independent microbicidal activities, e.g. the action of lysozyme [32]; the action of lactoferrin, which can have a microbiostatic effect [33]; lowering of the intraphagosomal pH [34]; and the activity of cationic proteins, which can be antimicrobial [35–39].

Most micro-organisms are killed by the microbicidal systems described above; however, some of the so-called intracellular micro-organisms (i.e. Mycobacteria, Salmonellae species, *Listeria monocytogenes, Legionella pneumoniae*) can survive inside the phagocytes. Optimal killing of these micro-organisms requires activation of macrophages [40,41]. How activated macrophages kill ingested organisms, is not known; an indication may be that the ability of these macrophages to kill bacteria correlates with the extracellular generation of H_2O_2 after triggering of the membranes [42–44].

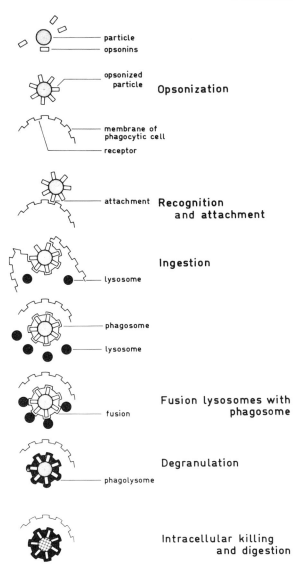

Fig. 46.2. Schematic representation of the various stages of phagocytosis and intracellular killing of micro-organisms.

Methods to measure phagocytosis and intracellular killing

In vivo *methods for the assessment of phagocytosis*

A number of *in vivo* methods to assess the phagocytic capacity of the organism are described. These methods mainly depend on measurement of the clearance from the circulation of intravenously injected material (e.g. colloids, bacteria, macromolecules, opsonized red

cells) [45–48]. These studies on clearance from the circulation can provide information about the functional state of the macrophages of the liver (Kupffer cells) and, to a lesser extent, of the macrophages of the lung and spleen. It has become clear, however, that the interpretation of the results is difficult, because the blood clearance of particulate matter is influenced by other factors as well, such as the flow rate of the blood, the presence or absence of opsonizing factors, 'stickiness' of the particles which may adhere to vessel walls, and changes in the population of phagocytic cells in the liver [48,49].

In vitro *methods for the assessment of phagocytosis*

The advantage of the measurement of phagocytosis *in vitro* is that cell populations, particles, opsonizing factors, and other conditions are well defined. To make certain that ingestion of particles is measured with the various methods developed, each method has to fulfil the following criteria:
(1) non-ingested cell-associated particles must be distinguished from those which have been ingested;
(2) ingestion must be zero at time zero;
(3) the rate as well as the degree of ingestion must reach zero-order kinetics when the particle:cell ratio is increased.

Methods to study ingestion by phagocytes that fulfil these criteria can be divided into two groups: methods which measure the increase in the number of intracellular particles; and methods in which the decrease in the number of extracellular particles is taken as a measure of ingestion.

Determination of phagocytosis as an increase in the number of intracellular particles

The number of particles ingested by phagocytes can be determined by light and/or electron microscopy, provided that a clear distinction can be made between extra- and intracellular particles [7,50–53]. This is often impossible by light microscopy, excluding methods in which xylol is used to dissolve extracellular latex particles attached to the cells [52], water or an ammonium chloride solution is used to lyse extracellular red cells [52], or lysostaphin is applied to lyse extracellular *S. aureus* [52,54].

The investigation of phagocytosis by microscopical methods is time-consuming, and reliable data on the rate and kinetics of the phagocytic process are difficult to obtain [50].

To determine the rate and kinetics of the phagocytic process, the method used must allow studies to be performed at different particle:phagocyte ratios, time intervals, and temperatures. These methods usually

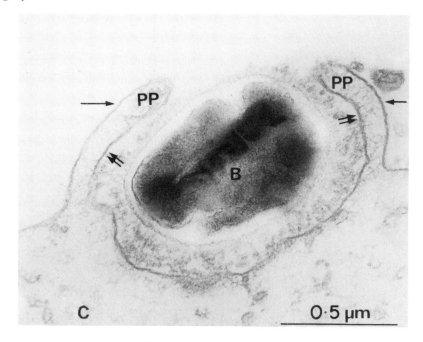

Fig. 46.3. Human granulocytes phagocytosing *S. aureus*. After incubation of the bacteria–cell suspension for 15 min, a bacterium (B) is partially enveloped by two pseudopods (PP) limited by the plasma membrane of the granulocytes (arrow). An invaginated part of the plasma membrane (double arrows) surrounds the bacterium; C, cytoplasm.

employ particles labelled with a fluorescent or radioactive probe, latex particles, or oil droplets [53,55–60]. The use of labelled particles permits rapid determination of the amount of intracellular label, but application of this method is restricted by the activity of the label, which may hamper measurements at low or high particle:phagocyte ratios. For the quantitative determination of intracellular latex particles or oil droplets, this material must be extracted from the phagocytes; therefore these methods have the disadvantage of destroying the phagocytes [61,53].

Since opsonization with antibodies and/or complement is necessary for optimal ingestion of microorganisms, it is relevant to study the kinetics of phagocytosis in a way that reflects the conditions that occur in infections, i.e. with the use of live microorganisms, (specific) antibodies, and/or activation of complement.

Determination of phagocytosis as a decrease in the number of extracellular particles

The decrease in the number of extracellular particles is used for investigation of the rate of phagocytosis of micro-organisms and immune complexes. The number of extracellular micro-organisms can be determined directly by microbiological methods or indir-

ectly with radiolabelled organisms [62–67]. The use of the latter has the drawback that the label only represents an average number of micro-organisms. The average number of bacteria per unit label can change due to bacterial division when viable labelled micro-organisms are used, or due to decay of the label in the case of storage of killed labelled microorganisms. Furthermore, methods using radioactivity provide no information about any microbicidal activity of serum factors or of factors released by the phagocytes during the assay.

These disadvantages can be avoided by making use of viable, non-labelled bacteria. Determination of the number of viable intracellular bacteria is inadequate, because this number is not solely the result of phagocytosis but includes also the intracellular killing during the ingestion interval studied [62,64,68–70]. Assessment of phagocytosis as decrease in the number of extracellular micro-organisms requires separation of the extracellular non-phagocytosed micro-organisms from the phagocytes. Moreover, the results of these experiments are influenced by bactericidal factors in the extracellular medium, agglutination of microorganisms, and the proliferation of extracellular bacteria. Therefore this approach requires appropriate control experiments for each kind of phagocyte, species of micro-organisms, and serum used for opsonization, to assess whether separation of phagocytes and non-phagocytosed bacteria is adequate and to exclude the presence of bactericidal or agglutination factors.

Methods to measure the microbicidal activity of phagocytes

To investigate the microbicidal activity of phagocytes, two approaches are commonly used: (1) direct, taking the decrease in the viability of micro-organisms as a measure of the bactericidal activity, and (2) indirect, with measurement of, for example, O_2 consumption, H_2O_2 production, or nitroblue tetrazolium (NBT) reduction, all of which are thought to reflect the microbicidal activity of phagocytes.

(1) Direct measurement of the microbicidal activity of phagocytes

The methods generally used for determination of the microbicidal activity of phagocytes are based on the decrease in the total number of viable micro-organisms during incubation of micro-organisms with phagocytes, or on the course of the number of viable cell-associated bacteria [62,71–76]. These methods have the disadvantage that the results are influenced by other factors besides microbicidal activity of the phagocytes. For example, in this assay the rate of intracellular killing measured depends on the rate at which the micro-organisms are ingested. Furthermore, the presence of extracellular bactericidal factors, agglutination of bacteria, and extracellular proliferation of the micro-organisms will interfere with interpretation of the results.

To avoid this problem and to gain insight into the process of intracellular killing of micro-organisms *per se*, methods have been developed to separate the ingestion phase from the phase of intracellular killing. To this end, after ingestion of micro-organisms by phagocytes for a specified period and washing of the cells to remove extracellular micro-organisms, an antibiotic or some other bactericidal agent was added to prevent the growth of extracellular bacteria [54,77,78]. However, consensus has not been reached concerning the penetration of these agents into phagocytic cells, and their functional activity inside [79–82]; therefore the results obtained employing such agents are questionable.

(2) Indirect measurement of the microbicidal activity of phagocytes

Since there is a correlation between the metabolic burst accompanying phagocytosis—in which O_2 is consumed and converted into $O_2^{-.}$ and H_2O_2—and the capacity of phagocytes to kill micro-organisms, methods including measurement of the intermediate or final products of the metabolic burst can be used to determine the microbicidal activity of phagocytes [24,43,44,83,84].

All these methods, however, provide information only about the functioning of the O_2-dependent microbicidal mechanisms of phagocytes. Therefore these methods cannot fully replace the microbiological assays.

Present method

Based on the arguments described above the authors feel that the best methods to establish the rate of phagocytosis and intracellular killing by phagocytic cells are microbiological assays. The present chapter, based in principle on the methods described by Maaløe [65], Cohn & Morse [62], and Mackaness [78], gives a detailed description of the technique for the *in vitro* determination of the phagocytosis and intracellular killing of micro-organisms by granulocytes and mononuclear phagocytes.

Materials

Media and sera

The media and sera employed in both phagocytosis and intracellular killing experiments are as follows.

1   Phosphate-buffered saline (PBS), pH 7.2, is prepared from Bacto haemagglutination Sörensen buffer (Difco Laboratories, Detroit, Michigan).

2   The heparin-saline solution for washing and harvesting of granulocytes, monocytes, and macrophages is made by adding appropriate amounts of heparin without preservative to sterile PBS.

3   Hanks' balanced salt solution (HBSS) (Oxoid, Ltd., London) is made according to the manufacturers description. The pH is adjusted to 7.2 with sodium bicarbonate.

4   The gelatin-Hanks' solution (0.1% gelatin-HBSS) is made by dissolving 100 mg gelatin (Difco) in 5 ml sterile HBSS under gentle heating and adding this solution to 95 ml sterile HBSS. Gelatin is added to protect the micro-organism, since HBSS alone is bactericidal [85].

5   The bovine albumin solution (0.01%) in distilled water, used for disrupting the leucocytes in the intracellular killing experiments, is prepared by adding 10 mg bovine albumin (Poviet N.V., Amsterdam) to 100 ml sterile bi-distilled water; the pH is adjusted to 7.3 with 0.1 M NaOH. Bovine albumin is

added to protect the bacteria against the bactericidal effect of bi-distilled water [62].

6 Serum from normal AB donors is used. Blood is clotted for 1 h at room temperature, centrifuged at 1100 *g* for 20 min, and stored at -70 °C for a maximum of 3 months. New born calf serum (NBCS) is obtained from Grand Island Biological (Grand Island, New York). Heat-inactivated serum is obtained by heating the serum for 30 min at 56 °C.

7 Lysostaphin (Sigma Chemical Co., St. Louis, Mo.) is dissolved in PBS and stored in small aliquots at -20 °C until use.

Tubes

Capped plastic tubes (16 × 100 mm; Falcon Plastics, Los Angeles, California) are used in experiments with granulocytes. To prevent adherence of cells, all experiments with monocytes and macrophages are done in siliconized glass tubes closed with non-toxic silicon rubber stoppers.

Cells

Human polymorphonuclear leucocytes

Blood is collected in a sterile tube containing 300 u heparin solution per 10 ml blood. The erythrocytes are sedimented with a 5% (w/v) solution of dextran in buffered saline (Mr 200 000); 3 ml solution to 10 ml blood) for 30 min at 37 °C. The leucocyte-rich supernatant fluid is then removed and centrifuged for 10 min at 110 *g*. The sedimented leucocytes are washed twice with heparin-saline, concentrated by centrifugation (10 min at 110 *g*), counted with a Bürker haemocytometer and suspended in gelatin HBSS to a concentration of $1–2 \times 10^7$ granulocytes/ml.

Human blood monocytes

For the study of the functional capacities of peripheral blood monocytes, a leucocyte-rich suspension is prepared by density centrifugation of blood on a Ficoll-Hypaque suspension (12 parts Ficoll 400, Pharmacia, Uppsala, Sweden, and 5 parts sodium metrizoate Isopaque, Nyegaard & Co., Oslo) [86]. Five millilitres of heparin blood is layered on 4 ml of the Ficoll-Hypaque suspension and centrifuged for 20 min at 400 *g* at room temperature. After collection of the monocyte–lymphocyte interphase, the cells are washed three times with heparin-saline, and adjusted to a concentration of $5–6 \times 10^7$ cells/ml. The percentage of monocytes in the cell suspension is determined in a Giemsa-stained cytocentrifuge preparation. Pure monocyte suspensions (i.e. more than 90% of the cells are monocytes) can be obtained by elutriation centrifugation [87,88].

Murine peritoneal macrophages

To obtain peritoneal macrophages of normal mice, mice are killed with chloroform. The skin is reflected over the abdomen and 2 ml PBS with 50 u heparin/ml injected into the peritoneal cavity. The abdomen is kneaded gently and after 1 min the cell-rich fluid is removed and placed in a siliconized glass tube at 0 °C (crushed ice). Peritoneal cell suspensions from various mice are pooled and centrifuged for 4 min at 110 *g*. The sedimented leucocytes are washed twice with heparin-saline and then suspended in gelatin HBSS to a concentration of $1–2 \times 10^7$ macrophages/ml.

Phagocytic cells from other sources

Although methods for assessing phagocytosis and intracellular killing of micro-organisms are described for populations of human peripheral blood leucocytes and mouse peritoneal macrophages, these methods can also be applied for the study of phagocytic cells from other sources. Methods to obtain reasonably homogeneous populations of phagocytic cells are described elsewhere [89,90].

Viability of cells

The viability of granulocytes, monocytes and macrophages is checked by exclusion of trypan blue dye [91].

Micro-organisms

Bacteria, e.g. *Staphylococcus epidermis*, *Staphylococcus aureus* (type 42 D), *Pseudomonas aeruginosa* (types P_2AB and P_{14}), *Salmonella typhimurium* (type I 505), *Candida albicans*, and *Escherichia coli* (054), are grown and kept on a slope of solid agar medium, and transferred at monthly intervals. All strains are serum-resistant, i.e. are not killed *in vitro* during incubation for 120 min at 37 °C with 90% serum. Before use, micro-organisms are cultured in 100 ml 2.5% Nutrient Broth (Oxoid) for about 18 h at 37 °C. To obtain a *Candida* suspension of single yeast cells, *Candida albicans* is cultured for 7–8 days at 30 °C in Nutrient Broth with 1% glucose [92]. After culture the bacteria are centrifuged for 10 min at 1500 *g*, washed twice with PBS, and resuspended in gelatin-HBSS to a concentration of $1–2 \times 10^7$ bacteria/ml. To determine the exact number present during each experiment the number of viable bacteria is determined microbiologically.

Pre-opsonization of bacteria is carried out by incubation of a bacterial suspension (5×10^6 bacteria/ml) with AB serum for 25 min at 37 °C under slow rotation (4 rev./min). The bacteria are centrifuged for 10 min at 1500 g and washed twice with gelatin-HBSS. Before use, the bacteria are resuspended in gelatin-HBSS to about 10^7 bacteria/ml.

Methods

Microbiological assay for the phagocytosis of micro-organisms

Phagocytes are incubated together with live micro-organisms in the presence of serum under continuous rotation (4 rev./min) at 37 °C, and at specified time points the number of viable non-ingested bacteria is determined. An outline of the method is given in Fig. 46.4.

The ratio of bacteria to cells routinely used for the phagocytosis assay is one. For this purpose 2 ml of the cell suspension ($1–2 \times 10^7$ cells/ml), 2 ml of the suspended bacteria ($1–2 \times 10^7$ micro-organisms/ml), and 0.4 ml serum (or $1–2 \times 10^7$ pre-opsonized bacteria/ml without serum) are combined and incubated at 37 °C under continuous rotation (4 rev./min). At several time points, a 0.5 ml aliquot of the suspension is removed and added to 1.5 ml ice-cold gelatin-HBSS to stop phagocytosis. This sample is centrifuged for 4 min at 110 g. Under this condition the non-ingested

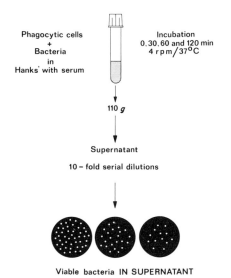

Fig. 46.4. Outline of the technique for assessing phagocytosis *in vitro*.

bacteria remain in the supernatant fluid [69,75]. With the supernatant fluid, serial tenfold dilutions in saline are made over a range ensuring that at least one dilution contains between 100 and 1000 viable bacteria/ml. Aliquots of 0.1 ml of the three highest dilutions are pipetted on to each of two DST agar plates (Diagnostic Sensitivity Medium Agar, Oxoid, Ltd., London) and immediately spread with a fine wire loop. The plates are incubated at 37 °C for 18–24 h, and the colonies are counted with a colony counter (Montagne, Bagneux, France). The number of viable bacteria/ml is calculated from the means of the colony counts of duplicate plates of the two highest dilutions, providing the plate contains less than 500 colonies.

Phagocytosis of *Candida albicans* is also measured as the decrease in the number of extracellular micro-organisms. For *Candida albicans* differential centrifugation does not separate non-ingested *Candida* from the phagocytes since *Candida* and phagocytic cells have about the same specific density. However, counting in a haemocytometer of extracellular *Candida* in samples at various time points provides a reliable measure for the phagocytosis of the micro-organisms [91].

Morphological assessment of phagocytosis

To determine the percentage of phagocytes that have ingested bacteria, a 0.5 ml sample of the bacteria-cell suspension is taken and added to 1.5 ml ice-cold gelatin-HBSS, centrifuged (4 min at 110 g), and washed three times with the same solution, after which 1 ml gelatin-HBSS is added. Next, cytocentrifuge preparations are made, cells are fixed with methanol and stained with Giemsa stain. The percentage of cells that have ingested bacteria is determined from counts of at least 200 phagocytic cells. The mean number of ingested bacteria/cell is determined by counting the number of bacteria per cell in 100 cells that have phagocytosed.

To distinguish between the number of *S. aureus* attached to the cells and the number of these bacteria actually ingested, extracellular *S. aureus* are lysed with lysostaphin. For this purpose cell suspensions are incubated after phagocytosis with 1 u lysostaphin/ml for 5 min at 37 °C, then washed three times with gelatin-HBSS, after which cytocentrifuge preparations are made [52].

Assay for the intracellular killing of micro-organisms

To measure the rate of intracellular killing independent from the rate of ingestion, phagocytic cells are allowed to ingest bacteria for a short period, washed thoroughly to remove all extracellular bacteria, and

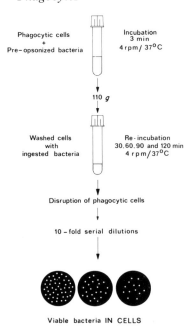

Fig. 46.5. Outline of the technique for assessing intracellular killing *in vitro*, after phagocytosis *in vitro*.

reincubated at 37 °C. During the period of re-incubation the number of viable intracellular bacteria is determined, thus providing data on the rate of intracellular killing. An outline of the method used to assess intracellular killing by phagocytes is given in Fig. 46.5.

The initial part of this test, i.e. the phagocytosis of bacteria, is done as described in the preceding section. On the basis of a bacterium:phagocytic cell ratio of one, 1.5 ml of a cell suspension ($1–2 \times 10^7$ phagocytes/ml) is added to an equal volume and equal concentration of pre-opsonized bacteria. After a short period (e.g. 3 min for granulocytes and monocytes, 20 min for peritoneal macrophages), phagocytosis is stopped by placing the tube in crushed ice and shaking it for 1 min. Extracellular bacteria are removed by differential centrifugation (4 min at 100 *g*) and two washes with gelatin-HBSS; next, the phagocytes are resuspended in HBSS with 10% serum and incubated at 37 °C. At various time points a 0.5 ml sample of the suspension is removed and added to 0.5 ml ice-cold HBSS to stop the intracellular killing. This sample is centrifuged for 4 min at 110 *g*, and 1 ml ice-cold distilled water with bovine albumin is added to the cell-pellet. Lysis of granulocytes is achieved by mixing the suspension on a vortex mixer and lysis of monocytes and macrophages by alternately freezing the suspension with liquid nitrogen (-170 °C) and thawing it rapidly in a water bath (± 37 °C) three times.

Finally, the number of viable micro-organisms is determined microbiologically, as described in the section on the phagocytosis assay.

The intracellular killing of *Candida* must be determined from the decrease in the total number of viable yeast cells during a 60 min period, since differential centrifugation does not separate non-ingested yeast cells from the phagocytes [91].

Micro-method for the determination of phagocytosis and intracellular killing

The methods described above to measure phagocytosis and intracellular killing have the disadvantage that relatively large numbers of phagocytes, i.e. about $2–4 \times 10^7$ are necessary, which hampers a functional assay requiring the blood of children or patients with low leucocyte numbers. To overcome this problem the phagocytosis assay has been adjusted by reducing the volume of both the cell and bacteria suspensions to 200 μl. Furthermore, during the incubation of cells and bacteria the samples taken have been reduced to 50 μl at the various time points [92].

For the intracellular killing assay similar adaptations have been applied, i.e. cell and bacteria suspensions (concentration 10^7/ml) are reduced to volumes of 200 μl, and the assays performed as described [92].

In vivo/in vitro *method to determine the intracellular killing by macrophages*

Intracellular killing of micro-organisms by peritoneal macrophages can be measured as described above. However, because phagocytosis by macrophages must proceed for 20 min before the peak number of viable intracellular bacteria is reached, the rate of intracellular killing can only be determined after a relative long period of phagocytosis. When peritoneal macrophages are allowed to phagocytose bacteria *in vivo*, enough bacteria for optimal determination of intracellular killing *in vitro* are ingested within a very short time, e.g. 3–5 min. An outline of this method is given in Fig. 46.6. One millilitre of a suspension of $1–2 \times 10^6$ bacteria/ml in gelatin-HBSS with 10% NBCS is injected intraperitoneally into living non-anaesthetized mice. After exactly 3 min the animals are killed by cervical dislocation, and 1 min later 2 ml PBS saline with heparin is injected, and peritoneal cells collected. To remove the extracellular bacteria, the cell suspension is washed three times with ice-cold gelatin-HBSS, centrifuged for 4 min at 110 *g* and the macrophage concentration adjusted to $6–8 \times 10^6$ cells/ml. Macrophages containing bacteria are re-incubated at 37 °C,

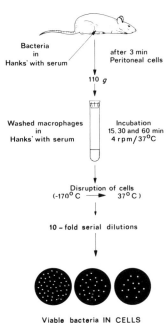

Bacteria
in
Hanks' with serum

after 3 min
Peritoneal cells

110 *g*

Washed macrophages
in
Hanks' with serum

Incubation
15, 30 and 60 min
4 rpm/37°C

Disruption of cells
(-170° C ⟶ 37°C)

10 – fold serial dilutions

Viable bacteria IN CELLS

Fig. 46.6. Outline of the technique for assessing intracellular killing *in vitro*, after phagocytosis *in vivo*.

and at various time points the number of viable intracellular bacteria determined as described above.

Calculations

Phagocytosis at a given time-point is expressed as the percentage decrease in the initial number of viable extracellular bacteria according to the following formula:

$$P(t) = (1 - N_t/N_0) \times 100 \tag{1}$$

where $P(t)$ is the phagocytic index at time $t = t$; N_0 and N_t are the number of viable extracellular bacteria at time $t = 0$ and $t = t$, respectively. To correct the number of viable extracellular bacteria for the growth of extracellular bacteria, the following formula (2) is used:

$$NC_t = N_t \times B_0/B_t \tag{2}$$

where NC_t is the corrected number of extracellular bacteria at time $t = t$; B_0 and B_t are the number of bacteria during incubation of bacteria and serum at time $t = 0$ and $t = t$, respectively. Substitution of formula 2 in formula 1 gives a corrected phagocytic index according to the following formula:

$$P(t) \text{ corrected} = \left(1 - \frac{N_t \times B_0}{B_t \times N_0}\right) \times 100 \tag{3}$$

The rate of phagocytosis (v_p) during the interval of exponential decrease is calculated according to the formula

$$v_p = k_p \times N_0 \tag{4}$$

where k_p is the rate constant calculated according to the formula

$$k_p = (\ln N_0 - \ln N_t)/t_0 \tag{5}$$

or after correction for the extracellular growth according to the formula

$$k_{\text{corrected}} = (\ln N_0 - \ln \frac{N_t \times B_0}{B_t})/t \tag{6}$$

The killing index $K(t)$ is calculated using the formula $K(t) = (1 - N_t/N_0) \times 100$, where N_0 and N_t are the numbers of viable intracellular bacteria at time $t = 0$ and $t = t$, respectively. The rate of intracellular killing v_k is calculated with the formula $v_k = k_k \times N_0$, in which k_k is the rate constant of killing, calculated according to the formula $k_k = (\ln N_0 - \ln N_t)/t$.

Notes, recommendations and results

Phagocytosis

Each experiment has three components: (1) incubation of cells, bacteria, and serum under continuous rotation; (2) incubation of bacteria and serum under continuous rotation, serving as a control on the initial number of bacteria and on the bacterial growth during the experiment; (3) stationary incubation of cells and bacteria, (standing control), serving as a rough check on bactericidal effects of serum or substances released by the cells. The release of bactericidal products from the cells can be checked more accurately by preparing bacteria- and cell-free supernatants after 60 or 120 min of phagocytosis and then re-incubation of bacteria with the supernatant for 2 h at 37 °C at 4 rev./min. In this way the growth of bacteria in the presence of these supernatants can be compared with the normal growth curve.

As an example of a phagocytosis experiment, *S. aureus* were incubated with granulocytes, both in final concentration of 5×10^6/ml, in the presence of 10% serum under slow rotation (4 rev./min) at 37 °C. The results (Fig. 46.7) show an exponential decrease in the number of viable extracellular micro-organisms—determined at intervals of 5 min—during the first 20–30 min. During this period more than 80% of the initial number of micro-organisms were ingested, whereas during the remaining 90 min this percentage rose to 99. After correction for the extracellular growth of bacteria in the suspension, an exponential

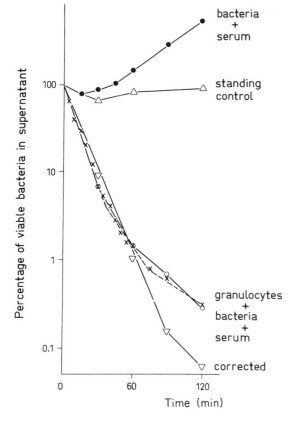

Percentage of viable bacteria in supernatant

bacteria + serum

standing control

granulocytes + bacteria + serum

corrected

Time (min)

Fig. 46.7. The kinetics of phagocytosis of *S. aureus* by human granulocytes; 5×10^6 granulocytes/ml were incubated with 5×10^6 *S. aureus* in the presence of 10% serum at 37 °C and 4 rev./min. Control experiments consisted of incubation of bacteria and serum, and of incubation of granulocytes, bacteria and serum without rotation (standing control).

decrease in the number of viable extracellular bacteria over the total period of 90 min is observed (Fig. 46.7). The rate constant calculated after correction for the outgrowth of extracellular bacteria over this 90 min interval did not differ from the constant obtained from the first 30 min without correction (data not shown). These results indicate that the difference between the uncorrected rates of phagocytosis during 30 and 90 min incubation is due to the multiplication of extracellular *S. aureus*, and that information on the rate of phagocytosis obtained during the first 30 min is representative for the entire experimental period.

Incubation of a bacterial suspension without granulocytes in the presence of serum showed an increase in the number of micro-organisms (Fig. 46.7). Incubation of the micro-organisms with granulocytes in the presence of 10% serum at 37 °C without rotation

showed no decrease in the number of extracellular micro-organisms (Fig. 46.7). Supernatants free from granulocytes and bacteria prepared after 60 or 120 min of phagocytosis showed no bactericidal activity for *S. aureus* when incubated with bacteria for 2 h at 37 °C. Together these results show that the decrease in the number of viable extracellular bacteria is not due to extracellular killing of micro-organisms.

Kinetics of phagocytosis

When 5×10^6 granulocytes were incubated with various concentrations of *S. aureus* (5×10^4–5×10^9/ml) in the presence of serum, a decrease in the rate constant of phagocytosis is observed when bacteria:granulocyte ratios higher than 10:1 were used (Fig. 46.8). Incubation of granulocytes and bacteria at ratios of 100:1 and 1000:1 only gave reliable information about the kinetics of phagocytosis for periods of 90 and 60 min, respectively, due to disruption of granulocytes saturated with bacteria. The results of the morphological assessment of phagocytosis are summarized in Table 46.1. Bacteria concentrations of 10^{10}/ml or more were not used because of clumping of bacteria. Investigation of the effect of various granulocyte concentrations (5×10^4–5×10^7/ml) on the kinetics of phagocytosis showed that incubation of 5×10^4 granulocytes with bacteria at 37 °C and 4 rev./min did not lead to any detectable decrease in the number of extracellular micro-organisms. Phagocytosis during incubation of 5×10^5–5×10^7 granulocytes with various concentrations of bacteria was characterized by an initial rate of phagocytosis depending on the bacteria:cell ratio and the number of granulocytes [69,70]. These results demonstrate that the rate of phagocytosis *in vitro* depends on the bacteria:cell ratio, and the concentration of both bacteria and granulocytes.

From the present experiments it is concluded that phagocytosis experiments carried out over a period of 120 min and using a bacteria:cell ratio of 1:1 (concentration 5×10^6/ml) give reliable information about the rate of ingestion. Results of phagocytosis experiments with granulocytes of healthy donors with *Staphylococcus aureus*, *S. epidermidis*, *E. coli*, *Streptococcus pyogenes*, *Group B streptococci*, *Candida albicans*, and *Pseudomonas aeruginosa* are summarized in Table 46.2.

Phagocytosis by human peripheral blood monocytes

An example of the decrease in the number of viable extracellular *S. aureus* during incubation with blood monocytes (concentration of both: 5×10^6/ml) in the presence of 10% serum at 37 °C and 4 rev./min is

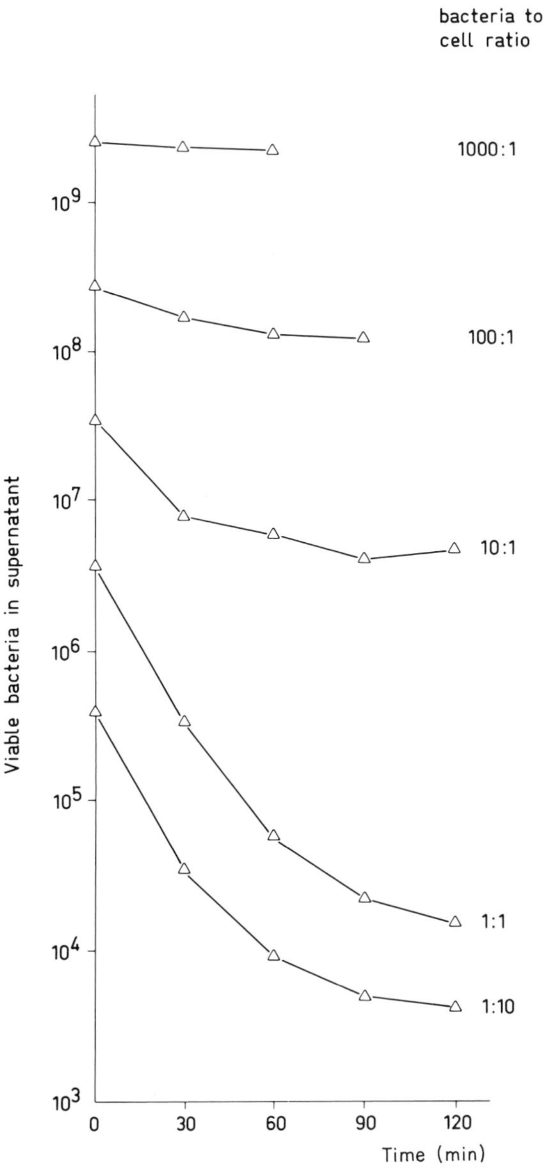

bacteria to
cell ratio

Table 46.1. Morphological assessment of phagocytosis of *S. aureus* by granulocytes*

Bacteria:cell ratio	Percentage of cells containing *S. aureus*	Mean number of bacteria per ingesting cell
1:10	39	1
1:1	91	3
10:1	100	9
100:1	100	†

* After 60 min phagocytosis.
† Too numerous for an accurate count.

Table 46.2. Phagocytosis of bacteria by human granulocytes*

	Percentage phagocytosis	
	at 60 min	at 120 min
Staphylococcus albus	98.1	99.8
Staphylococcus aureus	97.5	99.4
Escherichia coli	98.3	99.6
Streptococcus pyogenes	99.0	99.0
Group B streptococci	97.6	98.9
Pseudomonas aeruginosa	97.4	99.6
Candida albicans	96.0	N.D.

* Phagocytosis was measured at a bacteria:cell ratio of 1:1 at 37 °C. Values represent the means of at least ten experiments.
N.D. = not determined.

Fig. 46.8. Phagocytosis of *S. aureus* by human granulocytes at various bacteria:cell ratios; 5×10^6 granulocytes/ml were incubated with various concentrations *S. aureus* at 37 °C and 4 rev./min.

shown in Fig. 46.9. The results reveal a rapid ingestion of *S. aureus* during the first 60 min, after which about 92% of the initial number of bacteria are ingested. Comparison of the rate of phagocytosis by granulocytes and monocytes showed that granulocytes ingest *S. aureus* at a higher rate than monocytes do. Results of phagocytosis experiments done with monocytes and

various micro-organisms are summarized in Table 46.3.

Phagocytosis by murine peritoneal macrophages

An example of the ingestion of *S. aureus* by peritoneal macrophages during incubation of macrophages and *S. aureus* in a ratio of 1:1, in the presence of 10% NBCS at 37 °C under rotation, is given in Fig. 46.9. During 120 min of incubation 70% of the bacteria were ingested. The phagocytic activity of murine macrophages proved to be lower than that of the human granulocytes and monocytes; this applies not only to *S. aureus* but also to the ingestion of other micro-organisms (Tables 46.2, 46.3, 46.4).

Opsonic activity of serum

Incubation of *S. aureus* and granulocytes or monocytes (ratio of 1:1) in the presence of various concen-

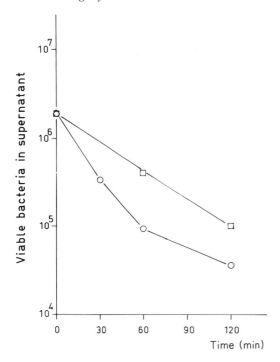

Fig. 46.9. Phagocytosis of *S. aureus* by human monocytes (○) and murine peritoneal macrophages (□) in the presence of 10% AB-serum and murine serum respectively at a bacteria:cell ratio of 1:1 (concentrations: 5×10^6/ml).

Table 46.3. Phagocytosis of bacteria by human monocytes*

	Percentage phagocytosis	
	at 60 min	at 120 min
Staphylococcus albus	91	96
Staphylococcus aureus	90	92
Escherichia coli	92	96
Streptococcus pyogenes	95	98
Group B streptococci	94	96
Candida albicans	95	N.D.

* Phagocytosis was measured at a bacteria:cell ratio of 1:1 at 37 °C. Values represent the means of at least ten experiments.
N.D. = not determined.

trations of serum at 37 °C revealed that both the rate and the maximal degree of phagocytosis depends on the serum concentration. These experiments showed that at least 2.5% serum is necessary to obtain optimal phagocytosis of *S. aureus* by granulocytes (Fig.

Table 46.4. Phagocytosis of bacteria by murine macrophages

	Percentage phagocytosis	
	at 60 min	at 120 min
Staphylococcus albus	77	94
Staphylococcus aureus	61	68
Pseudomonas aeruginosa	85	92

Phagocytosis was measured at a bacteria:cell ratio of 1:1 at 37 °C.

46.10a) and 1% by monocytes (Fig. 46.10b). Similar experiments performed with *E. coli* instead of *S. aureus* clearly demonstrate a different requirement for opsonins for the ingestion of *E. coli* by both types of phagocytes, as compared to this requirement for *S. aureus* (Fig. 46.10).

These results indicate that to obtain insight into the opsonic activity of an unknown serum, a choice must be made as to which micro-organism the opsonic activity is determined for, as well as which kind of phagocytic cell is responsible for ingestion. The opsonic activity of an unknown serum must therefore be compared to the opsonic activity of various concentrations of a pool of sera of healthy donors.

Intracellular killing of micro-organisms by human granulocytes

The number of viable intracellular bacteria during incubation of phagocytic cells and micro-organisms depends on two different processes: the ingestion and intracellular killing of the bacteria. Therefore, prior to the measurement of intracellular killing, the optimal period of ingestion giving the maximum recovery of viable intracellular bacteria has to be determined.

Incubation of 5×10^6 granulocytes/ml with 5×10^6 pre-opsonized *S. aureus* at 37 °C under rotation showed that a maximum number of viable intracellular bacteria was obtained at about 3–5 min (Fig. 46.11). Incubation of granulocytes with non-opsonized *S. aureus* in the presence of 10% fresh serum gave the maximum number of viable intracellular *S. aureus* in the period between 10 and 15 min (Fig. 46.11). Incubation of granulocytes and *S. aureus* in the presence of 10% serum and 2 mg phenylbutazone/ml, which does not affect ingestion but inhibits intracellular killing [75], resulted in a continuous increase in the number of viable intracellular bacteria (Fig. 46.11). Comparison of the number of viable intracellular *S. aureus* under the various incubation conditions indi-

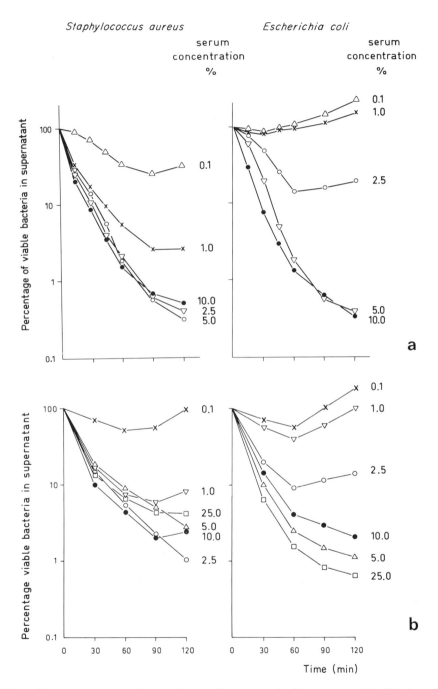

Fig. 46.10 (a) Effect of the serum concentrations on the rate of phagocytosis of *S. aureus* and *E. coli* by human granulocytes; 5×10^6 granulocytes/ml were incubated with 5×10^6 bacteria/ml in the presence of various concentrations of serum at 37 °C. (b) Effect of serum concentration on the rate of phagocytosis of *S. aureus* and *E. coli* by human monocytes; 5×10^6 monocytes/ml were incubated with 5×10^6 bacteria/ml in the presence of various concentrations serum at 37 °C.

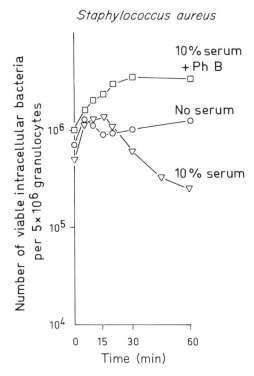

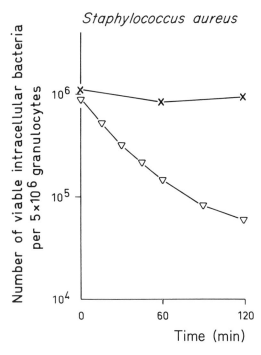

Fig. 46.11. Determination of the optimal time of ingestion for use in the intracellular killing test. 5×10^6 granulocytes/ml were incubated at 37 °C in the presence of the following material: (1) 5×10^6 pre-opsonized bacteria/ml (O); (2) 5×10^6 bacteria/ml and 10% serum ($\triangledown$); (3) 5×10^6 bacteria/ml, 10% serum plus 2 mg phenylbutazone/ml ($\square$). At various time points the number of viable intracellular bacteria was determined.

Fig. 46.12. Kinetics of intracellular of *S. aureus* by human granulocytes at 37 °C and 4 °C. After 3 min phagocytosis at a bacteria:cell ratio of 1:1, 5×10^6 granulocytes/ml containing bacteria were incubated in the presence of serum at 4 °C (x) and 37 °C ($\triangledown$).

cated that a 3 min ingestion period of pre-opsonized bacteria yields a maximal recovery of viable intracellular *S. aureus*. Similar results were obtained for other species of bacteria [70,75].

Giemsa-stained preparations and electron-microscopical observations showed that granulocytes no longer carry any bacteria on their surface after 3 min phagocytosis of pre-opsonized bacteria and after being washed twice. On the basis of these findings the killing assay was performed after 3 min of phagocytosis of pre-opsonized bacteria, at which point the highest number of viable intracellular bacteria is obtained.

An example of intracellular killing of *S. aureus* by granulocytes is given in Fig. 46.12. These results show that during the first 60 min, 85% of the ingested bacteria are killed. When the assay is performed at 4 °C instead of 37 °C no killing occurs. Results of intracellular killing experiments performed with var-

ious micro-organisms summarized in Table 46.5 indicate a rapid rate of intracellular killing of all these species.

To compare the results obtained with the present method for the assessment of intracellular killing to those determined with the original technique, experiments were performed according to the original description [62]. Three millilitres of a *S. aureus* suspension (1.5×10^7 bacteria/ml) and 3 ml of a granulocyte suspension (1.7×10^7 cells), in the presence of 10% serum, were incubated at 37 °C and 4 rev./min. After various intervals the following determinations were done.

1 The total number of viable bacteria, i.e. the number of viable non-ingested bacteria plus the number of viable cell-associated bacteria (a 0.2 ml sample of the suspension is added to 2.5 ml ice-cold distilled water with bovine albumin to disrupt the granulocytes, after which the number of viable bacteria is determined microbiologically).

2 The number of viable extracellular bacteria, i.e. bacteria in suspension and adherent to the cells (0.5 ml of the suspension is added to 1.5 ml ice-cold gelatin

Table 46.5. Intracellular killing of bacteria by human granulocytes*

	Killing index	
	at 60 min	at 120 min
Staphylococcus aureus	95.8	94.4
Staphylococcus epidermidis	86.1	98.6
Escherichia coli	99.0	99.5
Streptococcus pyogenes	97.0	99.3
Group B streptococci	96.3	98.9
Pseudomonas aeruginosa	93.2	95.2
Candida albicans	60	N.D.

* Values represent the means of ten experiments.

HBSS, not disrupting the granulocyte, and the viable bacteria determined).

3 The number of viable cell-associated bacteria (0.5 ml of the suspension is added to 1.5 ml ice-cold gelatin HBSS then centrifuged for 4 min at 110 *g*, the supernatant fluid is carefully withdrawn, and 1 ml ice-cold HBSS is added; next the number of viable bacteria determined).

4 The number of viable bacteria within the granulocytes (a 0.5 ml aliquot is added to 0.5 ml ice-cold HBSS, then centrifuged for 4 min at 110 *g*, the supernatant discarded, 1.0 ml ice-cold water containing albumin added, and after disruption of the granulocytes the number of viable bacteria determined).

The results of this experiment show that during the first 60 min of incubation the rate of decrease in the number of viable extracellular bacteria (supernatant) is identical with the rate of decrease in the number of viable extracellular bacteria plus cell-associated bacteria (total) (Fig. 46.13). This indicates that during this period the ingestion of *S. aureus* is rapidly followed by intracellular killing. Comparison of the results obtained with both methods showed identical patterns for the decreases in the numbers of viable cell-associated bacteria (sediment) and viable intracellular bacteria, indicating that both techniques measure the number of viable bacteria within the cells.

The rate of intracellular killing measured with the original method depends largely on the rate of phagocytosis and gives only information when the rate of

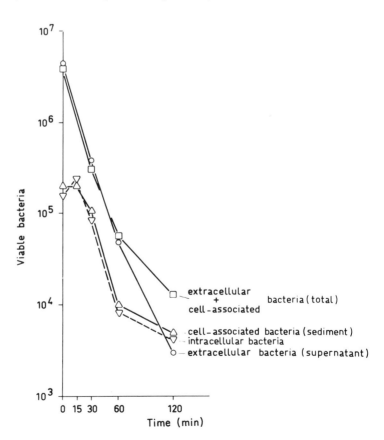

Fig. 46.13. Determination in one experiment of phagocytosis and intracellular killing, according to Cohn & Morse [62].

killing is lower than the rate of ingestion; the rate of intracellular killing determined with the present method provides information which is totally independent of the rate of phagocytosis. Furthermore, the present method allows experiments on the effects of extracellular factors (e.g. antibiotics, serum proteins) on the intracellular survival of micro-organisms without possible effects on extracellular bacteria and on the ingestion phase.

Mathematical analysis of the phagocytic process

Assuming that both the rate of ingestion and intracellular killing, as determined independently of each other, also hold true during incubation of phagocytic cells and bacteria in the presence of 10% sera at a bacteria:cell ratio of 1:1, and because intracellular killing occurs after the ingestion of bacteria, it is possible to describe both processes mathematically, assuming the following scheme of events:

$$(B_{ext}) \ ^{k_1} \ (B_{int}) \ ^{k_2} \ (B_{killed})$$

in which B_{ext} is the number of viable extracellular (not yet ingested) bacteria, B_{int} the number of viable intracellular bacteria, and B_{killed} the number of bacteria killed intracellulary. k_1 is the initial rate constant of phagocytosis, and k_2 the rate constant of the intracellular killing. This leads to the following reaction equations:

$$\frac{d(B_{ext})}{dt} = -k_1 \times B_{ext} \qquad (i)$$

which leads to:

$$B_{ext} = B_{ext_{t=0}} \cdot e^{-k_1 t} \qquad (ia)$$

$$\frac{d(B_{int})}{dt} = k_1 \times B_{ext} - k_2 \times B_{int} \qquad (ii)$$

which leads to:

$$B_{int} = \frac{k_1}{k_2 - k_1} B_{ext_{t=0}} \{e^{-k_1 t} - e^{-k_2 t}\} \qquad (iia)$$

$$\frac{d(B_{killed})}{dt} = k_2 \times B_{int} \qquad (iii)$$

which leads to:

$$B_{killed} = B_{ext_{t=0}} \left\{ 1 - \frac{k_2}{k_2 - k_1} \times e^{-k_1 t} + \frac{k_1}{k_2 - k_1} \times e^{-k_2 t} \right\}$$
$$(iiia)$$

Incubation of 5×10^6 *Staphyloccus aureus*/ml with 5×10^6 granulocytes/ml, in the presence of 10% serum

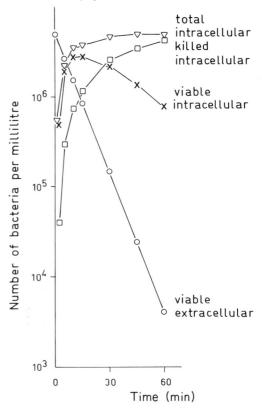

Staphylococcus aureus

Fig. 46.14. Theoretical curves for the numbers of viable extracellular, viable intracellular, and total intracellular bacteria during incubation of 5×10^6 granulocytes/ml and 5×10^6 *S. aureus*/ml in the presence of 10% serum at 37 °C under rotation.

at 37 °C, resulted in a k_1 value of 0.118 min^{-1} [69] and a k_2 value of 0.026 min^{-1}. Under the assumption of an initial number of 5×10^6 viable extracellular *S. aureus* at $t = 0$, taken together with both k values, the authors obtained the curves for the number of viable extracellular, viable intracellular, and killed bacteria, as shown in Fig. 46.14.

Intracellular killing by human monocytes

An example of the intracellular killing of *S. aureus* by monocytes from normal healthy donors, after 3 min of phagocytosis of pre-opsonized bacteria—which was determined as the optimal phagocytosis time—is given in Fig. 46.15. The results of this experiment show a rapid decrease in the number of viable *S. aureus* during the first hour of incubation of monocytes containing bacteria in the presence of serum. Comparison of the

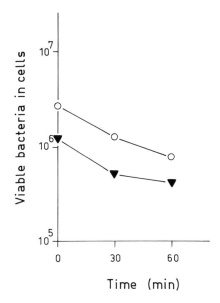

Fig. 46.15. Intracellular killing of *S. aureus* by human monocytes after 15 min of ingestion of the bacteria with serum present (▼) and after 3 min of phagocytosis of pre-opsonized bacteria (○).

rate of intracellular killing by granulocytes and monocytes revealed that granulocytes kill ingested bacteria at a higher rate than monocytes.

Intracellular killing by peritoneal macrophages

Examples of three intracellular killing experiments by peritoneal macrophages are given in Fig. 46.16. These results show the clearance in the numbers of viable intracellular bacteria after *in vitro* phagocytosis of *S. aureus* for 20 min or 30 min at 37 °C, and after *in vivo* phagocytosis for only 3 min. After all ways of ingestion, during re-incubation of macrophages containing bacteria at 37 °C, the number of viable intracellular *S. aureus* decreased by about 70% within 1 h, indicating that the rate of intracellular killing is not influenced by the way of ingestion.

Stimulation of intracellular killing by extracellular serum

Incubation of phagocytes containing ingested bacteria in the presence of extracellular serum resulted (for granulocytes, monocytes, and peritoneal macrophages) in rapid decreases in the number of viable intracellular bacteria (Fig. 46.17); if, however, serum was omitted from the suspension different results were obtained. No intracellular killing was observed for

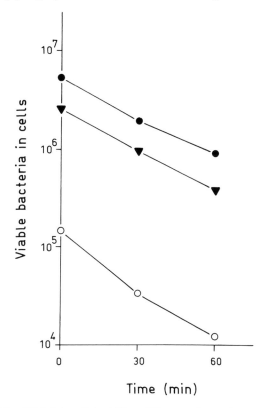

Fig. 46.16. Intracellular killing of *S. aureus* by murine macrophages after 30 min ingestion of bacteria with serum present (▼), 20 min phagocytosis of pre-opsonized bacteria (●), and 3 min *in vivo* phagocytosis after intraperitoneal injection of the bacteria (○).

monocytes, whereas the killing by peritoneal macrophages and granulocytes was suboptimal, indicating the requirement of extracellular serum factors for an optimal intracellular killing. Detailed investigations revealed that phagocytes must be stimulated by extracellular IgG, C3/C3b, and B/Bb interacting via the respective receptors on the cell membrane [94,95].

Concluding remarks

The procedures described in this chapter provide methods for the separate evaluation of the phagocytosis and intracellular killing of micro-organisms by granulocytes, monocytes, and macrophages. Studying the functional capacities of other phagocytes and using other micro-organisms and sera requires appropriate control experiments, as indicated for the various methods to ascertain that valid conclusions are drawn.

Indications for the use of these methods to obtain insight in the functional activities of granulocytes and

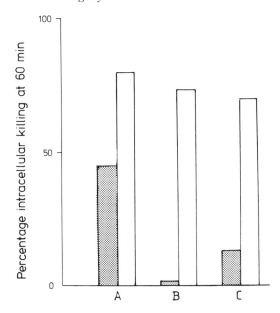

Fig. 46.17. Intracellular killing of *S. aureus* by human granulocytes (A) human monocytes (B) and murine peritoneal macrophages (C) in the presence (open bars) and absence (stippled bars) of extracellular serum. Granulocytes and monocytes, containing *S. aureus* were incubated in the presence of 10% AB-sera; peritoneal macrophages containing *S. aureus* were incubated in 10% murine serum.

mononuclear phagocytes, as well as the activities of humoral factors involved in these processes should be obtained from detailed clinical observation in which a case history with severe infection may be most valuable.

References

1 WALKER R.I. & WILLEMZE R. (1980) Neutrophil kinetics and the regulation of granulopoiesis. *Rev. infect. Dis.* **2**, 282.

2 GOUD TH.J.L.M. & VAN FURTH R. (1975) Proliferative characteristics of monoblast grown *in vitro. J. exp. Med.* **142**, 1200.

3 VAN FURTH R. & DIESSELHOFF-DEN DULK M.M.C. (1970) The kinetics of promonocytes and monocytes in the bone marrow. *J. exp. Med.* **132**, 812.

4 VAN FURTH R., VAN DER MEER J.W.M., BLUSSÉ VAN OUD ALBLAS A. & SLUITER W. (1982) Development of mononuclear phagocytes. In *Self-defense mechanisms. Role of macrophages*, (eds. Mizuno D., Cohn Z.A., Takeya K. & Ishida N.), p. 25. University of Tokyo Press/Elsevier Biomedical Press, New York, Amsterdam.

5 HAECKEL E. (1862) *Die Radiolaren*, p. 104. Druck und Verlag von Georg Reimer, Berlin.

6 METCHNIKOFF E. (1892) Leçons sur la pathologie compatu de l'inflammation. G. Masson, Paris.

7 WRIGHT A.E. & DOUGLAS S.R. (1904) An experimental investigation of the role of the blood fluids in connection with phagocytosis. *Proc. Roy. Soc. Lond.* **72**, 357.

8 ALEXANDER M.D. (1980) Specificity of Fc receptors on human monocytes for IgG1 and IgG3. *Int. Archs Allergy appl. Immunol.* **62**, 99.

9 AREND W.P. & MANNIK M. (1975) Quantitative studies on IgG receptors on monocytes. In *Mononuclear Phagocytes in Immunity, Infection and Pathology*, (ed. Van Furth R.), p. 303. Blackwell Scientific Publications, Oxford.

10 HUBER H., POLLEY M.J., LINSCOTT W.D., FUDENBERG H.H. & MÜLLER-EBERHARD H.J. (1968) Human monocytes: distinct receptor sites for the third component of complement and for immunoglobulin G. *Science*, **162**, 1281.

11 MESSNER R.P. & JELINEK J. (1970) Receptors for human γG globulin on human neutrophils. *J. clin. Invest.* **49**, 2165.

12 BIANCO C. (1977) Plasma membrane receptors for complement. In *Biological Amplification Systems in Immunity*, (eds. Day V.K. & Good R.A.), p. 69. Plenum Press, New York.

13 EHLENBERGER A.G. & NUSSENZWEIG V. (1977) The role of membrane receptors for C3b and C3d in phagocytosis. *J. exp. Med.* **145**, 357.

14 VAN FURTH R., RAEBURN J.A. & VAN ZWET T.L. (1979) Characteristics of human mononuclear phagocytes. *Blood*, **54**, 485.

15 GRIFFIN F.M., GRIFFIN J.A., LEIDER J. & SILVERSTEIN S.C. (1975) Studies on the mechanism of phagocytosis. (I) Requirements for circumferential attachment of particle-bound ligands to specific receptors in the macrophage plasma membrane. *J. exp. Med.* **142**, 1263.

16 GRIFFIN F.M., GRIFFIN J.A. & SILVERSTEIN S.C. (1976) Studies on the mechanism of phagocytosis. (II) The interaction of macrophages with anti-immunoglobulin IgG-coated bone marrow derived lymphocytes. *J. exp. Med.* **144**, 788.

17 RABINOVITCH M. (1968) Phagocytosis: the engulfment stage. *Semin. Hematol.* **5**, 134.

18 BEVILACQUA M.P., AMRANI D., MOSESSON M.W. & BIANCO C. (1981) Receptors for cold-insoluble globulin (plasma fibronectin) on human monocytes. *J. exp. Med.* **153**, 42.

19 CZOP J.K., FEARON D.T. & AUSTEN K.F. (1978) Opsonin-independent phagocytosis of activators of the alternative complement pathway by human monocytes. *J. Immunol.* **120**, 1132.

20 SABA T.M., NICHANS G.D. & DILLON B.C. (1981) Reticuloendothelial response to shock and trauma; its relationship to disturbances in fibronectin and cardiopulmonary function. In *Pathophysiology of the reticuloendothelial system*, (eds. Altura B.M. & Saba T.M.), p. 131. Raven Press, New York.

21 WEIR D.M. & ÖGMUNDSDOTTIR H.M. (1980) Cellular recognition by phagocytes: role of lectin-like receptors. In *Mononuclear Phagocytes—Functional Aspects. Part I*, (ed. Van Furth R.), p. 865. Nijhoff (Martinus) Publishers B.V.

22 VAN OSS C.J. (1978) Phagocytosis as a surface phenomenon. *Ann. Rev. Microbiol.* **32**, 19.

23 SHAW D.R. & GRIFFIN F.M. jun. (1981) Phagocytosis requires repeated triggering of macrophage phagocytic receptors during particle ingestion. *Nature*, **289**, 409.

24 BABIOR B.M. (1978) Oxygen-dependent microbial killing by phagocytes. *New Engl J. Med.* **298**, 659, 721.

25 JOHNSTON R.B. jun., LEYMEYER J.E. & GUTHRIE L.A. (1976) Generation of superoxide anion and chemiluminescence by human monocytes during phagocytosis and on contact with surface-bound immunoglobulin G. *J. exp. Med.* **143**, 1551.

26 KAPLAN E.L., LAXDALL T. & QUIE P.G. (1968) Studies of polymorphonuclear leucocytes from patients with chronic granulomatous disease of childhood; bactericidal capacity for streptococci. *Pediatrics*, **41**, 591.

27 ROSSI F., ROMEO D. & PATRIARCA P. (1972) Mechanism of phagocytosis-associated oxidative metabolism in polymorphonuclear leukocytes and macrophages. *J. Reticuloendothel. Soc.* **12**, 127.

28 KLEBANOFF S.J. & CLARK R.A. (1977) Iodination by human polymorphonuclear leukocytes: a re-evalution. *J. Lab. Clin. Med.* **89**, 675.

29 ROOT R.K. & STOSSEL T.P. (1974) Myeloperoxidase-mediated iodination by granulocytes: intracellular site of operation and some regulating factors. *J. clin. Invest.* **53**, 1207.

30 QUIE P.G. (1972) Clinical manifestations of chronic granulomatous disease of childhood: a congenital defect in phagocyte function. In *Phagocyte mechanisms in health and disease*, (eds. Williams R.C. & Fudenberg H.D.), p. 139. Intercontinental Medical, New York.

31 RODEY G.E., PARK B.H., WINDHORST D.B. & GOOD R.A. (1969) Defective bactericidal activity of monocytes in fatal granulomatous disease. *Blood*, **33**, 813.

32 SPITZNAGEL J.K., DALLDORF F.G., LEFELL M.S., FOLDS J.D., WELSH I.R.H., COONEY M.H. & MARTIN L.E. (1974) Characterization of azurophilic and specific granules purified from human polymorphonuclear leukocytes. *Lab. Invest.* **30**, 774.

33 ORAM J.D. & REITER B. (1968) Inhibition of bacteria by lactoferrin and other non-chelating agents. *Biochim. Biophys. Acta*, **170**, 351.

34 MANDELL G.L. (1970) Intraphagosomal pH of human polymorphonuclear neutrophils. *Proc. Soc. exp. Biol. Med.* **134**, 447.

35 HIRSCH J.G. (1956) Phagocytin: a bactericidal substance from polymorphonuclear leukocytes. *J. exp. Med.* **103**, 589.

36 HIRSCH J.G. (1960) Further studies on the preparation and properties of phagocytin. *J. exp. Med.* **111**, 323.

37 LEHRER R.I. (1972) Functional aspects of a second mechanism of candidacidal activity by human neutrophils. *J. clin. Invest.* **51**, 2566.

38 ODEBERG H. & OLSSON I. (1975) Antibacterial activity of cationic proteins from human granulocytes. *J. clin. Invest.* **56**, 1118.

39 WEISS J., FRANSON R.C., BECKERDITE S., SCHMEIDLER K. & ELSBACH P. (1975) Partial characterization and purification of a rabbit granulocyte factor that increases permeability of *E. coli. J. clin. Invest.* **55**, 33.

40 MACKANESS G.B. (1962) Cellular resistance to infection. *J. exp. Med.* **116**, 381.

41 COHN Z.A. (1978) The activation of mononuclear phagocytes. Fact, fancy and future. *J. Immunol.* **121**, 813.

42 MURRAY H.W. (1981) Interaction of Leishmania with a macrophage cell line. Correlation between intracellular killing and the generation of oxygen intermediates. *J. exp. Med.* **153**, 1690.

43 NATHAN C., NOGUEIRA N., JUANGBHANICK C., ELLIS J. & COHN Z. (1979) Activation of macrophages *in vivo* and *in vitro*. Correlation between hydrogen peroxide release and killing of *Trypanosoma cruzi. J. exp. Med.* **149**, 1056.

44 WILSON C.B., TSAI V. & REMINGTON J.S. (1980) Failure to trigger the oxidative metabolic burst by normal macrophages. Possible mechanism for survival of intracellular pathogens. *J. exp. Med.* **151**, 328.

45 BOUVENG R., SCHMIDT B. & SJÖGVIST J. (1975) Estimation of RES phagocytosis and catabolism in man by the use of ^{125}I-labeled micro-aggregates of human serum albumin. *J. Reticuloendothel. Soc.* **18**, 151.

46 KAVET R.J. & BRAIN J.D. (1980) Methods to quantify endocytosis. *J. Reticuloendothel. Soc.* **27**, 201.

47 NORMANN S.J. (1973) The kinetics of phagocytosis. *J. Reticuloendothel. Soc.* **14**, 587.

48 STIFFEL C., MOUTON D. & BIOZZI G. (1970) Kinetics of the phagocytic function of reticuloendothelial macrophages *in vivo*. In *Mononuclear Phagocytes*, (ed. Van Furth R.), p. 335. Blackwell Scientific Publications, Oxford.

49 SABA T.M. & DILUZIO M.R. (1966) Kupffer cell phagocytosis and metabolism of a variety of particles as a function of opsonization. *J. Reticuloendothel. Soc.* **2**, 437.

50 BRANDT L. (1967) Studies on the phagocytic activity of neutrophilic leukocytes. *Scand. J. Haematol.* (suppl. 2).

51 CAPO C., BONGRAND P., BENOLIEL A.M. & DEPIEDS R. (1979) Non-specific recognition in phagocytosis: ingestion of aldehyde-treated erythrocytes by rat peritoneal macrophages. *Immunology*, **36**, 501.

52 VAN FURTH R. & DIESSELHOFF-DEN DULK M.M.C. (1980) Method to prove ingestion of particles by macrophages with light microscopy. *Scand. J. Immunol.* **12**, 265.

53 WEISSMAN R.A. & KORN E.D. (1967) Phagocytosis of latex beads by acanthamoeba. (I) Biochemical properties. *Biochemistry*, **6**, 485.

54 TAN J.S., WATANAKUNAKORN C. & PHAIR J.P. (1971) A modified assay of neutrophil function: use of lysostaphin to differentiate defective phagocytosis from impaired intracellular killing. *J. Lab. Clin. Med.* **78**, 316.

55 HÄLLGREN R. & STALENHEIM G. (1976) Quantification of phagocytosis by human neutrophils. The use of radiolabeled staphylococcal protein A-IgG complexes. *Immunology*, **30**, 755.

56 MICHELL R.H., PANCAKE S.J., NOSEWORTHY J. & KARNOVSKY M.L. (1969) Measurement of rates of phagocytosis. The use of cellular monolayers. *J. Cell Biol.* **40**, 216.

57 STOSSEL T.P., MASON R.J., HARTWIG J. & VAUGHAN M. (1972) Quantitative studies of phagocytosis by polymorphonuclear leukocytes: use of emulsions to measure the initial rate of phagocytosis. *J. clin. Invest.* **51**, 615.

58 VERHOEF J., PETERSON P.K. & QUIE P.G. (1977) Kinetics

of staphylococcal opsonization, attachment, ingestion and killing by human polymorphonuclear leukocytes: a quantitative assay using ³H-thymidine labeled bacteria. *J. immunol. Meth.* **14**, 303.

59 VRAY B., HOEBEKE J., SAINT-GUILLAIN M., LELOUP R. & STROSBERG A.D. (1980) A new quantitative fluorimetric assay for phagocytosis of bacteria. *Scand. J. Immmunol.* **11**, 147.

60 YAMAMURA M., BOLER J. & VALDIMARSSON H. (1977) Phagocytosis measured as inhibition of uridine uptake by *Candida albicans. J. immunol. Meth.* **14**, 19.

61 STOSSEL TH.P. (1974) Phagocytosis. *New Engl J. Med.* **290**, 717, 774 & 833.

62 COHN Z.A. & MORSE S.I. (1959) Interactions between rabbit polymorphonuclear leucocytes and staphylococci. *J. exp. Med.* **110**, 419.

63 GRANGE M.J., ECKE F., DRESCH C. & NAJEAN Y. (1975) A new method for measuring simultaneously the phagocytic and bactericidal capacity of human leukocytes. *Biomedicine*, **23**, 414.

64 LI J.W., MUDD J. & KAPRAL F.A. (1963) Dissociation of phagocytosis and intracellular killing of *Staphylococcus aureus* by human blood leukocytes. *J. Immunol.* **90**, 805.

65 MAALØE O. (1946) *On the relation between alexin and opsonin.* Thesis, Munksgaard, Copenhagen.

66 PITT J. & BERNHEIMER H.P. (1974) Role of peroxide in phagocytic killing of pneumococci. *Infect. Immun.* **9**, 48.

67 YAMAMURA M., BOLER J. & VALDIMARSSON (1976) A ⁵¹chromium release assay for phagocytic killing of *Candida albicans. J. immunol. Meth.* **13**, 227.

68 CRAIG C.P. & SUTER E. (1966) Extracellular factors influencing staphylocidal capacity of human polymorphonuclear leukocytes. *J. Immunol.* **97**, 287.

69 LEIJH P.C.J., VAN DEN BARSELAAR, VAN ZWET TH.L., DUBBELDEMAN-REMPT Y. & VAN FURTH R. (1979) Kinetics of phagocytosis of *Staphylococcus aureus* and *Escherichia coli* by human granulocytes. *Immunology*, **37**, 453.

70 LEIJH P.C.J., VAN DEN BARSELAAR M.TH. & VAN FURTH R. (1981) Kinetics of phagocytosis and intracellular killing of *Staphylococcus aureus* and *Escherichia coli* by human monocytes. *Scand. J. Immunol.* **13**, 159.

71 CASCIATO D.A., BLUESTONE R. & GOLDBERG L.S. (1977) Comparison of killing of bacteria by guinea pig neutrophils and monocytes. *J. Lab. Clin. Med.* **90**, 273.

72 ORLOWSKI J.P., SIEGER L. & ANTHONY B.F. (1976) Bactericidal capacity of monocytes of newborn infants. *J. Pediat.* **89**, 797.

73 PETERSON P.K., VERHOEF J., SABATH L.D. & QUIE P.G. (1976) Extracellular and bacterial factors influencing staphylococcal phagocytosis and killing by human polymorphonuclear leukocytes. *Infect. Immun.* **14**, 496.

74 STEIGBIGEL R.T., LAMBERT L.H. & REMINGTON J.S. (1974) Phagocytic and bactericidal properties of normal human monocytes. *J. clin. Invest.* **53**, 131.

75 LEIJH P.C.J., VAN DEN BARSELAAR M.TH., DUBBELDE-MAN-REMPT I. & VAN FURTH R. (1980) Kinetics of intracellular killing of *Staphylococcus aureus* and *Escherichia coli* by human granulocytes. *Eur. J. Immunol.* **10**, 750.

76 LEIJH P.C.J., VAN DEN BARSELAAR M.TH., VAN ZWET TH.L., DAHA M.R. & VAN FURTH R. (1979) Requirement of extracellular complement and immunoglobulin for

intracellular killing of micro-organisms by human monocytes. *J. clin. Invest.* **4**, 772.

77 HOLMES B., QUIE P.G., WINDHORST D.B., POLLARA B. & GOOD R.A. (1966) Protection of phagocytized bacteria from the killing action of antibiotics. *Nature*, **210**, 1131.

78 MACKANESS G.B. (1960) The phagocytosis and inactivation of staphylococci by macrophages of normal rabbits. *J. exp. Med.* **112**, 35.

79 BRUMFITT W., GLYNN A.A. & PERCIVAL A. (1965) Factors influencing the phagocytosis of *Escherichia coli.* *Br. J. Path.* **46**, 213.

80 COLE P. & BROSTOFF J. (1975) Intracellular killing of *Listeria* monocytogenes by activated macrophages (Mackaness system) is due to antibiotic. *Nature*, **256**, 515.

81 EASMON C.S.F. (1979) The effect of antibiotics on the intracellular survival of *Staphylococcus aureus in vitro. Br. J. exp. Path.* **60**, 24.

82 VAN DEN BROEK P.J., DEHUE F.A.M., LEIJH P.C.J., VAN DEN BARSELAAR M.TH. & VAN FURTH R. (1982) The use of lysostaphin in *in vitro* assays of phagocyte functions: adherence to and penetration into granulocytes. *Scand. J. Immunol.* **15**, 467.

83 KARNOVSKY M.L., SIMMONS S., GLASS E.A., SHAFER A.W. & D'ARCY P. (1970) Metabolism of macrophages. In *Mononuclear Phagocytes*, (ed. Van Furth R.), p. 103. Blackwell Scientific Publications, Oxford.

84 KLEBANOFF S.J. & CLARK R.A. (1978) *The neutrophil. Function and Clinical Disorders.* North–Holland Publishing Co., Amsterdam, New York, Oxford.

85 ROBERTS R.B. (1967) The interaction *in vitro* between group B meningococci and rabbit polymorphonuclear leukocytes. Demonstration of type specific opsonins and bactericidins. *J. exp. Med.* **126**, 795.

86 BØYEM A. (1968) Separation of leucocytes from blood and bone marrow. *Scand. J. clin. Lab. Invest.* **21**, (suppl. 97).

87 LEIJH P.C.J., VAN DEN BARSELAAR M.R., DAHA M.R. & VAN FURTH R. (1982) Stimulation of the intracellular killing of *Staphylococcus aureus* by monocytes: regulation by immunoglobin G and complement components C3/C3b and B/Bb. *J. Immunol.* **129**, 322.

88 FIGDOR C.G., BONT W.S., DE VRIES J.E. & VAN ES W.L. (1981) Isolation of large numbers of highly purified lymphocytes and monocytes with a modified centrifuged elutiation technique. *J. immunol. Meth.* **40**, 275.

89 ADAMS D.O., EDELSON P.J. & KOREN H.S. (1981) *Methods for studying mononuclear phagocytes.* Academic Press, New York, London.

90 HERSCOWITZ H.B., HOLDEN H.T., BELLANTI J.A. & GHAFFEN A. (1981) *Manual of Macrophage Methodology, collection, characterization and function.* Marcel Dekker Inc., New York, Basel.

91 LEIJH P.C.J., VAN DEN BARSELAAR M.TH. & VAN FURTH R. (1977) The kinetics of phagocytosis and intracellular killing of *Candida albicans* by granulocytes and monocytes. *Infect. Immun.* **17**, 313.

92 MARÓDI L., LEIJH P.C.J. & VAN FURTH R. (1983) A Micromethod for the separate evaluation of phagocytosis and intracellular killing of *Staphylococcus aureus* by human monocytes and granulocytes. *J. immunol. Meth.* **57**, 353.

93 LEIJH P.C.J., VAN ZWET TH.L. & VAN FURTH R. (1980)

Effect of extracellular serum in the simulation of intracellular killing of streptococci by human monocytes. *Infect. Immun.* **30**, (no. 2), 421.

94 LEIJH P.C.J., VAN DEN BARSELAAR M.TH., DAHA M.R. & VAN FURTH R. (1981) Participation of immunoglobulins and complement components in the intracellular killing of *Staphylococcus aureus* and *Escherichia coli* by human granulocytes. *Infect. Immun.* **33**, 714.

Chapter 47
Secreted proteins of resting and activated macrophages

ZENA WERB, M. J. BANDA, R. TAKEMURA & S. GORDON

Macrophages as secretory cells, 47.1

Markers for resting, inflammatory, and activated macrophages, 47.6

Regulation of secretion by macrophages, 47.7

General concepts for identification and assay of specific secretion products of macrophages, 47.8

Method for biosynthetic radiolabelling of cellular and secreted proteins of mononuclear phagocytes, 47.9

Method for SDS-polyacrylamide gradient gel electrophoresis of labelled macrophage proteins, 47.10

Methods for the assay of plasminogen activator, 47.14

Method for the assay of macrophage elastase, 47.21

Methods for the assay of macrophage lysozyme, 47.24

Macrophages are specialized phagocytic cells, collectively known as the mononuclear phagocyte system, that originate in bone marrow and are then widely distributed in tissues such as liver and spleen [1–3]. The mononuclear phagocytes play an important role in the ability of the host to respond to injury and infection and in resistance to tumour cells. Macrophages are long-lived, actively endocytic cells that display a remarkable responsiveness to various stimuli in their environment. In particular, in the course of certain infections such as listeriosis, tuberculosis and trypanosomiasis, macrophages may become metabolically activated, show increased plasma membrane and phagocytic activity, and acquire an enhanced microbicidal capacity for the infectious agents and for unrelated organisms [4–8]. As biochemical markers suitable for study are made available, the mechanism and regulation of the macrophage phenotypes are being elucidated.

Macrophages as secretory cells

While early studies of macrophages emphasized their prominent endocytic activity, the importance of the secretory activities of macrophages has been recognized only in the past decade. Macrophages secrete into their milieu a large variety of biologically active substances that are important in many macrophage functions, such as immunoregulation and the killing of microbes and tumours [124]. The secretory products of macrophages are not all secreted by a single macrophage simultaneously but are regulated as cells display distinct secretion phenotypes under developmental or environmental control [9,10]. Some products are constitutively secreted (e.g. lysozyme [11]), others are secreted by inflammatory and activated macrophages (e.g. plasminogen activator [12–14]), some are secreted only by activated macrophages (e.g. H_2O_2 [14–16]), and others are secreted in response to specific stimuli (e.g. angiogenesis factor from hypoxic macrophages [17]).

Macrophages secrete a variety of enzymes that participate in a wide range of functions, such as accelerating inflammation, clearing up the debris in inflammation sites, killing tumours, and metabolizing lipoproteins (Table 47.1).

Most of the secreted proteinases of macrophages are active at physiologic pH (Table 47.2) [18,19,125]. In general, these proteinases have a small intracellular compartment and are continuously secreted by inflammatory and activated macrophages, whereas unstimulated macrophages have low rates of proteinase secretion [14]. Although there seems to be some co-ordination in the regulation of secretion of different enzymes, the precise regulation differs.

Three types of collagenase that differ in specificity are secreted by macrophages. One collagenase similar to other classic mammalian collagenases cleaves types I, II, and III collagen (interstitial collagens) specifically into one-quarter and three-quarter fragments [18,20]. This collagenase is a metalloproteinase and is secreted mostly in a latent form, from which the active enzyme can be generated by proteinases such as plasmin or trypsin. Secretion of this collagenase is low compared to that from fibroblasts, and purification has not been achieved. A second metalloproteinase,

Table 47.1 Enzymes secreted by macrophages

Product	Synonyms	Regulation*	Function
Plasminogen activators	Urokinase	B^1, G	Inflammatory
Collagenase I, II, III		B^1	Inflammatory
Collagenase IV		B^1	Inflammatory
Collagenase V		B^1	Inflammatory
Elastase	Proteoglycan-degrading enzyme, myelin basic protein-degrading enzyme	B^2, G	Inflammatory
Cytolytic proteinase		B^3	Tumoricidal
Complement components C1, C2 Factor B Factor D Factor I		E	Antimicrobial, inflammatory opsonic
Coagulation factors Factor VII Factor IX Factor X		D	Coagulation, tissue repair
Angiotensin-converting enzyme		F^1	Activation of angiotensin
Acid hydrolases	Lysosomal enzymes, acid glycosidases, cathepsin	B^1	Inflammatory
Arginase		B^1	Antimicrobial, tumoricidal, immunoregulatory
Lysozyme		A	Antimicrobial
Lipoprotein lipase		A	Metabolism of lipoproteins

* A, constitutive; B^1, increased in inflammatory or activated macrophages; B^2, increased in inflammatory but not activated macrophages; B^3, increased in activated but not inflammatory macrophages; D, not determined; E, various; F^1, increased by glucocorticoids; G, varies during differentiation of mononuclear phagocytes.

which cleaves type V collagen, can be separated from classic collagenase by ion-exchange chromatography [21]. A third macrophage enzyme degrades basement membrane type IV collagen [22].

Macrophage elastase is a metalloproteinase, whereas pancreatic and polymorphonuclear leucocyte elastases are serine proteinases [23,24]. The proteolytic cleavage of elastin by macrophage elastase is more limited than cleavage by other mammalian elastases, and elastinolytic activity in macrophage culture medium is activated by sodium dodecyl sulphate [13, 24]. Macrophage elastase is capable of limited proteolysis of immunoglobulin G, fibrinogen, cartilage proteoglycan, myelin basic protein, and α_1-proteinase inhibitor [24–29]. This elastase constitutes approximately 0.1% of the total protein secreted by thioglycollate-elicited mouse macrophages. Elastase secretion is increased in inflammatory macrophages but is decreased in activated macrophages [13,14].

Macrophage plasminogen activators are serine proteinases [12]. There are several mammalian plasminogen activators, including urokinase and tissue activator [30]. The predominant mouse macrophage plasminogen activator has a relative molecular mass of 48 000 [12], similar to the enzyme secreted by virally transformed fibroblasts, and is probably urokinase-like. In addition to the secreted form, macrophage plasminogen activator is also located on the cell surface and can be isolated in membrane fractions [31, 32]. A proteinase cytolytic to neoplastic cells has been reported to be secreted by activated macrophages but not by stimulated macrophages and is therefore likely to differ from the other proteinases [33]. Macrophage secretions contain a number of serine esterases that have not been characterized [12,34].

Macrophages also secrete angiotensin-converting enzyme, an exopeptidase that cleaves the carboxyl-terminal dipeptide of angiotensin I to form an active vasoconstrictor, angiotensin II [35]. It is actively secreted by glucocorticoid-treated macrophages [35], whereas secretion of the neutral proteinases is decreased by glucocorticoids [36]. Secretion of angioten-

Table 47.2. Classification of macrophage proteinases

Proteinase class	Enzyme	pH Optimum
Aspartic (EC 3.4.23)	Cathepsin D	3–5
Cysteine (EC 3.4.22)	Cathepsin B	4–7
	Cathepsin N (collagenolytic)	
Serine (EC 3.4.21)	Plasminogen activator	7–9
	C1	
	C2	
	C3	
	C5	
	Factor B	
	Factor D	
	Casein-degrading proteinase	
Metallo (EC 3.4.24)	Collagenase (types I, II, III)	7–9
	Type V-specific collagenase	
	Macrophage elastase	
Not classified	Prothrombinase	Neutral
	Amyloid-degrading proteinase	Neutral

sin-converting enzyme is increased in certain pathologic conditions, such as sarcoidosis, Gaucher's disease, and leprosy; however, the role of this enzyme in these diseases is not clear.

Macrophage acid hydrolases are usually contained within the cells in lysosomes, but they can be secreted under certain conditions [37]. The secreted hydrolases are mainly the enzymically active precursor forms of acid glycosidases (unpublished observation). The function of extracellularly secreted acid hydrolases is not clear. Their activity in the extracellular environment is likely to be limited when the pH is neutral. Under some conditions, when the pH of the environment surrounding the cells becomes acidic, these enzymes may degrade extracellular macromolecules [13].

Arginase is secreted by activated macrophages, and it has been suggested that the depletion of arginine by arginase is responsible for some of the cytotoxic activity of macrophages against malignant cells [38, 39]. The arginase secreted by macrophages may also suppress lymphocyte immune function [39] and may be cytotoxic to *Schistosoma mansoni* [40].

Lysozyme (relative molecular mass 14 000) is an enzyme that hydrolyses the N-acetylmuramic-$\beta(1\rightarrow4)$-N-acetylglucosamine linkages of peptidoglycan in the bacterial cell wall. It is a major, constitutive secretory product of macrophages and is secreted by unstimulated and inflammatory macro-

phages to a similar extent [11]. Lysozyme may participate in the extracellular killing of micro-organisms. Macrophage lysozyme is indistinguishable from lysozyme of polymorphonuclear leucocytes in its substrate specificity, size, and inhibition of activity by specific antisera [11]. Macrophages secrete lipoprotein lipase, which cleaves triglyceride in triglyceride-rich lipoproteins, such as chylomicrons or very low density lipoproteins, releasing fatty acids and monoglycerides [41].

Macrophages secrete or release a group of protein enzyme inhibitors [42,126], including α_2-macroglobulin, a major plasma proteinase inhibitor of broad specificity [43]. The significance of macrophage-derived enzyme inhibitors is not known. However, they may be important in the regulation of enzyme activities within the environment surrounding macrophages. Although secretion of both enzymes and enzyme inhibitors by the same cell may be puzzling, it is reasonable that cells possess mechanisms to regulate the activities of their own secretory products [19,44]. Macrophages have a plasma membrane receptor for α_2-macroglobulin-proteinase complexes that participates in clearing proteinases inactivated by α_2-macroglobulin from the extracellular milieu [45].

Macrophages secrete a number of plasma proteins that participate in inflammation, tissue repair, immunoregulation, and molecular transport, including some of the complement components, coagulation factors, opsonins, transport proteins, and enzyme inhibitors (Table 47.3). The complement system consists of about twenty plasma proteins. Although the sites of biosynthesis of these proteins seem to be distributed among various cell types and organs [46], the liver is probably the primary site of synthesis of C3, C6, C8, properdin, and factor B. Macrophages synthesize C3, C4, C5, factor B, factor D, properdin, and factor H (β1H), as well as the enzymes C1, C2, factor B, factor D, and factor I (C3b inactivator) [47,48, 127,128]. Macrophages secrete coagulation factors VII, IX, X, and V [49,50] and, in addition, have procoagulant activity on their cell surfaces [51]. Through these secretory products macrophages may contribute to the deposition of fibrin, which is important in tissue repair and immunologically induced tissue injuries.

Apolipoprotein E is one of the major secretory products of macrophages [14,52]. Its secretion is stimulated when resident macrophages ingest large quantities of cholesterol [52]. As a component of plasma lipoproteins, apolipoprotein E may participate in cholesterol and triglyceride transport to the liver [52]. Apolipoprotein E also is suppressive for lymphocyte function [53,54]. It is interesting that after activation of macrophages with Gram-negative

Table 47.3. Plasma proteins secreted by macrophages

Product	Synonyms	Regulation*	Function
Complement components C1 C2 C3 C4 C5 Factor B Factor D		E	Antimicrobial, inflammatory, opsonic
Factor I	C3b inactivator, C3b INA		
Factor H	β1H		
Properdin			
Fibronectin		E, G	Opsonic, adhesive
Apolipoprotein E	Apoprotein E	C^1, F^2, G	Transport of cholesterol from macrophage to liver, immunoregulatory
Transcobalamin II		B^1	Transport of vitamin B12 to tissues
Coagulation factors Factor VII Factor IX Factor X Factor V		D	Coagulation, tissue repair
α_2-Macroglobulin		G	Regulation of plasma enzyme activities
Thrombospondin		C^1, G	Adhesive
α_1-Proteinase inhibitor			

* B^1, increased in inflammatory or activated macrophages; C^1, decreased in activated macrophages; D, not determined; E, various; F^2, increased by cholesterol; G, varies during differentiation of mononuclear phagocytes.

organisms or endotoxin, apolipoprotein E secretion is suppressed [14,55], and that under these conditions cellular and humoral immunity may be stimulated. Apolipoprotein E synthesis is also developmentally regulated [56].

Fibronectin accounts for up to 5% of the secreted proteins of macrophages [14,57,58]. It is not secreted by monocytes, but its secretion is initiated once these cells differentiate to mature macrophages [57]. Monocytes have receptors for fibronectin on their surface and can use these for attachment [59]. Fibronectin also serves as an opsonin for phagocytosis by macrophages [60,124]. Macrophages secrete a variety of other plasma proteins, including transcobalamin II, a vitamin B12 transport protein [61], and thrombospondin, an adhesive molecule also contained in platelet granules [121].

Macrophages secrete a variety of factors, most likely polypeptides, that participate in body defence mechanisms by regulating functions of other cells (Table 47.4). These factors include interferon, an anti-viral factor [62,63]; factors cytotoxic to cells or microbes [64]; angiogenesis factor [17,65] and mitogens, which stimulate proliferation of fibroblasts and endothelial cells to promote wound healing [17, 66]; myeloid colony-stimulating factors [67]; tumour necrosis factor (cachectin) [130]; and interleukin 1 [68], which stimulates the immune response by acting on T cells [69]. Macrophages participate in acute phase response as well by generating fever via secretion of endogenous pyrogen [70] and promoting synthesis by the liver of acute phase proteins such as amyloid A and haptoglobin [71,72]. Because the biochemical nature of every factor is not yet well defined, some of the factors described by different functions may turn out to be the same molecule. It is already becoming apparent that interleukin 1, a polypeptide of relative molecular mass 14 000, plays multiple roles. Endo-

Table 47.4. Substances secreted by macrophages that regulate function or growth of other cells

Product	Synonyms	Regulation*	Function
Interferon	Non-immune interferon	B[1]	Anti-viral
Interleukin 1	Lymphocyte-activating factor	B[1]	Immunoregulatory, acute phase response (fever, acute phase protein synthesis)
	Endogenous pyrogen		
	Acute phase protein synthesis factor		
Tumour necrosis factor	Cachect	—	Anti-tumour, decreases triglyceride stores
Angiogenesis factor		F[3]	Tissue repair
Mitogen for fibroblasts	Interleukin 1	B[1]	Tissue repair, regulates fibroblasts
Mitogen for endothelial cells		B[1]	Tissue repair, regulates endothelial cells
Serum amyloid A synthesis stimulating factor	Interleukin 1	B[1]	Acute phase response, regulates hepatocytes
Haptoglobulin synthesis stimulating factor	Interleukin 1	B[1]	Acute phase response regulates hepatocytes
Collagenase and prostaglandin E stimulating factor	Interleukin 1	B[1]	Inflammatory, regulates rheumatoid synovial cells
Listeria growth inhibitory factor		B[1]	Antimicrobial
Erythropoietin			Regulates erythroid differentiation
G/M-CSF			Regulates myeloid differentiation

* B[1], increased by activation; F[3], increased by hypoxia.

Table 47.5. Low molecular weight substances secreted by macrophages

Product	Synonyms	Regulation*	Function
O_2^- (superoxide)		B[1]	Microbicidal, tumoricidal
H_2O_2 (hydrogen peroxide)		B[1]	Microbicidal, tumoricidal
OH· (hydroxylradical)		B[1]	Microbicidal, tumoricidal
$^1O_2$ (singlet oxygen)		B[1]	Microbicidal, tumoricidal
Prostaglandin E1		D	Inflammatory, immunoregulatory
Prostaglandin E2		C[2]	Inflammatory, immunoregulatory
6-Ketoprostaglandin F1α		D	Inflammatory, immunoregulatory
Thromboxane B2		D	Inflammatory, immunoregulatory
Leucotriene C	Slow-reacting substance of anaphylaxis	D	Inflammatory, immunoregulatory
12-Hydroxyeicosatetranoic acid		D	Inflammatory, immunoregulatory
Platelet-activating factor		D	Inflammatory, activates platelets
cAMP		F[4]	Cellular regulation for many types of cells
Thymidine		D	Tumoricidal
Uracil		D	Not known
Uric acid		D	Not known
Pteroyl metabolite		D	Not known

* B[1], increased in inflammatory or activated macrophages; C[2], decreased in inflammatory or activated macrophages; D, not determined; F[4], induced by prostaglandin E1.

genous pyrogen, which acts on the hypothalamus to change the set point of body temperature [73], and acute phase protein synthesis promotion factor [74] both seem to be interleukin 1. Interleukin 1 also promotes synthesis of collagenase and prostaglandin E by rheumatoid synovial cells [75] and promotes synthesis of collagen by fibroblasts [76]; therefore it may be involved in rheumatoid arthritis as well. Interleukin 1 has recently been cloned [131]. Erythropoietin, a factor promoting differentiation of erythroid precursors, is also secreted by macrophages [122].

In addition to the other proteins described, macrophages secrete at least two kinds of low molecular weight substances—reactive metabolites of oxygen [15,16,77–79], bioactive derivatives of arachidonate [80–84], and purine, pyrimidine and pteroyl metabolites [85–87] (Table 47.5). These are not truly secretory products, because they are not secreted by the fusion of secretory vesicles to plasma membranes, but they are released extracellularly or may diffuse out from macrophages. These products are dealt with in detail in other Chapter 50.

Table 47.6. Inflammatory macrophages compared to quiescent resident macrophages

---

Non-specific inflammatory events
    Increased size
    Increased rate of spreading
    Increased adherence to glass
    Increased rate and extent of phagocytosis
        IgG-coated particles
        C3b-coated particles
    Modification of plasma membrane ectoenzymes
        Decreased 5′-nucleotidase
        Increased alkaline phosphodiesterase
    Increased rate of fluid-phase pinocytosis
    Secreted proteins
        Increased plasminogen activator
        Increased elastase
        Increased collagenase
    Increased cellular ATP
    Increased O_2 consumption, glucose, O_2^- release
    Increased prostaglandin release
    Decreased leucotriene C production

Lymphokine-mediated events
    Decreased 18A rRNA
    Decreased protein secretion
    Increased microbicidal activity
    Increased tumour cytostasis and killing
    Increased H_2O_2 release
    Decreased secretion of apolipoprotein E
    Increased amount of Fc_{2a}-receptor
    Decreased size
    Decreased spreading

Markers for resting, inflammatory, and activated macrophages

Broadly speaking, serous macrophages display three functionally distinct but apparently interconvertible phenotypes, each of which is characterized and defined by a set of markers [6–8]: (1) unstimulated *resident* macrophages, (2) non-specifically *inflammatory* macrophages (e.g. thioglycollate-elicited), and (3) immunologically *activated* macrophages (e.g. bacillus Calmette-Guerin [BCG]-activated) (Table 47.6). Examples of eliciting stimuli that yield macrophages with these characteristics are shown in Table 47.7. For example, an intraperitoneal injection of thioglycollate

Table 47.7. Stimuli for obtaining inflammatory and activated macrophages from animals

Non-specific inflammatory eliciting stimuli	Immunologically activating stimuli
Brewer's thioglycollate broth	Living mycobacteria (BCG)
$NaIO_4$	
Protease peptone broth	γ-interferon
Concanavalin A	Living *Trypanosoma cruzi*
Starch	Killed *Corynebacterium parvum*
Mineral oil	Lipopolysaccharide
	Pyran copolymer

broth elicits a vigorous inflammatory exudate in the mouse and serves as a potent, non-specific method for increasing the yield of inflammatory macrophages (Table 47.8). In culture thioglycollate-elicited macrophages secrete high levels of several proteinases, such as plasminogen activator(s) (PA) and elastase, which are absent or only barely detectable in cultures of untreated resident macrophages (Table 47.8). In contrast, BCG-activated macrophages secrete PA but little elastase. The following evidence shows that proteolytic activities are synthesized and secreted in culture. Total net activity increases up to 50-fold during two days in culture, and progressive extracellular accumulation for as long as two weeks has been demonstrated. The continued release of proteolytic activities is blocked by cycloheximide. Intracellular levels of activity represent less than 20% of total activity produced per day and are usually negligible. Direct evidence for synthesis and secretion of other specific proteins, including elastase, apolipoprotein E, fibronectin, and factor B has been obtained [24,52,57, 88]. Fixed tissue macrophages such as Kupffer cells may be deficient in generating reactive oxygen intermediates [132,133]

Table 47.8. Cellular and secreted proteins of mouse macrophages elicited by various inflammatory stimuli*

Stimulus	Relative ApoE secretion rate‡	Secreted plasminogen activator	5'-Nucleotidase	Secreted elastase	β-Glucuronidase		Macro-phages recovered per mouse
					Cellular	Secreted at 48 h	
		(U/48 h/10^6 cells)	(nmol/min/10^6 cells)	(U/48 h/10^6 cells)	(nmol/min/10^6 cells)		($\times 10^{-6}$)
None	1.0	18	10.1	6.2	45	23	2.1
Concanavalin A, 750 μg	1.5	155	0.4	23.4	256	144	7.4
Thioglycollate,							
0.2 ml	2.0	N.D.§	0.4	26.6	98	92	3.2
1.0 ml	2.0	121	0.5	27.2	114	92	8.1
2.0 ml	1.5	54	1.1	27.2	200	148	20.9
C. parvum, pyridine							
extract, 1 mg	1.0	24	0.4	8.8	34	78	3.3
NaIO$_4$, 0.5 ml of 5 mM	0.5	87	5.7	28.3	155	75	6.6
Complete Freund's							
adjuvant, 0.1 ml	0.4	24	1.0	9.8	44	31	5.6
Pristane, 0.1 ml	0.2	N.D.	0.5	5.0	34	27	3.1
Pyran copolymer, 25 mg/kg	>0.1	116	0.3	1.8	39	38	6.8
Endotoxin, 10 μg	>0.1	108	0.1	1.6	120	93	5.8
BCG, 5×10^6 organisms	>0.1	136	0.1	6.8	52	20	4.8
C. parvum, whole, 1 mg	>0.1	53	>0.5	4.7	N.D.	N.D.	4.9

* Data represent the means of 2–8 experiments, each with duplicate or triplicate determinations.
‡ ApoE secretion, as determined from gels of labelled secreted proteins after 2 h in culture, was normalized for cell protein and resident macrophage secretion was rated 1.
§ N.D., not determined.
Reprinted from ref. 14, with permission of The Rockefeller University Press.

Regulation of secretion by macrophages

In addition to regulation of macrophage secretion by inflammatory stimuli, secretion can be regulated by various effectors in culture. For example, PA can also be induced by allowing macrophages from mice injected with lipopolysaccharide endotoxin to ingest a load of latex particles *in vitro* [89]. The use of such a two-stage induction procedure has made it possible to independently study the role of cell activation *in vivo* and phagocytosis *in vitro*. Macrophage priming is not confined to endotoxin but is also observed after treatment with various other intraperitoneal inflammatory irritants, such as mineral oil. A spectrum of enhanced macrophage fibrinolysis is generally observed, in parallel with the intensity of the inflammatory reaction elicited (Table 47.9). Latex and a variety of other ingested particles, such as *Micrococcus lysodeikticus*, aggregated immunoglobulin G, and immune complexes, all enhance the fibrinolytic activity of macrophages primed by endotoxin. The initial phagocytic trigger is, therefore, not specific for the particular substance used, but the ability to induce a sustained response does depend on the persistence of the phagocytized particle within the cell. Prolonged secretion of PA and other proteolytic activities continues at high levels for many days after uptake of latex, which cannot be digested, whereas PA is secreted only transiently after ingestion of particles that are rapidly degraded, such as *M. lysodeikticus*.

Secretion of PA can also be induced in macrophages by an immunologically specific mechanism. Peritoneal cells from mice infected with BCG or *Trypanosoma cruzi* show a striking enhancement of fibrinolytic activity after challenge with purified protein derivative [90] or heat-killed *T. cruzi* [91], respectively. PA can be induced by exposing unstimulated macrophages to pure, sensitized, specifically challenged lymphocytes or their cell-free products. A high level of PA inducer is found in supernatants from primary and secondary spleen, mixed-leucocyte culture reactions. The PA inducer is closely related to migration inhibition factor [92], which depends on T lymphocytes for its production. Lymphokines have also been reported to enhance release of macrophage collagenase [93]. Recent evidence suggests that the predominant macrophage activating factor is interferon-γ [134,135]. In contrast, apolipoprotein E secretion is down-regulated by macrophage activation [14,55]. Secretion of PA, elastase, and collagenase is decreased by glucocorticoids [36].

Table 47.9. Enhancement of macrophage plasminogen activator

In vivo	BCG infection
	T. cruzi infection
	Thioglycollate broth
	Endotoxin
In vitro	Phagocytosis—latex, micro-organisms, immune complexes
	Lymphokines—mixed leucocyte cultures, BCG, *T. cruzi*
	Plasma (?Hageman factor)
	Concanavalin A
	Phorbol myristate acetate
	N-formyl met-met-met
	EGTA

The induction of the proteinases is regulated independently of that of some other enzymes of macrophages (Table 47.9). Lysozyme is secreted as a bulk product by all macrophages, independent of exogenous stimulation [11], and only partial secretion of acid hydrolases, which are predominantly intracellular digestive enzymes, is induced by activation [14,37]. Compounds such as steroids and colchicine also differentiate among these products [29,36,94]. For example, whereas elastase and collagenase (Fig. 47.1) and PA

[36] are all decreased by glucocorticoids, secretion of lysozyme and acid β-glucuronidase are unaffected [36].

General concepts for identification and assay of specific secretion products of macrophages

A complete description of the protein synthetic phenotype of mononuclear phagocytes involves defining all the biochemical and functional properties of the cells. One approach is to measure enzyme and protein activities of the cells. Another approach is to examine the pattern of mRNA present in a macrophage at any given time. This can be achieved by using specific cloned complementary DNA probes, by translating isolated mRNA in cell-free systems (a process that requires a large number of cells and is unsuitable for examination of many samples), or by studying the translation of mRNA into proteins using the machinery of a live cell. If radiolabelled amino acids are present during translation in live cells, the resulting biosynthesized proteins can be analysed by polyacrylamide gel electrophoresis to give detailed 'fingerprints' of specific macrophage phenotypes [14,95]. These procedures offer high resolution and specificity, require small numbers of cells (as few as 1×10^5), and are applicable to a wide variety of mononuclear phagocytes from man, mouse, rat, rabbit, and guinea-pig. In conjunction with other methods, such as

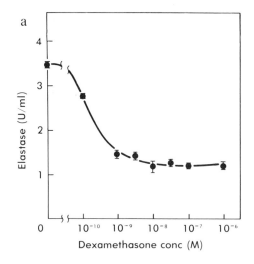 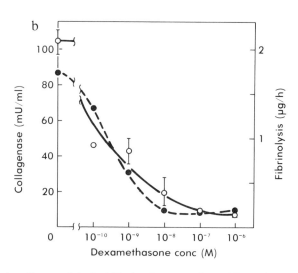

Fig. 47.1. Effect of dexamethasone on secretion of proteinases by adjuvant-elicited rabbit alveolar macrophages. Macrophages were plated at 1.4×10^6 cells/2-cm^2 well. (a) Secretion of elastase was studied by incubating macrophages in DME-LH containing dexamethasone for 96 h; conditioned culture media were then assayed for activity with ^{3}H-elastin-SDS as substrate. Values are shown as mean $\pm$ s.D. (n = 3). (b) Secretion of collagenase and fibrinolytic neutral proteinase was examined by performing enzyme assays on conditioned culture media after 48 h incubation with dexamethasone. Values are shown as mean $\pm$ s.D. (n = 3). Collagenase activity ($\bigcirc$) was determined with radioactive collagen fibrils as substrate. Fibrinolytic activity ($\bullet$) was determined with ^{125}I-fibrin as substrate. Reproduced from ref. 36, with permission of The Rockefeller University Press.

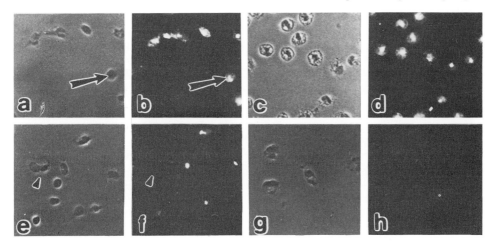

Fig. 47.2. Immunocytochemical localization of apolipoprotein E in mouse peritoneal macrophages cultured for 2 h. (a, b) Resident; (c, d) thioglycollate-elicited; (e, f) sodium periodate-elicited; and (g, h) pyran copolymer-elicited macrophages. Note the macrophages containing extracellular apolipoprotein E (arrows), and macrophages negative for apolipoprotein E (arrowheads). (a, c, e, g) Phase-contrast microscopy; (b, d, f, h) fluorescence microscopy, × 300. Reproduced from ref. 14, with permission of The Rockefeller University Press.

specific immunoprecipitation of labelled proteins and radioimmunoassays, it is possible to examine in detail changes in the properties of macrophages that may not be seen with a single assay such as receptor binding or quantification of a secreted proteolytic enzyme. Some secreted proteins are present in sufficient concentrations intracellularly to be detected by immunolocalization (e.g. apolipoprotein E, Fig. 47.2). Such methods can also be used to assess heterogeneity in macrophage populations. In addition, these methods can be used to detect contamination by other cell populations by searching for biosynthesized proteins specific for those cells. Further study, using the methods described here, should establish the role of these proteins in the protective and injurious effects of cell-mediated immunity.

Method for biosynthetic radiolabelling of cellular and secreted proteins of mononuclear phagocytes

Materials

Tissue culture media are obtained from standard suppliers and stored at 4 °C except where noted. Culture plastic ware is available from standard suppliers.
Heat-inactivated fetal calf serum: thaw to room temperature and heat in a 56 °C water bath for 30–60 min. Lactalbumin hydrolysate (extra-soluble, tissue culture grade) (LH): sterilize a 10% stock solution in water by filtration through a 22 μm filter; store at

−20 °C. Dulbecco's modified Eagle's medium (DME) is supplemented with heat-inactivated fetal calf serum to a final concentration of 10% (DME-10%) or with 0.2% LH (DME-LH). RPMI-1640 or minimal essential medium can be substituted for DME. Methionine-free medium can be purchased as a custom order from most suppliers, or minimal essential medium and RPMI can be mixed free of any amino acids from 'select-amine' kits available from Grand Island Biological Co.
^{35}S-Methionine (> 1000 Ci/mmol), stored at −80 °C until needed. Labelling medium is made up fresh at 25 μCi/ml in methionine-free medium.
M. lysodeikticus dried cell walls (Sigma Chemical Co.). Wash once with saline and then make up to 2 mg/ml with saline. The suspension is stored at 4 °C and should be prepared fresh every two weeks.
Trichloroacetic acid (45%). Use for precipitation of labelled proteins.
2X Laemmli sample buffer (see below).
Screw-capped cryotubes, 2 and 5 ml sizes (Nunc and Cooke) or screw-capped microfuge tubes (1.5 ml polypropylene).

Procedure

1 Plate macrophages in DME-10% at $5 \times 10^5 – 10^6$ cells per well (16 mm diameter). Allow cells to adhere for 2–24 h at 37 °C in 5% CO_2 in humidified air. Wash the cells at least three times with DME to remove non-adherent cells. The macrophages can be treated with various agents in 0.5–1.0 ml of DME-LH or DME-10% for the desired time period.

2 Wash the macrophages three times with methionine-free DME and add 0.5–1.0 ml methionine-free DME containing 25 μCi ^{35}S-methionine/ml; usually any agent used during pre-treatment is also added. Macrophages are generally radiolabelled for 2–4 h, although periods as short as 10 min are feasible for special purposes. Up to 300 μCi ^{35}S-methionine/ml can be used for very short labelling times. At the end of the labelling period, collect the conditioned medium in 1.5 ml microfuge tubes with Pasteur pipettes. Wash the cells 3–4 times with saline and lyse (in the plate) with 0.2 to 0.5 ml of 1X sample buffer or 0.1% sodium dodecyl sulphate (SDS) followed by an equal volume of 2X sample buffer. Freeze plates at $-80\,°C$ in zip-lock plastic bags. Just before electrophoresis, check for complete lysis by microscopy and transfer the lysates to tubes for boiling. Spin the collected medium for 2.5 min in a Beckman microfuge B (about 8730 *g*) to remove any loose cells and debris. This step is of utmost importance for analysis of macrophage secretion products; otherwise, minor cellular contaminants will appear in the fluorographs along with proteins from the medium. The presence of actin (Mr 42 000) in conditioned medium is a marker for contamination by cell debris. With a Pasteur pipette carefully transfer all but the bottom 10 μl of medium to another microfuge tube; no pellet will be visible.

3 To each sample, add 150 μg (75 μl) *M. lysodeikticus* cell suspension (kept stirring on a magnetic stirrer). This carrier was chosen because, unlike protein carriers such as bovine serum albumin, it does not enter the gel during electrophoresis, and there is consequently less chance for interference with the electrophoretic run. Precipitate protein with ice-cold trichloroacetic acid (150 μl of 45%, w/v) to a final concentration of 5–7%. Cap and shake tubes and allow to stand in an ice-bath for at least 20 min. Centrifuge, wash, and vortex the pellet containing *M. lysodeikticus* 1–2 times with 1 ml 5% trichloroacetic acid or 1 ml acetone. Remove as much supernatant as possible with a Pasteur pipette and discard the supernatant as radioactive waste.

An alternative concentration method uses quinine sulphate. This method is also suitable for concentrating media for two-dimensional gel electrophoresis. Adjust sample volume to 0.5 ml with H_2O. Add 10 μl of 10% (w/v) SDS and vortex. Add 100 μl 0.1 M-quinine sulphate solution (which is prepared by weighing an appropriate amount of quinine sulphate to give a 0.1 M final concentration, dissolving in 1.0 M HCl, then diluting with distilled water to the final volume). Pellet in a microcentrifuge and wash pellet with 80% acetone [123].

4 Resuspend the pellet in 50–100 μl of 1X sample buffer; if necessary, adjust to alkaline pH with 1–5 μl 1 M NaOH (yellow acid sample becomes blue when basic). Caution: when boiled, excessively high concentrations of NaOH (pH > 10) will result in hydrolysis of the protein sample, *M. lysodeikticus*, and stacker gel. Freeze the samples at $-80\,°C$ until the day of electrophoresis. Determine incorporation by putting 5 μl samples into counting vials containing scintillant. (Work should be done in the fume hood.) Rinse out the pipette tip with the scintillant. This precaution is necessary because the sample tends to adhere to the walls of the tip, resulting in incorrect counts. Positive displacement tips are best.

Trichloroacetic acid precipitation can be used to quantify protein incorporation in samples containing unincorporated counts. Place a GF/C glass fibre filter, labelled by scissor notches, on a piece of aluminum foil. Drip 3 drops of 10% trichloroacetic acid into the middle of the filter from a Pasteur pipette. Immediately spot 1–10 μl of sample on to a soaked part of the filter and air-dry for about 10 min. Transfer filter to a 500 ml disposable beaker (on ice) containing about 200 ml 10% trichloroacetic acid. Swirl occasionally for a total of 15 min. As many as 10 filters can be treated in a single beaker. Pour off acid, then wash with 200 ml cold 5% trichloroacetic acid, swirl occasionally for a total of 5 min and pour off. Repeat this wash once more. Pour off 5% wash, and wash twice with ice-cold 95% ethanol. Transfer filters to aluminum foil, air-dry for 30 min, or dry under heat lamp for 5 min, then count.

Method for SDS-polyacrylamide gradient gel electrophoresis of labelled macrophage proteins

Principle

Samples are electrophoresed on 7–18% polyacrylamide–0.1% SDS gradient slab gels, using the Tris-glycine-SDS buffer system of Laemmli [96]. The resolving power of gradient gels is far superior to that of uniform percentage gels, which tend to yield diffuse bands, especially with proteins in the conditioned medium. For some types of analysis it may be helpful to add 2 M-urea to gels and sample buffer.

Low plating efficiencies and short labelling periods will obviously result in lower incorporation. The fluorographic methods are presented to increase the efficiency of detection of bands up to tenfold for ^{35}S and ^{14}C and to allow visualization of ^{3}H-labelled proteins. Enhancing screens (e.g. Dupont Chromex) increase ^{125}I and ^{32}P efficiency up to fivefold.

Materials

All electrophoresis stock solutions are made from electrophoretic grade reagents from Bio-Rad. Many designs of electrophoresis apparatus can be used; a suitable design is available from Bio-Rad.

30% Acrylamide-*N*-*N*′-methylenebisacrylamide. Dissolve 29.2 g acrylamide and 0.8 g bisacrylamide in triple distilled water, adjust the volume to 100 ml, and filter through No. 1 Whatman filter paper. Store at 4 °C in a brown bottle. Avoid contact with skin; acrylamide in solution is a neurotoxin.

4X Lower gel buffer. 1.5 M-Tris-HCl, pH 8.8, with 0.4% SDS. Store at 4 °C.

4X Upper gel buffer. 0.5 M-Tris-HCl, pH 6.7, with 0.4% SDS. Store at 4 °C.

10% Ammonium persulphate. Make up fresh in water.

N,*N*,*N*′,*N*′-Tetramethylethylenediamide (TEMED). Store at 4 °C. Prolonged gelling time may be due to weak or old TEMED.

10X Electrode buffer. 0.25 M-Tris, 1.9 M-glycine, and 1% SDS. Store at room temperature. Dilute with water before use.

2X Laemmli sample buffer. 1% *β*-mercaptoethanol, 0.1% Bromophenol blue, 0.625 M-Tris-HCl, pH 6.8, 50% glycerol, and 2% SDS. Store at room temperature. For 1X sample buffer, dilute with water.

[14]C-Methylated protein markers (Amersham). Contains myosin, phosphorylase B, bovine serum albumin, ovalbumin, carbonic anhydrase, and lysozyme.

Kodak X-Omat AR X-ray film.

Procedure

1 Gradient slab gels are prepared the day before electrophoresis. The volumes needed depend on the design of the electrophoresis apparatus; best results are obtained with gels that are 0.75 mm thick and 10–20 cm long. For each slab gel containing 0.375 M-Tris-HCl, pH 8.8, and 0.1% SDS, prepare one volume each of 7% and 18% acrylamide gel solution according to the following recipe. Mix gently in a beaker of ice 0.25 vol. lower gel buffer, 0.75 vol. acrylamide-water (dilute stock acrylamide with appropriate volume of water to give a final concentration of 7% or 18%), 0.00145 vol. 10% ammonium persulphate, and 0.0005 vol. TEMED. A few grains of Bromophenol blue are added to the 7% solution to aid in visualization of gradient formation and water overlaying. Pour the gradient gel with a linear gradient maker at a rate of 1 ml/min. Gently overlay the surface with water from a 22-gauge, bevelled, two-inch needle and syringe. Allow to polymerize undisturbed for 20–30 min. Prolonged polymerization time indicates old TEMED, and fresher catalyst should be used. Wash the surface twice with fresh water. The gel can be left at room temperature overnight. For longer storage (2–3 days) use 1X lower gel buffer to overlay the gel.

Pour off the water and gently blot the surface with bibulous paper before adding the stacking gel solution. For a 3% stacker gel containing 0.125 M-Tris-HCl, pH 6.8, and 0.1% SDS, mix gently in a beaker: 0.25 vol. upper gel buffer, 0.1 vol. acrylamide, 0.64 vol. water, 0.01 vol. 10% ammonium persulphate, and 0.0005 vol. TEMED. Quickly pipette the solution on to the gradient gel and insert the sample-well comb, without forming any air pockets. Sample wells 1.8–2.8 cm long and 0.45–0.9 cm wide (10- or 20-well combs) are usually used. Allow to polymerize. Wash the wells twice with 1X electrode buffer.

2 Apply samples to the wells with either equivalent counts or proportionate volumes. Equivalent counts will show changes in incorporation by particular bands, whereas proportionate volumes will show overall changes in the secretory pattern. Reserve one well for ^{14}C-labelled protein markers (diluted 1 to 40 with 1X sample buffer and boiled for 3 min). If different volumes are applied, a more even run is achieved by equalizing the volumes in each well with half-strength sample buffer before overlaying with electrode buffer. Electrophorese at 20 mA per gel. A typical run time for $10 \times 14 \times 0.75$ mm gels is 3 h.

3 Fix the gels in 50% trichloroacetic acid for 1 h or overnight. Staining is usually eliminated because there is not enough protein to be detected visually; any stain would be extracted during preparation for fluorography.

One of two procedures can be used to fluorograph gels. The method of Bonner & Laskey [97] involves (1) replacement of water in the gel with dimethyl sulphoxide, (2) impregnation with the fluor, 2,5-diphenyloxazole, followed by (3) precipitation with water. The second procedure eliminates steps (1) and (2) and consists of soaking the gel for 1 h in a commercial fluorographic solution (e.g. EN[3]HANCE, New England Nuclear), or in 22% 2,5-diphenyloxazole in glacial acetic acid, followed by precipitation with water for 1 h, then drying the gel under vacuum in a standard drying apparatus.

4 Expose Kodak X-Omat AR or equivalent X-ray film to a flash of light before exposure to the gel. According to Laskey & Mills [98], the absorbance of the fluorographic image is not linear with the amount of radioactivity or with exposure time. Pre-exposure of the film to a suitably filtered flash unit corrects for this non-linearity and increases the efficiency of detection. Place the film against the gel and seal them inside the film envelope with photographic tape. If necessary, wrap the envelope with lead foil to prevent exposure from any stray radioactive sources. Secure between

two boards with clamps and expose at $-80\,°C$. Fluorographs can be scanned in a gel densitometer (LKB, Hoefer, etc.) to determine relative molecular masses and relative incorporation by individual bands.

Notes and recommendations

Incorporation of ^{35}S-methionine into cell-associated and secreted proteins varies with cell number and labelling time, as well as time in culture. Protein patterns from 10^6 macrophages can be detected in as little as 15 min of labelling; however, it should be noted that the exposure time will be longer than that for cells labelled for 2–4 h (Fig. 47.3). If fewer cells are available, e.g. 10^5, the incorporation time can be increased to 4 h and fluorographs can be readily examined after only 10 days of exposure at $-80\,°C$.

Incorporation of label into the secreted proteins of macrophages varies from 1.5 to 20% of the total incorporated label. Typical labelling of 5×10^5 thioglycollate-elicited macrophages for 2 h under the conditions described here is approximately 2.3×10^4 c.p.m.

in the secreted proteins and about 1×10^6 c.p.m. in the cell-associated proteins. For similar numbers of resident macrophages, approximately 1×10^4 c.p.m. are seen in the secreted proteins and about 1.2×10^5 c.p.m. in the cell-associated proteins.

The reproducibility of incorporation depends on the age and specific activity of ^{35}S-methionine and on the time in culture of the macrophages. Because the half-life of ^{35}S is only 87.5 days, the concentration of the isotope is recalculated with each use to maintain a constant concentration from one experiment to another. Macrophages change their pattern of protein synthesis with adherence and with time in culture in various media (Fig. 47.4).

Differences in synthesis and secretion patterns of mononuclear phagocytes from different sources

The procedures outlined here are powerful tools for tracing the history of mononuclear phagocytes. The gel patterns of both cell-associated and secreted proteins of macrophages from various inbred mouse strains, including the recombinant resistant strains,

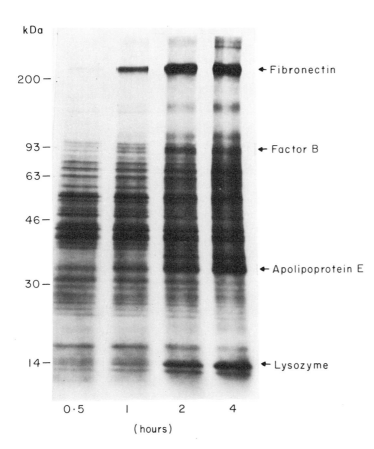

Fig. 47.3. Time course of incorporation of ^{35}S-methionine into thioglycollate-elicited macrophages. The cells were incubated with 25 μCi ^{35}S-methionine/ml for the times indicated. Relative molecular mass standards and identity of some major products are shown.

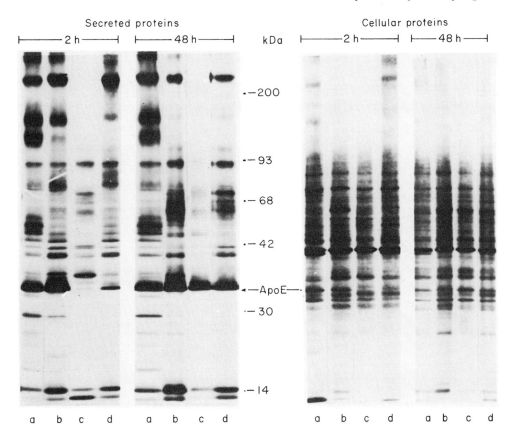

Fig. 47.4. Autoradiogram of secreted (left) and cellular (right) proteins of mouse peritoneal macrophages after 2 h or 48 h in culture. (a) Resident; (b) thioglycollate-elicited; (c) pyran copolymer-elicited; and (d) sodium periodate-elicited macrophages labelled for 2 h with 25 μCi ^{35}S-methionine/ml [14]. Migration of relative molecular mass standards and apolipoprotein E (ApoE) is indicated.

exhibit significant differences that cannot be attributed to differences in the H-2 haplotype of the mice (Fig. 47.5). The most striking distinctions between resident and inflammatory (e.g. thioglycollate-, endotoxin-, or pyran copolymer-elicited) macrophages can be seen by radiolabelling with ^{35}S-methionine and ^{3}H-mannose (Fig. 47.6). There are similarities between species: rat, rabbit, human, and mouse macrophages share some major secreted proteins but also differ significantly in others. Similarly, proliferating tumour-derived macrophages share some major proteins with macrophages from normal mice. However, in this case, major differences are possibly due to the biosynthesis and secretion of viral proteins by the tumour cells. Radiolabelling can also be used to examine modulation of macrophage function. For example, new proteins are biosynthesized in response to treatment of mouse macrophages with glucocorticoids, prostaglandins, and antibody-coated erythrocytes.

Another important use of radiolabelling is to help

evaluate the contamination of macrophages or other cell populations by other cells. For example, the presence of radiolabelled plasma proteins such as albumin and fibrinogen in the gel patterns of secreted proteins from Kupffer cell populations indicates hepatocyte contamination. Similarly, fibroblast-specific proteins (e.g. collagens) can be used to evaluate fibroblast contamination in inflammatory macrophage monolayers, and similar evaluations can be made for thymocytes and B cells.

The procedures outlined here involve the use of ^{35}S-methionine as the biosynthetic label of choice. However, other labels, such as ^{3}H-glucosamine, other amino acids, ^{32}PO$_4^{3-}$ or ^{35}SO$_4^{2-}$, can be used in this way. Indeed, the most dramatic differences between resident and inflammatory macrophages appear to be specific to the secreted glycoproteins (Fig. 47.6). Incorporation of monosaccharides into glycoconjugates is particularly useful in this regard.

Specific labelled proteins can be immunoprecipi-

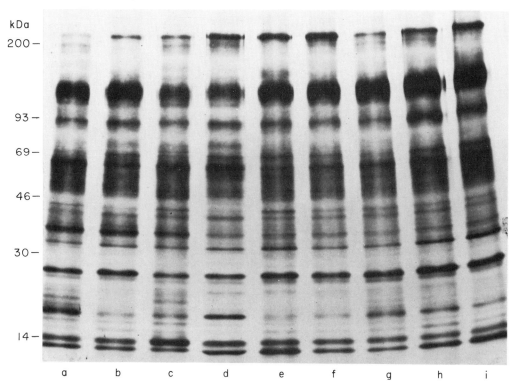

Fig. 47.5. Secreted proteins of resident mouse peritoneal macrophages obtained from various inbred strains differing in H-2 haplotype. Cells were cultured for 24 h, then labelled with ^{35}S-methionine for 4 h. (a) BALB/c (H-2^d); (b) AKR/J (H-2^k); (c) A/J (H-2^a); (d) DBA/2J (H-2^d); (e) C57BL/6J (H-2^b); (f) B10D2/nSn (H-2^d); (g) B10BR/SgSn (H-2^k); (h) B10A(5R)/SgSn (H-2^{i5}); and (i) B10A(2R)/SgSn (H-2^{h2}).

tated directly with immune serum or indirectly with specific immunoglobulins followed by protein A or a second antibody or by 'Western' immunoblotting methods. These techniques have been used to investigate macrophage apolipoprotein E [14,56] (Fig. 47.7), complement factor B [88], α_2-macroglobulin [43], fibronectin [57], and β-glucuronidase [99]. Labelling procedures can also be used to study the regulation of the various proteins secreted by macrophages. Several agents, including phagocytic stimuli, endotoxin, colchicine, prostaglandins, and steroids, alter secretion of specific macrophage proteins (Fig. 47.8) [55].

Additional details about the synthesis and processing of macrophage proteins can be obtained by peptide mapping of specific proteins as described by Cleveland *et al.* [100] and Johnson *et al.* [101]. These techniques have been applied to studies of lysosomal enzymes, complement, proteins, and apolipoprotein E.

Methods for the assay of plasminogen activator

Principle

Plasminogen activators that are secreted by cells or present in plasma in an inactive form convert plasminogen, a serum zymogen, to plasmin, a potent fibrinolytic enzyme. Astrup *et al.* originally developed a simple procedure to assay plasmin activity from zones of lysis in fibrin plates, but the use of ^{125}I-labelled fibrin plates by Unkeless *et al.* [102] has greatly increased the sensitivity and versatility of the assay. Tissue culture dishes are coated with a thin film of ^{125}I-fibrinogen, which is dried and converted to fibrin by thrombin. The generation of plasmin by PA is then measured from solubilization of the ^{125}I-fibrin. This assay has been adapted to measure PA secretion by intact cells and also to estimate PA concentrations in cell-free conditioned media and cell lysates.

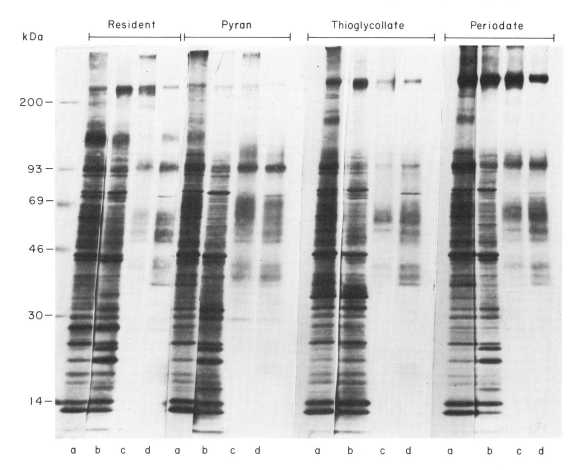

Fig. 47.6. Comparison of the incorporation of various radiolabelled amino acids and sugars into secreted proteins of resident and inflammatory macrophages. The cells were radiolabelled for 24 h with (a) ^{35}S-methionine, (b) ^{3}H-labelled mixed amino acids, (c) ^{14}C-glucosamine, or (d) ^{3}H-mannose.

Methods for preparation of assay reagents and samples

Purification of fibrinogen

Bovine fibrinogen (Calbiochem) is further purified to reduce contamination with plasminogen.

Dissolve 4 g fibrinogen in 400 ml 0.1 M phosphate buffer, pH 6.4; add 200 ml distilled water, and leave on ice for 6–18 h. Filter and discard precipitate. Make filtrate, 1/3 final concentration, with ammonium sulphate, pH 7.0, and stir for 2 h at room temperature. Centrifuge precipitate. Take up precipitate in about 50 ml 0.5 M NaCl, pH 7.0, and dialyse three times in the same buffer at room temperature. Measure fibrinogen concentration by the Lowry method. Add 5 vol. 5 mM-Na$_2$PO$_4$, 0.12 M-lysine, pH 7.0, to 10 mg/ml fibrinogen in 0.6 M NaCl, pH 7.0. Bring to 0 °C. Add

ethanol to 7% final concentration. Stir for 30 min at 4 °C. Centrifuge. Dissolve the precipitate in 10–20 ml 0.6 M NaCl, pH 7.4, and dialyse in same buffer. Pass through filter paper and sterilize by Millipore filtration. Measure protein concentration and freeze at −20 °C.

Comments

Use plastic containers to minimize clotting. Repeat ethanol precipitation if significant plasmin concentration remains.

Iodination of fibrinogen

Iodination of fibrinogen is performed by the chloramine T method [103], using mild conditions to prevent denaturation of fibrinogen.

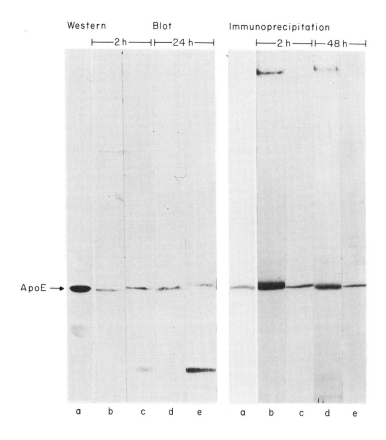

Western   Blot   Immunoprecipitation

├──2 h──┤├─24 h──┤   ├──2 h──┤├─48 h──┤

ApoE →

    a   b   c   d   e   a   b   c   d   e

Fig. 47.7. Comparison of the detection of apolipoprotein E (ApoE) in thioglycollate-elicited macrophages in culture by Western immunoblotting procedures (left) and immunoprecipitation of ^{35}S-methionine-labelled proteins (right). (a) Mouse very-low-density lipoprotein standard, ^{125}I-labelled; (b) conditioned medium and (c) cell lysates at 2 h in culture; (d) conditioned medium and (e) cell lysates at 24 h (Western blot) or 48 h (immunoprecipitation) in culture. The 220 kDa band in immunoprecipitates is fibronectin binding to *Staphylococcus aureus*, used as a source of protein A. See ref. 14 for details.

Add 0.5 mCi ^{125}I-Na (carrier free), 50 μl chloramine T (2 mg/ml in 0.3 M phosphate-buffered saline, pH 7.4) and up to 250 μl fibrinogen (8–14 mg/ml in 0.3 M phosphate-buffered saline, pH 7.4) and mix at room temperature for 2 min. Add 150 μl of saturated tyrosine and 200 μl of 5% bovine serum albumin, pH 7.4, and pass the mixture over a small column (2 ml) of Sephadex G-25 to separate the ^{125}I-fibrinogen from the bulk of unincorporated ^{125}I. Pool the labelled fibrinogen and filter through a 0.22 μm filter, adding bovine serum albumin (5%) to minimize losses. Determine acid-precipitable radioactivity. Typical incorporation efficiency is 30% (5×10^5 c.p.m./μg protein). The labelled fibrinogen can be stored frozen at -20 °C, although the proportion of acid-precipitable protein may decrease rapidly after several weeks' storage.

Preparation of ^{125}I-fibrin plates

Tissue culture plates (24 wells, 16 mm diameter) are especially useful, although 35 mm tissue culture dishes can also be used. Dilute the desired amount of ^{125}I-fibrinogen and unlabelled fibrinogen with sterile distilled water so that 0.3 ml of the final solution contains approximately 10^5 acid-precipitable c.p.m. and 20 μg unlabelled fibrinogen. Keep the solution warm to prevent precipitation of fibrinogen and dispense 0.3 ml samples with automatic dispenser to each well. A glass rod is needed to distribute fibrinogen over the surface of 35 mm dishes. Dry at 45 °C in an incubator under sterile conditions for a minimum of 3 days. The radioactive plates can then be stored for several weeks at room temperature or in the cold.

Activation of plates before use

Incubate each well with 1 ml Dulbecco's medium plus 10% fetal bovine serum (FBS) for 2 h at 37 °C to convert fibrinogen to fibrin. Thrombin solutions can also be used. The action of thrombin in the serum releases 10–15% of ^{125}I-fibrinogen. Wash twice with Hanks' balanced salt solution (HBSS). Plates can also be activated overnight and may be kept for 1 day after activation. Wash again before use.

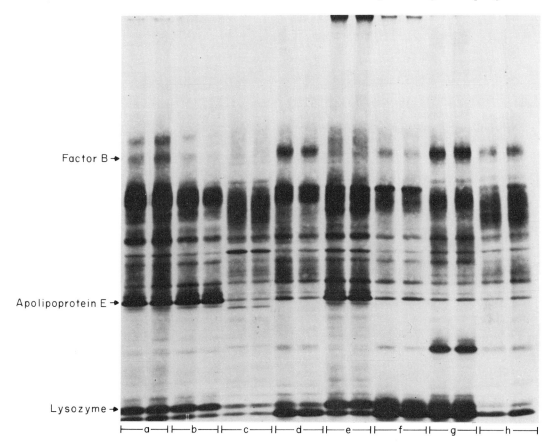

Fig. 47.8. Effects of various agents on secretion of proteins from mouse bone marrow-derived macrophages [56] labelled with 25 μCi ^{35}S-methionine/ml. Cultures (12 day) were incubated with agents for 24 h before radiolabelling and during the 4 h labelling period. (a) Control cells; (b) dexamethasone, 1 μM; (c) colchicine, 1 μM; (d) endotoxin, 10 μg/ml; (e) prostaglandin E2, 1 μM; (f) prostaglandin E2, 1 μM, plus endotoxin, 10 μg/ml; (g) dexamethasone, 1 μM, plus endotoxin, 10 μg/ml; (h) colchicine, 1 μM, plus endotoxin, 10 μg/ml. The migration of some secreted proteins is indicated on the left.

Purification of plasminogen

Purify plasminogen from human plasma or dog serum by affinity chromatography on lysine-Sepharose (Pharmacia) or lysine-agarose (Miles Labs) according to the method of Deutsch & Mertz [104]. Serum (10–20 ml) is run through a 5 cm column of adsorbent, the adsorbed protein is washed thoroughly with saline in 0.01 M phosphate buffer, pH 7.4, and the plasminogen is then eluted with 0.2 M-ε-aminocaproic acid. The ε-aminocaproic acid is removed by gel filtration on Sephadex G-25 or by dialysis. The plasminogen is assayed with urokinase (Sigma; Leo Pharmaceutical Products, Denmark) or macrophage-conditioned medium containing PA to determine the optimal concentration required for assay. Filter, subdivide, and store frozen at −20 °C.

Acid-treated serum

Acid treatment of serum is designed to destroy inhibitors of proteinase activity, such as α_2-macroglobulin, without affecting plasminogen. Slowly add 2 M HCl in 0.14 M-saline to fetal bovine or dog serum and leave at pH 2.0 at room temperature for 30 min. Then carefully neutralize the acid-treated serum with 2 M NaOH in 0.15 M-saline, filter to sterilize, subdivide, and store frozen at −20 °C until used. Because a precipitate may form in dog serum after reneutralization, filtration is made easier by dilution to 5% in Dulbecco's medium. Fetal bovine serum retains more antiplasmin activity than dog serum after acid treatment.

Macrophage sources

The authors have used specific pathogen-free mice of either sex, weighing 25–30 g. Peritoneal cells are harvested by standard methods from unstimulated animals or from mice 4 days after intraperitoneal injection of 1 ml Brewer's thioglycollate medium (Difco Labs; 'complete'; prepared and stored according to the manufacturer's instructions). Lipopolysaccharide endotoxin (LPS) from *Salmonella typhimurium* (RIBI Immunochem, Inc.) is particularly potent. The LPS is suspended in sterile saline (1 mg/ml), sonically disrupted briefly, and can be stored frozen ($-20\,°C$) for up to 2 months. The LPS is insoluble and should be resuspended carefully before injection. Peritoneal cells are harvested after 4–5 days. The potency of a particular batch of LPS should be determined by dose–response experiments. The authors have obtained optimal macrophage spreading and fibrinolysis after injection of 10–30 μg LPS.

Cell culture

Standard procedures of macrophage cultivation are modified as follows. Peritoneal cell suspensions are plated at $2–5 \times 10^5/cm^2$ on regular or ^{125}I-fibrin-coated tissue culture dishes, unless stated otherwise. The culture medium consists of Dulbecco's modified medium (H-21, Gibco), penicillin and streptomycin supplemented as follows: for culture on uncoated dishes, with 15% acid-treated FBS; for culture on ^{125}I-fibrin-coated dishes, with 10% FBS and 60 μg/ml soybean trypsin inhibitor (Sigma), to suppress fibrinolysis, unless stated otherwise. The plates are washed free of lymphocytes and the cells are fed fresh medium of the same composition after 4 and 24 h incubation.

Collection of conditioned medium

The same procedure is followed for all the proteolytic activities discussed. Conditioned medium is routinely prepared after 48 h cultivation on non-radioactive dishes in medium containing acid-treated serum. Wash the monolayers carefully at least three times with HBSS to remove inhibitors and incubate in serum-free Dulbecco's medium supplemented with 0.2% LH for 1–4 days. Neumann-Tytell medium (Gibco) is a more expensive but particularly rich serum-free medium that may be preferred for certain purposes. After 4–24 h cultivation in medium with serum, macrophages can be exposed to repeated cycles of serum-free medium for up to 3 weeks without loss of viability or decrease in lysozyme secretion, but cells may display reduced concentrations of other activities,

such as plasma membrane 5′-nucleotidase. Collect the conditioned medium, spin in microfuge to remove cell debris, and store the supernatant at $-20\,°C$ until assay.

Preparation of conditioned medium for assay

Although the secreted proteinase activities described in this chapter are stable for several cycles of freezing and thawing, the enzymes are sticky and easily lost on precipitates and surfaces when dilute solutions in serum-free medium are handled. PA and elastase activities can be measured directly or after concentration. Thioglycollate-elicited macrophages secrete rather small amounts of collagenase. Large amounts of conditioned medium that have been appropriately concentrated are needed for a collagenase assay (details are described elsewhere [18]). To amplify dilute proteinase activities, conditioned medium is dialysed against three changes of 20 vol. of 10 mM-NH$_4$HCO$_3$, a volatile salt, and lyophilized. The lyophilized material is then reconstituted in the appropriate assay buffer.

Cell lysates

Wash the monolayers twice with HBSS, then add 0.5–1 ml of 0.1–0.2% Triton X-100, scrape from the dish with a rubber policeman, and store at $-20\,°C$. Cells can also be harvested by scraping in isotonic saline and collected by centrifugation before treatment with Triton X-100. The nuclei can then be removed by low-speed centrifugation before freezing. Triton X-100 stimulates PA activity by approximately 30%.

Procedure for assay of fibrinolysis

Intact cells

Various cell concentrations and appropriate controls without cells are added to ^{125}I-fibrin-coated wells. Adherent cells attach and spread well on this substrate. Fibrinolysis is either measured directly or after cultivation in the presence of inhibitors: 10–20% FBS with or without 60 μg/ml soybean trypsin inhibitor for thioglycollate-elicited macrophages, 2% FBS for unstimulated cells. Media are monitored for fibrin solubilization before each change. It is usually possible to maintain cells for no longer than 4–5 days on these plates because of gradual solubilization of the fibrin.

To initiate the fibrinolytic assay the monolayer is washed 3 times with HBSS to remove inhibitors and incubated in Dulbecco's medium (0.5 or 2.5 ml for Linbro wells or 35 mm dishes, respectively) plus 5% acid-treated FBS; 5% acid-treated dog serum is used

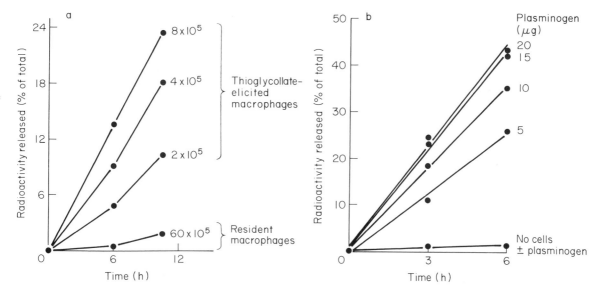

Fig. 47.9. Fibrinolysis by mouse peritoneal macrophages. (a) Comparison of living thioglycollate-elicited and resident macrophages assayed in Dulbecco's medium supplemented with 5% acid-treated fetal bovine serum. (b) Effect of various concentrations of purified dog plasminogen on fibrinolysis by endotoxin-elicited macrophages. The incubation medium was Dulbecco's medium supplemented with 0.1% lactalbumin hydrolysate and various amounts of plasminogen.

for less active cells. Samples are removed at various intervals and counted in a gamma spectrometer to measure solubilization of fibrin. Cells are observed by phase-contrast microscopy during the assay, which can be extended to 24 h to detect low levels of activity. Results are expressed as the percentage of total radioactivity released by trypsin. Thioglycollate-elicited macrophages are at least ten times as fibrinolytic as unstimulated macrophages (Fig. 47.9a). No activity is demonstrable with acid-treated FBS depleted of plasminogen by lysine-Sepharose chromatography and the plasminogen dependence of fibrinolysis has been confirmed by reconstitution with purified plasminogen.

Notes

The assay can be made considerably more sensitive by adding purified plasminogen to intact cells, with endotoxin-stimulated macrophages. Unstimulated macrophages that have been cultivated for 24 h will also show significant fibrinolytic activity with plasminogen. This type of assay is useful for detection of PA secretion by unstimulated human monocytes but requires plasminogen uncontaminated with plasmin. The results of assays with various concentrations of plasminogen are shown in Fig. 47.9b.

Activated macrophages show marked adherence and spreading in the course of the fibrinolytic reaction, especially in the presence of purified plasminogen.

Other cell types may become detached from their substrate as a result of the action of plasmin.

Cell-free fractions

Cultivation of macrophages in acid-treated serum results in higher levels of proteolytic activity in serum-free conditioned medium. Acid treatment may also be performed on conditioned media collected in the presence of serum. The conditioned medium and cell lysates are assayed, in duplicate, in a final reaction volume of 0.4 (Linbro wells) or 1.0 ml (35 mm dishes), in 0.1 M-Tris-HCl buffer, pH 8.0, containing 125 μg bovine serum albumin, 2–5 μg plasminogen, and 10–100 μl of the test fraction. The plates are incubated at 37 °C for 1–6 h and the solubilized radioactivity is measured at two or three time points. Appropriate controls for all reagents and media are included and the plasminogen-dependent fibrinolysis is determined. Total releasable counts are obtained by incubation in trypsin. The radioactivity released should be proportional to enzyme concentration and time of incubation as long as the solubilization does not exceed approximately 30%.

Notes and recommendations

The ^{125}I-fibrin plate assay is a rapid, sensitive, and versatile assay that can be used to detect PA, plasminogen, or plasmin in culture fluids, column effluents, and SDS gels. To detect the presence of PA, it is necessary to show that fibrinolysis depends on added plasminogen; to use this indirect assay quantitatively, it is necessary to determine conditions such that substrate digestion is proportional to the amount of PA or number of cultivated macrophages added. It is important to exclude direct fibrinolysis, independent of plasminogen, in assays with intact cells as well as with cell-free fractions. Optimal plasminogen concentration should also be determined; plasminogen is relatively labile to heating at 56 °C (30–60 min). Different batches of serum differ in their antiplasmin activity and should be standardized; the use of acid-treated dog serum and acid-treated FBS makes it possible to adjust the sensitivity of the assay and the rate of fibrinolysis as required for a particular system. Cell-free controls should be included in all assays and should be suitably low, provided the reagents are purified and stored with care to prevent generation of plasmin.

One drawback of the ^{125}I-fibrin plate assay is the lack of standardization that makes it difficult to compare results from different batches of reagents. Arbitrary units can be used to compare results, e.g. 1 unit represents 5% of the trypsin-releasable radioactivity solubilized in 1 h at 37 °C. Urokinase reference standards can also be useful. Activity of different cell lines can be normalized to the number of cells required to cause release of 50% of available radioactivity, under standard conditions.

In populations of activated macrophages, it is especially important to ensure that any fibrinolysis observed is not due to contamination with highly active polymorphonuclear leucocytes. Since polymorphonuclear leucocytes die within 6–12 h of cultivation, it is essential to pre-incubate these cultures for at least 1 day in the presence of high concentrations of serum supplemented with soybean trypsin inhibitor before assay of macrophage fibrinolytic activity.

For some purposes it may be helpful to demonstrate conversion of plasminogen to plasmin directly. This is done by SDS-polyacrylamide gel electrophoresis of ^{125}I-plasminogen after incubation with PA in the presence of bovine pancreatic trypsin inhibitor, which stabilizes the ^{125}I-plasmin formed [105]. The two polypeptide chains of plasmin, which are linked by a disulphide band, are smaller, after reduction, than the single-chain parent molecule (Fig. 47.10).

Enhancement of macrophage fibrinolysis

Phagocytosis can be used to enhance fibrinolysis by endotoxin-stimulated macrophages [89]. Polystyrene latex particles (1.01 μm, Dow Diagnostics) are washed thoroughly by centrifugation, resuspended in Dul-

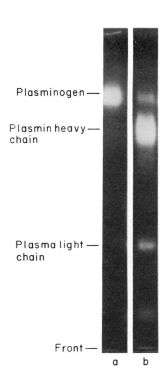

Fig. 47.10. SDS-polyacrylamide gel analysis of the direct cleavage of ^{125}I-plasminogen to plasmin by plasminogen activator. (a) Control; (b) incubation with plasminogen. Note the cleavage of intact plasminogen to the heavy and light chains of plasmin [102,105].

becco's medium, and irradiated with ultraviolet light. Macrophages are generally cultivated for 24 h before phagocytosis. Monolayers are washed twice and incubated in medium containing 5% FBS. Particulate preparations are resuspended in serum-free medium by passage through a syringe and 26-gauge needle and carefully distributed in the culture medium. Soybean trypsin inhibitor (60 μg/ml) is included in the medium during phagocytosis in experiments on radioactive plates. Phagocytosis is observed by phase-contrast microscopy and is stopped when more than 95% of cells have ingested 20–50 particles per cell. The cells are then washed and placed in fresh medium, as required. Macrophages are normally cultivated in medium containing serum for one day after phagocytosis before collection of conditioned medium.

PA can be induced in unstimulated macrophages by products in lymphocyte-conditioned medium. Conditioned medium should be prepared by incubating the appropriate spleen or lymphocyte culture in medium containing 2–5% FBS or horse serum for 2–3 days [90–92]. The conditioned medium must be filtered before use to prevent phagocytosis of lymphocyte membrane fragments. Unstimulated macrophages (5×10^5/well) are prepared on ^{125}I-fibrin plates in 2% FBS and exposed to various dilutions of the lymphocyte-conditioned medium in Dulbecco's medium with FBS (~ 0.1 ml conditioned medium per 0.4 ml with FBS, final concentration 2%). After 2–3 days' incubation the cells are washed 3 times and assayed in 5% acid-treated dog serum to enhance sensitivity. High concentrations of FBS during the induction period depress subsequent fibrinolysis, probably because of the persistence of serum inhibitors.

Methods for the assay of macrophage elastase

Principle

Macrophage elastase has little if any activity when assayed with synthetic substrates; thus elastin must be used to screen for this enzyme. The ^{3}H-elastin assay, which is representative of the more sensitive elastin assays [106–109], takes advantage of the ability of aldol, isodesmosine, and desmosine cross-links to be reduced and labelled with ^{3}H-NaBH$_4$. Because these cross-links are distributed throughout the elastin structure and retain the label even after autoclaving, the ^{3}H-elastin can be added to cell cultures if necessary. The solubilization of label from these cross-links is a reliable indication of proteolytic degradation of elastin.

Methods for preparation of ^{3}H-elastin substrate

1   Because ^{3}H$_2$ gas is a by-product of the reaction, all work must be carried out in a well-ventilated fume hood. The reaction vessel should be a 500-ml Erlenmeyer flask, preferably placed in a clear, non-breakable, two litre plastic beaker. The flask and beaker assembly should be placed on a magnetic stirring plate in the fume hood.

2   Suspend 2.5 g elastin (< 400-mesh elastin E60 from Elastin Products Co.) in 50 ml of distilled H$_2$O in a 500-ml Erlenmeyer flask. (Wet the elastin powder with ethanol before mixing with H$_2$O.) Adjust pH to 9.2 with NaOH.

3   Dissolve 25 mCi ^{3}H-NaBH$_4$ (New England Nuclear) in a minimal volume of 0.003 M NaOH and add to the elastin.

4   After 10 min, add 250 mg non-radioactive NaBH$_4$ dissolved in a minimal volume of 0.003 M NaOH. Allow to mix in hood for 2 h.

5   Adjust pH to 3 by carefully adding glacial acetic acid. Check pH with paper. Be careful of foaming; a few drops of antifoam B emulsion (Sigma) will suppress foaming. If the flask must be removed from

the beaker, wait until foaming has stopped. Mix for an additional 30 min.

6   Collect the elastin by centrifuging at 10 000 g for 30 min and wash repeatedly by resuspending in cold H$_2$O and recentrifuging until the activity of the supernatant is 1800–2000 d.p.m./100 μl. It is advisable to pool the elastin into one 50-ml centrifuge tube after the first two or three washes. If the labelling procedure is carried out in the early afternoon, four or five washes can be done and the elastin can be left in the 50-ml tube stirring on a magnetic stirrer overnight at 4 °C. This will allow much of the non-covalently bound radioactivity to leach out of the elastin particles.

7   Resuspend the elastin in H$_2$O at 16 mg/ml, stirring constantly on a magnetic stirring plate. Put 5 ml (80 mg) into 50 ml sterile screw-capped tubes (Corning) and keep frozen at -80 °C until needed. Use a pipette with a wide mouth when dispensing the elastin. *Do not pipette by mouth.*

8   To determine specific radioactivity, incubate a measured portion of the ^{3}H-elastin with pancreatic elastase (Sigma) at an enzyme : substrate ratio of 1 : 100 in 0.1 M-Tris, pH 8.0, with 0.05 M-CaCl$_2$. Allow the reaction to proceed at 37 °C until all of the substrate is degraded, usually 3–4 h for 100–300 μg. The total radioactivity incorporated should be about 600–1000 d.p.m./μg.

9   Any non-elastin protein contamination of the ^{3}H-elastin substrate can be a substrate for non-specific proteinases. To determine non-specific labelling, incubate the elastin for 16 h with trypsin-TPCK (Worthington) in 0.05 M-Tris-HCl buffer, pH 8.1, containing 0.012 M-CaCl$_2$ at an enzyme : substrate ratio of 1 : 100. After 16 h the released radioactivity should not exceed 2% of the total available radioactivity.

Procedure for assay of elastinolysis

Reagents

3X assay buffer (0.3 M-Tris-HCl buffer containing 0.015 M-CaCl$_2$ and 0.02% NaN$_3$); pancreatic elastase from porcine pancreas (E-1250, Sigma).

Substrate

Thaw a tube of ^{3}H-elastin, resuspend in 10 ml of H$_2$O, and centrifuge at 2000 g for 15–20 min. Discard the supernatant and resuspend to 40 ml with 3X assay buffer. This will give 2 mg/ml of ^{3}H-elastin substrate.

1   Reagent blank. To a 400 μl microfuge tube, add 200 μl of DME-LH or appropriate solvent. Add 100 μl of substrate suspension in 3X assay buffer.

2   Total lysis control. To a 400 μl microfuge tube, add 200 μl of DME-LH or appropriate solvent plus 2 μl of

pancreatic elastase. Add 100 μl of substrate suspension in 3X assay buffer.

3   Sample tubes. To a 400 μl microfuge tube, add up to 200 μl of sample (e.g. conditioned medium). Adjust volume to 200 μl with solvent (DME-LH) if necessary. Add 100 μl of substrate suspension in 3X assay buffer.

4   Cap or cover all tubes and incubate at 37 °C for 16 h. If a large number of tubes are being assayed, it may be more convenient not to cap the tubes but simply to cover the entire rack of tubes with cellophane or Parafilm.

5   After incubation, centrifuge for 3 min in a Beckman microfuge (or equivalent). Remove 100 μl of supernatant from each tube to a scintillation vial. Add scintillant and count; a counting time of 1 min is usually sufficient.

Calculation of data

A unit of elastinolytic activity is defined as the amount of enzyme that degrades 1.0 μg of elastin/h. In each assay there is an internal set of controls to determine non-enzymatic release of radioactivity (blank) and the total counts in 200 μg (100 μl) of elastin.

Dispensing elastin substrate

When dispensing particulate elastin substrate of any kind, be certain that the suspension is constantly stirring on a magnetic stirring plate. When pipetting samples of the suspension, use a Gilson Pipetman P-200, or equivalent, that has had 1–2 mm cut from the end of the disposable plastic tip. This will enlarge the bore of the tip, preventing obstruction of the tip and inadvertent sieving of the elastin particles.

Reagent blank

Care must be taken to maintain low radioactivity in the reagent blank. Should the activity of the blank exceed approximately 1–2% of the total radioactivity (determined with pancreatic elastase), the elastin should be centrifuged, washed once with H_2O, recentrifuged, and reconstituted in fresh 3X assay buffer. Generally, high values in the blank are the result of either insufficient washing after the labelling procedure or enzymatic contamination during sampling.

Substrate concentration

The maximum substrate concentration, determined from double reciprocal plots, suggests the use of several milligrams of elastin per assay tube. This would prove to be impractical and rather expensive. The assay is sufficiently sensitive not to warrant the routine use of higher substrate concentrations. The use of an insoluble substrate does not permit the Michaelis-Menten-type interpretation of kinetic data and thus the assignment of an absolute substrate optimum.

Effect of sample volume and assay time

In comparative studies of elastase from mouse macrophage-conditioned medium, it is important always to assay the same volume of sample. Frequently, the relationship between volume assayed and activity is not linear. An assay volume of 25 μl will indicate more units per millilitre than 200 μl of the same material. The authors interpret these observations to be the possible dilution of an uncharacterized proteinase inhibitor.

Elastase activity is linear with time for 18 h. A minimum assay time of 8 h is recommended for active samples.

Notes and recommendations

The macrophage elastase is a stable enzyme accumulated to high levels of specific activity in medium conditioned by thioglycollate-elicited macrophages and by macrophage cell lines, such as P388D1, but differs from PA in its striking enhancement after treatment of cells with colchicine [94]. The elastinolytic assay is less sensitive than that for PA but may be easier to standardize. No simple quantitative assays suitable for use with intact cells are available. While macrophages can be incubated with autoclaved ^{3}H-elastin particles, some particles are ingested, making it difficult to determine mechanism. Living macrophages in culture can degrade an extracellular matrix containing insoluble elastin in their immediate vicinity (Fig. 47.11); detailed methods for such analyses are described elsewhere [13,22,29,110].

Macrophage elastase is an endopeptidase with a broad range of substrates, including immunoglobulins [28], α_1-proteinase inhibitor [27], myelin basic protein [24,25], plasminogen, fibrinogen, and fibrin [111,112]. The proteolysis of these substrates can be detected by polyacrylamide gel electrophoresis of the purified protein substrates after incubation with conditioned medium. That macrophage elastase will also degrade fibrinogen and fibrin means that this proteinase may be responsible for the plasminogen-free, EDTA-suppressible direct fibrinolysis seen in PA assays. Despite this broad substrate specificity, elastin is a very useful substrate because it provides an unambiguous assay: macrophage elastase is the only secreted or cellular macrophage proteinase that will directly degrade elastin.

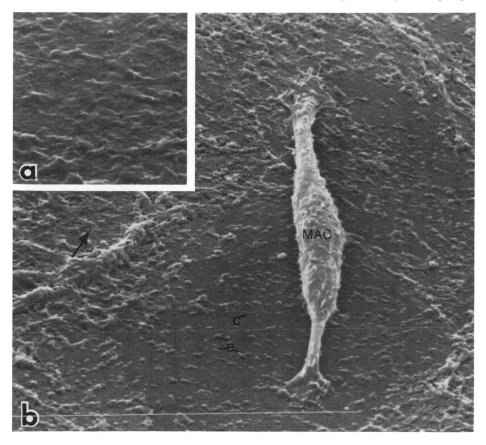

Fig. 47.11. Scanning electron micrograph showing degradation of an elastin-rich extracellular matrix by a thioglycollate-elicited macrophage. (a) Control matrix; (b) degraded matrix, concentrated in the pericellular area of the macrophage (MAC), showing some residual elastin fibres (e) and collagen (c). At a distance from the cell there is also some degradation evident by the friable appearance of the matrix surface (arrow). The incubation medium was Dulbecco's medium supplemented with 0.2% lactalbumin hydrolysate and 10 µg/ml plasminogen. × 2850. Reproduced from ref. 29, with permission of The Rockefeller University Press.

Enhancement of elastinolysis with SDS

SDS will enhance elastase activity two- to tenfold, depending on the source and treatment of the sample [106–108,113,114]. Typically, the SDS-elastin assay will give elastase activity of 6–8 (U/10^6 cells for resident macrophages, 15–20 U/10^6 cells for thioglycollate-elicited macrophages (Table 47.8), and 5–11 U/10^6 cells for P388D1. Although the precise ratio of SDS:elastin (w/w) must be determined for each batch of elastin substrate by a dose–response experiment, the authors found the optimal ratio to be 0.2. The mechanism of SDS enhancement is not clear. Some investigators have suggested that SDS changes the conformation of the molecule and renders the substrate more accessible to degradation [108], whereas others suggest that SDS increases the binding of enzyme to substrate [113,114]. Another possible role of SDS is to interfere with the action of an endogenous elastase inhibitor. Whatever the mode of action, care must be taken when interpreting data collected with the SDS-elastin assay. For example, macrophage-conditioned medium has an eight- to tenfold increase in elastase activity when SDS is included in the elastin assay. When the medium is first dialysed against 10 mM-NH$_4$HCO$_3$, there is no change in activity in the SDS-elastin assay. However, in the non-SDS-elastin assay, dialysis enhances the activity up to eightfold. Thus some effects are masked by SDS. The authors suggest that, for each investigation, dialysed and non-dialysed conditioned medium be assayed with SDS- and non-SDS-modified substrate to determine the most informative assay for the particular study. SDS-elastin is especially useful in the detection of low-level elastase activity from crude conditioned medium.

The authors strongly recommend that elastin without SDS be used for the evaluation of biological inhibitors of elastase. α_2-Macroglobulin will readily inhibit macrophage elastase in a non-SDS-elastin assay but not in SDS-elastin [24]. The free SDS concentration (99 μg/ml; ratio of bound to free is 0.34) of an SDS:elastin ratio of 0.2 is sufficient to dissociate α_2-macroglobulin–enzyme complexes. Again, careful interpretation of data from the SDS-elastin assay is in order.

If the SDS-elastin assay blank shows increased radioactivity it should be discarded, because the addition of fresh SDS assay buffer will change the ratio of bound to free SDS.

Methods for the assay of macrophage lysozyme

Principle

Lysozyme (EC 3.2.1.17), a constitutive secretory enzyme of all macrophages, hydrolyses the *N*-acetyl-muramic-$\beta(1\rightarrow4)$-*N*-acetylglucosamine linkages of peptidoglycan in Gram-positive bacterial cell walls. Several assay methods have been described for quantifying lysozyme activity. They are all based on the lysis of a suspension of freeze-dried *Micrococcus luteus* or *M. lysodeikticus*. These methods, which have been reviewed elsewhere [115], include a spectrophotometric assay [116] as well as non-enzymatic assays, such as a radioimmunoassay [117] and an immunolocalization assay [118, 119]. The authors will describe a lysozyme plate assay [120] that quantifies activity by the clearing of a suspension of *M. lysodeikticus* that has been immobilized in agarose.

Method for preparation of lysozyme plates

Melt 1.0 g of agarose in 80 ml of 50 mM-Tris-HCl (phosphate buffer may also be used), pH 6.5–7.0, and let the solution cool to 50 °C. In a separate container, suspend 30 mg of *M. lysodeikticus* in 20 ml of the Tris buffer. Add the suspension of bacteria to the cooled agarose and quickly mix. Sodium azide, as a bacteriostat, can be added to the cooled agarose to give a final concentration of 0.02%. Do not boil or add the azide to the boiling agarose. Pipette 15 ml of the agarose-*M. lysodeikticus* suspension into each of six 100 × 15 mm square plastic Petri dishes, using a levelling table if necessary. After the plates have solidified, they should be stored at 5 °C in plastic bags to retard evaporation.

Assay of lysozyme activity

Just before use, make sample wells 15–20 mm apart in the agarose plate, using a 2–3 mm cannula. Add a measured volume (10–20 μl) of conditioned medium or standard solution to each well. Do not allow the solution to overfill the wells. A standard curve can be constructed with a series of samples containing 0.03–10 μg of egg-white lysozyme (Sigma).

Incubate the plates at room temperature for 1–10 h or until clear lysis zones with well-defined edges appear. Determine the area of lysis of each well. A reticule and an indirect light box are particularly useful for this. The area of the lysis zone is proportional to the log of the egg-white lysozyme concentration.

Notes and recommendations

The lysozyme plate assay may not be as precise as the spectrophotometric assay, but it is sufficiently quantitative for routine determinations. The plate assay has the advantage of not requiring a spectrophotometer or recording equipment. It is also convenient to have the plates made up ahead of time, stored at 5 °C, as well as a 1 mg/ml egg-white lysozyme stock solution stored at -20 °C. Punching wells and adding several samples to a few plates takes very few minutes. The lysozyme plate method, therefore, is a rapid means of assaying several samples at once.

Concluding remarks

Cell culture provides a closed system that makes it possible to account accurately for the extracellular and intracellular distribution of any activities produced during continued cultivation. A constituent of macrophage-conditioned medium may be secreted or shed by viable cells, released by damaged cells, or derived from serum or other cell sources after modification or activation by macrophages. Adherence of products to cells or the culture vessel and uptake by endocytosis should be accounted for. The study of neutral proteinase secretion from macrophages is complicated yet further. The methods described measure only activity, not enzyme protein. In some cases individual enzyme activities have not been purified and characterized, and the role of enzyme precursors, activation and degradation, and of cellular inhibitors remains obscure. Macrophages from different sources within the same animal or from different species may secrete different proteins or different proportions of proteins.

Note added in proof

Recently, a new, sensitive method for analysing macrophage proteolytic enzymes and their inhibitors has been developed [136,137]. In this procedure a protein substrate, such as casein or soluble elastin, is incorporated into an SDS-gel. Enzymes present in lysates of as few as 2×10^4 cells, or in 10 ml of conditional culture medium, are detected as zones of clearing. The detailed method will appear elsewhere [138].

Acknowledgements

The authors thank Jennie R. Chin for technical assistance, and Dr Michael McKinley, Department of Neurology, University of California, San Francisco, for introducing them to the quinine sulphate procedure of Durbin & Manning [123]. This work was supported in part by the U.S. Department of Energy (#DE-AM03-76-SF01012), the U.S. Public Health Service (#HL26323), and the Medical Research Council (UK).

References

1 VAN FURTH R. (ed.) (1975) *Mononuclear Phagocytes in Immunity, Infection, and Pathology.* Blackwell Scientific Publications, Oxford.

2 NELSON D.S. (ed.) (1976) *Immunobiology of the Macrophage.* Academic Press, New York.

3 VAN FURTH R. (ed.) (1980) *Mononuclear Phagocytes: Functional Aspects.* Nijhoff (Martinus) Publishers B.V.

4 NELSON D.S. (1972) Macrophages as effectors of cell-mediated immunity. *CRC Crit. Rev. Microbiol.* **1**, 353–384.

5 MACKANESS G.B. (1970) Cellular immunity. In *Mononuclear Phagocytes*, (ed. van Furth R.), pp. 461–477. Davis, Philadelphia.

6 COHN Z.A. (1978) The activation of mononuclear phagocytes: fact, fancy, and future. *J. Immunol.* **121**, 813–816.

7 KARNOVSKY M.L. & LAZDINS J.K. (1978) The biochemical criteria for activated macrophages. *J. Immunol.* **121**, 809–813.

8 NORTH R.J. (1978) The concept of the activated macrophage. *J. Immunol.* **121**, 806–809.

9 TAKEMURA R. & WERB Z. (1984) Secretory products of macrophages and their physiologic functions. *Am. J. Physiol.* **246** (Cell Physiology, 15), C1–C9.

10 WERB Z. (1983) How the macrophage regulates its extracellular environment. *Am. J. Anat.* **166**, 237–256.

11 GORDON S., TODD J. & COHN Z.A. (1974) *In vitro* synthesis and secretion of lysozyme by mononuclear phagocytes. *J. exp. Med.* **139**, 1228–1248.

12 UNKELESS J.C., GORDON S. & REICH E. (1974) Secretion of plasminogen activator by stimulated macrophages. *J. exp. Med.* **139**, 834–850.

13 WERB Z., BANDA M.J. & JONES P.A. (1980) Degradation of connective tissue matrices by macrophages. (I) Proteolysis of elastin, glycoproteins, and collagen by proteinases isolated from macrophages. *J. exp. Med.* **152**, 1340–1357.

14 WERB Z. & CHIN J.R. (1983) Apoprotein E is synthesized and secreted by resident and thioglycollate-elicited macrophages but not by pyran copolymer- or bacillus Calmette-Guerin-activated macrophages. *J. exp. Med.* **158**, 1272–1293.

15 NATHAN C. & COHN Z. (1980) Role of oxygen-dependent mechanisms in antibody-induced lysis of tumor cells by activated macrophages. *J. exp. Med.* **152**, 198–208.

16 NATHAN C., NOGUEIRA N., JUANGBHANICH C., ELLIS J. & COHN Z. (1979) Activation of macrophages *in vivo* and *in vitro*: correlation between hydrogen peroxide release and killing of *Trypanosoma cruzi. J. exp. Med.* **149**, 1056–1068.

17 KNIGHTON D.R., HUNT T.K., SCHEUENSTUHL H., HALLIDAY B.J., WERB Z. & BANDA M.J. (1983) Oxygen tension regulates the expression of angiogenesis factor by macrophages. *Science*, **221**, 1283–1285.

18 WERB Z. & GORDON S. (1975) Secretion of a specific collagenase by stimulated macrophages. *J. exp. Med.* **142**, 346–360.

19 WERB Z. (1981) Characterization and classification of macrophage proteinases and proteinase inhibitors. In *Methods for Studying Mononuclear Phagocytes*, (eds. Adams D.O., Edelson P. & Koren H.S.), pp. 561–575. Academic Press, New York.

20 WERB Z. (1978) Pathways for the modulation of macrophage collagenase activity. In *Mechanisms of Localized Bone Loss*, (Special Supplement to *Calcified Tissue Abstracts*), (eds. Horton J.E., Tarpley T.M. & Davis W.F.), pp. 213–228. Information Retrieval, Inc., Washington D.C.

21 MAINARDI C.L., SEYER J.M. & KANG A.H. (1980) Type-specific collagenolysis: a type V collagen-degrading enzyme from macrophages. *Biochem. biophys. Res. Commun.* **97**, 1108–1115.

22 JONES P.A. & WERB Z. (1980) Degradation of connective tissue matrices by macrophages. (II) Influence of matrix composition on proteolysis of glycoproteins, elastin, and collagen by macrophages in culture. *J. exp. Med.* **152**, 1527–1536.

23 WERB Z. & GORDON S. (1975) Elastase secretion by stimulated macrophages: characterization and regulation. *J. exp. Med.* **142**, 361–377.

24 BANDA M.J. & WERB Z. (1981) Mouse macrophage elastase: purification and characterization as a metalloproteinase. *Biochem. J.* **193**, 589–605.

25 CAMMER W., BLOOM B.R., NORTON W.T. & GORDON S. (1978) Degradation of basic protein in myelin by neutral proteases secreted by stimulated macrophages: a possible mechanism of inflammatory demyelination. *Proc. natn. Acad. Sci. U.S.A.* **75**, 1554–1558.

26 HAUSER P. & VAES G. (1978) Degradation of cartilage proteoglycans by a neutral proteinase secreted by rabbit bone-marrow macrophages in culture. *Biochem. J.* **172**, 275–284.

27 BANDA M.J., CLARK E.J. & WERB Z. (1980) Limited proteolysis by macrophage elastase inactivates human α_1-proteinase inhibitor. *J. exp. Med.* **152**, 1563–1570.

28 BANDA M.J., CLARK E.J. & WERB Z. (1983) Selective proteolysis of immunoglobulins by mouse macrophage elastase. *J. exp. Med.* **157**, 1184–1196.

29 WERB Z., BAINTON D.F. & JONES P.A. (1980) Degradation of connective tissue matrices by macrophages. (III) Morphological and biochemical studies on extracellular, pericellular, and intracellular events in matrix proteolysis by macrophages in culture. *J. exp. Med.* **152**, 1537–1553.

30 LEVIN E.G. & LOSKUTOFF D.J. (1982) Cultured bovine endothelial cells produce both urokinase and tissue-type plasminogen activators. *J. Cell Biol.* **94**, 631–636.

31 CHAPMAN H.A. jun., VAVRIN Z. & HIBBS J.B. jun. (1982) Macrophage fibrinolytic activity: identification of two pathways of plasmin formation by intact cells and of a plasminogen activator inhibitor. *Cell*, **28**, 653–662.

32 SOLOMON J.A., CHOU I.-N., SCHRODER E.W. & BLACK P.H. (1980) Evidence for membrane association of plasminogen activator activity in mouse macrophages. *Biochem. biophys. Res. Commun.* **94**, 480–486.

33 ADAMS D.O., KAO K.-J., FARB R. & PIZZO S.V. (1980) Effector mechanisms of cytolytically activated macrophages. (II) Secretion of a cytolytic factor by activated macrophages and its relationship to secreted neutral proteases. *J. Immunol.* **124**, 293–300.

34 WIENER E. & LEVANON D. (1968) Macrophage cultures: an extracellular esterase. *Science*, **159**, 217–219.

35 SILVERSTEIN E., FRIEDLAND J. & SETTON C. (1979) Angiotensin converting enzyme: induction in rabbit alveolar macrophages and human monocytes in culture. *Adv. exp. Med. Biol.* **121(A)**, 149–156.

36 WERB Z. (1978) Biochemical actions of glucocorticoids on macrophages in culture. Specific inhibition of elastase, collagenase, and plasminogen activator secretion and effects on other metabolic functions. *J. exp. Med.* **147**, 1695–1712.

37 SCHNYDER J. & BAGGIOLINI M. (1980) Secretion of lysosomal enzymes by macrophages. In *Mononuclear Phagocytes: Functional Aspects*, (ed. van Furth R.), pp. 1369–1384. Nijhoff (Martinus) Publishers B.V.

38 CURRIE G.A. (1978) Activated macrophages kill tumour cells by releasing arginase. *Nature*, **273**, 758–759.

39 KUNG J.T., BROOKS S.B., JAKWAY J.P., LEONARD L.L. & TALMAGE D.W. (1977) Suppression of *in vitro* cytotoxic response by macrophages due to induced arginase. *J. exp. Med.* **146**, 665–672.

40 OLDS G.R., ELLNER J.J., KEARSE L.A. jun., KAZURA J.W. & MAHMOUD A.A.F. (1980) Role of arginase in killing of schistosomula of *Schistosoma mansoni*. *J. exp. Med.* **151**, 1557–1562.

41 KHOO J.C., MAHONEY E.M. & WITZTUM J.L. (1981) Secretion of lipoprotein lipase by macrophages in culture. *J. Biol. Chem.* **256**, 7105–7108.

42 REMOLD-O'DONNELL E. & LEWANDROWSKI K. (1983) Two proteinase inhibitors associated with peritoneal macrophages. *J. Biol. Chem.* **258**, 3251–3257.

43 HOVI T., MOSHER D. & VAHERI A. (1977) Cultured human monocytes synthesize and secrete α_2-macroglobulin. *J. exp. Med.* **145**, 1580–1589.

44 MURPHY G. & SELLERS A. (1980) The extracellular regulation of collagenase activity. In *Collagenase in Normal and Pathological Connective Tissues*, (eds. Wooley D.E. & Evanson J.M.), pp. 65–81. Wiley (John) & Sons Ltd., New York.

45 KAPLAN J. (1980) Evidence for reutilization of surface receptors for α-macroglobulin protease complexes in rabbit alveolar macrophages. *Cell*, **19**, 197–205.

46 FEY G. & COLTEN H.R. (1981) Biosynthesis of complement components. *Fedn Proc.* **40**, 2099–2104.

47 SUNDSMO J.S. & FAIR D.S. (1983) Relationships among the complement, kinin, coagulation, and fibrinolytic systems in the inflammatory reaction. *Clin. physiol.* *Biochem.* **1**, 225–284.

48 BENTLEY C., ZIMMER B. & HADDING U. (1981) The macrophage as a source of complement components. In *Lymphokines*, Vol. 4, (ed. Pick E.), pp. 197–230. Academic Press, New York.

49 OSTERUD B., BOGWARD J., LINDAHL U. & SELJELID R. (1981) Production of blood coagulation factor V and tissue thromboplastin by macrophages *in vitro*. *FEBS Lett.* **127**, 154–156.

50 OSTERUD B., LINDAHL U. & SELJELID R. (1980) Macrophages produce blood coagulation factors. *FEBS Lett.* **120**, 41–43.

51 LEVY G.A. & EDGINGTON T.S. (1980) Lymphocyte cooperation is required for amplification of macrophage procoagulant activity. *J. exp. Med.* **151**, 1232–1244.

52 BASU S.K., BROWN M.S., HO Y.K., HAVEL R.J. & GOLDSTEIN J.L. (1981) Mouse macrophages synthesize and secrete a protein resembling apolipoprotein E. *Proc. natn. Acad. Sci. U.S.A.* **78**, 7545–7549.

53 AVILA E.M., HOLDSWORTH G., SASAKI N., JACKSON R.L. & HARMONY J.A.K. (1982) Apoprotein E suppresses phytohemagglutinin-activated phospholipid turnover in peripheral blood mononuclear cells. *J. Biol. Chem.* **257**, 5900–5909.

54 CURTISS L.K. & EDGINGTON T.S. (1979) Differential sensitivity of lymphocyte subpopulations to suppression by low density lipoprotein inhibitor, an immunoregulatory human serum low density lipoprotein. *J. clin. Invest.* **63**, 193–201.

55 WERB Z. & CHIN J.R. (1983) Endotoxin suppresses expression of apoprotein E by mouse macrophages *in vivo* and in culture: a biochemical and genetic study. *J. Biol. Chem.* **258**, 10642–10648.

56 WERB Z. & CHIN J.R. (1983) Onset of apoprotein E secretion during differentiation of mouse bone marrow-derived mononuclear phagocytes. *J. Cell Biol.* **97**, 1113–1118.

57 ALITALO K., HOVI T. & VAHERI A. (1980) Fibronectin is produced by human macrophages. *J. exp. Med.* **151**, 602–613.

58 VARTIO T., HOVI T. & VAHERI A. (1982) Human macrophages synthesize and secrete a major 95,000-dalton gelatin-binding protein distinct from fibronectin. *J. Biol. Chem.* **257**, 8862–8866.

59 BEVILACQUA M.P., AMRANI D., MOSESSON M.W. & BIANCO C. (1981) Receptors for cold-insoluble globulin

(plasma fibronectin) on human monocytes. *J. exp. Med.* **153**, 42–60.

60 VAN DE WATER L. III, SCHROEDER S., CRENSHAW E.B. III & HYNES R.O. (1981) Phagocytosis of gelatin-latex particles by a murine macrophage line is dependent on fibronectin and heparin. *J. Cell Biol.* **90**, 32–39.

61 RACHMILEWITZ B., RACHMILEWITZ M., CHAOUAT M. & SCHLESINGER M. (1978) Production of TCII (vitamin B$_{12}$ transport protein) by mouse mononuclear phagocytes. *Blood*, **52**, 1089–1098.

62 FLEIT H.B. & RABINOVITCH M. (1981) Production of interferon by *in vitro* derived bone marrow macrophages. *Cell. Immunol.* **57**, 495–504.

63 SMITH T.J. & WAGNER P.R. (1967) Rabbit macrophage interferons. (I) Conditions for biosynthesis by virus-infected and uninfected cells. *J. exp. Med.* **125**, 559–577.

64 BAST R.C. jun., CLEVELAND R.P., LITTMAN B.H., ZBAR B. & RAPP H.J. (1974) Acquired cellular immunity: extracellular killing of *Listeria monocytogenes* by a product of immunologically activated macrophages. *Cell. Immunol.* **10**, 248–259.

65 POLVERINI P.J., COTRAN R.S., GIMBRONE M.A. jun. & UNANUE E.R. (1977) Activated macrophages induce vascular proliferation. *Nature*, **269**, 804–806.

66 MARTIN B.M., GIMBRONE M.A. JUN., UNANUE E.R. & COTRAN R.S. (1981) Stimulation of nonlymphoid mesenchymal cell proliferation by a macrophage derived growth factor. *J. Immunol.* **126**, 1510–1515.

67 RALPH P., BROXMEYER H.E., MOORE M.A.S. & NAKOINZ I. (1978) Induction of myeloid colony-stimulating activity in murine monocyte tumor cell lines by macrophage activators and in a T-cell line by concanavalin A. *Cancer Res.* **38**, 1414–1419.

68 MIZEL S.B. & MIZEL D. (1981) Purification to apparent homogeneity of murine interleukin 1. *J. Immunol.* **126**, 834–837.

69 ROSENWASSER L.J. & DINARELLO C.A. (1981) Ability of human leukocytic pyrogen to enhance phytohemagglutinin induced murine thymocyte proliferation. *Cell. Immunol.* **63**, 134–142.

70 BODEL P. (1974) Studies on the mechanism of endogenous pyrogen production. (III) Human blood monocytes. *J. exp. Med.* **140**, 954–965.

71 PALMER W.G. (1976) The serum haptoglobin response to inflammation in neonatal mice and its relationship to phagocytosis. *J. Reticuloendothel. Soc.* **19**, 301–309.

72 SIPE J.D., VOGEL S.N., RYAN J.L., McADAM K.P.W.J. & ROSENSTREICH D.L. (1979) Detection of a mediator derived from endotoxin-stimulated macrophages that induces the acute phase serum amyloid A response in mice. *J. exp. Med.* **150**, 597–606.

73 DINARELLO C.A. & WOLFF S.M. (1982) Molecular basis of fever in humans. *Am. J. Med.* **72**, 799–819.

74 SZTEIN M.B., VOGEL S.N., SIPE J.D., MURPHY P.A., MIZEL S.B., OPPENHEIM J.J. & ROSENSTREICH D.L. (1981) The role of macrophages in acute-phase response: SAA inducer is closely related to lymphocyte activating factor and endogenous pyrogen. *Cell. Immunol.* **63**, 164–176.

75 MIZEL S.B., DAYER J.-M., KRANE S.M. & MERGENHAGEN S.E. (1981) Stimulation of rheumatoid synovial cell collagenase and prostaglandin production by partially purified lymphocyte-activating factor (interleukin 1). *Proc. natn. Acad. Sci. U.S.A.* **78**, 2474–2477.

76 SCHMIDT J.A., MIZEL S.B., COHEN D. & GREEN I. (1982) Interleukin 1, a potential regulator of fibroblast proliferation. *J. Immunol.* **128**, 2177–2182.

77 JOHNSTON R.B. jun. (1978) Oxygen metabolism and the microbicidal activity of macrophages. *Fedn. Proc.* **37**, 2759–2764.

78 SASADA M. & JOHNSTON R.B. jun. (1980) Macrophage microbicidal activity. Correlation between phagocytosis-associated oxidative metabolism and the killing of *Candida* by macrophages. *J. exp. Med.* **152**, 85–98.

79 MURRAY H.W., NATHAN C.F. & COHN Z.A. (1980) Macrophage oxygen-dependent antimicrobial activity. (IV) Role of endogenous scavengers of oxygen intermediates. *J. exp. Med.* **152**, 1610–1624.

80 STENSON W.F. & PARKER C.W. (1980) Prostaglandins, macrophages, and immunity. *J. Immunol.* **125**, 1–5.

81 GEMSA D., SEITZ M., KRAMER W., TILL G. & RESCH K. (1978) The effects of phagocytosis, dextran sulfate, and cell damage on PGE$_1$ sensitivity and PGE$_1$ production of macrophages. *J. Immunol.* **120**, 1187–1194.

82 HUMES J.L., BURGER S., GALAVAGE M., KUEHL F.A. jun., WIGHTMAN P.D., DAHLGREN M.E., DAVIES P. & BONNEY R.J. (1980) The diminished production of arachidonic acid oxygenation products by elicited mouse peritoneal macrophages: possible mechanisms. *J. Immunol.* **124**, 2110–2116.

83 MENCIA-HUERTA J.M. & BENVENISTE J. (1979) Platelet-activating factor and macrophages. (I) Evidence for the release from rat and mouse peritoneal macrophages and not from mastocytes. *Eur. J. Immunol.* **9**, 409–415.

84 ROUZER C.A., SCOTT W.A., COHN Z.A., BLACKBURN P. & MANNING J.M. (1980) Mouse peritoneal macrophages release leukotriene C in response to a phagocytic stimulus. *Proc. natn. Acad. Sci. U.S.A.* **77**, 4928–4932.

85 CHAN T.-S. (1979) Purine excretion by mouse peritoneal macrophages lacking adenosine deaminase activity. *Proc. natn. Acad. Sci. U.S.A.* **76**, 925–929.

86 GEMSA D., STEGGEMANR L., MENZEL J. & TILL G. (1975) Release of cyclic AMP from macrophages by stimulation with prostaglandins. *J. Immunol.* **114**, 1422–1424.

87 STADECKER M.J. & UNANUE E.R. (1979) The regulation of thymidine secretion by macrophages. *J. Immunol.* **123**, 568–571.

88 OOI Y.M. & OOI B.S. (1982) Biosynthesis of membrane factor B by mouse peritoneal macrophages. *Nature*, **298**, 389–391.

89 GORDON S., UNKELESS J.C. & COHN Z.A. (1974) Induction of macrophage plasminogen activator by endotoxin stimulation and phagocytosis. Evidence for a two-stage process. *J. exp. Med.* **140**, 995–1010.

90 GORDON S. & COHN Z.A. (1978) Bacille Calmette-Guerin infection in the mouse. Regulation of macrophage plasminogen activator by T lymphocytes and specific antigen. *J. exp. Med.* **147**, 1175–1188.

91 NOGUEIRA N., GORDON S. & COHN Z. (1977) *Trypanosoma cruzi*: modification of macrophage function during infection. *J. exp. Med.* **146**, 157–171.

92 NOGUEIRA N., GORDON S. & COHN Z. (1977) *Trypano-*

soma cruzi: the immunological induction of macrophage plasminogen activator requires thymus-derived lymphocytes. *J. exp. Med.* **146**, 172–183.

93 WAHL L.M., WAHL S.M., MERGENHAGEN S.E. & MARTIN G.R. (1975) Collagenase production by lymphokine-activated macrophages. *Science*, **187**, 261–263.

94 GORDON S. & WERB Z. (1976) Secretion of macrophage neutral proteinase is enhanced by colchicine. *Proc. natn. Acad. Sci. U.S.A.* **73**, 872–876.

95 WERB Z. & CHIN J. (1981) Biosynthetic radiolabeling of cellular and secreted proteins of mononuclear phagocytes. In *Methods for Studying Mononuclear Phagocytes*, (eds. Adams D.O., Edelson P. & Koren H.S.), pp. 861–872. Academic Press, New York.

96 LAEMMLI U.K. (1970) Cleavage of structural proteins during the assembly of the head of bacteriophage T4. *Nature*, **227**, 680–685.

97 BONNER W.M. & LASKEY R.A. (1974) A film detection method for tritium-labelled proteins and nucleic acids in polyacrylamide gels. *Eur. J. Biochem.* **46**, 83–88.

98 LASKEY R.A. & MILLS A.D. (1975) Quantitative film detection of ^{3}H and ^{14}C in polyacrylamide gels by fluorography. *Eur. J. Biochem.* **56**, 335–341.

99 SKUDLAREK M.D. & SWANK R.T. (1979) Biosynthesis of two lysosomal enzymes in macrophages. Evidence for a precursor of β-galactosidase. *J. Biol. Chem.* **254**, 9939–9942.

100 CLEVELAND D.W., FISCHER S.G., KIRSCHNER M.W. & LAEMMLI U.K. (1977) Peptide mapping by limited proteolysis in sodium dodecyl sulfate and analysis by gel electrophoresis. *J. Biol. Chem.* **252**, 1102–1106.

101 JOHNSON E.F., ZOUNES M.C. & MULLER-EBERHARD U. (1979) Characterization of three forms of rabbit microsomal cytochrome P-450 by peptide mapping utilizing limited proteolysis in sodium dodecyl sulfate and analysis by gel electrophoresis. *Archs Biochem. Biophys.* **192**, 282–289.

102 UNKELESS J.C., TOBIA A., OSSOWSKI L., QUIGLEY J.P., RIFKIN D.B. & REICH E. (1973) An enzymatic function associated with transformation of fibroblasts by oncogenic viruses. (I) Chick embryo fibroblast cultures transformed by avian RNA tumor viruses. *J. exp. Med.* **137**, 85–111.

103 HUNTER W.M. & GREENWOOD F.C. (1962) Preparation of iodine-131 labelled human growth hormone of high specific activity. *Nature*, **194**, 495–496.

104 DEUTSCH D.G. & MERTZ E.T. (1970) Plasminogen: purification from human plasma by affinity chromatography. *Science*, **170**, 1095–1096.

105 WERB Z. & AGGELER J. (1978) Proteases induce secretion of collagenase and plasminogen activator by fibroblasts. *Proc. natn. Acad. Sci. U.S.A.* **75**, 1839–1843.

106 BANDA M.J., DOVEY H.F. & WERB Z. (1981) Elastinolytic enzymes. In *Methods for Studying Mononuclear Phagocytes*, (eds. Adams D.O., Edelson P. & Koren H.S.), pp. 603–618. Academic Press, New York.

107 GORDON S., WERB Z. & COHN Z. (1976) Methods for detection of macrophage secretory enzymes. In *In Vitro Methods in Cell-Mediated and Tumor Immunity*, (eds. Bloom B.R. & David J.R.), pp. 341–352. Academic Press, New York.

108 TAKAHASHI S., SEIFTER S. & YANG F.C. (1973) A new radioactive assay for enzymes with elastolytic activity using reduced tritiated elastin. The effect of sodium dodecyl sulfate on elastolysis. *Biochim. biophys. Acta*, **327**, 138–145.

109 STONE P.J., CROMBIE G. & FRANZBLAU C. (1977) The use of tritiated elastin for the determination of subnanogram amounts of elastase. *Analyt. Biochem.* **80**, 572–577.

110 JONES P.A. & WERB Z. (1981) Growth of macrophages on collagen-, elastin-, and glycoprotein-coated plates as a tool for investigating macrophage proteinases. In *Methods for Studying Mononuclear Phagocytes*, (eds. Adams D.O., Edelson P. & Koren H.S.), pp. 577–591. Academic Press, New York.

111 BANDA M.J., CLARK E.J. & WERB Z. (1981) The role of macrophage elastase in the proteolysis of plasma and interstitial proteins. In *Heterogeneity of Mononuclear Phagocytes*, (eds. Forster O. & Landy M.), pp. 286–288. Academic Press, New York.

112 BANDA M.J. & WERB Z. (1980) The role of macrophage elastase in the proteolysis of fibrinogen, plasminogen, and fibronectin. *Fedn Proc.* **39**, 1756.

113 KAGAN H.M., CROMBIE G.D., JORDAN R.E., LEWIS W. & FRANZBLAU C. (1972) Proteolysis of elastin–ligand complexes. Stimulation of elastase digestion of insoluble elastin by sodium dodecyl sulfate. *Biochemistry*, **11**, 3412–3418.

114 KAGAN H.M. (1978) Changes in the state of ionization of carboxyl groups in elastin in response to the binding of sodium dodecyl sulfate. *Connect. Tissue Res.* **6**, 167–169.

115 NERURKAR L.S. (1981) Lysozyme. In *Methods for Studying Mononuclear Phagocytes*, (eds. Adams D.O., Edelson P. & Koren H.S.), pp. 667–683. Academic Press, New York.

116 LITWACK, G. (1955) Photometric determination of lysozyme activity. *Proc. Soc. exp. Biol. Med.* **89**, 401–403.

117 PEETERS T.L., DEPRAETERE Y.R. & VANTRAPPEN G.R. (1978) Radioimmunoassay for urinary lysozyme in human serum from leukemic patients. *Clin. Chem.* **24**, 2155–2157.

118 KLOCKARS M., ADINOLFI M.C. & OSSERMAN E.F. (1974) Ontogeny of lysozyme in the rat. *Proc. Soc. exp. Biol. Med.* **145**, 604–609.

119 SPICER S.S., FRAYSER R., VIRELLA G. & HALL B.J. (1977) Immunocytochemical localization of lysozymes in respiratory and other tissues. *Lab. Invest.* **36**, 282–295.

120 OSSERMAN E.F. & LAWLOR D.P. (1966) Serum and urinary lysozyme (muramidase) in monocytic and monomyelocytic leukemia. *J. exp. Med.* **124**, 921–951.

121 SCHWARTZ B.S., DOYLE M.J., WESTRICK L.L. & MOSHER D.F. (1983) Human peripheral monocytes synthesize and secrete thrombospondin. *Blood*, **62** (suppl. 1), 87a.

122 RICH I.N., HEIT W. & KUBANEK B. (1982) Extrarenal erythropoietin production by macrophages. *Blood*, **60**, 1007–1018.

123 BOLTON D.C., McKINLEY M.P. & PRUISNER S.B. (1982) Identificaton of a protein that purifies with scrapie prions. *Science*, **218**, 1309–1311.

124 CIBA FOUNDATION SYMPOSIUM NO. 118 (1985) *Biochemistry of Macrophages* (in press).

125 GORDON S. & EZEKOWITZ R.A.B. (1985) Macrophage neural proteinases: nature, regulation, and role. In *The Reticuloendothelial System. A Comprehensive Treatise* (eds. Reichard S.M. & Filkins J.P.), Vol 7B, pp. 95–141.

126 PERLMUTTER D.H., COLE S.S., ROSSING P., KILBRIDGE P. & COLTEN H.R. (1985) Expression of α_1 proteinase inhibitor gene in human monocytes and macrophages. *Proc. natn. Acad. Sci. U.S.A.* **85**, 795–799.

127 SUNDSMO J.S., CHIN J.R., PAPIN R.A., FAIR D.S. & WERB Z. (1985) Factor B, the complement alternative pathway serine proteinase, is a major constitutive protein synthesized and secreted by resident and elicited mouse macrophages. *J. exp. Med.* **161**, 306–322.

128 EZEKOWITZ R.A.B., SIM R.B., HILL M. & GORDON S. (1984) Local opsonization by secreted macrophage complement components. Role of receptors for complement in uptake of zymosan. *J. exp. Med.* **159**, 244–260.

129 WRIGHT S.D., LICHT M.R., CRAIGMYLE L.S. & SILVERSTEIN S.C. (1984) Communication between receptors for different ligands on a single cell. Ligation of fibronectin receptors induces a reversible alteration in the function of complement receptors on cultured human monocytes. *J. Cell Biol.* **99**, 336–339.

130 BEUTLER B., MAHONEY J., LE TRANG N., PEKALA P. & CERAMI A. (1985) Purification of cachectin , a lipoprotein lipase-suppressing hormone secreted by endotoxin-induced RAW 264.7 cells. *J. exp. Med.* **161**, 984–995.

131 LOMEDICO P.T., GUBLER U., HELLMANN C.P., DUKOVICH M., GIRI J.G., PAN Y.-C.E, COLLIER K., SEMIONOW R., CHUA A.O. & MIZEL S.B. (1984) *Nature*, **312**, 458–462.

132 LEPAY D.A., NATHAN C.F., STEINMAN R.M., MURRAY H.W. & COHN Z.A. (1985) Murine Kupffer cells. Mononuclear phagocytes deficient in the generation of reactive oxygen intermediates. *J. exp. Med.* **161**, 1079–1096.

133 LEPAY D.A., STEINMAN R.M., NATHAN C.F., MURRAY H.W. & COHN Z.A. (1985) Liver macrophages in murine listeriosis. Cell-mediated immunity is correlated with an influx of macrophages capable of generating reactive oxygen intermediates. *J. exp. Med.* **161**, 1503–1512.

134 SCHREIBER R.D., HICKS L.J., CELADA A., BUCHMEIER N.A. & GRAY P.W. (1985) Monoclonal antibodies to murine γ-interferon which differentially modulate macrophage activation and antiviral activity. *J. Immunol.* **134**, 1609–1618.

135 MURRAY H.W., SPITALNY G.L. & NATHAN C.F. (1985) Activation of mouse peritoneal macrophages *in vitro* and *in vivo* by interferon-γ. *J. Immunol.* **134**, 1619–1622.

136 CHIN J.R., MURPHY G. & WERB Z. (1985) Stromelysin, a connective tissue-degrading metalloendopeptidase secreted by stimulated rabbit synovial cells in parallel with collagenase. Biosynthesis, isolation, characterization, and substrates. *J. Biol. Chem.* **260**, in press.

137 MCKERROW J.H., PINO-HEISS S., LINDQUIST R. & WERB Z. (1985) Purification and characterization of an elastinolytic proteinase secreted by cercariae of *Schistosoma mansoni*. *J. Biol. Chem.* **260**, 3703–3707.

138 WERB Z., BANDA M.J. & MCKERROW J.H. (1986) Degradation of elastin. *Meth. Enzym.* (in press).

Chapter 48
Macrophage membrane receptors

J. STEWART, ELIZABETH J. GLASS, D. M. WEIR & M. R. DAHA

Receptors for the Fc fragment of immunoglobulins (FcR), 48.2
Methods for detecting FcRs, 48.2
Receptors for complement components, 48.5
Methods for detecting complement receptors, 48.6
'Lectin-like' receptors for bacterial cell wall sugars, 48.9
Methods for detecting 'lectin-like' receptors, 48.9
Ia antigens on macrophages, 48.9
Methods for the detection of Ia antigens on macrophages, 48.10
Appendix, 48.11

The detection and study of macrophage membrane receptors have proved of central importance in cell lineage studies and for the determination of the functional activities of these cells. Recognition of the wide variety of receptors (probably more than 30) has placed the macrophage as the central cell in initiating immune responsiveness as an antigen presenting cell (APC), and in regulating the activities of other cells of the immune system. At the same time, but often overlooked by immunologists, by receptor ligand interaction the macrophage takes part in wound healing, lipid metabolism, and regulation of granulocyte and macrophage pools through the production of colony stimulating factors. These various processes operate through complex feedback loops [for review, see 1].

To the immunologist interested in studying the macrophage the most widely used assays are those for the various Fc receptors, usually those for IgG subclasses, for complement receptors and for other surface structures including products of the major histocompatibility complex (MHC) and 'lectin-like' receptors.

In general these assays are performed *in vitro* and the results may not reflect the true *in vivo* situation. In addition assays carried out on adherent cells may give different results than cell suspensions. It has been reported that human blood monocytes as monolayers bind ^{125}I-lactoferrin with approximately 100-fold lower affinity as compared to cells in suspension [2]. For tests in suspension the problem of adherence of monocytes/macrophages to the container with the likely selection of subpopulations can be reduced by the use of polyethylene tubes (Minisorb, Nune, Denmark) or by treating the container with siliconizing fluid (Dimethyldichlorosilane solution, BDH, Poole, Dorset). It has been pointed out that assays using adherent cell preparations are more likely to represent the *in vivo* environment where macrophages would spread out on interstitial tissue and in these conditions the cells can show altered functional activities [3]. The process of tissue homogenization, as well as other disruptive methods to prepare cell suspensions, can lead to possible damage to cells with changes in receptor expression, as a result of the enzyme treatment destroying or uncovering the receptor or the selection of particular subpopulations of cells. Another consideration when assaying receptor ligand interactions stems from the physical nature of the ligand and whether it is in a state that is likely to lead to endocytosis or phagocytosis. In studies of the C3b receptor, a complex of C3b and a red cell membrane preparation was found to bind 15–80 times more effectively than free ^{125}I-labelled C3b [4] and the complex is also found to be phagocytosed quite readily by resident guinea-pig peritoneal macrophages.

Methods available for the estimation and detection of monocyte/macrophage receptor ligand interactions fall into three general categories.

1 Where the ligand is particulate, e.g. bacterium, yeast, and red blood cells, the attachment can be detected visually [5,6,7] or an appropriate isotope can be used to label the particle [8], and binding detected radioactively.

2 Where the ligand is in a soluble or an aggregated form, it can be labelled with ^{125}I for direct detection [9,10]. Alternatively, receptors for these types of ligand can be investigated by attachment to carrier particles such as red blood cells. An erythrocyte (E), can be coated with a purified preparation of a particular immunoglobulin class or subclass (EA) for Fc receptor detection [11] or with IgM and C3b (EAC3b) for complement receptor identification [12] or chemicals (histamine) by appropriate reagents [13]. Disrupted erythrocyte membranes with attached C3b labelled with ^{125}I have also been used [14]. A hapten such as dinitrophenol can be attached to the ligand and bound ligand detected using ^{125}I-labelled antibody directed against the hapten [3,15,16].

3 Where the receptor is exposed to anti-receptor antibodies, conventional or monoclonal, they are usually radioactively labelled [17] but they can also be attached to an appropriate carrier particle. Anti-receptor antibodies bound to the cell surface can also be detected by simple rosette assays [18], immuno-fluorescence [19], immunoperoxidase [20], and fluorimetry [21].

Receptors for the Fc fragment of immunoglobulins (FcR)

Macrophage Fc receptors are involved in the selective binding and ingestion of foreign material [22] and effete autologous material [23]. These receptors bind to the Fc portion of immunoglobulins which have been produced against and bind to foreign antigens. Apart from their involvement in phagocytosis, Fc receptors are also important in antibody-dependent cell-mediated cytotoxicity (ADCC) [24,25,26].

Inflammatory mediators, including prostaglandins (particularly PGE_2), are released after ingestion of antibody–antigen complexes or antibody-coated red cells [27,28]. Fc receptor interaction also stimulates the secretion of superoxide anion [29] and various enzymes [30,31].

In man peripheral blood monocytes express receptors that recognize the Fc portion of IgG1, IgG3, and IgG4. There are reported to be $14.5–19 \times 10^3$ receptors/cell for IgG with cross-species reactivity for rabbit IgG which binds to the receptor with a lower affinity [9]. Human monocytes also express IgM [32] and IgE receptors [33,34]. The IgE receptor on the monocyte may be different from that on mast cells and basophils as IgE binds to these latter cells with a much higher affinity (10^8–10^{10} M^{-1}) [35]. Murine Fc receptors have been identified for IgG_{2a} (FcR_1), IgG1 and IgG_{2b} (FcR_2), and IgG3 (FcR_3) [36]. There are about 4.4×10^5 sites per cell for FcR_1 and 2.9×10^5 for FcR_2 [37]. Guinea-pig Fc receptors for IgG1 and IgG2 have been described on peritoneal macrophages [15,38]. Fc receptors are present on many cells apart from monocytes and macrophages, including lymphoid cells of the B,T and null lineage [39,40,41], neutrophils [42], eosinophils [43], basophils [44], and platelets [45]. It has been reported that IgG2 receptor on guinea-pig macrophages binds IgG2 some 50–70 times more effectively than the receptor on neutrophils [15].

Methods for detecting Fc receptors

Rosette assay

Equipment

Spectrophotometer.
Centrifuge.
Water-bath.
Microscope.
Conical centrifuge tubes.
Sixteen millimetre diameter tissue culture plates.
Thirteen millimetre diameter glass coverslips.
Glass microscope slides.

Materials

Mouse IgG_{2b} anti-sheep erythrocyte monoclonal antibody (Sera-Lab).
Sheep red cells.
0.15 M-NaCl.
Phosphate-buffered saline (PBS).
Methanol.
May Grunwald and Giemsa stains.
Alsever's solution.
10% formol-saline (10 ml formalin up to 100 ml with PBS).

Procedure

Preparation of indicator cells

1 Obtain sheep blood aseptically and dilute 1:1 with sterile Alsever's solution. Store at 4 °C for not longer than 2 weeks.
2 Wash the red cells (at 600 *g*) three times with PBS and then adjust the cell concentration to 1×10^9 cells/ml (see 'Notes and recommendations').
3 Mix an equal volume of antibody and red cells. The dilution of antibody required will depend on its titre (see 'Notes and recommendations').
4 Incubate the mixture for 30 min at 37 °C.
5 Wash the cells a further three times with PBS. The resultant cells coated with immunoglobulin are termed EA_G and can be stored at 4 °C for up to 5 days if they are washed daily with PBS.

Detection of Fc receptors on cells in suspension

1 Mix together 0.1 ml of EA_G (10^8 cells per ml) and 0.1 ml of macrophages (1×10^6 macrophages per ml) in conical centrifuge tubes.
2 Centrifuge at 100 *g* for 10 min at 4 °C and incubate the pellets for 30 min at 4 °C.
3 Remove supernatant, gently resuspend the pellet in

0.1 ml Eagles' medium containing 1% formol saline (final concentration) and smear the suspension on to clean glass slides.

4 Dry the smears quickly in air, fix in methanol (at least 10 min) and stain with May Grunwald/Giemsa. Macrophages with three or more adherent red cells are termed rosettes. In each slide count 200 cells and calculate the percentage of rosetted cells.

Detection of Fc receptors on cells in monolayers

1 Prepare monolayers by layering 2×10^5 macrophages in 1 ml on to 13 mm diameters (No. 1) glass coverslips in 16 mm diameter tissue culture plates. Incubate the cells for 1 h at 37 °C and remove non-adherent cells by washing with **PBS**.
2 Add 2 ml of EA_G (2.5×10^7 cells per ml) to each monolayer, centrifuge for 5 min at 100 g and incubate for 40 min at 37 °C.
3 Remove non-adherent red cells by very gently washing with **PBS**.
4 Dry the coverslips in air and fix and stain as above. Macrophages with two or more adherent red cells are termed rosettes. In each coverslip count 200 cells and calculate the percentage of rosetted cells.

Notes and recommendations

The concentration of sheep red blood cells can be determined in the conventional way using a haemocytometer or more easily and accurately using a spectrophotometer as follows.

Take a portion of the cells and make a 1:30 dilution with distilled water. Allow the cells to lyse. Read the optical density of the solution at either 541 nm or 414 nm. The concentration of the red cells can thus be calculated:

$$1 \times 10^9 \text{ red cells per ml:O.D.}_{541} = 0.350$$
$$5 \times 10^8 \text{ red cells per ml:O.D.}_{541} = 0.175$$
$$1 \times 10^8 \text{ red cells per ml:O.D.}_{414} = 0.286$$

The dilution of antibody used to sensitize the red cells has to be just below the agglutinating titre. The class and subclass of antibody can be varied, as can the source of erythrocyte. Bovine red blood cells can be coated with large amounts of antibody before they are agglutinated [46] and are useful for studying low avidity receptors.

After rosetting in suspension, a hair dryer or fan (no heat) can be used to speed up drying of smears. This reduces the chance of red cell lysis.

Monolayers are best washed by dipping the coverslip into a number of beakers containing buffer and finally dipping into Eagles' medium with 1% formol saline.

Binding of aggregated immunoglobulin

Equipment

Spectrophotometer.
Ultracentrifuge.
Microscope.
Microcentrifuge.
2.5×30 cm chromatography column.

Materials

Guinea-pig serum.
Ammonium sulphate.
DEAE-cellulose (Whatman, Kent, UK).
0.01 M-Tris-HCl, pH 8.0.
0.1 M-borate-buffered saline (BBS), pH 7.4.
Sucrose.
Reagent for iodination of proteins by chloroamine T [47].
0.01 M-Tris-buffered Hanks' solution (TBH), pH 7.4.
Sheep red blood cells (SRBC).
Twelve millilitre glass round-bottom tubes, lightly siliconized (Prosil 28™, PCR research chemicals Inc., Gainesville, Florida 32602).
Dibutyl phthalate (J.T. Baker Chemicals, Deventer, The Netherlands).
Dinonyl phthalate (Merck, Dormstadt, W. Germany).
Polypropylene micro-test-tubes.

Procedure

Preparation of aggregated IgG2 (AIgG2)

1 Isolate guinea-pig IgG_2 from 100 ml of normal Hartley strain guinea-pig serum by precipitation of globulins with 33% ammonium sulphate and subsequent anion-exchange chromatography on a 2.5×30 cm DEAE-cellulose (Whatmann, Kent, UK) column equilibrated in 0.01 M-Tris-HCl buffer (pH 8.0).
2 Pool the fall-through fractions containing IgG_2, dialyse against 0.1 M-borate-buffered saline and concentrate to 20 mg/ml.
3 Radiolabel 2 ml volumes of IgG_2 by the chloramine T method [47] to a specific activity of 0.1 mCi/mg protein.
4 Determine the concentrations of IgG by optical absorption at 280 nm using an extinction coefficient ($E^{1\%}_{1cm}$) of 14.7.
5 Incubate ^{125}I-IgG_2 (10.0 mg/ml) for 20 min at 63 °C.
6 Separate the aggregates of ^{125}I-IgG_2 ($AIgG_2$) of different sizes by ultracentrifugation for 2 h at 269 000 g in 10–30% (w/v) sucrose gradients.

Notes and recommendations

To preserve the homogeneity of the $AIgG_2$ make the
gradients in 0.5% bovine serum albumin (BSA)
[48,49], and store the fractionated $AIgG_2$ at $-80\,°C$ in
the same protein-containing buffer. Calculate the
approximate mean number of IgG molecules per
aggregate in each fraction from the sedimentation
coefficient (S-rate) as described [50]. Then calculate the
molar concentration of $(AIgG_2)_n$ (n is the average
number of IgG_2 per aggregate) for each fraction from
the relative molecular mass and specific activity.

Determination of the number of Fc receptors

1 Obtain peritoneal macrophages from healthy
Hartley strain guinea-pigs (300–400 g each) by lavag-
ing the peritoneal cavity of freshly sacrificed animals
with 50 ml of 0.01 M-Tris-buffered Hanks' solution (at
37 °C).
2 Centrifuge the cells at 1500 *g* for 10 min and
resuspend in TBH containing 0.5% BSA (TBH-BSA).
3 Pre-incubate 1 ml portions of cell suspension for 2
h at 37 °C in new, lightly siliconized, round-bottom 12
ml glass tubes to allow macrophages to adhere. The
cells were added at a concentration which from
preliminary experiments was known to give 0.5×10^6
macrophages per tube (see 'Notes and recommendations').
4 Agitate the tubes and aspirate the non-adherent
cells.
5 Add ^{125}I-$AIgG_2$ (0.01–10.0 μg) in 200 μl TBH-BSA
to each tube and incubate the tubes for 20 h at 4 °C
with continuous shaking.
6 Shake the contents of the tubes vigorously and
layer the cell suspension over 1 ml of a mixture of 7
vols. dibutyl phthalate (J.T. Baker Chemicals,
Deventer, The Netherlands) and 3 vols. dinonyl
phthalate (Merck, Darmstadt, Germany) in 1.5 ml
polypropylene micro-test-tubes.
7 Centrifuge for 45 s at room temperature in a
Beckman microcentrifuge at 8000 *g* to sediment the
particles.
8 Remove the aqueous phase together with the
upper four-fifths of the oil mixture to quantify free
^{125}I-$AIgG_2$.
9 Cut the tubes just above the cell pellets and count
the sections containing the pellets to measure the
amount of ^{125}I-$AIgG_2$ bound by the macrophages.

Notes and recommendations

Fig. 48.1 shows the results obtained with
^{125}I-$(AIgG_2)_{10}$ expressed as a percentage of the maximum bindable AIgG to an excess of macrophages. The

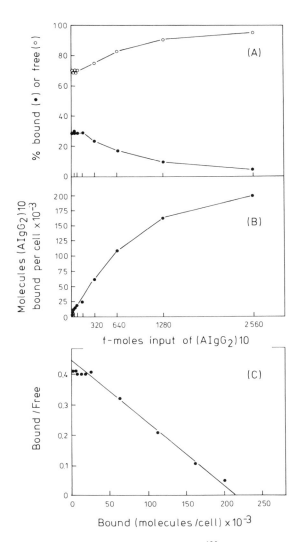

Fig. 48.1. Binding during 20 h at 4 °C of ^{125}I-$(AIgG_2)_{10}$ to
0.5×10^6 adherent peritoneal macrophages (panel A). In
panel B the results are expressed as number of molecules
$(AIgG_2)_{10}$ bound per cell in relation to the input of
^{125}I-$(AIgG_2)_{10}$. In panel C the data are plotted in a
Scatchard plot in which the number of molecules of
^{125}I-$(AIgG_2)_{10}$ bound per cell are shown versus the bound
over free ligand ratio.

maximum bindable $(AIgG_2)_{10}$ in the ^{125}I-$AIgG_{10}$ preparation is 80.1%. As expected an increase in the dose of
^{125}I-$(AIgG_2)_{10}$ results in an increase in the amount of
ligand bound to the cells (Fig. 48.1a and b). These
results were plotted in a Scatchard [51] plot and from
Fig. 48.1c it is computed that the maximum number of
$(AIgG_2)_{10}$ bound per cell is 215 000. Using the formula
$B/F = nK_a - BK_a$, the K_a is calculated to be 0.61×10^{10}

M^{-1} (B stands for bound ^{125}I-$AIgG_2$; F for free ^{125}I-$AIgG_2$; n is the number of ^{125}I-$AIgG_2$ bound per cell; and K_a is the association constant). In parallel experiments, data were obtained for the binding of $(AIgG_2)_{40}$, $(AIgG_2)_{20}$, $(AIgG_2)_5$ and monomeric IgG_2 by macrophages. The maximum numbers of molecules of these ligands bound to the cells are presented in Table 48.1. It can be concluded from the data that the numbers of $AIgG_2$ which are bound per macrophage decreases as the size of the aggregate increases. On the other hand, aggregates are bound with greater affinity to the Fc receptors on the peritoneal macrophages than are monomeric IgG_2. Although slightly fewer molecules of $(AIgG_2)_5$ or $(AIgG_2)_{10}$ are bound per macrophage as compared to the binding of monomeric IgG_2, the relatively more avid binding of $(AIgG_2)_5$ and $(AIgG_2)_{10}$ permits better washing of the cells at the end of the experiments, which results in lower backgrounds in the assays. The cells can therefore be washed in the same tubes with ice-cold TBH-BSA rather than centrifuging them through an oil phase.

By counting the aspirated cells it was established that in the authors' system $40.1 + 4.8\%$ of the cells adhered. Hence it can be assumed that 40.1% of the added cell suspensions adhere, allowing the results to be calculated on a per macrophage basis. Studies with similar preparations show that greater than 90% of the adherent cells ingested latex and are positive for α-naphthyl butyrate esterase [52]. In addition, more than 90% of the adherent cells are able to ingest sheep erythrocytes (SRBC) sensitized with subagglutinating concentrations of IgG_2-anti SRBC. Pre-incubate control tubes, which are included in all experiments, with buffer alone or with 5×10^6 SRBC and otherwise treat

Table 48.1. Maximum number of various sized aggregates or monomeric IgG_2 bound per macrophage and the mean equilibrium constants, K_a.

	Maximum ^{125}I-$(AIgG_2)_n$ bound per cell	Equilibrium constant, $K_a \times 10^{10}$ M^{-1}
$(AIgG_2)_{40}$	146 000	1.48
$(AIgG_2)_{20}$	165 200	1.32
$(AIgG_2)_{10}$	215 000	0.61
$(AIgG_2)_5$	236 000	0.21
Monomeric IgG_2	251 000	0.09

The maximum number of ^{125}I-$AIgG$ bound per cell was calculated by multiplying the moles of $AIgG$ bound at saturation (abscissa intercept) and dividing by the number of cells. Equilibrium constants were determined from the scope of the straight line fitted to the data.

exactly as the macrophage-containing tubes. Lightly siliconized glass tubes are used to allow the macrophages to adhere but stop non-specific binding of ^{125}I-$AIgG_2$ to the glass. Tubes are immersed in siliconizing solution, 15 ml of PROSIL-28™ added to ten litres distilled water, and dried upside down.

The above method can be used for macrophages prepared by different techniques or any other cell type by starting at step 5.

Receptors for complement components (CR)

Complement receptors are involved in the selective elimination of invasive pathogens by macrophages. Their biological importance is evidenced by patients with hereditary C3 metabolism. These patients, whose serum opsonizing capacity is diminished [53], have an increased susceptibility to life-threatening recurrent infections which can be controlled by phagocytes in normal serum. Both complement and Fc receptors are important in bacterial killing by human monocytes [54].

C3b receptor stimulation causes lysosomal enzyme release from macrophages, presumably by interacting with C3b receptors [55] and it has been suggested that this may play an important role in certain chronic inflammatory conditions [56]. These receptors may play a role in antigen presentation to B lymphocytes by enhancing the approximation of different cell types involved in co-operation [57].

Human leucocytes express three types of C3 receptors; CR1, 205 000 Mr, specific for a c region site in C3b, iC3b, and C3c; CR2, 72 000 Mr, specific for a d region site in iC3b, C3d-g, and C3d; CR_3, 90 000 and 105 000 Mr (in mouse), specific for the g region of C3d-g [58].

The CR1 receptor is expressed on a number of different cell types including human monocytes, lymphocytes, and granulocytes. The CR2 is only present on B lymphocytes, and the CR3 is detectable on 95% monocytes, 99% neutrophils, and 40% of large granular lymphocytes, with good correlation of expression with Mac-1 and OKM-1 antigens [59]. Ross & Lachmann [59] have provided evidence that the CR3 receptor may be a lectin-like molecule as the binding of its ligand was inhibited by N-acetyl-D-glucosamine and EDTA.

The human CR1 C3b/C4b receptor on red cells, phagocytes and lymphocytes has been shown to be a polymorphic membrane glycoprotein of approximately 200 kDa (Mr) and exists in four codominantly expressed allotypic variants [97]. These forms are stable phenotypic characters [60]. Human, swine and rabbit C3b receptors share common antigenic sites, as detected by a monoclonal antibody, and this suggests that the C3b receptor molecule has been conserved through evolution [61].

Methods for detecting complement receptors

Rosette assay

Equipment

See Fc receptor rosette assay.

Materials

See Fc receptor rosette assay.
Dulbecco's phosphate-buffered saline (DPBS) (PBS contains 0.9 mM Ca^{2+} ions and 0.5 mM Mg^{2+} ions).
Mercaptoethanol.
Iodoacetamide.
Azide.

Preparation of indicator cells (EAC) using zymosan depleted serum (R3) as a source of complement

The cells were prepared as for Fc receptors except that IgM was used to coat the red cells instead of IgG. The resultant red cells are termed EA_M.

1   Obtain fresh AB serum from a suitable donor (see 'Notes and recommendations').
2   Mix equal volumes of yeast (prepared as described below) and AB serum, and incubate for 30 min at 37 °C.
3   Centrifuge to remove yeast (400 *g* for 10 min). The resulting supernatant is termed R3 and is used as a source of complement. This method activates the alternate pathway of complement and turns over the terminal components of complement C5 to C9. Although when using human serum a considerable proportion of C3 is also used up, it is still possible to coat the sheep cells (EA_M) with more C3, without causing lysis, than would be the case if the highest possible concentration of AB serum was used.
4   Mix equal volumes of R3 diluted to a suitable concentration with DPBS and EA_M (1×10^8 cells per ml).
5   Incubate for 30 min at 37 °C.
6   Wash the cells once with DPBS and resuspend to give a final concentration of 1×10^8 cells per ml. The resultant cells are termed EAC.

Preparation of yeast

The method is modified from that of Hadding [62].
1   Suspend 250 g of fresh baker's yeast in one litre of PBS and autoclave for 30 min at 120 °C.
2   Wash with PBS (600 *g*) until the supernatant is clear and finally resuspend in 250 ml PBS containing 0.1 M-mercaptoethanol.
3   Incubate the mixture at 37 °C for 2 h with frequent stirring and wash once with 0.15 M-NaCl to remove most of the mercaptoethanol.
4   Stir the yeast at room temperature for 2 h in 250 ml of 0.15 M-NaCl containing 20% w/v 0.2 M-phosphate buffer (pH 7.2) and 20 mM-iodoacetimide. The pH should be checked periodically.
5   Wash three times with PBS and resuspend the yeast in one litre of the same buffer.
6   Re-autoclave for 30 min at 120 °C.
7   Wash until the supernatant is clear.
8   Finally resuspend the yeast in 500 ml DPBS containing 0.01% azide and store at 4 °C.

Titration of yeast

1   Wash yeast twice with DPBS and incubate various dilutions of suspension with an equal volume of AB serum for 30 min at 37 °C.
2   Centrifuge the suspension at 400 *g* for 10 min and collect the supernatants.
3   Add 0.1 ml of the above supernatants to an equal volume of EA_M (1×10^8 cells per ml) and incubate for 30 min at 37 °C. The dilution that is just below that which gives detectable lysis should be used to generate R3 (using IgM anti-sheep erythrocyte antibody from Sera-Lab, 1/5 dilution of stock was correct).

Notes and recommendations

The AB serum must be checked for the presence of Forssmann's antibody by incubating neat serum with sheep red blood cells. If lysis occurs, absorb the serum with sheep erythrocytes at 4 °C with frequent shaking for at least 3 h. Centrifuge the serum to remove the red cells, aliquot and store at −70 °C for not longer than 6 months. For each experiment use a fresh ampoule and do not refreeze.

Preparation of indicator cells (EAC) using purified complement components

Equipment

See Fc receptor rosette assay.

Materials

See Fc receptor rosette assay.
Purified complement components (Cordis Laboratories, Miami, U.S.A.).
Five Times Veronal (5XV). Mix 52.5 g NaCl, 1.875 g

sodium barbitone and 2.875 g barbitone and make up to one litre with distilled water.

Gelatin-Veronal buffer (GVB^{2+}). Mix together 200 ml 5XV, 10 ml 10% gelatin, 5 ml 0.03 M-CaCl$_2$ and 5 ml 0.1 M-MgCl$_2$ and adjust the volume to one litre with distilled water.

5% Dextrose (D5W^{2+}). Mix together 50 g D-glucose, 5 ml 0.03 M CaCl$_2$ and 5 ml 0.1 M-MgCl$_2$ and adjust the volume to one litre with distilled water.

Dextrose-gelatine-Veronal buffer (DGVB^{2+}). Mix together equal volumes of GVB^{2+} and D5W^{2+}.

Procedure

1 Mix EA$_M$ (1×10^8 cells per ml) with 400 effective molecules of human C1 per red cell (to determine the number of effective molecules—see Chapter 39) and incubate for 15 min at 37 °C.
2 Wash twice with DGVB^{2+} and resuspend at the above concentration.
3 Add 6 000 molecules of C4 per red cell and incubate for 30 min at 37 °C.
4 Wash twice with DGVB^{2+} and resuspend at 1×10^8 cells per ml. (C4b receptors on human monocytes can be detected using these indicator cells).

Preparation of EA1423b

1 Prepare EA1 as described above.
2 Add 400 effective molecules of C4 per cell and incubate the mixture for 30 min at 37 °C.
3 Wash twice with DGVB^{2+}.
4 Add a further 400 molecules per cell of C1 to EA14 and incubate for 15 min at 37 °C.
5 Wash the cells twice with DGVB^{2+}.
6 Incubate with 50 molecules of C2 per cell for 10 min at 30 °C. Without washing add C3 to EA142 (the amount will depend on the cell type; 200 molecules of C3 per cell will detect about 20% rosettes on human blood monocytes) and incubate for 30 min at 37 °C.
7 Wash twice with DGVB^{2+} and resuspend the EA1423b to 10^8 cell per ml.

Preparation of inactivated EA1423b

Two methods for preparing these indicator cells are possible.

Factor I (C3b inactivator)

1 Prepare EA1423b cells as described above.
2 Incubate with Factor I, at a concentration which reduces immune adherence (see below) by 95%, for 1 h at 37 °C.

3 Wash twice with DGVB^{2+} and resuspend to 1×10^8 cells per ml.

Immune adherence assay can be used to demonstrate the presence of C3b. Human red cells have receptors for C3b and not for iC3b or C3d. Mix 50 μl human O red cells (10^8 cells per ml) and 50 μl of test sheep red cells (10^8 cells per ml) in V-shaped microtitre plate and incubate at 37 °C for 2 h. From the settling pattern it is possible to determine which complement coated sheep red cells have C3b deposited on their surface. If the cells spread out over the bottom of the well, immune adherence has occurred, whereas if the cells pellet the test cells do not have C3b on their membranes.

EDTA-chelated AB serum

1 Incubate EA1423b cells with neat AB serum chelated with 10 mM-EDTA (inhibit both classical and alternate pathway) for 15 min at 37 °C.
2 Wash the cells twice with DGVB^{2+} and resuspend at 10^8 cells per ml.

Preparation of EA1423d

1 Incubate inactivated EA1423b (made by either of the above two methods) with 0.25 mg trypsin per 10^8 cells for 2.5 min at 37 °C.
2 Stop the reaction by adding ice-cold DGVB^{2+} and wash the cells twice with DGVB^{2+}.
3 Resuspend to 1×10^8 cells per ml.

Detection of complement receptors on cells in suspension or on monolayers

The procedure is exactly the same as for Fc receptors, using any of the above red cell preparations, except that for macrophages in suspension the pellets are incubated for 40 min at 37 °C.

Binding of dimeric C3b

Equipment

Chromatography columns.
Amicon filtration equipment.
Ultracentrifuge.

Materials

Fresh human plasma.
Polyethylene glycol.
Lysine-Sepharose 4B.
DEAE-Sephacel.
SP-C50 Sephadex.

Sephacyl-S300.
Sephadex G-75 superfine.
Sephadex G-25.
1% Trypsin.
0.1 M-phosphate buffer containing 0.1 M-NaCl, pH 7.5.
N-Succinimidyl-3-(2-pyridyldithio) propionate (SPDP, Pharmacia, Zoetermeer, The Netherlands).
Ethanol.
Biogel-A1.5 (Biorad, Woerden, The Netherlands).
Materials for labelling proteins by solid-phase lactoperoxidase [63].

Procedure

1   Prepare C3 from fresh human plasma by polyethylene glycol precipitation, lysine-Sepharose 4B, DEAE-Sephacel, SP-C50 Sephadex, and Sephacyl-S300 chromatography [64].
2   Convert the purified C3 to C3b by treatment for 1 min at 37 °C with 1% (w/w) trypsin and pass down a Sephadex G-75 superfine column.
3   Pool the C3b containing fractions, concentrate to 4.4 mg/ml by Amicon filtration and dialyse against 0.1 M-phosphate buffer containing 0.1 M-NaCl, pH 7.5.
4   Incubate 1 ml C3b for 1 h at 20 °C with 60 µg of the heterobifunctional reagent *N*-succinimidyl-3-(2-Pyridyldithio) propionate dissolved in 10 µl 96% ethanol.
5   Separate the SPDP treated C3b from non-reacted SPDP by G-25 gel filtration in 0.1 M-phosphate buffer containing 0.1 M-NaCl.
6   Pool fractions containing activated C3b, concentrate to 2 ml and add to another 1 ml of C3b (4.4 mg/ml) in the same buffer [65].
7   Incubate for 18 h at room temperature and apply the whole mixture to a 2.5×90 cm Biogel-A 1.5 (Biorad, Woerden, The Netherlands) column (Fig. 48.2).
8   Pool fractions containing the dimeric form of C3b, and concentrate to 0.5 mg/ml.
9   Label 50 µg portions of this dimeric C3b with the solid-phase lactoperoxidase method [63] to specific activities of 0.05 mCi/mg protein, and store in aliquots at −80 °C in TBH-BSA.
10   Incubate 0.05–5.0 µg ^{125}I-(C3b)$_2$ with 0.5×10^6 adherent peritoneal macrophages in a final volume of 250 µl TBH-BSA for 20 h at 4 °C.
11   Assess the bound and free ligand as with the ^{125}I-AIgG.
12   Convert the results into a Scatchard plot and the number of ^{125}I-(C3b)$_2$ bound per macrophage computed.

Notes and recommendations

Ultracentrifugation showed that the ^{125}I-(C3b)$_2$ preparation was contaminated with less than 5% monomeric C3b. In addition, larger aggregates were not detectable.

A maximum of 62 000 molecules of ^{125}I-(C3b)$_2$ are bound per macrophage with a calculated K_a of 1.1×10^{-9} M^{-1} (Fig. 48.3). Treatment of adherent cells with 1 mg/ml of trypsin at 37 °C followed by washing and subsequent determination of the number of molecules of ^{125}I-(C3b)$_n$ bound per cell revealed that within 5 min more than 90% of the binding sites for ^{125}I-(C3b)$_2$ are destroyed (Table 48.2). The binding of ^{125}I-(C3b)$_2$ to the adherent peritoneal macrophages could also be fully inhibited by prior incubation of the adherent phagocytes with 20 mg/ml of monomeric

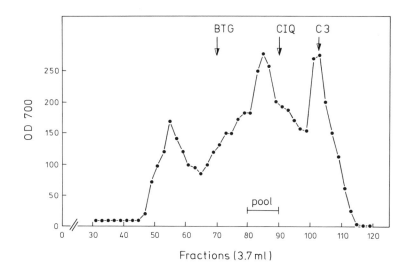

Fig. 48.2. Biogel-A1.5 gel filtration of SPDP-cross-linked C3b on a 2.5×90 cm column equilibrated in veronal-buffered saline, pH 7.5. The filtration volumes of bovine thyroglobulin (600 000), C1*q* (400 000) and C3 (180 000) obtained from a separate run are shown. Fractions 80–90 were pooled, concentrated and radiolabelled with ^{125}I.

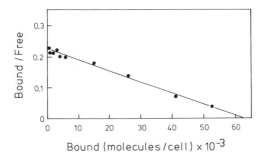

Fig. 48.3. Equilibrium binding at 4 °C of ^{125}I-(C3b)$_2$ to 0.5×10^6 adherent peritoneal macrophages.

Table 48.2. Maximum number of ^{125}I-(C3b)$_2$ bound per macrophage before and after treatment of the adherent phagocytes for different time periods with 1 mg/ml of Trypsin

Trypsin treatment (min at 37 °C)	Maximum number of ^{125}I-(C3b)$_2$ bound per cell	Percentage inactivation
0	62 600	0
2.5	20 250	68
5	6 100	91
10	2 000	97
20	1 500	98

Adherent peritoneal macrophages (0.5×10^6) in triplicate were incubated with 1 mg/ml of Trypsin for the indicated time periods at 37 °C, washed and the maximum number of ^{125}I-(C3b)$_2$ bound per cell was determined subsequently after incubation of the cells with ^{125}I-(C3b)$_2$ for 20 h at 4 °C.

C3b. These results indicate that ^{125}I-(C3b)$_2$ can be used as a probe for the determination of the relative number of C3b-receptors on cells and also permits the characterization of the functional activity of C3b-receptors on cells.

'Lectin-like' receptors for bacterial cell wall sugars

'Lectin-like' receptors for bacterial cell wall sugars have been described on mouse macrophages and other phagocytes of various species including human monocytes. These receptors mediate the attachment to the phagocyte membrane of various bacteria including *Staphylococcus albus*, *E. coli*, *S. typhimurium*, *N. gonorrhoeae*, *K. aerogenes*, and *C. parvum* [66–70].

An association between the lectin-like receptor for *S. albus* and I-A products of the MHC has recently been established [71], these observations point to a possible role for these carbohydrate-recognizing receptors in antigen presentation by macrophages. The expression of the lectin-like receptors has been found to be decreased in the *in vivo* inflammatory response [72] and *in vitro* on exposure of murine macrophages to chemotactic peptides [73].

Methods for detecting 'lectin-like' receptors

Equipment

See Fc receptor rosette assay (page 48.2).
Sterile flasks.

Materials

See also Fc receptor rosette assay.
Sterile nutrient broth.
Bacteria.

Procedure

Preparation of bacteria

The following bacteria have been used to detect lectin-like receptors: *Corynebacterium parvum*, *Escherichia coli*, and *Staphylococcus albus*. Grow these as required; kill by 24 h exposure to 0.5% formalin in 0.15 M-NaCl; store at 4 °C for not more than two weeks.

Bacterial binding to cell monolayers

1   Prepare monolayers as described above.
2   Add 1 ml bacteria in DPBS and incubate for 2 h at 4 °C.
3   Remove non-attached organisms by repeated washing with DPBS.
4   Air-dry coverslips, fix in methanol, and stain with May Grunwald/Giemsa. Macrophages with bacteria attached at two or more discrete points are positive.

Inhibition of bacterial binding by sugars

1   Make an isotonic solution of the sugar required with distilled water, filter, and store at 4 °C.
2   Dilute as necessary with DPBS.
3   Incubate cell monolayers with 0.5 ml of sugar solutions for 20 min at 4 °C.
4   Wash the monolayers once and perform the bacterial binding assay as described above.

Ia antigens on macrophages

Ia antigens, expressed on macrophages acting as antigen presenting cells, appear to regulate immune responsiveness. Such antigens also appear as differentiation markers during haematopoietic development with the stem cells lacking detectable Ia [65]. Mature macrophages in peritoneal exudates or spleen contain Ia^+ and Ia^- subpopulations and this expression is subject to environmental regulation [72,75,76].

Techniques for detection of Ia alloantigens include serological detection by complement mediated cytotoxicity, immunofluorescence, immunoperoxidase staining, absorption analysis, and direct or indirect antibody binding. Both conventional antisera and monoclonal antibodies have been used in these assays. The mouse I region has been subdivided into the subregions I-A, I-J and I-E, and an extensive series of MHC congenic and recombinant mice bred on the C57BL/10 background has allowed the production of alloantisera specific for the Ia antigens I-A, I-J and I-E from various mouse haplotypes.

Methods for the detection of Ia antigens on macrophages

Rosette assay

Equipment

pH meter.
Centrifuge.
Spectrophotometer.
Microscope.

Materials

Chromic chloride ($CrCl_3.6H_2O$; it must be hydrated).
0.15 M Sodium chloride.
Phosphate-buffered saline (PBS).
Rabbit anti-mouse-immunoglobulin (or species of interest).
Anti-'Ia' antibody.
Fetal calf serum (FCS).
Sheep red blood cells.
Methyl violet.

Procedure

1 Prepare stock solution of chromic chloride by dissolving $CrCl_3.6H_2O$ at 1% (w/v) in 0.15 M-NaCl and immediately bring pH to 4.5 with 0.1 M-NaOH. Store at room temperature and for the first three weeks readjust to pH 4.5 once a week. After this curing, keep at room temperature and it will be stable indefinitely. For coupling dilute 1/10 with 0.15 M-NaCl; store this for up to 6 months at room temperature or until it tends to agglutinate red cells.
2 Wash sheep red blood cell four times with 0.15

M-NaCl (600 **g** for 7 min) and finally resuspend in 0.15 M-NaCl to give 10^9 cells per ml (see previous section on Fc receptors, page 48.3).
3 Mix 1 ml of sheep red blood cells at 10^9 cells per ml with anti-immunoglobulin and immediately add $CrCl_3$ with constant shaking.
4 Leave mixture for 5 min at room temperature and then stop reaction by adding 2 ml PBS.
5 Centrifuge coupled red cells (400 **g** for 5 min) and wash with PBS. Finally resuspend pellet in PBS/5% FCS at 2×10^8 cells per ml.
6 Prepare macrophages at 2×10^6 cells per ml in PBS/5% FCS.
7 Add 50 μl cells along with 50 μl of anti-Ia antibody to V-well microtitre plate and incubate at 0 °C for 30 min.
8 Wash twice with PBS/5% FCS by centrifugation (200 **g** for 7 min at 4 °C) and resuspend in 50 μl PBS/5%.
9 To cells add 50 μl coupled red cells, centrifuge at 120 **g** for 8 min at 4 °C and incubate on ice for 45 min.
10 Add 50 μl of 0.1% methyl violet. (Stock 1% in distilled water. Dilute with 0.15 M-NaCl/0.5% FCS pre-warmed to 37 °C and filter prior to use.) Resuspend gently, transfer to haemocytometer, and count percentage of cells which bind more than three erythrocytes.

Notes and recommendations

This method can be adopted to detect any surface antigen to which there is antibody and in any species to which there is anti-immunoglobulin. The anti-immunoglobulin must be dissolved in saline since the presence of buffer solutions inhibits the coupling reaction. The chromic chloride must be the hexahydrate and care must be taken when adjusting the pH since it precipitates at pH 6.0. The appropriate amounts of antibody and chromic chloride must be determined prior to assay. As a general rule about 0.4 mg of antibody should be added to 10^9 sheep red blood cells in 1 ml. The amount of $CrCl_3$ required will vary between 20 and 80 μl. Choose an amount where agglutination is just noticeable but does not interfere with counting. The coupled red cells will keep for 4 days if washed every second day and readjusted to 2×10^8 cells per ml, using a spectrophotometer, before use.

As an alternative, protein A can be used in the detection system. This method has the advantage over the use of anti-immunoglobulin that the spleen cells' surface immunoglobulin does not require to be capped. In this case 50 μg protein A is added to 2 ml sheep red blood cells (10^9 ml^{-1}) in saline. This mixture is incubated with 40 μl of 0.1% CrCl$_3$ at room temperature for 7 min, and treated as above.

Normal serum of different species can be added to block the binding of the first antibody to Fc receptors or aggregated antibody can be spun out prior to use. If B cells are being investigated, surface immunoglobulin should be capped prior to adding antibody to leucocytes.

The assay can also be carried out on monolayers which are prepared as detailed before. If coverslips are used, invert the monolayer on to the antibody (0.1–0.2 ml). The coupled red cells are added at 2×10^7 in 2 ml, spun on to the coverslips (100 *g* for 5 min) and incubated for 45 min at 4 °C. The coverslips are then washed gently by multiple dipping and treated as for Fc receptor assay.

Complement mediated cytotoxicity

Equipment

Microscope.
Water bath.
Centrifuge.

Materials

Dulbecco's phosphate-buffered saline (DPBS).
Anti-Ia antibody.
0.05% Trypan blue.

Procedure

1 Prepare macrophage monolayers as previously described.
2 Invert coverslips on to 0.2 ml of alloantibody and incubate for 45 min on ice.
3 Wash coverslips gently by dipping into DPBS and place on to 0.2 ml of guinea-pig serum (1/20 dilution, mouse spleen cell absorbed) and incubate for 30 min at 37 °C.
4 Immerse the coverslips in 0.2 ml of 0.05% trypan blue (stock of 1% trypan blue in distilled water; dilute to 0.05% with saline to use; filter if necessary) and count 200 cells and determine the percentage of dead cells.

Notes and recommendations

The concentration of antibody used has to be the lowest concentration which gives highest detectable binding to cell. The procedure can also be carried out in suspension. Use cells at 2×10^6 cells per ml and incubate with antibody at 4 °C for 45 min. Centrifuge to pellet cells, discard supernatant and resuspend in DPBS containing guinea-pig serum, as above. Incubate for 30 min at 37 °C add 100 μl of 0.05% trypan blue and examine in a haemocytometer.

Appendix

Obtaining mononuclear phagocytes

Mononuclear phagocytes originate from precursor pro-monocytes of the bone marrow, circulate in the blood as monocytes, and emigrate into the tissues where they differentiate into macrophages [77]. Macrophages play a central role in the immune system. They are actively involved in resistance to intracellular infections [78]; they act as accessory cells in the immune response [79,80], function as cytotoxic cells acting against tumour cells [81] or virally infected cells [82], and play a part in homeostatic processes [83]. Their ability to perform these various roles is related to their functional state.

Exposure of resident macrophages to a variety of agents leads to changes in the functional activities of the cells that include alterations in enzyme content and secretion and enhanced phagocytic, bactericidal, and tumoricidal effects. Mackaness [84,85] described the functional changes that occur in macrophages in animals infected with intracellular bacteria and used the term 'activated' to describe their enhanced bactericidal properties. Evans & Alexander [81] have also used this term to describe macrophages that show cytotoxic activity against tumour cells. Macrophages that have been exposed to irritants such as thioglycollate or casein show less marked functional changes that do not include bactericidal effects and are usually termed 'stimulated' [86; see also Chapter 50].

Intraperitoneal injections of irritant substances have been used for many years to increase the yield of inflammatory cells. The most commonly used stimulating agents include mineral oil, thioglycollate, casein, protease peptone broth, and glycogen. The changes induced in peritoneal macrophages exposed to such substances include increase in size, increased rate and extent of spreading on surfaces, changes in levels of certain enzymes and surface markers, increased ruffling of the cell membrane, and prominence of pseudopodia as well as cytoplasmic granules and vacuoles [86].

Activation of macrophages was originally described in animals infected with intracellular pathogens such as *Mycobacterium*, *Listeria* and *Brucella* [85,87], and *Toxoplasma*, *Trichinella* and *Trypanosoma* [88,89]. This activation is dependent on T cells [90] and can be induced *in vitro* by T cell products [91]. However, certain other agents such as polyanions, extracts of *Mycobacterium* and possibly immune complexes can

cause activation without a requirement for lymphocytes.

Sources, preparation, and induction of mononuclear phagocytes

Macrophages can be easily obtained from the serous
cavities (peritoneum, pleural sac) but they can also be
isolated from lung, spleen, lymph node, liver, and
thymus. Peripheral blood monocytes can be obtained
from human donors and various laboratory animals
although those from the latter tend to be more difficult
to purify.

Peritoneal cells

Except in mice and rats the number of resident cells
obtained from the peritoneal cavity is very low and not
really economical. Therefore various agents have been
used to provoke a peritoneal exudate rich in macrophages. It must be remembered that these cells show
various chemical and morphological changes (see
above) from the non-induced cells.

Equipment

Dissection kit (scissors, artery clamps, forceps,
syringes and needles).

Materials

Glycogen: (ex-oyster pure AR, Koch-Light Laboratories Ltd., Colnbrook, Bucks, UK) causes a moderate
increase in the number of macrophages 3 days after i.p.
injection in mice and guinea-pigs. Prepare at 1 mg
ml^{-1} in 0.15 M-saline. Inject 20 ml into a guinea-pig
weighing 500–800 g and 1 ml into mice.
Thioglycollate: (Brewer Thioglycollate Medium,
Difco Laboratories, West Molesey, Surrey, UK).
Prepare as 10% solution and autoclave at 103.5 kPa
for 15 min with slow exhaust. After cooling, store in
the dark for at least 2 months before use. For mice
inject 1 ml i.p. 3–4 days before harvest.
Proteus peptone broth: (Proteose peptone, Difco
Laboratories, West Molesey, Surrey, UK). Prepare as
10% solution when required and inject 1 ml per mouse.
Collect cells 3–4 days later.
Mineral oil: Liquid paraffin is most commonly used
and gives a very large increase in the yield of
macrophages. Inject 0.1–0.5 ml for mice and 5 ml kg^{-1}
for larger animals 4–5 days before cells are required.
The cells obtained are contaminated by a large number
of dead cells and free oil which must be removed by
multiple centrifugation and washing. This procedure
tends to give rise to cells that are not clumpy or sticky

and is the method of choice for migration inhibition
tests.
Concanavalin A: 0.5–1 mg (for mice) of con A injected
i.p. 4–5 days before cells are required.
Corynebacterium parvum: inject 0.25 mg of formalin
killed *C. parvum* (Wellcome Research Labs., Becken-
ham, UK) per mouse and harvest cells 4 days later.
This produces a population of activated cells.
Others: other agents which have been used include
starch, casein, peptone water, and various heart and
brain extracts.
Phosphate-buffered saline (PBS).
70% Ethanol.

Procedure for mice

1 Kill animal by cervical dislocation and swab
abdomen with 70% ethanol.
2 Incise the skin upward from the anterior abdomen
wall with forceps and pull back.
3 Inject (26-gauge, $\frac{1}{2}''$ needle) 2.5 ml of sterile PBS
containing 10 U heparin per ml into the peritoneal
cavity through the mid-anterior line (heparin can be
omitted and any balanced salt solution used).
4 Circulate the fluid gently by shaking and prodding.
5 Aspirate the cell suspension slowly by inserting a
needle (23-gauge, $1''$) into the left flank and applying
lateral traction so that a pocket of fluid forms behind
the spleen.
6 Remove needle and transfer cells to a sterile
container.
7 Repeat lavage process.

Notes and recommendations

If complete sterility is required, lavage only once with
5 ml of PBS.
    The number of cells obtained varies with strain, sex,
and age of mouse. Female mice tend to have higher
numbers of peritoneal cells. For 8–12-week-old female
C3H mice $2–4 \times 10^6$ resident peritoneal cells are
obtained of which 40–60% are macrophages. Stimulation with glycogen will give 3.5×10^6 cells while
injection with *C. parvum* gives $5–10 \times 10^6$ cells; both
procedures do not drastically affect the percentage of
macrophages. Up to 2.5×10^7 cells can be elicited with
con A and similar number of cells can be obtained with
thioglycollate. With the latter agent 80–90% of the
cells are macrophages.

Procedure for guinea-pigs

1 Kill animal by cervical dislocation or intracardiac
anaesthetic.
2 Soak the anterior abdomen with 70% ethanol.

3   Remove a wide strip of skin along the mid-anterior line.
4   Make a small incision in abdominal wall and hold opposite side with artery clamps.
5   Add 40–80 ml (depending on size of animal) of PBS containing 10 U heparin per ml.
6   Circulate the fluid carefully by prodding the abdominal wall or by mixing gently with a tongue depressor.
7   Increase the size of the opening to run most of the length of the abdomen.
8   Remove the cell suspension with a pipette or syringe (use tongue depressor to hold back mesentery).
9   Repeat washing procedure.

Notes and recommendations

There are very few resistant macrophages in the guinea-pig peritoneal cavity and it is therefore preferable to use an inducing agent such as glycogen or mineral oil. Between 2×10^7 and 4×10^7 cells, of which 90% are macrophages, can be obtained 3 days after injecting a 500–800 g guinea-pig with glycogen. Mineral oil produces an exudate which contains up to 2×10^8 cells.

Care must be taken not to damage the spleen during cervical dislocation. Intraperitoneal injection of anaesthetic results in a wash-out contaminated with erythrocytes.

Procedure for other species

Rabbits and rats are treated in the same fashion as guinea-pigs. However, the volume of lavage fluid must be increased or decreased as required. Rabbits require induction since a normal healthy rabbit's peritoneal cavity contains only about 3×10^6 cells. Rats have more cells, $1–2 \times 10^7$, of which approximately 10% are mast cells.

Human peritoneal cells can be obtained from peritoneal dialysis patients or from cadavers. However, these cells are difficult to obtain and are probably abnormal.

Alveolar macrophages

Alveolar macrophages can be collected from a number of species including man. For all laboratory species the technique is the same apart from the fluid and size of cannula.

Equipment

Dissection kit (scissors, curved forceps).
'Button' grade cotton thread.

Intravenous catheter tubing (Portex Ltd., Hythe, Kent, UK) with Luer fitting at one end.
Syringe.

Materials

70% Ethanol.
Phosphate-buffered saline.

Procedure

1   Inject a lethal dose of anaesthetic intraperitoneally.
2   Pin animal to cork board ventral aspect uppermost.
3   Swab neck area with 70% ethanol.
4   Remove the overlying skin and tissue to expose trachea, taking care to avoid adjacent blood vessels.
5   Tie off the trachea with cotton thread.
6   Position another piece of thread below the first.
7   Make a small incision between the cartilaginous rings just above second piece of thread.
8   Introduce an intravenous catheter tube and tie firmly in place with second piece of thread.
9   Dissect out the lungs carefully so as not to damage or pierce them and remove completely from animal.
10   Place lungs on a piece of benchkot (shiny side uppermost) and add lavage fluid pre-warmed to 37 °C with a syringe (use any isotonic buffered salt solution containing 10 U heparin per ml).
11   Gently withdraw fluid and wash four more times.

Notes and recommendations

Mice: use tubing with outside diameter 0.75 mm and 1 ml fluid to wash. Rats: use tubing with outside diameter 2.1 mm and 10 ml fluid to wash. Guinea-pigs: use tubing with outside diameter 2.7 mm and 20 ml fluid to wash.

If excess bleeding occurs during dissection, bleed out the animal first by cutting the vena cava. The authors always remove the lungs; the technique can be carried out with the lungs *in situ* but fewer cells are obtained. If difficulty is encountered in recovering the fluid, care must be taken to avoid subjecting the lungs to excess negative pressure as damage to tissue may occur. This is usually due to the trachea collapsing and may be overcome by gently stretching the trachea while withdrawing the fluid.

The number of cells obtained depends mainly on the size of the animal. Also, the larger the animal the easier the dissection. The cell populations obtained are usually 70–85% macrophages: guinea-pigs $2–5 \times 10^7$ cells, rats $5–10 \times 10^6$ cells and mice $0.4–0.8 \times 10^6$ cells.

Holt [92] has described a method of obtaining

increased number of cells by the use of the local anaesthetic lignocaine and other workers have obtained macrophages from whole macerated lung [93]. This latter procedure yields a substantial number of cells but a significant proportion cannot be alveolar in origin.

Tissue macrophages

Macrophages can be obtained from solid tissue, including tonsil, lymph node, spleen, and thymus, by surgical biopsy in humans or from experimental animals.

Equipment

Loose fitting homogenizer.
Dissection kit.
CO_2 incubator.

Materials

Petri dishes.
Sterile steel gauze.
Medium (199, Eagles' or equivalent with antibiotics and 10% fetal calf serum).
Deoxyribonuclease Type 1 (BDH, Poole, England).
Dispase (Boehringer Corp. London, UK).

Procedure for spleen, lymph node, tonsil, and other soft tissues

1 Place tissue in a Petri dish and cut into small pieces with sterile scissors.
2 Transfer to homogenizer containing about 5 ml of medium and grind gently to give a fine cell suspension.
3 Pass cell suspension through steel gauze.
4 Wash cells until supernatant is clear of fatty material.
5 Separate macrophages by adherence to glass coverslips or tissue culture Petri dishes, or by other available methods.

Notes and recommendations

Adherence can be carried out as follows.
1 Plate out at about $5-10 \times 10^6$ cells per ml in medium containing 10% fetal calf serum (10 ml to 60 mm Petri dish).
2 Incubate for 1 h at 37 °C.
3 Swirl plate to resuspend settled cells and pour off non-adherent population.
4 Wash plate three times with medium.
5 Remove adherent cells or use monolayer obtained.
  Macrophages can be recovered using a disposable cell scraper (Costar, Cambridge, Mass., U.S.A.). Slight loss of viability can occur, so it is better to prepare a monolayer in the vessel where the experiment is to be carried out. To avoid clumping of cells do not allow the cell number to rise above 5×10^7 cells per ml and add heparin to the medium at a final concentration of 10 U ml. In general, 1–5% of the starting population, depending on tissue, age and strain of mouse, will be adherent.

Procedure for neoplasms and tough tissue

1 Place tissue in Petri dish and cut into small pieces with scalpel blade.
2 Transfer to universal container and stir for 30 min at room temperature in Hanks' solution containing 0.05% Dispase and 0.001% deoxyribonuclease.
3 Allow undigested fragments to settle or pass through steel gauze.
4 Wash cells and treat as above.

Peripheral blood monocytes

Lymphoid cells can be separated by methods based on differences in cell size and density by gradient [94,95] or counter-current [96] centrifugation.

The efficiency of separation varies with different species and the density has to be adjusted by trial and error. However, human monocytes can be readily separated on a cushion of Ficoll/hypaque (density 1.078 gml^{-1}) and commercial separation fluids are also available (lymphocyte separation medium: Flow Laboratories, Irvine, Ayrshire, UK; Ficoll-Paque, Pharmacia, Uppsala, Sweden).

A good separation of murine mononuclear cells can be obtained using lymphocyte-M (Cedarlane Laboratories, Hornby, Ontario, Canada).

Equipment

Centrifuge.

Materials

0.15 M-saline.
Ficoll/hypaque (for human, density 1.078 g ml^{-1}) or equivalent.
15 ml plastic conical centrifuge tubes.

Procedure

1 Dilute heparinized blood (10 U ml^{-1}) 1/4 with 0.15 M-saline.
2 Layer diluted blood on to a cushion of separation fluid (3 ml Ficoll/hypaque for 10 ml of diluted blood).

3 Centrifuge at 400 *g* for 30 min.
4 Collect the interface cells (lymphocytes, monocytes, and platelets).
5 Wash cells once with PBS, at 15 *g* for 10 min to remove platelets, and then again at 200 *g* for 7 min.
6 Resuspend in medium at required volume for use, or further purify by adherence etc.

Notes and recommendations

One millilitre of blood yields about 10^6 mononuclear cells, of which 10–20% are monocytes.

References

1 GOLDE D.W. & HOCKING W.G. (1982) Monocyte and macrophage development. In *Advances in Host Defence Mechanisms*, Vol 1, (eds. Gallin J. & Fauci W.S.). Raven Press, New York.

2 BIRGENS H.S., HANSEN N.E., KARLE H. & KRISTENSEN L.O. (1983) Receptor binding of lactoferrin by human monocytes. *Br. J. Haematol.* **54**, 383.

3 FINBLOOM D.S. (1982) Assessment of Fc (IgG) receptor function in adherent murine peritoneal macrophages using soluble model immune complexes. *Cell. Immunol.* **74**, 294.

4 DE WATER R., GINSEL L.A., DAEMS W.TH. & DAHA M.R. (1983) Autoradiographical demonstration of C3b receptor activity on resident peritoneal macrophages. *Histochemistry*, **77**, 289.

5 GLASS E.J., STEWART J. & WEIR D.M. (1981) Presence of bacterial 'lectin-like' receptors on phagocytes. *Immunology*, **44**, 529.

6 KOLB H. & KOLB-BACHFEN V. (1978) A lectin-like receptor on mammalian macrophages. *Biochem. biophys. Res. Commun.* **85**, 678.

7 CAPO C., BONGRAND P., BENOLIEL A.M. & DEPIEDS R. (1979) Nonspecific recognition in phagocytosis: ingestion of aldehyde-treated erythrocytes by rat peritoneal macrophages. *Immunology*, **36**, 501.

8 SUGARMAN B. & DONTA S.T. (1979) Specificity of attachment of certain Enterobacteriaceae to mammalian cells. *J. gen. Microbiol.* **115**, 509.

9 RASMUSSEN J.M., BRANDSLUND I., LESLIE R.G.Q. & SEUHAG S.E. (1983) Quantitative studies of Fc receptors on human monocytes: characterisation by binding of homologous and heterologous monomeric IgG and soluble immune complexes of different composition. *Immunology*, **49**, 537.

10 CARTER S.D., LESLIE R.G.Q. & REEVES W.G. (1982) Human monocyte binding of homologous monomer and complement IgG. *Immunology*, **46**, 793.

11 GLASS E.J. & KAY A.B. (1980) Enhanced expression of human monocyte complement (C3b) receptors by chemoattractants. *Clin. exp. Immunol.* **39**, 768.

12 GRIFFIN F.M. JUN., BIANCO C. & SILVERSTEIN S.C. (1975) Characterization of the macrophage receptor for complement and demonstration of its functional independence

13 KEDAR E. & BONAVIDA B. (1974) Histamine receptor-bearing leukocytes (HRL). (I) Detection of histamine receptor-bearing cells by rosette formation with histamine-coated erythrocytes. *J. Immunol.* **113**, 1544.

14 FEARON D.T., KANEKO I. & THOMSON G.G. (1981) Membrane distribution and adsorptive endocytosis by C3b receptors on human polymorphonuclear leukocytes. *J. exp. Med.* **153**, 1615.

15 COUPLAND K. & LESLIE R.G.Q. (1983) The expression of Fc receptors on guinea pig peritoneal macrophages and neutrophils. *Immunology*, **48**, 647.

16 LESLIE R.G.Q. & ALEXANDER M.D. (1979) Cytolytic antibodies. *Curr. Top. Microbiol. Immunol.* **88**, 25.

17 FEARON D.T. (1980) Identification of the membrane glycoprotein that is the C3b receptor of the human erythrocyte, polymorphonuclear leukocyte, B lymphocyte and monocyte. *J. exp. Med.* **152**, 20.

18 PARISH C.R. & MCKENZIE I.F.C. (1978) A sensitive rosetting method for detecting subpopulations of lymphocytes which react with alloantisera. *J. immunol. Meth.* **20**, 173.

19 COWING C. (1981) Antisera against Ia antigens. In *Methods for studying mononuclear phagocytes*, (eds. Adams D.O., Edelson P.J. & Koren H.), Ch. 33, p. 315. Academic Press, New York.

20 MASON D.Y., FARRELL C. & TAYLOR C.R. (1975) The detection of intracellular antigens in human leukocytes by immunoperoxidase staining. *Br. J. Haematol.* **31**, 361.

21 HIGGINS T.J., O'NEILL H.C. & PARISH C.R. (1981) A sensitive and quantitative fluorescence assay for cell surface antigens. *J. immunol. Meth.* **47**, 275.

22 REYNOLDS H.Y. (1974) Pulmonary host defenses in rabbits after immunization with *Pseudomonas* antigens: the interaction of bacteria, antibodies, macrophages and lymphocytes. *J. infect. Dis.* **130S**, S134.

23 KAY M.M.B. (1975) Mechanism of removal of senescent cell by human macrophages *in situ*. *Proc. natn. Acad. Sci. U.S.A.* **72**, 3521.

24 WALKER W.S. (1977) Mediation of macrophage cytolytic and phagocytic activities by antibodies of different classes and class-specific Fc-receptors. *J. Immunol.* **119**, 367.

25 HASKILL J.S. & FETT J.W. (1976) Possible evidence for antibody-dependent macrophage-mediated cytotoxicity directed against murine adenocarcinoma cells *in vivo*. *J. Immunol.* **117**, 1992.

26 SHAW G.M., LEVY P.C. & LOBIGLIO A.F. (1978) Human monocyte cytotoxicity to tumor cells. (1) Antibody-dependent cytotoxicity. *J. Immunol.* **121**, 573.

27 KURLAND J.I. & BOCKMAN R. (1978) Prostaglandin E production by human blood monocytes and mouse peritoneal macrophages. *J. exp. Med.* **147**, 952.

28 BONNEY R.J., DAVIES P., KUEHL F.A. JUN. & HUMES J.L. (1980) Arachidonic acid oxygenation products produced by mouse peritoneal macrophages responding to inflammatory stimuli. *J. Reticuloendothel. Soc.* **28** (suppl.), 113s.

29 GOLDSTEIN I.M., ROOS D., KAPLAN H.B. & WEISSMANN G. (1975) Complement and immunoglobulins stimulate superoxide production by human leukocytes independently of phagocytosis. *J. clin. Invest.* **56**, 1155.

30 CORDELLA C.J., DAVIES P. & ALLISON A.C. (1974) Immune complexes induce selective release of lysosomal hydrolases from macrophages. *Nature*, **247**, 46.

31 PASSWELL J.H., DAYER J.-M., GASS K. & EDELSON P.J. (1980) Regulation by Fc fragments of the secretion of collagenase, PGE_2, and lysozyme by mouse peritoneal macrophages. *J. Immunol.* **125**, 910.

32 LAY W.H. & NUSSENZWEIG V. (1969) Ca^{++}-dependent binding of antigen-19S antibody complexes to macrophages. *J. Immunol.* **102**, 1172.

33 CAPRON A., DESSAINT J.-P. & CAPRON M. (1975) Specific IgE antibodies in immune adherence of normal macrophages to *Schistosoma mansoni* schistosomules. *Nature*, **253**, 474.

34 JOSEPH M., DESSAINT J.-P. & CAPRON A. (1977) Characteristics of macrophage cytotoxicity induced by IgE immune complexes. *Cell. Immunol.* **34**, 247.

35 MELEWICZ F.M., BOLTZ-NITULESCU G. & SPIEGELBERG H.L. (1981) Fc receptors for IgE on human monocytes and rat macrophages. In *Heterogeneity of Mononuclear Phagocytes*, (eds. Forster O. & Landy M.), p. 102. Academic Press, New York.

36 DIAMOND B. & BIRSHSTEIN B.K. (1981) Identification and fine specificity of Fc receptors on mouse macrophages. In *Heterogeneity of Mononuclear Phagocytes*, (eds. Forster O. & Landy M.), p. 97. Academic Press, New York.

37 UNKELESS J.C. & EISEN H.N. (1975) Binding of monomeric immunoglobulins to Fc receptors of mouse macrophages. *J. exp. Med.* **142**, 1520.

38 LESLIE R.G.Q. & COHEN S. (1976) Comparison of the cytophilic activities of guinea pig IgG_1 and IgG_2 antibodies. *Eur. J. Immunol.* **6**, 848.

39 BASTEN A., MILLER J.F.A.P., SPRENT J. & PYE J. (1972) A receptor for antibody on B lymphocytes. (I) Method of detection and functional significance. *J. exp. Med.* **135**, 610.

40 ANDERSON C.L. & GREY H.M. (1974) Receptors for aggregated IgG on mouse lymphocytes. Their presence on thymocytes, thymus-derived, and bone marrow-derived lymphocytes. *J. exp. Med.* **139**, 1175.

41 STOUT R.D. & HERZENBERG L.A. (1975) The Fc receptor on thymus-derived lymphocytes. (I) Detection of a subpopulation of murine T lymphocytes bearing the Fc receptor. *J. exp. Med.* **142**, 611.

42 MESSNER R.P. & JELINEK J. (1970) Receptors for human G globulin on human neutrophils. *J. clin. Invest.* **49**, 2165.

43 ANWAR A.R.E. & KAY A.B. (1977) Membrane receptors for IgG and complement (C4, C3b and C3d) on human eosinophils and neutrophils and their relation to eosinophilia. *J. Immunol.* **119**, 976.

44 SEGAL D.M., SHARROW S.O., JONES J.F. & SIRAGANIAN R.P. (1981) Fc (IgG) receptors on rat basophilic leukaemia cells. *J. Immunol.* **126**, 138.

45 PFUELLER S.L., WEBER S. & LÜSCHER E.F. (1977) Studies of the mechanism of human platelet release reaction induced by immunologic stimuli. (III) Relationship between the binding of soluble IgG aggregates to the Fc receptor and cell response in the presence and absence of plasma. *J. Immunol.* **118**, 514.

46 GLEESON WHITE M.H., HEARD D.H., MYNORS L.S. & COOMBS R.R.A. (1950) Factors influencing the agglutinability of red cells. (I) The demonstration of a variation in the susceptibility to agglutination exhibited by the red cells of individual oxen. *Br. J. Exp. Path.* **31**, 321.

47 MCCONAHEY P.J. & DIXON F.J. (1966) A method of trace iodination of proteins for immunologic studies. *Int. Archs Allergy*, **29**, 185.

48 KNUTSON D.W., KIJLSTRA A., LENTZ H. & VAN ES L.A. (1979) Isolation of stable aggregates of IgG by zonal ultracentrifugation in sucrose gradients containing albumin. *Immunol. Commun.* **8**, 337.

49 KAUFFMANN R.H., VAN ES L.A. & DAHA M.R. (1979) Aggregated human immunoglobulin G stabilized by albumin: a standard for immune complex detection. *J. immunol. Meth.* **31**, 11.

50 STEENSGAARD J. & FUNDING L. (1974) On the formulation of a reaction scheme for the interaction between antigen and its antibody. *Immunology*, **26**, 299.

51 PINCKARD R.N. & WEIR D.M. (1967) Equilibrium dialysis and preparation of hapten conjugates. In *Handbook of Experimental Immunology*, (ed. Weir D.M.). Blackwell Scientific Publications, Oxford.

52 VAN FURTH R. (1976) An approach to the characterization of mononuclear phagocytes involved in pathological processes. *Agents Actions*, **6**, 9.

53 ALPER C.A., COLTEN H.R., GEAR J.S.S., ROBSON A.R. & ROSEN F.S. (1976) Homozygous human C3 deficiency. The role of C3 in antibody production, CIs-induced vasopermeability and cobra venom-induced passive hemolysis. *J. clin. Invest.* **57**, 222.

54 LEIJH P.C.J., VAN DER BARSELAAR M. TH., VAN ZWET T.L., DAHA M.R. & VAN FURTH R. (1979) Requirement of extracellular complement and immunoglobulin for intracellular killing of micro-organisms by human monocytes. *J. clin. Invest.* **63**, 772.

55 SCHORLEMMER H.U. & ALLISON A.C. (1976) Effects of activated complement components on enzyme secretion by macrophages. *Immunology*, **31**, 781.

56 SCHORLEMMER H.U., BITTER-SUERMANN D. & ALLISON A.C. (1977) Complement activation by the alternative pathway and macrophage enzyme secretion in the pathogenesis of chronic inflammation. *Immunology*, **32**, 929.

57 PEPYS M.B. (1976) Role of complement in the induction of immunological responses. *Transplant Rev.* **32**, 93.

58 ROSS G.D. (1982) Structure and function of membrane complement receptors. *Fedn Proc.* **41**, 3089.

59 ROSS G.D. & LACHMANN P.J. (1983) Comparison of leukocyte membrane C-receptor type three (CR_3) and bovine serum conglutinin (K). *Immunobiology*, **164**, 290.

60 WONG W.W., WILSON J.G. & FEARON D.T. (1983) Genetic regulation of a structural polymorphism of human C3b receptor. *Immunobiology*, **164**, 238.

61 GERDES J., MASON D.Y. & STEIN H. (1983) Relationship between complement (C3b) receptors of different species determined with monoclonal antibody C3RTo5. *Immunobiology*, **164**, 245.

62 HADDING U. (1967) *Protides of the biological fluids*, Vol. 17, (ed. Peters H.). Elsevier/North–Holland Biomedical Press, Amsterdam.

63 TJORELL J.L. & LARSON I. (1974) Lactoperoxidase coupled to polyacrylamide for radio-iodination of proteins to high specific activity. *Immunochemistry*, **224**, 203.

64 TACK B.F. & PRAHL J.W. (1976) Third component of human complement: purification from plasma and characterization. *Biochemistry*, **15**, 4513.

65 SCHREIBER R.D., PANGBURN M.K., BJORNSON A.B., BROTHERS M.A. & MÜLLER-EBERHARD H.J. (1982) The role of C3 fragments in endocytosis and extracellular cytotoxic reactions by polymorphonuclear leukocytes. *Clin. Immunol. Immunopath.* **23**, 335.

66 OGMUNDSDOTTIR H.M. & WEIR D.M. (1976) The characteristics of binding of *Corynebacterium parvum* to glass adherent mouse peritoneal exudate cells. *Clin. exp. Immunol.*, **26**, 334.

67 FREIMER N.B., OGMUNDSDOTTIR H.M., BLACKWELL C.C., SUTHERLAND I.W., GRAHAM L. & WEIR D.M. (1978) The role of cell wall carbohydrates in binding of microorganisms to mouse peritoneal exudate macrophages. *Acta path. microbiol. scand.* (section B) **86**, 53.

68 GLASS E.J., STEWART J. & WEIR D.M. (1981) The presence of bacterial binding 'lectin-like' receptors on phagocytes. *Immunology*, **44**, 529.

69 WEIR D.M., STEWART J. & GLASS E.J. (1982) Phagocyte recognition by lectin receptors. *Immunobiology*, **161**, 334.

70 KINANE D.F., WEIR D.M., BLACKWELL C.C. & WINSTANLEY F.P. (1984) Binding of *Neisseria gonorrhoeae* by lectin-like receptors on human phagocytes. *J. Clin. Lab. Immunol.* **13**, 107.

71 STEWART J., GLASS E.J. & WEIR D.M. (1982) Macrophage binding of *Staphylococcus albus* is blocked by anti I-region antibody. *Nature*, **298**, 852.

72 GLASS E.J., STEWART J. & WEIR D.M. (1983) Membrane changes in murine macrophages after *in vivo* stimulation and activation. *Immunology*, **50**, 165.

73 GLASS E.J., STEWART J. & WEIR D.M. (1982) The influence of chemotactic factors on the expression of phagocyte receptors. *J. Clin. Lab. Immunol.* **7**, 39.

74 WINCHESTER R.J. & KUNKEL H.G. (1979) The human Ia system. *Adv. Immunol.* **28**, 221.

75 SCHER M.G., BELLER D.J. & UNANUE E.R. (1980) Demonstration of a soluble mediator that induces exudates rich in Ia-positive macrophages. *J. exp. Med.*, **152**, 1684.

76 EZEKOWITZ R.A.B. & GORDON S. (1982) Down regulation of mannosyl receptor mediated endocytosis and antigen F4/80 in bacillia calmette-guerin-activated murine macrophages. Role of T lymphocytes and lymphokines. *J. exp. Med.* **155**, 1623.

77 VAN FURTH R., COHN Z.A., HIRSCH J.G., HUMPHREY J.H., SPECTOR W.G. & LANGEVOORT H.L. (1972) The mononuclear phagocyte system: a new classification of macrophages, monocytes and their precursor cells. *Bull. Wld Hlth Org.* **46**, 845.

78 MACKANESS G.B. (1964) The immunological basis of acquired cellular resistance. *J. exp. Med.* **120**, 105.

79 UNANUE E.R. (1981) The regulatory role of macrophages in antigenic stimulation. Part two: symbiotic relationship between lymphocytes and macrophages. *Adv. Immunol.* **31**, 1.

80 HOWIE S. & MCBRIDE W.H. (1982) Cellular interactions thymus-dependent antibody responses. *Immunology Today*, **3**, 273.

81 EVANS R. & ALEXANDER P. (1976) Mechanisms of extracellular killing of nucleated mammalian cells by macrophages. In *Immunobiology of the Macrophage*, (ed. Nelson D.S.), p. 535. Academic Press, New York.

82 PROBERT M., STOTT E.J. & THOMAS L.H. (1977) Interactions between calf alveolar macrophages and parainfluenza-3 virus. *Infect. Immun.* **15**, 576.

83 SILVERSTEIN S.C. (1982) Membrane receptors and the regulation of mononuclear phagocyte effector functions. In *Advances in Experimental Medicine and Biology*, Vol. 155, (eds. Norman S.J. & Sorkin E.), p. 21. Plenum, New York.

84 MACKANESS G.B. (1962) Cellular resistance to infection. *J. exp. Med.* **116**, 381.

85 MACKANESS G.B. (1970) The monocyte in cellular immunity. *Semin. Hematol.* **7**, 172.

86 OGMUNDSDOTTIR H.M. & WEIR D.M. (1980) Mechanisms of macrophage activation. *Clin. exp. Immunol.* **40**, 223.

87 RUSKIN J., MCINTOSH J. & REMINGTON J.S. (1969) Studies on the mechanism of resistance to phylogenetically diverse intracellular organisms. *J. Immunol.* **103**, 252.

88 MCLEOD R. & REMINGTON J.S. (1977) Studies on the specificity of killing of intracellular pathogens by macrophages. *Cell. Immunol.* **34**, 156.

89 WING E.J., GARDNER I.D., RYMING F.W. & REMINGTON J.S. (1977) Dissociation of effector functions in populations of activated macrophages. *Nature*, **268**, 642.

90 KRAHENBUHL J.L., ROSENBERG L.T. & REMINGTON J.S. (1973) The role of thymus-derived lymphocytes in the *in vitro* activation of macrophages to kill *Listeria* monocytogenes. *J. Immunol.* **111**, 992.

91 DAVID J.R. & REMOLD H.G. (1976) Macrophage activation by lymphocyte mediators and studies on the interaction of macrophage inhibitory factor (MIF) with its target cells. In *Immunobiology of the Macrophage*, (ed. Nelson D.S.), p. 401. Academic Press, New York.

92 HOLT P.G. (1979) Alveolar macrophages. (1) A simple technique for the preparation of high numbers of viable alveolar macrophages from small laboratory animals. *J. immunol. Meth.* **27**, 189.

93 HUNNINGHAKE G.W. & FAUCI A.S. (1976) Immunological reactivity of the lung. (1) A guinea pig model for the study of pulmonary mononuclear cell subpopulations. *Cell. Immunol.* **26**, 89.

94 BOYUM A. (1968) Isolation of leukocytes from human blood. Further observations. Methyl cellulose, dextran and Ficoll as erythrocyte-aggregating agents. *Scand. J. clin. Lab. Invest.* **21** (suppl. 97), 31.

95 LOOS H., BLOK-SHUT B., VAN DOOM R., HOKSBERGEN R., BRUTEL, DE LA RIVIERE A. & MEARHOF L. (1976). A method for the recognition and separation of human blood monocytes on density gradients. *Blood*, **48**, 731.

96 SANDERSON R.J. & BIRD K.E. (1977) Cell separations by counterflow centrifugation. In *Methods in Cell Biology*, Vol. 15, (ed. Prescott D.M.), p. 1. Academic Press, New York.

97 ROSS G.D. & ATKINSON J.C. (1985) Complement receptors, structure and function. *Immunol. Today*, **6**, 115.

Chapter 49
Dendritic cells

R. M. STEINMAN, W. C. VAN VOORHIS & D. M. SPALDING

Principal features of dendritic
    cells, 49.1
Preparation of dendritic cells
    from mouse spleen and lymph
    node, 49.3

Preparation of dendritic cells
    from murine Peyer's patch,
    49.5
Dendritic cells from rats, 49.6
Dendritic cells from human
    blood, 49.6

Principal features of dendritic cells

Dendritic cells (DC) are specialized stimulator cells for the immune response. DC are often confused with macrophages. Therefore a short introduction is presented to summarize the principal features of DC.

What is a dendritic cell?

The term 'dendritic cell' is used here to describe a distinctive type of leucocyte that has been identified in rodents and man. The main properties of DC are outlined in Table 49.1. These irregularly shaped, non-phagocytic cells are derived from bone marrow and express class I and II products of the major histocompatibility complex (MHC) and the leucocyte common antigen. The frequency of DC in all tissues is small, less than 1%, but the cells have been detected in lymphoid and some non-lymphoid organs as well as blood and lymphatic circulations. DC lack the differentiation markers of all other cell types (Table 49.1) and in mouse react with a cell-specific monoclonal antibody, 33D1 [reviewed in 26]. The distinctive function of DC is their capacity to act as accessory or stimulator cells for many lymphocyte responses (see below).

DC can adhere to such substrates as glass, plastic, nylon wool, and Sephadex. For this reason, DC are sometimes considered to be 'macrophages' or 'macrophage-like'. Adherence is not a cell-specific marker and is exhibited to some degree by most cell types. Most DC from mouse spleen and human blood adhere initially but become non-adherent after overnight culture. However, most DC from mouse Peyer's patch and all rat tissues are non-adherent immediately upon isolation. Beyond adherence, there is little that DC have in common with mononuclear phagocytes, either tissue macrophages or blood monocytes. The two cell types exhibit stable differences in morphology, surface markers and function [reviewed in 27 and 28].

Approaches to the study of dendritic cells

DC are not simple to identify because they are present in such small numbers. Cytologic and cytochemical criteria, particularly phase contrast microscopy of glutaraldehyde-fixed or liver specimens, are most useful. DC are always irregular in shape. The types of process can vary from spiny dendrites, to bulbous pseudopods and large thin lamellipodia or veils. The cytoplasm has many phase dense mitochondria. The nucleus is often irregular in shape and has small nucleoli. Surface ruffles are absent, except at points where a new process is about to form. Few endocytic vacuoles and lysosomes are present. The latter can be documented with appropriate exogenous tracers and with acridine orange staining or acid phosphatase cytochemistry. In addition, DC lack Fc receptors and the differentiation antigens of other cell types, e.g. surface Ig for B cells, thy-1 for T cells, F4/80 antigen for macrophages. In mice, a DC specific monoclonal antibody, 33D1, is now available.

In mouse spleen several features allow identification of DC without multistep enrichment procedures. First, DC adhere firmly to glass and plastic, and removal of non-adherent cells leaves an adherent population that is 5–40% DC. Second, DC spread quickly so that their distinctive cytologic features are readily apparent. Third, DC can be selectively labelled (indirect immunofluorescence) or depleted (complement-mediated cytotoxicity) with the 33D1 monoclonal antibody. Antibody-mediated cytolysis enables one to compare the function of adherent DC and macrophages shortly after removal from the animal.

In other tissues and species, DC are far outnumbered by macrophages and/or lymphocytes even when they adhere to glass or plastic as in human blood. Therefore enrichment techniques must be employed. Features that are useful in enriching DC (Table 49.2) include the following: adherence properties; low buoyant density; failure to express Fc receptors and

Table 49.1. Features of dendritic cells

Features	References
Distinct cytologic features, especially cell processes	[1–6]
Cytochemistry: weak for non-specific esterase, acid phosphatase, membrane ATPase	[1,3,6,8]
Non-phagocytic, weak pinocytic activity	[3–8]
Low buoyant density	[2–8]
Adherent in some cases, non-adherent in others	[2–6,8,20]
Express class I and II MHC products, and the leucocyte common antigen	[2,4,6,8,9]
Express the 33D1 antigen in mice	[4,10–13]
Lack Fc receptors and the differentiation antigens of other cells, e.g.:	[2–8,18]
Macrophages: F4/80, mac-1, 63D3, 3C10/1D9	[3,12,14,15]
B cells: Ig and BA-1	[2,3,5–7,9,14,15]
T cells: thy-1; Lyt-1,2; OKT 3,4,6,8; Leu 1–3,7; OX19; W3/13	[2,3,5–7,9,14,15]
Potent stimulators of lymphocyte responses	
Allogeneic MLR	[8,16–18,22,24]
Graft rejection	[19,38]
Syngeneic MLR	[3,8,9,18,20]
Cytolytic T cells	[20–22]
Antibody forming responses	[13,36,37]
Contact sensitivity	[23]
Proliferation to soluble antigens	[24,39]
Oxidative mitogenesis	[3–5,8,9,12,25]
Aggregate with responding T cells and B cells	[4,20,29,36,37]

Table 49.2. Approaches to the purification of dendritic cells

Species	Organ	Traits permitting enrichment	Purity	References
Mouse	Spleen, node	Adherent then non-adherent; Low density; EA$^-$	90%	[2,7,20]
	Peyer's patch	Low density; Form clusters with T cells	60%	[4]
Rat	Spleen, node	Radioresistant; Low density; EA$^-$	70%	[5]
	Liver, skin, peritoneal cavity		50%	[8]
	Lymph		50%	[6]
Man	Blood	Adherent then non-adherent; Low density; EA$^-$, Ig$^-$, E$_N$; Lack antigens detected with monoclonals (3C10, BA-1, Leu 1)	70%	[3,15,18]

the differentiation markers of other cell types; radio-resistance; and ability to form clusters with T cells. Enrichment procedures are best monitored by cytology as described above.

The procedures described in this section should be performed only if one is prepared to monitor DC content. Even selective depletion experiments with specific monoclonal antibodies should be monitored to document the efficacy of killing.

What do dendritic cells do?

The dendritic cell is a potent stimulator or accessory cell for several responses (Table 49.1). Our group has drawn a distinction between the terms 'accessory or stimulator cell', and the more frequently used term, 'antigen presenting cell'. The term antigen presentation implies that nominal antigen must be *altered* or *processed* to expose or select a specific determinant, and/or the antigen must in some way *associate with* a class I or II MHC product. As a result the processed or associated antigen can be recognized by a T cell precommitted to respond to the new or 'altered self' determinant(s). Further definition is difficult, since there is little biochemical information describing processed or presented antigen. The authors use the term accessory cell to mean cells that are needed to stimulate responses, particularly the growth and differentiation of resting lymphocytes; they suspect that accessory cells do something beyond antigen presentation, i.e. accessory cells are required *in addition* to antigen and MHC products.

This concept of specialized accessory cells has emerged from data on the functional properties of DC in mouse, rat and man. In all species, DC are strong stimulators of lymphocyte responses (Table 49.1), e.g. the allogeneic and syngeneic mixed leucocyte reaction, and oxidative mitogenesis (the proliferation of periodate or neuraminidase/galactose oxidase-modified T cells). In mice, selective depletion of DC with 33D1 antibody and complement (C*) reduces stimulatory capacity 75–90% [4,11–13]. In many instances macrophages have been studied and shown to be weak or inactive stimulators [3,4,8,9,11–13,18–21]. The most detailed comparison of DC and Ia$^+$ macrophages has been carried out in man [9]. DC are strong stimulators of mixed leucocyte reactions, oxidative mitogenesis and the proliferative response to tetanus toxoid. Monocytes are weak stimulators as assessed by positive and negative selection techniques (cell sorting with fluorescent anti-monocyte antibody, and selective depletion with antibody and complement). Each T cell response is blocked by an Fab fragment of a monoclonal anti-MHC class II antibody. However, quantitative binding studies with this Fab indicate that DC and monocytes express similar levels of the required class II or Ia products. It appears then that MHC products are required for proliferation, but they become effective in generating T cell responses when present on DC. There is no known function for class II or Ia antigens other than to serve as restriction elements for T cells. Therefore Ia antigens on macrophages must be able to function in 'antigen presentation', but it is likely that additional features are present on DC that are needed to stimulate lymphocyte responses.

Preparation of dendritic cells from mouse spleen and lymph node

Equipment

Centrifuge: medium speed, swinging bucket rotor, refrigerated.
Microscope: inverted and routine, with phase contrast.
Tissue culture facilities: laminar flow hood, CO_2 incubators.

Materials

Collagenase: Worthington Biochemicals, Freehold, NJ.

Deoxyribonuclease: DNAase I, Sigma, St. Louis, Mo.
Culture medium: RPMI 1640.
Fetal calf serum.
Glutaraldehyde.
Poly-L-lysine (PLL): Type VII, Sigma.
33D1 anti-dendritic cell monoclonal antibody: Grand Island Biologicals (GIBCO).
Bovine plasma albumin (BPA): armour fraction V has been the only preparation that the authors have employed. For every 10 g of albumin powder, prepare solute consisting of 2.9 ml of 1 M NaOH, and 6.5 ml of glass distilled H_2O with either 18.6 ml ('dense BPA'; $\rho = 1.080$) or 38.6 ml ('dilute BPA'; $\rho = 1.060$) or phosphate-buffered saline (PBS). Sprinkle the powder on the solute in a wide beaker and leave at 4 °C to dissolve overnight. Do not attempt to speed the dissolution of the BPA by stirring. Check the density by refractive index and sterilize through a combination of a coarse prefilter and a 0.45 μm filter.
Complement: rabbits are selected for low background toxicity, i.e. no detectable killing at a final concentration of $2–3 \times 10^6$ cells per ml and 6–10% fresh rabbit serum. Fasted rabbits are bled every two weeks. The blood is allowed to clot for 45–60 min at room temperature and serum is collected following centrifugation on ice. Aliquots of 0.5–1.0 ml are quick frozen in an ethanol–dry ice bath with swirling to distribute the serum over the tube. The samples are lyophilized and stored at −70 °C. Several commercial sources have been used successfully, but on occasion the available lots reduce MLR stimulating capacity at the doses needed to support antibody-mediated lysis.
Cytotoxicity medium: antibody-mediated cytolysis is performed in a medium containing 0.3% BPA, 25 mM-HEPES and RPMI-1640. This medium avoids variability due to changes in pH or anticomplementary serum factors. DNAase (30 μg/ml final) is also included.
Antibody-coated erythrocytes (EA): hyperimmune rabbit anti-sRBC serum is titred in a haemagglutination assay using serial two dilutions of serum and 5% v/v packed red cells that have been washed three times in saline. The first subhaemagglutinating dose is used to opsonize the red cells. The EA are stored at 5% in RPMI-1640 at 4 °C and are active for at least 2–3 weeks.

Procedure

1 Dissociate the spleen or node: use teasing and/or grinding techniques. Treatment with collagenase, 0.5 mg/ml for 30 min at 37 °C, or Dispase (see next section, below) increases total cell yield, and releases a population of large macrophages (laden with haemosiderin in spleen) that is not otherwise obtained.

2 Prepare adherent cells: adhere the cell suspension outright, or preferably apply the suspension (2–4 spleens in 3–10 ml) to a column (25–40 ml) of medium with 10% fetal calf serum and centrifuge at 150 g for 10 min. Most of the debris, connective tissue fragments, and dead cells remain in the supernatant. Resuspend the cell pellet and plate at 37 °C for 1–3 h in medium containing serum (1–10% FCS) or 0.3% BPA. Cell loads are $3–5 \times 10^6$/16 mm diameter well, $25–40 \times 10^6$/60 mm dish, $100–200 \times 10^6$/100 mm dish. Dislodge the non-adherent cells with gentle Pasteur pipetting; swirling, shaking, and rocking will not remove lymphocytes adequately. Be sure to wash the rims of the culture vessel and use an inverted microscope to monitor the efficacy of washing. Properly washed spleen adherent cells represent just 1–2% of total spleen cells in pathogen free mice; much higher frequencies (N 1090) are obtained in mice infected with BCG or with *Listeria*.

A simpler procedure is to prepare DC from the low density subpopulation of spleen, rather than whole spleen. Suspend the spleen cells in dense BPA, 10×10^7/ml, overlay with 2 ml dilute BPA, and spin to equilibrium in a swingout bucket rotor at 10 000 g for 12 min at 4 °C. The low density or floating fraction represents 5–10% of total cells, but has $\geqslant \frac{2}{3}$ of the DC. Prepare adherent cells as above. The adherent cells from 4–6 mice are now present on a single 60 mm plate, rather than 2–4 sparse 100 mm plates as with whole spleen adherent cells. The high-density fraction from the BPA columns can be used to prepare macrophage-rich adherent cells (see below). Typical yields for 6 mice would be: 40×10^7 spleen, $2–3 \times 10^7$ low-density cells, $1–2 \times 10^6$ low-density adherent cells, $1–4 \times 10^6$ high-density adherent cells. The low-density adherent cells contain $\leqslant 2\%$ lymphocytes and consist primarily of DC and MØ.

3 Purify the DC from the DC-MØ adherent population: culture the adherent monolayers overnight in 5% FCS-medium. Most of the DC and some of the MØ can then be dislodged into a suspension of viable cells using the same gentle pipetting procedure employed for the initial preparation of the adherent population. The authors have not been successful in scraping or dislodging DC in a viable state on the first day of the experiment, i.e. 1–3 h after preparing the adherent cells. EA rosetting is one way to remove MØ from the suspension. Spin the EA and adherent cells (25–50 EA/white cell) into a pellet at 4 °C, leave for 20 min, gently resuspend (rosettes can then be counted on a hemocytometer), and centrifuge over a dense albumin column. The DC float; EA$^+$ white cells and some DC pellet. Alternatively, remove macrophages by applying the cell suspension in fresh medium to a plastic or glass surface. The macrophages readhere firmly over a

1–3 h period. Dislodge the DC by gentle pipetting over the surface.

Monitor the purity of the DC fraction by attaching an aliquot ($1–3 \times 10^4$ cells in 50–100 μl) to 12 mm circular coverslips that have been coated with 25–50 μg/ml PLL and washed in water. Viable cells adhere firmly. The percentage of DC is monitored by phase contrast. The DC extend processes in many directions, while contaminating macrophages and lymphocytes are usually round and will rosette EA.

4 To prepare spleen or node macrophages, begin with either low-density, high-density, or total spleen adherent cells. Macrophages can then be selected by one of the following methods.
(1) EA rosetting: this approach is not desirable. There is considerable toxicity if macrophages phagocytose any of the EA [30] and the rosetting fraction is contaminated with lymphocytes and DC.
(2) Readherence: this approach (see part 3 of the procedure, above) routinely provides >95% pure MØ, as assessed by cytology and EA rosetting, as long as one washes the readherent macrophage monolayer by gentle pipetting.
(3) Persistently adherent cells: some macrophages remain adherent after overnight culture. Generally one can only obtain sufficient numbers of macrophages by this method if infected mice are used.
(4) Deplete DC with the 33D1 monoclonal antibody and C* using spleen adherent cell suspensions or fresh adherent populations as described elsewhere [11]. Monitor killing by cytology.

Monitor the purity of the MØ population by showing that most of the cells bind and phagocytose EA. Place aliquots of the cells on coverslips in cylinders with medium, and spin on 15 μl of 5% EA. Rosettes form immediately at 4 °C. Phagocytosis occurs within 30 min at 37 °C. To visualize the rosettes, just shake the cylinders to rinse off non-bound EA. To visualize uptake, lyse extracellular EA with a water shock or with ammonium chloride.

Notes and recommendations

The EA depletion technique provides DC of the highest purity, but there is some loss of non-rosetting DC into the EA$^+$ fraction. Readherence is a simpler and higher yield procedure, but more macrophages can contaminate the DC fraction. In functional assays, DC prepared by either method behave similarly.

It may be useful to summarize how DC behave in the standard procedures that are used to enrich or deplete other populations of leucocytes. DC are enriched if B or T cells are depleted by panning or by treatment with lymphocyte-specific antibodies and C*. DC stick to Sephadex G10 and to nylon-wool.

One standard column passage depletes most DC. However, as DC are maintained in culture, the capacity to stick efficiently to these columns is lost.

Preparation of dendritic cells from murine Peyer's patch

Materials

Equipment and reagents are the same as for preparation from mouse spleen and lymph node, but add the following items.

Joklik's medium: GIBCO.

Dispase: Grade II, Boehringer Mannheim, Indianapolis, IN.

Dilute BPA: dilute the $\rho = 1.080$ stock (see previous section) with PBS to $\rho = 1.030$ and to 1.008 for use in making continuous BPA gradients (to isolate lymphocyte-DC aggregates from single cells); or dilute to $\rho = 1.068$, 1.063, and 1.040 for use in discontinuous gradients (to purify PP DC).

Gradient maker and peristaltic pump.

Beckmann L-50 refrigerated ultracentrifuge with SW 50.1 swinging bucket rotor.

Procedure

1 Dissociate the Peyer's patches (PP) with Dispase [31,32]. The latter is essential for obtaining suspensions with accessory activity comparable to spleen [4]. The nodules (20–100 from 2–10 mice, 6–8 weeks old) are incubated in 10–15 ml Joklik medium containing Dispase 1.5 mg/ml and DNAase (15 μg/ml) with constant stirring at 37 °C, but not in a CO_2 incubator. At 30 min intervals, remove the cells and add fresh medium for a total of 4–5 extractions. Following each extraction, wash the cells twice in RPMI 1640 and maintain at room temperature in medium with 5% serum until all 4 extractions are complete. Yield is 20–25 × 10^6 cells/mouse, and viability is > 95%. Remove debris by rapidly passing the suspension through a Pasteur pipette lightly packed with glass wool.

2 Allow the DC to form aggregates with responding T lymphocytes: the majority of DC in PP are non-adherent, so a distinctive enrichment procedure has been devised. Culture enzymatically dissociated PP cells with irradiated, periodate-treated spleen T cells (nylon wool non-adherent) for 16–20 h in 24-well culture dishes (generally 7.5 × 10^6 PP cells and 3–5 × 10^6 T cells per well). The irradiated T cells form clusters with DC comparable to that seen when DC and non-irradiated T cells are co-cultured. However, irradiated T cells do not blast transform, so that the DC is the principal cell in the cluster with a low buoyant density.

3 Isolate the clusters: use velocity sedimentation on preformed continuous gradients of BPA ($\rho = 1.030 \rightarrow 1.008$) constructed with a gradient maker, peristaltic pump, and 15 ml of BPA of each density. Gently aspirate the PP-spleen T cell cultures with a Pasteur pipette and transfer directly on to the BPA gradient. Load up to 200 × 10^6 cells in 10 ml, although the capacity may be higher. Centrifuge at 50 *g* for 5 min in a swinging bucket rotor. The clusters layer out on the bottom of the gradient, and the single cells are found near the top. Gently aspirate and discard the BPA leaving the pellet of clusters undisturbed. Save the 5 ml of the gradient just above the pellet and place a sample on a haemocytometer to verify that no single cells or clusters are detectable, i.e. that the separation of clusters and nonclusters is clean.

4 Retrieve the DC from the clusters: leaving the clusters in the tube, wash once in 50 ml ice-cold PBS and resuspend the clusters in 2–3 ml ice-cold PBS (calcium- and magnesium-free) in a 15 ml tube. Leave on ice 15 min and then disrupt the clusters into single cells with repeated Pasteur pipetting. It is essential to maintain the cells at 4 °C to prevent reaggregation. Inadequate disruption of the clusters decreases the yield of DC, while excessively vigorous disruption can fragment the DC. Now centrifuge at 4 °C for 10 min and resuspend the pellet with repeated pipetting into 2 ml of dense BPA, $\rho = 1.080$. Overlay with 1 ml each of BPA at 1.068, 1.063 and 1.040. Centrifuge at 10 000 *g* and 4 °C for 15 min. Aspirate the cells at the 1.063/1.040 and 1.068/1.063 interfaces. Evaluate DC content by morphology on PLL coated coverslips and/or by cytotoxicity with 33D1 and C*. Purity is 60–80% and yield is 0.8 to 1.1% of the original PP suspension.

Notes and recommendations

This procedure can also be employed with PP cells that have been enriched for DC by an initial flotation in dense BPA (see page 49.4). In this case, the authors generate DC-T cell clusters by culturing 2 × 10^6 low-density PP cells with 3–5 × 10^6 irradiated, periodate-treated spleen T cells.

Preformed continuous Percoll gradients can be utilized to isolate clusters, instead of continuous BPA gradients. Gradients are formed as described below (page 49.6). Generally 50 × 10^6 cells in 1–2 ml are loaded on to 10 ml of Percoll in a 15 ml round-bottomed tube. Centrifuge at 75 *g* for 10 min.

The PP enrichment procedure, which includes Dispase digestion and formation of DC-T cell clusters, has been used successfully to purify spleen DC. This approach is useful for comparative assays of PP and spleen DC, but the procedures outlined in the previous section are simpler.

Pathogen-free animals were utilized in the development of the above procedure. Subsequently, it has been found that use of non-pathogen free animals can result in variable B cell contamination of the DC-enriched population. To circumvent this the B cells were routinely removed by panning on anti-immunoglobulin coated dishes prior to cluster formation when using non-pathogen free animals.

Dendritic cells from rats

Klinkert *et al.* [5,8] and Pugh *et al.* [6] have published procedures for enriching DC from rats. The procedures will not be outlined here except to point out the differences in strategy that are required. Rat DC are non-adherent but have a low buoyant density. Most lymphocytes are high density, particularly if the cells are studied 1–5 days after high doses of ionizing irradiation *in vitro*, or 2–3 days after whole body irradiation *in situ*. The non-adherent population that retains a low buoyant density following irradiation is 50–80% DC.

The authors have attempted to purify mouse and human DC using the irradiation procedure. Unfortunately, the DC often do not survive for more than 24 h, and the irradiated low density fractions are heavily contaminated with lymphocytes. Presumably there are species differences in the ability of DC to survive high doses of ionizing irradiation. However, when mouse and human DC are irradiated and then tested immediately for functional activity, the irradiated DC function identically to non-irradiated cells.

Dendritic cells from human blood

Materials

Equipment and reagents as on page 49.3 but add the following items.
Ficoll-Hypaque: Sigma.
Monoclonal antibodies:
(1) 3C10 anti-monocyte (GIBCO)
(2) BA-1 anti-B cell (Hybritech)
(3) Leu-1 anti-T cell (Becton Dickinson).
Percoll: Percoll is purchased from Pharmacia and an isotonic stock solution is prepared by mixing 9 parts Percoll with 1 part 10X concentrated PBS. Continuous gradients for equilibrium density separation are prepared by mixing isotonic Percoll, PBS and fetal calf serum in a ratio of 57:40:3 and centrifuging at 38 000 g for 18 min. For velocity separation, mix isotonic Percoll, PBS, and fetal calf serum in a ratio of 45:31:24 and centrifuge at 18 000 g for 35 min. The preformed

gradients can be stored on ice for several hours until use.
Modified erythrocytes:
(1) EA (see page 49.3).
(2) E anti-human Ig [33]
(3) E neuraminidase [34].

Procedure

1   Prepare a mononuclear cell fraction from blood obtained by venipuncture (15 units/ml heparin) or from leucocyte-rich buffy coats obtained from a blood bank. Collect the mononuclear fraction from Ficoll-Hypaque columns. Wash by centrifugation three times with the aim of removing most platelets.

2   Prepare adherent cells: apply about 5×10^7 mononuclear cells to 100 mm plastic Petri dishes in 8 ml of RPMI-1640 supplemented with 5% FCS. After 1–3 h at 37 °C, rinse off the non-adherent cells with 4–6 washes in RPMI-1640, with rocking and swirling. In contrast to the preparation of mouse adherent cells, do not attempt to remove human blood non-adherent cells by pipetting over the monolayer. This results in large losses of monocytes and DC. The adherent fraction contains 50–70% monocytes, 20–40% lymphocytes and only a small percentage of DC ($\sim 2\%$). In general, human blood DC are not as well spread as their murine counterparts. One can obtain fresh adherent cells with higher percentages of DC by depleting monocytes and lymphocytes with cell-specific antibodies and C*. Treatment of whole mononuclear cells, however, requires a lot of antibody and C*, so we prefer to enrich DC from adherent subpopulations (see below).

3   Separate the adherent cells into firmly adherent and detached ('1X released') fractions. Following overnight culture, 50–80% of the adherent cells are in suspension or can be released by simple swirling. This detached '1X released' population contains most of the DC as well as most of the lymphocytes and many monocytes. The firmly adherent population is a highly enriched source of Ia$^+$ monocytes. The 1X released population can then be processed in two ways to provide enriched DC (Table 49.3). The 'physical' method provides DC as well as monocytes and B cells; the 'antibody-cytolysis' method provides DC only, but in higher purity and yield.

4   To purify the DC by the physical method, first readhere the 1X released population on plastic exactly as described above. The cells that reattach are primarily monocytes, while the cells that do not readhere (the '2X released') contain most of the DC and lymphocytes. Suspend the latter in dense BPA, $\rho = 1.080$ and spin to equilibrium, just as is done with mouse spleen cells. Alternatively, low- and high-density cells can be

Table 49.3. Enrichment of dendritic cells from human blood

	'Physical method'	'Cytolytic method'
Technique:	Isolate mononuclear cells	Isolate mononuclear cells
	Make adherent cells	Make adherent cells
	Culture overnight	Culture overnight
	Readhere to remove most monocytes; rosette with anti-immunoglobin coated erythrocytes, and centrifuge in dense albumin to pellet most lymphocytes	Remove most monocytes with anti-monocyte antibody and complement; remove lymphocytes and remaining monocytes with anti-monocyte, -B, and -T cell antibodies and complement; retrieve viable cells on dense albumin
Result:	DC purity: 20–60%	DC purity: 65–80%
	Monocyte and lymphocyte contamination (10% or more)	Less than 2% monocyte and B and T cell contamination

separated by equilibrium density separation in continuous gradients of Percoll, prepared as described above. Suspend up to 3×10^8 cells in 1–2 ml dense isotonic Percoll solution; with a long Pasteur pipette place the suspension under a 10 ml gradient in a 15 ml tube (diameter 15 mm), and spin to equilibrium at 1150 *g* for 20 min. High- and low-density bands are clearly resolved near the bottom and top of the gradients, respectively. The high-density cells ($\sim 80\%$ of the 2X released) are primarily B cells that are monocyte- and DC-depleted. The low-density cells are $\geqslant 20\%$ DC, but contain significant levels of monocytes (10–30%), T cells (5–20%), B cells (10–30%) as well as Ia$^+$ round cells that have not been classified. One can enrich DC further by depleting monocytes (with EA rosetting, or by another readherence), B cells (with E anti-Ig), or T cells (with E$_N$).

5 An alternative approach is to take the 1X released population and deplete monocytes, B cells and T cells using cytotoxic cell-specific antibodies. 3C10 anti-monocyte, BA-1 anti-B cell, and Leu-1 anti-T cell all kill their respective cell types in the presence of rabbit C*, but do not kill DC. Two cycles of cell killing are preferable. In the first, kill the monocytes with 3C10 and C*. In the second, use a cocktail of 3C10, BA-1 and Leu-1. In each case, mix the cells and antibody for 15 min on ice, add the C*, and then incubate for 60–70 min at 37 °C in the presence of 30 μg/ml DNAase. Wash off the reagents and culture the cells for 2 h in the presence of 20 μg/ml DNAase to allow damaged cells to die. Float the suspension in dense BPA; most of the viable cells float. The low-density fraction is highly (65–80%) enriched in DC, and there are few residual monocytes, B cells and T cells. A priori, the primary limitation to purity is the presence of other trace cell types that would not react with the cytolytic antibodies, e.g. NK cells, immature myeloid cells.

6 Monitor the purification procedure by cytologic criteria: spin aliquots on to coverslips coated with 100 μg/ml PLL in protein-free medium, and allow the cells to spread for 20 min at 37 °C. Under these conditions, DC form large numbers of processes, the cytoplasm has many mitochondria, and the nucleus is irregularly shaped. Monocytes spread circumferentially and have obvious pinocytic vesicles, lysosomes, and refractile lipid droplets. Lymphocytes remain round. Lymphoblasts can exhibit a single large pseudopod or many fine processes; however, a large transformed nucleus and nucleolus are diagnostic. Cytochemistry for nonspecific esterase [35] yields strong cytoplasmic staining on monocytes and weak, absent, or granular staining of DC and lymphocytes. Immunofluorescence with cell-specific antibodies is also helpful.

7 To enumerate rather than purify DC in small volumes of blood (e.g. 20–50 ml), plate 10×10^6 mononuclear cells per 60 mm plastic tissue culture plate, remove non-adherent cells, and culture the adherent monolayers overnight. The 1X released fraction is resuspended in 1 ml RPMI, overlaid on to dense BPA adjusted to $\rho = 1.075$, and centrifuged at 7000 *g* for 12 min. The low-density, interface cells are collected, washed free of BPA, and spun on to PLL-coated coverslips as above. The differential count of lymphocytes, monocytes and DC is determined by morphology. The yield of DC in this simplified method agrees well with that provided by the multistep procedures outlined above (Table 49.4).

Notes and recommendations

It may be useful to summarize the behaviour of DC in other protocols that are frequently used to enrich or deplete specific subpopulations of human blood leucocytes. The frequency of DC is increased relative to

Table 49.4. Comparison of dendritic cell isolation technique

Isolation technique	N	Total cells in DC fraction per ml blood	% DC	% DC in PBMC	DC/ml blood
Physical technique from buffy coats	30	7.6×10^3 $\pm 5.2 \times 10^3$	29 ± 8	0.14 ± 0.06	2.2×10^3 $\pm 1.5 \times 10^3$
Cytolytic technique	6	2.2×10^3 $\pm 0.7 \times 10^3$	73 ± 6	0.13 ± 0.09	1.6×10^3 $\pm 0.6 \times 10^3$
Crude fractions from small samples of blood	10	1.5×10^4 $\pm 1.1 \times 10^4$	11 ± 5	0.17 ± 0.12	1.7×10^3 $\pm 1.2 \times 10^3$

control if T cells are depleted by rosetting with SRBC (E$_n$-ve), B cells with RBC coated with anti-Ig (Ig-ve), and monocytes with RBC coated with anti-RBC (FcR-ve). However, some non-rosetting cells always contaminate the rosette-positive fraction, so that some DC may be present. Efficient methods for depleting DC are passage over nylon wool and Sephadex G10 columns, and treatment with monoclonal anti-Ia and complement. We have not studied how DC behave during monocyte depletion with carbonyl iron or silica.

Acknowledgements

Supported by grants AI 13013 and CA 30198 to R.M. Steinman from the N.I.H., and grant AI18958 to D.M. Spalding. R.M. Steinman is an Established Investigator of the American Heart Association. D.M. Spalding is an Investigator of the Arthritis Foundation.

References

1 STEINMAN R.M. & COHN Z.A. (1973) Identification of a novel cell type in peripheral lymphoid organs of mice. (I) Morphology, quantitation, tissue distribution. *J. exp. Med.* **137**, 1142–1162.
2 STEINMAN R.M., KAPLAN G., WITMER M.D. & COHN Z.A. (1979) Purification of spleen dendritic cells, new surface markers, and maintance *in vitro. J. exp. Med.* **149**, 1–16.
3 VAN VOORHIS W.C., HAIR L.S., STEINMAN R.M. & KAPLAN G. (1982) Human dendritic cells: enrichment and characterization from peripheral blood. *J. exp. Med.* **155**, 1172–1187.
4 SPALDING D.M., KOOPMAN W.J., ELDRIDGE J.H., McGHEE J.R. & STEINMAN R.M. (1983) Accessory cells in murine Peyer's Patch. (I) Identification and enrichment of a functional dendritic cell. *J. exp. Med.* **157**, 1646–1659.
5 KLINKERT W.E.F., LABADIE J.H., O'BRIEN J.P., BEYER C.F. & BOWERS W.E. (1978) Rat dendritic cells function as accessory cells and control the production of a soluble factor required for mitogen responses of T lymphocytes. *Proc. natn. Acad. Sci. U.S.A.* **77**, 5414–5418.
6 PUGH C.W., MACPERSON G.G. & STEER H.W. (1983) Characterization of nonlymphoid cells derived from rat peripheral lymph. *J. exp. Med.* **157**, 1758–1779.
7 STEINMAN R.M. & COHN Z.A. (1974) Identification of a novel cell type in peripheral lymphoid organs of mice. (II) Functional properties *in vitro. J. exp. Med.* **139**, 380–397.
8 KLINKERT W.E.F., LABADIE J.H. & BOWERS W.E. (1982) Accessory and stimulating properties of dendritic cells and macrophages isolated from various rat tissues. *J. exp. Med.* **156**, 1–19.
9 VAN VOORHIS W.C., VALINSKY J., HOFFMAN E. & STEINMAN R.M. (1983) The relative efficacy of human monocytes and dendritic cells as accessory cells for T cell replication. *J. exp. Med.* **158**, 174–191.
10 NUSSENZWEIG M.C., STEINMAN R.M., WITMER M.D. & GUTCHINOV B.A. (1982) A monoclonal antibody specific for mouse dendritic cells. *Proc. natn. Acad. Sci. U.S.A.* **79**, 161–165.
11 STEINMAN R.M., GUTCHINOV B., WITMER M.D. & NUSSENZWEIG M.C. (1983) Dendritic cells are the principal stimulators of the primary mixed leukocyte reaction in mice. *J. exp. Med.* **157**, 613–627.
12 AUSTYN J.M., STEINMAN R.M., WEINSTEIN D.E., GRANELLI-PIPERNO A. & PALLADINO M.A. (1983) Dendritic cells initiate a two stage mechanism for lymphocyte proliferation. *J. exp. Med.* **157**, 1101–1115.
13 INABA K.S., STEINMAN R.M., VAN VOORHIS W.C. & MURAMATSU S. (1983) Dendritic cells are critical accessory cells for thymus-dependent antibody responses in mouse and in man. *Proc. natn. Acad. Sci. U.S.A.* **80**, 6041–6045.
14 NUSSENZWEIG M.C., STEINMAN R.M., UNKELESS J.C., WITMER M.D., GUTCHINOV B. & COHN Z.A. (1981) Studies of the cell surface of mouse dendritic cells and other leukocytes. *J. exp. Med.* **154**, 168–187.
15 VAN VOORHIS W.C., STEINMAN R.M., HAIR L.S., LUBAN J., WITMER M.D., KOIDE S. & COHN Z.A. (1983) Specific anti-mononuclear phagocyte monoclonal antibodies: application to the purification of dendritic cells and the tissue localization of macrophages. *J. exp. Med.* **158**, 126–145.
16 STEINMAN R.M. & WITMER M.D. (1978) Lymphoid dendritic cells are potent stimulators of the primary mixed leukocyte reaction in mice. *Proc. natn. Acad. Sci. U.S.A.* **75**, 5132–5136.
17 MASON D.W., PUGH C.W. & WEBB M. (1981) The rat

mixed lymphocyte reaction: roles of a dendritic cell in intestinal lymph and T cell subsets defined by monoclonal antibodies. *Immunology*, **44**, 75–87.

18 KUNTZ-CROW M. & KUNKEL H.G. (1982) Human dendritic cells: major stimulators of the autologous and allogenic mixed leukocyte reactions. *Clin. exp. Immunol.* **49**, 338–341.

19 LECHLER R.I. & BATCHELOR J.R. (1982) Restoration of immunogenicity to passenger cell-depleted kidney allografts by the addition of donor strain dendritic cells. *J. exp. Med.* **155**, 31–41.

20 NUSSENZWEIG M.C. & STEINMAN R.M. (1980) Contribution of dendritic cells to stimulation of the murine syngeneic mixed leukocyte reaction. *J. exp. Med.* **151**, 1196–1212.

21 NUSSENZWEIG M.C., STEINMAN R.M., GUTCHINOV B. & COHN Z.A. (1980) Dendritic cells are accessory cells for the development of anti-trinitrophenyl cytotoxic T lymphocytes. *J. exp. Med.* **152**, 1070–1084.

22 ROLLINGHOFF M., PFIZENMAIER K. & WAGNER H. (1982) T–T cell interaction during cytotoxic T cell responses. (IV) Murine lymphoid dendritic cells are powerful stimulators for helper T lymphocytes. *Eur. J. Immunol.* **12**, 337–342.

23 BRITZ J.S., ASKENASE P.W., PTAK W., STEINMAN R.M. & GERSHON R.K. (1982) Specialized antigen-presenting cells: splenic dendritic cells, and peritoneal exudate cells induced by mycobacteria activate effector T cells that are resistant to suppression. *J. exp. Med.* **155**, 1344–1356.

24 SUNSHINE G.H., KATZ D.R. & FELDMAN M. (1980) Dendritic cells induce proliferation of synthetic antigens under Ir gene control. *J. exp. Med.* **152**, 1817–1822.

25 PHILIPS M.L., PARKER J.A., FRELINGER J.A. & O'BRIEN R.L. (1980) Characterization of responding cells in oxidative mitogen stimulation. (II) Identification of an Ia-bearing adherent accessory cell. *J. Immunol.* **124**, 2700–2707.

26 STEINMAN R.M., WITMER M.D., NUSSENZWEIG M.C., GUTCHINOV B. & AUSTYN J.M. (1983) Studies with a monoclonal antibody to mouse dendritic cells. *Transplant. Proc.* **15**, 299–310.

27 STEINMAN R.M. & NUSSENZWEIG M.C. (1980) Dendritic cells: features and fuctions. *Immunol. Revs.* **53**, 127–147.

28 VAN VOORHIS W.C., WITMER M.D. & STEINMAN R.M. (1983) The phenotype of dendiritic cells and macrophages. *Fed. Am. Soc. Exp. Biol.* **42**, 3114–3118.

29 STEINMAN R.M. & COHN Z.A. (1975) A novel adherent cell in mouse lymphoid organs. In *Immune Recognition*, (ed. Rosenthal A.S.), pp. 571–587. Academic Press, San Francisco.

30 MELLMAN I.S., PLUTNER H., STEINMAN R.M., UNKELESS J.C. & COHN Z.A. (1983) Selective internationalization and degradation of macrophage Fc receptors during receptor-mediated phagocytosis. *J. cell. Biol.* **96**, 887–895.

31 FRANGAKIS M.V., KOOPMAN W.J., KIYONO H., MICHALEK S.M. & MCGHEE J.R. (1982) An enzymatic method for preparation of dissociated murine Peyer's patch cells enriched for macrophages. *J. immunol. Meth.* **48**, 33–44.

32 KIYONO H., MCGHEE J.R., WANNEMUEHLER M.J., FRANGAKIS M.V., SPALDING D.M., MICHALEK S.M. & KOOPMAN W.J. (1982) *In Vitro* immune responses to a T-dependent antigen by dissociated murine Peyer's patch cultures. *Proc. natn. Acad. Sci. U.S.A.* **79**, 596–600.

33 GOTTLIEB A.B., FU S.M., YU D.T.Y., WANG C.Y., HALPER J.P. & KUNKEL H.G. (1979) The nature of the stimulatory cell in human allogeneic and syngeneic MLC reactions: role of isolated IgM bearing B cells. *J. Immunol.* **123**, 1497–1503.

34 HOFFMAN T. & KUNKEL H.G. (1976) The E rosette test. In In Vitro *Methods in Cell-Mediated Immunity*, (eds. Bloom B.R. & David J.R.), pp. 71–81. Academic Press, New York.

35 LI C.Y., LAM K.W. & YAM L.T. (1973) Esterases in human leukocytes *J. Histochem. Cytochem.* **21**, 1–12.

36 INABA K., GRANELLI-PIPERNO A. & STEINMAN R.M. (1983) Dendritic cells induce T lymphocytes to release B cell stimulating factors by an interleukin 2 dependent mechanism. *J. exp. Med.* **158**, 2040–2057.

37 INABA K., WITMER M.D. & STEINMAN R.M. (1984) The clustering of dendritic cells, helper T lymphocytes and histocompatible B cells during primary antibody responses *in vitro*. *J. exp. Med.* **169**, 858–876.

38 FAUSTMAN D., STEINMAN R.M., GREBEL H., HAUPTFELD V., DAVIE J. & LACY P. (1984) Presentation of rejection of murine islet allografts by pretreatment with anti-dendritic cell antibody. *Proc. natn. Acad. Sci. U.S.A.* **81**, 3864–3868.

39 SUNSHINE G.H., GOLD D.P., WORTIS H.H., MARRACK P. & KAPPLER J.W. (1983) Mouse spleen dendritic cells present soluble antigens to antigen-specific T cell hybridomas. *J. exp. Med.* **158**, 1745–1750.

Chapter 50
Reduction and excitation of oxygen by phagocytic leucocytes: biochemical and cytochemical techniques

J. A. BADWEY, J. M. ROBINSON, M. J. KARNOVSKY &

M. L. KARNOVSKY

Overview, 50.1
General aspects, 50.1

Biochemical methodologies for
active oxygen species, 50.4

Cytochemical methodologies for
active oxygen species, 50.8

Depending upon conditions, phagocytic leucocytes can undergo a rapid increase in oxygen consumption during phagocytosis or upon stimulation of their plasmalemma with a variety of agents. This increased respiration is accompanied by the production of superoxide (O_2^-) and hydrogen peroxide (H_2O_2), which may subsequently interact to form the hydroxyl radical ($OH\cdot$) and perhaps singlet oxygen ($^1O_2$). These products of oxygen reduction (i.e. O_2^-, H_2O_2, $OH\cdot$) and excitation (i.e. $^1O_2$) have been implicated in the destruction of bacteria, yeast, viruses, and mycoplasmas by leucocytes, and thus they constitute key components in the antimicrobial mechanisms of phagocytes. Unfortunately, untoward exposure of normal tissues to the extracellular release of 'active oxygen species' during chronic inflammation may effect a variety of pathological changes such as the destruction of neighbouring cells [for review, see 1–3].

Apart from the microbicidal and pathological properties mentioned, 'active oxygen species' have also been implicated recently in a variety of diverse biological processes. Examples include the cytolysis of tumour cells by various phagocytic systems [e.g. 4,5], suppression of the cidal activity of human natural killer cells [6], suppression of murine lymphocyte proliferation [7] and the inactivation of leucotrienes B_4, C_4, D_4, and E_4 [8]. Detection and quantification of these oxygen species is thus of interest to a broad spectrum of biologists.

In this chapter, procedures are described for monitoring the various active oxygen species and the concomitant phenomena associated with their production (i.e. oxygen consumption, chemiluminescence). The procedures are presented in a format that emphasizes the advantages and limitations of the various assays rather than as a list of detailed methodologies. This style was necessitated by the current state of flux of this area and by the broad scope of the approach taken. The authors have avoided discussions of the chemistry of the various active oxygen species since these are thoroughly covered in recent reviews [1–3].

Overview

The active oxygen species produced by phagocytes, and phenomena associated with their production (i.e. oxygen consumption, chemiluminescence), are listed in Table 50.1, along with the chemical and cytochemical assays and the equipment necessary for monitoring these phenomena. All of the chemicals required are commercially available. The advantages and limitations of each of these procedures, particularly as they pertain to whole cells, are discussed in the respective sections below. In later tables (Table 50.4 and 50.5) detailed lists of representative studies where these assays have been applied to phagocytes from a variety of species are given.

General aspects

Agents that stimulate leucocytes to produce active oxygen species

The oxidative metabolism of leucocytes can be triggered by a variety of 'particulate' and 'soluble' surface active agents. Most particulate agents require opsonization to be effective (e.g. zymosan, *S. aureus*) [27,28] and phagocytosis generally accompanies the phenomenon. Latex particles are the major exception which do not require opsonization. Particles are opsonized as

Table 50.1. Chemical and cytochemical methods for monitoring the production of active oxygen species and concomitant phenomena

Process	Indicator	Product monitored	Equipment or method of detection	Reference
Chemical assays				
Chemiluminescence				
(i) inherent light	—	—	Liquid scintillation counter	—
(ii) amplified light	Luminol	Aminophthalate ion	Liquid scintillation counter	[9,10]
Oxygen consumption	—	—	Oxygen electrode	—
Superoxide	Ferricytochrome c	Ferrocytochrome c	Spectrophotometer	[11]
Hydrogen peroxide	Scopoletin (reduced)	Scopoletin (oxidized)	Fluorimeter	[12,13]
Hydroxyl radical	Methional	Ethylene	Gas chromatograph	[14]
	2-Keto-4-thiomethylbutyrate	Ethylene	Gas chromatograph	[15]
	Dimethyl sulphoxide	Methane or formaldehyde	Gas chromatograph or fluorimeter	[16,17]
	7-^{14}C-Benzoate	$^{14}CO_2$	Liquid scintillation counter	[18]
	5,5-Dimethyl-1-pyrroline-*N*-oxide	5,5-Dimethyl-2-hydroxypyrolidine-*N*-oxide radical	Electron spin resonance spectrometer	[19]
Singlet oxygen	2,5-Diphenylfuran	*cis*-Dibenzoylethylene	Spectrophotometer, thin-layer chromatography	[20,21]
	1,3-Diphenylisobenzofuran	*o*-Dibenzoylbenzene	Spectrophotometer, thin-layer chromatography	[22,23]
Cytochemical assays				
Superoxide	Nitroblue tetrazolium	Formazan	Light microscope	[24,25]
Hydrogen peroxide	Cerium chloride ($CeCl_3$)	Cerium perhydroxide	Electron microscope	[26]

described in [29]. Antibody-coated 'target cells' (e.g. lymphoma cells [30]) and aggregated immunoglobulin fixed to solid surfaces [e.g. 31] are particulate agents which stimulate the oxidative metabolism of phagocytes but are not phagocytosed. These stimuli are employed to study the involvement of phagocytes in extracellular antibody-dependent cytotoxicity reactions and the pathogenesis of immune complex disorders.

The soluble stimuli comprise a remarkably diverse group of chemicals. These agents can be broadly divided on the basis of whether cytochalasins B or E are employed to augment their activity. Soluble agents which are utilized without cytochalasin include digitonin [32], deoxycholate [32], fatty acids [33–35] phorbol 12-myristate 13-acetate [36], and fluoride [37]. Soluble agents which generally are employed with cytochalasins include concanavalin A [e.g. 38,39], calcium ionophore A23187 [e.g. 40], complement (i.e. C3b, C5a) [41], and chemotactic peptides (e.g. *N*-formyl-L-methionyl-L-leucyl-L-phenylalanine)   [e.g. 40,42].

Various stimuli can exhibit marked differences in terms of the magnitude of a particular phenomenon (e.g. O_2^-) that they elicit at 'saturating' concentrations [35,43]. In addition, a particular oxidative phenomenon under study may also be highly dependent upon the stimulating agent utilized. For example, human neutrophils stimulated with latex particles exhibit high levels of oxygen consumption and H_2O_2 production, but release little O_2^- [44]. In contrast, these cells, when stimulated with opsonized zymosan to a level at which the oxygen consumption is identical to that observed with latex particles, release massive amounts of O_2^- [44]. Unfortunately, similar comparative studies on the balance between oxygen consumption and O_2^- and H_2O_2 release with other stimuli are not available.

Various types of phagocytes can respond differently to certain stimuli. For example, both saturated and unsaturated fatty acids stimulate a respiratory burst in elicited guinea-pig neutrophils [33,34], but only the latter compounds are active with human neutrophils [35]. Opsonized zymosan is an extremely effective stimulator with human neutrophils, but is rather poor with guinea-pig neutrophils [45].

Phorbol 12-myristate 13-acetate is in the authors' view the reagent of choice for stimulating the oxidative metabolism of phagocytes. This reagent is stable, does not require cytochalasins, and stimulates the oxidative metabolism of a wide variety of phagocytes to levels comparable with or superior to those observed with other stimuli. Receptors for this agent have been reported recently in human monocytes and neutrophils [46–48] and the biochemical events which occur when these receptors are occupied are now being illuminated for different cell types [e.g. 49].

Cell types and effects of elicitation procedures on the respiratory burst

The majority of studies concerning the oxidative metabolism of leucocytes have involved neutrophils since these cells are more abundant than other cells of the blood that are capable of producing O_2^- and H_2O_2 (i.e. eosinophils [50], monocytes [51], natural killer cells [52]). Neutrophils are also easily obtainable in large quantities and pure form (*c.* 90%) by elicitation. 'Elicited neutrophils' are cells which migrate into the peritoneum of animals (e.g. guinea-pig [53], mouse [54]) 4–18 h following the injection of a sterile inflammatory agent (e.g. casein, proteose-peptone). The ability of such cells to release O_2^- upon stimulation has recently been shown to be highly dependent upon the eliciting agent utilized and the time after injection at which the cells are harvested [54]. A number of striking biochemical changes occur when neutrophils leave the circulation to become exudate cells (e.g. loss of specific granules [55], glycogen accumulation [56]). The influence of elicitation conditions should therefore be considered when extrapolations are made in terms of the physiological relevance of particular effects.

The situation with respect to the oxidative metabolism of macrophages is even more complex. These cells may be broadly divided into three categories: *resident*, normal washout cells obtained by lavage alone; *elicited*, inflammatory cells; lymphokine *activated* cells. Elicited macrophages are cells obtained from the peritoneal cavities of animals *several days* after the injection of a sterile inflammatory agent (e.g. casein, thioglycollate). Activated macrophages are obtained from the peritoneum (or other locales) after infection of the host with an intracellular parasite (e.g. *Bacillus Calmette-Guérin, Listeria monocytogenes*). A number of biochemical differences have been described among the categories of macrophages [for review, see 57–59]. These differences include the ability to produce O_2^- and H_2O_2. Resident macrophages release little, if any, O_2^- and H_2O_2 upon stimulation [54,60–62]. Activated and elicited macrophages may release O_2^- and H_2O_2 [54,60–62]; the quantitites released are highly dependent upon the activating agents [for review, see 63], or the eliciting procedure itself [54], as was noted above for neutrophils. In addition, if the cells are cultured, the length of time macrophages are in culture as well as the culture conditions also influence oxidative activity [61,64,65].

Quantitative aspects of the respiratory burst

A survey of the recent literature indicates that some admonitory remarks are necessary when reporting cellular phenomena. The composition of the cell preparations employed (i.e. percentages of granulocytes, lymphocytes, etc.) should always be reported. Further, effects under study should be reported as maximal rates, i.e. rates obtained at saturating levels of stimuli under conditions of linearity with respect to both time and cell concentration. To facilitate comparison of data between different laboratories, rates should be expressed in terms of a fixed number of cells. If it is necessary to express rates in terms of the cellular protein concentration, factors for converting from protein concentration to cell number should be reported. These matters are not always observed in the field being covered here, but they do facilitate and illuminate when applied.

Biochemical methodologies for active oxygen species

Chemiluminescence

Allen *et al.* [66] observed in 1972 that phagocytosing granulocytes exhibit chemiluminescence and proposed that $^1O_2$ was responsible for this phenomenon. This report provided the first indication that oxygen species other than H_2O_2 (i.e. $^1O_2$, O_2^-) were produced by stimulated phagocytes. Oxidation of exogenous luminol by phagocytes to electronically excited states which strongly chemiluminesce was employed later to amplify the response for a variety of phagocytes [67]. Subsequent studies have shown that chemiluminescence results from a complicated series of reactions that may involve all of the oxygen species produced by granulocytes as well as components of the phagocytosed particles [68,69]. Chemiluminescence thus provides only a qualitative or comparative measure of oxidative metabolism that is rather non-specific. The simplicity and exactness of measuring cellular O_2^- and H_2O_2 release directly by chemical means has rendered this technique generally less desirable in the authors' view but special circumstances for employing it may pertain. Detailed procedures for measuring chemiluminescence of phagocytes, the use of luminol to amplify the response, and methods of data presentation are thoroughly reviewed elsewhere [70].

Oxygen consumption

Virtually all respirometric studies on phagocytes are now performed with a Clark oxygen electrode connected to an oxygen monitor and recorder [44,45,71,72,73]. Absolute calibration of the electrode can be conveniently performed by the phenylhydrazine-ferricyanide method [74]. The reaction mixtures must be thoroughly mixed throughout all measurements to prevent the probe from locally depleting oxygen from solution directly below the cathode. After temperature equilibration, oxygen uptake by cells is measured for several minutes before stimulation to determine the resting rate. The increased respiration upon stimulation is the maximal rate observed after the addition of the stimulating agent, minus the resting rate. Some studies now combine oxygen uptake and O_2^- and/or H_2O_2 measurements [28,75]. Superoxide and H_2O_2 are measured in the reaction mixture in those studies by endpoint procedures subsequent to determination of the rate of oxygen uptake (see below).

A major advantage of this technique (and the chemiluminescence method) is that it is a non-invasive procedure: no external reagents must be added for the determination *per se* and the phenomenon can be followed continuously. The disadvantage is that the values obtained are *net* values which result from several possible reactions of O_2 uptake and release in a cyclic series of reactions [76]. Thus differences between cell types are not always easily explained in terms of a single reaction or process. Another disadvantage of this method is that large quantities of cells are required because of the volume (1.0–3.0 ml) of the reaction chambers of most oxygen electrodes. This problem can now be circumvented by plastic wells which reduce the assay volume to 0.20 ml [see 77].

Superoxide release

Superoxide is easily measured spectrophotometrically at 550 nm by monitoring the ability of this anion to reduce exogenous ferricytochrome *c* [11; application to phagocytes 27,28]. Superoxide dismutase (SOD) specifically catalyses the decomposition of O_2^- ($O_2^- + O_2^- + 2H^+ \rightarrow H_2O_2 + O_2$) and therefore prevents the O_2^--mediated reduction of ferricytochrome *c* [11]. Addition of SOD to a sample containing all of the components of the reaction mixture thus provides a blank for subtracting out all of the ferricytochrome *c* reduction that may occur by agents other than O_2^- (e.g. by ascorbate) [11,79]. Advantages of this assay are that the reaction involves the transfer of single electrons (1:1 stoichiometry between O_2^- release and ferricytochrome *c* reduction); the product (ferrocytochrome *c*) is stable during assay, and the extinction coefficient for the reaction is quite large (20 000 $M^{-1}cm^{-1}$ [79]). These properties enable one to measure cellular O_2^- release by either an endpoint procedure (fixed time measurements [27,45,78]) or in a continuous fashion [80]. A double-beam spectrophotometer is required in the latter case where the SOD blank serves as the reference cuvette. In our experience the utility of the continuous assay is limited to studies with soluble stimulating agents since particulate agents, (e.g. opsonized zymosan), can cause problems associated with light-scattering at concentrations where the maximal effects are observed. Superoxide release under such circumstances is most accurately measured by an endpoint assay where the reaction is stopped by chilling and the particles and cells are removed by centrifugation prior to measuring, in a known aliquot, the amount of ferricytochrome *c* reduced.

Hydrogen peroxide release

The most widely accepted method now utilized for monitoring H_2O_2 release from cells is the fluorometric assay of Root *et al.* which measures the H_2O_2 mediated peroxidation of scopoletin [73]. Scopoletin (6-methoxy-7-hydroxyl-1,2-benzopyrone) is a fluorescent hydrogen donor that emits light at 450 nm with an intensity directly proportional to its concentration when excited by light at 360 nm [12,13]. This compound is oxidized stoichiometrically by H_2O_2 (1:1) in a peroxidase catalysed reaction with complete loss of fluorescence [12,13]. Cells are incubated in a spectrophotofluorometer in the presence of exogenous scopoletin and horseradish peroxidase for several minutes to determine the base-line extinction of fluorescence for scopoletin. This basal rate corresponds largely to H_2O_2 release by the non-stimulated cells. Cells are then stimulated and H_2O_2 release is measured continuously as the loss of fluorescence with a constant recording apparatus. The maximal rate of change of fluorescence intensity is converted to units of H_2O_2 by means of a standard curve constructed with an appropriate H_2O_2-generating system (e.g. xanthine plus xanthine oxidase, glucose plus glucose oxidase) [73]. Catalase specifically catalyses the decomposition of H_2O_2 ($2H_2O_2 \rightarrow 2H_2O_2 + O_2$), and if added to the reaction mixture inhibits scopoletin oxidation by competing with peroxidase for the H_2O_2 formed. This control is frequently employed to verify the specificity of the assay. The major advantages of this assay are its sensitivity (detection of 0.01 μM-H_2O_2) [73] and high specificity, since horseradish peroxidase is active with only hydrogen- and monoalkyl-hydrogen peroxides [81]. In addition, the optical geometry can be set such that the assay system is largely unaffected by problems associated with light scattering and quenching [see 73]. Unlike measurements of O_2^-, this enables one to monitor H_2O_2 release continuously from cells stimulated with particulate as well as soluble agents. This method can also be utilized

in an 'endpoint' fashion to measure H_2O_2 accumulation in the medium at fixed time points [e.g. 28].

Hydroxyl radical formation

As a result of the lack of a specific test for this species a number of methods have evolved to monitor $OH\cdot$ production by phagocytes. Hydroxyl radical is detected by measuring a chemical reaction effected by this species, along with the inhibition of the reaction by reagents which react with $OH\cdot$. These 'inhibitors' provide a degree of specificity to the assays but lack the certainty which superoxide dismutase, and catalase and/or peroxidase confer on the assays for O_2^- and H_2O_2 (see above).

Hydroxyl radical production by phagocytes is most commonly monitored by measuring the production of ethylene effected by $OH\cdot$ from thioethers: 3-thiomethylpropionaldehyde (methional) [82,83] or 2-keto-4-thiomethylbutyric acid [84,85] (reactions 1 and 2, Table 50.2). Cells are stimulated in sealed glass siliconized tubes in the presence of thioether and ethylene gas released into the vapour phase is quantified by gas chromatography. 2-Keto-4-thiomethylbutyric acid is preferred to 3-thiomethylbutyric acid because the latter reagent autoxidizes to produce ethylene under ambient conditions [84]. Unfortunately, both thioethers are converted to ethylene by a variety of agents other than $OH\cdot$. Thus reaction 1 may be effected by H_2O_2 [85], a variety of organic radicals such as alkoxy radicals ($RO\cdot$), peroxy radicals ($ROO\cdot$) [86] and peroxidase catalysed reactions [87]. Reaction 2 may be effected by $^1O_2$ [85], HOCl [85], alkoxy radicals [88] and peroxidase catalysed reactions [87].

Methane production from dimethyl sulphoxide has been employed as an assay for $OH\cdot$ production by phagocytes [16] (reaction 3, Table 50.2). Cells with dimethyl sulphoxide are stimulated in sealed glass siliconized tubes and methane gas released into the headspace is measured by gas chromatography. Advantages of this assay are that dimethyl sulphoxide is highly permeant to cells, non-toxic, stable and unreactive with H_2O_2 and $^1O_2$ [16]. Whether organic radicals or peroxidase catalysed reactions promote reaction 3 remains to be determined. It has been shown with a variety of $OH\cdot$ generating systems (but not phagocytes) that formaldehyde, rather than methane, is the *major* product of the interaction of $OH\cdot$ with dimethyl sulphoxide [17]. Formaldehyde was measured in the fluid phase of the reaction mixtures in those studies [17] by either spectrophotometric [89] or fluorometric [90] methods following deproteinization of the samples with trichloroacetic acid. The fluorometric method was noted to be very sensitive to the

Table 50.2. Chemical assays for hydroxyl radical

Reactant	Products

(1) 3-Thiomethylpropionaldehyde

$H_3C—S—CH_2—CH_2—CHO \rightarrow$ C_2H_4 + $\frac{1}{2}(H_3CS)_2$ + $COOH$
Ethylene   Methyldisulphide   Formic acid

(2) 2-Keto-4-thiomethylbutyric acid

$H_3C—S—CH_2—CH_2—C—COOH \rightarrow$ C_2H_4 + $\frac{1}{2}(H_3CS)_2$ + $COOH$ + CO_2
‖   Ethylene   Methyldisulphide   Formic acid   Carbon dioxide
O

(3) Dimethyl sulphoxide

$$\overset{\displaystyle O}{\underset{\displaystyle \|}{}}$$
$H_3C—S—CH_3 \rightarrow$ H_3CSO_2H + $H_3C\cdot$
Methylsulphonic acid   Methyl radical

$H_3C\cdot + RH$ $\rightarrow$ $CH_4 + R\cdot$
Methane

$2H_3C\cdot + 2O_2 \rightarrow 2$ $H_3COO\cdot$ H_3COH + $HCHO$
Methylperoxy   Methanol   Formaldehyde
radical

(4) 7-^{14}C—Benzoate

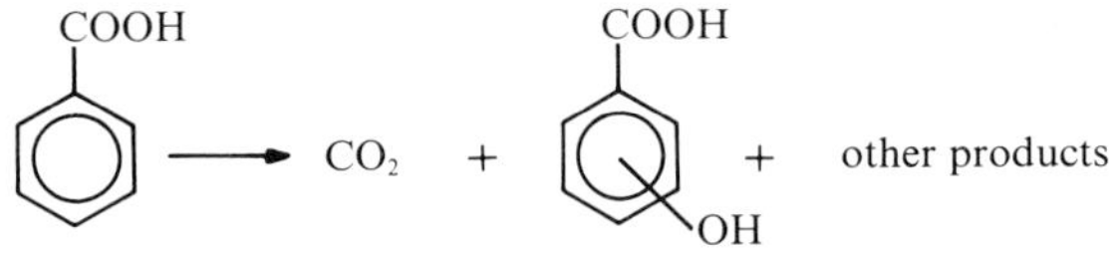

Hydroxybenzoic acids

(5) 5,5-Dimethyl-1-pyrroline-N-oxide (DMPO)

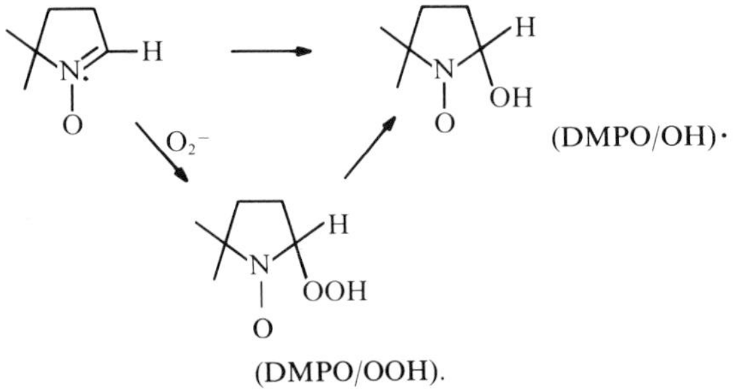

(DMPO/OH)·

(DMPO/OOH).

experimental conditions [17]. Formaldehyde formation from dimethyl sulphoxide may thus be a sensitive assay for OH· production by phagocytes provided that this aldehyde is not substantially metabolized by the cells.

Hydroxyl radical mediated decarboxylation of 7-^{14}C-benzoate to ^{14}CO$_2$ by stimulated phagocytes has been demonstrated (reaction 4, Table 50.2) [91]. This reaction was employed to measure cellular OH· production continuously by an ionization chamber electrometer system [91] and should be easily adapt-

able to an 'endpoint' assay [see 88]. Benzoate does not decompose spontaneously to produce CO$_2$ and produces no adverse effects on cells at the concentration utilized (i.e. 0.025 mM) [91]. Most importantly, studies with model systems show that this reaction is not effected by O$_2^-$, H$_2$O$_2$, ^{1}O$_2$, organic hydroperoxides or alkoxy radicals [88]. Thus, this reaction appears presently to be the most specific and simplest method of measuring OH·.

Hydroxyl radical reacts with the spin trap, 5,5-dimethyl-1-pyroline-N-oxide (DMPO) to yield the long-lived nitroxide adduct 5,5-dimethyl-2-hydroxy-pyrolidine-*N*-oxide radical (DMPO/OH)· which is easily identified by electron spin resonance spectroscopy [19]. This technique has been employed to detect OH· formation by stimulated granulocytes [92,93]. Those studies, however, have been questioned on the grounds that the (DMPO/OH)· adduct observed was not due to the trapping of OH·, but rather to the decomposition of the (DMPO/OOH)· adduct formed by trapping O_2^- [94]. A recent review has described straightforward procedures to resolve such ambiguities in model systems [95] and those procedures should now be applied to phagocytes.

As noted above, compounds which react with OH· are always utilized as 'inhibitors' of the reactions listed above to provide further evidence that OH· is being monitored. Substances which have been employed for this purpose with cells include benzoate (2–20 mM) (in methodologies which do not employ its decarboxylation as the indicator; see above) ethanol (20–100 mM), mannitol (5–60 mM), thiourea (1.5–15 mM), histidine (0.1 mM), methionine (1 mM), and tryptophan (1.0 mM) [16,82–85,91]. Additional inhibitors which have been employed in non-cellular systems include *p*-nitroso-dimethylaniline [96], *p*-aminobenzoate [97], dimethyl sulphoxide [97] (cf. case of benzoate above) and butanol [97]. It is, of course, necessary to show that these compounds do not adversely effect cells under the assay conditions employed.

Singlet oxygen formation

Production of $^1O_2$ by stimulated phagocytes has not been demonstrated by chemical means. Quenchers of $^1O_2$ are frequently employed, however, to implicate this species in the cidal activity of these cells [5,64,85,98]. Two laboratories have reported that $^1O_2$ is produced *in vitro* in reconstituted peroxidase-H_2O_2-halide systems [99,100]. Similar systems function in the antimicrobial armamentarium of certain phagocytes [reviewed in 2 and 3]. Singlet oxygen was detected in the reconstituted systems by its ability to react with 2,5-diphenylfuran [99] and 1,3-diphenylisobenzofuran [100] to yield *cis*-dibenzoylethylene and *o*-dibenzoylbenzene, respectively (Table 50.3). The disappearance of the former compounds in the reaction can be followed spectrophotometrically in model systems (2,5-diphenylfuran at 324 nm [20] and 1,3-diphenyliso-benzofuran at 390 nm [22]) and the products are easily identified by thin-layer chromatography [21,23,99]. The peroxidase catalysed reactions were inhibited by quenchers of $^1O_2$ (β-carotene [101], diazobicyclo-octane [102], bilirubin [103], and histidine [104]) and were stimulated by substitution of D_2O for H_2O in the medium. The latter effect was thought to be due to the longer lifetime of $^1O_2$ in D_2O [105,106], but other explanations are possible [e.g. 107].

Serious questions have been raised about the validity of this approach for detecting $^1O_2$ in peroxidase

Table 50.3. Chemical assays for singlet oxygen

Reactant	Product
(1) 2,5-Diphenylfuran	

cis-Dibenzoylethylene

(2) 1,3-Diphenylisobenzofuran

o-Dibenzoylbenzene

systems. These criticisms are equally relevant to studies involving phagocytes, particularly with regard to the use of quenchers of $^1O_2$. Hypochlorous acid (HOCl), a known product of the myeloperoxidase-H_2O_2-Cl^- system [108], reacts directly with 1,5-diphenylfuran, 1,3-diphenylisobenzofuran and $^1O_2$ quenchers and thus mimics the results of the peroxidase systems without involving $^1O_2$ *per se* [109–111]. A peroxy radical has also been shown to react with 2,5-diphenylfuran and $^1O_2$ scavengers [112]. Thus current methodologies for implicating $^1O_2$ in phagocyte function are extremely tenuous.

Cytochemical methodologies for active oxygen species

Biochemical measurements reflect the statistical view of a population of cells for a particular event. Cytochemical studies, in contrast, provide information about individual cells and subpopulations of cells. Together, both techniques lead to a better understanding of cellular phenomena. Advantages of cytochemical procedures are that relatively few cells are required and that the cells need not be purified. These procedures are therefore particularly suited for cells such as

natural killer cells and human alveolar macrophages where both the paucity of the cells available and contamination of the preparations may present problems. Further, ultrastructural cytochemistry provides information concerning structure-function relationships in cells under non-disruptive conditions (i.e. on intact cells). A disadvantage of cytochemistry is that the cellular 'threshhold' response necessary to effect a particular reaction is unknown for most assays. A critical review of the utility and limitations of cytochemistry appears elsewhere [113].

In the section below, the utility of various reagents and techniques have been assessed in the context of this discussion of phagocytic leucocytes and active oxygen species.

Reduction of nitroblue tetrazolium

The first cytochemical reaction to be used to address questions concerning the respiratory burst of neutrophils was the reduction of nitroblue tetrazolium (NBT) to the insoluble formazan reaction product [24,114]. When neutrophils are presented with phagocytosable particles and NBT and examined at the light

Table 50.4. Oxidative metabolism of phagocytic leucocytes. Representative studies of biochemical techniques

Cell type and species	Phenomena assayed				
	Chemiluminescence	O_2 uptake	O_2^- release	H_2O_2 release	OH· release
Neutrophils					
human	66–69, 146	44, 45, 72, 73, 156	27, 28, 37, 45, 78	28, 73	16, 82–85, 91–93
mouse	—	—	45, 54	60	—
guinea-pig	147, 148	45, 148, 157	34, 45, 80, 148	80	148
rat	149	—	164	164, 170	164
rabbit	67, 147	157	40	—	—
Eosinophiles					
human	150, 151	50	50, 150, 151	—	—
guinea-pig	—	—	—	—	85
Monocytes					
human	51, 146, 152	156	51, 156, 165	65	83, 16
Natural killer cells					
human	52	—	52	—	—
Alveolar macrophages					
human	153	158, 159, 160	158, 159, 160	—	16, 160
guinea-pig	147	157, 161	161, 166	—	—
rat	149	162	164	164, 170	164
rabbit	67, 147	157	167, 168	—	—
Peritoneal macrophages					
mouse	154	163	54, 61, 62	60, 64, 171, 172	—
guinea-pig	147	157	169	169	—
rat	—	—	164	164	164
rabbit	67, 147	157	—	—	—
Kupffer cells					
rat	155	155	155	—	—

Table 50.5. Oxidative metabolism of phagocytic leucocytes. Representative studies of cytochemical techniques

Cell type and species	Phenomena assayed	
	NBT reduction	Cerium precipitation
Neutrophils		
human	24*,115+,173*,174+	26,45,124,125
guinea-pig	—	45
rat	—	170
Eosinophils		
human	150	—
Monocytes and macrophages		
human	175+,176+,177*+,178*	—
Alveolar and macrophages		
rabbit	179+	—
rat	—	170,128
Peritoneal macrophages		
mouse	177*+,64	54
guinea-pig	180*,181+	—
rat	182+	—
rabbit	183*	—

* Cytochemical NBT reaction
+ Quantitative NBT reaction

microscope level, the reaction product is found within the phagosomes [24]. Reduction of NBT is indicative of the respiratory burst since neutrophils from patients suffering from chronic granulomatous disease (CGD) do not reduce this reagent to formazan [24,114]. Chronic granulomatous disease is an inherited condition in which neutrophils from the afflicted patients fail to exhibit a respiratory burst or to produce O_2^- and H_2O_2 [for review, see 2 and 3] upon stimulation.

This cytochemical reaction was subsequently modified to yield a quantitative assay of neutrophil function with special reference to screening for CGD [115]. In this assay the formazan reaction product is extracted from the cells and solubilized with dioxane or pyridine and quantified spectrophotometrically.

Baehner *et al.* [25] presented evidence that NBT reduction in neutrophils is oxygen-dependent and results from the formation of active oxygen species. They noted that O_2^- and not H_2O_2 is probably responsible for this reaction. It should be noted here that Seidler [116] has proposed a model for tetrazolium reduction which involves O_2^- both as a reductant and as an intermediate.

Based upon cell fractionation studies it was proposed that the NBT-reductase activity resides on the plasmalemma [117]. Presence of reduced NBT on the plasmalemma of phagocytosing neutrophils has been directly shown at the ultrastructural level [26]. The reduction of NBT to formazan by stimulated neutrophils is no doubt a consequence of the oxidative

metabolism in these cells; however, the exact chemical mechanisms underlying this reaction remain to be fully elucidated and the contention that O_2^- is the major reductant [25] remains to be verified.

Application of the 'NBT test' to clinical situations has had a chequered past. It was hoped that this test would provide a rapid means of distinguishing between pyogenic infection and other diseases. There followed a number of reports suggesting that the 'NBT test' did not always give clear cut results when applied to clinical situations [for review, see 118]. The quantitative NBT reaction [115] has only limited value since the reduction of ferricytochrome *c* is far better suited for determination of O_2^- (see above). At the cytochemical level the NBT reaction does have applications. It has been very useful in providing an indication of the percentage of cells that undergo a respiratory burst in bone marrow cultures [119,120], murine peritoneal macrophages [62] and in lymphokine treated macrophages infected with toxoplasmas [64]. In summary, the NBT reaction at the cytochemical level is rapid, easy, requires relatively little equipment, and can be done on very few cells.

Detection of hydrogen peroxide

With diaminobenzidine

The reagent 3,3'-diaminobenzidine (DAB) was introduced as a cytochemical probe by Graham & Karnovsky [121]. This reagent has been widely employed for both the cytochemical localization of endogenous peroxidatic activity as well as for exogenously applied peroxidase (i.e. tracer studies). The multiple uses of this reagent have been reviewed [122].

The first unequivocal demonstration that H_2O_2 is present in the phagosomes of neutrophils was achieved with the use of DAB [123]. Neutrophils were allowed to phagocytose latex beads in the presence of this reagent. Oxidized DAB reaction product was observed in the phagosomes at the ultrastructural level. Presence of reaction product was due to activity of cellular myeloperoxidase using endogenously produced H_2O_2 as substrate. Azurophil granules contain myeloperoxidase and fuse with the phagosomes during phagocytosis. While this method was very useful in demonstrating the presence of endogenously produced H_2O_2, a more direct method (below) was desirable for routine cytochemical studies.

With cerous salts

A cytochemical method for the direct ultrastructural detection of H_2O_2 produced by stimulated neutrophils was reported by Briggs *et al.* [26]. In this method cerium is used as the capture agent for metabolically produced H_2O_2. Cerous ions react with H_2O_2 to form cerium perhydroxide $[Ce(OH)_3OOH]$. The cerium perhydroxide reaction product has several characteristics which make it suitable as an ultrastructural probe for H_2O_2. It is (1) insoluble in aqueous solutions, (2) insoluble in the organic solvents routinely employed in electron microscopy, (3) very electron dense, and (4) stable under the beam of the electron microscope. The electron-dense cerium perhydroxide is not, however, visible at the light microscope level. Furthermore, no methods have been devised for the chemical conversion of cerium perhydroxide to a visible product.

Briggs *et al.* [26] found cerium perhydroxide on the inner face of the phagosome and on the outer face of the plasmalemma of glass-adherent human neutrophils. More recently, Ohno *et al.* [124,125] also found cerium perhydroxide on the inner face of phagosomes and on the plasmalemma at the points of attachment of aggregated neutrophils in suspension. Neutrophils stimulated with soluble agents such as phorbol myristate acetate, lectins, digitonin, and lipopolysaccharide also have cerium perhydroxide deposits; these deposits are localized to intracellular vacuoles and the plasmalemma [26,45,125]. Stimulated neutrophils from patients with chronic granulomatous disease were shown to deposit little or no cerium perhydroxide [126].

The actual presence of cerium in the electron dense reaction product in human neutrophils has been verified independently by two different groups using X-ray microanalysis [124,127].

The standard medium employed for the cytochemical detection of H_2O_2 in neutrophils is 0.1 M-Tris-maleate buffer (pH 7.5), 1 mM-$CeCl_3$, 10 mM 3-amino-1,2,4-triazole (an inhibitor of catalase), 1 mM-glucose, a reduced pyridine nucleotide, and 5% sucrose [26,124]. This medium can be used with no deleterious effects on unfixed *neutrophils*. When this medium is applied to unfixed *macrophages* attached to glass coverslips, the cells round up and no longer demonstrate their normal spreading morphology. Reduction of the concentration of Tris-maleate and $CeCl_3$ to 10 mM and 0.10 mM respectively eliminated this problem and still produced good staining results [54]. Mouse peritoneal macrophages stimulated with phorbol myristate acetate have also been examined cytochemically for H_2O_2 [54]. Resident macrophages exhibited very little reaction product. On the other hand, when elicited macrophages were examined, reaction product was readily observed within phorbol induced vesicles and channels, while little or no reaction product was formed on the cell surface. The majority of activated macrophages were similar to elicited macrophages in terms of staining for H_2O_2 and also exhibited a small population of cells ($\sim 2\%$) which had cerium perhydroxide reaction product on the cell surface. These observations agreed with biochemical observations [54].

Rat alveolar macrophages have been examined following stimulation with lipopolysaccharide and incubation in a cerium containing cytochemical medium [128]. The authors report that cerium perhydroxide was localized on the plasmalemma and in small vesicles which were presumed to be derived from the cell surface.

A precaution to be exercised in cerium based cytochemical experiments is to exclude inorganic phosphate from the medium. Cerium reacts with inorganic phosphate to form cerium phosphate which is insoluble and electron dense [129,130].

Since the introduction of cerium as an ultrastructural probe for H_2O_2 in neutrophils, methods for the cytochemical localization of several oxidative enzymes have been developed. These studies have served to verify the usefulness of the cerium method originally described for neutrophils. A partial survey of the literature on the use of cerium for the cytochemical detection of oxidative enzymes is included for the interested reader. Hydrogen peroxide produced by D-amino acid oxidase has been studied in kidney [131,132], neutrophils [133], liver [134], rat central nervous system [135], as well as the yeast *Hansenula polymorpha* [136–138]. Various other peroxisomal enzymes have also been studied; methanol oxidase and glycolate oxidase in yeast [136–138], urate oxidase in liver [134], and plant root nodules [139], and other α-OH acid oxidases in liver and kidney [134,140] and plant tissues [41]. An NAD(P)H oxidase has been reported on the apical surface of rat thyroid follicles [142]. Monoamine oxidase [143] and sites which may be lipid peroxide [144] have been described cytochemically in cardiac tissue by cerium deposition. The herbicide paraquat causes generation of O_2^- and H_2O_2 in green plants; the sites of H_2O_2 accumulation in paraquat treated plant tissue have recently been described [145] using this method.

It is thus clear that cerium-based techniques originally applied to phagocytic leucocytes have proved to be very useful in the more general cytochemical demonstration of sites of H_2O_2 production at the ultrastructural level for a variety of cells and tissues.

Acknowledgements

The authors wish to acknowledge with thanks help from Dr John T. Curnutte, as well as many stimulating discussions with him.

Work reported from these laboratories was supported by grants from the United States Public Health Service, N.I.H. Nos. AI-03260 and AI-17945.

References

1 BADWEY J.A. & KARNOVSKY M.L. (1980) Active oxygen species and the functions of phagocytic leukocytes. *Ann. Rev. Biochem.* **49**, 695.

2 BABIOR B.M. (1978) Oxygen-dependent microbial killing by phagocytes. *New Engl. J. Med.* **298**, 659.

3 KLEBANOFF S.J. & CLARK R.A. (1978) *The Neutrophil, Function and Clinical Disorders*, 1st edn. North–Holland Publishing Co., Amsterdam.

4 EDELSON P.J. & COHN Z.A. (1973) Peroxidase-mediated mammalian cell cytotoxicity. *J. exp. Med.* **138**, 318.

5 NATHAN C.F., SILVERSTEIN S.C., BRUKNER L.H. & COHN Z.A. (1979) Extracellular cytolysis by activated macrophages and granulocytes. (II) Hydrogen peroxide as a mediator of cytotoxicity. *J. exp. Med.* **149**, 100.

6 SEAMAN W.E., GINDHART T.D., BLACKMAN M.A., DALAL B., TALAL N. & WERB Z. (1982) Suppression of natural killing *in vitro* by monocytes and polymorphonuclear leukocytes. *J. clin. Invest.* **69**, 876.

7 METZGER Z., HOFFELD J.T. & OPPENHEIM J.J. (1980) Macrophage-mediated suppression. (I) Evidence for participation of both hydrogen peroxide and prostaglandins in suppression of murine lymphocyte proliferation. *J. Immunol.* **124**, 983.

8 HENDERSON W.R. & KLEBANOFF S.J. (1983) Leukotriene B_4, C_4, D_4 and E_4 inactivation by hydroxyl radicals. *Biochem. biophys. Res. Commun.* **110**, 266.

9 WHITE E.H., ZAFIRIOU O., KÄGI H.H. & HILL J.H.M. (1964) Chemiluminescence of luminol: the chemical reaction. *J. Am. chem. Soc.* **86**, 940.

10. WHITE E.H. & BURSEY M.M. (1964) Chemiluminescence of luminol and related hydrazines: the light emission step. *J. Am. chem. Soc.* **86**, 941.

11 McCORD J.M. & FRIDOVICH I. (1969) Superoxide dismutase. An enzymic function for erythrocuprein (hemocuprein). *J. Biol. Chem.* **244**, 6049.

12 ANDREAE W.A. (1955) A sensitive method for the estimation of hydrogen peroxide in biological materials. *Nature*, **175**, 859.

13 PERSCHKE H. & BRODA E. (1961) Determination of very small amounts of hydrogen peroxide. *Nature*, **190**, 257.

14 BEAUCHAMP C. & FRIDOVICH I. (1970) A mechanism for the production of ethylene from methional. The generation of the hydroxyl radical by xanthine oxidase. *J. Biol. Chem.* **245**, 4641.

15 HEIKKILA R.E., WINSTON B., COHEN G. & BARDEN H. (1976) Alloxan-induced diabetes—evidence for hydroxyl radical as a cytotoxic intermediate. *Biochem. Pharmac.* **25**, 1085.

16 REPINE J.E., EATON J.W., ANDERS M.W., HOIDAL J.R. & FOX R.B. (1979) Generation of hydroxyl radical by enzymes, chemicals, and human phagocytes *in vitro*. Detection with the anti-inflammatory agent, dimethyl sulfoxide. *J. clin. Invest.* **64**, 1642.

17 KLEIN S.M., COHEN G. & CEDERBAUM A.I. (1981) Production of formaldehyde during metabolism of dimethylsulfoxide by hydroxyl radical generating systems. *Biochemistry*, **20**, 6006.

18 MATTHEWS R.W. & SANGSTER D.F. (1965) Measurement by benzoate radiolytic decarboxylation of relative rate constants for hydroxyl radical reactions. *J. phys. Chem.* **69**, 1938.

19 HARBOUR J.R., CHOW V. & BOLTON J.R. (1974) An electron spin resonance study of the spin adducts of OH and HO_2 radicals with nitrones in the ultraviolet photolysis of aqueous hydrogen peroxide solutions. *Canad. J. Chem.* **52**, 3549.

20 PORTER D.J.T. & INGRAHAM L.L. (1974) Concerning the formation of singlet O_2 during the decomposition of H_2O_2 by catalase. *Biochim. biophys. Acta* **334**, 97.

21 KING M.M., LAI E.K. & McCAY P.B. (1975) Singlet oxygen production associated with enzyme-catalyzed lipid peroxidation in liver microsomes. *J. Biol. Chem.* **250**, 6496.

22 ADAMS D.R. & WILKINSON F. (1972) Lifetime of singlet oxygen in liquid solution. *J. chem. Soc.* Farady Transactions 2, **68**, 586.

23 PENDERSON T.C. & AUST S.D. (1973) The role of superoxide and singlet oxygen in lipid peroxidation promoted by xanthine oxidase. *Biochem. biophys. Res. Commun.* **52**, 1071.

24 NATHAN D.G., BAEHNER R.L. & WEAVER D.K. (1969) Failure of nitroblue tetrazolium reduction in the phagocytic vacuoles of leukocytes of chronic granulomatous disease. *J. clin. Invest.* **48**, 1895.

25 BAEHNER R.L., BOXER L.A. & DAVIS J. (1976) The biochemical basis of nitroblue tetrazolium reduction in normal human and chronic granulomatous disease polymorphonuclear leukocytes. *Blood*, **48**, 309.

26 BRIGGS R.T., DRATH D.B., KARNOVSKY M.L. & KARNOVSKY M.J. (1975) Localization of NADH oxidase on the surface of human polymorphonuclear leukocytes by a new cytochemical method. *J. Cell Biol.* **67**, 566.

27 CURNUTTE J.T. & BABIOR B.M. (1974) Biological defense mechanisms. The effect of bacteria and serum on superoxide production by granulocytes. *J. clin. Invest.* **53**, 1662.

28 ROOT R.K. & METCALF J.A. H_2O_2 release from human granulocytes during phagocytosis. Relationship to superoxide anion formation and cellular catabolism of H_2O_2: studies with normal and cytochalasin B-treated cells. *J. clin. Invest.* **60**, 1266.

29 HOHN D.C. & LEHRER R.I. (1975) NADPH oxidase deficiency in X-lined chronic granulomatous disease. *J. clin. Invest.* **55**, 707.

30 CLARK R.A. & KLEBANOFF S.J. (1977) Studies on the mechanism of antibody dependent polymorphonuclear leukocyte-mediated cytotoxicity. *J. Immunol.* **119**, 1413.

31 JOHNSTON R.B. & LEHMEYER J.E. (1976) Elaboration of toxic oxygen by-products by neutrophils in a model of immune complex disease. *J. clin. Invest.* **57**, 836.

32 GRAHAM R.C., KARNOVSKY M.J., SHAFER A.W., GLASS E.A. & KARNOVSKY M.L. (1967) Metabolic and morphological observations on the effect of surface-active agents on leukocytes. *J. Cell Biol.* **32**, 629.

33 KAKINUMA K. (1974) Effects of fatty acids on the oxidative metabolism of leukocytes. *Biochim. biophys. Acta*, **348**, 76.

34 KAKINUMA K. & MINAKAMI S. (1978) Effects of fatty acids on superoxide radical generation in leukocytes. *Biochim. biophys. Acta*, **538**, 50.

35 BADWEY J.A., CURNUTTE J.T. & KARNOVSKY M.L. (1981) *cis*-Polyunsaturated fatty acids induce high levels of superoxide production by human neutrophils. *J. Biol. Chem.* **256**, 12640.

36 REPINE J.E., WHITE J.G., CLAWSON C.C. & HOLMES B.M. (1974) Effects of phorbol myristate acetate on the metabolism and ultrastructure of neutrophils in chronic granulomatous disease. *J. Clin. Invest.* **54**, 83.

37 CURNUTTE J.T., BABIOR B.M. & KARNOVSKY M.L. (1979) Fluoride-mediated activation of the respiratory burst in human neutrophils. A reversible process. *J. clin. Invest.* **63**, 637.

38 COHEN M.S., METCALF J.A. & ROOT R.K. (1980) Regulation of oxygen metabolism in human granulocytes: relationship between stimulus binding and oxidative response using plant lectins as probes. *Blood*, **55**, 1003.

39 KITAGAWA S., TAKAKU F. & SAKAMOTO S. (1980) Evidence that proteases are involved in superoxide production by human polymorphonuclear leukocytes and monocytes. *J. clin. Invest.* **65**, 74.

40 BECKER E.L., SIGMAN M. & OLIVER J.M. (1979) Superoxide production induced in rabbit polymorphonuclear leukocytes by synthetic chemotactic peptides and A23187. *Am. J. Path.* **95**, 81.

41 GOLDSTEIN I.M., ROOS D., KAPLAN H.B. & WEISSMANN G. (1975) Complement and immunoglobulins stimulate superoxide production by human leukocytes independently of phagocytosis. *J. clin. Invest.* **56**, 1155.

42 LEHMEYER J.E., SNYDERMAN R. & JOHNSTON R.B. (1979) Stimulation of neutrophil oxidative metabolism by chemotactic peptides: influence of calcium ion concentration and cytochalasin B and comparison with stimulation by phorbol myristate acetate. *Blood*, **54**, 35.

43 McPHAIL L.C., HENSON P.M. & JOHNSTON R.B. (1981) Respiratory burst enzyme in human neutrophils. Evidence for multiple mechanisms of activation. *J. clin. Invest.* **67**, 710.

44 CURNUTTE J.T. & TAUBER A.I. (1983) Failure to detect superoxide in human neutrophils stimulated with latex particles. *Pediat. Res.* **17**, 281.

45 BADWEY J.A., CURNUTTE J.T., ROBINSON J.T., LAZDINS J.K., BRIGGS R.T., KARNOVSKY M.J. & KARNOVSKY M.L. (1980) Comparative aspects of the oxidative metabolism of neutrophils from human blood and guinea pig peritonea: magnitude of the respiratory burst, dependence upon stimulating agents, and localization of the oxidases. *J. cell Physiol.* **105**, 541.

46 LEHRER R.I. & COHEN L. (1981) Receptor-mediated regulation of superoxide production in human neutrophils stimulated by phorbol myristate acetate. *J. clin. Invest.* **68**, 1314.

47 GOODWIN B.J. & WEINBERG J.B. (1982) Receptor-mediated modulation of human monocyte, neutrophil, lymphocyte, and platelet function by phorbol diesters. *J. clin. Invest.* **70**, 699.

48 TAUBER A.I., BRETTLER D.B., KENNINGTON E.A. & BLUMBERG P.A. (1982) Relation of human neutrophil phorbol ester receptor occupancy and NADPH-oxidase activity. *Blood*, **60**, 333.

49 CASTAGNA M., TAKAI Y., KAIBUCHI K., SANO K., KIKKAWA U. & NISHIZUKA Y. (1982) Direct activation of calcium-activated, phospholipid-dependent protein kinase by tumor-promoting phorbol esters. *J. Biol. Chem.* **257**, 7847.

50 TAUBER A.I., GOETZL E., & BABIOR B.M. (1979) Unique characteristics of superoxide production by human eosinophils in eosinophilic states. *Inflammation*, **3**, 261.

51 JOHNSTON R.B., LEHMEYER J.E. & GUTHRIE L.A. (1976) Generation of superoxide anions and chemiluminescence by human monocytes during phagocytosis and on contact with surface-bound immunoglobulin. *J. exp. Med.* **143**, 1551.

52 RODER J.C., HELFAND S.L., WERKMEISTER J., McGARRY R., BEAUMONT T.J. & DUWE A. (1982) Oxygen intermediates are triggered early in the cytolytic pathway of human NK cells. *Nature*, **298**, 569.

53 DePIERRE J.W. & KARNOVSKY M.L. (1974) Ecto-enzymes of the guinea pig polymorphonuclear leukocyte. (I) Evidence for an ecto-adenosine monophosphatase, -adenosine triphosphatase, and -*p*-nitrophenyl phosphatase. *J. Biol. Chem.* **249**, 7111.

54 BADWEY J.A., ROBINSON J.M., LAZDINS J.K., BRIGGS R.T., KARNOVSKY M.J. & KARNOVSKY M.L. (1983) Comparative biochemical and cytochemical studies on superoxide and peroxide in mouse macrophages. *J. cell. Physiol.* **115**, 208.

55 WRIGHT D.G. & GALLIN J.I. (1979) Secretory responses of human neutrophils: exocytosis of specific (secondary)

granules by human neutrophils during adherence *in vitro* and during exudation *in vivo*. *J. Immunol.* **123**, 285.

56 ROBINSON J.M., KARNOVSKY M.L. & KARNOVSKY M.J. (1982) Glycogen accumulation in polymorphonuclear leukocytes and other intracellular alterations that occur during inflammation. *J. Cell Biol.* **95**, 933.

57 KARNOVSKY M.L. & LAZDINS J.K. (1978) Biochemical criteria for activated macrophages. *J. Immunol.* **121**, 809.

58 COHN Z.A. (1978) The activation of mononuclear phagocytes: fact, fancy, and future. *J. Immunol.* **121**, 813.

59 NORTH R.J. (1978) The concept of the activated macrophage. *J. Immunol.* **121**, 806.

60 NATHAN C.F. & ROOT R.K. (1977) Hydrogen peroxide release from mouse peritoneal macrophages. Dependence on sequential activation and triggering. *J. exp. Med.* **146**, 1648.

61 JOHNSTON R.B., GODZIK C.A. & COHN Z.A. (1978) Increases superoxide anion production by immunologically activated and chemically elicited macrophages. *J. exp. Med.* **148**, 115.

62 BRYANT S.M., LYNCH R.E. & HILL H.R. (1982) Kinetic analysis of superoxide production by activated and resident murine peritoneal macrophages. *Cell. Immunol.* **69**, 46.

63 SOBERMAN R.J. & KARNOVSKY M.L. (1981) Biochemical properties of activated macrophages. In *Lymphokines*, Vol. 3, (ed. Pick E.), p. 11. Academic Press, New York.

64 MURRAY H.W. & COHN Z.A. (1980) Macrophage oxygen-dependent antimicrobial activity. (III) Enhanced oxidative metabolism as an expression of macrophage activation. *J. exp. Med.* **152**, 1596.

65 NAKAGAWARA A., NATHAN C.F. & COHN Z.A. (1981) Hydrogen peroxide metabolism in human monocytes during differentiation *in vitro*. *J. clin. Invest.* **68**, 1243.

66 ALLEN R.C., STJERNHOLM R.L. & STEELE R.H. (1972) Evidence for the generation of an electronic excitation state(s) in human polymorphonuclear leukocytes and its participation in bactericidal activity. *Biochem. biophys. Res. Commun.* **47**, 679.

67 ALLEN R.C. & LOOSE L.D. (1976) Phagocytic activation of a luminol-dependent chemiluminescence in rabbit alveolar and peritoneal macrophages. *Biochem. biophys. Res. Commun.* **69**, 245.

68 ROSEN H. & KLEBANOFF S. (1976) Chemiluminescence and superoxide production by myeloperoxidase-deficient leukocytes. *J. clin. Invest.* **58**, 50.

69 CHESON B.D., CHRISTENSEN R.L., SPERLING R., KOHLER B.E. & BABIOR B.M. (1976) The origin of the chemiluminescence of phagocytosing granulocytes. *J. clin. Invest.* **58**, 789.

70 TRUSH M.A., WILSON M.E. & VAN DYKE K. (1978) The generation of chemiluminescence (CL) by phagocytic cells. *Meth. Enzym.* **57**, 462.

71 ROSSI F. & ZATTI M. (1964) Changes in the metabolic pattern of polymorphonuclear leukocytes during phagocytosis. *Br. J. exp. Path.* **45**, 548.

72 ROOT R.K. & STOSSEL T.P. (1974) Myeloperoxidase-mediated iodination by granulocytes. Intracellular site of operation and some regulating factors. *J. clin. Invest.* **53**, 1207.

73 ROOT R.K., METCALF J., OSHINO N. & CHANCE B. (1975) H_2O_2 release from human granulocytes during phagocytosis. (I) Documentation, quantitation, and some regulating factors. *J. clin. Invest.* **55**, 945.

74 MISRA H.P. & FRIDOVICH I. (1976) A convenient calibration of the Clark oxygen electrode. *Analyt. Biochem.* **70**, 632.

75 GREEN T.R., SCHAEFER R.E. & MAKLER M.T. (1980) Significance of O_2 availability and cycling on the respiratory burst response of human PMNs exposed to cytochrome *c* and superoxide dismutase. *Biochem. biophys. Res. Commun.* **94**, 1213.

76 BADWEY J.A., CURNUTTE J.T. & KARNOVSKY M.L. (1979) The enzyme of granulocytes that produces superoxide and peroxide. An elusive pimpernel. *New Engl. J. Med.* **300**, 1157.

77 NAKAMURA M., NAKAMURA M.A. & YANAI M. (1981) Polarographic micromethods for the rapid assay of phagocytosis-connected oxygen consumption by leukocytes in diluted peripheral blood. *J. Lab. Clin. Med.* **97**, 31.

78 BABIOR B.M., KIPNES R.S. & CURNUTTE J.T. (1973) Biological defense mechanisms. The production by leukocytes of superoxide, a potential bactericidal agent. *J. clin. Invest.* **52**, 741.

79 MCCORD J.M., CRAPO J.D. & FRIDOVICH I. (1977) Superoxide dismutase assays: a review of methodology. In *Superoxide and Superoxide Dismutase*, 1st edn. (eds. Michelson A.M., McCord J.M. & Fridovich I.), p. 1. Academic Press, New York.

80 COHEN H.J. & CHOVANIEC M.E. (1978) Superoxide generation by digitonin-stimulated guinea pig granulocytes: a basis for a continuous assay for monitoring superoxide production and for the study of the activation of the generating system. *J. clin. Invest.* **61**, 1081.

81 MAEHLY A.C. & CHANCE B. (1954) The assay of catalases and peroxidases. *Meth. biochem. Analysis*, **1**, 357.

82 TAUBER A.I. & BABIOR B.M. (1977) Evidence for the hydroxyl radical production by human neutrophils. *J. clin. Invest.* **60**, 374.

83 WEISS S.J., KING G.W. & LOBUGLIO A.F. (1977) Evidence for hydroxyl radical generation by human monocytes. *J. clin. Invest.* **60**, 370.

84 WEISS S.J., RUSTAGI P.K. & LOBUGLIO A.F. (1978) Human granulocyte generation of hydroxyl radical. *J. exp. Med.* **147**, 316.

85 KLEBANOFF S.J. & ROSEN H. (1978) Ethylene formation by polymorphonuclear leukocytes. Role of myeloperoxidase. *J. exp. Med.* **148**, 490.

86 PRYOR W.A. & TANG R.H. (1978) Ethylene formation from methional. *Biochem. biophys. Res. Commun.* **81**, 498.

87 YANG S.F. (1969) Further studies on ethylene formation from α-keto-δ-methylthiobutyric acid or β-methylthiopropionaldehyde by peroxidase in the presence of sulfite and oxygen. *J. Biol. Chem.* **244**, 4360.

88 WINSTON G.W. & CEDERBAUM A.I. (1982) Oxidative decarboxylation of benzoate to carbon dioxide by rat liver microsomes. A probe for oxygen radical produc-

tion during microsomal electron transfer. *Biochemistry*, **21**, 4265.

89 NASH T.C. (1953) The colorimetric estimation of formaldehyde by means of the Hantzsh reaction. *Biochem. J.* **55**, 416.

90 STEFFEN C. & NETTER K.J. (1979) On the mechanism of paraquat action on microsomal oxygen reduction and its relation to lipid peroxidation. *Toxic. appl. Pharmac.* **47**, 593.

91 SAGONE A.L., DECKER M.A., WELLES R.M. & DEMOCKO C. (1980) A new method for the detection of hydroxyl radical production by phagocytic cells. *Biochim. biophys. Acta*, **628**, 90.

92 GREEN M.R., O'HILL H.A., OKOLOW-ZUBKOWSKA M.J. & SEGAL A.W. (1979) The production of hydroxyl and superoxide radicals by stimulated human neutrophils–measurements by EPR spectroscopy. *FEBS Letts.* **100**, 23.

93 ROSEN H. & KLEBANOFF S.J. (1979) Hydroxyl radical generation by polymorphonuclear leukocytes measured by electron spin resonance spectroscopy. *J. clin. Invest.* **64**, 1725.

94 FINKELSTEIN E., ROSEN G.M. & RAUCKMAN E.J. (1979) Spin trapping of superoxide. *Mol. Pharmac.* **16**, 676.

95 FINKELSTEIN E., ROSEN G.M. & RAUCKMAN E.J. (1980) Spin trapping of superoxide and hydroxyl radical: practical aspects. *Archs. Biochem. Biophys.* **200**, 1.

96 KRALJIC I. & TRUMBORE C.N. (1965) p-Nitrosodimethylaniline as an OH radical scavenger in radiation chemistry. *J. Am. chem. Soc.* **87**, 2547.

97 DORFMAN L.M. & ADAMS G.E. (1973) *NSRDS-NBS*, No. 46, p. 46. U.S. Department of Agriculture, National Bureau of Standards.

98 ROSEN H. & KLEBANOFF S.J. (1979) Bactericidal activity of a superoxide anion-generating system. A model for the polymorphonuclear leukocyte. *J. exp. Med.* **149**, 27.

99 ROSEN H. & KLEBANOFF S.J. (1977) Formation of singlet oxygen by the myeloperoxidase-mediated antimicrobial system. *J. Biol. Chem.* **252**, 4803.

100 PIATT J.F., CHEEMA A.S. & O'BRIEN P.J. (1977) Peroxidase catalyzed singlet oxygen formation from hydrogen peroxide. *FEBS Letts.* **74**, 251.

101 FOOTE C.S. & DENNY R.W. (1968) Chemistry of singlet oxygen. (VII) Quenching by β-carotene. *J. Am. chem. Soc.* **90**, 6233.

102 OUANNES C. & WILSON T. (1968) Quenching of singlet oxygen by tertiary aliphatic amines. *J. Am. chem. Soc.* **90**, 6527.

103 FOOTE C.S. & CHING T.-Y. (1975) Chemistry of singlet oxygen. (XXI) Kinetics of bilirubin photooxygenation. *J. Am. chem. Soc.* **97**, 6209.

104 TOMITA M., IRIE M. & UKITA T. (1969) Sensitized photooxidation of histidine and its derivatives. Products and mechanism of the reaction. *Biochemistry*, **8**, 5149.

105 MERKEL P.B., NILSSON R. & KEARNS D.R. (1972) Deuterium effects of singlet oxygen lifetimes in solutions. A new test of singlet oxygen reactions. *J. Am. chem. Soc.* **94**, 1030.

106 MERKEL P.B. & KEARNS D.R. (1972) Radiationless decay of singlet molecular oxygen in solution. An experimental and theoretical study of electronic-to-vibrational energy transfer. *J. Am. chem. Soc.* **94**, 7244.

107 SWAIN C.G. & KETLEY A.D. (1955) The chlorinium ion as an intermediate in the chlorination of aromatic compounds by hypochlorus acid. *J. Am. chem. Soc.* **77**, 3410.

108 HARRISON J.E. & SCHULTZ J. (1976) Studies on the chlorinating activity of myeloperoxidase. *J. Biol. Chem.* **251**, 1371.

109 HELD A.M. & HURST J.K. (1978) Ambiguity associated with use of singlet oxygen trapping agents in myeloperoxidase-catalyzed oxidations. *Biochem. biophys. Res. Commun.* **81**, 878.

110 HARRISON J.E., WATSON B.D. & SCHULTZ J. (1978) Myeloperoxidase and singlet oxygen: a reappraisal. *FEBS Letts.* **92**, 327.

111 USHIJIMA Y. & NAKANO M. (1980) No or little production of singlet molecular oxygen in HOCl or HOCl/H_2O_2. A model system for myeloperoxidase/H_2O_2/Cl$^-$. *Biochem. biophys. Res. Commun.* **93**, 1232.

112 PACKER J.E., MAHOOD J.S., MORA-ARELLANO V.O., SLATER T.F., WILLSON R.L. & WOLFENDEN B.S. (1981) Free radicals and singlet oxygen scavengers: reaction of a peroxy-radical with β-carotene, diphenylfuran and 1,4-diazobicyclo (2,2,2)-octane. *Biochem. biophys. Res. Commun.* **98**, 901.

113 SHNITKA T.K. & SELIGMAN A.M. (1971) Ultrastructural localization of enzymes. *Ann. Rev. Biochem.* **40**, 375.

114 BAEHNER R.L. & NATHAN D.G. (1967) Leukocyte oxidase: defective activity in chronic granulomatous disease. *Science*, **155**, 835.

115 BAEHNER R.L. & NATHAN D.G. (1968) Quantitative nitroblue tetrazolium test in chronic granulomatous disease. *New Engl. J. Med.* **278**, 971.

116 SEIDLER E. (1979) Zum mechanismus der tetrazoliumsalzreduktion und wirkungsweise des phenazinmethosulfates. *Acta histochem.* **65**, 209.

117 BAEHNER R.L. (1975) Subcellular distribution of nitroblue tetrazolium reductase (NBT-R) in polymorphonuclear leukocytes (PMN). *J. Lab. Clin. Med.* **88**, 785.

118 SEGAL A.W. (1974) Nitroblue-tetrazolium tests. *Lancet*, **ii**, 1248.

119 NEWBURGER P.E., KRUSKALL M.S., RAPPEPORT J.M., ROBINSON S.H., CHOVANIEC M.E. & COHEN H.J. (1980) Chronic granulomatous disease. Expression of the metabolic defect by *in vitro* culture of bone marrow progenitors. *J. clin. Invest.* **66**, 599.

120 GREENBERG H.M., NEWBURGER P.E., PARKER L.M., NOVAK T. & GREENBERGER J.S. (1981) Human granulocytes generated in continuous bone marrow culture are physiologically normal. *Blood*, **58**, 724.

121 GRAHAM R.C. & KARNOVSKY M.J. (1966) The early stages of absorption of injected horseradish peroxidase in the proximal tubules of mouse kidney: ultrastructural cytochemistry by a new technique. *J. Histochem. Cytochem.* **14**, 219.

122 LITWIN J.A. (1979) Histochemistry and cytochemistry of 3,3′-diaminobenzidine. A review. *Acta histochem. cytochem.* **17**, 3.

123 BRIGGS R.T., KARNOVSKY M.L. & KARNOVSKY M.J. (1975) Cytochemical demonstration of hydrogen per-

oxide in polymorphonuclear leukocyte phagosomes. *J. Cell Biol.* **64**, 254.

124 OHNO Y.-I., HIRAI K.-I., KANOH T., UCHINO H. & OGAWA K. (1982) Subcellular localization of H2O2 production in human neutrophils stimulated with particles an effect of cytochalasin-B on the cells. *Blood*, **60**, 253.

125 OHNO Y.-I., HIRAI K.-I., KANOH T., UCHINO H. & OGAWA K. (1982) Subcellular localization of hydrogen peroxide production in human polymorphonuclear leukocytes stimulated with lectins, phorbol myristate acetate, and digitonin: an electron microscopic study using CeCl3. *Blood*, **60**, 1195.

126 BRIGGS R.T., KARNOVSKY M.L. & KARNOVSKY M.J. (1977) Hydrogen peroxide production in chronic granulomatous disease. A cytochemical study of reduced pyridine nucleotide oxidases. *J. clin. Invest.* **59**, 1088.

127 KARNOVSKY M.J., ROBINSON J.M., BRIGGS R.T. & KARNOVSKY M.L. (1981) Oxidative cytochemistry in phagocytosis: the interface between structure and function. *Histochem. J.* **13**, 1.

128 HIRAI K.-I., UENO S. & OGAWA K. (1980) Plasma membrane-associated NAD(P)H oxidase and superoxide dismutase in pulmonary macrophages. *Acta histochem. cytochem.* **13**, 113.

129 ROBINSON J.M. & KARNOVSKY M.J. (1983) Ultrastructural localization of 5′-nucleotidase in guinea pig neutrophils based upon the use of cerium as capturing agent. *J. Histochem. Cytochem.* **31**, 1190.

130 ROBINSON J.M. & KARNOVSKY M.J. (1983) Ultrastructural localization of several phosphatases with cerium. *J. Histochem. Cytochem.* **31**, 1197.

131 ARNOLD G., LISCUM L. & HOLTZMAN E. (1977) Cytochemistry of D-amino acid oxidase in rat cerebellum and kidney. *J. Cell Biol.* **75**, 202a.

132 VEENHUIS M. & WENDELAAR-BONGA S.D. (1977) The cytochemical demonstration of catalase and D-amino acid oxidase in the microbodies of teleost kidney cells. *Histochem. J.* **9**, 171.

133 ROBINSON J.M., BRIGGS R.T. & KARNOVSKY M.J. (1978) Localization of D-amino acid oxidase on the cell surface of human polymorphonuclear leukocytes. *J. Cell Biol.* **77**, 59.

134 VEENHUIS M. & WENDELAAR-BONGA S.D. (1979) Cytochemical localization of catalase and several peroxide-producing oxidases in the nucleoids and matrix of rat liver peroxisomes. *Histochem. J.* **11**, 561.

135 ARNOLD G., LISCUM L. & HOLTZMAN E. (1979) Ultrastructural localization of D-amino acid oxidase in microperoxisomes of the rat nervous system. *J. Histochem. Cytochem.* **27**, 735.

136 VEENHUIS M., VAN DIJKEN J.P. & HARDER W. (1976) Cytochemical studies on the localization of methanol oxidase and other oxidases in peroxisomes of methanol-grown *Hansenula polymorpha*. *Archs Microbiol.* **111**, 123.

137 VEENHUIS M., VAN DIJKEN J.P., PILON S.A.F. & HARDER W. (1978) Development of crystalline peroxisomes in methanol-grown cells of the yeast *Hansenula polymorpha* and its relation to environmental conditions. *Archs Microbiol.* **117**, 153.

138 VEENHUIS M., KEIZER I. & HARDER W. (1979) Characterization of peroxisomes in glucose-grown *Hansenula polymorpha* and their development after transfer of cells into methanol-containing media. *Archs Microbiol.* **120**, 167.

139 VAUGHN K.C., DUKE S.O., DUKE S.H. & HENSON C.A. (1982) Ultrastructural localization of urate oxidase in nodules of *Sesbania exaltata*, *Glycine max*, and *Medicago satina*. *Histochemistry*, **74**, 309.

140 ARNOLD G., & HOLTZMAN E. (1980) Ultrastructural localization of α-OH acid oxidase in peroxisomes with the CeCl3 technique. *J. Histochem. Cytochem.* **28**, 1025.

141 THOMAS J. & TRELASE R.N. (1981) Cytochemical localization of glycolate oxidase in microbodies (glyoxysomes and peroxisomes) of higher plant tissues with the CeCl3 technique. *Protoplasma*, **108**, 39.

142 BJORKMAN U., EKHOLM R. & DENEF J.-F. (1981) Cytochemical localization of hydrogen peroxide in isolated thyroid follicles. *J. Ultrastr. Res.* **74**, 105.

143 FUJIMOTO T., INOMATA K. & OGAWA K. (1982) A cerium method for the ultrastructural localization of monoamine oxidase activity. *Histochem. J.* **14**, 87.

144 CHRISTIE K.N. & STOWARD P.J. (1982) The cytochemical reactivity of cerium ions with cardiac muscle. *Acta histochem. cytochem.* **15**, 656.

145 VAUGHN K.C. & DUKE S.O. (1983) *In situ* localization of the sites of paraquat action. *Pl. Cell. Envir.* **6**, 13.

146 SAGONE A.L., KING G.W. & METZ E.N. (1976) A comparison of the metabolic response to phagocytosis in human granulocytes and monocytes. *J. clin. Invest.* **57**, 1352.

147 HATCH G.E., GARDNER D.E. & MENZEL D.B. (1978) Chemiluminescence of phagocytic cells caused by N-formylmethionyl peptides. *J. exp. Med.* **147**, 182.

148 TAKANAKA K. & O'BRIEN P.J. (1980) Generation of activated oxygen species by polymorphonuclear leukocytes. *FEBS Letts.* **110**, 283.

149 WELCH W.D., GRAHAM C.W., ZACCARI J. & THRUPP L.D. (1980) Analysis and comparison of the luminol-dependent chemiluminescence responses of alveolar macrophages and neutrophils. *J. Reticuloendothel. Soc.* **28**, 275.

150 DECHATELET L.R., SHIRLEY P.S., MCPHAIL L.C., HUNTLEY C.C., MUSS H.B. & BASS D.A. (1977) Oxidative metabolism of human eosinophil. *Blood*, **50**, 25.

151 KLEBANOFF S.J., DURACK D.T., ROSEN H. & CLARK R.A. (1977) Functional studies on human peritoneal eosinophiles. *Infect. Immun.* **17**, 167.

152 NELSON R.D., MILLS E.L., SIMMONS R.L. & QUIE P.G. (1976) Chemiluminescence response of phagocytizing human monocytes. *Infect. Immun.* **14**, 129.

153 BEALL G.D., REPINE J.E., HOIDAL J.R. & RASP E.L. (1977) Chemiluminescence by human alveolar macrophages: stimulation with heat-killed bacteria or phorbol myristate acetate. *Infect. Immun.* **17**, 117.

154 SCHLEUPNER C.J. & GLASGOW L.A. (1978) Peritoneal macrophage activation indicated by enhanced chemiluminescence. *Infect. Immun.* **21**, 886.

155 BHATNAGAR R., SCHIRMER R., ERNST M. & DECKER K. (1981) Superoxide release by zymosan-stimulated rat Kupffer cells *in vitro*. *Eur. J. Biochem.* **119**, 171.

156 REISS M. & ROOS D. (1978) Differences in oxygen metabolism of phagocytosing monocytes and neutrophils. *J. clin. Invest.* **61**, 480.

157 ROSSI F., ZABUCCHI G. & ROMEO D. (1975) Metabolism of phagocytosing mononuclear phagocytes. In *Mononuclear Phagocytes in Immunity, Infection and Pathology.* 1st edn. (ed. Van Furth R.), p. 441. Blackwell Scientific Publications, Oxford.

158 HOIDAL J.R., REPINE J.E., BEALL G.D., RASP F.L. & WHITE J.G. (1978) The effect of phorbol myristate acetate on the metabolism and ultrastructure of human alveolar macrophages. *Am. J. Path.* **91**, 469.

159 HOIDAL J.R., FOX R.B. & REPINE J.E. (1979) Defective oxidative metabolic responses *in vitro* of alveolar macrophages in chronic granulomatous disease. *Am. Rev. resp. Dis.* **120**, 613.

160 HOIDAL J.R., BEALL G.D. & REPINE J.E. (1979) Production of hydroxyl radical by human alveolar macrophages. *Infect. Immun.* **26**, 1088.

161 HOLIAN A. & DANIELE R.P. (1979) Stimulation of oxygen consumption and superoxide anion production in pulmonary macrophages by N-formyl methionyl peptides. *FEBS Letts.* **108**, 47.

162 DRATH D.B., KARNOVSKY M.L. & HUBER G.L. (1979) Tobacco smoke. Effects on pulmonary host defense. *Inflammation*, **3**, 281.

163 KARNOVSKY M.L., LAZDINS J.K. & SIMMONS S.R. (1975) Metabolism of activated mononuclear phagocytes at rest and during phagocytosis. In *Mononuclear Phagocytes in Immunity, Infection and Pathology.* 1st edn., (ed. Van Furth R.), p. 423. Blackwell Scientific Publications, Oxford.

164 DRATH D.B., KARNOVSKY M.L. & HUBER G.L. (1979) Hydroxyl radical formation in phagocytic cells of the rat. *J. Appl. Physiol.* **46**, 136.

165 KITAGAWA S., TAKAKU F. & SAKAMOTO S. (1980) Evidence that proteases are involved in superoxide production by human polymorphonuclear leukocytes and monocytes. *J. clin. Invest.* **65**, 74.

166 HOLIAN A. & DANIELE R.P. (1982) Formyl peptide stimulation of superoxide anion release from lung macrophages: sodium and potassium involvement. *J. cell. Physiol.* **113**, 413.

167 STOKES S.H., DAVIS W.B. & SORBER W.A. (1978) Effect of phagocytosis on superoxide anion production and superoxide dismutase levels in BCG-activated and normal rabbit alveolar macrophages. *J. Reticuloendothel. Soc.* **24**, 101.

168 LEW P.D. & STOSSEL T.P. (1981) Effect of calcium on superoxide production by phagocytic vesicles from rabbit alveolar macrophages. *J. clin. Invest.* **67**, 1.

169 PICK E. & KEISARI Y. (1981) Superoxide anion and hydrogen peroxide production by chemically elicited peritoneal macrophages—induction by multiple nonphagocytic stimuli. *Cell. Immunol.* **59**, 301.

170 BIGGAR W.D. & STURGESS J.M. (1978) Hydrogen peroxide release by rat alveolar macrophages: comparison with blood neutrophils. *Infect. Immun.* **19**, 621.

171 TOMIOKA H. & SAITO H. (1980) Hydrogen peroxide-releasing function of chemically elicited and immunologically activated macrophages: differential response to wheat germ lectin and concanavalin A. *Infect. Immun.* **29**, 469.

172 SAITO H. & TOMIOKA H. (1979) Enhanced hydrogen peroxide release from macrophages stimulated with streptococcal preparations OK-432. *Infect. Immun.* **26**, 779.

173 O'DONNEL M.J., JABS A.D., HORITA M., REGAN M. & YOKOYAMA A. (1979) The application of antibody coated polyacrylamide gel (immunobead) in the NBT test for the detection of ingestion and killing functions in human neutrophils. *Immunol. Commun.* **8**, 539.

174 STOSSEL T.P. (1973) Evaluation of opsonic and leukocyte function with spectrophotometric test in patients with infection and with phagocytic disorders. *Blood*, **42**, 121.

175 JARSTRAND C. & EINHORN S. (1981) Interferon enhances NBT-reduction and phagocytosis by human monocytes. *J. Clin. Lab. Immunol.* **6**, 211.

176 WESTON W.L., DUSTIN R.D. & HECHT S.K. (1975) Quantitative assays of human monocyte-macrophage function. *J. immunol. Meth.* **8**, 213.

177 WILSON C.B., TSAI V. & REMINGTON J.S. (1980) Failure to trigger the oxidative metabolic burst by normal macrophages. Possible mechanisms for survival of intracellular pathogens. *J. exp. Med.* **151**, 328.

178 VILDE J.L. & VILDE F. (1976) Nitroblue tetrazolium reduction by human macrophages: studies in chronic granulomatous disease. *Adv. exp. Med. Biol.* **73A**, 139.

179 BOXER L.A., ISMAIL G., ALLEN J.M. & BAEHNER R.L. (1979) Oxidative metabolic responses of rabbit pulmonary alveolar macrophages. *Blood*, **53**, 486.

180 KRUEGER G.G., OGDEN R.E. & WESTON W.L. (1976) *In vitro* quantitation of cell-mediated immunity in guinea pigs by macrophage reduction of nitro-blue tetrazolium. *Clin. exp. Immunol.* **23**, 517.

181 PICK E., CHARON J. & MIZEL D. (1981) A rapid densitometric microassay for nitroblue tetrazolium reduction and application of the microassay to macrophages. *J. Reticuloendothel. Soc.* **30**, 581.

182 DREXHAGE H.A., van der GAAG R.D. & NAMAVAR F. (1978) Nitroblue tetrazolium-dye reduction by rat peritoneal macrophages during the uptake of *Diplococcus pneumoniae*, type VI. *Antonie van Leeuwenhoek* **44**, 377.

183 ANDO M., SUGA M., SHIMA K., TAKENAKA S. & TOKUOMI H. (1976) Nitroblue tetrazolium reduction by macrophages Its possible role in cell-mediated antibacterial immunity. *Kumamoto Med. J.* **29**, 88.

184 ALFOLDY P. & LEMMEL E.-M. (1979) Reduction of nitroblue tetrazolium in the cell-mediated immune reaction. *Clin. Immunol. Immunopath.* **12**, 263.

Chapter 51
Locomotion and chemotaxis of leucocytes

P.C. WILKINSON

Forms of locomotor behaviour, 51.1

Method for the micropore filter assay, 51.5

Method for the agarose assay, 51.8

Method for the orientation assay, 51.9

Method for time-lapse cinematography of moving leucocytes, 51.11

The study of chemotactic and other locomotor responses of leucocytes to attractants has become popular in recent years. Several methods are available, and a voluminous literature describes variants on these. However, much of the literature still shows confusion about reactions such as chemotaxis and chemokinesis, and therefore the methods here are introduced by giving some background about what these and other terms mean. The locomotor responses of cells to environmental stimuli may be quite subtle, and it is probable that our categories are simplistic. Nevertheless, some classification is clearly needed, even if it will need to be modified when our understanding improves.

Forms of locomotor behaviour

Random locomotion

In order to understand the reactions that cause cell locomotion to be directed, we should start by discussing what we mean by random locomotion. Some definitions of random and directed locomotory responses have been published [1] which, though not definitive, have been widely accepted. The interested reader is also referred to a good discussion [2] of the theoretical background to random and directed cell behaviour.

The most familiar example of random displacement is the Brownian random walk in which, if the path of the particle is represented as a series of straight line segments separated by turns, the direction of any segment of path is independent of the direction of the previous segment. It is now clear that cells, moving in the absence of any directional cue, do not move like this. In a study of random movement of neutrophils [3], the mean angle of turn between segments, each representing the cell displacement during 40 s, was

about 40°, which is much smaller than would be expected by chance. From this it follows that when cells are studied over brief time intervals (a minute or two for neutrophils), their paths show persistence in a particular direction. However, if cells are studied during longer intervals, then as the sampling interval increases, so the path approximates to a random walk in which mean square displacement is proportional to time [4]. This 'persistent random walk' is characteristic of all tissue cells that have been studied. This is what would be expected given the flowing nature of cell movement, which would be inconsistent with a strictly Brownian random walk.

A definition of random locomotion of cells is difficult, but the one that fits most closely to leucocyte behaviour is that given by Keller et al. [1] as follows: 'Motion in which the cell or organism shows a tendency to move along a path that can be represented by a line segment, but that is randomly orientated in relation to the environment', or, to put it another way [2], 'Random locomotion . . . is that in which the cell displacements during any single time interval are random vectors'.

The random locomotion of cells can be modified by a variety of cues from the environment. These cues may have effects on the speed of cells, on their turning behaviour or on the direction of their locomotion *inter alia*. The cues themselves may be very diverse and include chemical substances, and a wide variety of physical properties of the environment, including adhesiveness and the geometry and mechanical properties of the surface with which the cells are in contact. Obviously some classification is needed and the next section runs briefly through some of the common responses that leucocytes show to such environmental properties.

Kinesis

Kineses are responses in which the magnitude of cell motility is related to the magnitude of some property of the environment. *Chemokinesis* has been defined as 'a reaction by which the speed or frequency of locomotion and/or the frequency and magnitude of turning (change of direction) of cells or organisms moving at random is determined by substances in the environment' [1]. Chemokinesis is a response to chemical substances in the environment. It is also probable that other features of the environment, e.g. physical features such as adhesiveness or temperature, influence the speed or turning behaviour of cells. Responses to these properties would be classified as kineses, but not necessarily as chemokineses.

Apart from classifying kineses according to the determinant property of the environment, e.g. chemokinesis, photokinesis, etc. another useful classification is based on the change in behaviour of the cells evinced by that property. Thus *orthokinesis* is 'a reaction by which the speed or frequency of locomotion is determined by the intensity of the stimulus'; *klinokinesis* is 'a reaction by which the frequency or amount of turning per unit time is determined by the intensity of the stimulus' [1]. These two reactions are actually very different and lead to different end results, as discussed below.

Cells in a uniform concentration of a chemokinetic factor would be expected to move randomly and would not accumulate at particular loci. However, kinetic factors whose concentration is not uniform may cause the cells to become distributed non-randomly. The most striking example of this is klinokinesis stimulated by factors to which cells show adaptation. Bacteria (*Escherichia coli*) move in a tumbling motion, and show much tumbling (turning) when moving down an attractant gradient. However, increasing the attractant concentration causes a cessation of tumbles, so that cells move up-gradient in straight runs. Adaptation leads to tumbling again. There is no change in speed of the bacteria whether moving up- or down-gradient, and the effect of the attractant is solely on the amount of turning per unit time. However, the end-result is accumulation of cells at the gradient source. Thus 'klinokinesis with adaptation' in bacteria is really synonymous with chemotaxis. As Dunn [2] points out, kineses can be defined as responses to scalar properties of the environment, and taxes as responses to vector properties. Using this definition, the behaviour of bacteria should properly be called chemotaxis and is usually so called. If nothing else, this illustrates some of the difficulties that nomenclature can lead us into.

Klinokinetic responses are still to be explored in leucocytes under physiological conditions. However, a major effect of anti-tubulin drugs such as colchicine on locomotion of neutrophils is to cause the cells to turn more frequently [3] and therefore probably to reduce the persistence of the random walk. A very similar behavioural defect is seen in clinical microtubular defects such as the 'immotile cilia syndrome' [5]. In leucocytes, chemotactic factors have not been shown to affect the frequency of turning; rather they influence the angle of turn. Thus the behaviour of chemotactically responding leucocytes is quite different from that of bacteria described above.

Most of the chemokinesis seen in neutrophils and other leucocytes is, in fact, orthokinesis. Many chemotactic factors, e.g. formyl-met-leu-phe, have effects not only on cell direction but also on cell speed, causing the cells to accelerate [6]. Other factors produce orthokinetic reactions through effects on the substratum. Neutrophils and lymphocytes move faster on glass surfaces or in micropore filters if these surfaces are coated with serum albumin than without, and this effect is dose-related [7,8]. This is an accelerated random locomotion. Native albumin has no effect on the direction of locomotion. The available evidence suggests that the positive orthokinetic effect of albumin is mediated by modifying the cell-to-substratum adhesion in a way that optimizes locomotion. The importance of such positive orthokinetic effects *in vivo* is uncertain since they are usually studied *in vitro* on non-ideal substrata. *In vivo* many substrata may be optimally kinetic. It is possible that *negative* orthokinetic effects are more important *in vivo* since these can lead to cell accumulation. A good example is the behaviour of neutrophil leucocytes on surfaces coated with immune complexes. In recent experiments [37], glass coverslips were coated with BSA, then anti-BSA IgG was added to one side of the coverslip as a surface coat, so that a sharp boundary was present between the antigen-coated glass and the immune complex-coated glass. Neutrophils were placed on the coverslip (without serum, i.e. in the absence of a chemotactic stimulus) and their movement at the boundary was filmed. The experiment showed that cells moved well on the albumin coat but more slowly on the immune complexes. There was no change in turning behaviour and (since no serum was present) no chemotaxis on either side of the boundary, and the immune complexes seemed to have a pure negatively orthokinetic effect (reduction of cell speed), probably because the cells became tethered to solid-phase immunoglobulin by their Fc receptors. In such a circumstance, one would expect cells to cross the boundary from BSA to BSA–anti-BSA more frequently than in the converse direction. This proved to be so. Thus a negative orthokinesis can cause cell accumulation in the absence of a chemotactic factor, and the cells accumulate where they move most slowly. This may be quite important *in vivo*, and one can imagine other factors, e.g. leucocyte immobilizing lymphokines, that may have similar effects.

The major points to be emphasized from this section therefore are (1) that orthokinesis and klinokinesis are very distinct reactions, (2) that kineses can cause cells to accumulate provided the kinetic factor is non-randomly distributed, and (3) that *negative* orthokinesis may result in leucocyte accumulation, i.e. the cells accumulate where they move most slowly. Locomotion-inhibitory factors may act in this way.

Chemotaxis

Chemotaxis is 'a reaction by which the direction of locomotion of cells or organisms is determined by substances in their environment' [1]. In leucocytes, the chemotactic response shows two essential features. First, morphological *orientation* of cells in gradients, so that cells previously in rounded non-polarized morphology, when exposed to a chemotactic gradient, put out a leading lamellipodium in the direction facing the gradient source. Typically the lamellipodium is hyaline, phase-dark, ruffled and motile. Behind the lamellipodium is the cell body, which includes all the organelles, and which may remain rounded or tapered and refractile. Thus the polarized cells change from a rounded to a wedged or triangular shape. Note that this change in shape is a feature of all locomotion, whether directed or not, and that what the chemotactic gradient does essentially is to determine the direction in which the leading lamellipodium is protruded. There has been much debate about whether cells detect chemotactic gradients by a spatial sensing mechanism (detecting different concentrations of attractant at different points of the cell) or by a temporal sensing mechanism (detecting concentration differences at different points in time). It was first suggested by Zigmond [9] that detection was spatial, since the cell responded accurately to the gradient (by protruding a lamellipodium) before it started moving. However, more recently adaptation has been observed in leucocytes [6] and adaptation is a feature of temporal sensing, so that the idea has gained ground that gradient detection is temporal and due to the capacity of receptors moving in the cell membrane, e.g. moving forwards as the extending lamellipodium moves forwards, to detect concentration differences at different points in time.

The second characteristic of the chemotactic response, following morphological polarization in the gradient, is directional locomotion up the gradient. If this is analysed by plotting cell paths in segments as described above, it can be established that the major effect of the chemotactic gradient is to narrow the angles between segments, so that the cells follow a nearly straight path in which deviations of more than 30° from the perpendicular to the gradient source (in a good gradient) are rare [9]. An early measure of the straightness of this path, which is still useful, was the 'chemotactic ratio' of McCutcheon [10] i.e. displacement to source/total distance travelled to source. In a perfect chemotaxis, i.e. if the cells moved in a straight line to the chemotactic source, this ratio would be 1.0.

Chemotaxis is a phenomenon in which cells require to detect signals precisely and to perceive differences in the strength of the signal at different points around the cell. It is now clear that accurate signal detection requires recognition of ligands (e.g. formyl peptides or C5a) by cell surface receptors. Zigmond [11] has calculated that neutrophils are able to detect and respond to differences in attractant concentration down to 1% across the length of the cell and Lauffenburger [12] has discussed the problem of how the cells discriminate between signals and noise. Following signal perception, the cell must make an appropriate response, i.e. it must orient and move towards the gradient source. This requires a transduction system to transmit information to the locomotor apparatus: the cytoskeletal actin microfilament network. This is not the place to discuss the details of stimulus-response coupling in neutrophils, many of which are still not well understood, or to discuss how locomotor force is generated. These topics are reviewed in refs. 13–15.

Chemotaxis is an excellent mechanism for causing cells to accumulate, but it must be emphasized that it is not the only one, as discussed above. A corollary of this is that observations that cell accumulation has occurred either *in vivo* or *in vitro* do not justify the conclusion that the cells got where they did by chemotaxis. Since many methods for studying cell locomotion both *in vivo* (e.g. the skin window) and *in vitro* (e.g. the micropore filter assay) rely on an endpoint measure of the position of cell populations, this point is not trivial. Even worse than these are capillary tube assays in which often neither the mechanism of cell movement, nor the disposition of factors influencing the movement, nor even the nature of the moving cells, are precisely defined.

Contact guidance

Under the heading 'contact guidance' [16] have been grouped a number of responses in which the direction of locomotion of cells is determined by the shape, alignment, curvature or other structural or mechanical properties of the substratum. The author has studied contact guidance of leucocytes moving through 3-D fibrous gels of collagen or fibrin which had been aligned by stretching, so that parallel fibres of collagen or fibrin could easily be seen in the microscope. When neutrophils were filmed moving through such aligned gels [17], it was seen that locomotion was biased in favour of the axis of fibre alignment. Cells spent much more time moving up and down the fibres than crossing them. Thus the cells were moving directionally, but, unlike chemotaxis, this was not a unidirectional but a bidirectional response. Later experiments have shown similar guidance responses in monocytes and lymphocytes. Contact guidance can reinforce or interfere with chemotactic responses [18]. It may therefore be an important determinant of how leucocytes move through aligned or patterned tissues and so one would expect that tissue architecture might be quite an important factor in determining the efficiency of inflammatory responses. The mechanisms for contact guidance are still not clear, and there may be several different mechanisms. These have been reviewed by Dunn [19]. Contact guidance is likely to be determined by physical features of the environment, and probably does not require a specialized sensory system, as chemotaxis does.

To summarize this section, Fig. 51.1 shows in schematic form how the reactions discussed above, chemokinesis, chemotaxis and contact guidance, would be expected to affect the displacement of a population of cells if each were acting in isolation. It is more likely, in living tissues, that the distribution of cells is determined by one or more of these reactions acting together.

Choice of method

Cell locomotion and chemotaxis are complex phenomena in which the cells are moving through space and time, and in which the movement responds and changes continuously as the environment changes. A chemotactic gradient is usually a changing environment. Thus to assay these phenomena accurately, or to determine any single parameter that gives a useful measure of them is not straightforward. The different assays that are available at present are useful in different contexts, and choice of an assay depends on what the investigator wants to find out. Full information about a particular problem in cell locomotion may only be obtained by using more than one assay.

Assays of locomotion and chemotaxis can be separated into two categories. The first includes those in which a large population of cells is allowed to move in the presence or absence of locomotor stimulants or chemotactic factors. After an arbitrary interval, the movement is stopped and the distribution of the cell

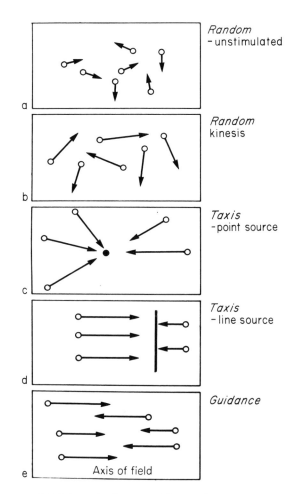

Fig. 51.1. Schematic diagram to illustrate locomotor responses of cells. The arrows represent the extent and direction of cell displacements, not detailed cells' tracks. The kinesis shown (b) is orthokinesis which increases the extent but not the direction of displacement. Chemotaxis (c and d) and guidance (e) influence the direction of cell displacement as detailed in the text. Illustration from ref. 31, by courtesy by Plenum Press.

population is examined, i.e. these are endpoint assays. They are the most widely used and they include the micropore filter assay and the agarose assay. The second category includes those in which the behaviour of individual cells exposed to locomotor or chemotactic stimuli is examined. These are visual analyses and include time-lapse cinematography and other visual assays such as the orientation assay [11]. In these assays, the behaviour of the cells can be followed through the whole experimental time; thus much detail can be studied. However, it is only practicable to make such detailed analyses on small populations of cells. Bearing this in mind, the following guidelines may be useful.

Endpoint assays, e.g. the micropore filter assay, give little information about locomotor behaviour. They are not good assays of locomotion *per se*, but provide an easy and reproducible method for detecting that locomotion has been altered by the introduction of chemical stimulants or inhibitors into the assay system. Micropore filters and wells in agarose allow chemotactic gradients to be set up and it is easy to show that the cell population moves towards the chemotactic factor, but not so easy to show that this movement is really chemotaxis and not some form of chemokinesis. Because they are easy to use and large numbers of tests can be done in a short time, these assays are useful for the identification, dose–response characterization and monitoring of chemotactic factors and inhibitors. Thus, for the biochemist or pharmacologist interested in identifying chemotactic factors, studying structure–activity relationships between different molecules, studying the modification of the response with drugs or physiological inhibitors or potentiators, this type of assay offers the best tool. They are also useful for the clinician trying to assess the functions of leucocytes in patients, and have been widely used for this purpose. However, from all the clinical studies that have been done, little insight has been gained into mechanisms of disordered leucocyte locomotion. This is certainly due in part to the lack of information that studies using these methods have yielded about cell behaviour.

Visual assays give much information about cell behaviour and allow direct measurement of the speed, turning behaviour, directional responses and detailed shape changes of individual cells in movement. They allow detailed study of interactions between different cells and how they respond to contact with homotypic cells or with heterotypic cells in culture, such as endothelium. They allow study of cell behaviour in contact with substrata varying in adhesiveness, coated with various materials, or varying in geometry, e.g. 3-D gels of fibrous proteins such as collagen or fibrin. They allow unequivocal distinctions to be made between chemokinesis, chemotaxis and contact guidance. They require more sophisticated apparatus than the endpoint assays, e.g. time-lapse cine-cameras or video systems, and analytical projectors, and are thus likely to appeal only to those who wish to make a major commitment to the study of locomotory behaviour. They would probably be cumbersome as assays for measuring the dose–response of cells to a stimulant and, since the number of cells studied in any film sequence is usually small (< 100), there is higher chance of statistical error in comparing several samples than with an assay that uses large populations of cells.

Method for the micropore filter assay

This assay, introduced by Boyden [20], is still the most popular assay for measuring leucocyte chemotaxis. The principle is simple. A porous filter separates two compartments. In the upper compartment are cells; in the lower one, an attractant. The attractant diffuses up through the pores of the filter, forming a gradient. The cells then respond by migrating through the pores of the filter (which must be large enough to let this happen) towards the lower surface. The experiment is stopped by fixing the filter and staining it. Then the locomotion of the cells is measured in one of a number of ways, e.g. by estimating the distance travelled by a sample of the cells, usually the leading front, or by counting the cells which have reached or passed a fixed point. The principles, advantages and disadvantages of the various modifications of this assay have been discussed in considerable detail elsewhere [13] and one of a number of alternative methods shall be outlined simply here, together with some caveats.

Materials

Chemotaxis chambers: There are too many variants of these to describe in detail. They all consist of an upper chamber in which the cell suspension is placed, which is separated by a micropore filter from the lower chamber, in which the chemotactic factor is placed. The author uses a simple apparatus in which the lower chamber is a multiwell compartment placed in a sandwich box with holes bored in its lid, and the upper chamber is a sawn-off tuberculin syringe with the filter glued (Uhu glue) to its lower end (Fig. 51.2).

Filters: Cellulose ester filters (thickness, c. 150 μm) are recommended. Pore sizes: for neutrophils, 3 μm; for macrophages or monocytes, 8 μm or 12 μm. A number of firms supply these. Those from Sartorius, Göttingen, Germany, are satisfactory. Note that, though polycarbonate filters are widely used, especially for studies of monocytes, this author does not recommend them. They are only 12 μm thick and little discrimination can be gained from an assay in which cells are only required to migrate a single cell diameter.

Cells: Human blood cells (neutrophils, monocytes, lymphocytes) can be separated by a variety of standard procedures. Neutrophils are the most commonly studied cells and are usually prepared by dextran-sedimentation of the blood followed by centrifugation on Ficoll-Hypaque (Sp. G. 1.078). Cells are suspended in Hanks-HEPES or Hanks-Mops buffer at 7.2 at a concentration of 10^6 per ml. Cells do not migrate on

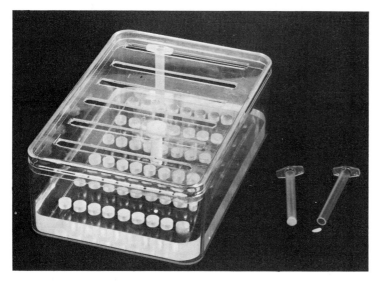

Fig. 51.2. An apparatus for the micropore filter assay. This consists of a perspex block machined to contain a series of wells. Chemotactic factor is placed in the wells (170 μl per well). The block fits into a sandwich box and the upper chambers containing the cells (100 μl) are suspended into the wells through slits in the lid of the box. The upper chambers are made from sawn-off tuberculin-syringe barrels with a filter glued to the lower end. This apparatus was modified by Dr J.M. Lackie from earlier versions.

protein-free substrata; therefore the cells should be suspended in protein (e.g. serum albumin) at any preferred concentration between 1 and 20 mg/ml.
Chemotactic factors: Many can be used. Details are given for only two: (1) *Casein* (Alkalilöslich, Merck) in Hanks-HEPES solution. The optimal dose varies from batch to batch between 500 μg/ml and 5 mg/ml and should be established by doing a dose–response curve. This casein is not easily soluble. The suspension needs to be taken at pH 12, left a few minutes and then brought back carefully to pH 7.2. Casein is a cheap and stable material to use as a positive control. (2) *Formyl-methionyl-leucyl-phenylalanine* (f-Met-Leu-Phe) (Miles): Make up a stock solution at 10^{-2} M in dimethyl sulphoxide in the presence of 2×10^{-2} M-2-mercaptoethanol. The mercaptoethanol is to prevent oxidation of the methionine sulphur which causes gradual inactivation of the peptide. Use at 10^{-8}–10^{-9} M (dilute in Hanks-HEPES solution with especial care for accuracy). Tests with f-Met-Leu-Phe *must* be done in the presence of albumin. Add HSA (Behringwerke) at any preferred concentration between 1 and 20 mg/ml both to the peptide solution and to the cells. The negative control (no peptide) must also contain albumin. Sera: if it is wished to test the chemotaxis-generating activity of a patient's or other serum, this serum may be activated by incubation at 37 °C for 30 min with endotoxin and used as a chemotactic agent against the patient's own cells and normal control cells. A normal control serum should be tested at the same time in the same way. The optimal dilution at which such sera should be used is 1:10 to 1:20. Certain sera may contain inhibitors and pre-incubation of normal cells in the patient's serum may be a worthwhile test to detect such inhibitors.

Procedure

1   Prepare cells in Hanks-HEPES solution at about 10^6 cells/ml. Make sure the cell concentration is roughly the same in the test and control samples.
2   Fill the lower compartments of the chemotaxis chambers with appropriate chemotactic reagents and controls pre-adjusted to a pH of 7.2. For the apparatus shown in Fig. 51.2, 170 μl are required.
3   Fill the upper compartments with the cell suspension, ensuring that the fluid level in the upper chamber is the same as in the lower, otherwise the gradient will be disturbed (100 μl in the tuberculin syringes used above).
4   Allow the filters to wet from the top before putting them in the lower compartments. When the upper compartments are placed in the lower compartments the concentration of chemotactic factor throughout the filter is zero and, as soon as the filter is placed in the chemotactic solution, the gradient begins to form from the bottom of the filter. If the filter is allowed to wet from below, a good gradient will not be obtained. Put up each test in duplicate or triplicate.
5   Incubate the tests at 37 °C in air. Do not allow them to be disturbed until the end of the experiment, lest the gradient be destroyed.
Times of incubation: for neutrophils—60–75 min; for monocytes, macrophages, lymphocytes—2 h.
6   At the appropriate time, depending on the method used for measuring migration, take the tests out of the incubator, remove the upper compartments and invert them to empty fluid out of them.
7   Fix by immersing the filters in 70% ethanol or methanol. After a few minutes in the alcohol, the glue will melt and the filter will become loose from the

bottom of the syringe barrel. It can then be picked off with dental packing forceps, taking care to touch only the rim and to avoid the surface with cells on.

8 Staining: it is obviously important when staining many small filters to avoid getting them mixed up. Sterilin plastic dishes (Repli 103) containing 25 compartments each of 1.8 cm² can be easily adapted. Small holes are punched into the bottom of each compartment so that fluid can flow in and out freely. The filters for each sample are separated from those for other samples by placing each set into one of these compartments. The dish containing all the filters is then lowered into a glass staining dish. A simple staining procedure is as follows.

Transfer filters from ethanol to distilled water.

Distilled water	1 min
Haematoxylin	30 s to 1 min
Distilled water	1 min
Tap water	10 min
70% ethanol	2 min
95% ethanol	3 min
80% ethanol ⎱ mixture	5 min
20% butanol ⎰	
Xylene	10 min

(Methanol can be substituted for ethanol throughout.) Mount under a coverslip using any common mountant. Measure cell migration microscopically as detailed below.

9 Procedure for assessing cell migration.

(i) Measuring distance travelled: the 'leading front' method. The cells are allowed to incubate for a length of time such that the fastest moving cells have migrated a good distance into the filter but no cells have reached the lower surface. The filters are mounted topside up and the fine adjustment is racked down past the leading front of cells. Using the ×40 objective it is then racked back up to the leading plane in which the nuclei of two or more cells are in focus together in a field. A micrometer reading is then taken. If a single cell appears in front of the others, it is ignored. The fine adjustment is then racked up to the top of the filter and a second micrometer reading is taken. The difference between the two readings gives a measure of the distance migrated by the leading front of cells. Five readings are taken at different planes in each filter. The leading front method is accurate and reproducible and can be used for 'chequerboard' assays (see below). One of its disadvantages is that it is relatively insensitive to changes in the proportion of cells in any population that are able to translocate and, since chemical agents or diseases may change this proportion, it should ideally be used in conjunction with some measure of the population of migrating cells.

(ii) Counting cells at or beyond a given level. The easiest level at which to count cells is the lower surface of the filter. A major disadvantage of this is that cells which have reached the lower surface may not stick there, but drop off. This makes the method inaccurate, and alternative procedures are recommended. One is to use a two-filter method. Cells that drop off the top filter are trapped by a second filter and can be counted there [21,22]. Another way is to count cells that have entered the filter, but not reached its lower surface. The number of cells per field which have passed a predetermined depth (e.g. 40 μm or 60 μm) in the filter can be counted. This achieves much the same thing as the lower-surface count but without the disadvantage of cell loss due to detachment.

Various devices are now available for automating cell counts in filter assays [24,25]. These require a mechanism for automatic focusing of the microscope objective at 10 μm intervals of depth in the filter. The microscope is connected to an image analyser which does the counting. Such a procedure gives very full information, so that an estimate of the total population entering the filter, the population which has passed any depth or the leading front measure, can all be obtained. However, it is not cheap to set up.

Notes: distinguishing chemotaxis from changes in locomotor rate into filters

Obviously the fact that cells have moved in response to a chemotactic gradient at higher speeds or in greater numbers than in a control medium is not sufficient evidence that the cells have moved chemotactically. They may simply have accelerated orthokinetically. The procedure that is usually adopted to distinguish these two reactions is the chequerboard assay. This requires that a series of chambers be set up in which the cells are exposed (1) to a range of positive gradients, (2) to a range of negative gradients, and (3) to a range of absolute concentrations (with no gradient) of the factor. Series (3) should give an orthokinetic dose–response curve. If the cells in (1) are clearly moving farther, and those in (2) less far than would be expected from (3), this constitutes indirect evidence for chemotaxis. The problem has been how to quantify this impression. The paper of Zigmond & Hirsch [23] outlined a procedure for doing this based on the leading-front assay. From curve (3) a series of velocities for cells moving in any given concentration of attractant was obtained; therefore accelerations between any two concentrations could easily be calculated (assuming a linear gradient between the two concentrations). These calculations gave the figure for migration between any two attractants in the series (1) or (2) that would be expected on the assumption that the cells responded only by accelerating or decelerating in response to the change in absolute concentration, and not by a directional response to the gradient. Then the difference between the experimental value for cell migration and the above calculated migration would be an indication of chemotaxis. This procedure, despite the assumptions it makes about linearity of gradients, homogeneity of cell behaviour, etc., actually works quite well when carried out properly with neutrophils, though there have been numerous chequerboards published in which the above calculations were omitted, or even using polycarbonate filters which were only 12 μm thick. One limitation until recently was that it could only be used with the leading-front assay. However, a recent paper [26] has demonstrated how the same principle can also be applied to cell-counting assays.

Note also that an increase or decrease in the 'leading-front' measure or in the number of cells counted in a filter may be due neither to chemotaxis nor chemokinesis, but simply to an increase or decrease in the proportion of the cell population that is moving. To evaluate this, it is necessary to count the number of cells entering the filter, i.e. to do counts at a series of depths (10 μm apart) from the top of the filter. This is tedious if done by hand, and facilitated by the automated methods discussed above.

Method for the agarose assay

Measurement of locomotion of neutrophil leucocytes under agarose has become popular recently, particularly in clinical laboratories. It has the advantages of being simple, rapid and cheap. The principle is similar to that of gel diffusion tests. In its simplest form, three circular wells are cut into agarose on a glass or plastic slide. The central well is filled with cells, one of the outer wells is filled with a control solution and the other with a chemotactic solution. The chemotactic factor diffuses radially through the agar and attracts cells from the central well. The cells migrate out

between the agarose and the slide, and, after a period of incubation, take up an egg-shaped distribution (Fig. 51.3). Various measures of the difference between A and B can be taken as indices of the attractant effect. The presence of protein is required for optimal chemotaxis under agarose and many workers have used serum. However, this may add some variables that are difficult to control, and the author therefore describes below a modification using gelatin [27].

Materials

Clean glass slides; agarose (Sigma Chemical Co., Poole, Dorset), template for cutting wells in agarose (see Fig. 51.4), neutrophils prepared as above, chemotactic solutions as desired (e.g. f-Met-Leu-Phe, Sigma Chemical Co. Poole, Dorset), gelatin (Plasmagel).

Procedure [27]

1 Dip clean glass slides in 0.5% gelatin, rinse in distilled water and dry by draining in air.
2 Dissolve agarose (2%) and gelatin (0.5%) in distilled water in a boiling water bath. Cool to 48 °C in a water bath and add one volume of Hanks-HEPES buffer per volume of agarose (final concentration of agarose: 1%).
3 Pour 5 ml of the agarose on to a gelatin-coated glass slide and allow to set at 4 °C for 30 min.
4 Punch wells in the agarose with a metal template, as shown in Fig. 51.4. Remove agarose plugs with a hypodermic needle or with a Pasteur pipette attached to a vacuum pump.
5 Put slides in a damp-chamber.
6 Add test solutions: (i) to central well, neutrophil suspension prepared as previously described and made up to 2.5×10^7 cells per ml; add 10 μl (2×10^5 cells) of this suspension; (ii) add chemotactic solution (10 μl) to one outer well. Note that the best results are obtained from the agarose assay using concentrations of chemotactic factor (f-Met-Leu-Phe, C5a, etc.) about an order of magnitude higher than in other assays. This is because of the way the gradient diffuses in a system

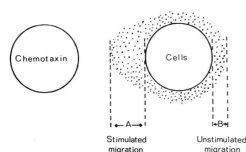 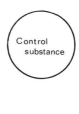

Fig. 51.3. Schematic diagram to illustrate the under-agarose assay. Stimulated locomotion is usually measured by some comparison of A with B (see text). From ref. 31.

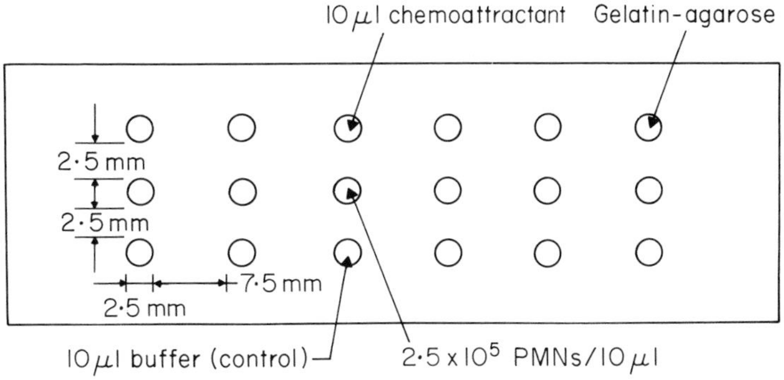

Fig. 51.4. Plan for setting up the agarose assay. A metal template is used to punch six series of 3 holes each into the agarose. Each series of 3 holes is used as shown in Fig. 51.3. Method of Chenoweth *et al.* [27].

with the dimensions of the agarose assay [28]. (iii) Add control solution (Hanks-HEPES buffer, 10 μl) to the other outer well.

7 Incubate at 37 °C for 2 h.

8 Fix in absolute alcohol for 30 min, then replace with fresh absolute alcohol and leave overnight. The agarose can then be floated off or gently removed. The cells are stained with any appropriate stain for counting (e.g. May-Grünwald Giemsa).

9 Using a squared eyepiece graticule and a ×40 objective, chemotaxis is measured microscopically in the line that joins the centres of the wells. This can be done by measuring the distance reached by the leading front of cells (3 cells per square) in the direction both of the attractant and of the control. Alternatively, the number of cells in each square of the graticule from the cell well outwards can be counted. In both cases, migration towards the attractant is compared with migration towards the control. A number of indices have been described that can be used to evaluate the attractant effect [27,29,30].

Notes and recommendations

Defining chemotaxis by the above procedures is subject to the same caveats as mentioned in discussing the leading-front and cell-count methods for measuring chemotaxis in filter assays. However, the agarose assay has the advantage that it can also be used as a visual assay. Thus orientation of cells can easily be scored visually (though it is preferable to use glutaraldehyde 1.25% as a fixative since this does not distort cell shape) or time-lapse films of cells moving under agarose can be taken, using an inverted microscope. The author has seen very good directional locomotion of cells in f-Met-Leu-Phe gradients by such filming [13]. Monocyte locomotion can also be studied under agarose by similar procedures. Nelson [29] uses a long incubation period (18 h), but the author has had satisfactory results using a 3 h incubation. In his

experience, results with monocytes are more variable than those with neutrophils.

Method for the orientation assay

A very convenient and simple way of assessing whether neutrophils really are responding by chemotaxis is to study their morphological orientation in gradients. A very simple perspex chamber for doing this was described by Zigmond [11] and is shown in Fig. 51.5. This assay has not been used much yet in clinical studies but in patients whose cells show locomotor defects in filter assays, study of their ability to orient would be useful in determining whether the defect was due to inability to respond to the gradient or to some other cause. The ability of serum from patients to generate gradients (e.g. of C5a) which would cause normal neutrophils to orient could be studied by the same means.

The chamber

The chamber (Fig. 51.5) is a $1'' \times 3'' \times 1/8''$ perspex slide cut to form two wells 1 mm deep and 5 mm wide separated by a bridge 1 mm wide. A coverslip (22 × 32 mm) is held in place over the bridge by two brass spring-clips screwed into the perspex on either side. There should be sufficient spring in the clips to hold the coverslip down firmly—hence their shape shown in the figure.

Procedure

1 Coverslips (22 × 32 mm) are cleaned by washing in detergent followed by very thorough rinsing in distilled water and drying with a cloth.

2 A drop of neutrophil preparation (c. 200 μl) is spread across the middle of the coverslip so that the cells will cover the bridge. A neutrophil concentration of 2×10^6/ml gives sufficient cells to make counting

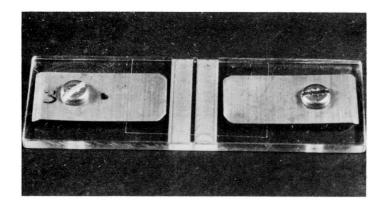

Fig. **51.5.** The orientation chamber [11]. Illustration from ref. 36.

easy. The neutrophils are allowed to attach for 5 min, then the coverslip is washed in Hanks-HEPES and inverted over the bridge of the perspex chamber. Air bubbles can be avoided by placing a drop of Hanks-HEPES on the bridge before inverting the coverslip over it. Clean the cell-free surface of the coverslip with a tissue moistened with water before inverting it over the bridge, otherwise salts will crystallize on it during incubation. Fasten the clips in place and tighten (not too tight or the cells will be squashed). A few trial runs are useful here.

3   One well is then filled with a control solution, the other with f-Met-Leu-Phe at 10^{-8} M. A gradient will then be formed across the bridge. Place the perspex slide in a damp chamber for 30–40 min.

4   At the end of this time, examine under the $\times 40$ objective of a microscope (preferably phase-contrast). Normal neutrophils should show strong orientation ($> 90\%$) towards the well into which the peptide was placed (Fig. 51.6). Orientation is scored by counting 100–200 cells and assessing the percentage polarized in the 180° arc towards the gradient and in the 180° arc away from the gradient. Disregard rounded-up cells or cells oriented parallel to the edge of the bridge i.e. not oriented to or away from the gradient.

Notes and recommendations

Tests should be done in duplicate. If the clips are not screwed down tightly enough, currents across the bridge may disturb the gradient; if they are too tight the cells may be damaged. An ideal gap between coverslip and bridge is 10 μm; thus there is a certain amount of chance in achieving a good result. This diminishes with experience. Note that the solutions in the wells may dry out, but this is not a problem if the

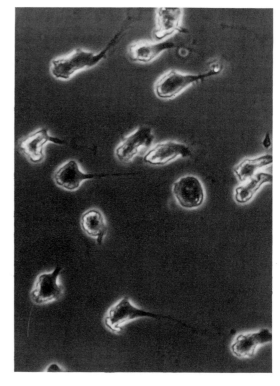

Fig. **51.6.** Orientation of human blood neutrophils in a gradient of f-Met-Leu-Phe (0–10^{-8} M) in the chamber shown in Fig. 51.5. The cells are polarized with broad fronts facing the gradient source (on the left) and posterior tails with retraction fibres. From ref. 13, courtesy of Churchill-Livingstone.

tests are maintained in a moist environment during the necessary 30–40 min of incubation.

Method for time-lapse cinematography of moving leucocytes

Taking the film

The speed of locomotion of vigorously moving neutrophils or lymphocytes is around 20 μm (or two cell diameters) per minute. Though it is just about possible to follow a single cell moving at that speed by eye for a short time, it is quite impossible to follow a population of 100 or so cells in a single field directly, and some sort of filmed record has to be made. This is done by time-lapse cinematography, using a lapse interval that allows the film, when run, to show events happening faster than they did in actual time. For several decades now, this has been done using a cine-camera. At the present time, videotape is coming into increasing use for the same purpose since it is now economically competitive with cinematography.

Time-lapse cinematography can be used as an accurate and quantitative technique for the study of cell behaviour. It has acquired an unjustified reputation of being a poorly quantitative, anecdotal method, capable of providing pretty films for showing at meetings, but not very rigorous. This is because many people who make such films never analyse them. Analysis of cell movement by cinematography is laborious, but well worthwhile, since it provides useful and precise information that can be obtained in no other way. Methods for analysis are discussed below.

Equipment

The basic requirements for taking time-lapse films are listed below.

A microscope with, as a minimum, good phase-contrast optics. Something is always lost when an image is filmed, and the better the original image, the better the film will be. Details of microscopic requirements will vary depending on what is under study. Low magnifications (e.g. × 10 or × 20 objectives) may be all that is required for charting the paths of a cell population, and this may not require high quality optics. On the other hand, for studying detailed shape changes in individual cells, high magnifications and sharp focussing are needed. Differential interference-contrast ('Nomarski') optics are very suitable for such studies.

A heated microscope stage. Naturally, mammalian cells move best at or near 37 °C, and some means of maintaining them at this temperature during filming is needed. The best way is to use an air curtain. We use an apparatus devised by Dr Graham Dunn consisting of a fan-heater that blows warm air across the stage. The temperature is controlled thermostatically by a miniature-bead thermistor placed on the stage in the path of the warm air and set at 37 °C. Control is quite precise. Various microscope firms supply water-heated stages, but temperature regulation with these is not as good. The specimen should be mounted in such a way as to reach and maintain physiological temperature without drying out. Metals conduct heat well, so metal specimen-holders are preferable to those of glass or plastic. The stainless steel chamber used in the author's laboratory is shown in Fig. 51.8.

A cine-camera (or video-camera) with time-lapse attachments. Most people use 16 mm cine-cameras. The camera used by the author is the Bolex H16 reflex with automatic exposure and an automatic timer (Nikon) on which a range of desired frame intervals (from 4 frames per second to one frame per 30 min) can be selected. The camera may be mounted over a conventional microscope, or alongside an inverted microscope, in both cases being connected via a camera attachment over an eyepiece (Fig. 51.7). An important requirement is for a beam splitter, so that the field that is seen by the camera can, at the same time, be seen by the eye. This is essential for field selection and focussing. The beam splitter eyepiece should contain cross hairs (for focussing and centring) and an indication of frame size. For time-lapse filming, a slow, reversal film (e.g. Kodak Plus-X reversal) is suitable for most purposes, though for filming rapid shape changes, a faster film (e.g. Kodak Tri-X reversal) may be preferable.

As an alternative to the cine-camera, a television camera and a time-lapse videotape recorder may be used, together with a television monitor. Apart from the cost, another advantage of video-recording is that it can be played back immediately. There is no need to wait for the film to be developed. A time-date generator is necessary to give a record of 'real' time, for analysis, since the time base provided by film frames is not provided by videotape. Further discussion of videotape *vis-à-vis* cine-film will be found in ref. 31. The quality of image obtained with videotape is still inferior to that obtained from cine-films.

Examples of use of visual assays

Method for chemotaxis assay using Candida albicans

As an example of a time-lapse film assay of chemotaxis that we have found useful, details are given below of a method using *Candida albicans* as a gradient source [3].

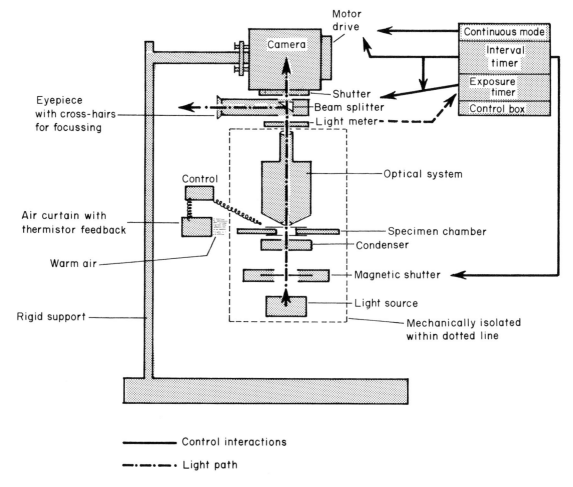

Control interactions

—·—·—· Light path

Fig. 51.7. Schematic diagram of the apparatus for time-lapse cinematography. From ref. 31, courtesy of Plenum Press.

Materials

Candida albicans cultured on dextrose-peptone agar, a medium which allows growth of blastospores about 3 μm in diameter, but not of pseudomycelial forms. A suspension of *Candida* (10^6 spores/ml) is made in Hanks' solution by picking a colony off the plate with a loop.

Leucocytes: neutrophil leucocytes are prepared from blood by any appropriate method and a suspension of 2×10^6 cells is made up in Hanks' solution + HSA (10 mg per ml).

The stainless-steel filming chamber shown in Fig. 51.8 is used. This chamber measures $76 \times 25 \times 1$ mm and has a circular hole of 19 mm diameter drilled into the middle. A clean (detergent-washed) coverslip is attached by surrounding the hole with silicone grease, then pressing the slide down over the hole. The chamber is then inverted.

Procedure

1   One drop of the leucocyte suspension is placed on the coverslip and the leucocytes are allowed to settle and adhere for 5 min. Unattached cells are washed off with Hanks' solution.

2   The well is filled with 0.35 ml of a mixture of 25 parts fresh human serum (as a complement source), 20 parts *Candida albicans* suspension and 55 parts Hanks' solution. This mixture should have been pre-heated at 37 °C for 20 min to activate complement.

3   The well is then sealed by lowering a coverslip, ringed with silicone grease, over the top, avoiding the presence of air-bubbles in the sealed preparation.

4   The chamber is placed on the microscope stage, pre-warmed to 37 °C. An appropriate field is chosen in which neutrophils are sufficiently far from each other, and from the nearest *Candida* spore, for them to have to migrate 30–50 μm to reach the spore. In this way,

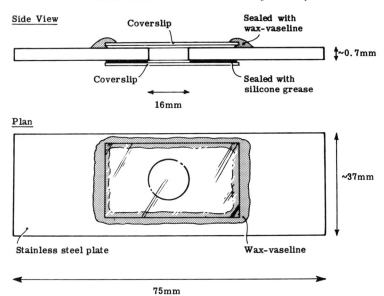

Fig. 51.8. Side and plan views of the stainless-steel filming chamber used in our laboratory for time-lapse filming. From ref. 31, courtesy of Plenum Press.

good chemotactic responses should be observed. The author uses an *inverted* microscope for this assay, so that the cells and *Candida* are on the lower of the two coverslips. This is because *Candida* are non-adherent to glass and will detach if the *specimen* is inverted.

5 Filming is carried out at a magnification of × 100, which gives a field with quite a large number of cells. Neutrophils are filmed at 15 frames a minute, though, for more slowly-moving cells such as mononuclear phagocytes, a slower filming speed (7.5 frames per minute) is preferable.

6 After the film is developed, cell paths are tracked by dotting in the cell position every 10 frames (i.e. 40 s for neutrophils; 80 s if a macrophage population is being studied). These intervals allow enough cell displacement for the cell centre to be positioned with fair accuracy, but are not too long to give details of the cell path. Further details of analysis for this and other visual assays are discussed below.

Use of collagen and fibrin gels for filming locomotion in 3-D

Studies of cell locomotion through 3-D fibrous gels are becoming increasingly popular, since these provide a near approach to a physiological substratum and, for example, allow good locomotion of lymphocytes [32,33], a cell-type that moves poorly on 2-D surfaces. Type I collagen may be prepared from rat tail tendon by the method of Elsdale & Bard [34] and stored in soluble form in aqueous, weakly acid medium. The collagen forms a gel within a few minutes of being restored to physiological pH and ionic strength. A

collagen gel can easily be cast in the filming chamber described above. The optimum collagen concentration for cells to invade and move freely is 1–2 mg per ml. Fibrin can be cast in the same way by adding 1 part of thrombin (Sigma, Poole, Dorset: 10 NIH units per ml) to 9 parts of fibrinogen (Sigma, human fraction I at 1.5 mg per ml). Neutrophils or lymphocytes placed on the upper surfaces of such gels rapidly invade them. Thus the gels can be used rather like micropore filters (a chemotactic source can be placed below them), but with the advantage that they are transparent and cell locomotion can be watched. Alternatively, the gels can be stretched by placing slight tension on each end [17] so that the fibres align in one axis. Aligned gels can be used for assays of contact guidance.

Analysing the film

Equipment

For analysis of cine-film, a 'stop-action' or analytical projector (e.g. Lafayette, John Hadland Ltd. Bovingdon, Herts) is essential. This is a projector which allows the film to be moved forwards or backwards, either continuously at 16 or 24 frames per minute, or step-by-step either manually or automatically at set intervals (1, 2, 4, 6, 8, 12 frames per second).

Procedure

The film is projected on to a piece of paper and cell paths can be traced on to the paper. This is usually done by dotting the cell position in at preselected intervals, then joining the dots. The intervals must not be too long, or the path drawn will only be a crude approximation to the real path. Likewise it must not be so short that the cell has moved too little to plot its displacement accurately. Having obtained a series of tracks on the paper, the tracks must be analysed, and how this is done depends on what information is required. As a minimum, the following are the requirements for analysis of taxis, kinesis and guidance, as discussed above:

(1) an estimate of the speed of each cell and the mean speed (or better the root-mean-square speed) of the whole cell population;

(2) an estimate of turning behaviour, i.e. if the cell path is tracked as a series of segments, the angle of turn between each segment, and from this, the mean angle of turn for the whole cell path and for the whole cell population;

(3) an estimate of directional locomotion, or deviation from random locomotion. Is the cell population moving in one direction, as in chemotaxis? Is it moving in two opposite directions, but in a single axis as in a guidance? This information may be derived from the analysis of turning behaviour in relation to a given axis (i.e. the perpendicular to a gradient source or the axis of alignment of a guidance field) or from plots of displacements of all the cells in a population, and comparison with displacements expected if locomotion were random.

To make all these calculations from the paths of cells drawn on paper by using a ruler and protractor requires much patience, though the author has done quite a lot of this. Fortunately the procedure can be accelerated by tracing the cell paths out on to a digitizer tablet (e.g. Summagraphics: Bit Pad One $11'' \times 11''$) by touching each point in the path on to the tablet with the stylus. The digitizer tablet is connected to a microcomputer (e.g. Superbrain, Intertec Data Systems, Columbia, SC) and sends the rectangular coordinates of each point to the computer. The digitizer tablet has to be calibrated and an axis defined by marking the ends of a scale bar of known length in μm. The computer is appropriately programmed to measure the lengths of track segments, the angles between segments, angles of each segment related to the defined axis, net cell displacements, etc. according to the information that is required.

Establishing the presence of a chemotactic response

Time-lapse cinematography is the most direct way to demonstrate chemotaxis. How this is done depends on the nature of the chemotactic gradient source. If this is a point source, such as a micro-organism, cells can be seen to move directly to the source (see *Candida*

albicans assay above). The McCutcheon ratio, displacement/distance travelled to source, can be estimated for each cell and should be near unity. In comparing McCutcheon ratios for two cell populations, non-parametric statistics should be used, since the distribution of such ratios is not normal.

If the chemotactic source is distant, e.g. a linear source in a trough, the whole cell population should move in the same direction. In this case, the easiest way to establish a chemotactic response is to plot the displacements of the cells on a vector scatter diagram in which one of the axes is the perpendicular to the source (see Fig. 51.9). Then displacement of the whole cell population can be tested for non-randomness by measuring the mean and standard error of the mean for both the x- and y-components of the displacements and using Student's t-test, or the probability of a non-random displacement can be tested by calculation directly from random walk theory by applying the formula

$$p = \exp\left[-\{(\Sigma x)^2 + (\Sigma y)^2\}/(\Sigma x^2 + \Sigma y^2)\right]$$

where x and y are the displacements of each cell in the

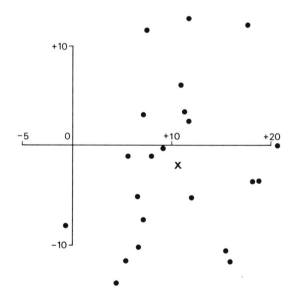

Fig. 51.9. A vector scatter diagram to show displacement of human blood neutrophils under agarose in a gradient of f-Met-Leu-Phe diffusing from a well placed in the line of the x-axis to the right of the field. Cell displacements were plotted taking the zero point as the starting point of each cell. A field was filmed between the cell well and the attractant well (see Fig. 51.3) in which cells had an equal possibility of moving in any direction. Almost all the cells show displacement to the right. The cross shows the mean displacement for the cell population (p < 0.001). From ref. 13, courtesy of Churchill-Livingstone.

x- and y-axes. The rationale for this is outside the scope of the present discussion, but is well outlined by Dunn [2].

The analysis of chemokineses and guidance responses

The visual analysis of orthokinesis and klinokinesis is quite complex, and beyond the range of the present chapter. The theoretical background for this analysis is discussed by Gail & Boone [4] and Dunn [35]. Such analyses are being carried out in the authors's laboratory and those interested could contact either him or Dr John Lackie, Cell Biology Department, University of Glasgow. Contact guidance is simpler to analyse. Some methods are given in refs. 17 and 18.

Note added in proof

A useful assay, not described above, to measure the immediate response of leucocytes to locomotor stimulation, e.g. by chemotactic factors, which is quick, easy and accurate, is to measure the shape-change from spherical to locomotor which occurs once the chemotactic factor is added. The assay is done on cells in suspension and is independent of secondary adhesive shape-changes. A method is outlined by Haston W.S. & Shields J.M. [38].

References

1 KELLER H.U., WILKINSON P.C., ABERCOMBIE M., BECKER E.L., HIRSCH J.G., MILLER M.E., RAMSEY W.S. & ZIGMOND S.H. (1977) A proposal for the definition of terms related to locomotion of leucocytes and other cells. *Clin. exp. Immunol.* **27**, 377.
2 DUNN G.A. (1981) Chemotaxis as a form of directed cell behaviour; some theoretical considerations. In *Biology of the Chemotactic Response*, (eds. Lackie J.M. & Wilkinson P.C.), p. 1. Cambridge University Press.
3 ALLAN R.B. & WILKINSON P.C. (1978) A visual analysis of chemotactic and chemokinetic locomotion of human neutrophil leucocytes. *Expl Cell Res.* **111**, 191.
4 GAIL M.H. & BOONE C.W. (1970) The locomotion of mouse fibroblasts in tissue culture. *Biophys. J.* **10**, 980.
5 ENGLANDER L.L. & MALECH H.L. (1981) Abnormal movement of polymorphonuclear neutrophils in the immotile cilia syndrome: cinemicrographic analysis. *Expl Cell Res.* **135**, 468.
6 ZIGMOND S.H. & SULLIVAN S.J. (1979) Sensory adaptation of leucocytes to chemotactic peptides. *J. Cell Biol.* **82**, 517.
7 WILKINSON P.C. & ALLAN R.B. (1978) Assay systems for measuring leukocyte locomotion: an overview. In *Leukocyte Chemotaxis*, (eds. Gallin J.I. & Quie P.G.), p. 1. Raven Press, New York.
8 KELLER H.U., WISSLER J.H., HESS M.W. & COTTIER H. (1978) Distinct chemokinetic and chemotactic responses in neutrophil granulocytes. *Eur. J. Immunol.* **8**, 1.
9 ZIGMOND S.H. (1974) Mechanisms of sensing gradients by polymorphonuclear leukocytes. *Nature*, **249**, 450.
10 McCUTCHEON M. (1946) Chemotaxis in leukocytes. *Physiol. Rev.* **26**, 319.
11 ZIGMOND S.H. (1977) Ability of polymorphonuclear leukocytes to orient in gradients of chemotactic factors. *J. Cell Biol.* **75**, 606.
12 LAUFFENBURGER D.A. (1982) Influence of external concentration fluctuations on leukocyte chemotactic orientation. *Cell Biophys.* **4**, 177.
13 WILKINSON P.C. (1982) *Chemotaxis and Inflammation*, 2nd edn. Churchill-Livingstone, Edinburgh.
14 SHA'AFI R.I. & NACCACHE P.H. (1981) Ionic events in neutrophil chemotaxis and secretion. In *Advances in Inflammation Research*, Vol. 2, (eds. Weissmann G., Samuelsson B. & Paoletti R.). Raven Press, New York.
15 HARTWIG J.H., YIN H.L. & STOSSEL T.P. (1980) Contractile proteins and the mechanism of phagocytosis in macrophages. In *Mononuclear Phagocytes: Functional Aspects*, (ed. van Furth R.), p. 971. Nijhoff (Martinus) Publishers B.V.
16 WEISS P. (1961) Guiding principles in cell locomotion and cell aggregation. *Expl Cell Res.* (Suppl. 8), 260.
17 WILKINSON P.C., SHIELDS J.M. & HASTON W.S. (1982) Contact guidance of human neutrophil leukocytes. *Expl Cell Res.* **140**, 55.
18 WILKINSON P.C. & LACKIE J.M. (1983) The influence of contact guidance on chemotaxis of human neutrophil leukocytes. *Expl Cell Res.* **145**, 255.
19 DUNN G.A. (1982) Contact guidance of cultured tissue cells: a survey of potentially relevant properties of the substratum. In *Cell Behaviour*, (eds. Bellairs R., Curtis A.S.G. & Dunn G.A.), p. 247. Cambridge University Press.
20 BOYDEN S.V. (1962) The chemotactic effect of mixtures of antibody and antigen on polymorphonuclear leukocytes. *J. exp. Med.* **115**, 453.
21 KELLER H.U., BOREL J.F., WILKINSON P.C., HESS M. & COTTIER H. (1972) Reassessment of Boyden's technique for measuring chemotaxis. *J. immunol. Meth.* **1**, 165.
22 GALLIN J.I., CLARK R.A. & KIMBALL H.R. (1973) Granulocyte chemotaxis: an improved *in vitro* assay employing ⁵¹Cr-labelled granulocytes. *J. Immunol.* **110**, 233.
23 ZIGMOND S.H. & HIRSCH J.G. (1973) Leukocyte locomotion and chemotaxis. New methods for evaluation, and demonstration of a cell-derived chemotactic factor. *J. exp. Med.* **137**, 387.
24 VAN DYKE T.E., REILLY A.A., HOROSZEWICZ H., GAGLIARDI N. & GENCO R.J. (1979) A rapid, semi-automated procedure for the evaluation of leukocyte locomotion in the micropore filter assay. *J. immunol. Meth.* **31**, 271.
25 TURNER S.R. (1979) Acdas: an automated chemotaxis data acquisition system. *J. immunol. Meth.* **28**, 355.
26 LAUFFENBURGER D. (1983) Measurement of phenomenological parameters for leukocyte motility and chemotaxis. *Agents Actions* (Suppl.), **12**, 34.
27 CHENOWETH D.E., ROWE J.G. & HUGLI T.E. (1979) A modified method for chemotaxis under agarose. *J. immunol. Meth.* **25**, 337.
28 LAUFFENBURGER D.A. & ZIGMOND S.H. (1981) Chemo-

tactic factor concentration gradients in chemotaxis assay systems. *J. immunol. Meth.* **40,** 45.

29 NELSON R.D., QUIE P.G. & SIMMONS R.L. (1975) Chemotaxis under agarose: a new and simple method for measuring chemotaxis and spontaneous migration of human polymorphonuclear leukocytes and monocytes. *J. Immunol.* **115,** 1650.

30 ORR W. & WARD P.A. (1978) Quantitation of leukotaxis in agarose by three different methods. *J. immunol. Meth.* **20,** 95.

31 WILKINSON P.C., LACKIE J.M. & ALLAN R.B. (1982) Methods for measuring leukocyte locomotion. In *Cell Analysis*, (ed. Catsimpoolas N.), p. 145. Plenum Press, New York.

32 HASTON W.S., SHIELDS J.M. & WILKINSON P.C. (1982) Lymphocyte locomotion and attachment on two-dimensional surfaces and in three-dimensional matrices. *J. Cell Biol.* **92,** 747.

33 SCHOR S.L., ALLEN T.D. & WINN B. (1983) Lymphocyte migration into three-dimensional collagen matrices: a quantitative study. *J. Cell Biol.* **96,** 1089.

34 ELSDALE T. & BARD J. (1972) Collagen substrata for studies on cell behaviour. *J. Cell Biol.* **54,** 626.

35 DUNN G.A. (1983) Characterising a kinesis response: time-averaged measures of cell speed and directional persistence. *Agents Actions* (Suppl.), **12,** 14.

36 WILKINSON P.C. (1981) Neutrophil leucocyte function tests. In *Techniques in Clinical Immunology*, 2nd edn., (ed. Thompson R.A.), p. 273. Blackwell Scientific Publications, Oxford.

37 WILKINSON P.C., LACKIE J.M., FORRESTER J.V. & DUNN G.A. (1984) Chemokinetic accumulation of human neutrophils on immune-complex-coated substrata: analysis at a boundary. *J. Cell Biol.* **99,** 1761.

38 HASTON W.S. & SHIELDS J.M. (1985) Neutrophil leucocyte chemotaxis: A simplified assay for measuring polarising responses to chemotactic factors. J. immunol. Meth. (in press).

Chapter 52
Assays for phagocyte ecto-enzymes

P. J. EDELSON

Ecto-enzymes, as originally defined by Karnovsky and his students [1], are plasma membrane enzymes whose active sites are accessible to the external milieu. They may be considered special examples of the more general class of plasma membrane ecto-proteins, i.e. hormone receptors, neurotransmitter binding sites, microbial receptor sites, and other proteins whose ligand binding sites are oriented toward the extracellular medium [2]. Such enzymes appear on many cell types, but have been most extensively studied on neutrophils and macrophages. Examples of phagocyte ecto-enzymes include an ATP-ase [3], 5'-nucleotidase [4,5], alkaline phosphodiesterase I [6,7], a protein kinase [8], leucine aminopeptidase [9], and α-naphthyl butyrate esterase [10]. However, it is important to appreciate that expression of these enzymes can vary among species, among cell types, and, in some cases, among physiologic states of the cells themselves [11].

In this chapter, techniques are presented for assaying several of the more widely studied ecto-enzymes. In addition, various working criteria are discussed that have been used to identify ecto-enzymes, and a method is presented for preparing and assaying a reagent that has been very useful in establishing activities as resulting from ecto-enzymes.

Criteria for ecto-enzymes

In their original description of guinea-pig neutrophil ecto-enzymes, DePierre & Karnovsky used two major criteria for assigning to these enzymes an 'ecto' orientation [12,13]. First, they showed that exposure of intact cells to a non-penetrating reagent could lead to irreversible inhibition of the 5'-nucleotidase activity. The reagent they used, the diazonium salt of sulphanilic acid (DASA), had been originally developed as a tool for selectively probing the external membrane proteins of red blood cells [14]. They confirmed that under appropriate conditions, this reagent does not gain access to the leucocyte cytoplasm by showing that the cytoplasmic enzyme lactate dehydrogenase (LDH) is not inhibited when intact cells are exposed to the reagent. LDH is not, however, intrinsically insensitive to this compound, and is readily inactivated when a cell lysate is exposed to the diazotizing reagent. As an additional control, 5'-nuc-

leotidase was shown to be as sensitive to the DASA in cell lysates as it was in intact cells. This eliminated the possibility that the inhibition of 5'-nucleotidase was an indirect one, resulting from an effect of the DASA on putative plasma membrane mechanisms responsible for transporting nucleotides into the cells where they are then hydrolysed by 5'-nucleotidase.

Their second criterion for identifying 5'-nucleotidase as an ecto-enzyme was that the activity was readily demonstrated in intact cells, and that no increase in activity was demonstrable in broken cell preparations, i.e. there was no enzyme latency. Appropriate controls were used in these studies to rule out inward transport of substrate and outward transport of product.

Following Karnovsky's approach, the author used DASA to identify the mouse macrophage ecto-enzymes 5'-nucleotidase [4], alkaline phosphodiesterase I [7], and leucine aminopeptidase [9]. This technique not only allows a qualitative assessment of enzyme location, it also allows a quantification of plasma membrane and intracellular pools. This makes it possible to look at the quantitative effects of endocytosis on membrane markers, and to compare the relative fraction of enzyme and of plasma membrane lipid internalized, in order to assess enrichment or deprivation of vacuolar membrane for the particular enzyme [15].

Salem et al. [16] have applied a panel of impermeant enzyme inactivators to study the outward orientation of 5'-nucleotidase, acetylcholinesterase, and an ATPase on cultivated neural cells. They make two methodologically interesting observations. First, they note that enzyme sensitivities to the various inactivators can be quite varied so that, for example, under conditions where the ecto-ATPase is completely inactivated by the reagent 1-fluoro-2,4-dinitrobenzene, the 5'-nucleotidase is nearly fully active. A second observation they make is that substrates can protect enzymes from inactivation. Edelson & Duncan (unpublished observations) have made a similar observation, that 5'-AMP protects 5'-nucleotidase from inactivation by DASA, and have used this reversible protection as the basis for differentially labelling the enzyme prior to its isolation.

In addition to the use of impermeant enzyme

inactivators, several other techniques have also been successfully applied to identify various ecto-enzymes. Obviously, each approach has its own particular advantages and disadvantages. For example, reagents with highly reactive functional groups are often quite easy to use, but under certain conditions they may react so extensively with various plasma membrane components that the membrane integrity is impaired and cell viability declines. Again, measurement of enzyme activity in whole cell preparations may be a relatively straightforward matter, but the results may be difficult to interpret if optimal assay conditions are incompatible with the requirements for cell viability.

Histochemical techniques have been applied to the localization of a number of phagocyte plasma membrane enzymes (Table 52.1). Obviously the resolution of these techniques is such that they cannot, strictly speaking, distinguish the orientation of a given enzyme (i.e. outward-facing vs. inward-facing) except inferentially, when there is accompanying evidence that the cells remained impermeable to the substrate. Histochemical localization has been used by two groups to study the α-naphthyl butyrate esterase present in human monocytes [10,17]. A plasma membrane Mg^{2+}-dependent ATPase has also been histochemically demonstrated on guinea-pig macrophages [3], as well as on mouse cells [18,19]. Several reports have been published describing histochemical techniques for demonstrating 5′-nucleotidase (see, for

Table 52.1. 5′-Nucleotidase activity of selected cell types

Cell type	Species	5′-Nucleo-tidase activity	Reference
Neutrophil	Guinea-pig	Present	[2]
	Human	Absent[a]	[8]
Monocyte	Mouse	Absent	[9]
	Human	Absent[b]	[10]
Alveolar macrophage	Mouse	Present	[9]
Peritoneal macrophage			
Resident	Mouse	Present	[11,12]
Thioglycollate-stimulated	Mouse	Absent	[12]
BCG/PPD-stimulated	Mouse	Absent	[13]
Granuloma macrophage	Mouse	Absent	[14]
Platelet	Human	Absent	[15]
Erythrocyte	Human	Absent	[15]
Lymphocyte			
B lymphocyte	Human	Present	[16]
T lymphocyte	Human	Present	[16]

[a] See text
[b] Activity develops over 24–48 h in culture.
(From ref. 28, with permission.)

example, ref. 20). A major methodologic problem in demonstrating this enzyme has been that because 5′-nucleotidase is a metalloenzyme, the lead used as a capture reagent to precipitate the phosphate group freed by enzymatic hydrolysis can poison the enzyme, inhibiting all activity. Thus the results of biochemical measurements of enzyme activity, under the chosen staining conditions, must be presented in parallel with the histochemical studies [20] to ensure that the histochemical reaction is not being ascribed to an activity not actually present during the procedure. Other necessary controls should be carried out to rule out non-enzymatic hydrolysis of substrate [21], or artifactual precipitation of a reaction product which may actually be generated in solution, but which then subsequently accumulates on the cell surface [22].

Another series of approaches has used neutralizing antibodies or lectins, neither of which would be expected to traverse the plasma membrane, as impermeant reagents. Duncan & Edelson (unpublished observations) have confirmed the 'ecto' orientation of 5′-nucleotidase by showing that any one of a panel of monoclonal antibodies to the enzyme could neutralize the enzyme activity in intact cells. In addition to such biochemical studies, it is also possible to label these reagents and examine their distribution on the cell surface at either the light or the electron microscopic level. Again, such microscopic techniques would not necessarily demonstrate the location of the active site, but could at least verify that the enzyme is present at the outer face of the plasma membrane. Irreversible enzyme inhibitors which can be labelled might be used in a similar way.

Another approach involves the use of proteolytic enzymes. Here, evidence of enhanced inactivation in intact cells exposed to these enzymes can also be used as an argument for an 'ecto' orientation. Of course, failure of a particular enzyme or panel of enzymes to accomplish this should not be taken as evidence against an outward orientation, as there are many examples of plasma membrane components with selective protease sensitivity, including 5′-nucleotidase [4] and the macrophage C3bi receptor [23].

In a few studies, the effect of endocytosis on an enzyme has been used as evidence of plasma membrane localization [5,24]. In these studies, a considerable amount of plasma membrane was internalized by allowing the cell to ingest a substantial number of latex beads. It has been possible in this system to show both an immediate displacement of enzyme from the plasma membrane to an internal compartment, as judged by the effect of detergent lysis or impermeant inhibitors on enzyme activity, followed by a slower decay of enzyme activity in this compartment over the next 4–8 h. These studies have been interpreted to mean that, at least under certain conditions, a given plasma membrane activity may be internalized in association with the phagocytic vacuole, and will subsequently be degraded by lysosomal hydrolases delivered when the phagosome fuses with lysosomal granules.

Finally, techniques for cell fractionation have been used for defining plasma membrane enzymes for both the neutrophil [25,26] and the macrophage [27]. This method has, for example, confirmed the assignment of both 5'-nucleotidase and alkaline phosphodiesterase I to the plasma membrane of the mouse peritoneal macrophage [27].

It should be pointed out that even when a particular protein has been localized to the plasma membrane, it is still necessary to be sure that the protein is in fact a product of the cell, and not simply associated with the cell membrane as the result of adsorption of plasma proteins to the phagocyte surface. Such evidence can be obtained either by studying the endogenous incorporation of a labelled precursor, or by demonstrating turnover of the protein *in vitro*.

Method for the assay of 5'-nucleotidase

Introduction

5'-Nucleotidase (EC3.1.3.5) is widely distributed throughout the body [29] and has been used as a marker for the plasma membrane in a variety of cell fractionation studies [30]. Antisera have been prepared to the rat [29] and the mouse enzyme [31] and a partial purification scheme has been presented [32].

Werb & Cohn [24] have reported on some characteristics of the mouse macrophage enzyme. The enzyme is relatively labile to repeated freeze-thaw cycles, but if kept at -20 °C, it maintains its activity for up to six months. Only 5'-nucleotides will serve as substrates, with 5'-UMP and 5'-IMP hydrolysed as rapidly as 5'-AMP. 5'-dAMP is hydrolysed to 25–33% the extent of 5'-AMP. 2',3'-AMP and β-glycerophosphate (an excellent substrate for the 'non-specific' acid and alkaline phosphatese) are not hydrolysed at all.

Although it has been claimed that 5'-nucleotidase has two pH optima, one at 5.0 and another above pH 8.0, the characteristics of the activities under the two conditions are markedly different. The sensitivity of the pH 5.0 activity to tartrate suggests that this activity is due to the non-specific acid phosphatase [33] present in substantial levels in macrophages. The enzyme is routinely assayed at an alkaline pH. In cells with substantial activities of alkaline phosphatase, one may either include tartrate (10 mM) as an inhibitor, or, as the author routinely does, use the preferred substrate β-glycerophosphate.

The enzyme appears to be a metallo-enzyme, with marked inhibition by EDTA (30 mm), Zn^{2+} (0.1 mm). It may also be inhibited by ADP, or by α,β-methylene ADP, though these are neither substrates nor capable of binding to the enzyme active site.

Expression of 5'-nucleotidase by phagocytic cells is quite complex. There is substantial species-to-species variability for expression of the enzyme by neutrophils. Guinea-pig neutrophils do display the enzyme [1] while mouse neutrophils do not (Edelson P.J., unpublished observations). There has been considerable disagreement about the human neutrophil, with some workers claiming that the activity reported was actually due to the granule-associated alkaline phosphatase [35], while others claim that human neutrophils do express specific 5'-nucleotidase [36].

While circulating monocytes generally do not express 5'-nucleotidase, they may develop the activity over several days in culture [37]. 5'-Nucleotidase is expressed on resident mouse peritoneal macrophages, but is not present on inflammatory cells [5] or on cells activated immunologically [38], and we have proposed that the failure to express this enzyme is a characteristic of the activated macrophage [31].

Several other groups have also used 5'-nucleotidase expression as a marker for activation, as summarized in Table 52.1.

Principle

5'-Nucleotidase hydrolyses the phosphoester linkage of selected 5'-monophosphate nucleotides to yield inorganic phosphate and the corresponding nucleoside. Assays may be based on a measurement of the rate at which the substrate disappears, or, more frequently, on the rate of appearance of either of the two products. This assay, originally developed by Avruch & Wallach [39], uses a (^{3}H)-AMP substrate. The labelled substrate is separated from the product by precipitation with barium sulphate, and the amount of free (^{3}H)-adenosine in the supernate is measured in a scintillation counter.

Equipment

37 °C shaking water bath.
Centrifuge capable of producing a force of 1500 g.
Scintillation counter optimized for counting tritium.

Materials

(^{3}H)-AMP stock (25 μCi/ml in 50% ethanol) (10 ml); add 9.75 ml ice-cold 50% ethanol to one vial adenosine 2-(^{3}H)-5'-monophosphate, ammonium salt, 250 μCi in 0.250 ml, 2000 mCi/mmol (Amersham Corp., Arlington Heights, IL, Catalog #TRK.344). (^{3}H)-AMP stock can be used for approximately four months if stored at -20 °C. 0.25 M-ZnSO$_4$ (100 ml). Add distilled water to 7.19 g ZnSO$_4$.7 H$_2$O to make 100 ml of solution. This may be stored indefinitely at room temperature.

0.25 M-Ba(OH)$_2$ (100 ml) 7.89 g Ba(OH)$_2$.8 H$_2$O. Add distilled water to make 100 ml of solution. Ba(OH)$_2$ may be stored indefinitely at room temperature. This is a saturated solution and should be filtered through coarse paper (e.g. Whatman #1) immediately before use.

Substrate (25 nCi 5'-(^{3}H)-AMP/ml, 0.15 mM-5'-AMP, 6 mM-*p*-NP) (100 ml) 5.8 mg adenosine-5'-monophosphoric acid, sodium salt, from yeast, crystalline, Type II (Sigma Chemical Corp., St. Louis, MO, Catalog #A-1752) (Mr = 388.4); 222.6 mg *p*-nitrophenyl phosphate, disodium (Sigma Chemical Corp., St. Louis, MO, Catalog #104.0); 0.1 ml (^{3}H)-AMP stock; 100 ml Tris-HCl buffer. Substrate should be prepared immediately prior to assay and kept on ice.

Procedure

1   Place 0.1 ml aliquots of sample (e.g. cell lysate prepared in fresh 0.05% Triton X-100), or of the appropriate enzyme blank (e.g. 0.05% Triton X-100 alone) in glass test-tubes (culture tubes, disposable glass, 12 × 75 mm, Curtin, Matheson Scientific, Inc., Houston, TX, Catalog #339–275) on ice.

2   Add 0.5 ml substrate, shake well, and incubate in a 37 °C water bath for 30 min.

3   Stop the reaction by returning the tubes to an ice bath and adding 0.2 ml 0.25 M-ZnSO$_4$. Vortex briefly.

4   Add 0.2 ml freshly filtered 0.25 M-Ba(OH)$_2$ and vortex thoroughly.

5   Centrifuge at 1500 *g* for 20 min at room temperature (or 4 °C).

6   Add 0.5 ml supernatant to 5 ml Aquassure (New England Nuclear, Boston, MA, Catalog #NEF-965) in 6 ml plastic minivials (Plastic Sampule liquid scintillation vials, Wheaton Scientific, Millville, NJ, Catalog #986624) and mix well.

7   Prepare counting standards (equivalent of 100% hydrolysis) by diluting 1.0 ml substrate with 1.0 ml water. Add 0.5 ml to 5 ml Aquassure, as above.

Count for 10 min in a liquid scintillation counter (Packard Instrument Co., Inc., Downers Grove, IL). Typical settings for ^{3}H for a Tricarb counter are: A-B channel; 70% gain; 50–4000 gate setting; external standard off.

Calculations

0.5 ml of 0.15 mM-5'-AMP substrate = 75 nmol and 5'-AMP per sample. Thus specific activity can be

expressed as mU/mg protein = nmol 5'-AMP hydro-lysed/min/ng protein

$$\frac{(\text{c.p.m.}_{\text{EXP}} - \text{c.p.m.}_{\text{BL}})/(\text{c.p.m.}_{\text{STD}} - \text{c.p.m.}_{\text{BL}})}{(30 \text{ min}) \times (\text{mg protein}/0.1 \text{ ml})} \times 75 \text{ nmol}$$

Protein concentration can be determined by any routine method [40].

Notes and recommendations

This is a fairly simple and highly reproducible assay, with a range of sensitivity wide enough to detect activity of between 5×10^4 and 1×10^6 resident mouse peritoneal macrophages. The activity present in 5×10^5 resident macrophages is about 44.2 mU/mg protein.

This method presents a convenient alternative to spectrophotometric assays for 5'-nucleotidase or protocols using ^{32}P-labelled nucleotides. It requires no second enzyme for product conversion as some spectrophotometric protocols do, and offers the greater sensitivity inherent in assays using radioactive tracers without the hazard of using ^{32}P. It is also relatively rapid; a typical assay takes about three hours.

It is important to establish that the activity observed is actually due to 5'-nucleotidase, rather than a non-specific phosphatase. *p*-Nitrophenyl phosphate is used here as a competitive inhibitor of other phosphatases. At pH 9.0, acid phosphatase activity is not of concern and 5 mM-β-glycerophosphate may be used in place of *p*-NPP as an effective inhibitor of alkaline phosphatase in situations where confusion with other intracellular phosphatases (e.g. glucose 6-phosphate phosphatase) is not an issue. Tartrate (10 mM) inhibits phosphatases active at pH 5.0. 5'-Nucleotidase shows peaks in activity at pH 5.5 and 7.0, with an additional peak occurring at about pH 9.2 when MgCl$_2$ is included in the reaction mix. Removal of divalent cations with 20 mM-EDTA reduces activity more than 95% at pH 9.0. Addition of 0.1 mM-Zn^{2+} completely eliminates nucleotidase activity. One should be cautioned, however, that EDTA interferes with the BaSO$_4$ precipitation and a different assay method must be used [28].

Method for the assay of alkaline phosphodiesterase I

Principle

Phosphodiesterase I (EC 3.1.4.1) hydrolyses polyribonucleotides or oligodeoxyribonucleotides in a stepwise manner, starting at the free 3'-OH end of the chain, and liberating 5'-nucleotides.

This protocol uses an artificial substrate, originally designed by Razzell & Khorana [50], in which a single nucleotide has been coupled at its 5′ end to a *p*-nitrophenyl group through a phosphate ester linkage. When the 5′-nucleotide is liberated by the enzyme, the *p*-nitrophenyl group can be detected by its strong yellow colour in alkaline solutions.

The assay may be carried out on cell lysates, cell fractions or extracellular fluid. The method easily detects the activity present in 10^6 mouse resident peritoneal macrophages.

Equipment

37 °C shaking water bath.
Spectrophotometer capable of reading at 400 nm.

Materials

Substrate solution (thymidine-5′-phosphate-*p*-nitrophenol, 1.5 mmol) is prepared by dissolving 8.11 mg TMP-*p*-NP (Calbiochem-Behring Corp., La Jolla, CA, Catalog #48786), Mr 537.5, in 10 ml Sorensen's glycine II-zinc acetate buffer (pH 9.6).

Substrate should be stored desiccated, refrigerated, and protected from light. Substrate solution should be prepared daily, but may be held on ice for several hours if protected from light.

Procedure

1 Place 50 μl aliquots of cell lysates (prepared in 0.05% Triton X-100) or 0.05% Triton X-100 alone (for enzyme blank) in small disposable glass test-tubes (culture tubes, disposable glass, 12 × 75 mm, Curtin, Matheson Scientific, Inc., Houston, TX, Catalog #339–275).
2 Add 0.5 ml substrate, pre-warmed to 37 °C.
3 Shake briskly, cover rack with aluminium foil, and incubate tubes in 37 °C water bath for 30 min.
4 At end of incubation, immediately place tubes on ice, and stop reaction with 1.0 ml 0.1 M NaOH.
5 Vortex each tube thoroughly.
6 Read absorbance within 30 min at 400 nm.

Calculation

One unit equals that amount of enzyme which hydrolyses 1 μmol of substrate per minute under above assay conditions.
mU/mg protein = {absorbance (sample) − absorbance (blank)} × (1/protein conc^n) × 6.5. Protein concentration is measured in mg/ml.
The factor 6.5 is derived as follows.
Molar extinction coefficient of *p*-nitrophenol $= 12 \times 10^3$ OD U/1 M (at 400 nm).

Then, specific activity in mU/mg = nmol/min/mg protein =

$$\frac{\text{absorbance/ml}}{\text{protein conc}^n/\text{mg per ml}} \times (10^3/12) \times (1/30 \text{ min})$$

$$\times 1.5 \times 1.55 = \frac{\text{absorbance/ml}}{\text{protein conc}^n/\text{mg per mol}} \times 6.5$$

Notes and recommendations

This is a simple, straightforward, and highly reliable assay. Because it is based on a colorimetric measurement, it is about an order of magnitude less sensitive than assays using radioactive substrates, but even so it readily detects the activity present in 10^6 resident mouse peritoneal macrophages; i.e. about 1.43 mU/mg.

Method for the assay of leucine aminopeptidase activity

Leucine aminopeptidase (EC3.4.1.2.), an enzyme widely distributed in many tissues [41,42], has been particularly studied in man, where it occurs on monocytes and granulocytes, but not lymphocytes, basophils or promyelocytes [42], and in the mouse, where it appears to be restricted to the monocyte and tissue macrophage [42,43]. Wachsmuth has proposed that this enzyme is an ecto-enzyme because of its sensitivity to papain under conditions where cell integrity is preserved [44]. The activity is easily measured in cell lysates by following the hydrolysis of leucine *p*-nitroanilide to *p*-nitroaniline, as described by Wachsmuth & Stoye [45], and Morahan [46].

Equipment

37 °C shaking water bath.
Spectrophotometer capable of reading at 405 nm.

Materials

10 mM-Leucine *p*-nitroanilide substrate (Sigma L-9125). Prepare by dissolving 28.8 mg in 10 ml of absolute methanol. Store at 4 °C and prepare fresh every week. About twice the specific activity is obtained with the substrate prepared in methanol rather than dimethylsulphoxide.
Standard microsomal leucine aminopeptidase enzyme (Sigma L-6007). Hydrate the lyophilized enzyme in 1 ml distilled water. To prepare the stock, dilute the enzyme 1:100 in phosphate-buffered saline containing 0.1% bovine serum albumin as protein carrier. Store the material at 4 °C. Do not freeze, as activity will be rapidly lost. The standard remains stable for about three months.

Procedure

1 Prepare the standard enzyme by placing in a small glass tube 25 μl of the 1 : 100 stock enzyme solution and 75 μl of 0.05% Triton X-100 in distilled water.
2 Prepare blank tubes with 100 μl of 0.05% Triton X-100 in distilled water.
3 To each of the above tubes, add 800 μl of the phosphate buffer. A repetitive micropipettor can be used. Warm at 37 °C for 10 min.
4 Rapidly add 100 μl of leucine *p*-nitroanilide substrate to each tube, to provide a final 1 mM concentration. A repetitive micropipettor can be used. Reincubate in 37 °C water bath for 15 min.
5 Stop the reaction by placing the tubes on ice, after vortexing each tube. Read the concentration of *p*-nitroaniline at 405 nm. Read within one hour.

Calculation of data

1 The specific activity is calculated using a molar extinction coefficient of 9600 for *p*-nitroaniline at 405 nm.
2 The specific activity, in nmol/mg protein/min at 37 °C is calculated by:

$$SA = \frac{OD \text{ for the } 100 \ \mu l \text{ cell lysate}}{mg \text{ protein in that volume}} \times$$
$$\frac{1000}{min \text{ of reaction} \times 9.6}$$

The SA can, of course, also be based on DNA content or number of cells in the sample.
3 The standard enzyme is used as a check on the sensitivity and reproducibility of the system.

Notes and recommendations

This assay is sensitive enough to detect the activity of $0.5–1.5 \times 10^6$ resident mouse peritoneal macrophages. One should aim to achieve an absorbance (OD) in the range 0.1–0.7. In this range, and with 1 mM substrate concentration, the reaction is linear for up to 20 min incubation.

A histochemical assay which can be used to study single cells in cytocentrifuge preparations has been described by Wachsmuth & Stoye [44] using leucine-4-methoxy-2-naphthylamide as substrate and fast blue B salt. Other substrates, including alanine-*B*-naphthylanide [41] and angiotensin [47] have also been successfully used as the enzyme appears to have a broad terminal specificity.

Method for the preparation and assay of the diazonium salt of sulphanilic acid (Berg's reagent)

Preparation of reagent

This method is as described previously [5] based on the indirect method of DePierre & Karnovsky [12].

Equipment

Centrifuge, low-speed, table-top model (GLC-1 or equivalent).
Vortex mixer.
Glass stirring rod.

Materials

$NaNO_2$, 11.5 mg.
Sulphanilic acid, 19.5 mg (100 mmol).
Concentrated HCl.

Procedure

1 Place reagents in separate, clean, dry, glass, disposable test-tubes.
2 Chill 4–5 ml distilled water in a third glass test-tube on ice.
3 Add 1 ml iced water to $NaNO_2$. Vortex briefly to dissolve the powder completely.
4 Using a Pasteur pipette, transfer the $NaNO_2$ solution to the sulphanilic acid. Vortex vigorously until all acid has dissolved and solution is bright yellow. Return tube to ice.
5 Add 25 nl concentrated HCl. Vortex briefly. Colour of solution will become pale yellow.
6 Scratch the inside bottom of the test-tube with a glass rod until solution loses colour and begins to cloud.
7 Leave tube on ice for 15–20 min to allow product to precipitate.
8 Spin precipitate down at top speed for 3 min in table-top centrifuge.
9 Discard supernate. Add no more than 0.5 ml iced water. Resuspend pellet and spin again.
10 Dissolve pellet in 20 ml sodium phosphate buffer (0.1 M, pH 7.5) and use promptly. Nominal concentration is 5 mM.

Resorcinol assay of DASA

This protocol is based on the methods of Koltun [48] and Goldstein *et al.* [49], as used in ref. 5.

Equipment

Spectrophotometer capable of reading at 385 nm.

Materials

Resorcinol (Aldrich Chemical Co., Milwaukee, WI, Catalog #R.40–6).
Acetate buffer (pH 4.5).

Procedure

Prepare a 0.01 M solution of resorcinol (Mr = 110) in acetate buffer (pH 4.5) by dissolving 55 ng resorcinol in 50 ml acetate buffer. The assay is performed by mixing 0.9 ml resorcinol solution and 0.1 nl solution to be assayed (using 1/10 and 1/100 dilutions of DASA solution). The mixture is held at room temperature for 30 min and the absorbance is read at 385 nm.

Calculation of data

Molar concentration of the DASA is computed as

$$\text{Conc}^n = (OD_{385}/21.5 \times 10^3) \times \text{dilution factor}$$

Dilution factor refers to the dilution of DASA solution used (10 for 1/10 dilution: 100 for the 1/100 dilution).

Notes and recommendations

Colour development is maximal at 15 min and is stable for 2 h at room temperature.

Media

Tris-HCl buffer with 13 mM-MgCl₂ (pH 9.0)

Dissolve 6.51 g Trizma Base (Sigma Chemical Co., St. Louis, MO, Catalog #T-1503) and 2.44 g MgCl₂.6 H₂O in sufficient distilled water to make one litre of solution. Adjust to pH 9.0 with 2 M HCl. May be stored indefinitely at 4 °C.

Sorensen's glycine II buffer with 2 mM-zinc acetate (pH 9.6)

Solution A (0.1 M-glycine + 0.1 M-NaCl): 7.5 g glycine; 5.85 g NaCl.
Dissolve in sufficient distilled water to make one litre of solution.
Solution B (0.1 M NaOH): 4 g NaOH.
Dissolve in sufficient distilled water to make one litre of solution.
Combine 732 ml solution A + 238 ml solution B. Add 440 mg zinc acetate to one litre of buffer. Adjust pH to 9.6. Store refrigerated. Buffer can be stored indefinately.

0.1 M-Sodium phosphate buffer, pH 7.5

Prepare by mixing approximately 500 ml of 0.1 M-Na₂HPO₄ with 80 ml of 0.1 M-KH₂PO₄ to a pH of 7.5. If filter-sterilized, the buffer can be kept at 4 °C for months.

Triton X-100 (10.05%)

Prepare by adding 1 ml of a previously prepared stock solution of Triton X-100 (2%) (Mallinckrodt Chemical Co. #3555) to 39 ml distilled water. This working solution should be prepared fresh daily.

Acetate buffer, pH 4.5 (μ = 0.20)

Solution A: 0.2 M-acetic acid (1.14 ml concentrated acetic acid and 98.86 ml water).
Solution B: 0.2 M sodium acetate (use either 1.64 g/100 ml anhydrous sodium acetate or 2.72 g/100 ml sodium acetate-3H₂O).

Acknowledgements

The author is grateful to Rob Duncan, Katy Gass, and Dr. Page Morahan for permission to include material from their contributions to *Methods for Studying Mononuclear Phagocytes*, (1981) (eds. Adams D.O., Edelson P.J. & Koren H.). Academic Press, New York.

This work is supported by a grant from the National Science Foundation.

References

1 DePierre J.W. & Karnovsky M.L. (1974) Ecto-enzyme of granulocytes 5'-nucleotidase. *Science*, **183**, 1096.
2 Edelson P.J. (1980) Macrophage ecto-enzymes: their identification, metabolism, and control. In *Mononuclear Phagocytes: Functional Aspects*, (ed. van Furth R.), p. 665. Martinus Nijhoff Publishers, The Hague.
3 North R.J. (1966) The localization by electron microscopy of nucleoside phosphatase activity in guinea pig phagocyte cells. *J. Ultrastr. Res.* **16**, 83.
4 Edelson P.J. & Cohn Z.A. (1976) 5'-nucleotidase activity of mouse peritoneal macrophages. (I) Synthesis and degradation in resident and inflammatory populations. *J. exp. Med.* **144**, 1581.
5 Edelson P.J. & Cohn Z.A. (1976) 5'-nucleotidase activity of mouse peritoneal macrophages (Cellular distribution and effects of endocytosis). *J. exp. Med.* **144**, 1596.
6 Wachsmuth E.D. (1975) Aminopeptidase as a marker for macrophage differentiation. *Expl Cell Res.* **96**, 409.
7 Edelson P.J. & Erbs C. (1978) Plasma membrane localization and metabolism of alkaline phosphodiesterase I in mouse peritoneal macrophages. *J. exp. Med.* **147**, 77.

8 REMOLD-O'DONNELL E. (1978) Protein kinase activity associated with the surface of guinea pig macrophages. *J. exp. Med.* **148**, 1099.

9 MORAHAN P.S., EDELSON P.J. & GASS K.C. (1980) Changes in macrophage ectoenzymes upon *in vivo* or *in vitro* activation for antitumor activity. *J. Immunol.* **125**, 1312.

10 BOZDECH M.J. & BAINTON D.E. (1981) Identification of alpha-naphthyl butyrate esterase as a plasma membrane ecto-enzyme of monocytes and as a discrete intracellular membrane-bounded organelle in lymphocytes. *J. exp. Med.* **153**, 182.

11 MORAHAN P.S. (1980) Macrophage nomenclature: where are we going? *J. Reticuloendothel. Soc.* **27**, 223.

12 DEPIERRE J.W. & KARNOVSKY M.L. (1974) Ecto-enzymes of the guinea pig polymorphonuclear leukocyte I. Evidence for an ecto-adenosine monophosphatase, -adenosine triphosphatase, and -*p*-nitrophenyl-phosphatase. *J. Biol. Chem.* **249**, 7111.

13 DEPIERRE J.W. & KARNOVSKY M.L. (1974) Ecto-enzymes of the guinea pig polymorphonuclear leukocyte II—Properties and suitability as markers for the plasma membrane. *J. Biol. Chem.* **249**, 7121.

14 BERG H.C. (1969) Sulfanilic acid diazonium salt: a label for the outside of the human erythroycyte membrane. *Biochim. biophys. Acta,* **1983**, 65.

15 EDELSON P.J. (1980) Monocytes and macrophages: aspects of their cell biology. In *Cell Biology of Inflammation,* (ed. Weissmann G.), p. 469. Elsevier/North–Holland, Amsterdam.

16 SALEM N., LAUTER C.J. & TRANS E.G. (1981) Selective chemical modification of plasma membrane ectoenzymes. *Biochim. biophys. Acta,* **641**, 366.

17 MONAHAN R.A., DVORAK H.P. & DVORAK A.M. (1981) Ultrastructural localization of nonspecific esterase activity in guinea pig and human monocytes, macrophages, and lymphocytes. *Blood,* **58**, 1089.

18 GORDON S. & COHN Z.A. (1970) Macrophage–melanocyte heterokaryons (I) Preparation and properties. *J. exp. Med.* **131**, 981.

19 EDELSON P.J. & COHN Z.A. (1974) Effects of concanavalin A on mouse peritoneal macrophages. I—enhancement of endocytosis and inhibition of phago-lysosome formation. *J. exp. Med.* **140**, 1364.

20 UUSITALO R.J. & KAVNOVSKY M.J. (1977) Surface localization of 5′-nucleotidase on the mouse lymphocyte. *J. Histochem. Cytochem.* **25**, 87.

21 ROSENTHAL A.S., MOSES H.L., BEAVER D.L. & SCHUFFMAN S.S. (1966) Lead ion and phosphatase histochemistry (I) Nonenzymatic hydrolysis of nucleoside phosphatases by lead ion. *J. Histochem. Cytochem.* **14**, 698.

22 MOSES H.L. & ROSENTHAL A.S. (1968) Pitfalls in the use of lead ion for histochemical localization of nucleoside phosphatases. *J. Histochem. Cytochem.* **16**, 530.

23 BIANCO C., GRIFFIN F.M. & SILVERSTEIN S.C. (1975) Studies of the macrophage complement receptor. Alteration of receptor function upon macrophage activation. *J. exp. Med.* **141**, 1278.

24 WERB Z. & COHN Z.A. (1972) Plasma membrane synthesis in the macrophage following phagocytosis of polystyrene latex particles. *J. Biol. Chem.* **247**, 2439.

25 BAGGIOLINI M., BRETZ U. & DEWALD B. (1978) Subcellular localization of granulocyte enzymes. In *Neutral Proteases of Human Polymorphonuclear Leukocytes,* (eds. Havemann K. & Janoff A.), p. 3. Urban & Schwarzenberg, Inc., Baltimore.

26 KANE S.P. & PETERS T.J. (1975) Analytical subcellular fractionation of human granulocytes with reference to the localization of vitamin B_{12}-binding proteins. *Clin. Sci. Mol. Med.* **49**, 171.

27 DARTE C. & BEAUFAY H. (1983) Analytical subcellular fractionation of cultivated mouse resident peritoneal macrophages. *J. exp. Med.* **157**, 1208.

28 EDELSON P.J. & DUNCAN R.A. (1981) 5′-nucleotidase assay. In *Methods for Studying Mononuclear Phagocytes,* (eds. Adams D.O., Edelson P.J. & Koren H.), p. 461. Academic Press, New York.

29 RIEMER B.L. & WIDNELL C.C. (1975) The demonstration of a specific 5′-nucleotidase activity in rat tissues. *Archs Biochem. Biophys.* **171**, 343.

30 DEPIERRE J.W. & KARNOVSKY M.L. (1973) Plasma membranes of mammalian cells: a review of methods for their characterization and isolation. *J. Cell Biol.* **56**, 275.

31 EDELSON P.J. (1981) Plasma membrane ectoenzymes. Macrophage differentiation markers. In *Heterogeneity of Mononuclear Phagocytes,* (eds. Forster O. & Landy M.), p. 127. Academic Press, New York.

32 WIDNELL C.C. (1974) Purification of rat liver 5′-nucleotidase as a complex with sphingomyelin. In *Methods in Enzymology,* Vol. 32, part B, (eds. Fleischer S. & Pacher L.), p. 368. Academic Press, New York.

33 SMITH J.K. & WHITBY L.G. (1968) The heterogeneity of prostatic acid phosphatase. *Biochim. biophys. Acta,* **151**, 607.

34 BURGER R.M. & LOWENSTEIN J.M. (1970) Preparation and properties of 5′-nucleotidase from smooth muscle of small intestine. *J. Biol. Chem.* **245**, 6247.

35 SHIRLEY P.S., WANG P., DECHATELET L.R. & WAITE B.R. (1975) Absence of the membrane marker enzyme 5′-nucleotidase in human polymorphonuclear leukocytes. *Analyt. Biochem.* **64**, 624.

36 SMITH G.P., MACGREGOR R.R. & PETERS T.J. (1983) Subcellular localisation of leucine aminopeptidase in human polymorphonuclear leukocytes. *Biochim. biophys. Acta,* **728**, 222.

37 JOHNSON W.D., MEI B. & COHN Z.A. (1977) The separation, long-term cultivation, and maturation of the human monocyte. *J. exp. Med.* **146**, 1613.

38 EDELSON P.J. & ERBS C. (1978) Biochemical and functional characteristics of the plasma membrane of macrophages from BCG-infected mice. *J. Immunol.* **120**, 1532.

39 AVRUCH J. & WALLACH D.F.H. (1976) Preparation and properties of plasma membrane and endoplasmic reticulum fragments from isolated rat fat cells. *Biochim. biophys. Acta,* **233**, 334.

40 EDELSON P.J. & DUNCAN R.A. (1981) Lowry and Bradford Assays for Protein. In *Methods for Studying Mononuclear Phagocytes,* (eds. Adams D.O., Edelson P.J. & Koren H.), p. 337. Academic Press, New York.

41 ACKERMAN G.A. (1960) Histochemical demonstration of aminopeptidase activity in leukocytes of blood and bone marrow. *J. Histochem. Cytochem.* **8**, 386.

42 WACHSMUTH E.D. (1968) Lokalisation von aminopeptidase in gewebschnitten init einer enven immunoflureszenztechnik. *Histochemie*, **14**, 282.

43 WACHSMUTH E.D. & STABER F.G. (1977) Changes in membrane-bound amino peptidase on bone-marrow derived macrophages during their maturation *in vitro*. *Expl Cell Res.* **109**, 269.

44 WACHSMUTH E.D. & STOYE J.P. (1977) Aminopeptidase on the surface of differentiating macrophages: concentration changes on individual cells in culture. *J. Reticuloendothel. Soc.* **22**, 485.

45 WACHSMUTH E.D. & STOYE J.P. (1977) Aminopeptidase on the surface of differentiating macrophages: induction and characterization of the enzyme. *J. Reticuloendothel. Soc.* **22**, 469.

46 MORAHAN P.S. (1981) Quantitation of leucine aminopeptidase of mononuclear phagocytes. In *Methods for Studying Mononuclear Phagocytes*, (eds. Adams D.O., Edelson P.J. & Koren H.), p. 473. Academic Press, New York.

47 KURTZ A.B. & WACHSMUTH E.D. (1960) Identification of plasma angiotensinase as aminopeptidase. *Nature*, **224**, 92.

48 KOLTUN N.L. (1957) Physicochemical properties of *p*-carboxyphenylazoinsulins. *J. Am. chem. Soc.* **79**, 5681.

49 GOLDSTEIN I.M., CERQUEIRA M., LUND S. & KAPLAN H.B. (1977) Evidence that the superoxide-generating system of human leukocytes is associated with the cell surface. *J. clin. Invest.* **59**, 249.

50 RAZZELL W.E. & KHORANA H.G. (1959) Studies of polynucleotides (III) Enzymic degradation. Substrate specificity and properties of snake venom phosphodiesterase. *J. Biol. Chem.* **234**, 2105.

Chapter 53
Overview: Lymphocytes and their relations

H. S. MICKLEM

Monoclonal antibodies and
related techniques, 53.1
Molecular genetics, 53.2

T lymphocyte clones *in vitro*, 53.3
Cells, 53.3
Cell lineages, 53.5

Tissues, 53.5
Concluding remarks, 53.6

'The small lymphocyte seems a poor sort of cell . . .' [1]

A review looks back over what has happened, analyses and synthesizes. It is less clear what an overview is supposed to do, although the word itself suggests that the author should occupy an Olympian position some way above the general fray. Such a position, even if attainable, is precarious and constantly threatens to precipitate its occupant into the mire. The results of any such mishap may, one hopes, be ignored or forgiven. The author's assumption is that anyone who reads what is in essence an experimental methods book is about to roll up his or her sleeves and get down to some bench work; he will already have read some of the numerous reviews and will not wish to see another. The author, therefore, takes an eclectic approach (i.e. one that omits more worthwile things than it includes) to the changes that have come about since the last edition of this handbook appeared in 1978, and tries to draw attention to some of the problems that appear to offer a hope of solution before the next edition appears. The range of possible subjects is large; their number guarantees a superficial approach. The author makes no attempt to achieve a historical perspective and for the most part chooses to cite recent papers and, when available, reviews.

Monoclonal antibodies and related techniques

Although hybridomas are mentioned in the previous edition of the handbook, their metastasis from the primary site in Cambridge [2] to the thousands of secondary locations where they now grow has taken place largely in the last 5 years. Monoclonal antibodies have now come of age. More than any other single technical development, they have revolutionized the study of lymphocytes and their progenitors. They have also added impetus to the development of techniques for analysing and separating cells, including mass methods such as panning [3] and rosetting [4] and more refined but smaller-scale methods such as fluorescence activated cell sorting [5]. Cell sorters remain exasperatingly slow as sorters, but their operation has gained greatly in sophistication, assisted not only by the wealth of monoclonal reagents now available but also, latterly, by the arrival of new fluorochromes. Three- and even four-colour analysis and sorting are now becoming practicable, and the possibilities of cell subset definition are correspondingly enhanced [6].

These new techniques have contributed to the understanding of cells in several ways: (1) the identification of cell surface antigens; (2) the separation and analysis of the antigenic molecules, using one- and two-dimensional polyacrylamide gel electrophoresis; (3) identification of cell subsets defined by their membrane macromolecules; (4) functional studies of the subsets so defined; (5) delineation of the functions of the membrane macromolecules themselves. Of these, the last two have lagged some way behind the rest. Recent studies of the quantitative co-expression of two or three macromolecules, which can now be achieved with a two-laser cell sorter, have led to an increase in the apparent number of distinct cell populations in the immune system [7–10]. This trend seems likely to continue and much effort will be required to sort out which of the differences mark genuinely distinct subsets with different functions. However, a fairly comprehensive map of the cells of the immune system should emerge within the next few years, linking phenotype and function in a coherent way. The functions of many membrane macromolecules remain quite obscure. Surface immunoglobulin carried by B cells is, of course, the medium by which they are able to recognize antigens. Even here, however, all is not clear. In particular, the relative roles of IgM and IgD in antigen recognition and cell activation have still to be revealed [11–12] (see 'Cells' below).

For the rest, molecules whose presence had already been inferred from their function, such as receptors for Ig-Fc, complement and transferrin, have been identified by means of monoclonal antibodies. Conversely, plausible (and testable) hypotheses are emerging for the functions of several macromolecules known to be present on the surface of T cells, including Leu-1,2,3 and 4 (OKT-1, 5/8,4 and 3 respectively) in man [13].

Our perception of the roles of class I and class II molecules encoded by the major histocompatibility locus has changed dramatically in recent years. The long-standing association of the MHC locus with allograft recognition and rejection has proved somewhat misleading and it is now clear that MHC-coded molecules play a more general role in promoting appropriate interactions between cells of the immune system. Possibly they may also be important as interaction molecules in non-immune contexts, but this has not been firmly established [14]. Some of the other cell surface glycoproteins of T cells (in man, Leu-2 and Leu-3; in the mouse, Lyt-2 and L3T4 [15]) appear to function as part of the same guidance system, interacting with class I and class II MHC molecules respectively. It has long been thought that expression of Lyt-2 is correlated with cytotoxic and suppressor function, while its absence betokens helper function. It may be that the real correlation is with MHC reactivity and that the functional status of the cell is a secondary, non-obligatory correlate [16–17].

Molecular genetics

Genetic mapping of the murine MHC has revealed that K, I and D regions, which have occupied the attention of immunogeneticists for so long, form a relatively small part of what can be regarded, by virtue of sequence homologies, as a family of MHC-related genes on chromosome 17 [18]. The main question at present is how interesting the other members of the family, some 30 genes located in the Qa/Tla region distal to H-2D, will prove to be. It is possible that many of them are not expressed or are expressed at very low levels. However, Qa molecules (which, like Tla, are structurally class I molecules) are already known to be differentially expressed on T cell subsets [19, 20] and are beginning to turn up on other haematopoietic cells [21]. A very interesting pattern of cellular reactivity has been reported for a monoclonal antibody to Qa-m2; positive cells include a highly self-renewing subset of haematopoietic spleen colony-forming cells, although fluorescence activated cell sorter (FACS) analysis shows that the level of expression on the cell surface is indeed low [22]. Tla molecules, too, are present in embryonic tissues, but so far have not been found in the adult except in cortical thymocytes (and T cell leukaemias). Recently, SV-40 infection has been stated to lead to the expression of a Tla molecule in adult mice [23]. These observations suggest that products of at least some of the genes of the Qa/Tla region may emerge as elements in intercellular recognition and perhaps especially in embryonic development. Klein *et al.* [24], however, view such ideas with scepticism and prefer to think of the Qa/Tla region as a kind of 'laboratory' for the MHC, a large depot of genetic material whose products can be tried out in small quantities and eventually contribute to the polymorphism and functional adaptability of the MHC. There is evidence that it can provide DNA sequences for 'gene conversion' of H-2 genes and hence be involved directly in the extensive polymorphism of the H-2 region [25]. It is of interest that polymorphism seems to be largely restricted to certain parts of the MHC, namely H-2K, H-2DL, I-A and part of the I-E regions, while others (I-E$_\alpha$, Qa and Tla) are more conserved [26].

Molecular genetics has begun, and will certainly continue, to make a revolutionary impact not only on the analysis of the MHC but also on other aspects of cellular immunology. This impact has been particularly evident in three diverse contexts. First, it has drawn attention to the sequence homology, and hence the presumed common evolutionary descent between several of immunology's best-loved molecules, including immunoglobulins, MHC class I and II and Thy-1 (the last still, incidentally, lacking a known function) [27]. Very recently, the list has extended to the receptor for transepithelial transport of IgA and IgM across glandular epithelia [28]. Moreover, the protomolecules from which these appear to be derived may be of extraordinary antiquity since apparent homologues have been identified by serological cross-reactivity in diverse invertebrate groups, including insects [29], and by amino-acid sequencing in squids [30]. Their presence in insects and molluscs, two highly evolved groups whose ancestors diverged from those of the vertebrates several hundred million years ago, attests to their universal utility. Since allorecognition phenomena have been reported in such a primitive group as the coelenterates [31], it is conceivable that the molecules played a role in cellular interactions from the beginning. Second, it is now possible to look at the DNA of highly defined cell populations. This approach has been used to time the occurrence of immunoglobulin gene rearrangements at specific stages of pre-B cell development as defined by monoclonal antibodies [32]. Third, and perhaps most important, it has begun to throw new light on the nature of T cell receptors for antigen. This last development has been made possible by another recent advance—the ability to grow clones of T cells [33, and see below]. Such clones may manifest one or several particular T cell functions and display appropriate membrane macromolecules; in addition, they show antigen specificity via clonotypic receptor molecules which, like immunoglobulins, are glycoproteins composed of two polypeptide chains, α and β, each of 40–50 kDa molecular weight [34–36].

The identification of clone-specific DNA rearrangements has already led to detailed characterization of the β-chain gene. These studies, which have recently been reviewed [96], partly resolve the long-standing uncertainty over whether or not specific antigen recognition by T cells is based on the same systems of diversification that operate for immunoglobulins—namely, evolution of multiple variable-region genes, somatic mutation and variable V–(D)–J–C segment joining [97]. The answer is a qualified 'yes', the strongest qualification being that the T cell receptor β chain and immunoglobulins do not use the *same* V-region genes. The β-chain gene has, however, considerable similarities to an Ig light-chain gene: there are V, J and C segments, hypervariable regions within V, and substantial sequence homologies. There are also important differences: greater diversity of V sequences, more hypervariable regions, the presence of D segments as in Ig heavy chains and, at least in principle, less restriction on the ways in which V, D and J segments can combine [97]. It remains to be seen whether somatic mutation makes any contribution to β-chain diversity. As far as can be inferred from the organization of the β-chain gene, therefore, the repertoire of T cell receptors may be at least as large as that of immunoglobulins. It has been suggested that not all the hypervariable parts of the chain may be involved in antigen binding, the 'extra' ones functioning in the recognition of MHC determinants [98]. The β chain seems to have no isotypes; only two virtually identical C genes have been identified. The α chain, the gene for which has been characterized more recently, may owe much of its variability to multiple J segments and only a single C-region gene is present [99,112–113]. The role of another gene [100], now known to encode a third (γ) variable polypeptide [103–104], still has to be clarified, as does the precise function of the 'T3' molecule which is loosely associated with the antigen receptor and probably involved in transmembrane signalling [36,105–108]. Membrane macromolecules encoded by genes closely linked to the Igh locus on chromosome 12 have been identified on murine T cells by means of monoclonal antibodies [37,102]. Their association with particular subsets and maturational stages of T cells suggests that they may represent different isotypes of a T receptor C region [38]. However, the genes for α, β and γ chains all turn out to be located on chromosomes other than 12 [101,109], so the nature of the Igh-linked molecules remains enigmatic.

In a quite different context, mapping of the murine MHC has shown that there is not sufficient DNA in the right places to code for all the molecules whose existence has been postulated [26]. Specifically, the genes of the 'I-B' and 'I-J' regions cannot be located between the I-A and I-E regions, where immunogenetic analysis would have them. This is particularly remarkable for I-J, for the existence of which a wealth of functional (though little biochemical) evidence has been reported from many laboratories [39]. It is not yet clear how this paradox should be resolved. One suggestion is the I-J antigenic determinants are located on the I-E$_\beta$ chain after the latter has been conformationally modified by association with the antigen-binding chain of T suppressor factor [40]. Another, strongly supported by recent work, is that I-J determinants are idiotypes associated with inducible receptors for self class II MHC antigens [41,110,111].

Finally, the techniques of molecular genetics promise to stitch together several areas of enquiry that are now largely separate. For example, we may hope to see an exploration of the roles of cellular oncogenes in the normal ontogeny of lymphocytes and other cells and, conversely, of the unexpected expression of MHC molecules and Igh-V-related molecules on certain transformed cells [42].

T lymphocyte clones *in vitro*

The first reports of successful cloning of T cells were appearing while the last edition of this handbook was in preparation and this has been another area of active growth in the intervening years. Cloned lines can now be achieved in several different ways and continue to be an extremely important tool for studying the phenotypic and functional diversity of T cells, their repertoire of reactivities to antigens, the nature of T cell receptors and other topics. This field has been the subject of several recent reviews [33,43] and is beyond the scope of further discussion in the present chapter (see Chapter 75).

Cells

The availability of new techniques and reagents has been leading to a rapid increase in the apparent number of sets and subsets into which lymphocytes and other haematopoietic cells can be divided. Perhaps the so-called 'natural killer' cells and their relatives [44,45] have shown the most remarkable ascent to popular favour during the currency of the 3rd edition of this handbook. When it went to press, these cells still had the dubious status of a nuisance that impeded attempts to study antigen-specific cytotoxic reactions. NK cells first made their appearance in the literature at about the time when the idea of anti-tumour surveillance by T cells was becoming untenable [46]. Later it became possible to see them as rescuers of the surveillance concept. It seems fair to say that little has happened recently to strengthen the case for NK surveillance as a general anti-tumour mechanism. The opinion of many workers has hardened against such a role, although there is evidence for NK involvement in tumour resistance in certain specific cases [47]. Perhaps, in any event, immunologists and tumour biologists alike have been over-enamoured of surveillance as an idea. The proposal that tumours would, in the absence of surveillance, be a serious menace to young individuals of a species, and hence that natural selection might favour the evolution of surveillance, remains speculative. Increasing attention is now being directed towards other possible regulatory functions of NK cells. Cells carrying a membrane antigen believed to be present on at least some NK cells in man (Leu-7) have been described in germinal centres by several groups [48, 49]; there they are found at higher frequency than in other areas of lymphoid tissue. What are they doing there? Are they, for example, limiting lymphocyte proliferation [50], perhaps by attacking cells that carry transferrin receptors, the presence of which is characteristic of rapidly dividing cells [51]? Or do they limit immune responses less directly via an effect on antigen-presenting cells [52]? An NK-like cell can inhibit the proliferation of certain foreign murine haematopoietic stem cells *in vivo* [53], and of autologous or allogeneic human granulocyte/macrophage progenitor cells *in vitro* [54], but it is not clear whether they can act as haematopoietic regulators under normal conditions. It may continue to be difficult to disentangle real physiological functions from the adventitious by-products of experimental manipulation, but some homeostatic function in normal haematopoietic tissues currently seems to be the most plausible *raison d'être* for NK cells. That NK cells can interact in various ways with other cells is suggested by the evidence that some cloned NK lines secrete such molecules as interleukin-1, interleukin-2 and interferons [47].

Several categories of cell are now known to be able to present antigen to T and/or B cells. These include macrophages, or at least some of them (for they are a heterogeneous class both in Ia expression and in other respects) [55,56]. The Langerhans' cells of skin, veiled cells of lymph and interdigitating cells of lymphoid tissue represent another class of cell that presents antigen to T cells in association with MHC class II molecules [57]. More than one kind of dendritic, antigen-presenting cell seems to be present in lymphoid tissues [58,59], including some that bind antigen–antibody–complement complexes and probably act as a focus for B memory cells [60]. Cells capable of presenting antigen are also present in the mouse thymus from the fourteenth day of gestation, i.e.

about the time when lymphocytes first appear in the organ [61]. It may be speculated that they promote the expansion and functional maturation of the T cell system; several ways in which they might do this can be envisaged, but their precise function awaits clarification [61]. It is still not clear how closely these various antigen-presenting cells are related to each other, either in lineage or in function. Recent work by several groups has shown that tumour cells, hybridoma cells and lymphoblastoid cells of B lineage can present antigen to T cells [62–64], but it is doubtful how significant a B cell activity this is *in vivo* since so few B cells have the equipment (specific Ig receptors) to bind any particular antigen in the first place.

T cell subsets, too, have been proliferating. The 'old' classification allowed for two T cells (T-helper and T-suppressor) affecting B cells and antibody formation and two active in cell-mediated immunity (T-amplifier and T-cytotoxic). These two pairs had much in common, especially in their membrane antigenic markers, and one still frequently reads of the 'helper-inducer' and 'suppressor-cytotoxic' subsets, loosely based, in man, on their expression of Leu-3 (T4) and Leu-2 (T5/8) markers respectively. However, true helpers (for B cells) are now reported to form a small subset of the helper-inducer population in both man and the rat [65,66]. The monoclonal antibody-defined antigen Lym-22 distinguishes between suppressor and cytotoxic cells in the mouse [67]. The helper and suppressor categories themselves seem to be subdivisible functionally—according to target (antigen, allotype, idiotype) and different positions in the help–suppression–contrasuppression circuits— and phenotypically, e.g. in the expression of Qa antigens [68].

Relatively little attention has been paid until recently to the heterogeneity of B cells, although variable expression of Ig isotypes, particularly IgM and IgD, has been recognized for several years. Recently, quantitative immunofluorescence analysis with anti-μ and anti-δ antibodies has identified at least three categories of B cell in normal mouse spleen [7]. The varied occurrence of these cell types in respect of age, tissue (spleen vs. lymph node) and genotype (normal vs. X-linked immunodeficient) and the presence of the Ly-1 antigen on one of them [69] combine to suggest that the phenotypic variation has functional significance. Further subdivisions have now been reported on the basis of membrane antigens identified by two monoclonal antibodies, 30-E1 and 53-10.2 [8]. Other studies indicate that there are certain anatomical localities—germinal centres [70] and the marginal zone of spleen [71]— where IgD is absent or very poorly expressed on the B cell surface. IgD has been reported to be lost from memory B cells with high affinity receptors for the immunizing antigen [72]. In contrast, studies on mice that have been repeatedly exposed from birth to anti-δ antibodies and consequently lack IgD-expressing cells, suggest that no specific deficiences of immune competence are present [12]. The function(s) of IgD as a receptor distinct from IgM, therefore, remain(s) uncertain.

Cell lineages

We are still remarkably ignorant about many of the details of haematopoietic differentiation, which of course includes all the cells mentioned above and others besides. Ground may even have been lost in recent years because many fresh cell types have been identified or established as being part of the haematopoietic system. Stem cells are a case in point. It is common to talk of 'the pluripotent' stem cell, frequently equating it with 'the spleen colony-forming cell', and this tends to conceal a large area of uncertainty. 'Pluripotent' is a conveniently foggy word, implying that a cell can differentiate in several directions, not necessarily all, and failing to specify which the directions are. One rarely hears the term 'plenipotent stem cell', implying the ability to give rise to the whole gamut of haematopoietic cells, and for good reason: there is little evidence for the existence of such a cell except in the early embryo. Even pluripotency means different things to different people. In particular, the extent to which T and B lymphocytes are produced independently of other lineages (and/or each other) is still a matter of controversy [73,74]. Related to this is the question of 'prothymocytes', i.e. cells in the bone marrow that are committed to enter the thymus and beget thymocytes [75,76]: do such cells really exist or can the data be explained on the basis of a subset of pluripotent stem cells? There seems to be general agreement at least that there is no simple correspondence between prothymocytes and spleen colony-forming cells (CFU-S).

Even if plenipotent stem cells exist, that does not say anything about the frequency with which they feed cells into any particular lineage; there is little evidence to contradict the notion that lympho-committed progenitor cells exist with extensive powers of self-renewal, and such a compartment might be able to maintain itself for long periods without any input from a pluripotent precursor. *In vivo* studies in this area are hampered by the fact that members of a single clone may not appear and disappear synchronously in each differentiated compartment: long-lived T cells, for example, might be representatives of clones that had disappeared from compartments (e.g. erythrocytic and granulocytic) with a higher rate of turnover. *In vitro* studies are hampered by the fact that no one set of

culture conditions is conducive to the growth of B and T cells as well as other haematopoietic types. It has become clear that the CFU-S compartment itself is heterogeneous, including cells with very limited clonogenic capacity and hence little claim to be called stem cells [77]. Many workers subscribe to the idea of a hierarchical or 'generation-age' structure in the CFU-S population, according to which the cells, as they pass through successive divisions, become progressively more susceptible to mitogenic stimuli [78–80] and perhaps also less pluripotent [81]. From an immunological point of view, it would now be particularly interesting to know more about the progenitors of lymphocytes; and also to understand what positions antigen-presenting cells (other than macrophages whose close lineage relationship to neutrophil granulocytes is well established) and NK cells (variously believed to belong to the T cell lineage, the macrophage lineage or neither) really occupy in the haematopoietic edifice. The tools—new population markers, antibodies to membrane determinants, improved separation and *in vitro* culture methods, and the techniques of molecular genetics—are now at hand to approach such questions with some hope of success.

Tissues

Thymus

Although the thymus has long been established as a source of T lymphocytes, many things remain obscure about its structure, including the diversity and interrelationships of its thymocytes, its function, and the cell flows that exist into it, within it and out of it [82]. In particular, the scale of immigration of progenitor cells, which may well be different in the fetus and the adult, needs to be clarified. On the one hand, a considerable number of *in vitro* labelled bone marrow cells migrate into the thymus in the short term [83]. On the other hand, longer-term repopulation experiments have suggested that the rate of entry of progenitors is slow [84]. If there are few progenitors and they undergo extensive clonal proliferation within the thymus, that would allow receptor diversity to be generated, probably as a consequence of gene rearrangements analogous to those that give rise to Ig diversity, within the thymus itself; but it would be difficult to reconcile with recent suggestions that receptor specificity may be acquired at a prethymic stage [85,86]. If both receptor diversification and MHC restriction do indeed occur prethymically, that would leave little for the thymus to do, other than foster clonal expansion and maturation. Such a view seems quite implausible. What does now seem to be clear is that the thymus, at least in the adult, releases fully functional, differentiated T cells, not immature 'post-thymic precursors' that require further, extrathymic maturation [87].

Bone marrow

Many of the lineage questions posed above involve study of the bone marrow or of its haematopoietic equivalent (mainly the liver) in the fetus. Relatively few laboratories have been interested in the bone marrow from a standpoint that is primarily immunological. This state of affairs has probably resulted to some extent from technical constraints: neither the spleen colony technique nor long-term marrow cultures, which have dominated *in vivo* and *in vitro* studies of haematopoiesis for many years, have proved readily adaptable to the study of T or, until recently, B [87] lymphopoiesis. Similarly, while *in vitro* cloning methods have been developed for the early progenitors of other haematopoietic cell types, this has not been possible for lymphocytes. Given these constraints, impressive progress has been made in elucidating B lymphocyte development in both fetus and adult [89]. It is mainly at two stages that uncertainty persists: the grey area between pluripotent stem cells and the earliest recognizable B lineage cells (those that contain cytoplasmic μ-chains) and the stage at which apparently distinct B cell subsets diverge from each other (assuming that they are not simply different maturational stages of a single B cell lineage).

The role of T cells in the economy of the bone marrow deserves further analysis. The number of T cells normally present in the marrow is small, but there have been numerous reports that haematopoietic repopulation of irradiated recipients by injected marrow cells may be more effective if thymocytes are injected at the same time [90]. The fairly normal haematopoietic development of congenitally thymus-deficient nude mice makes it difficult to believe that T cells have any indispensible stimulatory or regulatory function in haematopoiesis, but they may be one source of stimulatory factors—perhaps a minor one under normal conditions. In this context, the identification of several factors produced by cloned T cells and acting upon various haematopoietic cell types *in vitro* is of particular interest [91].

Other lymphoid tissues

Most considerations of peripheral lymphoid tissues concern themselves in some way with lymphocyte recirculation. Here some important advances have been made possible by two techniques—the use of isolated and perfused lymphoid organs [92] and the frozen section method for observing adherence of lymphocytes to vascular endothelium [93]. A very

interesting recent development has been the monoclonal antibody Mel-14 which inhibits the binding of lymphocytes to lymph node vascular endothelium and appears to react with a specific recognition molecule on the lymphocyte [94]. It does not inhibit binding to the endothelium of Peyer's patches and this may indicate a molecular basis for selective localization of lymphocytes in different tissues.

Not all lymphocytes recirculate. In particular, a substantial B lymphocyte compartment has recently been identified in the splenic marginal zone (surrounding the lymphoid follicles proper). These B cells differ from most follicular B cells in not being depleted by thoracic duct drainage, although being derived apparently from recirculating precursors, and in carrying little or no surface IgD [95]. It seems possible that they correspond to the Ly-1-carrying B cells referred to earlier, but this does not seem to have been established.

Concluding remarks

Several new technologies are transforming our perceptions of the cells of the immune system. These include the use of monoclonal antibodies to cell surface antigens, the study of T cell clones, and the techniques of molecular genetics. Along with these go a number of other recently developed methods, especially those concerned with cell surface analysis, cell separation and *in vitro* cell culture. Many parts of the immunocytological map have been redrawn in the past 5 years. Many more will be redrawn, or drawn for the first time, in the next 5. It is satisfying to see so many interesting questions awaiting answers. If lymphocytes and their relatives still feel themselves to be 'poor' [1], it can only be because of the unremitting zeal with which they are pestered by the readers of this book.

This chapter is dedicated to the memory of Dr W. L. Ford. Bill Ford's untimely death has deprived immunology of a fine scientist and many immunologists of a valued friend.

References

1 TROWELL O.A. (1958) The lymphocyte. *Int. Rev. Cytol.* **7,** 236.

2 KÖHLER H. & MILSTEIN C. (1975) Continuous cultures of fused cells secreting antibody of predefined specificity. *Nature,* **256,** 495.

3 MAGE M.G., McHUGH L.L. & ROTHSTEIN T.L. (1977) Mouse lymphocytes with and without surface immunoglobulin: preparative scale separation in polystyrene tissue culture dishes coated with specifically purified anti-immunoglobulin. *J. immunol. Meth.* **15,** 47.

4 PARISH C.R. & HAYWARD J.A. (1974) The lymphocyte

surface. (II) Separation of Fc receptor, C3 receptor and surface immunoglobulin bearing lymphocytes. *Proc. R. Soc.* Series B: Biological Sciences, **187**, 65.

5 HERZENBERG L.A. & HERZENBERG L.A. (1978) Analysis and separation using the fluorescence-activated cell sorter (FACS). In *Handbook of Experimental Immunology*, 3rd edn., Chapter 22, (ed. Weir D.M.). Blackwell Scientific Publications, Oxford.

6 PARKS D.R., HARDY R.R. & HERZENBERG L.A. (1984) Three-color immunofluorescence analysis of mouse B lymphocyte subpopulations. *Cytometry*, **5**, 159.

7 HARDY R.R., HAYAKAWA K., HAAIJMAN J.J., HERZENBERG L.A. & HERZENBERG L.A. (1982) B cell subpopulations identified by two-color fluorescence analysis. *Nature*, **297**, 589.

8 HARDY R.R., HAYAKAWA K., PARKS D.R. & HERZENBERG L.A. (1983) Demonstration of B cell maturation in X-linked immunodeficient mice by simultaneous three-colour immunofluorescence. *Nature*, **306**, 270.

9 LANIER L.L., LE A.M., PHILLIPS J.H., WARNER N.L. & BABCOCK G.F. (1983) Subpopulations of human natural killer cells defined by expression of the Leu 7 (HNK-1) and Leu 11 (NKP-15) antigens. *J. Immunol.* **131**, 1789.

10 LANIER L.L. & LOKEN M.R. (1984) Human lymphocyte subpopulations identified by using three-color immunofluorescence and flow cytometry analysis. Correlation of Leu-2, Leu-3, Leu-7, Leu-8 and Leu-11 cell surface antigen expression. *J. Immunol.* **132**, 151.

11 SKELLY R.S., BAINE Y., AHMED A., XUE B. & THORBECKE G.J. (1983) Cell surface phenotype of lymphoid cells from normal mice and mice treated with monoclonal anti-IgD from birth. *J. Immunol.* **130**, 15.

12 METCALF E.S., MOND J.J. & FINKELMAN F.D. (1983) Effects of neonatal anti-δ antibody on the murine immune system. (II) Functional capacity of a stable sIg$^+$sIa$^+$sIgD$^-$ B cell population. *J. Immunol.* **131**, 601.

13 REINHERZ E.L., MEUER S.C. & SCHLOSSMAN S.F. (1983) The delineation of antigen receptors on human T lymphocytes. *Immunology Today*, **4**, 5.

14 EDIDIN M. (1983) MHC antigens and non-immune functions. *Immunology Today*, **4**, 269.

15 SWAIN S.L., DIALYNAS D.P., FITCH F.W. & ENGLISH M. (1984) Monoclonal antibody to L3T4 blocks the function of T cells specific for class 2 major histocompatibility complex antigens. *J. Immunol.* **132**, 1118.

16 SWAIN S.L. (1983) T cell subsets and the recognition of MHC class. *Immunol. Revs.* **74**, 128.

17 RAO A., ALLARD W.J., HOGAN P.G., ROSENSON R.S. & CANTOR H. (1983) Alloreactive T cell clones. Ly phenotypes predict both function and specificity for major histocompatibility complex products. *Immunogenetics*, **17**, 147.

18 HOOD L., STEINMETZ M. & MALISSEN B. (1983) Genes of the major histocompatibility complex of the mouse. *Ann. Rev. Immunol.* **1**, 529.

19 STANTON T.H., CALKINS C.E., JANDINSKI J., SCHENDEL D.J., STUTMAN O., CANTOR H. & BOYSE E.A. (1978) The Qa antigenic system. Relation of Qa-1 phenotypes to lymphocyte sets, mitogen responses and immune functions. *J. exp. Med.* **148**, 963.

20 SULLIVAN K.A. & FLAHERTY L. (1979) The Qa-2 antigen on lymphocyte subpopulations. Mixed lymphocyte culture and cell-mediated lympholysis. *J. Immunol.* **123**, 2920.

21 HOGARTH P.M., CREWTHER P.E. & MCKENZIE I.F.C. (1982) Description of a Qa-2 like alloantigen (Qa-m2). *Eur. J. Immunol.* **12**, 374.

22 HARRIS R.A., HOGARTH P.M., WADESON L.J., COLLINS P., MCKENZIE I.F.C. & PENINGTON D.G. (1984) An antigenic difference between cells forming early and late haematopoietic spleen colonies (CFU-S). *Nature*, **307**, 638.

23 BRICKELL P.M., LATCHMAN D.S., MURPHY D., WILSON K. & RIGBY P.W.J. (1984) Activation of a Qa/Tla class I major histocompatibility antigen gene is a general feature of oncogenesis in the mouse. *Nature*, **306**, 756.

24 KLEIN J., FIGUEROA F. & NAGY Z.A. (1983) Genetics of the major histocompatibility complex: the final act. *Ann. Rev. Immunol.* **1**, 119.

25 FLAVELL R.A., WEISS E.H. & MELLOR A.L. (1984) The generation of polymorphism in H-2 genes. *Prog. Immunol.* **5**, 215.

26 HOOD L., FISHER D., GOODENOW R., GOVERNMAN J. & 11 OTHERS (1984) MHC genes of the mouse. *Prog. Immunol.* **5**, 223.

27 WILLIAMS A.F. (1984) The immunoglobulin superfamily takes shape. *Nature*, **308**, 12.

28 MOSTOV K.E., FRIEDLANDER M. & BLOBEL G. (1984) The receptor for transepithelial transport of IgA and IgM contains multiple immunoglobulin-like domains. *Nature*, **308**, 37.

29 SHALEV A., PLA M., GINSBURGER-VOGEL T., ECHALIER G., LÖGDBERG L., BJÖRCK L., COLOMBANI J. & SEGAL S. (1983) Evidence for β_2-microglobulin-like and H-2-like antigenic determinants in *Drosophila*. *J. Immunol.* **130**, 297.

30 WILLIAMS A.F. & GAGNON J. (1982) Neuronal cell Thy-1 glycoprotein: homology with immunoglobulin. *Science*, **216**, 696.

31 HILDEMANN W.H. (1979) Immunocompetence and allogeneic polymorphism among invertebrates. *Transplantation*, **27**, 1.

32 COFFMAN R.L. & WEISSMAN I.L. (1983) Immunoglobulin gene rearrangement during pre-B cell differentiation. *J. Mol. cell. Immunol.* **1**, 31.

33 FATHMAN C.G. & FRELINGER J.G. (1983) T lymphocyte clones. *Ann. Rev. Immunol.* **1**, 633.

34 KAPPLER J., KUBO R., HASKINS K., WHITE J. & MARRACK P. (1983) The mouse T cell receptor: comparison of MHC-restricted receptors on two T cell hybridomas. *Cell*, **34**, 727.

35 MCINTYRE B.W. & ALLISON J.P. (1983) The mouse T cell receptor: structural heterogeneity of molecules of normal T cells defined by xenoantiserum. *Cell*, **34**, 739.

36 MEUER S.C., FITZGERALD K.A., HUSSEY R.E., HODGDON J.C., SCHLOSSMAN S.F. & REINHERZ E.L. (1983) Clonotypic structures involved in antigen-specific human T cell function. Relationship to the T3 molecular complex. *J. exp. Med.* **157**, 705.

37 OWEN F.L. & RIBLETT R. (1984) Genes for the mouse T cell alloantigens T$_{pre}$, T$_{thy}$ and T$_{su}$ are closely linked near Igh on chromosome 12. *J. exp. Med.* **159**, 313.

38 OWEN F.L. (1983) T cell alloantigens encoded by the IgT-C region of chromosome 12 in the mouse. *Adv. Immunol.* **34,** 1.

39 TANIGUCHI M., TOKUHISA T., KANNO M. & HONJO T. (1982) An antigen-specific T cell factor controlled by two genes in the immunoglobulin heavy chain linkage group and in the I-J region of the H-2 complex. *Curr. Top. Microbiol. Immunol.* **100,** 33.

40 KLEIN J., NAGY Z.A., BAXEVANIS C.N. & IKEZAWA Z. (1984) The major histocompatibility complex and the specificity of suppressor T cells. *Prog. Immunol.* **5,** 935.

41 TADA T. (1984) Points of contact between network and circuit. *Prog. Immunol.* **5,** 595.

42 FLOOD P.M., DELEO A.B., OLD L.J. & GERSHON R.K. (1983) Relation of cell surface antigens on methylcholanthrene-induced fibrosarcomas to immunoglobulin heavy chain complex variable region-linked T cell interaction molecules. *Proc. natn. Acad. Sci. U.S.A.* **80,** 1683.

43 MÖLLER G. (ed.) (1983) T lymphocyte clones. *Immunol. Revs.* **76.**

44 MÖLLER G. (ed.) (1979) Natural killer cells. *Immunol. Revs.* **44.**

45 STUTMAN O., LATTIME E.C. & FIGARELLA E.F. (1981) Natural cytotoxic cells against solid tumours in mice: a comparison with natural killer cells. *Fedn Proc.* **40,** 2699.

46 MÖLLER G. (ed.) (1975) Experiments and the concept of immunological surveillance. *Transplant. Rev.* **28.**

47 HERBERMAN R.B. (1984) Immune surveillance hypothesis: updated formulation and possible effector mechanisms. *Prog. Immunol.* **5,** 1157.

48 RITCHIE A.W.S., JAMES K. & MICKLEM H.S. (1983) The distribution and possible significance of cells identified in human lymphoid tissue by monoclonal antibody HNK-1. *Clin. exp. Immunol.* **51,** 439.

49 SI L. & WHITESIDE T.L. (1983) Tissue distribution of human NK cells studied with anti-Leu-7 monoclonal antibody. *J. Immunol.* **130,** 2149.

50 NABEL G., ALLARD W.J. & CANTOR H. (1982) A cloned cell line mediating natural killer function inhibits immunoglobulin secretion. *J. exp. Med.* **156,** 658.

51 VODINELICH L., SUTHERLAND R., SCHNEIDER C., NEWMAN R. & GREAVES M. (1983) Receptor for transferrin may be a 'target' structure for natural killer cells. *Proc. natn. Acad. Sci. U.S.A.* **80,** 835.

52 ABRUZZO L.V. & ROWLEY D.A. (1983) Homeostasis of the antibody response: immunoregulation by NK cells. *Science,* **222,** 581.

53 CUDKOWICZ G. & HOCHMAN P.S. (1979) Do natural killer cells engage in regulated reactions against self to ensure homeostasis? *Immunol. Revs.* **44,** 13.

54 HANSSON M., BERAN M., ANDERSSON B. & KIESSLING R. (1982) Inhibition of *in vitro* granulopoiesis by autologous and allogeneic human NK cells. *J. Immunol.* **129,** 126.

55 UNANUE E.R. (1981) The regulatory role of macrophages in antigenic stimulation. Part Two: symbiotic relationship between lymphocytes and macrophages. *Adv. Immunol.* **31,** 1.

56 SUN D. & LOHMANN-MATTHES M.-L. (1982) Functionally different subpopulations of mouse macrophages

57 SILBERBERG-SINAKIN I., GIGLI I., BAER R.L. & THORBECKE G.J. (1980) Langerhans cells: role in contact hypersensitivity and relationship to lymphoid dendritic cells and to macrophages. *Immunol. Revs.* **53,** 203.

58 STEINMAN R.M. & NUSSENZWEIG M.C. (1980) Dendritic cells: features and functions. *Immunol. Revs.* **53,** 127.

59 MANDEL T.E., PHIPPS R.P., ABBOT A. & TEW J.G. (1980) The follicular dendritic cell: long term antigen retention during immunity. *Immunol. Revs.* **53,** 29.

60 KLAUS C.G.B., HUMPHREY J.H., KUNKL A. & DONGWORTH D.W. (1980) The follicular dendritic cell; its role in antigen presentation in the generation of immunological memory. *Immunol. Revs.* **53,** 3.

61 ROBINSON J.H. (1983) The ontogeny of antigen-presenting cells in the thymus evaluated by MLR stimulation. *J. Immunol.* **130,** 1592.

62 CHESNUT R.W. & GREY H.M. (1981) Studies on the capacity of B cells to serve as antigen-presenting cells. *J. Immunol.* **126,** 1075.

63 KAPPLER J., WHITE J., WEGMANN T., MUSTAIN E. & MARRACK P. (1982) Antigen presentation by Ia⁺ B cell hybridomas to H-2 restricted T cell hybridomas. *Proc natn. Acad. Sci. U.S.A.* **79,** 3604.

64 ISSEKUTZ T., CHU E. & GEHA R. (1982) Antigen presentation by human B cells: T cell proliferation induced by Epstein-Barr virus B lymphoblastoid cells. *J. Immunol.* **129,** 1446.

65 REINHERZ E.L., MORIMOTO C., FITZGERALD K.A., HUSSEY R.E., DALEY J.F. & SCHLOSSMAN S.F. (1982) Heterogeneity of human T4⁺ inducer T cells defined by a monoclonal antibody that delineates two functional subpopulations. *J. Immunol.* **128,** 463.

66 SPICKETT G.P., BRANDON M.R., MASON D.W., WILLIAMS A.F. & WOOLLETT G.R. (1983) MRC OX-22, a monoclonal antibody that labels a new subset of T lymphocytes and reacts with the high molecular weight form of the leukocyte-common antigen. *J. exp. Med.* **158,** 795.

67 CHAN M.M., TADA N., KIMURA S., HOFFMANN N.K., MILLER R.A., STUTMAN O. & HÄMMERLING U. (1983) Characterization of T lymphocyte subsets with monoclonal antibodies: discovery of a distinct marker, Ly-m22, of T suppressor cells. *J. Immunol.* **130,** 2075.

68 GREEN D.R., FLOOD P.M. & GERSHON R.K. (1983) Immunoregulatory T cell pathways. *Ann. Rev. Immunol.* **1,** 439.

69 HAYAKAWA K., HARDY R.R., PARKS D.R. & HERZENBERG L.A. (1983) The 'Ly-1B' cell subpopulation in normal, immunodefective and autoimmune mice. *J. exp. Med.* **157,** 202.

70 KRAAL G., WEISSMAN I.L. & BUTCHER E.C. (1982) Germinal center B cells: antigen specificity and changes in heavy chain class expression. *Nature,* **298,** 377.

71 KUMARATNE D.S., BAZIN H. & MACLENNAN I.C. (1981) Marginal zones: the major B cell component of rat spleens *Eur. J. Immunol.* **11,** 858.

72 BLACK S.J., TOKUHISA T., HERZENBERG L.A. & HERZENBERG L.A. (1980) Memory B cells at successive stages of

differentiation: expression of surface IgD and capacity for self-renewal. *Eur. J. Immunol.* **10**, 846.

73 ABRAMSON S., MILLER R.G. & PHILLIPS R.A. (1977) The identification in adult bone marrow of pluripotent and restricted stem cells of the myeloid and lymphoid systems. *J. exp. Med.* **145**, 1567.

74 WU CHU-TSE & LIU MIN-PEI (1984) Characteristics of proliferation and differentiation of spleen colony-forming cells from bone marrow. *Int. J. Cell Cloning*, **2**, 69.

75 BOERSMA W., BETEL I., DACULSI R. & VAN DER WESTEN G. (1981) Post-irradiation thymocyte regeneration after bone marrow transplantation. (I) Regeneration and quantitation of thymocyte progenitor cells in the bone marrow. *Cell Tissue Kinet.* **14**, 197.

76 GREINER D.L., GOLDSCHNEIDER I. & BARTON R.W. (1982) Identification of thymocyte progenitors in hemopoietic tissues of the rat. (II) Enrichment of functional prothymocytes on the fluorescence-activated cell sorter. *J. exp. Med.* **156**, 1448.

77 SCHOFIELD R. (1978) The relationship between the spleen colony-forming cell and the haematopoietic stem cell. *Blood Cells*, **4**, 7.

78 MICKLEM H.S. & OGDEN D.A. (1976) Ageing of haematopoietic cell populations in the mouse. In *Stem Cells of Renewing Cell Populations*, (eds. Cairnie A.B., Lala P.K. & Osmond D.G.), p. 331. Academic Press, New York.

79 BOTNICK L.E., HANNON E.C. & HELLMAN S. (1979) Nature of the hemopoietic stem cell compartment and its proliferative potential. *Blood Cells*, **5**, 195.

80 ROSENDAAL M., HODGSON G.S. & BRADLEY T.R. (1979) Organization of haemopoietic stem cells: the generation-age hypothesis. *Cell Tissue Kinet.* **12**, 17.

81 LORD B.I. (1983) Haemopoietic stem cells. In *Stem Cells*, (ed. Potten C.S.), p. 118. Churchill Livingstone, Edinburgh.

82 SCOLLAY R. (1983) Intrathymic events in the differentiation of T lymphocytes: a continuing enigma. *Immunology Today*, **4**, 282.

83 LEPAULT F. & WEISSMAN I.L. (1981) An *in vivo* assay for thymus-homing bone marrow cells. *Nature*, **293**, 151.

84 MICKLEM H.S., OGDEN D.A., EVANS E.P., FORD C.E. & GRAY J.G. (1975) Compartments and cell flows within the mouse haemopoietic system. (II) Estimated rates of interchange. *Cell Tissue Kinet.* **8**, 233.

85 CHERVENAK R., COHEN J.J. & MILLER S.D. (1983) Clonal abortion of bone marrow T cell precursors: T cells acquire specific antigen reactivity prethymically. *J. Immunol.* **131**, 1688.

86 WAGNER H. (1984) Where is MHC restriction determined? *Prog. Immunol.* **5**, 809.

87 SCOLLAY R., CHEN W.-F. & SHORTMAN K. (1984) The functional capabilities of cells leaving the thymus. *J. Immunol.* **132**, 25.

88 WHITLOCK C.A. & WITTE O.N. (1982) B lymphocytes, at all stages of maturation, in modified Dexter-like cultures. *Proc. natn. Acad. Sci. U.S.A.* **79**, 3608.

89 KINCADE P.W. (1981) Formation of B lymphocytes in fetal and adult life. *Adv. Immunol.* **31**, 177.

90 GOODMAN J.W. & GOODMAN D.R. (1983) Involvement of cells of the immune system in regulation of erythropoiesis. In *Current Concepts in Erythropoiesis*, (ed. Dunn C.D.R.), p. 59. Wiley (John) & Sons, Chichester.

91 SCHRADER J.W., CLARK-LEWIS I., CRAPPER R.M. & WONG G.W. (1983) P-cell stimulating factor: characterization, action on multiple lineages of bone marrow derived cells and role in oncogenesis. *Immunol. Revs.* **76**, 77.

92 SEDGLEY M. & FORD W.L. (1976) The migration of lymphocytes across specialized vascular endothelium. (I) The entry of lymphocytes into the isolated mesenteric lymph node of the rat. *Cell Tissue Kinet.* **9**, 231.

93 STAMPER H.B. & WOODRUFF J.J. (1976) Lymphocyte homing into lymph nodes: *in vitro* demonstration of the affinity of recirculating lymphocytes for high-endothelial venules. *J. exp. Med.* **144**, 828.

94 GALLATIN W.M., WEISSMAN I.L. & BUTCHER E.C. (1983) A cell surface molecule involved in organ-specific homing of lymphocytes. *Nature*, **304**, 30.

95 KUMARATNE D.S. & MACLENNAN I.C. (1981) Cells of the marginal zone of the spleen are lymphocytes derived from recirculating precursors. *Eur. J. Immunol.* **11**, 865.

96 ROBERTSON M. (1984) Receptor gene rearrangement and ontogeny of T lymphocytes. *Nature*, **311**, 305.

97 HONJO T. (1983) Immunoglobulin genes. *Ann. Rev. Immunol.* **1**, 499.

98 PATTEN P., YOKOTA T., ROTHBARD J., CHIAN Y., ARAI K. & DAVIS M.M. (1984) Structure, expression and divergence of T cell receptor β-chain variable regions. *Nature*, **312**, 40.

99 Robertson M. (1984) The capture of the snark. *Nature*, **312**, 16.

100 SAITO H., KRANZ D.M., TAKAGAKI Y., HAYDAY A.C., EISEN H.N. & TONEGAWA S. (1984) Complete primary structure of a heterodimeric T cell receptor deduced from cDNA sequences. *Nature*, **309**, 757.

101 LEE N.E., D'EUSTACHIO P., PRAVTCHEVA D., RUDDLE F.H., HEDRICK S.M. & DAVIS M.M. (1984) Murine T cell receptor beta chain is encoded on chromosome 6. *J. exp. Med.* **160**, 905.

102 OKUMURA K., KARASUYAMA H., KIM M. & TADA T. (1984) Igh-linked allotypic markers on cloned T cells. *Progr. Immunol.* **5**, 791.

103 HAYDAY A.C., SAITO H., GILLIES S.D., KRANZ D.M., TANIGAWA G., EISEN H.N. & TONEGAWA S. (1985) Structure, organization and somatic rearrangement of T cell gamma genes. *Cell*, **40**, 259.

104 SNODGRASS H.R., DEMBIC Z., STEINMETZ M. & VON BOEHMER H. (1985) Expression of T cell antigen receptor genes during fetal development in the thymus. *Nature*, **315**, 232.

105 OETTGEN H.C., TERHORST C., CANTLEY L.C. & ROSOFF P.M. (1985) Stimulation of the T3-T cell receptor complex induces a membrane-potential-sensitive calcium influx. *Cell*, **40**, 583.

106 IMBODEN J.B. & STOBO J.D. (1985) Transmembrane signalling by the T cell antigen receptor. Perturbation of the T3-antigen receptor complex generates inositol phosphates and releases calcium ions from intracellular stores. *J. exp. Med.* **161**, 446.

107 ALLISON J.P. & LANIER L.L. (1985) Identification of

antigen receptor associated structures on murine T cells. *Nature*, **314**, 107.

108 SAMELSON L.E., HARFORD J., SCHWARTZ R.H. & KLAUSNER R.D. (1985) A 20-kDa protein associated with the murine T cell antigen receptor is phosphorylated in response to activation by antigen or concanavalin A. *Proc. natn. Acad. Sci. U.S.A.* **82**, 1969.

109 KRANZ D.M., SAITO H., DISTECHE C.M., SWISSHELM K., PRAVTCHEVA D., RUDDLE F.H., EISEN H.N. & TONEGAWA S. (1985) Chromosomal locations of the murine T-cell receptor alpha-chain gene and the T-cell gamma gene. *Science*, **227**, 941.

110 SUMIDA T., SADO T., KOJIMA M., ONO K., KAMISAKU H. & TANIGUCHI M. (1985) I-J as an idiotype of the recognition component of antigen-specific suppressor T-cell factor. *Nature*, **316**, 738.

111 URACZ W., ASANO Y., ABE R. & TADA T. (1985) I-J epitopes are adaptively acquired by T cells differentiated in the chimaeric condition. *Nature*, **316**, 741.

112 HAYDAY A.C., DIAMOND D.J., TANIGAWA G., HEILIG J.S., FOLSOM V., SAITO H. & TONEGAWA S. (1985) Unusual organization and diversity of T-cell receptor α-chain genes. *Nature*, **316**, 828.

113 ARDEN B., KLOTZ J.L., SIU G. & HOOD L.E. (1985) Diversity and structure of genes of the α family of mouse T-cell antigen receptor. *Nature*, **316**, 783.

Chapter 54
Physical methods for separation of lymphocyte subpopulations

R. G. MILLER

Design and analysis of cell
  separation experiments, 54.1
Preparation of cell suspension,
  54.4

Counting and size analysis, 54.4
Sedimentation separation, 54.5
Density separation, 54.8
Other methods, 54.9

To the eye, the lymphocyte is a nondescript, small, round cell with a large, nearly-round nucleus. Despite decades of study, microscopists failed completely to recognize the division of these cells into two main groups, B cells and T cells, which were, in fact, first recognized on the basis of differences in function. As the human eye is a remarkably sensitive instrument, we might expect any differences between B cells and T cells to be either very small or not obvious to the eye. Physically based separation technologies exploit the small differences that do exist. To the extent that these differences correlate with function, the separations are useful. Alternatively, one can make use of the biological differences between subpopulations to tag the cells in such a way that they can then be separated physically.

Physical separation procedures underwent their most active development during the late 1960s and early 1970s. Two procedures, sedimentation separation and density separation, with many variations of each, have since entered into widespread use and this chapter will be largely limited to these two procedures. The procedures are often complementary, so that a separation problem not solvable with either alone can often be solved by using the two sequentially. In more recent years, development of new technology has largely centred on procedures which can exploit biological differences, the one in most widespread use being fluorescence-activated cell sorting. This procedure can often give much better separation than one achievable with any strictly physically based procedure. However, a principal disadvantage of this procedure is its relatively slow rate of separation (typically no more than 3000 cells/s) so that, for example, to process 10^9 cells would take three continuous days of sorting. If the cells of interest could be enriched tenfold using sedimentation or density separation, an expectation which is often realistic, the sorting time could also be reduced tenfold.

There are several different reasons why one might want to use cell separation: to enrich for a particular cell of interest (e.g. dendritic cells), to prepare one cell type free of another (e.g. B cells free of T cells) or to use the separation procedure itself to investigate a biological problem (e.g. to see whether a particular cell type and a particular biological function distribute the same way with respect to the separation variable). Simple physical procedures are still often the best way to handle these problems. In this review, some general considerations valid for all cell separation technologies will be discussed first. This will be followed by a description of sedimentation and density methods and finally a brief survey of some other procedures.

Design and analysis of cell separation experiments

A cell separation experiment can have quite different objectives. Thus one might wish to obtain a 'pure' population of B cells or a population of B cells free of macrophages, or to follow some physical change in the B cell population (e.g. blast transformation) as a result of some treatment. The particular objective will have a major influence on how one performs and analyses the experiment. Most commonly, one is looking for enrichment of a cell type of interest. Routinely, investigators with this objective will measure enrichment as a function of the separation variable being used (e.g. density, sedimentation velocity). Unfortunately, this often produces very misleading results. Consider a fictitious example (but an example which mimics a number of experiments that the author has seen reported in the literature). One wishes to enrich for cell type E. A cell suspension from, say, bone marrow is fractionated into fifteen equal-sized fractions by, for example, velocity sedimentation or density separation and the relative number of E cells per fraction is determined by either functional or morphological criteria. The results of this analysis are

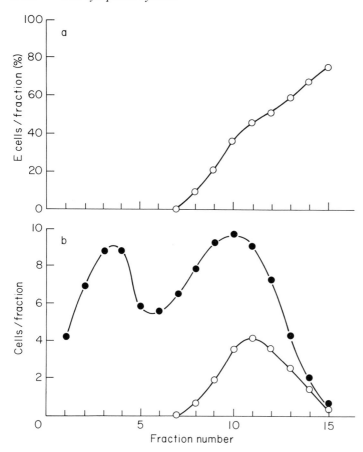

Fig. 54.1. Results of a hypothetical cell separation study of cell type 'E'. In (a), results are expressed as an enrichment profile (O) and in (b) as the actual profile of number of E cells with respect to the separation variable (O). Total cells per fraction are also shown (●).

shown in Fig. 54.1a. They indicate that fraction 15 is most enriched in cell type E. The investigator then uses this fraction in subsequent tests. He may find, for example, that some treatment of the donor of the cell suspension increases or decreases the enrichment seen in fraction 15 and draw conclusions from this observation. These conclusions might be completely erroneous, as a closer examination of the above procedure reveals.

A more appropriate analysis of the experiment of Fig. 54.1 would proceed as follows.
1 Determine the number of cells in each of the fractions. The profile obtained for the fictitious experiment being discussed is shown in Fig. 54.1b.
2 Determine the total number of E cells in each of the fractions. If cell type E can be directly counted by morphological or functional criteria, this is most easily done by multiplying the differential count by the total number of cells in the fraction. The profile so obtained for the fictitious experiment is also shown in Fig. 54.1b.

We now see that although fraction 15 is more

enriched in type E cells than any other fraction, it only contains a very small percentage (<2%) of all of the type E cells. These cells, being on the tail of the separation distribution, might not be typical of the population as a whole. Note as well that changes in enrichment measured for fraction 15 could as easily reflect changes in the contaminating cell population as in the type E cell population.

It is often not possible to count directly a cell type of interest. Instead, its relative frequency in the different fractions of a cell separation experiment must be determined in a functional assay. Let us consider another fictitious experiment. Cell type G cannot be directly identified by morphological criteria but can be detected in a functional assay (e.g. ^{3}HTdR incorporation following appropriate stimulation, or release of radiolabel following incubation with appropriate target cells). The procedure would then be as follows.
1 Fractionate the cell suspension containing G cells into equal-sized fractions as in Fig. 54.1.
2 Count the number of cells in each fraction.
3 Measure the functional activity in a series of

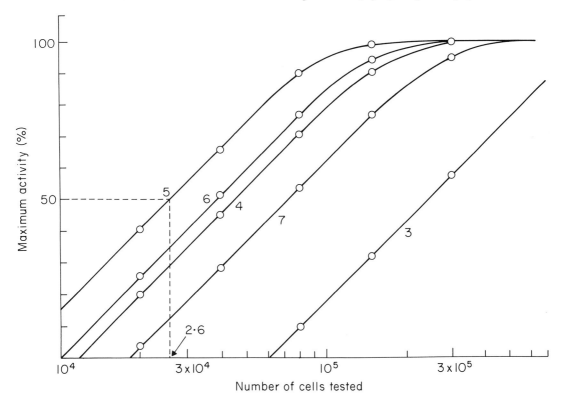

Fig. 54.2.   Functional assay for cell type 'G' in fractions 3–7 of a hypothetical cell separation experiment. See text.

dilutions of each fraction (e.g. 3×10^5, 1.5×10^5, 8×10^4, etc.). Results as shown in Fig. 54.2 might be obtained.

4   Define a certain activity level as containing one activity unit (e.g. 50% of maximum response).

5   Determine from the curves the number, n, of cells in each fraction required to produce one activity unit (e.g. 2.6×10^4 for fraction 5 in Fig. 54.2), and calculate the total number of activity units in the fraction, given by N/n where N is the total number of cells in the fraction. The results obtained from Fig. 54.2 are shown in Fig. 54.3.

6   As a check on procedures, compare the total activity recovered from the separation with the activity in an unseparated control. In the profile of Fig. 54.3, there are a total of 44×10^5 cells containing a total of 64 units of activity. Thus an unfractionated control should contain $64/44 = 1.5$ units of activity per 10^5 cells.

An alternative to the procedure just outlined would be to measure the activity in a set of dilutions of each fraction (e.g. 1/3, 1/10, 1/30,. . . of the volume of each fraction) instead of expressing everything in terms of cell number. The separation variable (fraction

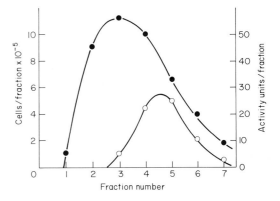

Fig. 54.3.   Activity profile (○) for cell type G found from the curves of Fig. 54.2. Total cell number per fraction is also shown (●).

number) is the only independent variable in the system so this is theoretically the best approach. However, the actual cell number used often has an important effect on the functional assay, so the procedure outlined above is usually safest. The essential feature of the curves of Fig. 54.2 is that they are all isomorphic, i.e. they are all identical to each other except for their relative position on the (logarithmic) x-axis. This will always be true if a single cell type is responsible for the function of interest and if the response of this cell type in the functional assay is independent of the bystander cells cultured with it. If non-isomorphic curves are obtained, the procedure described above is not valid. Such a result implies one of two things:

(1) bystander cells are having an enhancing or inhibitory effect on the functional assay; this effect might be overcome by judicious choice of feeder cells;

(2) the functional assay depends upon cell interactions; if so, it might be possible to provide one of the cells in excess so that the profile of the other can be measured.

Particular examples of these approaches as applied to cytotoxic T lymphocytes and to cells mediating ADCC are given elsewhere [ref. 1; see particularly Figs. 11 and 13 of this reference].

Preparation of cell suspensions

The results obtained in a cell separation experiment can be greatly affected by the method used to prepare the cell suspension. All procedures are best done starting with a cell suspension free of cell aggregates, cell debris and dead cells. For a solid organ such as spleen, lymph node or thymus, the author has found the following mechanical disruption and clean-up procedure, modified from Shortman *et al.* [2], to be most effective.

Equipment

Saucer-shaped wire screen (60 mesh), approximately 3 cm in diameter, soldered to a stainless steel rim and handle 10–15 cm long. The author makes his own in large numbers and always has an autoclaved supply on hand.
Sharp scissors.
Small glass syringe.
Plastic Petri dish and plastic tubes.
Clinical centrifuge.

Materials

Filtered (0.2 μm Millipore) stock solution of 6% bovine serum albumin (BSA, Cohn Fraction V) in PBS.
Phosphate-buffered saline (PBS).

Procedure

1 Place the organ in the middle of a saucer-shaped wire screen (60 mesh) and cut it into several hundred pieces with sharp scissors.

2 Hold the screen over a Petri dish containing 0.2% BSA (diluted from stock solution) in PBS and rub the tissue pieces through the screen with a glass pestle (from, for example, a small glass syringe), keeping the screen centre immersed in the PBS.

3 Transfer suspension into a plastic tube and allow large aggregates to settle out for 3–5 min. Discard aggregates.

4 Layer cell suspension over a few millilitres of 6% BSA in PBS (Shortman *et al.* use 100% FCS) in a plastic tube. Within 10–15 min, many of the remaining aggregates will settle into the 6% BSA.

5 Remove overlay with a Pasteur pipette and gently layer it into a second tube containing a few millilitres (2–3 cm deep) of 6% BSA in PBS.

6 Centrifuge cells through the BSA solution at a force not exceeding 250 g for the minimum time required to pellet all of them.

7 Resuspend pellet in the solution to be used for cell loading in the cell separation procedure. The resulting suspension is typically more than 90% viable by dye exclusion test and contains less than 2% cell aggregates.

Cell suspensions with similar viability can be made using enzymatic digestion and the author has occasionally used a procedure modelled on one developed by Meistrich [3]. The tissue is cut into several hundred pieces in PBS in a Petri dish and incubated with trypsin (0.25%, w/v) and deoxyribonuclease (20 μg/ml) at room temperature for a short period of time (less than 3 min). Cells are spun out of the enzyme mixture and washed by the procedure outlined above. The two advantages of this procedure are that there is less probability of damaging large cells (e.g. dendritic cells) and that the procedure destroys many, sometimes all, non-viable cells with no apparent loss of viable cells. The principal disadvantage is that the procedure is certain to digest off many surface structures—absolutely disastrous if the cell separation procedure to be used depends upon these structures.

Counting and size analysis

In many types of cell separation procedures, one produces a large number of fractions and wants to determine the cell concentration in each. Some kind of an automated cell counter is called for. The best currently available is an electronic cell detector of the Coulter type [4]. The heart of this instrument is a small aperture, typically about 100 μm in diameter, which is mounted in a glass tube and immersed in saline containing the cells to be counted. Electrodes are mounted on either side of the aperture and electrical current flows from one electrode to the other through the aperture. To count cells, a known volume of fluid (typically 0.5 ml) is sucked through the aperture. Each time a cell goes through the aperture, it increases the electrical resistance of the aperture and a pulse is generated, which can be amplified and counted in appropriate electronics.

The Coulter counter allows very rapid determination of cell concentrations per fraction. Measurement of one sample requires 5–10 ml of cell suspension; ideally at a concentration of 10^4/ml, and takes less than 1 min. Accurate counts of cell suspensions containing debris are not possible. However, if debris is present, it is often removed from the samples as part of the cell separation procedure. The author typically dilutes cells for counting in PBS. Particularly for very dilute cell suspensions, background counts in the PBS can give a falsely high reading. Filtration of the PBS (0.2 μm Millipore filter) can reduce these to well under 100 per ml.

Using the Coulter counter, it is possible to get much more information than just the cell concentration. The magnitude of the signal produced by a cell traversing the aperture is proportional, over a restricted but useful range [5], to the volume of the cell detected. One can get a direct measure of the volume distribution of the cells in the sample by connecting the Coulter counter to a pulse-height analyser. This instrument analyses each pulse and adds the count to one of a set of serially arranged memory locations ('channels') according to the size of the pulse. At the completion of the run, the memory can be displayed visually or printed out to produce a graph of pulse number versus pulse size, i.e. cell number versus cell volume.

The detailed shape of the volume distribution measured with a Coulter counter is affected by a number of complex artefacts [6–9]. However, for cells which are spherical or nearly so, the mode of the measured volume distribution is an accurate indicator of the actual modal volume of the cell suspension.

Sedimentation separation

The concept of the separation procedure is very simple. A thin layer of cell suspension is put on top of a fluid column and the cells are allowed to settle through the column under the action of either the earth's gravitational field ($1 \times g$) or of the larger forces available in a centrifuge. The sedimentation rate is given by

$$s = 2\,(\rho - \rho')\,\mathbf{g}r^2/9\eta \qquad (1)$$

where s is the sedimentation rate, $\mathbf{g}$ is the acceleration due to gravity ($1 \times \mathbf{g}$ separation) or the centrifugal acceleration (centrifugal separation), ρ is the density of the cell, ρ' is the density of the supporting fluid column, r is the radius of the cell, and η is the viscosity of the supporting medium. Typically, ρ' has a value of about 1.01 g/cm³, whereas ρ ranges from 1.05 to 1.10 g/cm³. Thus density variations alone will produce about a twofold variation in sedimentation rate. For lymphocyte populations (including progenitors and progeny), r may vary from 3 to 10 μm. Thus size variations may produce up to a tenfold variation in sedimentation rate, and sedimentation produces separation primarily on the basis of differences in cell size. Note that η depends strongly on temperature so that temperature must be maintained constant if reproducible results are to be obtained. For lymphoid populations separated gravitationally at 4 °C in a fluid column whose physical properties are similar to those of water, equation 1 reduces approximately to

$$s = r^2/4 \qquad (2)$$

where s is the sedimentation rate in mm/h and r is the radius of the cell in microns [10]. Within broad limits, the sedimentation rate is independent of cell shape [10].

The major technical problems are three in number. The first concerns the fluid column through which the cells sediment. Clearly, this must be isotonic or nearly so to prevent osmotic effects. In addition, to prevent the column from being unstable to either convection or small mechanical disturbances, the column must contain a mild density gradient, constructed such that $(\rho - \rho')$ is as large and nearly constant as possible throughout the column. Under these conditions, separation remains based primarily on differences in size. The same problems in choice of material as discussed later under density separation will apply here. However, the problems will be much less acute, since the amount of gradient material required to achieve the necessary stabilization is about tenfold less than that needed for density separation.

The second problem involves a poorly understood phenomenon called 'streaming'. If the concentration of cells in the starting band exceeds a certain critical concentration, called the streaming limit, local density inversions apparently occur, and small sections of the starting band sediment into the underlying fluid column, carrying the cells with them at a very high sedimentation rate. Below the streaming limit, all cells appear to sediment individually according to equation 1. Above the streaming limit, useful separation is seldom achieved. For mouse lymphoid cells, the streaming limit is about 10^7 cells/ml, the exact value being influenced by the shape of the gradient [10]. The resolution obtained in a sedimentation separation will be largely determined by the thickness of the starting cell band. Thus, to process large numbers of cells and achieve good resolution, one must use a starting band of large area. This is one major advantage of using the earth's gravitational field as the sedimenting force; it is simple to provide a uniform force over a large area. For $1 \times g$ separation, the third technical problem concerns a method for forming a thin layer of cells on top of the fluid column. This problem has been solved in a number of different ways by appropriate design of the sedimentation chamber, with appropriate procedures for filling and emptying it. One way [10] is now described.

Equipment

The apparatus ('staput'), illustrated in Fig. 54.4, has three main parts: the sedimentation chamber, the gradient maker, and a small intermediate vessel. It is a big advantage to have the sedimentation chamber

transparent so that one can see cell bands during the separation process. Sedimentation chambers made of Lucite, polycarbonate or glass have been used. The last two may be steam sterilized. The angle in the cone of the sedimentation chamber is nominally 30 °C but this is not critical and cone angles as low at 15 °C have been used. Tubing interconnections are best made using silicone tubing (Silastic, Dow Corning) because of the very low tendency for cells to stick to silicone rubber. Cells are loaded into the chamber through C and are lifted into their starting position (indicated by K in Fig. 54.4) by the gradient (loaded via gravity) introduced through the gradient maker (B). The small stainless steel baffle (G) at the bottom of the chamber is used to deflect incoming fluid during the loading procedure. Without this baffle, it is very difficult to load a gradient without mixing. The chamber has a lid (H). The screw (J) mounted in the lid has a sharpened point. Using this screw, one can reproducibly fill the chamber to the same volume by stopping the filling process when the screw tip just touches the rising

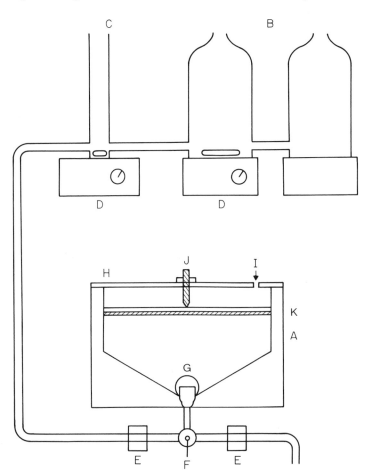

Fig. 54.4. Set up for velocity sedimentation cell separation using 'staput' chamber: A, sedimentation chamber; B, gradient maker; C, intermediate vessel; D, magnetic stirrers; E, flow-rate regulators; F, three-way valve; G, flow baffle; H, chamber lid; I, vent hole in chamber lid; J, screw; K, cell band shortly after loading is completed.

gradient. After the cells have sedimented for an appropriate length of time (2–4 h usually), fractions are collected through the bottom of the chamber. As discussed above, streaming limits the maximum cell concentration in the starting band. To process more cells and maintain resolution, one must use a chamber of larger diameter. Chambers varying from 5 to 39 cm in diameter have been used successfully.

A complete cell separation apparatus of the above type, made of glass, with chamber diameters of approximately 11, 17 or 25 cm is available from O.H. Johns Scientific (175 Hanson St., Toronto, Canada M4C 1A7). Alternatively, it can be easily assembled from readily available glassware or readily machined from plastic.

Materials

Stock solution of filtered (0.2 μm Millipore) 6% bovine serum albumin (BSA, Cohn Fraction V) in PBS.
Phosphate-buffered saline (PBS).
Collection tubes.
Fifty millilitre syringe with piece of tubing attached.

Procedure (chamber 12 cm in diameter).

1 Set up apparatus as in Fig. 54.4. The author routinely uses a 4 °C coldroom, as this is about the only place providing a constant temperature in his Institute. However, room temperature is satisfactory. Gradient bottles and an intermediate vessel with internal diameters of 7 and 2.2 cm, respectively, are used.
2 Prepare at least 300 ml each of 1% and 2% BSA in PBS. Bring to a temperature of 4 °C.
3 Fill all connecting tubing on the chamber side of C with PBS, making sure to get rid of air bubbles.
4 Centre the flow baffle (G) inside the cone of the sedimentation chamber. It is important that this be centred carefully.
5 Clamp the lines between all three gradient chambers. Load 300 ml of 1% BSA into the left-hand bottle of (B) and 300 ml of 2% BSA into the right-hand bottle.
6 Load top layer (30 ml of saline) into the sedimentation chamber through the intermediate vessel. Note that the total volume of the top layer will be whatever fluid is put in (C) plus the volume of the tubing between (C) and the sedimentation chamber (typically less than 5 ml). Check that the flow baffle is still correctly centred. The function of this top layer is to prevent disturbance of the cell band by erratic movements of the rising fluid meniscus as the chamber is filling.
7 Load cells in 20 ml of 0.2% BSA in PBS through

(C). The cell concentration must be below the streaming limit for the cells being loaded (10^7 cells/ml for murine lymphoid cells and the gradient described here). Clamp the line the instance the buffer chamber empties.
8 Rinse the buffer chamber twice with 0.2% BSA in PBS. Use a 50 ml syringe and a piece of tubing to do this. Check that no air bubbles entered the line during the rinse.
9 Fill (C) with 0.35% BSA in PBS to the level of the fluid in the gradient bottles. Adjust the needle valve for a flow of 2–3 ml/min. Turn on magnetic stirrers.
10 Remove all clamps and record time (t_1); the gradient will load itself. It will rise rapidly from 0.35 to 1% BSA and slowly thereafter to 2% BSA. The reasons for using a gradient of this shape are described elsewhere [10]. Once the cells have been lifted off the bottom, the flow rate can be increased. Continuously adjust by eye to a rate just below that at which the cell band is disturbed. Small disturbances will settle out. Loading should be as rapid as possible (10–15 min). The time elapsed between loading cells and starting gradient should also be as short as possible (4–8 min).
11 Record time cell band reaches top of cone (t_2).
12 After an appropriate sedimentation time (typically 3–4 h), unload chamber through the bottom at a rate of about 30 ml/min. Record start time (t_3) and discard cone volume.
13 Collect remainder of gradient in equal-sized fractions (e.g. 15 ml). Record time first fraction (N = 1) started (t_4) and last fraction finished (t_5). Also record number (N_f) and volume (V_f) of last fraction.
14 Measure cell concentration in each fraction, most easily done using a Coulter counter.
15 Calculate sedimentation velocity of each fraction. This is given by

$$s(N) = \frac{(N_f - N - 1/2)v - (V_o + \frac{1}{2}V_{cb} - V_f)}{a\,\{(t_4 - t_1) - 0.4(t_4 + t_2 - t_3 - t_1) + N(t_5 - t_4)/N_f\}}$$

(3)

The times t_1 to t_5 (in hours) are as defined above; V_o, V_{cb}, and V_f are the volumes above the cell band, the cell band, and the last fraction respectively; v is the volume per fraction. The parameter a is the millilitres of fluid per mm of chamber height in the cylindrical portion of the chamber. For a chamber 12 cm in diameter, a is 11.3 ml/mm. The quantity $s(N)$ is then the sedimentation velocity of fraction N in units of mm/h.

Occasionally, one wishes to separate very large or very sticky cells. There is a reasonable probability that some of these will sediment on to the cone or, in passing, stick to it during the loading procedure. These cells may either be permanently lost or, even worse, come off randomly during the draining procedure. To avoid these possibilities, it is desirable to have a procedure in which cells can be layered on top of a preformed gradient. The author has developed such a procedure, described in full detail elsewhere [11,12]. This procedure gives results directly comparable to those obtained using the apparatus described above.

The time required for a sedimentation separation can be greatly decreased by using a centrifugal elutriator, a device involving a specially designed centrifuge and rotor (manufactured by Beckman) which greatly increases the sedimentation rate. The principal advantage is the greater speed of separation. The principal disadvantage is the need for expensive equipment which takes some experience to learn how to use effectively. However, it can give useful results [e.g. ref. 13] and may be the method of choice if a particular sedimentation separation is to be performed in a routine and preparative manner.

Density separation

There are a large number of different procedures for separating cells on the basis of differences in buoyant density. Collectively, they almost certainly represent the most widely used set of cell separation procedures. The basic concept is very simple. One constructs a gradient, either continuous or step, covering the expected range in cell densities. The cells are loaded on the top, on the bottom, or dispersed throughout the gradient, which is then centrifuged with sufficient force for sufficient time (typically a few thousand times g for about 1 h) to enable all the cells to reach an equilibrium in that region of the gradient corresponding to their buoyant density. However, the procedures for achieving this are all different and very different results can be obtained with apparently similar procedures.

Cell buoyant density differences are small; the total range is typically no more than 1.05 to 1.10 g/cm^3. These differences reflect variations in both the composition of a cell and in its local environment. Cell membranes are readily permeable to water so that cells approach osmotic equilibrium with a new environment very rapidly (in less than 1 min) as the result of loss or gain of water but they are less permeable to electrolytes and relatively impermeable to solutes of high relative molecular mass. It can be shown [14] that

$$\rho = 1 + (1 - \Phi_d)m_d/V$$

where ρ, m_d, and V are the density, dry mass, and volume of the cell, respectively and Φ_d is the apparent specific volume of the dry matter (i.e. volume per gram dry mass). The quantities m_d and Φ_d are almost independent of the environment but V can vary widely as material, primarily water, is taken up or lost to maintain osmotic and hydrostatic equilibrium. Differences in ρ can be due to independent variations in each of the three parameters. One special case is worthy of comment. For at least some established cell lines in tissue culture, Φ_d is a constant, and m_d is proportional to V, so that cell density is a constant independent of position in the cell cycle [11,14]. These cell lines, when in exponential growth, form a single narrow peak when analysed on a density gradient. The same might be expected for a lymphoid cell population if it is truly a homogeneous population.

The most powerful density separation procedures are the analytic procedures, in which one obtains not only separation of different cell classes but also a direct measurement of the density profile of each class. The first truly analytic procedure was that of Leif & Vinograd [15,16], who used continuous bovine serum albumin (BSA) gradients at neutral pH to study the buoyant density distribution of human erythrocytes and found that erythrocyte density was correlated with the age of the cell.

There are several technical problems which must be overcome. The most critical one involves the choice of a suitable gradient material and its preparation before use. The material should be non-toxic to cells and have a high relative molecular mass. A common problem is that the density gradient may also form a significant tonicity gradient, either because the gradient material itself is light (making sucrose an unsuitable material for cell density separation) or because the gradient material used contains a significant amount of water or salt impurity. High relative molecular mass preparations often contain large salt impurities. In a gradient made with such material, as a cell moves into a region of higher density, it also moves into a region of higher tonicity. Osmotic forces will cause the cell to shrink, which, in turn, will increase its density, and so on. In the extreme case, the cells will all be pelleted on the bottom of the tube.

The most popular choice for the gradient material has been BSA. The results obtained depend critically upon the procedure used to prepare the BSA; different treatment procedures give different and often not very reproducible results. The procedure of Shortman *et al.* [17,18] results in an isotonic gradient and is highly reproducible but does not give completely satisfactory results on a rebanding experiment, i.e. cells of a particular density on a first separation do not return to precisely the same position if re-separated on a second gradient. Rebanding appears to be significantly better if the tonicity of the medium used is strictly iso-osmotic with respect to the species of origin of the cells [18]. Ficoll gradients, if properly deionized, appear to give satisfactory rebanding results [19], but these gradients are not isotonic at high Ficoll concentrations, probably due to interactions of Ficoll with water [18].

Both BSA and Ficoll tend to enhance cell aggregation, particularly with increasing cell load. This problem can be reduced by lowering the pH and/or by the use of a dispersing agent such as 2-naphthol-6,8-disulphonic acid [17]. Initial dispersion of the cells throughout the gradient reduces the probability of aggregation and also reduces both wall effects and cell streaming, which can be serious problems when the cells are loaded on the top of the gradient. Marbrook has recently provided a detailed description of the Shortman procedure [20].

Studies of colloidal silica as a gradient material date back more than 20 years [21–23]. The principal advantage of this material is that high densities can be achieved with little increase in tonicity or viscosity and without inducing cell aggregation. The principal disadvantage is that the colloidal silica is toxic. This toxicity can be at least partly overcome by incorporating a polymer of high relative molecular mass in the gradient [23,24,25]. Polyvinyl pyrrolidone (PVP) appears to be best for this purpose [24,25]. Percoll (Pharmacia), in which the silica is actually coated with PVP, may be even better, and this material has become extremely popular in recent years.

Discontinuous step gradients have been widely used for density separation. Two of the more popular procedures are those of Dicke *et al*. [26] and Raidt *et al*. [27]. These procedures have several intrinsic disadvantages compared to a continuous gradient: (1) the number of cells that can be processed before there is aggregation at the step interfaces is much lower than on a continuous gradient; (2) unless the number of steps is very large, one does not obtain a measure of the density profile of the cell of interest; (3) even if one's aim is solely to achieve high enrichment of the cell of interest, optimization of enrichment requires a large number of experiments with different density increments; and (4) a procedure suitable for one application is difficult to generalize to another. Despite these major drawbacks, step gradients continue to be extremely popular, perhaps because of their relative ease of preparation and collection. Raidt has recently provided detailed instructions for his procedure [28].

A popular preparative method for obtaining enriched populations of lymphocytes from blood is the 'Ficoll-Hypaque' method, originally developed by Böyum [29], in which a diluted suspension of whole blood is layered over a mixture of sodium diatrizoate (Hypaque) and Ficoll and is spun to equilibrium. Lymphocytes (contaminated with platelets) collect at the interface, whereas all other cells are found in the bottom layer. This procedure may be thought of as a two-step density gradient, although tonicity probably also plays a role.

Other methods

Several procedures have been developed which produce cell separation on the basis of differences in cell surface properties, e.g. electrophoresis [30,31], counter-current [32,33] and adherence to glass beads [34]. Of these, electrophoresis has probably been most widely used. It has been particularly useful for separating B cells and T cells [35]. Nylon wool columns can also be used to separate B and T cells [36]. B cells are retained on the column while T cells pass through.

In addition to fluorescence-activated cell sorting, a number of procedures with direct biological specificity have been developed. All of these use antibodies specific for a cell surface marker of interest but differ in the manner in which cells recognized by this antibody are separated from the others. In all of these procedures, the Fc portion of the antibody is bound to some substrate. It can be bound to glass beads in a column [37]. When cells are passed through the column those with the marker are retained. The antibody can be bound to a plastic dish and cells added [38]. Those carrying the marker will stick. Or, finally, the antibodies can be bound to erythrocytes which will then form rosettes with cells carrying the marker [39]. The rosettes can then be separated from other cells by either sedimentation or density.

References

1 MILLER R.G., GORCZYNSKI R.M., LAFLEUR L., MACDONALD H.R. & PHILLIPS R.A. (1975) Cell separation analysis of B and T lymphocyte differentiation. *Transplant. Rev.* **25**, 59.

2 SHORTMAN K., WILLIAMS N. & ADAMS P. (1972) The separation of different cell classes from lymphoid organs. (V) Simple procedures for the removal of cell debris, damaged cells and erythroid cells from cell suspensions. *J. immunol. Meth.* **1**, 273.

3 MEISTRICH M.L. (1972) Separation of mouse spermatogenic cells by velocity sedimentation. *J. cell. Physiol.* **80**, 299.

4 COULTER W.H. (1953) U.S. Patent No. 2,656,508.

5 KUBITSCHEK H.E. (1960) Electronic measurement of particle size. *Research*, **13**, 122.

6 HARVEY R.J. (1968) Measurement of cell volumes by electric sensing zone instruments. In *Methods in Cell Physiology III*, (ed. Prescott D.M.), p. 1. Academic Press, New York.

7 TAYLOR W.B. (1970) A versatile cell detector for cell volume measurements. *Med. biol. Eng.* **8**, 281.

8 GROVER N.B., NAAMAN J., BEN-SASSON S. & DOLJANSKI F. (1969) Electrical sizing of particles in suspensions. (I) Theory. *Biophys. J.* **9**, 1398.

9 MILLER R.G. & WUEST L.J. (1972) Volume analysis of human red cells. (II) The nature of the residue. *Ser. Haematol.* V, **2**, 128.

10 MILLER R.G. & PHILLIPS R.A. (1969) Separation of cells by velocity sedimentation. *J. cell. Physiol.* **73**, 191.

11 MacDONALD H.R. & MILLER R.G. (1970) Synchronization of mouse L-cells by a velocity sedimentation technique. *Biophys. J.* **9**, 834.

12 MILLER R.G. (1976) Separation of cells by velocity sedimentation. In In Vitro *Methods in Cell-Mediated and Tumour Immunity*, (eds. Bloom B.R. & David J.R.), p. 283. Academic Press, New York.

13 MEISTRICH M.L., MEYN R.E. & BARLOGIE B. (1977) Synchronization of mouse L-P59 cells by centrifugal elutriation. *Expl Cell Res.* **105**, 169.

14 ANDERSON E.C., PETERSEN D.F. & TOBEY R.A. (1970) Density invariance of cultured Chinese hamster cells with stage of the mitotic cycle. *Biophys. J.* **10**, 630.

15 LEIF R.C. & VINOGRAD J. (1964) The distribution of buoyant density of human erythrocytes in bovine albumin solutions. *Proc. natn. Acad. Sci. U.S.A.* **51**, 520.

16 LEIF R.C. (1970) Buoyant density separation of cells. In *Automated Cell Identification and Cell Sorting*, (eds. Wied G.L. & Bahr G.F.), p. 2. Academic Press, New York.

17 SHORTMAN K. (1968) The separation of different cell classes from lymphoid organs. (II) The purification and analysis of lymphocyte populations by equilibrium density gradient centrifugation. *Aust. J. exp. Biol. Med. Sci.* **46**, 375.

18 WILLIAMS N., KRAFT N. & SHORTMAN K. (1972) The separation of different cell clases from lymphoid organs. (VI) The effect of osmolarity of gradient media on the density distribution of cells. *Immunology*, **22**, 885.

19 GORCZYNSKI R.M., MILLER R.G. & PHILLIPS R.A. (1970) Homogeneity of antibody-producing cells as analyzed by their buoyant density in gradients of Ficoll. *Immunology*, **19**, 817.

20 MARBROOK J. (1980) Linear isopyknic BSA gradients. In *Selected Methods in Cellular Immunology*, (eds. Mishell B.B. & Shiigi S.M.), p. 188. W.H. Freeman, San Francisco.

21 MATEYKO G.M. & KOPAC M.J. (1959) Isopyknic cushioning for density gradient centrifugation. *Expl Cell Res.* **17**, 524.

22 MATEYKO G.M. & KOPAC M.J. (1963) Cytophysical studies. *Ann. N.Y. Acad. Sci.* **105**, 183.

23 PERTOFT H., BACK O. & LINDAHL-KIESSLING K. (1968) Separation of various blood cells in colloidal silica-polyvinylpyrrolidone gradients. *Expl Cell Res.* **50**, 355.

24 WOLFF D.A. (1975) The separation of cells and subcellular particles by colloidal silica density gradient centrifugation. In *Methods in Cell Biology*, Volume X, (ed. Prescott D.M.), p. 85. Academic Press, New York.

25 DETTMAN G.L. & WILBUR S.M. (1979) Colloidal silica-aluminium modified-PVP density gradient centrifuga-tion: centrifuge tube wall cell adherence, aggregation, separation properties and comparison to BSA and Ficoll. *J. immunol. Meth.* **27**, 205.

26 DICKE K.A., VAN HOOFT J.I.M. & VAN BEKKUM D.W. (1968) The selective elimination of immunologically competent cells from bone marrow and lymphatic cell mixtures. *Transplantation*, **6**, 562.

27 RAIDT D.J., MISHELL R.I. & DUTTON R.W. (1968) Cellular events in the immune response. Analysis and *in vitro* response of mouse spleen cell populations separated by differential flotation in albumin gradients. *J. exp. Med.* **128**, 681.

28 RAIDT D.J. (1980) Discontinuous BSA gradients. In *Selected Methods in Cellular Immunology*, (eds. Mishell B.B. & Shiigi S.M.), p. 193. W.H. Freeman, San Francisco.

29 BÖYUM A. (1968) Separation of leucocytes from blood and bone marrow, with special reference to factors which influence and modify sedimentation properties of hematopoietic cells. *Scand. J. clin. Lab. Invest.* (Suppl. 97) **21**, 1.

30 HANNIG K. (1971) Free-flow electrophoresis. In *Methods in Microbiology*, Vol. 5B, (eds. Norris J.R. & Ribbons D.W.), p. 513. Academic Press, London.

31 HÄYRY P., NORDLING S. & ANDERSSON L.C. (1976) Charge fractionation of lymphoid cells. In In Vitro *Methods in Cell-Mediated and Tumour Immunity*, (eds. Bloom B.R. & David J.R.), p. 309. Academic Press, New York.

32 BRUNETTE D.M., McCULLOCH E.A. & TILL J.E. (1968) Fractionation of suspensions of mouse spleen cells by counter current distribution. *Cell Tissue Kinet.* **1**, 319.

33 WALTER H. (1975) In *Methods in Cell Biology*, (ed. Prescott D.M.), p. 25. Academic Press, New York.

34 SHORTMAN K., WILLIAMS N., JACKSON H., RUSSELL P., BYRT P. & DIENER E. (1971) The separation of different cell classes from lymphoid organs. (IV) The separation of lymphocytes from phagocytes on glass bead columns, and its effect on subpopulations of lymphocytes and antibody forming cells. *J. Cell. Biol.* **48**, 566.

35 ZEILLER K., HOLZBERG E., PASCHER G. & HANNIG K. (1972) Free flow electrophoretic separation of T and B lymphocytes. Evidence for various subpopulations of B cells. *Hoppe-Seyler's Z. physiol. Chem.* **353**, 105.

36 JULIUS M.H., SIMPSON E. & HERZENBERG L.A. (1973) A rapid method for the isolation of functional thymus-derived murine lymphocytes. *Eur. J. Immunol.* **3**, 645.

37 WIGZELL H. (1976) Specific affinity fractionation of lymphocytes using glass or plastic bead columns. *Scand. J. Immunol.* **5**, 23.

38 WYSOCKI L.J. & SATO V.L. (1978) 'Panning' for lymphocytes: a method for cell selection. *Proc. natn. Acad. Sci. U.S.A.* **75**, 2844.

39 PARISH C.R. (1975) Separation and functional analysis of subpopulations of lymphocytes bearing complement and Fc receptors. *Transplant. Rev.* **25**, 98.

Chapter 55
Preparative immunoselection of lymphocyte populations

S.V. HUNT

Immunotoxicity, 55.3
Nylon wool columns, 55.5
Immunoadhesion, 55.5
Affinity columns for cells, 55.6
Affinity separation in dishes ('panning'), 55.7

Rosetting ('immunogravitation'), 55.8
Separation of rosettes from non-rosetted cells, 55.10
Metrizoate-Ficoll separation, 55.11

Aggregation (rosetting the rosettes), 55.12
Immunomagnetic methods, 55.12
Antigen-binding cells, 55.13
Prospects, 55.13

A legitimate aim of the experimentalist joining battle with the complexity of interactions between different lymphocytes is to classify the cells by their surface phenotypes. For the pragmatic purposes of experimental investigation it does not really matter whether the surface property is a narrowly defined differentiation antigen (Chapter 22), specific for one stage within one cell lineage, or simply a distinguishing marker that permits the analysis of the form and function of a population. The advent of monoclonal antibodies, with their power to precisely and reproducibly define discrete molecular determinants, has given added impetus to this approach, complementing and extending straightforward physical means of separation (Chapter 54). Singly or in combination, monoclonal antibodies promise the ultimate in selective discrimination between cell subpopulations. This is not to imply that conventional polyclonal antisera are now inevitably outdated. In some cases, e.g. anti-immunoglobulin antibodies, their widespread availability and clear characterization continue to make them reagents of first choice. They avoid the questions of isotype and antibody affinity which can complicate selection of the right monoclonal for a particular separation. It is beyond the scope of this chapter to recommend particular reagents (see instead Chapters 58 and 61, and refs. 1 and 2). Nonetheless the predominant problems in immunoselection separations are nowadays not so much to find suitable antibodies but to choose and make reliable a particular separation procedure. This chapter aims to compare different methods, and to suggest detailed protocols for those with which the author is directly familiar. It extends slightly beyond a consideration of only antibody-mediated procedures. Because of its common application in separating T cells from B cells, the use of nylon-wool columns will be described. Also included is a summary of developments in techniques for isolating specific antigen-binding lymphocytes since this too relies on affinity purification.

Some general comments apply to all these methods. First, each method has its own detection threshold. It is very rare to find a cell surface marker in which each labelled cell bears a constant number of molecules and every unlabelled cell bears none. In the rat the antigen W3/25 [3], present on T-helper cells, most closely approaches this ideal and the wide gap in labelling between W3/25-positive and W3/25-negative cells makes it more likely that the same discrimination between marked and unmarked will be made by any technique regardless of its 'sensitivity'. Whether judged by fluorescence, rosetting, panning or cytotoxicity, identical frequencies should be found analytically and obtained preparatively for W3/25-positive cells. Much more common though is the situation where the antigenic site density (Chapter 38) is disperse, giving a gradation of labelling. Then the frequency of cells detected as 'positive' may well vary according to the technique. An example of a discrepancy between cytotoxicity and immunofluorescence in identifying Lyt-1 positive cells is discussed further below. The most reliable separation methods will be those whose threshold falls in the trough of the labelling profile for site densities as revealed for instance by FACS analysis. This theoretical requirement has only very rarely been subjected to direct experimental test and it is not yet possible to draw sensible practical conclusions as to relative sensitivities. One great merit of the FACS is the ability to define precisely the threshold for separation.

In connection with the choice of the right threshold the cut-off of antigen density per cell as determined by the *biological* assay of the cell's activity should be considered. The immunological performance of a mixture of cells may perhaps be due to only a minor fraction among any of the subpopulations being separated. In this case it may not necessarily be true that the distinction between positive and negative cells when looking at the total population overall, e.g. as in the FACS analytical profile, corresponds to the *functional* distinction between positive and negative made by the biological assay. The threshold revealed by function may be different from any of the thresholds of the various separation procedures. Failure to obtain a separation with one method may therefore not necessarily mean failure with another. The example of finding Thy-1 on mouse spleen colony-forming units by immuno-fluorescence but not by cytotoxicity [4] illustrates this.

Antigens at the cell surface can be labelled by direct (one-stage) or indirect (two-stage, using an anti-immunoglobulin second step) procedures. Direct labelling carries the advantages of minimum cell handling, of greater speed, since one incubation step is omitted, and of better specificity, since no problems with the second layer anti-immunoglobulin reacting directly with cells can arise. On the other hand, the extra step in the indirect procedure can be more economical of a valuable reagent (the antibody to the cell surface); it can lower the detection threshold by an amplification of the binding produced by just a single layer of antibody; and it can be more convenient to employ when several different first layers are being used in different stainings with a common second layer. In practice, indirect procedures are more widespread except with complement-mediated cytotoxicity where the complement cascade brings its own built-in amplification with it.

In some studies proof that a particular subpopulation underwrites a particular function rests on the demonstration that removal of that population of cells by an antibody ablates the function, but is taken no further. This is especially true of complement-mediated cytotoxicity procedures where there is no way to recover labelled cells because they have been killed. To rely on this interpretation is to run the risk that the removed population may be acting in some accessory but not direct role. The complementary experiment should be performed in which marker positive cells are isolated as pure as possible and the defect caused by ablation is shown to be put right. In other words a balance-sheet of functional activity as well as overall cell number should be drawn up just as enzymologists do in their purifications. Hidden collaborative processes may thereby be revealed. All this puts a premium on separation methods in which both the enriched and depleted fraction are recovered. Positive as well as negative selection should be carried out.

In calculating the audit of functional activity it is the activity per entire fraction that matters so that the sum of activity recovered after separation can be compared with that put in. The alternative means of expressing activity on a per cell (or per million cells) basis is suitable for monitoring enrichment and allows an estimate of how many-fold purification has been achieved. A population purified to homogeneity will ideally show a constant specific activity whatever separation is performed upon it, showing that each cell in it is equally active. This distinction between 'activity' and 'enrichment' separation profiles is discussed further in ref. 5. Its practical importance is that it may influence the choice of cell dose in setting up assays for functional activity.

Choosing finally which procedure to use requires striking a balance between convenience, purity, and yield. How convenient a technique is will strongly depend on how many cells must be processed, on the availability of reagents, and on whether sterility must be maintained. Purity is in general inversely related to yield and both depend heavily on the fraction of marked cells in the input. Obviously, more contamination in a positively selected population is to be expected when the initial proportion is only 1% rather than, say, 30%. Table 55.1 summarizes the characteristics of each of the methods to be described in this chapter apart from magnetic methods of which only limited experience is available. It applies to a situation where at least 25% of the starting population carries the marker of interest, such as would occur for instance in most T cell–B cell separations. There may sometimes be a case for repeating a cycle of purification when the initial proportion is very low. It may make good sense to combine two methods such as first rosetting, because of the large number of cells that can be processed, followed by sorting on a FACS to capitalize on its good purities.

The descriptions that follow are based on typical procedures applied to suspensions of lymphoid cells prepared as in Chapter 57. Attention must be paid throughout to minimizing trauma to cells, e.g. by not blowing bubbles through cell suspensions. Except where indicated, the choice of handling medium is open to the user's preference but it should contain bland protein (0.2% w/v deionized bovine albumin [6] or 2% newborn calf serum) and, normally, 10 mM-NaN$_3$ to prevent capping. (For testing function subsequently *in vivo* scrupulous washing-out of the azide is unnecessary; even 0.5 ml of 10 mM-NaN$_3$ intravenously is not toxic to a 200 g rat, though giving this amount is not recommended as a routine.)

Table 55.1. Rough yields, capacities, and purities of different methods[1]

Method	Capacity (input cells × 10⁻⁶)	Depleted fraction		Enriched fraction Purity %	Fate of input dead cells
		Purity %	Recovery %		
Complement-mediated cytotoxicity	Unlimited	>95	80–90	Not possible	Not removed[2]
Nylon wool	80–100 per column	95	50–80	Rarely tried	Largely removed
Immunoadhesion					
Panning	30 per 50 mm dish	Varies[3]	70–80	Can be 95–98	Not removed
Not removed					
Columns	100 per 10 mm column	90–95	60–70	Rarely tried	Not removed
Rosetting	100 per tube	>95[4]	70–80	>95	Eliminated from depleted fraction
Fluorescence-activated cell sorting	15 per hour	99	30–40	95–98	Removed

[1] To be taken as a very approximate guide when peripheral lymphocytes (lymph node, spleen, blood) are separated containing an initial marked subpopulation that consists of at least 25% of the total. 'Recovery' refers to yield of viable cells as a proportion of the input viable cells lacking the marker used for separation; it does not include cell losses during labelling with antibodies.

[2] Except with additional step and consequent lower yield.

[3] Depends on particular antibody. Can be 95–98%, but less predictable than other methods.

[4] Can be over 99% with a little experience.

Immunotoxicity

Ever since the discovery of bacteriolysins and haemolysins the value of antibodies as specific cytotoxic reagents has been turned to account to remove unwanted cell populations. Almost always it is complement that has been used to provide the amplification that needs to puncture the target cell. In rare cases [e.g. 7], procedures using antibody alone without complement have been tried in order to avoid the alleged unreliability of some batches of complement. These depend on the opsonising properties of some antibodies to remove cells following *in vivo* transfer. However, the gay abandon with which immunologists sort and transfer antibody-stained cells (Chapter 29) and still generally observe adequate function suggests that opsonisation is an uncertain way to remove unwanted cells from a mixture. More promising, but outside the scope of this chapter [see 8], are a variety of ways of attaching drugs or toxins to antibodies for the therapy of tumours (Chapters 36 and 37). By far the most popular methods, however, for cellular immunological experiments are those using classical complement-dependent cytotoxicity.

Using complement has the following advantages. One hit by a single antibody molecule on an erythrocyte can cause lysis [9]. This encourages the idea that the procedure is very 'sensitive', though it is not clear that the one-hit theory can necessarily be extrapolated to nucleated cells [10]. The procedure for lysis is simple. The antibody is first added at 4 °C, with sodium azide present to inhibit capping (10 mM), then washed off before addition of complement at 37 °C. Finally, and optionally, dead cells can be removed on a density gradient (Chapter 54). It has the merit also of simple scaling-up to handle large numbers of cells.

Both monoclonal and conventional polyclonal antibodies work. As examples of the former, antibodies to T cell antigens have been used: anti-Thy.1 (mouse; many different clones including 30H12, 6/68 Ho.13.4., JIJ, F7D5); anti-Lyt.1 and anti-Lyt.2 (mouse); W3/13 (rat); OKT3,4,8,11 (human, but OKT6,9 and 10 are reportedly ineffective [11]): to B cell antigens, anti-Ia (10.2.16, mouse; OKIa1, human): and to monocytes, OKMI (human). The concentration of antibody to be used should be guided by the results of a preliminary titration, which should include a measurement of the residual functional activity remaining after treatment. In scaling-up, the aim should be to retain the same final concentration of antibody in the incubation mixture as in the pilot experiment, allowing for the greater absorptive capacity of the larger number of cells in the preparative procedure which will remove some of the antibody. To test whether enough was used, the supernatant left after treatment should still be able to kill target cells in a repeat of a pilot scale experiment equally as well as the fresh antibody.

As for the source of the complement the preference of many workers for rabbit serum rests on a comparative study [12] demonstrating an eightfold higher titre of complement from this species than from guinea-pig, using mouse spleen cells as targets. Another study [13] on erythrocyte lysis showed that homologous complement (in particular components C8 and C9) was markedly less efficient than heterologous complement in comparing human, rat, rabbit and guinea-pig sources. Just as important as the titre, however, is the need to avoid natural antibody in the complement which can give spontaneous high background lysis. In certain cases absorption of guinea-pig serum with agar can reduce this [14]. If possible it is better to screen the sera from several different individuals and discard unacceptable preparations rather than attempt to absorb the unwanted antibody. To be effective, absorption needs a large amount of tissue and it is hard to avoid a reduction in the complement titre even in an absorption performed at 0–4 °C under ideal conditions. Complement should be stored at −20 °C in small aliquots to eliminate more than one cycle of freezing and thawing.

Despite its simplicity and popularity, and accepting that it can only ever be a negative selection technique, there are several strong objections to the use of complement-mediated cytotoxicity. The most compelling is that the antigen density on a cell surface necessary to initiate lysis is not defined and instead varies from one stage of the cell cycle to another [15], from one cell type to the next [16], from one antigen to the next on a given target cell (lysis of B cells by anti-immunoglobulin is not always successful, while lysis by anti-Ia antibodies often works), and perhaps even from one determinant to the next on a given antigen on a given cell [17]. Considering that the technique relies on amplification by the complement cascade of an initial local event on a slippery cell surface from which antigens are prone to disappear by capping, it is perhaps not surprising that some cells escape that 'ought' to be lysed [18]. So while there may be a rough relationship between antigen density and susceptibility to lysis under the best conditions (two-stage procedure, in the presence of azide) [19] it is by no means exact [20]. The phenomenon of antibody-mediated modulation of susceptibility to lysis [21] shows that two opposing tendencies are at work when antibodies bind to cell surfaces: complement activation, leading to lysis, and modulation, protecting against it. Modulation can occur with only mild redistribution of antigen, long before capping proper [22]. The reason for employing a two-stage procedure under non-capping conditions rather than a single-stage procedure is to minimize antigen redistribution as far as possible though even so it is impossible to stop

it completely. In the future, another way to circumvent the modulation problem may be to use monoclonal antibodies prepared either by careful proteolytic digestion [146] or by 'hybrid hybridomas' [147]. At the heart of the problem lies the fact that a cell tested for exclusion of a vital dye is either dead or not dead: there is no halfway house. Antigen density on the other hand is continuously variable within a cell population. A widely-publicized example where lysis and antibody-binding studies gave different answers is Lyt-1, which was described as a helper T cell marker in the mouse as judged by cytotoxicity, but proved by analysis on a cell sorter to be present in low amounts on B cells also [23]. The glycoprotein variously called T200 [24] (mouse), leucocyte common antigen [25] (rat; man) is found on all lymphocytes, yet in many circumstances antibodies to it behave as specifically anti-T cell cytotoxic reagents [26]. Complement-mediated cytotoxicity may provide a valid operational definition of a lymphocyte subset if it is performed under reproducible conditions, but it should not be used as an arbiter of the presence or absence of a cell surface antigen.

Another warning is perhaps more obvious. The method for checking that the unwanted population really has been destroyed by the cytotoxic treatment must include a test of function. The test must be within a range of the assay able to detect levels of contamination that would matter if they interfered in the experiment. It is no good relying just on a dye-exclusion viability test. When they were selecting Thy-1 loss variants of a leukaemic cell line by treatment with anti-Thy-1 plus complement, Buxbaum *et al.* [27] found about a quarter of their clones remained Thy-1 positive in the face of 99.9% killing as judged by trypan blue uptake. Just as the specificity of antibodies should be checked by the detection method to be employed in the experiment itself (i.e. by cytotoxicity for a cytotoxic experiment), so also the function of cell subpopulations prepared by lysis should be checked by the assay of performance to be used in the experiment proper. So, for example, when B cells are being prepared to assay T-helper function, the criterion for effective cytotoxicity of an anti-T cell reagent should be no detectable T-help remaining, not just the number of cells with helper T phenotype.

Cytotoxicity is sometimes followed by another round of purification, e.g. panning in the preparation of 'standard' mouse spleen B cells [28]. In preparing normal B cells from mouse spleen Leibson *et al.* [148] found it necessary for thorough depletion of T cells first to inject anti-T cell globulin 2 days before sacrifice and then to use a cocktail of monoclonal anti-T cell reagents *in vitro*. This belt-and-braces approach sounds attractive but the severe upset to normal physiology, together with the possibility that contaminating antibodies may directly affect the B cells [149], should inspire some caution in applying it. The alternative of two rounds of cytoxicity *in vitro* is often performed, though without good theoretical justification if the antibody and the complement have been titrated before use.

Nylon wool columns [29]

Even though specific antibody is not used in nylon wool column separations, it is convenient to include the technique here for comparison with other immunoselective methods of preparing T lymphocytes. An empirical procedure, it relies on the greater non-specific adhesion of B cells and pre-B cells to solid supports [30–32] and the mechanism of adsorption combines 'active' and 'physical' adherence [33,34]. First devised for mouse spleen and lymph nodes [29,35], it has since been extended to other species (human [36,37], rabbit [38], guinea-pig [39], rat [40]). Dead cells and phagocytic cells tend to stick, so the passed fraction is rich in viable, relatively uncontaminated T cells (purity around 95–98%; yield around 50–80% of input T cells—the higher the initial viability the better the yield and purity). There is some dispute whether the procedure is selective for different T cell subpopulations [37,41,42] and one report [43] suggests there may be biochemical alterations in the T cells due to column passage, but with these reservations the great simplicity of the method justifies its continuing popularity. Attempts to recover the B cells by compressing the wool after separation have been reported [40,44,45] but they are seriously contaminated with T and dead cells.

Materials and procedure

1 Thoroughly wash wool (0.6 g) from a Leuko Pak filter (Fenwall Laboratories) by boiling in four changes of distilled water to remove a contaminant toxic in subsequent tissue culture.
2 Pack it in a 10 ml plastic syringe barrel to the 5 ml mark and wash with about 20 ml tissue culture medium (e.g. RPMI 1640 containing 5% v/v inactivated newborn or fetal calf serum).
3 Equilibrate the column to 37 °C.
4 Load up to 10^8 cells in 1 ml of the same medium and incubate at 37 °C for 20–40 min.
5 Elution is by three successive applications of 2 ml warm medium.

Immunoadhesion

If antibody to a cell surface molecule is bonded to a solid support, then cells may be separated by affinity chromatography on the same principles as if they were macromolecules undergoing conventional biochemical purification. In this case the variations between cell populations in their natural adhesion, such as those that were exploited in the nylon-wool columns described above, work against a clean separation and ought to be minimized. Instead we rely on the specificity of the antigen–antibody interaction. This interaction can be very strong relative to the forces acting on a cell in aqueous suspension. If the calculations of Bell [46] are right, then the force required to separate just one antigenic determinant from an antibody of moderate affinity for it (10^6 l mol^{-1}) can support a cell against at least two hundred times its net weight in saline solution, quite putting to shame any trapeze artiste suspending herself by her teeth. Of course the forces acting on a cell undergoing affinity chromatography are likely to be more powerful than those due simply to gravity alone because of the shear caused by the surrounding liquid flowing past it. However, the point of this calculation is that when a cell membrane antigen meets an antibody-coated support, presumably many hundreds or thousands of times over for each cell with a reasonable antigenic site number (see Chapter 38), there is no difficulty in making a strong enough attachment to immobilize the cell. Rather, the problems are to reduce the non-specific (i.e. non-antibody-related) background binding, and to detach the cell afterwards.

Reducing the background binding is aided by working at 4 °C instead of room temperature or 37 °C, and employing a metabolic inhibitor such as 10 mM-NaN$_3$; both these measures lower the cell's metabolism and membrane fluidity so that active adherence is minimised. The choice of the material of which the solid support is made may influence non-specific binding. Cross-linked dextran ('Sephadex') and agarose ('Sepharose') and polyacrylamide, all hydrophilic substrates, have good reputations for low non-specific cell entrapment. However, even the hydrophobic plastics like polystyrene and polymethylmethacrylate or glass with its negatively charged surface can show little non-specific binding if they are pre-treated with a bland protein solution like serum albumin. During the separation there ought to be some protein present, either albumin (0.2% w/v) or serum (say 2% v/v) [47]. So although various studies [48,49] have considered theoretical and practical correlations between cell adhesion and surface wettability in different solid support materials, such differences are probably relatively insignificant in practice.

Perhaps more important in deciding the material for the solid phase is the ease of conjugation with antibody. A firm bond is of course essential; otherwise the cell will spontaneously dissociate, the antibody now being attached to it instead of the support. A variety of procedures have been devised for derivatizing the saccharides of dextran or agarose (usually by cyanogen bromide activation [50]), polyacrylamide [51], polyamides [52], and collagen [53]. Some ingenious methods (to be discussed later) for releasing bound cells introduce chemically cleavable covalent bonds. One disadvantage of coupling antibody to a porous bead such as agarose is that much of it is wasted inside the bead while cell binding occurs only at the surface. With hydrophobic supports a covalent bond is unnecessary. Physical adsorption is much simpler and adequate for the job. Proteins such as immunoglobulins bind to plastic surfaces like untreated polystyrene, for example, by immersing the plastic in a solution of protein at moderately alkaline pH (9.0 to 9.5). When the coating solution is removed, a small amount of protein, say 5%, may desorb within 30 minutes or so, but the majority leaches away only very slowly, around 1% a day, perfectly acceptable for cell chromatography (Hunt, unpublished). Any remaining adsorption sites on the plastic are covered by exposure to bland protein. The simplicity of this method of bonding antibody to a solid phase makes it the method of choice.

One further broad choice must now be made, whether to use a column method with the antibody supported on spherical beads, or to go instead for a batch method using a flat surface ('panning'). Historically, column methods were developed first, no doubt because of the ingrained habits of biochemists accustomed to molecular separations. In principle, continuous flow methods such as those afforded by a column should be very controllable, leading to populations with steadily varying properties (e.g. surface antigen density) as an elution gradient is applied. In practice, elution of cells is too difficult to control in such a precise manner and only a coarse all-or-none elution really proves possible. The only genuine advantage remaining for column methods is ready adaptability to scaling-up to handle large numbers of cells reasonably conveniently. This is done by lengthening or widening the column. For each millimetre depth of column packed with beads of a typical diameter of say 200 μm, the surface area available for adsorbing cells is roughly three to five times as great as a flat dish of the same cross-sectional area as the column cross-section. Most columns are of course packed several centimetres deep. High capacity columns can therefore be relatively compact.

On the other hand, panning methods have several features in their favour. Chief among these is the opportunity they offer of direct microscopic observation of the progress of the separation, never a bad thing to counter the tendency to examine cells as plain electronic blips on a screen. This is invaluable especially when devising appropriate methods for removing bound cells. A monolayer of cells is more accessible to physical stripping of bound cells with a jet of liquid or a rubber policeman than cells attached to beads. The shear forces applied during this stripping can generally be applied more evenly across the whole plate than those generated by liquid flowing round beads which are sure to have 'dead spots' where there is no liquid flow. It is also easier to keep sterile the solutions and dishes used in panning, whereas it is more difficult to maintain sterility for subsequent tissue culture with column methods.

Affinity columns for cells

Columns are best suited for depleting large numbers of cells, say 10^8 or more of a particular subpopulation bearing a given antigen and are therefore a rival for rosette-depletion. Unless a chemically cleavable bond such as mercury-sulphur bridge [54], or a disulphide bond [55] has been introduced during the coupling of antibody to the bead, it is usually difficult to elute the bound cells. Chromatography with lectins is an apparent exception (reviewed by Pereira & Kabat [56]; detailed descriptions in refs. 57 and 58 (wheat germ agglutinin) and in the manufacturer's instructions accompanying the commercially-available lectin-Sepharose conjugates). In this case the lectin-saccharide union can be dissociated by high concentrations of free sugar, up to 1 mg ml^{-1}. For an antigen–antibody reaction however, the equivalent procedure is only possible where a hapten like Flu (fluorescein) [51,59,60] or Ars (arsanyl) [61] has been introduced as part of an indirect, two-stage, antibody bridge. It is not usually possible to obtain other determinants in adequate concentration to elute cells competitively (but see ref. 62 for a method of eluting B cells from anti-immunoglobulin columns using a high immunoglobulin concentration). Beads that can be digested with enzymes have been used (dextranase for Sephadex [63]; collagenase for a gelatin bridge [64]).

The procedure outlined below is adapted from ref. 65 for depleting B cells using an anti-immunoglobulin column. In the more general case as noted in the introduction, any affinity technique may employ either direct or indirect labelling. A direct method needs antibody against the surface antigen of the cells being separated. In the more versatile indirect method the column is coated with antibody against immunoglobulin of species X or with staphylococcal protein A

[66] while the cells are coated with antibody raised in species X against the component on the cell membrane [67,68, reviewed in 69].

Materials and equipment

Polymethylmethacrylate beads, 200–400 μm diameter (e.g. Degalan V26; Degussa Wolfgang Ag., Hanau am Main, Germany). Remove fines by repeated decantation in water and store at 4 °C under water. Can be re-used by washing twice in 5% v/v HCl and thorough rinsing.

Glass column, 15 mm diameter, plugged with nylon mesh (200 μm) or cotton wool. Equip with flow adjuster.

Anti-immunoglobulin reagent, IgG fraction. Antibody purified by elution from a specific immunoadsorbent is preferable, so as to give a high density of reactive molecules on the column. In the Uppsala procedure [70] this immunoadsorbent purification is performed *in situ*, by first coating the beads with IgG against which the anti-Ig is raised, and then passing whole serum anti-Ig to extract the specific antibody. Excess antibody must run through to provide free valencies able to bind cells applied subsequently. These columns may extract cells carrying Fc receptors as well [71] so it is worth checking that this is not giving unwanted interference. The way to obviate the difficulty would be to make (Fab′)$_2$ fragments of the material coating the beads and of the anti-Ig antibody.

Procedure

1 Rinse beads (autoclaved if necessary) in balanced salts solution. Coat with IgG by incubation of about 2.5 mg IgG per ml beads at 45 °C for 1 h, followed by 4 °C overnight. Rinse at least twice in a fivefold volume excess of balanced salts solution and incubate at room temperature for 1 h in medium containing 10% v/v serum that is unreactive with the anti-immunoglobulin.

2 Pour column to a depth of about 250 mm ($\pm$ 100 mm) in a column of such a diameter as to yield a cross-sectional area of about 100 mm^2 per 10^8 cells to be loaded. Rinse column with at least two column volumes of medium containing 10% v/v serum, and equilibrate at 4 °C. Washed cells in suspension at 2×10^7 to 2×10^8 per ml are loaded at a flow rate of 2–2.5 ml/min and immediately eluted at the same rate, without interruption, with medium containing 10% serum.

Notes and recommendations

A single passage should remove around 90% of cells carrying surface immunoglobulin; about 60–70% of the viable cells not bearing immunoglobulin pass through, the remainder being trapped non-specifically. Higher purities can be achieved with further passages through fresh columns, but at the expense of more non-specific loss. Recovery of the retained cells from these Degalan columns has not been attempted.

The non-specific loss when using Degalan can be ameliorated with the more hydrophilic Sephadex or Sepharose. Duffey *et al.* [72] recommend treating the CNBr-derivatized Sepharose with albuminated blue dextran to reduce non-specific binding yet further. At 37 °C it has been reported that T-suppressor cells may be selectively retained by a non-specific process [73], but when checked at 4 °C [74] there was no evidence for selectivity by Sephadex.

Affinity separation in dishes ('panning')

Panning [75,76,77] is used for both enrichment and depletion of subpopulations. The opportunity it provides to monitor directly the separation using a microscope should be welcomed and exploited at every stage of the procedure: check for an even monolayer of cells spaced optimally to use the binding area most economically: obtain the ratio of binders to non-binders by dislodging the unbound cells with a gentle stream of medium, maintaining continuous observation to gain an impression of how firmly attached the bound cells are: check how many residual cells are left after elution.

The following procedure is based on ref. 78 and the author's own unpublished observations, with suggestions from S. Bell [79] and M. Dyer (unpublished).

Materials and equipment

Bacteriological grade polystyrene Petri dishes: a 90 mm diameter plate will accommodate 2–3×10^7 cells. Plates which have been treated for tissue culture are unsatisfactory; they do not permit adequate adsorption of coating antibody. Larger plates become unwieldy, smaller ones accentuate edge effects due to the meniscus of the liquid (see 'Notes'). Some workers prefer enclosed flat-sided flasks to help maintain sterility.

Anti-immunoglobulin, IgG fraction. As in the case of beads (see above) antibody affinity-purified to Ig is preferable in order to give a high density of binding sites on the plate, but successful procedures using high-titred antibody without affinity purification have been devised [76]. Again, similar observations regarding Fc receptor binding apply equally in this case as with beads.

Rubber policeman (rubber tubing stretched over suitably bent glass or stainless steel rod about 3 mm diameter).

Vaseline/paraffin wax (50/50 w/w) (optional).

Procedure

1 Coating the plate: with IgG solution in 50–100 mM-Tris, pH 9.0–9.5 at 5–50 μg ml^{-1}, cover the whole area of the plate (10 ml for 90 mm plate). Substantial adsorption will occur within 2 h, and will be virtually completely saturating at the higher concentration with an overnight soaking. This can be done either at 4 °C or room temperature. Pour off and retain solution for later re-use. One square millimetre adsorbs approximately 1 ng IgG so the solution can be employed several times. Wash the plate in PBS/azide and soak for 30 min in balanced salt solution containing 0.1% albumin or 1% serum to block any residual protein-adsorbing sites on the dish. For tissue culture work the azide may be omitted, the dishes should be sterile, the solutions filtered through 0.45 μm filters and the procedure should be performed in a laminar flow hood.

2 Introduce 2×10^7 cells in about 3 ml solution containing 10 mM-NaN$_3$ with the plate on a levelling table to encourage an even distribution of cells (Note 1).

Leave to stand for 30 min. There is no agreement as to whether 4 °C or room temperature is better for this step; this must be decided in advance by trial and error for the particular antibody. Very gently swirl the plate with the aim of dislodging cells stacked on top of each other so that they all have access to the surface of the dish. Leave for a further 30 min.

3 Remove unbound cells. Most simply, tilt the plate to drain the liquid into one 'corner' and remove with a Pasteur pipette. Then rinse, very gently running medium down the walls of the dish; repeat twice. A variant of this stage [80] is to fill the dish carefully right to the top and replace the lid without trapping an air bubble. Then invert the whole dish to allow unbound cells to sediment away from the surface. After about 30 min restore the plate to its original position and draw off the supernatant liquid. This procedure is probably more controlled in the forces applied to the bound and unbound cells.

To recover bound cells either direct a vigorous jet of medium from a Pasteur pipette across the whole surface several times and collect the liquid [81,82]; or scrape the cells away with a rubber policeman (it is awkward to retrieve the cells near the edge by this technique); or add the local anaesthetic lignocain

hydrochloride (4 mg ml^{-1} in PBS free of Ca^{2+} and Mg^{2+}) and allow to stand for 10–15 min at room temperature [83]. This helps to release the cells which can be harvested by Pasteur pipette.

Some contamination of the unbound cells recovered in the first fraction by adherent cells is common (often no more than 3–4%, sometimes much worse, depending on the antibody). The purity of the adherent fraction can approach 95–100%, again depending on the antibody. If better purities are important it may be worth considering repeating the procedure, though at the cost of some cell loss.

Notes

The walls of the dish cause a raised meniscus to form and cells tend to concentrate around the edge. This may be accentuated if the base of the dish is bowed upwards. Some *aficionados* prevent the meniscus effect by making the walls non-wettable by dipping them in molten Vaseline/wax mixture before starting, but sterility is then difficult to maintain and it may not be worth the trouble.

Variations employing staphylococcal protein A [84] are common. One short-cut is to use the bacteria themselves, without purifying the protein A [85].

Rosetting ('immunogravitation')

Lymphocyte subpopulations can be separated by gravity or in a centrifuge if cell agglutinates can be formed so as to make one subpopulation effectively larger or denser than the other. The commonest way to do this is to coat erythrocytes with antibody or other reagent to bind to a lymphocyte surface ligand, making a rosette in which the lymphocyte is surrounded by many red cells. Then if the mixture is subjected to rate sedimentation (size separation) or equilibrium sedimentation (density separation) (see Chapter 54), the rosettes separate. Usually the lymphocyte in the centre can be recovered after lysis of the erythrocytes, but the particular merit of the procedure is to obtain the non-rosetted cells, i.e. as a depletion method with the capacity to handle easily large numbers of cells (Table 55.1). Rosetting can be either direct, with an antibody recognizing a cell surface molecule being conjugated straight to the erythrocyte, or indirect, using anti-immunoglobulin as a second stage antibody (Fig. 55.1). Avidin–biotin conjugation systems have also been employed [150].

In one particular circumstance it is possible to avoid the need to coat the erythrocytes. The very widely used E-rosette technique for depleting T cells takes advantage of the natural affinity of some as yet unidentified component of the sheep red cell surface for the

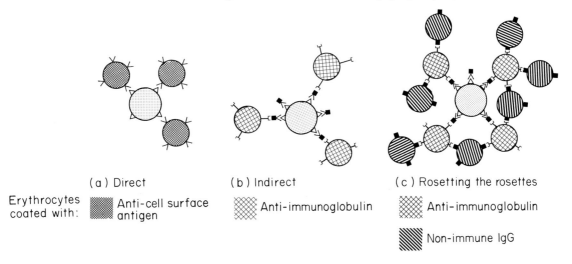

(a) Direct   (b) Indirect   (c) Rosetting the rosettes

Erythrocytes
coated with: ▨ Anti-cell surface antigen ▨ Anti-immunoglobulin ▨ Anti-immunoglobulin

▨ Non-immune IgG

Fig. 55.1. Principles of three variations of rosetting. In (c) the antibody to the cell surface and the non-immune IgG must both be recognized by the anti-immunoglobulin and should therefore be from the same species.

OKT11A antigen [86,87,88] on human T cells. The T cells of other species, pig [89,90], primates and strangely even sheep themselves [91] also form these rosettes. E-rosettes formed by normal peripheral blood lymphocytes are labile at 37 °C, though thymocytes and mitogen-activated T cells make E-rosettes that are stable at 37 °C [92]. To obtain firmly-bound rosettes the incubation should be done at 4 °C, using erythrocytes that have been pre-treated with either the reducing agent 2-aminoethylisothiouronium bromide [93] or desialylated with neuraminidase [94]. A detailed protocol is given in [95].

A situation which avoids the need for erythrocytes at all is when a cell suspension contains a very high proportion of cells bearing a particular marker which are to be depleted. Then the antibody acts as a straight agglutinating reagent and the clumped cells settle faster. This has been applied to the fractionation of mouse thymocytes using peanut agglutinin [96,97] and to the preparation of natural killer cells from mouse spleen with wheatgerm agglutinin [98]. The beauty of these lectin-induced agglutination reactions [56] is that the aggregates after separation are readily dispersed by incubation with the appropriate competing sugar: galactose for peanut and *N*-acetylglucosamine for wheatgerm. This very simple separation procedure probably only works well in a limited range of antigen- or ligand-positive cells. If too small a proportion is able to bind the antibody or lectin then the chances of an effective interaction to form an aggregate are too slight and there is interference by the negative cells. On the other hand, if the frequency is too high, over 95%

say, then losses of the negative cells due to non-specific entrapment become unacceptably severe.

Apart from these two cases, erythrocytes must be prepared by coating with antibody or other reagent detecting the membrane ligand on the lymphocyte. To prepare erythrocytes for detection of Fc receptors or complement receptors requires reaction with anti-erythrocyte antibody of the appropriate isotype respectively without or with complement (see also Chapter 48). For conjugation with antibodies to detect cell surface antigens, either IgG or (Fab')$_2$ to avoid problems of Fc binding, can be coupled using one of a variety of reagents, just as for coating erythrocytes for passive haemagglutination assays. A quick, cheap and easily stored reagent is 'matured' chromic chloride [99], for which a detailed protocol follows. Other linking agents [100] include bis-diazotized benzidine (carcinogenic) [101], carbodiimides [102,103], tannic acid [104] and tolylene diisocyanate [105]. The IgG to be coupled should contain a substantial proportion of specific antibody, over 50% if possible. Ascites for monoclonal antibodies, or anti-immunoglobulin as second-step (indirect) reagents prepared by affinity immunoadsorbent purification are suitable.

Materials

Erythrocyte preparation

The source of erythrocytes in rosetting procedures is usually sheep blood within 4 weeks of collection being preserved in Alsever's solution. To avoid unpredictable polymorphisms which can upset reproducibility through a series of experiments, many workers either pool blood from a large group of donors (more than 20, say) or reserve a single donor. Bovine erythrocytes are used where interference by the E-rosette receptor is possible. When washing blood to obtain erythrocytes, care should be taken to remove the buffy-coat cells overlying the cell pellet so as to avoid spontaneous rosette formation by the sheep leucocytes themselves [106].

For E-rosettes

Either suspend 20% erythrocytes in 0.14 M-2-aminoethylisothiouronium bromide at pH 9.0 for 15 min at 37 °C and wash four times [93,107], *or* treat erythrocytes suspended at 5% with neuraminidase (0.005 to 0.12 units ml^{-1} in different authors' hands) for 20–60 min at 37 °C [94] and wash.

For complement-receptor rosettes ('EAC') [108,109,110]

Incubate erythrocytes (final 2.5% v/v in phosphate-buffered saline) with a just sub-agglutinating dose of anti-erythrocyte antibody (e.g. serum from a day 5 bleed after a single intravenous injection with 1 ml 1% v/v erythrocytes) for 30 min at 37 °C. Wash once and remove one-fifth to provide control cells, not coated with complement. To the remaining four-fifths at 2.5% v/v in phosphate-buffered saline add C5-deficient serum to a final concentration of 10% v/v for a further 30 min at 37 °C (serum from selected rabbits or from DBA or AKR mice; serum from other sources may be used to provide complement, but careful titration to avoid haemolysis is then needed). Wash twice.

For Fc receptor rosettes ('EA')

The coating antibody here depends on the kind of Fc receptor, i.e. which heavy chain isotype it recognizes. Just sub-agglutinating doses of antiserum are added to erythrocytes at 2.5–5% v/v for 30 min at 4 °C, then washed twice.

For rosettes detecting cell surface antigens, including immuno-globulin or Ia antigens [111] on B cells

Mix, in the order stated, with vigorous stirring (e.g. vortex mixer):
0.85% (w/v) Unbuffered NaCl (3 ml). Packed erythrocytes, washed in unbuffered NaCl (0.15 ml).
Immunoglobulin (or Fab')$_2$ (0.15 mg) in about 0.15 ml unbuffered saline.
'Matured' chromic chloride, 0.1% w/v (volume deter-

mined by experiment—should be about 75 μl); continue addition in small (10 μl) aliquots until agglutination of erythrocytes is just visible to the naked eye. Stand for 5 min at 20 °C. Dilute in phosphate-buffered saline containing 2% serum or 0.1% w/v bovine albumin and wash once.

'Matured' chromic chloride

To a solution of 0.1 g CrCl$_3$.6H$_2$O in 100 ml 0.85% (w/v) unbuffered saline add 1 M-NaOH to bring pH to 5.0 (vigorous mixing during addition: if pH exceeds 6.0, precipitation occurs). Continue to adjust pH to 5.0 three times a week for three weeks and then do not adjust pH further. Solution is stable at room temperature for over two years [99].

Procedure

1   Both the lymphocytes and erythrocytes should be washed immediately before they are mixed, especially after storage, so as to prevent soluble material which may have leached away from the cell surface from inhibiting the reaction at the cell surface.
2   The cell concentration in the rosetting mixture should be between 5 and 10×10^6 ml^{-1} and the ratio of erythrocytes to cells should be 50 or 100:1 (1% v/v sheep erythrocytes is about 2×10^8 ml^{-1}). In the case of 'strong' rosettes (for complement-receptors, and most antigen–antibody interactions including anti-immunoglobulin reactions) the reaction mixture should be enclosed in a capped tube, trapping a small air bubble to mix the cell suspension as the tube turns end-over-end on a Matburn rotator at about 30 rev./min. For 'weak' rosettes (E-rosettes and many of the various Fc receptor rosettes) it may be better after a thorough initial mixing of the cells with the erythrocytes to pellet them gently together in the bottom of a centrifuge tube. For B cell Fc receptors and C3 receptors rosetting at 37 °C is recommended [108]: for all other receptors the rosetting itself should be done at 4 °C, though various pre-treatments of the cells at 37 °C are sometimes suggested for E-rosettes and Fc-receptors on T cells. Twenty to sixty minutes suffice, the shorter time being enough for the 'strong' rosettes.

Separation of rosettes from non-rosetted cells [112]

The most widely used separation procedure is density gradient centrifugation over metrizoate-Ficoll, which derives from the work of Böyum [113] on leucocyte preparation from human blood. For rosettes with human cells the same medium can be used as in the original leucocyte preparation (density = 1.076 g ml^{-1}) but in other species it can be worth experimenting with the density to minimize the leakage of non-rosetted cells [114]. In the rat, for example, a higher density (1.087 g ml^{-1}) is better. The density is raised by altering the concentration of Ficoll, since this does not affect the osmolarity significantly. This way of separating rosettes will probably be the method of choice for most people because of its familiarity and simplicity and because it yields clean populations of non-rosetted cells which are usually almost 100% viable because dead cells sink through the metrizoate-Ficoll. One sensible variant when rosettes are prepared by pelleting together the lymphocytes with the erythrocytes arranges for the dense medium to be laid over the pellet, thus causing the non-rosetted cells to float upwards during centrifuging, rather than the customary sedimentation downwards of the rosetted cells [95]. In this particular case the dense medium was colloidal silica, 'Percoll', adjusted to 1.078 g ml^{-1}, whose low viscosity is a convenient advantage [115].

It has been proposed [116] that rosettes could be separated by virtue of their greater size than non-rosetted cells, employing 1 g sedimentation (Chapter 54). The disadvantage of the extra time necessary for the separation makes this an unattractive competitor to density separation. However, one development of the rosetting technique does allow a very simple size separation and will be described below. This is based on the creation of very large aggregates, to rosette the rosettes with appropriately-coated erythrocytes and simply to allow them to settle for a short time (10 min or so) in the tube in which they are made [117]. This method can give purities almost as good as Isopaque-Ficoll separation, but it only works with indirect rosettes (Fig. 55.1).

Metrizoate-Ficoll separation

Work at 20–25 °C and bring all reagents (the density gradient, and the rosetted mixture) to this temperature before use, e.g. by a five-minute immersion in a water bath. A refrigerated centrifuge may be necessary if the friction generated by a relatively high-speed spin is not to cause overheating. A temperature of 4 °C ruins the separation.

Materials and equipment

Straight-sided centrifuge tube 100 × 15 mm, siliconed, or polycarbonate equivalent. Greater cell losses can be expected if other plastics are used.
Metrizoate-Ficoll: 10 parts by volume 'Isopaque' (= 32.8% w/v sodium metrizoate solution, Nyegaard, Oslo; or equivalent) plus 24 parts by volume Ficoll solution in distilled water (9% w/v for final density 1.078 g ml^{-1}; 14% w/v for final density 1.087 g ml^{-1}).

Procedure

1 Introduce 4 ml metrizoate-Ficoll into tube, with sterile precautions if necessary. Carefully layer rosette suspension with as little disturbance to the interface as possible (use a Pasteur pipette bent to 90° at the tip). Centrifuge with maximum acceleration at 20 °C for 20 min at 1700 g (at interface). Allow to stop without braking.
2 Discard the supernatant. Suck the top layer cells from the interface and retain them, taking all but about 1 ml of the metrizoate-Ficoll mixture, and including the cells that may have adhered to the walls of the tube. Dilute these with at least twice the volume of handling medium to recover non-rosetted cells by centrifugation. Discard the remaining metrizoate-Ficoll. The lower layer pellet may be rid of its red cells by brief exposure to buffered ammonium chloride, or in the case of complement-receptor lymphocytes by incubation at 37 °C in excess guinea-pig serum to cause complement-mediated lysis, or in the case of human E-rosettes by incubation in the patient's autologous serum [93].

Notes and recommendations

The overall cell recovery (interface plus pellet) can be expected to be 85–90%. The purity of the fractions can be checked by re-rosetting; in the top layers, less than 1% contamination is usual with the immunoglobulin and complement receptor separations. Fc receptor rosettes are more labile, and this degree of purity is less easy to achieve reproducibly.

The major hazard is non-specific leakage. Dead cells pass through the metrizoate-Ficoll layer but even with inputs of high viability some live cells also pass through. With thoracic duct lymphocytes the leakage is usually about 10% and may go up to 30% when depleting with chromic chloride treated erythrocytes; with bone marrow cells leakages as high as 60% have been noted. The leakage is less when the erythrocytes have not been coupled with chromic chloride; the presence of azide helps considerably and pre-incubation of the lymphoid cells at 37 °C instead of 4 °C may improve it slightly. However, a certain irreducible minimum still gets through, perhaps 'swept along' by unreacted erythrocytes present in considerable excess. Not even an initial purification of cells before rosetting over metrizoate-Ficoll eliminates this leakage. Hence the method is a powerful depletion technique, but less good as an enrichment technique.

Cell loads up to 10^8 are possible, increasing the

volume of the input, but above this the efficiency of the separation shows signs of deterioration. It is not difficult to set up several tubes in parallel to increase the total number of cells processed.

Aggregation (rosetting the rosettes) [117]

Materials

Erythrocytes coated with normal immunoglobulin; coat the same number of erythrocytes as were coated with anti-immunoglobulin via CrCl₃ coupling (see p. 55.10) with a crude IgG fraction (preparation by $(NH_4)_2 SO_4$ precipitation is pure enough) from normal, non-immune individuals of the species in which the antibody to the lymphocyte surface was raised (e.g. mouse Ig in the case of mouse antisera) (Fig. 55.1). It is particularly important to ensure that enough CrCl₃ is added to initiate small clumps of erythrocytes during the coupling reaction. Wash once.

Procedure

1 Work at 0–4 °C.
2 Add a suspension of these Ig-coated erythrocytes to the rosettes already prepared and mix end-over-end for 5 min.
3 Allow to settle. If good aggregates have formed, then within 5 min there should be a clear boundary between them and the non-rosetted cells plus unbound erythrocytes, which can be transferred to a separate tube. This separation can be accelerated by very gentle centrifugation (60 s at 160 *g*).
4 Some non-rosetted cells may become entrapped in the aggregates, so to improve the yield it is worth resuspending the aggregates gently in fresh medium and repeating the settling process once. After recovery of the non-rosetted cells by normal centrifugation, the surplus erythrocytes can be lysed with ammonium chloride solution.

Immunomagnetic methods

Cell separations using magnetic fields have been tried with two main advantages in prospect. First, they may be able to handle larger numbers of cells (up to 10^{10} have been tried) than centrifugation or solid-phase adsorption methods. For example, the removal of tumour cells from bone marrow by depleting tumour-specific surface antigen-bearing cells has begun to be explored clinically [118]. Second, because the magnetic field is easily applied or removed, there may be great potential in enrichment procedures since the method of release is so simple and it may not be difficult to strip magnetic marker particles from the cell surface by the

re-application suddenly of a high field [119]. Enthusiasm for magnetic separations no doubt prospers the more because of the well-established application in removing phagocytic cells that have ingested finely-divided iron [120].

The principle of the method has been established in practice and workable combinations of magnetic particles and suitable field strengths have been found. While it has proved possible to employ the weak magnetism of iron as methaemoglobin in red blood cells to separate rosetted from non-rosetted cells magnetically, very high field strengths are required, such as those generated by high-power conventional or superconducting electromagnets [121–123]. The method of choice in future is more likely to lie with the preparation of synthetic particles incorporating relatively large amounts of iron or cobalt and conjugated subsequently with antibody. Then it becomes possible to use permanent magnets, of the high strength cobalt-samarium kind if necessary, though perfectly satisfactory separations have been obtained with the older and widely available alloys. In many protocols the field is distributed throughout the column or tube being used for the separation by packing it with ferromagnetic, preferably stainless, wire. It remains to be judged which sort of magnetic particle will prove the most effective for labelling the cell surface. The main contenders at the moment are, first, polymeric beads of styrene, methacrylate or acrolein formed in the presence of colloidal iron [124,125] and, second, iron-dextran polymers [126]. The plastic beads may be conjugated to antibody by simple physical adsorption (see 'panning' earlier). They should be as monodisperse as possible so as to minimize differences in magnetic properties of the bead-cell conjugates: in one successful protocol beads of 2 μm diameter were used at a bead:cell ratio of 100:1 (roughly 1 mg beads per 5×10^6 cells) [119]. In a model system separating chicken from sheep red blood cells, very striking enrichments and depletions were recorded [125]. With some cell types there may be problems of non-specific binding and spontaneous aggregation of the beads [126]. The alternative iron-dextran ferromagnetic polymers are much smaller, around 40 nm, and can be coupled covalently and therefore permanently to proteins like staphylococcal protein A by periodate oxidation of the dextran. The particle size is suitable in addition for use as a tracer in electron microscopy. Recovery of cells in a small scale separation (10^6 cells) was good, but the purity was not documented [126]. Microspheres of cotton-seed oil–protein mixtures have also been reported [127–129] but their use is likely to be limited to heat resistant proteins since the method of preparation involves heating to 120 °C. Further experiments will have to decide the balance between ease of preparation, stability, and reproducibility in order to test the promise of these recent developments.

Antigen-binding cells

Because of their very low frequency among mature peripheral lymphocytes (approximately 10^{-4} to 10^{-5}) specific cells reactive to a single antigen must be purified with enrichment factors 3 or 4 orders of magnitude greater than in the methods discussed so far. The main requirements are the reduction of non-specific background binding and the capacity to handle large numbers of cells. Of the wide variety of ingenious techniques that were initially devised [130] the only methods apart from the FACS [131] (Chapter 29) to have provided highly enriched, functional cells are those based on panning in a flat dish. Rosetting methods [132] and columns [133] give disappointing recovery of B cell activity. In the dish technique, antigen is chemically coupled to gelatin adhering to the dish to lower non-specific background binding. The early development of this gelatin-coated plate procedure [134–136] is comprehensively reviewed in [137]. Neither cytotoxic nor helper T cells but only B cells and suppressor T cells show convincing binding [138].

Two similar panning protocols have been described. They differ mainly in the method of release of attached cells. In the Australian version [139] the gelatin is melted and any that remains adherent to the cell is digested with collagenase. This necessitates incubation at 37 °C, thus introducing the possibility of premature antigen-induced alterations in the cell. In the North Carolina version [55], the cells are preserved throughout at 4 °C by including a disulphide bridge between the antigen and gelatin which can later be reduced by thiol groups (dithiothreitol or simply 20% serum). Enrichment by better than 100-fold can be achieved, though the yield is not reported. Judged by limiting dilution analysis the frequency of specific antigen-reactive cells can be increased to between 1/10 and 1/25 by a single round of purification. Applications of these methods are discussed in refs. 140, 141 and 149.

Prospects

Two recent developments illustrate that not every biophysical or biochemical possibility has been explored. In one, a cytotoxic procedure has been devised that effectively inverts the results of conventional complement-mediated cytotoxicity. Cells are killed by a toxic agent, hydrogen peroxide, *unless* they have bound an antibody conjugate to shield them from it. Thus antibody–catalase complexes degrade

H_2O_2 in the immediate vicinity of the cell and convert cytotoxicity into a positive selection method for labelled cells [142,143]. The dividing line between protection and death is a fine one and the technique needs further development. The principle is attractive, however, and may lend itself to ready scaling-up if the correct conditions can be found.

Preparative electrophoresis of cells is another potentially valuable immunoselective technique. Normally the natural differences in net electrical charge on the cell form the basis for electrophoretic separation but the charge can also be affected if a cell population combines with antibody [144,145]. The procedure has advantages in yield, high cell throughput ($1–3 \times 10^8$ per hour) and in grading cells into different fractions according to surface antigen density. No other technique enjoys this combination of benefits and they may well justify the capital cost of the electrophoresis apparatus.

In the year of the discovery of the W-particle there is sure to be a broad-minded physicist somewhere conceiving a plan to make antibodies and therefore the cells to which they can attach susceptible to the action of a beam of intermediate vector bosons. However, with the wide range of procedures using gravitons and photons described in this chapter and already available, the 'immuno-weak force' will face strong competition for a place in the cellular immunologist's armoury.

Acknowledgements

The author is a Research Fellow of Keble College, Oxford. He is very grateful to Susan Bell and John Kemshead for their comments on parts of the manuscript, and to Paula Gaskel and Pam Woodward for typing it.

References

1 KENNETT R.H., McKEARN T.J. & BECHTOL K.B. (1980) *Monoclonal antibodies*. Plenum Publishing Corporation, New York.

2 McMICHAEL A.J. & FABRE J.W. (1982) *Monoclonal antibodies in clinical medicine*. Academic Press, New York.

3 MASON D.W., BRIDEAU R.J., McMASTER W.R., WEBB M., WHITE R.A.H. & WILLIAMS A.F. (1980) In *Monoclonal antibodies*, p. 251. Plenum Publishing Corporation, New York.

4 BASCH R.S. & BERMAN J.W. (1982) Thy-1 determinants are present on many murine hematopoietic cells other than T cells. *Eur. J. Immunol.* 12, 359.

5 MILLER R.G. (1973) Separation of cells by velocity sedimentation. In *New Techniques in Biophysics and Cell Biology*, (eds. Pain R.H. & Smith B.J.), p. 87. Wiley (John) & Sons Ltd., London.

6 SHORTMAN K. (1971) The density distribution of thymus, thoracic duct and spleen lymphocytes. *J. cell. Physiol.* **77**, 319.

7 ONOE K., YASUMIZU R., OH-ISHI T., KAKINUMA M., GOOD R.A., FERNANDES G. & MORIZAWA K. (1982) Specific elimination of the T lineage cells: effects of *in vitro* treatment with anti-Thy-1 serum without complement on the adoptive cell transfer system. *J. immunol. Meth.* **49**, 315.

8 MÖLLER G. (ed.) (1982) Antibody carriers of drugs and toxins in tumor therapy. *Immunol. Revs.* **62**, 1.

9 BORSOS T., RAPP H.J. & MAYER M.M. (1961) Studies on the second component of complement I. *J. Immunol.* **87**, 310.

10 LOSKI C.L., RAMM L.E., HAMMER C.H., MAYER M.M. & SHIN M.L. (1983) Cytolysis of nucleated cells by complement cell death displays multi-hit characteristics. *Proc. natn. Acad. Sci. U.S.A.* **80**, 3816.

11 GOTO M. & ZVAIFLEUR N.J. (1983) Characterization of the killer cell generated in the autologous mixed leukocyte reaction. *J. exp. Med.* **157**, 1309.

12 KOENE R.A.P. & McKENZIE I.F.C. (1973) A comparison of the cytolytic action of guinea pig and rabbit complement on sensitised nucleated mouse cells. *J. Immunol.* **111**, 1894.

13 HANSCH G.M., HAMMER C.H., VANGURI P. & SHIN M.L. (1981) Homologous species restriction in lysis of erythrocytes by terminal complement proteins. *Proc. natn. Acad. Sci. U.S.A.* **78**, 5118.

14 COHEN A. & SCHLESINGER M. (1970) Absorption of guinea pig serum with agar. *Transplantation,* **10**, 130.

15 KERBEL R.S. & DOENHOFF M.J. (1974) Resistance of mitotic B lymphocytes to cytotoxic effects of anti-Ig serum. *Nature,* **250**, 342.

16 LESLEY J., HYMAN R. & DENNERT G. (1974) Effect of antigen density on complement-mediated lysis, T-cell mediated killing and antigenic modulation. *J. Nat. Cancer Inst.* **53**, 1759.

17 GORDON J., ANDERSON V.A. & STEVENSON G.T. (1982) Loss of surface-bound antibody accompanying the anti-complementary modulation of leukemic B cell immunoglobulin: contrasting effects of antibodies directed against idiotypic and constant regions. *J. Immunol.* **128**, 2763.

18 OHANIAN S.H., BORSOS T. & RAPP H.J. (1970) Lysis of tumor cells by antibody and complement. (1) Lack of correlation between antigen content and susceptibility. *J. Nat. Cancer Inst.* **50**, 1313.

19 MÖLLER E. & MÖLLER G. (1962) Quantitative studies of the sensitivity of normal and neoplastic mouse cells to the cytotoxic action of isoantibodies. *J. exp. Med.* **115**, 527.

20 GORDON J., ANDERSON A., ROBINSON D.S.F. & STEVENSON G.T. (1982) The influence of antigen density and a comparison of IgG and IgM antibodies in the anti-complementary modulation of lymphocytic surface immunoglobulin. *Scand. J. Immunol.* **15**, 169.

21 OLD L.J., STOCKERT E., BOYSE E.A. & KIM J.H. (1967) Antigenic modulation. Loss of TL antigen from cells exposed to TL antibody. Study of the phenomenon *in vitro. J. exp. Med.* **127**, 523.

22 GORDON J. & STEVENSON G.T. (1981) Antigenic modulation of lymphocytic surface immunoglobulin yielding resistance to complement-mediated lysis. (II) Relationship to redistribution of the antigen. *Immunology,* **42**, 13.

23 LEDBETTER J.A., ROUSE R.V., MICKLEM H.S. & HERZENBERG L.A. (1980) T cell subsets defined by expression of Lyt-1,2,3 and Thy-1 antigens. Two parameter immunofluorescence and cytotoxic analysis with monoclonal antibodies modify current views. *J. exp. Med.* **152**, 280.

24 DENNERT G., HYMAN R., LESLEY J. & TROWBRIDGE I.S. (1980) Effects of cytotoxic monoclonal antibody specific for T200 glycoprotein on functional lymphoid cell populations. *Cell. Immunol.* **53**, 350.

25 CARTER P.B. & SUNDERLAND C.A. (1980) Biochemical identification of rat ART-1 and Ly-1 alloantigens. *Immunogenetics,* **10**, 583.

26 ELY J.M., GREINER D.L., LUBAROFF D.M. & FITCH F.W. (1983) Characterization of monoclonal antibodies that define rat T cell alloantigens. *J. Immunol.* **130**, 2798.

27 BUXBAUM J.N., BASCH R.S. & SZABADI R.R. (1977) Analysis of Thy-1 variants of murine lymphoma cells. *Somatic Cell Genet.* **3**, 1.

28 NAKANISHI K., HOWARD M., MURAGUCHI A., FARRAR J., TAKATSU K., HAMAOKA T. & PAUL W.E. (1983) Soluble factors involved in B cell differentiation: identification of two distinct T cell replacing factors (TRF). *J. Immunol.* **130**, 2219.

29 JULIUS M.H., SIMPSON E. & HERZENBERG L.A. (1973) A rapid method for the isolation of functional thymus-derived murine lymphocytes. *Eur. J. Immunol.* **3**, 645.

30 HUNT S.V. (1973) Separation of thymus-derived and marrow-derived rat lymphocytes on glass bead columns. *Immunology,* **24**, 699.

31 ADAMS P.B. (1973) A physical adherence column method for the preparation of T and B lymphocytes from normal mouse spleen. *Cell. Immunol.* **8**, 356.

32 DESLAURIERS-BOISVERT N., MERCIER G. & LAFLEUR L. (1982) The nylon wool adherence marker of the B cell lineage appears at the resting pre-B cell stage. *Eur. J. Immunol.* **12**, 285.

33 SHORTMAN K. (1972) Physical procedures for the separation of animal cells. *Ann. Rev. Biophys. Bioeng.* **1**, 93.

34 SHORTMAN K., WILLIAMS N., JACKSON H., RUSSELL P., BYRT P. & DIENER E. (1971) The separation of different cell classes from lymphoid organs. (IV) The separation of lymphocytes from phagocytes on glass bead columns and its effect on subpopulations of lymphocytes and antibody-forming cells. *J. Cell Biol.* **48**, 566.

35 TRIZIO D. & CUDCOWICZ G. (1974) Separation of T and B lymphocytes by nylon wool columns: evaluation of efficacy by functional assays *in vivo. J. Immunol.* **113**, 1093.

36 GREAVES M.F. & BROWN G. (1974) Purification of human T and B lymphocytes. *J. Immunol.* **112**, 420.

37 MASUCCI G., MASUCCI M.G. & KLEIN E. (1982) Human blood lymphocyte subsets separated on the basis of nylon adherence, sRBC and EA rosetting: natural cytotoxicity and characterization with monoclonal reagents. *Cell. Immunol.* **69**, 166.

38 REDELMAN D., SCOTT C.B., SHEPPARD H.W. & SELL S. (1976) *In vitro* studies of the rabbit immune system: (II)

Functional characterisation of rabbit T and B populations separated by adherence to nylon wool or lysis with anti-thymocyte serum and complement. *Cell. Immunol.* **24**, 11.

39 LIPSKY P.E., ELLNER J.J. & ROSENTHAL A.S. (1976) Phytohaemagglutinin-induced proliferation of guinea pig thymus-derived lymphocytes. (I) Accessory cell dependence. *J. Immunol.* **116**, 868.

40 WOAN M.C. & MCGREGOR D.D. (1981) T cell-mediated cytotoxicity induced by *Listeria monocytogenes*. (I) Activation of *Listeria* antigen-responsive cells. *J. Immunol.* **127**, 2319.

41 INDIVERI F., HUDDLESTONE J., PELLEGRINO M.A. & FERRONE S. (1980) Isolation of human T lymphocytes: comparison between nylon-wool filtration and rosetting with neuraminidase (YCN) and 2-aminoethyl isothiouronium bromide (AET)-treated sheep red blood cells (SRBC). *J. immunol. Meth.* **34**, 107.

42 YODOI J., TAKABAYASHI A. & MASUDA T. (1978) Immunological properties of Fc receptor on lymphocytes. (4) Fc receptor of ConA induced suppressor and helper T cells. *Cell. Immunol.* **39**, 225.

43 CORRIGAN A., O'KENNEDY R. & SMYTH H. (1979) Lymphocyte membrane alterations caused by nylon wool column separation. *J. immunol. Meth.* **31**, 177.

44 HANDWERGER B.S. & SCHWARTZ R.H. (1974) Separation of murine lymphoid cells using nylon wool columns. Recovery of the B cell enriched populations. *Transplantation*, **18**, 544.

45 WONG D.M. & MITTAL K.K. (1981) HLA-DR typing: a comparison between nylon wool adherence and T cell rosetting in the isolation of B cells. *J. immunol. Meth.* **46**, 177.

46 BELL G.I. (1978) Models for the specific adhesion of cells to cells. *Science*, **200**, 618.

47 HASTON W.S., SHIELDS J.M. & WILKINSON P.C. (1982) Lymphocyte locomotion and attachment on two-dimensional surfaces and in three-dimensional matrices. *J. Cell Biol.* **92**, 747.

48 GINGELL D. & VINCE S. (1980) Long-range forces and adhesion: an analysis of cell substratum studies. In *Cell Adhesion and Motility*, (eds. Curtis A.S.G. & Pitts J.D.), p. 1. Cambridge University Press.

49 MANLY R.S. (ed.) (1970) *Adhesion in Biological Systems*. Academic Press, New York.

50 AXEN R., PORATH J. & ERNBACK S. (1967) Chemical coupling of peptides and proteins to polysaccharides by means of cyanogen halides. *Nature*, **214**, 1302.

51 BARAN M.M., ALLEN D.M., RUSSELL S.R., SCHEETZ M.E. & MONTHONY J.F. (1982) Cell sorting using a universally applicable affinity chromatography matrix; solid-phase anti-fluorescein isothiocyanate antibody. *J. immunol. Meth.* **53**, 321.

52 KIEFER H. (1975) Separation of antigen specific lymphocytes. A new general method of releasing cells bound to nylon mesh. *Eur. J. Immunol.* **5**, 624.

53 WEBB C., TEITELBAUM D., RAUCH H., MAOZ A., ARNON R. & FUCHS S. (1975) Fractionation of functional lymphocytes sensitized to basic encephalitogen on derivatized collagen and gelatin gels. *J. Immunol.* **114**, 1469.

54 BONNAFOUS J.C., DORNAND J., FAVERO J., MIRIELLE S.,

BOSCHETTI E. & MANI J.-C. (1983) Cell affinity chromatography with ligands immobilised through cleavable mercury-sulphur bonds. *J. immunol. Meth.* **58**, 93.

55 CAMBIER J.C. & NEALE M.J. (1982) Isolated phosphorylcholine binding lymphocytes. (I) Use of a cleavable cross linking reagent for solid-phase adsorbent isolation of functional antigen-binding cells. *J. immunol. Meth.* **51**, 209.

56 PEREIRA M.E.A. & KABAT E.A. (1979) Immunochemical studies of lectins and their application to the fractionation of blood group substances and cells. *Crit. Rev. Immunol.* **1**, 33.

57 PEREIRA M.E.A. & KABAT E.A. (1979) A versatile immunoadsorbent capable of binding lectins of various specificities and its use for the separation of cell populations. *J. Cell Biol.* **82**, 185.

58 NICOLA N.A., BURGESS A.W., METCALF D. & BATTYE F.L. (1978) Separation of mouse bone marrow cells using wheat germ agglutinin affinity chromatography. *Aust. J. exp. Biol. Med. Sci.* **56**, 663.

59 FONG S., TSOUKAS C.D., PASQUALI J.-L., FOX R.I., ROSE J.E., RAIKLEN D., CARSON D.A. & VAUGHAN J.H. (1981) Fractionation of human lymphocyte subpopulations on immunoglobulin coated Petri dishes. *J. immunol. Meth.* **44**, 171.

60 FONG S., FOX R.I., ROSE J.E., LIU J., TSOUKAS C.D., CARSON D.A. & VAUGHAN J.H. (1981) Solid phase selection of human T lymphocyte subpopulations using monoclonal antibodies. *J. immunol. Meth.* **46**, 153.

61 CLARK N.W.T., PARKHOUSE R.M.E. & SIMMONDS R.G. (1982) Positive and negative selection of cells by hapten-modified antibodies. *J. immunol. Meth.* **51**, 167.

62 CRUM E.D. & MCGREGOR D.D. (1976) Functional properties of T and B cells isolated by affinity chromatography from rat thoracic duct lymph. *Cell. Immunol.* **23**, 211.

63 SCHLOSSMAN S.F. & HUDSON L. (1973) Specific purification of lymphocyte populations on a digestible immunoadsorbent. *J. Immunol.* **111**, 313.

64 THOMAS D.B. & PHILLIPS B. (1973) The separation of human B lymphocytes on a digestible immunoadsorbent column. *Eur. J. Immunol.* **3**, 740.

65 CAMPBELL P.A. & GREY H.M. (1972) Removal of immunoglobulin-bearing lymphocytes by anti-immunoglobulin-coated columns. *Cell. Immunol.* **5**, 171.

66 GHETIE V., MOTA M. & SJOQUIST J. (1978) Separation of cells by affinity chromatography on SpA Sepharose 6MB. *J. immunol. Meth.* **21**, 133.

67 JENSENIUS J.C. & WILLIAMS A.F. (1974) Total immunoglobulin of rat thymocytes and thoracic duct lymphocytes. *Eur. J. Immunol.* **4**, 98.

68 CANTOR H., SHEN F.W. & BOYSE E.A. (1976) Separation of helper T cells from suppressor T cells expressing different Ly component. (II) Activation by antigen: after immunization, antigen specific suppressor and helper activities are mediated by distinct T-cell subclasses. *J. exp. Med.* **143**, 1391.

69 SHARMA S.K. & MAHENDROO P.P. (1980) Affinity chromatography of cells and cell membranes. *J. Chromatog.* **184**, 471.

70 WIGZELL H. (1976) Specific affinity fractionation of lymphocytes using glass or plastic bead columns. *Scand. J. Immunol.* **5** (suppl.) 23.

71 ELDER M.E. & MACLAREN N.K. (1983) Identification of profound peripheral T lymphocyte immunodeficiencies in the spontaneously diabetic BB rat. *J. Immunol.* **130**, 1723.

72 DUFFEY P.S., DROUILLARD D.L. & BARBE C.P. (1981) Lymphocyte sorting on albuminated CIBA blue dextran-staphylococcal protein A-conjugated sepharose 6MB affinity columns. *J. immunol. Meth.* **45**, 137.

73 HOFFMAN M.K., POLLACK S., KROWN S.E. & MITTLER R.S. (1982) Deletion of active human suppressor T lymphocytes from peripheral blood by Sephadex G-10 filtration. *J. immunol. Meth.* **55**, 327.

74 KANSKI A., SPENCER J. & EREMIN O. (1981) Sephadex G-10 columns do not retain selectively T or B lymphocyte subpopulations. *J. immunol. Meth.* **42**, 147.

75 MAGE M.G., McHUGH L.L. & ROTHSTEIN T.L. (1977) Mouse lymphocytes with and without surface immunoglobulin: preparative scale separation in polystyrene tissue culture dishes coated with specifically purified anti-immunoglobulin. *J. immunol. Meth.* **15**, 47.

76 WYSOCKI L.J. & SATO V.L. (1978) 'Panning' for lymphocytes: a method for cell selection. *Proc. natn. Acad. Sci. U.S.A.* **75**, 2844.

77 MAGE M., MATHIESON B., SHARROW S., McHUGH L., HAMMERLING U., KANELLOPOULOS-LANGEVIN C., BRIDEAU D. & THOMAS C.A. (1981) Preparative nonlytic separation of Lyt-2$^+$ and Lyt 2$^-$ T lymphocytes, functional analyses of the separated cells and demonstration of synergy in graft vs. host reaction of Lyt 2$^+$ and Lyt 2$^-$ cells. *Eur. J. Immunol.* **11**, 228.

78 LEWIS G.K. & KAMIN R. (1980) In *Selected methods in cellular immunology*, (eds. Mishel B.B. & Shiigi S.M.), p. 227. W.H. Freeman, San Francisco.

79 BELL S.M., ASPINALL R. & STERN P.L. (1984) Enrichment of rat NK cytotoxicity for H2-negative murine embryonal carcinoma cells by panning and short-term culture in TCGF. *Immunology*, **53**, 23.

80 HOANG T., GILMORE D., METCALF D., COBBOLD S., WATT S., CLARK M., FURTH M. & WALDMANN H. (1983) Separation of hemopoietic cells from adult mouse marrow by use of monoclonal antibodies. *Blood*, **61**, 580.

81 TSOI M.-S., APRILE J., DOBBS S., GOEHLE S. & STORB R. (1982) Enrichment (and depletion) of human suppressor cells with monoclonal antibodies and immunoglobulin-coated plates. *J. immunol. Meth.* **53**, 293.

82 BUTTKE T.M., MALLET G.S. & CUCHENS M.A. (1983) Positive selection of mouse B and T lymphocytes and analysis of isolated populations by flow cytometry. *J. immunol. Meth.* **58**, 193.

83 WODA B.A., YGUERABIDE J. & FELDMAN J.D. (1980) The effect of local anaesthetics on the lateral mobility of lymphocyte membrane proteins. *Expl Cell Res.* **12**, 327.

84 NASH A.A. (1976) Separation of lymphocyte subpopulations using antibodies attached to staphylococcal protein A coated surfaces. *J. immunol. Meth.* **12**, 149.

85 RANDALL R.E. (1983) Preparation and use of immunoabsorbent monolayers in the purification of virus proteins and separation of cells on the basis of their cell surface antigens. *J. immunol. Meth.* **60**, 147.

86 VERBI W., GREAVES M.F., SCHNEIDER C., KOUBEK K., JANOSSY G., STEIN H., KUNG P.C. & GOLDSTEIN G. (1982) Monoclonal antibodies OKT11 and OKT11a have pan-T cell reactivity and block sheep erythrocyte receptors. *Eur. J. Immunol.* **12**, 81.

87 VAN WAUWE J., GOOSSENS J., DECOCK W., KUNG P. & GOLDSTEIN G. (1981) Suppression of human T-cell mitogenesis and E-rosette formation by the monoclonal antibody OKT11A. *Immunology*, **44**, 865.

88 KAMOUN M., MARTIN P.S., HANSEN J.A., BROWN M.A., SIADAK A.W. & NOWINSKY R.C. (1981) Identification of a human T lymphocyte surface protein associated with the E-rosette receptor. *J. exp. Med.* **153**, 207.

89 BINNS R.M. (1980) Pig lymphocyte behaviour, distribution and classification. *Monogr. Allergy*, **16**, 19.

90 OUTTERIDGE P.M., BINNS R.M. & LICENCE S.T. (1982) Subpopulations of pig blood E-rosette forming lymphocytes and thymus-dependent null cells: separation by nylon wool columns, rosette formation and macrophage-dependent mitogen and antigen responsiveness. *Int. Archs Allergy appl. Immunol.* **67**, 18.

91 OUTTERIDGE P.M., FAHEY K.J. & LEE C.S. (1981) Lymphocyte surface markers in sheep blood and lymph. *Aust. J. exp. Biol. Med. Sci.* **59**, 143.

92 WAUWE J. van & GOOSSENS J. (1982) E-rosette formation at 37 °C: analysis with monoclonal antibodies. *Cell. Immunol.* **68**, 181.

93 MADSEN M., JOHNSEN H.E., HANSEN P.W. & CHRISTIANSEN S.E. (1980) Isolation of human T and B lymphocytes by E-rosette gradient centrifugation. Characterisation of the isolated sub-populations. *J. immunol. Meth.* **33**, 323.

94 WEINER M.S., BIANCO C. & NUSSENZWEIG V. (1973) Enhanced binding of neuraminidase-treated sheep erythrocytes to human T lymphocytes. *Blood*, **42**, 939.

95 OWNBY D.R. & McCULLOUGH J. (1983) An improved technique for separating rosetted from non-rosetted lymphocytes. *J. immunol. Meth.* **56**, 281.

96 REISNER Y., LINKER-ISRAELI M. & SHARON N. (1976) Separation of mouse thymocytes into two subpopulations by the use of peanut agglutinin. *Cell. Immunol.* **25**, 129.

97 REISNER Y., RAVID A. & SHARON N. (1976) Use of soybean agglutinin for the separation of mouse T and B lymphocytes. *Biochem. biophys. Res. Commun.* **72**, 1586.

98 SARON M.-F., TRUFFA-BACHI P. & GUILLON J.-C. (1983) Rapid enrichment of mouse natural killer cells by use of wheat germ agglutinin. *J. immunol. Meth.* **59**, 151.

99 GODING J.W. (1976) The chromic chloride method of coupling antigens to erythrocytes: definition of some important parameters. *J. immunol. Meth.* **10**, 61.

100 HERBERT W.J. (1976) Passive haemagglutination with special reference to the tanned cell technique. In *Handbook of Experimental Immunology*, 3rd edn., (ed. Weir D.M.), p. 20.1. Blackwell Scientific Publications, Oxford.

101 PRESSMAN D., CAMPBELL D.H. & PAULING L. (1942) The agglutination of intact azoerythrocytes by antisera homologous to the attached groups. *J. Immunol.* **44**, 101.

102 JOHNSON H.M., BRENNER K. & HALL H.E. (1966) The use of a water soluble carbodiimide as a coupling reagent in the passive haemagglutination test. *J. Immunol.* **97**, 971.

103 JOHNSON H.M., SMITH B.G. & HALL H.E. (1968) Carbodiimide haemagglutination: a study of some of the variables of the coupling reaction. *Int. Archs Allergy appl. Immunol.* **33**, 511.

104 WALKER S.M., MEINKE G.C. & WEIGLE W.O. (1979) Separation of various B-cell subpopulations from mouse spleen. (I) Depletion of B-cells by rosetting with glutaraldehyde-fixed, anti-immunoglobulin-coupled red blood cells. *Cell. Immunol.* **46**, 158.

105 GYENES L. & SEHON A.H. (1964) The use of tolylene di-isocyanate as a coupling reagent in the passive haemagglutination reaction. *Immunochemistry*, **1**, 43.

106 O'NEILL P.A., WOODSON D.L. & MACKLER B.F. (1978) EAC-rosette-forming lymphocytes in commercial preparations of sheep erythrocytes. *J. Immunol.* **121**, 2586.

107 KAPLAN M.E. & CLARK C. (1974) An improved rosetting assay for the detection of human T lymphocytes. *J. immunol. Meth.* **5**, 131.

108 PARISH C.R. & HAYWARD J.A. (1974) The lymphocyte surface. (I) Relation between Fc receptor, C′3 receptors and surface immunoglobulin. *Proc. R. Soc.* Series B, **187**, 47.

109 GORDON J. & ANDERSON V.A. (1980) Isolation and characterization of leukaemic B lymphocytes: influence of anticoagulant on C3-receptor detection, humoral killing and capping of cell surface immunoglobulin. *J. immunol. Meth.* **38**, 295.

110 LINDSTEN T. & ANDERSSON B. (1981) Studies on functional subpopulations of B cells in mice. Correction of the immune defect of CBA/N mice by transfer of C3-receptor bearing B cells. *Cell Immunol.* **61**, 386.

111 HARADA H., OGATA K., KASAHARA T., SHIORI-NAKANO K. & KAWAI T. (1983) Isolation of Ia positive human leukocytes by a direct rosette assay. *J. immunol. Meth.* **59**, 189.

112 PARISH C.R. & HAYWARD J.A. (1974) The lymphocyte surface. (II) Separation of Fc receptor, C3 receptor and surface immunoglobulin-bearing lymphocytes. *Proc. R. Soc.* Series B, **187**, 65.

113 BÖYUM A. (1968) Separation of leucocytes from blood and bone marrow. *Scand. J. clin. Lab. Invest.* **21**, Suppl. 97.

114 PARISH C.R., KIROV S.M., BOWERN N. & BLANDEN R.V. (1974) A one-step procedure for separating mouse T and B lymphocytes. *Eur. J. Immunol.* **4**, 808.

115 FEUCHT H.E., HADAM M.R., FRANK FR. & RIETH-MÜLLER G. (1980) Efficient separation of human T lymphocytes from venous blood using PVP-coated colloidal silica particles (Percoll). *J. immunol. Meth.* **38**, 43.

116 KARNSTROM U. & HALLBERG T. (1983) Separation of lymphocyte subsets by expanding velocity sedimentation of E-rosettes at unit gravity. *J. immunol. Meth.* **59**, 349.

117 MASON D.W. (1981) Subsets of T cells in the rat mediating lethal graft-versus-host disease. *Transplantation*, **32**, 222.

118 POYNTON C.H., DICKE K.A., CULBERT S., FRANKEL L.S., JAGANNATH S. & READING S.L. (1983) Immunomagnetic removal of CALLA positive cells from human bone marrow. *Lancet*, **i**, 524.

119 KEMSHEAD J. Personal communication.

120 MISHELL B.B. & SHIIGI S.M. (1980) In *Selected methods in cellular immunology*, p. 179. W.H. Freeman, San Francisco.

121 OWEN C.S., WINGER L.A., SYMINGTON F.W. & NOWELL P.C. (1979) Rapid magnetic purification of rosette-forming lymphocytes. *J. Immunol.* **123**, 1778.

122 OWEN C.S. (1981) High gradient magnetic separation of rosette-forming cells. *Cell. Biophys.* **3**, 141.

123 OWEN C.S., BABU U.M., COHEN S.W. & MAURER P.H. (1982) Magnetic enrichment of antibody-secreting cells. *J. immunol. Meth.* **51**, 171.

124 MOLDAY R.S., YEN S.P.S. & REMBAUM A. (1977) Application of magnetic microspheres in labelling and separation of cells. *Nature*, **268**, 437.

125 REMBAUM A., YEN R.C.K., KEMPNER D.H. & UGELSTAD J. (1982) Cell labelling and magnetic separation by means of immunoreagents based on polyacrolein microspheres. *J. immunol. Meth.* **52**, 341.

126 MOLDAY R.S. & MacKENZIE D. (1982) Immunospecific ferromagnetic iron-dextran reagents for the labelling and magnetic separation of cells. *J. immunol. Meth.* **52**, 353.

127 WIDDER K.J. (1979) Magnetic protein A microspheres: a rapid method for cell separation. *Clin. Immunol. Immunopath.* **14**, 395.

128 KAUDZIA J., ANDERSON M.J.D. & MÜLLER-RUCHHOLTZ W. (1981) Cell separation by antibody-coupled magnetic microspheres and their application in conjunction with monoclonal anti HLA antibodies. *J. Cancer Res. clin. Oncol.* **101**, 165.

129 OVADIA H., CARBOUE A.M. & PATERSON P.Y. (1982) Albumin magnetic microspheres: a novel carrier for myelin basic protein. *J. immunol. Meth.* **53**, 109.

130 HUNT S.V. (1978) The separation of lymphocyte subpopulations. In *Handbook of Experimental Immunology*, 3rd edn., (ed. Weir D.M.), p. 24.14. Blackwell Scientific Publications, Oxford.

131 JULIUS M.H. & HERZENBERG L.A. (1974) Isolation of antigen-binding cells from unprimed mice. *J. exp. Med.* **140**, 904.

132 WALKER S.M. & WEIGLE W.O. (1979) Separation of various B-cell subpopulations of mouse spleen. (II) Depletion of antigen-specific B cells by rosetting with glutaraldehyde fixed antigen-coupled red blood cells. *Cell. Immunol.* **46**, 170.

133 SCOTT D.W. (1976) Antifluorescein affinity columns. Isolation and immunocompetence of lymphocytes that bind fluoresceinated antigens *in vivo* or *in vitro*. *J. exp. Med.* **144**, 69.

134 HAAS W., SCHRADER J.W. & SZENBERG A. A new, simple method for the preparation of lymphocytes bearing specific receptors. *Eur. J. Immunol.* **4**, 565.

135 HAAS W. & LAYTON J.E. (1975) Separation of antigen-specific lymphocytes. (1) Enrichment of antigen-binding cells. *J. exp. Med.* **141**, 1004.

136 HAAS W. (1975) Separation of antigen-specific lympho-

cytes. (II) Enrichment of hapten-specific antibody-forming cell precursors. *J. exp. Med.* **141,** 1015.

137 HAAS W. & VON BOEHMER H. (1978) Techniques for separation and selection of antigen-specific lymphocytes. *Curr. Top. Microbiol. Immunol.* **84,** 3.

138 JENSENIUS J.C. & WILLIAMS A.F. (1982) The T lymphocyte antigen receptor—paradigm lost. *Nature,* **300,** 583.

139 NOSSAL G.J.V., PIKE B.L. & BATTYE F.L. (1978) Sequential use of hapten-gelatin fractionation and fluorescence-activated cell sorting in the enrichment of hapten-specific B lymphocytes. *Eur. J. Immunol.* **8,** 151.

140 VAUX D.L., PIKE B. & NOSSAL G.J.V. (1981) Antibody production by single, hapten-specific B lymphocytes: an antigen-driven cloning system free of filler or accessory cells. *Proc. natn. Acad. Sci. U.S.A.* **78,** 7702.

141 PIKE B.L., VAUX D.L., CLARK-LEWIS I., SCHRADER J.W. & NOSSAL G.J.V. (1982) Proliferation and differentiation of single hapten-specific B lymphocytes is promoted by T-cell factors distinct from T-cell growth factor. *Proc. natn. Acad. Sci. U.S.A.* **79,** 6350.

142 LAKOW E. & BASCH R.S. (1981) Positive immunoselection using antibody–enzyme complexes. *J. immunol. Meth.* **44,** 135.

143 BASCH R., BERMAN J.W. & LAKOW E. (1983) Cell separation using positive immunoselective techniques. *J. immunol Meth.* **56,** 269.

144 HANSEN E. & HANNIG K. (1982) Antigen-specific electrophoretic cell separation: (ASECS): isolation of human T and B lymphocyte subpopulations by free-flow electrophoresis after reaction with antibodies. *J. immunol. Meth.* **51,** 197.

145 DUMONT F. & HABBERSETT R.C. (1982) Electrophoretic fractionation of murine lymphoid cells. (1) Enrichment of peripheral T lymphocyte subsets with distinct surface phenotypes. *J. immunol. Meth.* **53,** 233.

146 GLENNIE M.J. & STEVENSON G.T. (1982) Univalent antibodies kill tumour cells *in vitro* and *in vivo. Nature,* **295,** 712.

147 COBBOLD S.P. & WALDMANN H. (1984) Therapeutic potential of monovalent monoclonal antibodies. *Nature,* **308,** 460.

148 LEIBSON H.J., MARRACK P. & KAPPLER J.W. (1981) B cell helper factors. 1. Requirements for both interleukin 2 and another 40 000 Mol. Wt. factor. *J. exp. Med.* **154,** 1681.

149 PIKE B.L. & NOSSAL G.J.V. (1984) A reappraisal of T-independent antigens. *J. Immunol.* **132,** 1687.

150 WORMMEESTER J., STIEKEMA F. & DE GROOT K. (1984) A simple method for immunoselective cell separation with the avidin–biotin system. *J. immunol. Meth.* **67,** 389.

Chapter 56
Genetic markers for following cell populations

J. D. ANSELL & H. S. MICKLEM

Marked animals, 56.1
Cytological markers, 56.2

Biochemical markers, 56.7
Immunological markers, 56.13

Use of markers in combination, 56.14

Cell markers have been used extensively by developmental biologists for determining the origins, lineages and spatial arrangements of cells in developing organisms and also more indirectly for estimating the numbers of cells founding particular tissues during differentiation and organo-genesis. Whilst the haematologist or developmental biologist may have slightly different requirements for cell markers for analysis of, say, B-cell ontogeny, the fate of lymphoid cells after transplantation or the production of blood cells from their bone marrow precursors, the principles governing the choice of markers for any particular purpose are essentially the same.

Whether cell markers are endogenous or have been inserted into an animal artificially, they should ideally meet the six criteria discussed by McLaren [1], Oster-Granite & Gearhart [2] and West [3]. Such a marker would be: (1) fixed and localized to the cell—not secreted; (2) autonomous—not transferred to neighbouring cells or otherwise affecting them; (3) stable for the lifetime of the cell and in its daughters; (4) ubiquitous—in all cells under study and at all stages of development; (5) easy to detect and, where applicable, to measure with some precision; and (6) developmentally neutral—not affecting a cell's behaviour or conferring any physiological advantage or disadvantage. In addition, the marker should be readily accessible without recourse to complex preparation of animals (e.g. interspecies chimaeras).

As West [3] rightly points out, the ideal marker does not exist nor does every experiment demand its full range of attributes. For example, the potential scope of the Igh allotype markers is enhanced by their presence on serum immunoglobulin (Ig) molecules as well as on the B-cell surface. One's choice of system depends on the questions being asked, the cell type under study and the degree of precision required.

The purpose of this chapter is to outline the choices and suitability of some of the markers available to immunologists and some of the techniques for their use. The authors do not attempt a comprehensive listing of all the markers available. For the mouse such a list has been made by Green, in *Genetic Strains and Variants of the Laboratory Mouse* [4]. Brief mention only is made of those markers that are covered elsewhere within these volumes, e.g. the antigens of the T-cell series. The systems discussed fall into four broad categories: (1) cytological—both nuclear and cytoplasmic; (2) biochemical; (3) immunological; (4) combinations of markers and strategies for their use.

Marked animals

Natural occurrence

Natural cell markers occur by virtue of tissue mosaicism. In mammals, the majority of mosaics exist as a result of X-chromosome inactivation [5]. Early in development one of the two X-chromosomes in female cells is inactivated; these cells and their daughters will then express the products of genes on one X-chromosome or the other but not both. This event is apparently irreversible [6]. Consequently, when an animal is heterozygous for the alleles of any particular X-chromosome encoded gene, its tissues are composed of clones of cells expressing one or other allelic product, sometimes localized in patches. The size and number of these patches relate to the number of cells founding the tissue and the number of divisions required for the final differentiated state. The number of polymorphisms encoded on the X-chromosome is small, but these have many applications.

Mosaicism also exists for (autosomally encoded) immunoglobulin gene products. In this case the phenomenon is called allelic exclusion; only the products of one chromosome for both heavy and light chain genes are expressed [7]. Thus, as with X-chromosome mosaics, cellular mosaicism exists for the immunoglobulin allotypes. Somatic mutations early in embryogenesis, which are developmentally neutral, also give rise to uniquely marked clones of cells. These may be useful, especially those with chromosome rearrangements, but they are difficult to induce or study in a systematic way.

Individuals classed as naturally occurring chimaeras may also arise. These are derived from more than one zygote and may be either primary or secondary in character. Primary chimaeras can putatively arise by a number of different mechanisms (see McLaren [1]) and can result in individuals containing both male and female cell lines and/or a variety of different markers. Secondary chimaeras arise after cross-tranfusions between fetus and mother [8,9] or between embryos sharing a common placenta, e.g. freemartins in cattle [10]. In secondary chimaeras, marked cell lines carrying different histocompatibility phenotypes or red blood cell antigens are normally found only in the blood and haematopoietic tissues.

Artificial construction

Naturally occurring mosaics and chimaeras will only provide a limited number of marker systems and, more often than not, chimaeric animals containing appropriately marked cells will have to be constructed. These again may be regarded as primary or secondary [1]. Primary chimaeras or tetraparental animals are generated by association of pre-implantation embryos of up to 16 cells [11,12,13] or by directly injecting inner cell mass cells from one blastocyst into another [14]. Pre-implantation stage embryos will tend to stick together and aggregate. After a short time in culture the aggregated embryos can be transferred back into the uteri of foster mothers and a chimaera containing cell contributions from its constituent embryos will develop. Up to sixteen embryos, as well as isolated blastomeres or parts of embryos, have been combined in this way [13]. Techniques of making chimaeras by injection of inner cell mass cells into the blastocol cavity of the blastocyst are especially useful if interspecies chimaeras are needed [14]. Xenogeneic inner cell mass cells aggregate and develop with host inner cell mass cells surrounded by an intact trophoblast layer of the host embryo: in this way the usual graft rejection problems of interspecies crosses are avoided [15].

The construction of primary chimaeras is technically demanding, the expertise for it lying in the hands of relatively few people. The detailed techniques are described elsewhere [16] and will not be covered here.

In the context of this chapter, artificially constructed secondary chimaeras are those derived by transplantation of bone marrow or isolated haematopoietic (including lymphoid) cell populations into normal, X-irradiated or otherwise preconditioned recipients [17]. Bone marrow, intravenously injected as a single-cell suspension, will establish itself and contribute to the formation of blood cells in the transplanted individual. The degree of repopulation by donor bone marrow will depend on the source and number of cells injected and the degree to which the host's marrow has been ablated. Lethally irradiated mice can be repopulated with less than 10^5 syngeneic bone marrow cells [18], whereas 10^8 such cells are required to achieve up to 30% repopulation in a non-irradiated individual [19].

A variety of markers can be included in this type of chimaera. Normally, donor and host are histocompatible unless the aim of the experiments is to study graft-versus-host or host-versus-graft reactions. Binomial statistical analysis of mosaicism can be used (in both natural and artificial chimaeras) to estimate the numbers of cell clones contributing to tissues. Detailed discussions of this type of statistical treatment can be found in refs. 99–103.

Cytological markers

Chromosomal markers

The earliest use of chromosomally marked cells in bone marrow transplantation experiments was that of the stable radiation-induced T6 reciprocal chromosome translocation (T14:15/6Ca) between chromosomes 14 and 15 [20,21,22]. The translocation is unequal, one of the two products being about half the length of the shortest pair of normal autosomes and easily identifiable in a mitotic preparation by its size and characteristic shape. The translocation was subsequently back-crossed on to the CBA/H mouse background and a congenic stock derived carrying two small T6 chromosomes. The translocation appears to be neutral and competitive repopulation experiments showed that possession of T6 chromosomes conferred no proliferative advantage or disadvantage on haematopoietic cells [23]. T6 chromosome markers have been used extensively in investigations of haematopoietic differentiation either to distinguish between host and a single donor, or in the establishment of radiation chimaeras injected with two differentially marked cell populations [23]. For example, mixtures of cells carrying one or two chromosomally marked populations from different sources may be used to repopulate a host carrying no such marker.

In this context, 'unique' chromosome markers have also been used to follow cell populations after transplantation. The sources of such clones are the occasional animals that survive radiation close to the LD_{100}. In these animals surviving bone marrow stem cells display one or more uniquely rearranged, but apparently viable karyotypes [17]. With such substantial chromosomal abnormalities, the standard Giemsa or lacto-acetic orcein stains of mitotic figures are sufficient to identify the chromosome rearrangements. A more recent staining method [26] has been used to identify with certainty the Y chromosome as a marker in male–female or female–male bone marrow transplantation [19].

The following methods for chromosome spreading and staining are largely based on those of Ford [22].

Methods

Preparation of mice

Colchicine or its derivative demecolcine (Sigma D7385) is injected intraperitoneally at 4 μg/g body weight. Mice are killed 1–2 h after injection—a longer interval yields more mitoses but of lower overall quality.

Preparation of tissues

1   Tissues are dissected with a minimum of adhering fat into a balanced salt solution such as Hanks'. Bone marrow is obtained by removing the epiphyses of the bones and flushing out the marrow with a 23-gauge needle, taking care to avoid air bubbles. It has been reported [24,25] that increased yields of stem cells with different self-renewal characteristics can be obtained from the marginal areas of the bone by more vigorous flushing with a 21-gauge needle. Cell clumps are broken up by aspiration through the syringe needle. Other tissues are teased apart in a watch-glass or small Petri dish with fine forceps. If it is undesirable for mice to have been exposed to colchicine because some of its cells are to be used for other purposes, aliquots of single-cell suspensions obtained from untreated mice at this stage may be exposed to colchicine *in vitro* in a suitable medium at 37 °C. This procedure generally results in fewer mitoses.
2   Cell suspensions are left undisturbed for 5 mins to allow macroscopic clumps and debris to settle, transferred to round-bottomed tubes and centrifuged at 50 *g* for 5 min. Quantity of tissue and tube size should be such that centrifugation forms a hemispherical pellet about 1 mm thick.

Hypotonic treatment

After centrifugation the supernatant is removed, the cells are resuspended gently in hypotonic (0.75%) KCl, and left for 8–12 min. The longer time may be more suitable for spleen and lymph node cells and the shorter for thymus and bone marrow. The cells are centrifuged again at 50 *g* for 5 min.

Fixation

Fixation is the most critical stage and requires several steps.
1   Immediately after centrifugation, KCl is carefully removed from the cell pellet.
2   Ice-cold freshly prepared fixative (3:1, absolute ethanol (or methanol): glacial acetic acid) is run gently down the side of the tube so as not to disturb the pellet.
3   With the tip of the pipette just above the meniscus the tube is *carefully* filled to above the level previously reached by the KCl to remove water from the sides of the tube, still leaving the pellet undisturbed.
4   This fixative is immediately removed and replaced with 0.2–0.5 ml fresh fixative.
5   After 3–5 min, the fixative is again removed. The cells are gently resuspended in fresh fixative and left on ice for 10 min.
6   The cells are then centrifuged and resuspended again in fresh fixative.

Spreading

Spreading may be performed immediately, but if the results are unsatisfactory a further 1–2 h fixation (on ice), followed by a further change of fixative, may help. Clean, grease-free microscope slides are essential. They should be cleaned in chromic acid solution rinsed, thoroughly with distilled water and dried before use. Clean slides can also be stored indefinitely in ethanol.
1   A droplet of fixed cell suspension is placed on the slide. It should then spread out evenly towards the edge of the slide.
2   The slide is examined under a bench lamp; when contraction of the edge begins (indicated by the presence of Newton's rings), final evaporation is hastened by blowing gently on the surface.

The slide is examined under phase-contrast illumination at ×100 total magnification. Ideally cells should be well spaced, interphase cells non-refractile and dark grey in appearance. Mitotic cells should be numerous, with chromosomes adequately spread to avoid overlap but not so dispersed that they get lost or mixed with other cells. The attainment of these ideals is still less a matter of science than of art and good luck, but the authors have found this method to give generally consistent results. Other authors favour spreading in 60% acetic acid and/or the use of cooled slides. These methods may be tried if particular cells fail to spread satisfactorily with the method given above.

Staining

Many more or less sophisticated staining techniques

are available for chromosomes. Two are described here which are adequate for substantial chromosomal translocations and the Y chromosome respectively.

Orcein staining: a stock solution of orcein is prepared by grinding 1 g natural or synthetic orcein in a mortar with the addition of 2 ml of a 1:1 mixture of 70–80% DL-lactic acid and glacial acetic acid. Thirty millilitres of lactic acid is stirred into this mixture. The stain is prepared by adding 0.8–1 ml of distilled water to 2 ml stock and filtering or centrifuging immediately before use. A drop of the stain is placed on to a coverslip and lowered on to the slide. Such preparations may be used for 2 or 3 days, and may, if necessary, be rejuvenated by soaking in 75% acetic acid and restaining. Overstaining can be reduced by adding more water to the stock, pale chromosomes and overstaining of the cytoplasm may be overcome by adding less water to the stock.

Giemsa staining for the C-banding technique [26]: this particular technique was kindly communicated by Drs J.H. Tjio and G. Brecher.

Materials

1 N-Hydrochloric acid.
0.3 M-Barium hydroxide.
Hypertonic citrate saline (0.03 M-sodium citrate and 0.3 M-NaCl).
Gurr's Giemsa solution and Gurr's buffer solution, pH 6.8 (BDH Chemicals Ltd., Poole, U.K.).

Procedure

1 Dried chromosome spreads are incubated in freshly prepared 0.2 N-HCl for 1 h and then rinsed in deionized water.
2 Further incubation is carried out in freshly prepared barium hydroxide solution (10–20 ml of stock diluted to 50 cm^3 with water) for 1.5–2 min and then rinsed in deionized water. Slides spread more than 2 days previously require a longer incubation than freshly prepared slides.
3 The slides are incubated in hypertonic citrate saline at 60 °C for a further hour and rinsed once more.
4 They are stained for 15 min in Giemsa freshly made up by adding 2 ml Gurr's Giemsa to 48 ml Gurr's buffer solution and filtering.
5 Finally, the slides are rinsed and dried.

If chromosomes are too heavily stained, the incubation time in barium hydroxide or its concentration should be reduced. Too little contrast requires longer in barium hydroxide. Room temperature may also affect staining. If it is very warm, it is effective to decrease the HCl concentration from 0.2 N to 0.15 N. If

it is cold, the incubation time in barium hydroxide should be increased.

Examples of orcein-stained T6 marked cells and Giemsa-stained male cells are shown in Figs. 56.1 and 56.2 respectively.

Scoring of chromosome spreads

It is easy to be misled by chromosome analyses in any of several ways. Some sources of error are inherent in the method itself and are largely unavoidable; others arise from bias in the scoring procedure and can be minimized by careful attention to technique.

Inherent sources of error

Since only mitotic cells can be analysed, a slowly cycling cell population will be under-represented

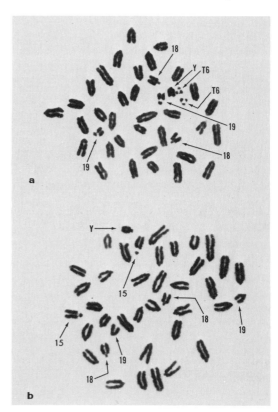

Fig. 56.1. Mitotic figures of chromosomally marked CBA/T6T6 (a) and normal CBA/Ca (b) male mouse nuclei, stained with lacto-acetic orcein. The marked nucleus has two T6 chromosomes, which are smaller than the Y-chromosome and the smallest autosomes. The tripartite shape of the T6 chromosomes is characteristic, but not so clearly visible in all metaphase spreads. (Photographs by C.E. Ford, previously published in ref. 20.)

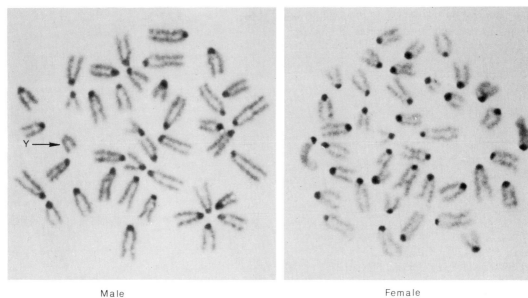

Male   Female

NORMAL

Fig. 56.2. Mitotic figures of male and female nuclei from DBA/2 mice, stained with Giemsa. The Y-chromosome is easily identified by the absence of darkly stained centromeric heterochromatin. Photographs kindly provided by Dr J.-H. Tjio.

compared to a rapidly cycling one. Irrespective of cycle time, different types of cell may be unequally represented. Since single-cell suspensions are used, cells that are part of the supporting stroma may be scarce or absent, as may any relatively fragile cells. Moreover, good fixation and spreading of the chromosomes, resulting in scorable mitotic figures, may be more easily achieved with some cells than with others.

Avoidance of scoring bias

This is not a simple matter. Bias can arise both from the scorer's expectations of the outcome of the experiment and from insufficient care. The following routine measures help to minimize such errors. (1) Preparations from each cell suspension should be scored by at least two observers, and chi-square tests should be used to monitor inconsistencies. (2) Slides should be coded, although the value of this procedure should not be exaggerated: it is too easy to get a 'feel' for how an experiment is turning out and this can only be avoided completely if coded material from several experiments is being scored concurrently. (3) Slides should be scanned at a magnification ($\sim 100 \times$) great enough to evaluate the quality of each mitotic spread, but too low to identify individual chromosomes. At this stage, a firm decision is made whether or not to score a cell before switching to a high-power objective.

Marker (e.g. T6 or Y) chromosomes can often be seen under high power even in technically poor spreads. Unless this procedure is followed, there is a danger of accepting marked cells into the record, while rejecting as unscorable cells of comparable quality in which no marker can be seen. (4) The chromosomes should be counted and presence of the correct number (40 in the mouse) verified. An apparent count of 39, or even 38, may be obtained if 1 (or 2) T6 chromosomes are obscured by an adjacent larger chromosome (where more careful study may reveal them). Conversely, the Y chromosome may divide prematurely and the separated chromatids mimic T6 in size (though not shape).

Attention to the above points is particularly necessary when three or more distinguishable cell populations are present (e.g. 2T6, 1T6 and normal) or when one is dealing with unique clonal markers.

For most purposes, enzyme markers (see below) seem likely to replace chromosome markers since the techniques are far less laborious. At present, however, they are still limited to distinguishing between two or three cell populations in a single specimen. By combining T6 and Y chromosome markers, on the other hand, one could theoretically distinguish six populations. Such a system would be demanding to work with and probably of limited utility; but multiple markers of this kind, or multiple clonal markers based on unique translocations, may be the only context in which chromosomes can now compete with enzymes.

A considerable number of chromosome markers are now available on inbred backgrounds in the mouse (see review by Searle [27]). However, T6 has been most commonly used in immunological and haematological studies and is probably at least as satisfactory in practice as any other.

DNA markers

Obviously the use of chromosome analysis is restricted by two disadvantages: (1) it only takes account of dividing cells and hence may not be representative of the whole tissue under study; (2) it cannot be used *in situ* since the procedure involves destruction of the tissue. The search for cytological markers that could be analysed *in situ* led Le Douarin and her colleagues to exploit the difference between the heterochromatic chromatin of chick and quail nuclei [28,29]. While chick cells do not show any identifiable masses of centromeric heterochromatin, in quail cells two such masses are visible after Feulgen–Rossbeck staining or electron microscopy. This phenomenon enabled most cells to be identified as chick or quail and made possible a series of elegant studies on cell migration during embryogenesis in chick–quail chimaeras, particularly to the thymus and bursa of Fabricius [30,31,32]. Cells do vary in their expression of this phenotype; e.g. in about a third of quail osteoclasts the marker is undetectable [33].

Another potentially valuable DNA marker has been developed by Rossant *et al.* [34]. It utilizes the interspecies polymorphism in satellite DNA between the species *Mus musculus* and *Mus caroli*. A radiolabelled cloned DNA probe identified *M. musculus* nuclei in both tissue sections and cell spreads after DNA–DNA *in situ* hybridization. This particular probe showed little cross-hybridization with *M. caroli* DNA satellite sequences, so that *M. caroli* nuclei appeared virtually unlabelled after *in situ* hybridization. The probe has been used to distinguish cells of these species in both embryonic and adult tissues of chimaeras between *musculus* and *caroli* (Fig. 56.3, [35,36]).

More recently, the satellite probe has been biotinylated and stained with a streptavidin–horse-radish peroxidase complex on tissue sections (Dr J. Rossant, personal communication). This modification reduces the problems of background staining and thus allows more accurate localization of cells within a tissue. Since the marker is ubiquitous, it satisfies most of the criteria for an ideal marker discussed in the introduction and may prove a very powerful tool in analysing, both *in situ* and in isolated blood cells, the clonal

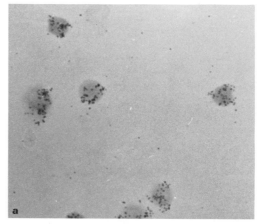
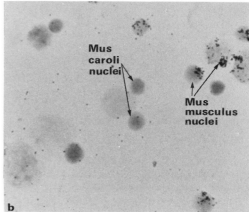

Fig. 56.3. *In situ* hybridization of *Mus musculus* (a) and chimaeric *Mus musculus–Mus caroli* (b) bone marrow spreads with a radioactively labelled, cloned DNA probe to *Mus musculus* satellite DNA. All bone marrow nuclei from the *Mus musculus* preparation are labelled, but only a proportion from the chimaera. The proportion of labelled to unlabelled nuclei in this bone marrow preparation was found to correspond to the proportion of GPI enzymes from each species. (Unpublished data of Dr J. Rossant, who kindly provided these photographs.)

relationships between cells of the haematopoietic/immune system in the mouse. These chimaeras are, however, difficult to produce and the probe is not yet commercially available. Conceivably the discovery of DNA polymorphisms within *M. musculus* may in future provide similar markers for transplantation studies. Polymorphisms in the length of restriction fragments of DNA in the X-linked gene, hypoxanthine ribosyl transferase (HPRT), have recently been used to determine the clonal origins of human tumours [104]. This technique uses endonuclease digests to distinguish between maternal and paternal X-chromosome activity of cell clones on the basis of different patterns of digestion. The active X-chromosome can then be identified by methylation changes [105] in the restriction fragments.

Cytoplasmic structural markers

Several cytoplasmic inclusions have been used to identify cells, of which probably the most notable are those seen in the beige (*bg/bg*) mouse mutant. At the cellular level this mutation has the general effect of clumping and/or enlarging cytoplasmic granules. Melanin granules, granules in mast cells (seen after Toluidine blue staining), granules in granulocytes (seen after Sudan black staining) and in osteoclasts are all enlarged. Enlargement of lysosomes visualized with the histochemical stain for acid phosphatase has been seen in fifteen different tissues in the mouse [37,38,39]. This mutant has been used extensively in studies of mast cell differentiation and distribution [40,41,42]. Beige mutants are also reported to be deficient in natural killer (NK) cells, thus providing a potentially useful combination of morphological and immunologically functional markers [43].

Biochemical markers

In this group a wealth of different options is available. Proteins may be assayed after tissue homogenization, providing indirect evidence for cell types present, or as histochemical markers *in situ*. Allelic variants of enzymes (alloenzymes) have been found in a variety of species, including the mouse; several are now available on congenic backgrounds. This section will deal with some of the biochemical markers under two headings—electrophoretic and histochemical. In the former, one particular enzyme, phosphoglycerate kinase (PGK-1) will be considered in some detail.

Electrophoretic markers

Electrophoretic techniques can be used to separate allelomorphs of many enzymes and other proteins. Under some circumstances the relative quantities present can be measured with reasonable accuracy. The techniques are indirect in the sense that they require tissue destruction and homogenization, and so provide no information about the spatial arrangements of cells in the tissues studied. On the other hand, they can tell one about the proportions of cells of different origins in tissues or indeed whether or not a particular cell lineage is contributing to a tissue. If the cells of interest are accessible in the blood, they (and by inference their precursors in haemopoietic tissues) can be assayed repeatedly over long periods.

Phosphoglycerate kinase

Phosphoglycerate kinase is an enzyme of the glycolytic pathway, catalysing the conversion of 1,3-diphosphoglyceric acid to 3-phosphoglyceric acid with the production of ATP. The structural locus for the somatic form of the enzyme PGK-1 in the mouse is on the X-chromosome [44,45]. The testicular form of the enzyme, PGK-2, is controlled by a locus on chromosome 17 [46], but does not concern us here. An electrophoretic variant of PGK-1 was found in a wild mouse population in Denmark and designated PGK-1A [47,48]. The common form was designated PGK-1B. The respective alleles *Pgk-1^a* and *Pgk-1^b* now exist on several inbred backgrounds. PGK-1A and B are similar biochemically, except for their differential electrophoretic migration and a somewhat higher thermolability of PGK-1B at 49 °C. Since no significant differences in tissue levels of PGK activity were found between *Pgk-1^a* and *Pgk-1^b* mice, it is likely that at the cellular level the activity of PGK-1A and PGK-1B is identical [49]. This is not to say, however, that the overall levels of PGK-1A and 1B in any tissue are the same. This will obviously depend on the variance of X-chromosome inactivation patterns in the tissue progenitors [50,51,52,53,54], and on genetic factors. A gene very closely linked to *Pgk-1*—the X-chromosome controlling element (*Xce*)—influences X-chromosome inactivation. Three alleles of this gene are known: *Xce^c*, introduced with *Pgk-1^a* from the wild mouse population, increases the frequency with which the chromosome carrying it remains active compared to the other two alleles, *Xce^b* and *Xce^a* [55,56,57]. In practice, mice heterozygous for *Pgk-1* in the C3H or CBA (*Xce^a*) strains have a mean ratio of 70% PGK-1A to 30% PGK-1B. Heterozygotes in the C57BL/10 (*Xce^b*) strain have a mean ratio of 60% PGK-1A to 40% PGK-1B, although in this case if the *Xce^b* gene is maternal in origin [58], the ratio is nearer to 50:50 [92].

Pgk-1 alleles are expressed in all tissues and their X-chromosome linkage and existence on congenic backgrounds make them good markers for estimation of the clonal composition of tissues and also for transplantation studies. Several electrophoretic systems exist for this enzyme and those currently in use in the authors' laboratory are described in detail. These are based on the technique first described by Bücher *et al.* [59] and subsequently used for mosaic analysis [53, 106], but do not rely (as does that technique) on the visualization of PGK bands by fluorescence. Electrophoresis is carried out on cellulose acetate membranes and PGK visualized either by reduction of a tetrazolium salt to formazan, or by autoradiography after incorporation of a ^{14}C-labelled substrate [60] (Fig. 56.4). The apparent complexity of the system is due to

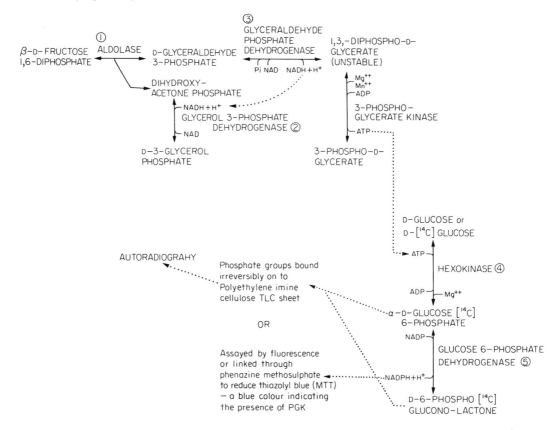

Fig. 56.4. The biochemical basis for the phosphoglycerate kinase assay. The substrate for PGK-1 is unstable and has to be generated *in situ* on the electrophoresis membrane. This is achieved by using fructose 1,6-diphosphate as the primary substrate and by the addition of enzymes 1, 2, and 3, NAD and inorganic phosphate. (The reaction catalysed by enzyme 2 provides a sink for NADH, which might otherwise cause a background colour reaction.) The ATP generated by PGK-1 action on its substrate is utilized in the phosphorylation of glucose by hexokinase. The NADPH produced during the subsequent conversion to phosphogluconolactone may be measured by its fluorescence or the colour produced by the reduction of thiazolyl blue to formazan. If ^{14}C-labelled glucose is included in the reaction mixture, the radiolabelled products of glucose phosphorylation may be assayed by autoradiography after their adsorption on to a thin-layer chromatographic membrane.

the fact that the substrate for PGK, 1,3-diphosphoglycerate, is unstable and has to be synthesized *in situ*. The ATP produced by PGK action is used in the production of 6-phosphogluconolactone (catalysed by hexokinase and glucose 6-phosphate dehydrogenase), with the accompanying production of NADPH. In practice, the following methods despite their rather labyrinthine appearance, are quite straightforward.

Electrophoresis equipment

The 'Helena' (Helena Laboratories, Beaumont, Texas, USA) electrophoresis system is used. Samples are applied to Titan III cellulose acetate membranes. Satisfactory results may be obtainable with other systems, but appropriate adjustments of electrophoresis buffer and/or separation time may be required.

Buffers

Electrophoresis buffer:
20 mM-sodium barbital (Sigma B0500);
10 mM-tri-sodium citrate;
5 mM-magnesium sulphate;
2 mM-ethylenediaminetetraacetate (EDTA).
The buffer is pH 8.8 at 4 °C.
Sample buffer: to 50 mM-triethanolamine hydrochloride (Sigma T1502) are added:
0.3 mg/ml dithioerythritol (Sigma D 8255);
0.5 mg/ml bovine serum albumin;
2 mg/ml digitonin (Sigma D 5628).

Staining reagents

Indicator stock: to 100 mM-triethanolamine hydrochloride are added:
magnesium sulphate to 130 mM;
glucose to 150 mM;
adenosine diphosphate (ADP) to 25 mM (Sigma A 8146);
NADP(TPN) to 40 mM (Sigma N 0505).
The solution is adjusted to pH 7.6 with 2 N-NaOH, and 100 μl aliquots are stored at $-20\,^{\circ}$C.

Assay stock: to electrophoresis buffer (see above) are added:
NAD (DPN) to 12 mM (Sigma N 7004);
trisodium fructose 1,6-diphosphate to 40 mM (Sigma 752-1);
K_2HPO_4 to 40 mM.
400 μl aliquots are stored at $-20\,^{\circ}$C.

Staining reagents:
MTT (thiazolyl blue) 10 mg/ml distilled H_2O (Sigma M 2128);
PMS (phenazine methosulphate) 2.5 mg/ml distilled H_2O (Sigma P 9625).

Radioactive substrate:
U-^{14}C glucose (New England Nuclear, Southampton, Cat. no. NEC-042X);

Enzymes:
glucose 6-phosphate dehydrogenase (G6PDH) E.C.1.1.1.49 (Sigma G 8878);
hexokinase E.C.2.7.1.1 (Sigma H 5625);
aldolase E.C.4.1.2.13 (Boehringer Mannheim Cat. no. 102644);
glucose dehydrogenase (GDH) E.C.1.1.1.47 (Sigma G 6751);
glyceraldehyde 3-phosphate dehydrogenase (GAPDH) E.C.1.2.1.12 (Boehringer Mannheim Cat. no. 105686).

Preparation of tissues

Samples are homogenized and stored at $-60\,^{\circ}$C in sample buffer, which keeps the lysate in a reduced condition and helps to stabilize the enzyme. Storage for up to 6 months in these conditions is satisfactory, but longer storage tends to decrease preferentially activity of the 1B form. PGK activity per cell varies. For example, there is approximately ten times less activity in erythrocytes than in granulocytes. The final concentration in sample buffer has to be determined by trial and error.

Electrophoresis

1 Titan III cellulose acetate membranes are soaked in electrophoresis buffer for 20 min.
2 Fifty milligrams of adenosine 5'-monophosphate (AMP; Sigma A 2127) are added to 200 ml electrophoresis buffer and divided equally between cathodal and anodal chambers of the electrophoresis tank.
3 The wicks are soaked in electrophoresis buffer and applied over the sides of the bridge.
4 Using the Helena applicator system (Super Z) samples are loaded at the cathodal end of the cellulose acetate membrane.
5 The membrane is placed, sample side down, on to the bridges of the electrophoresis chamber. A small weight (5–10 g: a coin is convenient) should be placed on to the membrane to ensure maximum contact between the cellulose acetate and the bridge.
6 A voltage is applied across the membrane and run at a constant current of 12.5 mA per membrane for 45 min.
7 The power pack is disconnected, the membrane removed and, after any excess fluid has been blotted off, placed on a levelling table.

Visualization of bands

About 10 min before the end of the run, the staining reagents should be prepared. The methods of staining are different for the tetrazolium and autoradiographic techniques and should be considered separately.

MTT staining: to 800 μl electrophoresis buffer are added: 75 μl sample buffer; 400 μl assay stock; 100 μl indicator stock; 10 μl G6PDH (300 u/ml); 10 μl aldolase (6.5 u/ml); 7.5 μl GAPDH (10 mg/ml); 5 μl hexokinase (6000 u/ml); 5 μl GDH (220 u/ml); 500 μl MTT.

The concentrations of enzymes in parenthesis are approximate. The actual volume of enzymes added to the staining mixture will need to be adjusted from time to time if the manufacturers' specifications alter significantly.

To the above mixture are added 500 μl PMS and the whole solution is quickly mixed with 2.4 ml of 1.2% agarose previously kept at 56 $^{\circ}$C. Pour evenly over the membrane, cover, and when set incubate at 37 $^{\circ}$C until bands appear. The membranes can be fixed in an aqueous solution of 15% glycerol and 3% acetic acid.

Autoradiographic preparation

1 A polyethylene imine (PEI) TLC plate (Bakerflex, Linton Products, Hysol, Harlow, UK) is soaked in distilled water for 20 min and blotted.
2 The 'staining' reagents are made up similarly to those for MTT staining except that the quantities or electrophoresis buffer and sample buffer are reduced to 600 μl and 30 μl respectively and MTT, PMS and agarose are omitted.
3 Immediately before staining, 15 μl (15 μCi) of

U-^{14}C glucose are added to the stain and the mixture is poured evenly on to the PEI sheet.

4 The cellulose acetate membrane is placed face down on to the PEI sheet, excluding air bubbles from the interface.

5 The PEI/membrane 'sandwich' is then incubated for 15 min at 37 °C.

6 The 'sandwich' is cooled at 4 °C for 5 min. The PEI sheet is separated from the membrane and rinsed with 500 ml 8 mM-Tris (Sigma T 1378).

7 The PEI sheet is soaked (with stirring) in 8 mM-Tris for 4 h.

8 The PEI sheet is dried and exposed to X-ray film (Kodak X-Omat S) for 3 days.

9 X-ray films are developed in a 1:5 solution of Kodak LX 24 developer for 2.5 min, washed in 2% acetic acid, fixed for 5 min in a 1:5 solution of Kodak FX-40 liquid fixer and washed for 20 min.

The autoradiographic method is approximately ten times more sensitive than the MTT system. If a further increase in sensitivity is required, the amount of unlabelled glucose in the indicator stock may be reduced by a factor of 10, thus increasing the proportion of labelled glucose in the stain.

Densitometry of bands

The proportions of the two PGK phenotypes in either system (Fig. 56.5) may be estimated after measurement of their intensities in a scanning densitometer (Chromoscan 3, Joyce-Loebl, Vickers Instruments, Gateshead, UK). Examples of the repeatability obtainable within and between runs are shown in Fig. 56.6. The experience of the authors' laboratory is that whole blood gives the largest spread of readings and thymus the smallest. Other haematopoietic tissues and cells are intermediate. There is little between tetrazolium and autoradiographic methods (except in sensitivity, although interference with background density by haemoglobin makes the former more difficult to use with erythrocytes or whole blood. In artificial mixtures of PGK-1A and PGK-1B cell lysates, the authors have found an approximately linear relationship between the proportions measured electrophoretically and

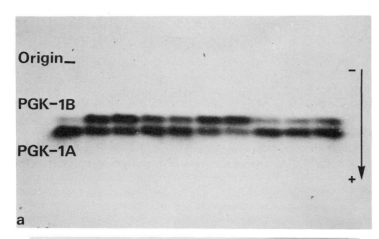

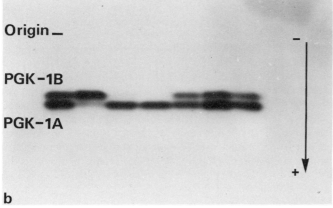

Fig. 56.5. Examples of PGK-1 electrophoreses visualized by ^{14}C autoradiography (a) and reduction of thiazolyl blue (b). Samples in (a) are artificial mixtures of lysates of PGK-1A and PGK-1B thymus cells. Samples in (b) are lysates of PGK-1AB bone marrow cells.

Fig. 56.6. Reproducibility of PGK-1 alloenzyme measurements on a single sample of lysed heterozygous blood cells, assayed by both autoradiographic and colorimetric methods. Aliquots (0.25 μl) of the sample were applied several times to each of a series of electrophoresis membranes. Each point represents a single track and each column a different membrane. The presence of haemoglobin in lysed blood sample tends to reduce the efficiency of electrophoretic separation and makes assays of blood more variable technically than those of other tissues. Interference by haemoglobin is also responsible for the apparently higher mean proportion of PGK-1A in the MTT preparations (71%; range 64–79) compared with the ^{14}C preparations (66%; range 58–73). Similar experiments on cell lysates containing little haemoglobin show less variation, with ranges that rarely exceed 8% with either method (cf. Fig. 56.7).

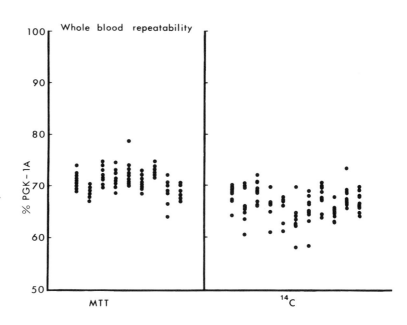

volumetrically (Fig. 56.7); this covers the range 20–80%, with minor components tending to be overestimated outside this range. It is possible to detect 1% or less of a minor component by overstaining/overexposing, but such a proportion cannot be measured accurately. Good reproducibility of measurement can only be achieved through rigorous quality control. In practice, this means rejecting any separations in which the total enzyme activity is too high or too low or in which bands show appreciable trailing or distortion.

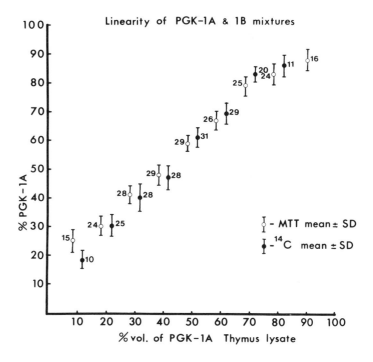

Fig. 57.7. Linearity of the PGK-1 alloenzyme assay for a range of artificial mixtures of PGK-1A and PGK-1B thymus lysates. Each lysate was prepared from a similar number of thymus lobes and made up to the same volume. Differences in original cell concentration and therefore in the concentration of enzyme in these lysates are probably sufficient to explain the excess of PGK-1A over the range studied. The numbers beside each symbol indicate the number of repeat analyses of each mixture.

To avoid bias, the decision to reject must be made before the densitometric scan has been made and without knowledge of the identity of the sample. The presence of large amounts of haemoglobin tends to prevent sharp separation of the bands. Correct sample dilution and consistent judgement in integrating the densitometric scans is necessary when handling such materials.

PGK analysis of blood leucocytes

A typical experimental protocol for PGK analysis of the granulocyte and lymphocyte populations of whole blood from a mouse heterozygous for PGK-1A and 1B is as follows.

1 Five drops of blood are collected from the retro-orbital sinus into 8 ml phosphate-buffered saline (PBS) containing 0.1% BSA, 0.2 mg/ml EDTA and 500 u heparin.

2 This is centrifuged at 200 *g* for 10 min.

3 The supernatant is discarded, the pellet resuspended, and 4.5 ml distilled water are added, to lyse red cells. After 12 seconds 0.5 ml 10 × concentrated PBS (or Hanks' solution) is added and the tube topped up with PBS.

4 The cells are centrifuged again and resuspended in 0.3 ml PBS.

5 Lymphocyte and granulocyte populations are separated on a cell sorter (Becton-Dickinson FACS IV) on the basis of their differential forward and 90° light scattering properties. If desired, lymphocyte subsets can be separated after staining with appropriate fluorochrome-labelled antibodies.

6 300 000 lymphocytes are collected, and spun down in a micro-haemocrit centrifuge. The supernatant is removed as completely as possible and 6 μl of sample buffer added. 50 000 granulocytes are prepared simi-larly in 5 μl of sample buffer, granulocytes having approximately five times greater activity of PGK-1 per cell than lymphocytes. These concentrations are good for PGK analysis after autoradiography using $\frac{1}{10}$ of the standard 'cold' glucose concentration (see above). Since the Helena system applies 0.25 μl of sample to the gel, the lysates of approximately 2500 granulocytes and 12 500 lymphocytes are being assayed.

Glucose 6-phosphate dehydrogenase (G6PDH)

Electrophoretic variants of the X-chromosome linked enzyme G6PDH have been found in man and in *M. caroli* but not in *M. musculus* [45]. The G6PDH markers have been used extensively in man to analyse the clonality of tumours and to establish founder cell numbers for different tissues [52,61,62]. G6PDH is a dimeric enzyme, each *Gpdx* allele coding for a monomeric unit. In normal tissues, the mosaicism for G6PDH in female heterozygotes is expressed as a two-banded phenotype after electrophoresis. If X-inactivation has not occurred (as in pre-meiotic germ cells [63]), or if a fusion has occurred between cells with different X-chromosomes active, a three banded phenotype, due to random association of monomeric units, is observed. This property has been used in the authors' laboratory to look for evidence of cell fusion in methylcholanthrene-induced fibrosarcomas in female *M. caroli* heterozygotes (Woodruff, Ansell & Hodson, unpublished). G6PDH variants can be run on the Helena electrophoresis system and stained with MTT similarly to PGK-1 [64]. In this case the electrophoresis buffer is 25 mM-Tris-glycine at pH 8.5.

Samples are run at 200 V for 35 min. The staining mixture consists of: 100 μl glucose 6-phosphate (141 mg/ml; Sigma G 7879); 1000 μl NADP (1 mg/ml); 50 μl

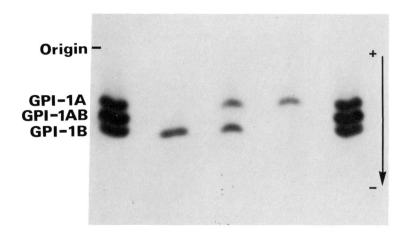

Fig. 56.8. A sample of GPI-1 electrophoresis after staining as described. Tracks 1 and 5 are lysates of a spleen cell suspension from a *Gpi-1ᵃᵇ* heterozygous mouse, showing the characteristic three-banded phenotype. Tracks 2 and 4 are from a *Gpi-1ᵃ* and a *Gpi-1ᵇ* homozygous mouse respectively. Track 3 is a mixture of the lysates used in tracks 2 and 4.

magnesium acetate (85.8 mg/ml); 600 μl 1.0 M-Tris–HCl, pH 8.0; 3 ml of 1.2% agarose; 150 μl MTT (10 mg/ml); 150 μl PMS (2.5 mg/ml).

Glucose phosphate isomerase (GPI-1)

The structural locus controlling electrophoretic variations of GPI-1 alloenzymes (*Gpi-1s*) is on chromosome 7. [65]. Four alleles have been identified, two of which, *Gpi-1s*[a] and *Gpi-1s*[b] exist in common inbred strains [4]. Like G6PDH, GPI is a dimeric enzyme, it is ubiquitous and has a high activity in most cells. Alleles of GPI-1 are commonly used as markers for mouse chimaeras [1]. Electrophoresis techniques allow detection of a minor component which is 1% or less in small pieces of tissue [66,67]. A recent electrophoretic microelution technique allows accurate quantification of variants of this enzyme [68]. Since GPI-1 is a dimeric enzyme and is autosomally encoded, normal somatic tissues of heterozygotes express a three-banded phenotype (cf. G6PDH).

The occurrence of three bands in GPI chimaeras has been used to detect cell fusions in skeletal muscle [66], and in determining the origins of multinucleate and polyploid cells in placental tissues [66,69]. The existence of the alleles a and b on CBA/Ca congenic backgrounds has enabled us to use GPI as a marker for host cell contributions to the haemopoietic tissues when marrow from a *Pgk-1* heterozygous, *Gpi-1s*[b] donor is transplanted into *Gpi-1s*[a] recipients.

GPI can also be measured on the Helena system using MTT. However, its use for quantitative work should be approached with some caution. Both the A and B alloenzymes of GPI-1 express a minor or secondary band which migrates more slowly on electrophoresis. The strength of this band apparently depends on the tissue being studied and/or the conditions of storage prior to electrophoresis. A large minor component of the B alloenzyme can confound the measurement of the A alloenzyme since they tend to migrate to a similar position. This problem can be minimized by ensuring that the tissues are stored for the shortest possible time before electrophoresis and that the minimum concentration of tissue lysate is applied to the electrophoresis membrane.

Method

Supraheme electrophoresis buffer (Helena Laboratories), pH 8.2–8.6. Samples are loaded at the anode and run for 1 h 20 min at 350 V. Membranes are stained with: 1000 μl 1.0 M-Tris–HCl, pH 8.0, containing 0.3 mg NADP and 6.5 mg; fructose 6-phosphate (Sigma F 3627); 15 μl G6PDH (300 u/ml); 500 μl MTT (10 mg/ml); 500 μl PMS (2.5 mg/ml); 400 μl 500 mM-Tris–HCl, pH 8.0; 2.4 ml 1.2% agarose.

Several other electrophoretic enzyme variants have been used as markers in other systems (see Green [4] for a comprehensive list of variants available in the mouse) but most suffer from the drawbacks of low activity, complex assays or restricted distribution. Electrophoretic variants of haemoglobin have also been used as markers for erythropoiesis after transplantation [70,71], but obviously they are not applicable to lymphoid cells.

Histochemical markers

There exist several enzyme variants which show differences in levels of enzyme activity or thermolability or which are for practical purposes inactive. The differences may be large enough to serve as *in situ* markers. For example, high and low activity variants of β-glucuronidase and β-galactosidase have been used in mouse chimaeras to study patch sizes in the liver and other tissues [72,73,74,75]. These approaches are largely unexplored for the haematopoietic system. Histochemical analyses are unsuitable for many tissues since levels of cellular activity are often too low to detect differences between variants [76]. Alkaline phosphatase, for example, has very little activity in mouse granulocytes. However, this property has been exploited for granulocyte identification in interspecies radiation chimaeras between rat and mouse, since the level of the enzyme in rat granulocytes is much higher [75]. The X-chromosome linked enzyme ornithine carbamoyl transferase has an abnormal form in the mouse mutant *spf* (sparse fur), which is not detected by a histochemical technique that demonstrates the enzyme in normal cells [77]. This variant has been used to study clonality in liver tumours [78,79]. The potential of other such markers, especially thermolabile variants is dealt with in detail by West [3].

Immunological markers

Antibodies to cell membrane alloantigens have been used in mouse chimaeras to follow the tissue distributions of cells. Such methods are described elsewhere in this volume by Butcher & Ford [80]. These techniques may make use of antigens such as Thy-1 or Ia, which are restricted to certain cell types, or universally expressed antigens such as H-2, and may be used on cells both in suspension and *in situ*. Histocompatibility antigen differences, for example, have been widely used as *in situ* markers on tissue sections from aggregation chimaeras, but may, for obvious reasons, be unsuitable as markers in transplantation experiments. Monoclonal antibodies (McAbs) that are specific for allelic variants of intracellular proteins may make *in situ* analysis of chimaeric tissues much more flexible in the future. An allele-specific antiserum has been developed against the B variant of GPI-1 and has been used histochemically, by conjugation to a peroxidase label, to identify cells in mouse chimaeras [81,82]. McAbs to antigens that have a restricted tissue distribution may also be used to follow cell lineages. Raff has elegantly used this approach to dissect developmental lineages in neural tissue [83,84]. McAbs to Igh allotypes of IgM and IgD in the mouse, and κ chain allotypes in the rat, are useful tools for studying B lymphocytes in chimaeric or F_1 animals. Plasma cells can be followed indirectly by measuring allotypic Ig [85] or specific antibodies [86] in the serum.

Use of markers in combination

The value of genetic markers, such as those described above, may be greatly enhanced by using them in conjunction with other resources: these include animals with mutations that affect haematopoiesis and the immune system in various ways [87,88,89] and modern techniques for identifying and separating cell populations [90]. A recent experiment by Mintz *et al.* was something of a *tour de force* in its use of several markers and haematopoietic mutants [91]. Fetal liver haematopoietic stem cells were injected into the placental circulation of fetal mice at 11 days of gestation. Since both the recipient fetus and the donor were immunologically immature, allogeneic combinations could be used without complications resulting from graft-versus-host or host-versus-graft reactions. With this technique it was shown that successful haematopoietic engraftment in a series of W mutants, with stem cell defects of various degrees of severity, could take place with very few, possibly even single pluripotent stem cells. These cells were shown to give rise to several lineages by including haemoglobin markers for erythrocytes, the beige marker for granulocytes, an Igh allotype marker for B cells and H-2 markers for T-cells.

Competition between a 'standard' and an 'experimental' cell population provides a useful experimental basis for many studies. This normally requires three distinct markers, or two markers in addition to the normal phenotype. This approach has been in use with the T6 chromosome markers for more than 20 years [93]. The arrival of the alloenzymes has greatly increased the possible scope of such experiments; these markers can more easily be used to study small numbers of cells and far more tests can be carried out in a given time. The cells themselves may be non-dividing and may have been isolated on the basis of their size, density or antigenic characteristics. For example,

Table 57.1. Example of chimaera construction, using alloenzyme-congenic mice, for comparative study of haematopoietic cell populations

	Gpi-1		*Pgk-1*	
	Genotype	Phenotype	Genotype	Phenotype
Donor 1	bb	B	aa or aY	A
Donor 2	bb	B	bb or bY	B
Host*	aa	A	bb or bY	B

chimaeras can be constructed as shown in Table 56.1, using alloenzyme-congenic mice on the CBA/Ca background. In view of the problems that may arise in quantifying GPI-1 on cellulose acetate, the host may with advantage be lethally irradiated; GPI-1 analysis then serves mainly to confirm the absence of host cells. If a GPI-1 variant is to be used to quantify host and donor cells in such an experiment, it must be borne in mind that GPI-1 and PGK-1 may exist in different proportions in different cell populations.

The mice can be bled at intervals and the contribution of the three components of the chimaera to the various blood cell populations (preferably separated on a cell sorter) determined electrophoretically. Alternatively, mice can be sacrificed serially for study of a wider range of tissue cells. In these experiments donor 1 or 2 can be a control—e.g. normal adult bone marrow cells—that functions as a yardstick for the performance of the other donor population. In this way it is practicable to study the long-term haematopoietic potential of stem cells selected for particular physical or antigenic properties. The ability to analyse small numbers of well characterized cells makes this a useful tool for the elucidation of haematopoietic lineages.

The alloenzyme markers can also be applied to a variety of analyses of genetic deficiencies or abnormalities in the immune system. An example is the X-chromosome linked immunodeficiency (*Xid*) mutant of CBA/N mice [94]. These mice are deficient in a B-lymphocyte subpopulation that expresses large quantities of IgD and small quantities of IgM on the cell surface [95,96]. By combining heterozygosity for *Xid* with heterozygosity for *Pgk-1*, the extent to which B lymphocytes and other cells express the genes on the *Xid*-carrying chromosome has been monitored [97,98].

These examples are chosen almost at random and readers who have persevered this far will find no difficulty in devising numerous other uses for cellular markers. Markers have been omitted from many past experiments that would have benefited from their use, usually because of the difficulties inherent in chromosome analysis. With the advent of the techniques for detecting enzyme variants described above, the difficulties of including markers in such experiments are significantly diminished. The authors envisage that enzyme variant markers will replace chromosome markers for most purposes.

Recently it has proved possible to introduce specific 'fingerprints' into the DNA of haematopoietic stem cells by means of random retroviral insertions [107]. These are detected by Southern blotting of restriction digests of DNA. This opens the way to the production of unique clonal markers.

The availability of markers for *in situ* analysis is still restricted. Probes for DNA polymorphisms may become more numerous, but their effective use will still depend on the construction of chimaeras. One desirable development would be the production of allele-specific monoclonal antibodies to X-chromosome linked products such as phosphoglycerate kinase, and their use in analysis of mosaicism *in situ*.

Acknowledgements

The authors' work with allozyme markers has been supported by the Cancer Research Campaign, the Medical Research Council and the Melville Trust.

Many people have made, directly or indirectly essential contributions to the genesis of this paper. The authors are particularly indebted to the following people: Drs J.F. Loutit and C.E. Ford, in whose laboratory one of the authors first learned the value of cell markers; Dr V.M. Chapman for his help in setting up assays for PGK allozymes; Drs J.D. West and M.J. Marshall for gifts of, respectively, *Pgk-1ᵃ* and CBA/Ca-*Gpi-1ᵃ* mice. In addition, the authors have recently enjoyed the benefit of many discussions with Drs G. Brecher, V.M. Chapman, L.A. Herzenberg and J.D. West and Sir Michael Woodruff. In their own laboratory, Mr D.A. Ogden provided cytological expertise and Mss D. Burton, L. Forrester and J. Wayman provided the congenic CBA/Ca-*Pgk-1ᵃ* strain. Specific contributions are acknowledged in the text.

References

1 McLaren A. (1975) *Mammalian Chimaeras.* Cambridge University Press, Cambridge and London.

2 Oster-Granite M.L. & Gearhart J. (1981) Cell lineage analysis of cerebellar Purkinje cells in mouse chimaeras. *Devl Biol.* **85**, 199.

3 West J.D. (1984) Cell Markers. In *Chimaeras in Developmental Biology*, (eds. Le Douarin N. & McLaren A.), p. 39. Academic Press.

4 Green M.C. (1981) Catalog of mutant genes and polymorphic loci. In *Genetic Variants and Strains of the Laboratory Mouse*, (ed. Green M.C.), p. 8. Gustav Fischer Verlag, Stuttgart, New York.

5 Lyon M.F. (1974) Mechanisms and evolutionary origins of variable X-chromosome activity in mammals. *Proc. R. Soc.* Series B: Biological Sciences, **187**, 243.

6 Chapman V.M., Kratzer P.G., Siracusa L.D., Quarantillo B.A., Evans R. & Liskay R.M. (1982) Evidence for DNA modification in the maintenance of X-chromosome inactivation of adult tissues. *Proc. natn. Acad. Sci. U.S.A.* **79**, 5357.

7 Herzenberg L.A., Herzenberg L.A., Black S.J., Loken M.R., Okumura K., van der Loo W., Osbourne B.A., Hewgill D., Goding J.W., Gutman G. & Warner N.L. (1976) Surface markers and functional relationships of cells involved in murine B lymphocyte differentiation. *Cold Spring Harb. Symp. quant. Biol.* **41**, 33.

8 Cohen F., Zuelzer W.W., Gustafson D.C. & Evans M.M. (1964) Mechanism of isoimmunisation. (1) The transplacental passage of fetal erythrocytes in homospecific pregnancies. *Blood*, **23**, 621.

9 Herzenberg L.A., Bianchi D.W., Schroder J., Cann H.M. & Iverson M.G. (1979) Fetal cells in the blood of pregnant women: Detection and enrichment by fluorescence-activated cell sorting. *Proc. natn. Acad. Sci. U.S.A.* **76**, 1453.

10 Short R.V. (1970) The bovine freemartin: a new look at an old problem. *Phil. Trans. Roy. Soc. Lond.* **259**, 141.

11 Mintz B. (1964) Formation of genetically mosaic mouse embryos, and early development of 'lethal (*t¹²/t¹²*)–normal' mosaics. *J. exp. Zool.* **157**, 273.

12 Bowman P. & McLaren A. (1970) Viability and growth of mouse embryos after *in vitro* culture and fusion. *J. Embryol. exp. Morph.* **23**, 693.

13 Mintz B. (1975) Experimental genetic mosaicism in the mouse. In *Preimplantation Stages of Pregnancy*, (eds. Wolstenholme G.E.W. & O'Connor M.), p. 194. Churchill London.

14 Gardner R.L. (1971) Manipulations on the blastocyst. *Adv. Biosci.* **6**, 279.

15 Gardner R.L. & Johnson M.H. (1973) Investigation of early mammalian development using interspecific chimaeras between rat and mouse. *Nature New Biol.* **246**, 86.

16 Papaioannou V.E. & Dieterlen-Lièvre F. (1984) Making Chimaeras. In *Chimaeras in Developmental Biology*, (eds. Le Douarin N. & McLaren A.), p. 3. Academic Press, New York, London.

17 Micklem H.S. & Loutit J.F. (1966) *Tissue Grafting and Radiation.* Academic Press, New York, London.

18 van Bekkum D.W. & Vos O. (1957) Immunological aspects of homo- and heterologous bone marrow transplantation in irradiated animals. *J. cell. comp. Physiol.* **50** (suppl. 1), 139.

19 Brecher G., Ansell J.D., Micklem H.S., Tjio J.-H. & Cronkite E.P. (1982) Special proliferative sites are not needed for seeding and proliferation of transfused bone marrow cells in normal syngeneic mice. *Proc. natn. Acad. Sci. U.S.A.* **79**, 5085.

20 Ford C.E., Hamerton J.L., Barnes D.W.H. & Loutit J.F. (1956) Cytological identification of radiation chimaeras. *Nature*, **177**, 452.

21 Carter T.C., Lyon M.F. & Phillips R.J.S. (1956)

Further genetic studies of eleven translocations in the mouse. *J. Genet.* **54**, 462.

22 FORD C.E. (1966) The use of chromosome markers. In *Tissue Grafting and Radiation*, (eds. Micklem H.S. & Loutit J.F.), p. 197. Academic Press, New York, London.

23 MICKLEM H.S., FORD C.E. EVANS E.P. & OGDEN D.A. (1975) Compartments and cell flows within the mouse haemopoietic system. (1) Restricted interchange between haemopoietic sites. *Cell Tissue Kinet.* **8**, 219.

24 LORD B.I. & HENDRY J.H. (1972) The distribution of haemopoietic colony-forming units in the mouse femur and its modification by X-rays. *Br. J. Radiol.* **45**, 110.

25 LORD B.I., TESTA N.G. & HENDRY J.H. (1975) The relative spatial distributions of CFU$_S$ and CFU$_C$ in the normal mouse femur. *Blood*, **46**, 65.

26 SUMNER A.T. (1972) A simple technique for demonstrating centromeric heterochromatin. *Expl Cell Res.* **75**, 304.

27 SEARLE A.G. (1981) Chromosomal Variants. In *Genetic Variants and Strains of the Laboratory Mouse*, (ed. Green M.C.), p. 324. Gustav Fisher Verlag, Stuttgart, New York.

28 LE DOUARIN N.M. (1973) A biological cell labelling technique and its use in experimental embryology. *Devl Biol.* **30**, 217.

29 LE DOUARIN N.M. (1980) The ontogeny of neural crest in avian embryo chimaeras. *Nature*, **286**, 663.

30 LE DOUARIN N.M. & JOTEREAU F.V. (1973) Origin and renewal of lymphocytes in avian thymuses studied in interspecific combinations. *Nature New Biol.* **246**, 25.

31 LE DOUARIN N.M., HOUSSAINT E., JOTEREAU F.V. & BELO M. (1975) Origin of haematopoietic stem cells in the embryonic bursa of Fabricius and bone marrow studied through interspecific chimaeras. *Proc. natn. Acad. Sci. U.S.A.* **72**, 2701.

32 HOUSSAINT E., BELO M. & LE DOUARIN N.M. (1976) Investigations in cell lineage and tissue interactions in the developing bursa of Fabricius through interspecific chimaeras. *Devl Biol.* **53**, 260.

33 JOTEREAU F.V. & LE DOUARIN N.M. (1978) The developmental relationship between osteocytes and osteoclasts. A study using the quail-chick nuclear marker in endochondrial ossification. *Devl Biol.* **63**, 253.

34 SIRACUSA L.D., CHAPMAN V.M., BENNET K.L., HASTIE N.D., PIETRAS D.F. & ROSSANT J. (1983) Use of repetitive DNA sequences to distinguish *Mus musculus* and *Mus caroli* cells by *in situ* hybridisation. *J. Embryol. exp. Morph.* **73**, 163.

35 ROSSANT J., VIJH M., SIRACUSA L.D. & CHAPMAN V.M. (1983) Identification of embryonic cell lineages in histological sections of *M. musculus–M. caroli* chimaeras. *J. Embryol. exp. Morph.* **73**, 179.

36 ROSSANT J. & CHAPMAN V.M. (1983) Somatic and germline mosaicism in interspecific chimaeras between *Mus musculus* and *Mus caroli*. *J. Embryol. exp. Morph.* **73**, 193.

37 OLIVER C. & ESSNER E. (1973) Distribution of anomalous lysosomes in the beige mouse. A homologue of Chediak–Higashi syndrome. *J. Histochem. Cytochem.* **21**, 218.

38 OLIVER C. & ESSNER E. (1975) Formation of anomalous lysosomes in monocytes, neutrophils and eosinophils from bone marrow of mice with Chediak–Higashi syndrome. *Lab. Invest.* **32**, 17.

39 ASH P., LOUTIT J.F. & TOWNSEND K.M.S. (1980) Osteoclasts derived from haemopoietic stem cells. *Nature*, **283**, 669.

40 KITAMURA Y., SHIMADA M., HATANAKA K. & MIYANO Y. (1977) Development of mast cells from grafted bone marrow cells in irradiated mice. *Nature*, **268**, 442.

41 KITAMURA Y., SHIMADA M., GO S., MATSUDA H., HATANAKA K. & SEKI M. (1979) Distribution of mast-cell precursors in haematopoietic and lymphopoietic tissues of mice. *J. exp. Med.* **150**, 482.

42 KITAMURA Y., SONODA T. & YOKOYAMA M. (1983) Differentiation of tissue mast cells. In *Haemopoietic Stem Cells. Characterization, Proliferation, Regulation.* Alfred Benzon Symposium 18, (eds, Killmann Sv.-Aa., Cronkite E.P. & Muller-Berat C.N.), p. 350. Munksgaard, Copenhagen.

43 RODER J.C. & DUWE A.K. (1979) The *beige* mutation in the mouse selectively impairs natural killer cell function. *Nature*, **278**, 451.

44 KOZAK L.P., MCLEAN G.K. & EICHER E.M. (1974) X linkage of phosphoglycerate kinase in the mouse. *Biochem. Genet.* **11**, 41.

45 CHAPMAN V.M. & SHOWS T.B. (1976) Somatic cell genetic evidence for X-chromosome linkage of three enzymes in the mouse. *Nature*, **259**, 665.

46 VAN DE BERG J.L.D. & BLOHM S.V. (1977) An allelic isozyme of mouse Pgk-2 with low activity. *J. exp. Zool.* **201**, 479.

47 NIELSEN J.T. & CHAPMAN V.M. (1977) Electrophoretic variation for X-chromosome-linked phosphoglycerate kinase (PGK-1) in the mouse. *Genetics*, **87**, 319.

48 WEST J.D. & CHAPMAN V.M. (1978) Variation for X-chromosome expression in mice detected by electrophoresis of phosphoglycerate kinase. *Genet. Res.* **32**, 91.

49 MUHLBACHER C., KUNTZ G.W.K., HAEDENKAMP G.A. & KRIETSCH W.K.G. (1983) Comparison of the two purified allozymes (1A and 1B) of X-linked phosphoglycerate kinase in the mouse. *Biochem. Genet.* **21**, 487.

50 MCLAREN A. (1972) Numerology of development. *Nature*, **239**, 274.

51 WEST J.D. (1975) A theoretical approach to the relation between patch size and clone size in chimaeric tissues. *J. theor. Biol.* **50**, 153.

52 FIALKOW P.J. (1973) Primordial pool size and lineage relationships of five human cell types. *Ann. Human Genet.* **37**, 39.

53 PAPPAIOANNOU V.E., WEST J.D., BÜCHER T. & LINKE I.M. (1981) Non-random X-chromosome expression early in mouse development. *Devl Genet.* **2**, 305.

54 MCMAHON A., FOSTEN M. & MONK M. (1983) X-chromosome inactivation mosaicism in the three germ layers and the germ line of the mouse embryo. *J. Embryol. exp. Morph.* **74**, 207.

55 CATTANACH B.M. (1972) X-chromosome controlling element (*Xce*). *Mouse News Letter*, **47**, 33.

56 JOHNSTON P.G. & CATTANACH B.M. (1981) Controlling elements in the mouse. (iv) Evidence of non-random X-inactivation. *Genet. Res.* **37**, 151.

57 CATTANACH B.M. & PAPWORTH D. (1981) Controlling elements in the mouse. (v) Linkage tests with X-linked genes. *Genet. Res.* **38**, 57.

58 RASTAN S. & CATTANACH B.M. (1983) Interaction between the *Xce* locus and imprinting of the paternal X chromosome in mouse yolk-sac endoderm. *Nature*, **303**, 635.

59 BÜCHER T., BENDER W., HOFNER H. & LINKE I. (1980) Quantitative evaluation of electrophoretic allo- and isozyme patterns. *FEBS Lett.* **115**, 319.

60 CHASIN L.A. & URLAUB G. (1976) Mutant alleles for hypoxanthine phosphoribosyltransferase, codominant expression, complementation and segregation in Chinese hamster cells. *Somatic Cell Genet.* **2**, 453.

61 FIALKOW P.J. (1976) Clonal origin of human tumours. *Biochim. biophys. Acta*, **458**, 283.

62 FIALKOW P.J. (1983) Hierarchical haematologic stem cell relationships studied with glucose-6-phosphate dehydrogenase enzymes. In *Haemopoietic Stem Cells. Characterisation, Proliferation, Regulation.* Alfred Benzon Symposium 18, (eds. Killmann Sv.-Aa., Cronkite E.P. & Muller-Berat C.N.) p. 174. Munksgaard, Copenhagen.

63 KRATZER P.G. & CHAPMAN V.M. (1981) X chromosome reactivation in oocytes of *Mus caroli. Proc. natn. Acad. Sci. U.S.A.* **78**, 3093.

64 MIGEON B.R. & KENNEDY J.F. (1975) Evidence for the activation of an X chromosome early in the development of the human female. *Am. J. Human Genet.* **27**, 233.

65 DE LORENZO R.J. & RUDDLE F.H. (1969) Genetic control of two electrophoretic variants of glucose phosphate isomerase in the mouse (*Mus musculus*). *Biochem. Genet.* **3**, 151.

66 CHAPMAN V.M., ANSELL J.D. & MCLAREN A. (1972) Trophoblast giant cell formation in the mouse. Expression of glucose phosphate isomerase (GPI-1) electrophoretic variants in transferred and chimeric embryos. *Devl Biol.* **29**, 48.

67 PETERSON A.C., FRAIR P.M. & WONG G.G. (1978) A technique for detection and quantitative analysis of glucose phosphate isomerase isozymes from nanogram tissue samples. *Biochem. Genet.* **16**, 681.

68 MARSHALL M.J. & WORSFOLD M. (1978) Analytical micro-preparative electrophoresis: quantitation of phosphoglucose isomerase enzymes. *Analyt. Biochem.* **91**, 283.

69 ANSELL J.D., BARLOW P.W. & MCLAREN A. (1974) Binucleate and polyploid cells in the decidua of the mouse. *J. Embryol. exp. Morph.* **31**, 223.

70 HARRISON D.E. (1973) Normal production of erythrocytes by mouse marrow continuous for 73 months. *Proc. natn. Acad. Sci. U.S.A.* **70**, 3184.

71 HARRISON D.E. & CHERRY M. (1975) Survival of marrow allografts in *W/W^v* anemic mice: effect of disparity at the Ea-2 locus. *Immunogenetics*, **2**, 219–229.

72 WEGMANN T.G. (1970) Enzyme patterns in tetraparental mouse liver. *Nature*, **225**, 462.

73 WEST J.D. (1976) Patches in the livers of chimaeric mice. *J. Embryol. exp. Morph.* **36**, 151.

74 DEWEY M.J. & MINTZ B. (1978) Direct visualisation, by β-glucuronidase activity, of differentiated normal cells derived from malignant teratocarcinoma in allophenic mice. *Devl. Biol.* **66**, 550.

75 VAN BEKKUM D.W. & DE VRIES M.J. (1967) *Radiation Chimaeras*, p. 17. Logos Press, Academic Press, London.

76 PAIGEN K. (1979) Acid hydrolases as models of genetic control. *Ann. Rev. Genet.* **13**, 417.

77 DE MARS R., LEVAN S.L., TREND B.L. & RUSSELL L.B. (1976) Abnormal ornithine carbomoyl transferase in mice having the sparse-fur mutation. *Proc. natn. Acad. Sci. U.S.A.* **73**, 1693.

78 WILLIAMS E.D., WAREHAM K.A. & HOWELL S. (1983) Direct evidence for the single cell origin of mouse liver cell tumours. *Br. J. Cancer*, **49**, 723.

79 WAREHAM K.A., HOWELL S., WILLIAMS D. & WILLIAMS E.D. (1983) Studies of X-chromosome inactivation with an improved histochemical technique for ornithine carbomoyl transferase. *Histochem. J.* **15**, 363.

80 BUTCHER E.C. & FORD W.L. (1985) Following cellular traffic: methods of labelling lymphocytes and other cells to trace their migration *in vitro*. In *Handbook of Experimental Immunology*, 4th edn., Chapter 57, (eds. Weir D.M., Herzenberg L.A., Blackwell C.C. & Herzenberg L.A.). Blackwell Scientific Publications, Oxford.

81 GEARHART J. & OSTER-GRANITE M.L. (1978) Antibodies to allozymes as potential cell markers for chimaeric mouse studies. In *Genetic Mosaics and Chimaeras in Mammals*, (ed. Russell L.B.), p. 111. Plenum Press, New York.

82 GEARHART J., OSTER-GRANITE M.L. & MUSSER J.M. (1979) Immunoreactivity of the two common allozymes of murine glucose phosphate isomerase. *Biochem. Genet.* **19**, 445.

83 TEMPLE S. & RAFF M.C. (1985) Differentiation of a bipotential glial progenitor cell in a single cell microculture. *Nature*, **313**, 223.

84 ABNEY E., WILLIAMS B.P. & RAFF M.C. (1983) Tracing the development of oligodendrocytes from precursor cells using monoclonal antibodies, fluorescence activated cell sorting and cell culture. *Devl Biol.* **100**, 166.

85 MICKLEM H.S., ANDERSON N., URE J. & JONES H.P. (1976) Long term immunoglobulin G production by transplanted thymus cells. *Eur. J. Immunol.* **6**, 425.

86 OKUMURA K., JULIUS M.H., TSU T., HERZENBERG L.A. & HERZENBERG L.A. (1976) Demonstration that IgG memory is carried by IgG-bearing cells. *Eur. J. Immunol.* **6**, 467.

87 RUSSELL E.S. (1979) Hereditary anemias of the mouse: A review for geneticists. *Adv. Genet.* **20**, 357.

88 RUSSELL E.S. (1983) Three distinct gene actions disturbing proliferation and function of hemopoietic stem cells. In *Haemopoietic Stem Cells. Characterisation, Proliferation, Regulation.* Alfred Benzon Symposium 18, (eds. Killmann Sv.-Aa., Cronkite E.P. & Muller-Berat C.N.), p. 108. Munksgaard, Copenhagen.

89 THOMPSON M.W., MCCULLOCH E.A., SIMINOVITCH L. & TILL J.E. (1966) The cellular basis for the defect in hemopoiesis in mice with Hertwig's anemia. *Genetics*, **54**, 366.

90 PARKS D.R., HARDY R.R. & HERZENBERG L.A. (1983)

Dual immunofluorescence—new frontiers in cell analysis and sorting. *Immunology Today*, **4**, 145.

91 FLEISCHMAN R.A., CUSTER R.P. & MINTZ B. (1982) Totipotent haematopoietic stem cells: normal self-renewal and differentiation after transplantation between mouse fetuses. *Cell*, **30**, 351.

92 FORRESTER L.M. & ANSELL J.D. (1985) Parental influences on X chromosome expression. *Genet. Res. Camb*. **45**, 95.

93 MICKLEM H.S. & FORD C.E. (1960) Proliferation of injected lymph node and thymus cells in lethally irradiated mice. *Transplant. Bull*. **28**, 436.

94 SCHER I. (1982) The CBA/N mouse strain: an experimental model illustrating the influence of the X chromosome on immunity. *Adv. Immunol*. **33**, 1.

95 HARDY R.R., HAYAKAWA K., HAAIJMAN J., HERZENBERG L.A. & HERZENBERG L.A. (1982) B cell subpopulations identified by two-color fluorescence analysis. *Nature*, **297**, 589.

96 HARDY R.R., HAYAKAWA K., PARKS D.R., HERZENBERG L.A. & HERZENBERG L.A. (1984) Murine B cell differentiation lineages. *J. exp. Med*. **159**, 1169.

97 NAHM M.H., PASLAY J.W. & DAVIE J.M. (1983) Unbalanced X chromosome mosaicism in B cells of mice with X-linked immunodeficiency. *J. exp. Med*. **158**, 920.

98 WITKOWSKI J., FORRESTER L.M., ANSELL J.D. & MICKLEM H.S. (1985) Influence of the *Xid* mutation on B lymphocyte development in adult mice. In *Microenvironments in the Lymphoid System*, (ed. Klaus G.), p. 47. *Adv. exp. Biol. Med*. **186.** Plenum Press, New York.

99 NESBITT M.N. (1971) X chromosome inactivation mosaics in the mouse. *Devl. Biol*. **26**, 252.

100 MCLAREN A. (1972) Numerology of development. *Nature*, **239**, 274.

101 STONE M. (1983) A general statistical model for clone-tissue studies, using X-chromosome inactivation data. *Biometrics*, **39**, 395.

102 STONE M. (1984) Variance-covariance modelling with chromosome markers. *J. theor. Biol*. **107**, 275.

103 ROSSANT J. (1984) Somatic cell lineages in mammalian chimaeras. In *Chimaeras in Developmental Biology*, (eds. Le Douarin N. & McLaren A.), p. 89. Academic Press, New York, London.

104 VOGELSTEIN B., FEARON E.R., HAMILTON S.R. & FEINBERG A.P. (1985) Use of restriction fragment length polymorphisms to determine the clonal origin of human trumors. *Science*, **227**, 642.

105 EHRLICH M. & WANG R.Y.-H. (1981) 5-Methylcytosine in eukaryotic DNA. *Science*, **212**, 1350.

106 WEST J.D., BÜCHER T., LINKE I.M. & DÜNNWALD M. (1984) Investigation of variability among mouse aggregation chimaeras and X-chromosome inactivation mosaics. *J. Embryol. exp. Morphol*. **84,** 309.

107 WILLIAMS D.A., LEMISCHKA I.R., NATHAN D.G. & MULLIGAN R.C. (1984) Introduction of new genetic material into pluripotent haematopoietic stem cells of the mouse. *Nature*, **310**, 476.

Chapter 57
Following cellular traffic: methods of labelling lymphocytes and other cells to trace their migration *in vivo*

E. C. BUTCHER & W. L. FORD

Counting cells in traffic streams, 57.2

The tracer sample principle, 57.3

Radioactive labels for lymphocytes and other cells, 57.5

Non-radioactive methods of cell tracing, 57.12

Intrinsic markers for cell tracing, 57.17

In vitro assay of lymphocyte binding to post-capillary high endothelial venules, 57.18

The lymphocytes in the bloodstream cross blood vessel walls with fine discrimination to enter mainly lymphatic tissues. After following partially defined routes through the interstitial spaces of the spleen, lymph nodes, and gut-associated lymphoid tissue, they return to the blood within a few hours or days depending on the organ and the class of lymphocytes. The recirculating pool of T lymphocytes in a young adult rat is described schematically in Fig. 57.1. B lymphocytes also recirculate, although they take much longer to traverse the spleen and lymph nodes to return to the blood. They leave the blood at about the same rate as do T lymphocytes and show preferential entry into certain organs such as Peyer's patches and the spleen. After arriving by the same portal of entry, the B lymphocytes segregate from the T lymphocytes to enter the follicular areas which are usually recognizable by the presence of germinal centres.

The term 'recirculation' refers to the complete, cyclical journey from blood to tissue and back to blood; 'migration' refers to the movement of cells from one location to another; 'localization' refers to the numbers of cells belonging to a defined population present at a given site at a particular time. The terms 'influx' and 'efflux' are appropriate for the rates at which cells enter or leave a given compartment. Thus increased localization in a compartment may be a consequence of increased influx or decreased efflux, i.e. retention.

There are two general reasons for studying lymphocyte traffic. The first is to gain understanding of immune responses *in vivo* since the stream of lymphocytes through a tissue provides a supply of antigen reactive cells [1]. The second is to clarify the mechanisms underlying the selective migration of leucocytes from the bloodstream and in an even broader context as a model for the cellular interactions underlying the organization of cells into tissues. Lymphocytes of different classes have a complicated relationship to vascular endothelia in different organs. Although it is at present incompletely understood, the tools required to unravel this pattern of interactions are becoming available.

Lymphocyte recirculation has been divided into four stages.

1 *Distribution by the bloodstream.* The fraction of cardiac output reaching an organ determines the supply of lymphocytes available for extraction. In the course of immune responses, local increases in blood flow contribute to a greater influx of lymphocytes. Blood flow to lymphatic organs has been measured by the embolization of radiolabelled microspheres [2]; the rubidium-86 clearance technique [3] and has been visualized by micro-angiography [4].

2 *Crossing vascular endothelium.* This stage can be subdivided into adhesion to the luminal face of the endothelial cell, followed by migration across the endothelium and through the basement membrane [5].

3 *Segregation of B and T cells* into distinctive compartments [6]. This can only be studied effectively by histological techniques.

4 *Movement through the tissues* and return to the bloodstream. This is not precisely delimited from stage 3.

The technical approaches used for studying lymphocyte traffic can be classified as: (1) counting cells in traffic streams within lymphatic channels; (2) the tracer sample principle by which a sample population of marked cells is followed over a period of time—the label may be applied *in vitro* or *in situ*; and (3) *in vitro*

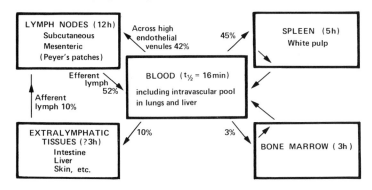

Fig. 57.1. The recirculating pool of T lymphocytes in the rat. Five compartments are represented although the lymph nodes and extra-lymphatic tissues could each be subdivided. The stated percentage refers to the fraction of T lymphocytes leaving the blood. Thus 45% of lymphocytes leaving the blood enter the spleen. The stated time refers to an approximate average transit time across the compartment.

The mesenteric lymph nodes probably receive many more lymphocytes via their afferent lymphatics than do subcutaneous lymph nodes, so that the 10% for afferent lymph is a loose approximation. The number of recirculating T lymphocytes in an adult rat of 200 g is approximately 10^9 but varies greatly according to strain and environment.

studies of the interaction of lymphocytes with the specialized endothelial cells that mediate their exit from the blood, in isolation from the complexities of the *in vivo* situation. These methods are considered below in terms of their usefulness for studies of lymphocyte migration but the techniques involved have wider applicability to the study of the migration, maturation and fate of many cell types.

Counting cells in traffic streams

The rate at which lymphocytes leave a lymph node under different circumstances can be estimated by cannulation of the efferent lymphatic from the lymph node, as has been done for several centuries [7]. Cells are collected over measured time intervals, enumerated usually by means of a Coulter counter and the cell flux is expressed as the number of cells per hour. The volume of lymph is also recorded since increased lymph flow can 'wash out' an increased number of cells although in the long term the traffic of cells in lymph appears to be independent of physiological fluctuations in the flow of lymph.

In recent years the most informative experiments using this approach have exploited the prominent lymphatic vessels of the sheep. The single efferent lymphatic from a lymph node such as the popliteal or prescapular can be cannulated and lymph can be collected over a period of weeks [8,9,10]. Larger animals such as sheep [11], pigs [12], and humans [13] also offer the opportunity of cannulating afferent lymphatics. If the cannula is pointed distally, peripheral lymph that has not passed through a lymph node can be collected. Such lymph has a low concentration of cells which include macrophages, mainly T lymphocytes and veiled cells which are probably the immediate precursors of interdigitating cells in lymph nodes.

The afferent lymphatic may be cannulated with the cannula pointing centrally—towards the lymph node—in order that drugs, mediators or antigens can be infused to reach the lymph node by the natural avenue. The efferent lymphatic may be cannulated at the same time to allow the flux of cells from the lymph node to be continuously monitored. Thus any change in the fourth stage of recirculation—the release of lymphocytes from the tissue—can be critically analysed in response to such agents. For example, the sheep lymph node with afferent and efferent lymphatics cannulated has yielded unique information on the biphasic changes in cell efflux following the injection of antigens into the lymph node. An early decrease in cell traffic is followed by an increased efflux of lymphocytes including a high proportion of lymphoblasts [9].

The great advantage of this approach is that recirculating lymphocytes do not have to be marked or modified in any way that may interfere with their ability to migrate. The flux of cells in a lymphatic channel can be studied under near to steady-state conditions since when only a single lymph node is cannulated the rate of depletion of the whole recirculating pool is very slow even if the cells are not replaced. The main disadvantage of simply measuring cell fluxes in a lymphatic channel is that it is limited in scope. Unless supplemented by other techniques it provides no direct information on the influx of lymphocytes from the blood or the segregation of B and T lymphocytes.

In experimental species more usually favoured by immunologists, namely mice and rats, cannulation of the efferent lymphatic from a single lymph node is too difficult to have become routine. Cannulation of the thoracic duct in the abdomen permits the collection of lymph from all the tissues below the diaphragm. Most of the lymphocytes in the collection will have recirculated through lymph nodes and Peyer's patches. A method for the cannulation of the thoracic duct of the rat was described in the previous two editions of this handbook [14] where references were given to the technique in the mouse [15] as well as other species. In rats and mice undergoing thoracic duct drainage the recirculating lymphocyte pool is rapidly depleted because of the loss of all the cells recirculating through the drainage area. Thus in the rat the thoracic duct output falls nearly exponentially with a halving time of 1.4 days [16]. The great advantages of thoracic duct cannulation in rodents are as a source of (predominantly) recirculating lymphocytes and in combination with the tracer sample principle (see below).

The tracer sample principle

A more versatile approach was pioneered by Gowans & Knight [17]. A sample of lymphocytes taken from a certain source is injected intravenously into one or more recipients in order that its fate and distribution can be followed over a period of time (Fig. 57.2). The main disadvantage is that the cells must be marked in some way, either by applying an extrinsic label such as fluorescence or radioactivity or they must bear an intrinsic label usually recognized as an antigen. The possibility that the marker may interfere with the cell traffic has to be recognized, and when a new method is introduced the effect of the labelling procedure on lymphocyte circulation should be assessed by comparison with an alternatively labelled population whose migratory behaviour is known from previous experiments or from the literature. This principle can be modified to study all stages of lymphocytes recirculation and is, therefore, considered in detail below.

General conditions

The starting population: the sample of lymphocytes to be followed in the recipient may be obtained from lymph, from blood after separating lymphocytes from other cells, or from lymphatic tissues—usually the lymph nodes but sometimes the spleen or other tissues. The sample may be fractionated, e.g. into T or B cells by the positive or negative selection techniques described in Chapter 55. The choice of starting population will of course depend on the questions being addressed by the experiment. If there is no special reason to use cells from lymphatic tissues, then to start with cells centrifuged from efferent lymph has a number of advantages. First, most of the cells are recirculating lymphocytes and second, the effect of Ficoll separation or the unavoidable trauma of producing a single cell suspension is avoided. Third, the cells were about to enter the venous blood and therefore injecting them intravenously comes close to the physiological situation. If lymphatic cannulation is a routine in a laboratory it represents little or no inconvenience.

Separation of mononuclear cells from the blood can be performed efficiently by the Ficoll-isopaque method of Bøyum [18]. Far fewer lymphocytes are obtained: an overnight collection of thoracic duct lymphocytes contains about 50 times as many lymphocytes as can be recovered from a 2 ml blood sample from a rat. In the case of humans the blood is the most convenient source of recirculating lymphocytes and leucocophoresis, using continuous flow centrifugation with a cell separator, offers a great advantage in cell numbers obtainable [19].

In experimental animals, especially mice, it is convenient to start with a suspension made from lymph nodes, Peyer's patches, or spleen. In this case, the possibility of trauma during cell suspension must be borne in mind, as well as the fact that these tissues

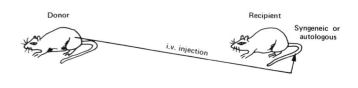

Fig. 57.2. The tracer sample principle, indicating the three areas in which consideration of the experimental design is important.

contain non-lymphocytic cells. For example, about 20% of the mononuclear cells in the adult mouse spleen are non-lymphocytic. Moreover the lymphocyte populations in these tissues (and in efferent lymph as well) are far from uniform. First, recirculating lymphocytes differ in their migratory behaviour and tissue preferences as a function of their class and state of differentiation; second, the migratory capacity of lymphocytes may be reversibly altered by the process of crossing the vascular endothelium [20]; and third, some lymphocytes in lymphoid organs seem to be transiently or permanently outside the recirculating pool.

Handling lymphocytes in vitro

Several enzymes, lectins, and antibodies applied to lymphocytes *in vitro* have been found to inhibit the ability of lymphocytes to cross high endothelial venules into lymph nodes [21,22]. Simply holding lymphocytes *in vitro*, either in lymph or in RPMI 1640, also profoundly depresses this delicate function. Similarly, the changes in temperature inherent in a radioactive labelling procedure significantly impair early localization in lymph nodes [16,20]. Fig. 57.3 shows the different tempo of localization in lymph nodes of thoracic duct cells, that have been collected conventionally overnight at 0 °C, labelled with ^{51}Cr and injected i.v., and thoracic duct cells similarly labelled but passaged from blood to lymph through an intermediate rat before injection. Selection of a subset of 'fast recirculators' is not the explanation of this difference [20]. The authors are not suggesting that every experiment on lymphocyte traffic requires the sample population to have been passaged from blood to lymph but this is a unique way of restoring labelled lymphocytes to their physiological state, as described in the sample experiment on page 57.12.

The recipients

Lymphocytes injected into an incompatible recipient are liable to rejection, as are other cell types. Even in recipients that have never been immunized, the elimination of allogeneic lymphocytes begins within a few hours [23,24]. Therefore tracer sample studies are usually performed in a syngeneic donor/recipient combination of inbred rats or mice. In larger animals, including man, lymphocytes are isolated, labelled *in vitro*, and reinfused autologously [19].

The next consideration is where and when to look for the injected cells in the recipients. The search should be as comprehensive as possible but, as with all scientific endeavour, a compromise must be struck between what is practicable and what is necessary to provide informative and interpretable data. After i.v. injection most of the changes in small lymphocyte localization occur in the first 30–60 min (Fig. 57.3); between 60 min and 24 h there is not a great deal of change except in the spleen, from whence there is a net redistribution of lymphocytes to the lymph nodes [16]. For many purposes, examining recipients at 30 min and 24 h is satisfactory but with lymphoblasts more time intervals are necessary because in general these cells take longer to leave the lungs and liver than do small lymphocytes [25].

The reason for recommending these time intervals is that at 30 min about three-quarters of the injected lymphocytes have left the blood but none have yet returned from the tissues. Thus the 30 min observations indicate the rate at which lymphocytes are leaving the blood and entering tissues. At 24 h the injected population is near to being evenly distributed throughout the recirculating pool so that the localization of the marked cells gives an indication of the fraction of the recirculating pool in that compartment. If it were necessary to confine a study of lymphocyte

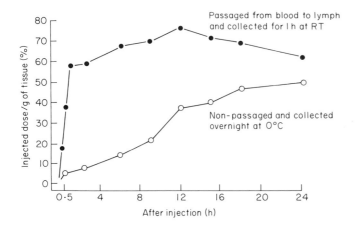

Fig. 57.3. Localization of thoracic duct lymphocytes (TDL) in the cervical lymph nodes after intravenous injection into a syngeneic rat. -O- TDL collected for 16 h at 0 °C, labelled with ^{51}Cr, and injected according to a conventional experimental procedure [25]. ● TDL collected for 16 h at 0°C, labelled with ^{51}Cr, passaged from blood to lymph through an intermediate and collected for 1 h at room temperature [16], according to the sample experiment described. The superior early localization of passaged TDL is due mainly to the conditions of collections and not to selection [20].

traffic to one time interval, 30 or 60 min would usually be a more rational choice than 24 h.

The organs examined obviously depend on the objective of the experiment but in order to understand the variables that may be operating in a whole animal it is suggested that the following should be included: (1) the spleen, (2) the cervical lymph nodes (generally other subcutaneous lymph nodes show similar patterns of localization), (3) mesenteric lymph nodes, (4) a liver sample to check against damage to the cells leading to excessive liver localization, (5) the lungs with the major bronchi removed, (6) the blood mononuclear cells separated from a measured sample of blood by Ficoll/hypaque [18], (7) Peyer's patches, (8) small intestine with Peyer's patches removed, and (9) bone-marrow. With ^{51}Cr-labelled lymphocytes a whole tibia or femur can be inserted into a vial for gamma counting.

In small rodents it is usual to inject a series of recipients to be killed at the chosen time intervals after i.v. injection. At the time of sacrifice the animal is anaesthetized, a large blood sample is taken from the vena cava into a heparinized syringe and the aorta is severed to minimize the blood content of other organs. If the recipients are very precious or limited in number, biopsies of spleen, cervical lymph nodes, and a blood sample can be taken under anaesthesia at an early time interval and the animal killed at a later time interval.

To study lymphocyte recirculation from blood to lymph in rodents, labelled lymphocytes are injected into a recipient that has been subjected to thoracic duct cannulation on the previous day and has recovered from the acute stress of operation. Lymph is collected using a standard fraction collector (e.g. an LKB ultrorac) set for 90 min intervals. Each 90 min lymph fraction is collected into a 12 ml plastic centrifuge tube with 3 ml of heparinized Dulbecco's solution. This enables the tempo of recirculation from blood to lymph to be charted in detail [e.g. 16].

The influence of blood flow in controlling the delivery of lymphocytes to antigenically stimulated lymph nodes has been studied by combining tracer sample experiments using ^{51}Cr-lymphocytes with rubidium-86 chloride estimation of the fractional blood flow [26,27]. This technique is included in the sample experiment at the end of the next section.

Radioactive labels for lymphocytes and other cells

All the methods for labelling lymphocytes produce uneven labelling of the cells and some methods label only certain sub-populations (Table 57.1). The choice of method depends on which lymphocytes are to be studied (e.g. large or small), whether the labelled lymphocytes are to be detected by autoradiography or

by counting whole organs, and sometimes on the practical question of the type of counting apparatus available.

Labelling in vitro *with isotopes which are mainly associated with intracellular protein*

Sodium (^{51}Cr) chromate

A simple, cheap and effective method for making lymphocytes radioactive is to incubate them in the presence of Na$_2$^{51}CrO$_4$. Radioactive chromium enters the cells and is bound principally to intracellular protein [28]. After a substantial loss in the first hour the isotope is lost from living lymphocytes at a low rate (probably about 1% per hour) which may reflect the metabolic turnover of protein [29]. An outstanding advantage of ^{51}Cr labelling is that it emits γ-radiation and therefore tissues containing ^{51}Cr need no preparation beyond putting them in a tube suitable for a deep well scintillation counter. Autoradiography of ^{51}Cr-labelled cells is possible by exploiting the internal conversion effect [30]. This method is satisfactory for methanol-fixed smears of lymphocytes but localization of cell-associated radioactivity in sections of lymphoid organs is poor for unknown reasons.

Equipment

Water bath at 37 °C.
Bench centrifuge.
Sterile 10 ml tubes or 25 ml Erlenmayer flasks.
One millilitre syringes.

Materials

Sodium (^{51}Cr) chromate (from Amersham International CJS.IP; specific activity 100–300 mCi/mg Cr).
HEPES buffered RPMI 1640 (Flow Labs.) plus 10% fetal calf serum or newborn calf serum.

Procedure (based on refs. 31 and 32)

1 Washed cells are suspended at a concentration of 5×10 cells per ml in medium RPMI 1640 plus 10% fetal calf serum.
2 Sodium (^{51}Cr) chromate is added to a concentration of 10 μCi/ml. Note that for labelling target cells for *in vitro* cytotoxicity assays much higher concentrations (100–200 μCi/ml) are conventionally used. However, radiocytotoxicity has been detected when lymphocytes were labelled *in vitro* at 100 μCi/ml and then tested *in vivo* by the popliteal lymph node assay [33].
3 The suspension is incubated at 37 °C for 60 min with frequent gentle resuspension.

Table 57.1. Summary of selected methods for radioactively labelling lymphocytes and other cells *in vitro*

Principal material labelled	Distribution of label among lymphocytes	Isotope	Compound	Suggested concentration in medium[1]	Suitability for auto-radiography[2]	Method of counting[3]	Re-utiliz-ation[4]	Toxicity[5]	References
Protein	All cells, large more than small	^{51}Cr	Sodium chromate	10 μCi/(5×10^7 cells per ml)	±	γ	±	+	[31,32,35]
		^{111}In	Indium oxine	5–20 μCi/(10^8 cells per ml)	+	γ	±	++	[36–43]
		^{114m}In	Indium oxine	1–5 μCi/(10^8 cells per ml)	+	β or γ	±	+++	–
		^{3}H	4,5-^{3}H-leucine	10 μCi/(5×10^7 cells per ml)	++	β	+++	+	[6]
		^{14}C	U-^{14}C-leucine	1–2 μCi/(5×10^7 cells per ml)	++	β	+++	+	[35]
RNA	Large more than small	^{3}H	5-^{3}H-uridine	5–25 μCi/(5×10^7 cells per ml)	+++	β	±	+	[50–52]
	In some species, small T more than small B	^{14}C	U-^{14}C-uridine	1–2 μCi/(5×10^7 cells per ml)	+++	β	±	+	[50–52]
DNA	Exclusively large lymphocytes (20–100% depending on time of incubation)	^{3}H	6-^{3}H-thymidine	0.1–0.3 μCi/(5×10^7 cells per ml)	+++	β	++	++	[17,55,65]
		^{14}C	U-^{14}C-thymidine	0.1 μCi/(5×10^7 cells per ml)	++	β	++	++	[69]
		^{125}I	Iododeoxy-uridine	0.01–0.1 μCi/(5×10^7 cells per ml)	++	γ	±	+++	[65–67]

[1] A suitable concentration of cells in the labelling medium is 5×10^7 cells per ml but concentrations of 10^7–10^8 cells per ml have been used.
[2] +++, excellent for autoradiographic tracing.
[3] β, liquid scintillation counter; γ, gamma counter.
[4] +++, extensively re-utilized; ±, re-utilization is very little. Note that isotopes that are not in the strict sense re-utilized may nevertheless be retained in the tissue in another form under certain circumstances, e.g. ref. 41.
[5] +++, toxicity is a major problem.

4 The cells are washed two or three times to remove excess isotope.

This method labels rat lymphocytes at about 2000 c.p.m. per 10^6 cells. Since usually $10–100 \times 10^6$ cells are injected into each recipient and tissue samples are counted for 10 min, the counts in the lymphatic organs at least are statistically adequate for most purposes, e.g. at 1 h after injecting 20×10^6 lymphocytes the average count in the spleen exceeds 10^5 in 10 min.

The method labels 98–99% of lymphocytes. However, the labelling is uneven; on autoradiographs it is clear that large lymphocytes take up most radioactivity and there is a close positive correlation between cell volume and ^{51}Cr uptake, as shown by sedimentation velocity analysis [34]. Erythrocytes take up at least as much ^{51}Cr as small lymphocytes and this can be misleading, especially if measurements are to be made on the blood of recipients. It may be necessary to remove them before labelling, preferably by Ficoll/Hypaque centrifugation.

After it is released from cells, ^{51}Cr is concentrated by the kidney and excreted quickly, which minimizes the potentially misleading effect of the persistence of isotope that is no longer associated with cells [35]. ^{51}Cr is not reutilized in the usual sense but when lymphocytes die in lymphatic tissues there is strong presumptive evidence that the ^{51}Cr is retained for long periods in non-lymphocytic cells [24]. The popularity of ^{51}Cr for following cells *in vivo* is deserved, although for some special purposes, especially autoradiography, other isotopes are better.

^{111}In-indium oxine

Indium-111 emits penetrating gamma rays of an energy that is especially suitable for external detection. Its half life of 2.8 days is near to ideal for studies in patients when it is important to minimize the cumulative dose of radiation. In order to enhance the uptake by cells *in vitro* McAfee & Thakur [36] chelated indium with oxine (hydroxyquinolone)—a lipophilic chelating agent. It has been consistently found that lymphocytes incubated at 10^8 per ml with ^{111}In-oxine take up 80–90% of the ^{111}In at room temperature in 10 min [37,38,39]. Another advantage of ^{111}In labelling is that under favourable conditions the spontaneous release of radioactivity from living cells is very slow, so that it can be used as an alternative to ^{51}Cr as a label for target cells for the quantification of cytotoxicity [40].

A number of methodological studies of the conditions labelling lymphocytes with ^{111}In have been published in recent years [37–41]. It has emerged that the low energy Auger electrons from ^{111}In are very damaging to radiosensitive cells like lymphocytes. Because of this and the high proportion of ^{111}In incorporated, radiation toxicity is a serious problem.

Labelling lymphocytes at 20 μCi/10^8/ml allows most of them to survive for 24 h [39,41] but six days later most of them were found to be dead [41], which stresses that the radiation damage to cells is cumulative, so that the shorter the experiment the less the danger of cell damage.

Materials

Quality controlled ^{111}In-oxine is available from Amersham International UK and Diagnostic Isotopes Ltd. Bloomfield, N.J. In the authors' laboratory and others, chemical toxicity has been evident when ^{111}In has been chelated with oxine under conditions that have allowed slight contamination with heavy metals [41].

Procedure

1 Glassware to be used for the labelling procedure is soaked overnight in 0.01 N HCl and exhaustively rinsed in distilled water to remove traces of metals.
2 Lymphocytes are washed twice in PBS (*without* serum) and resuspended for labelling in a glass tube at 10^8 cells per ml in PBS.
3 In-oxine is added to give a final concentration of 4–20 μCi of ^{111}In per ml.
4 The suspension is left at room temperature for 10 min with occasional swirling.
5 The tube is filled with Dulbecco's solution (DAB), centrifuged, washed once in DAB, and finally washed by layering the cell suspension on top of 10 ml
6 DAB:FCS (1:1) in a 35 ml conical tube. This removes any loosely attached indium by exploiting the avid binding capacity of the transferrin in FCS.

The cells are resuspended in DAB plus 2% FCS for injection.

Detection of ^{111}In

The labelled lymphocytes can be followed by (1) external detection devices such as the gamma camera or detectors placed over the spleen, lymph nodes etc., (2) gamma counting of tissue samples, and (3) autoradiography exploiting the Auger electrons of ^{111}In. For human studies it is usually best to separate leucocytes initially by continuous centrifugation of blood on a cell separator. The white cell concentrate is then subjected to Ficoll/isopaque purification as has been described in detail elsewhere [19]. After labelling about 5×10^8 cells at 20 μCi/10^8/ml approximately 100 μCi of ^{111}In are injected. This gives sufficient localization of radioactivity in the spleen and lymph nodes to produce satisfactory gamma camera images. Dynamic studies of lymphocyte migration can be obtained by taking gamma camera images at a succession of times up to 48 h. The early events after intravenous injection have been followed by placing a gamma camera over the patient from the time of injection [42].

In large and expensive experimental animals such as sheep the opportunity to use gamma camera imaging may be invaluable. Frost *et al.* produced excellent gamma camera images of the spleen and lymph nodes of the sheep by injecting 150 μCi of ^{111}In associated with autologous lymphocytes [43]. Another advantage of ^{111}In in precious recipients is that two populations of lymphocytes labelled alternatively with ^{51}Cr and ^{111}In can be followed independently by setting appropriate windows of a gamma counter [44,99].

In small rodents ^{111}In can be used as an alternative to ^{51}Cr labelling. Tissue samples can be counted in a gamma counter and autoradiography of labelled cells in sections is better than with ^{51}Cr-labelled cells although not as good as with ^{3}H-uridine. However, because of the short half-life, histological processing must be rapid. In conclusion, ^{51}Cr labelling remains more convenient than ^{111}In labelling for most experimental purposes, partly because its longer half-life means that new batches need be purchased only once every 4–6 weeks.

Current developments of indium labelling techniques

Tropolone is under trial as an alternative chelating agent to oxine. It effectively carries ^{111}In into polymorphs, and the labelling can be done in the presence of serum which may be a considerable advantage for lymphocytes as well as for polymorphs [45].

Another isotope of indium—[114m]In—has been chelated with oxine to label lymphocytes. It emits both energetic β and γ rays and has a half-life of 50 days. Its usefulness is being evaluated in Manchester.

4,5-^{3}H-leucine and U-^{14}C-leucine

Lymphocytes labelled with ^{3}H-leucine or ^{14}C-leucine can be detected autoradiographically or by liquid scintillation counting. If serum is added to the labelling mixture, then the endogenous leucine will reduce the uptake of radioactive leucine but this slight disadvantage is usually more than compensated for by the beneficial effect of serum on cell recovery.

Materials and equipment

As required for labelling with ^{51}Cr except 4,5-^{3}H-leucine (TRK.170, Amersham International) or U-^{14}C-leucine (CFB.67,A.I.).

Procedure

1   Washed lymphoid cells are suspended at a concentration of 5×10^7 cells per ml in a buffered medium (e.g. RPMI 1640 with bicarbonate buffer) plus 5% fetal or new-born bovine serum.
2   ^{3}H-leucine or ^{14}C-leucine is added to a concentration of 10 μCi/ml or 1–2 μCi/ml respectively.
3   The mixture is incubated at 37 °C for 1 h while the cells are kept in suspension.
4   The cells are washed two to three times to remove the excess isotope.

The loss of radioactivity from leucine-labelled cells after transfer to irradiated recipients is substantially faster than is the case with ^{51}Cr-labelled cells, and ^{3}H is lost faster than [14]C [35]. As would be expected, radioactive leucine is extensively reutilized and the proportion of lymphocyte-associated radioactivity to reutilized radioactivity varies between different tissues. The main application of leucine labelling may be for the autoradiographic localization of lymphocytes for up to 48 h [6]. For organ or tissue counting it is inferior to ^{51}Cr on several counts.

In the third edition of this book, methods for labelling lymphocytes with sodium pertechnetate (^{99m}Tc) and ^{75}Se-selenomethonine were described [14] but they have not proved to be popular.

Labelling in vitro *with radioactive RNA precursors*

A range of radioactive RNA nucleosides is available from Amersham International. The most suitable compounds for labelling lymphocytes are 5-^{3}H-uridine and U-^{14}C-uridine. Neither of these compounds is completely specific for RNA; both may be converted to DNA precursors to a limited extent. The labelled atom of 5-^{3}H-uridine is lost when it is converted to thymidylic acid by methylation at the 5 position [46], but it is retained when uridine is converted to cytidine nucleotides which are incorporated into both DNA and RNA [47].

5-^{3}H-uridine or U-^{14}C-uridine

Materials and equipment

As for labelling with ^{51}Cr except for radioactive uridine (see below).

Procedure

1   The cells are counted, centrifuged, and resuspended at 5×10^7 cells per ml in medium RPMI 1640 (Flow Laboratories) to which has been added 10% fetal bovine serum.
2   The suspension is transferred to a sterile 25 ml conical flask.

3 With a disposable 1.0 ml syringe 5-^{3}H-uridine (TRA.178, Amersham) is added to give a concentration of 5–10 μCi/ml. Alternatively, U-^{14}C-uridine (CFB.51) is added to a concentration of 1–2 μCi/ml.
4 The flask is incubated for 1 h at 37 °C. The cells are kept in suspension by gentle swirling every 15 min.
5 The cells need only be washed once before being injected into a recipient. The radioactivity per 10^6 cells injected is measured on an aliquot of the final cell suspension.

The absolute radioactivity associated with thoracic duct lymphocytes labelled in this way is about 20 000 d.p.m. for every 10^6 cells with 5-^{3}H-uridine (5 μCi/ml) and 5000 d.p.m. for every 10^6 cells with U-^{14}C-uridine (2 μCi/ml). These figures are only a rough guide because there is much day-to-day variation. If labelling is poor, it often helps to incubate the uridine at 80 °C for 10 min immediately prior to use.

Immediately after labelling, most of the radioactivity in lymphocytes is in the form of low molecular weight, acid-soluble material. Approximately half of the radioactivity is lost from the cells within 12 h of labelling and by that time most of the rest is present in RNA (acid-insoluble). After the early period of rapid loss, radioactivity is lost much more slowly from lymphocytes (very approximately 20% per day); this is mainly attributable to the metabolic turnover of RNA.

Radioactive uridine labels both large and small lymphocytes. The intensity of labelling is uneven among the small lymphocytes in rat thoracic duct lymph because T small lymphocytes take up about 10–15 times as much isotope as B small lymphocytes [34]. This useful difference in the labelling of B and T small lymphocytes is not present in mouse small lymphocytes [48]. The difference is detectable between human B and T lymphocytes [49] but whether it is large enough to be exploited is doubtful.

Although in the rat B lymphocytes are so much inferior to T lymphocytes in their uptake of radioactive uridine, they can be labelled for autoradiography at a concentration of 25 μCi/ml of ^{3}H-uridine with exposures of 2–4 weeks. This enables lightly labelled B lymphocytes to be distinguished from heavily labelled T lymphocytes, provided that the populations have segregated in the tissue. The main applications of labelling with radioactive uridine are for autoradiography and for organ localization studies by scintillation counting where it is an advantage to be able to detect alternatively labelled populations in the same tissue. By labelling one population with ^{3}H-uridine and a control population with ^{14}C-uridine it is possible to detect differences in localization between populations of the order of 1–2%. This principle was described independently by Thursh & Emeson [50] and

Ford & Simmonds [51]. Swapping the isotopes between the two populations enables compensation to be made for the fact that ^{3}H is lost from cells slightly faster than ^{14}C. The application of this method has been described in detail [52].

The disadvantages of ^{3}H- or ^{14}C-uridine labelling are the laborious sample preparation which is necessary for organ counting and the fact that the radioactivity which is released from living lymphocytes, although probably poorly reutilized for RNA synthesis, persists for some time in tissues and is therefore a source of quantitative error in localization studies. This persistence is much greater with ^{3}H-uridine than with ^{14}C-uridine and therefore the former is generally unsuitable for localization studies in non-lymphoid tissue where the released radioactivity may swamp the relatively small localization of lymphocyte-associated radioactivity. Theoretically this difficulty could be overcome by trichloracetic acid extraction [53] but in practice application of this procedure to solid tissues is uncertain in its effectiveness.

Labelling in vitro *with radioactive DNA precursors*

Proliferating cells such as large lymphocytes incorporate thymidine during the DNA synthesizing phase of their cell cycle. Small lymphocytes are non-proliferating cells and do not synthesize DNA unless activated and transformed to a blast cell by a mitogen or an appropriate antigen. Therefore when lymphocytes are incubated *in vitro* with a radioactive DNA precursor such as ^{3}H-thymidine or ^{14}C-thymidine, small lymphocytes are not labelled. However, those large lymphocytes which are in 'S'-phase do take up label and this may approach 50% as the 'S'-phase forms a relatively large part of the short cell cycle time of large lymphocytes [54]. Since the population is dividing asynchronously, the proportion of labelled large lymphocytes increases with the duration of incubation.

6-^{3}H-thymidine and U-^{14}C-thymidine

Labelling *in vitro* with radioactive thymidine has been used to trace the fate of large lymphocytes [17,55]. The procedure is identical to that described for radioactive uridine except that either 6-^{3}H-thymidine (TRA.61) or alternatively U-^{14}C-thymidine (CFB.77) is added to a concentration of 0.1–0.3 μCi/ml. Several difficulties must be considered in interpreting experiments with radioactive thymidine, including (1) release of label by dead cells and its reutilization by other cells [56–58], and (2) damage to the labelled cells due to intranuclear radiation [59,60]. In general, the concentration of radioactive thymidine should be kept at a minimum and when necessary reutilization can be reduced by giving an excess of non-radioactive thymidine.

5-¹²⁵I-iodo-2'-deoxyuridine (¹²⁵IUdR)

5-^{125}I-iodo-2'-deoxyuridine (^{125}IUdR)

This compound competes with thymidine for uptake during DNA synthesis because the iodine atom is sterically similar to the methyl group of thymidine. It has become popular as a label for DNA synthesizing cells because it is released from dead cells as ^{125}I so that reutilization is minimal [61,62] and because sample preparation for counting ^{125}I is easy.

Labelling with ^{125}IUdR *in vitro* has proved useful for at least two purposes: (1) labelling target cells for cytotoxic assays based on isotopic release from dead cells [63]; and (2) determining the fate of tumour cells after injection into recipients [64]. However, for lymphocyte tracing studies the serious toxicity of intranuclear radiation from ^{125}I is a considerable disadvantage. Hofer & Hughes [60] estimated that radiation from ^{125}IUdR is about 4–5 times as toxic as radiation from ^{3}H-thymidine and provided a physical explanation for this large factor. Several workers [65–67] have used ^{125}IUdR to label DNA-synthesizing lymphoid cells in order to follow their fate in recipients. Sprent [65] concluded that labelling at 1.0 μCi/ml or 0.1 μCi/ml was a useful method for short-term studies of T lymphocyte migration but he implied that even the lower concentration is toxic by 5 days after labelling. Both these points have been confirmed; a rat lymphoma showed evidence of radiation toxicity after labelling at 0.05 μCi/ml, but up to 1.0 μCi/ml can be used for short-term studies on activated lymphocytes (Haslett, Rannie & Ford, unpublished). In conclusion, labelling *in vitro* with ^{125}IUdR should usually be done at several isotopic concentrations. The results can only be regarded as reliable if it is evident that in the particular circumstance less than a seriously toxic concentration was employed.

Labelling in vivo *with radioactive DNA precursors*

Radioactive thymidine

The precursors of small lymphocytes are proliferating cells, and after a single injection of ^{3}H-thymidine is given to an intact animal some of them will take up radioactivity which will be retained in the DNA of the small lymphocytes they produce. When small lymphocytes in the blood of a rat are examined a week after a single pulse of ^{3}H-thymidine, approximately 1% are labelled. Although many large lymphocytes are labelled at a few hours after a single pulse of ^{3}H-thymidine, very few will be detectably labelled after a week because they 'dilute out' their label by repeated cell division.

The continuous infusion of ^{3}H-thymidine labels all the small lymphocytes that have been formed from their precursors since just after the start of the infusion. Labelled small lymphocytes accumulate in the blood, but even after 220 days of continuous i.v. ^{3}H-thymidine infusion, 10% of lymphocytes in the blood of rats were *not* labelled, indicating that some small lymphocytes have a very long life span [58]. The rate at which labelled small lymphocytes accumulate in the blood is higher (6–10% per day) during the first 5 days after continuous exposure to ^{3}H-thymidine infusion than later (about 1–2% per day [58,68]). This and other findings have suggested that some small lymphocytes have a much shorter life span than the majority. On the basis of studies with ^{3}H-thymidine, small lymphocytes have been classified as 'long-lived' and 'short-lived'. The latter have a mean life span of 5 days and a maximum life span of 2 weeks [68]. In the context of ^{3}H-thymidine studies 'life span' is used in a technical sense. Labelled small lymphocytes may disappear from the blood or other tissues because they die, but there are three other possibilities: (1) they divide and dilute out their label; (2) they transform into another cell-type and are no longer recognized as small lymphocytes; and (3) they migrate into another anatomical compartment.

As an alternative to continuous i.v. infusion, ^{3}H-thymidine may be given by repeated i.p. injections every 3, 6 or 12 h depending on how important it is to label all, as opposed to most, newly produced cells. If the object is simply to label some lymphocytes then daily injections are most convenient.

A regime for the rat which labels 'long-lived' lymphocytes is to give daily injections of ^{3}H-thymidine (6-^{3}H-thymidine, TRA.61) at a dose of 1 μCi/g of body weight per day for 20 days and to allow 17 days' interval before isolating thoracic duct or other lymphocytes. This allows time for large lymphocytes to dilute out their label and for 'short-lived' lymphocytes to disappear. If the injections are started in female rats of about 70 g, the cost of labelling each rat is about £50 (Amersham International, 1984). The intensity of the labelling is about 150 d.p.m. for every 10^6 thoracic duct lymphocytes, which is sufficient for autoradiography and for liquid scintillation counting. ^{14}C-thymidine has been injected into mice to label proliferating lymph node cells [69] but in most circumstances it is too expensive.

It is not possible to label exclusively short-lived lymphocytes, but an alternative regime which labels recently produced lymphocytes (i.e. 'short-lived' lymphocytes and young 'long-lived' lymphocytes) is to inject ^{3}H-thymidine daily or twice daily for 5 days and to allow a further 2-day period before isolating the cells to allow some dilution of the large lymphocyte label. A third regime is to administer ^{3}H-thymidine

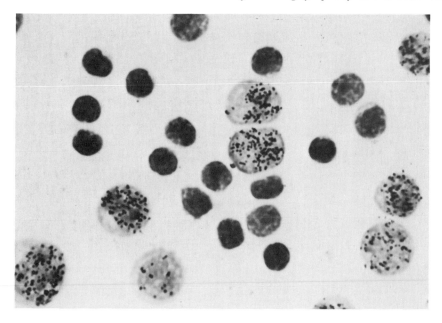

Fig. 57.4. Autoradiograph of thoracic duct lymphocytes from a rat which had received a continuous intravenous infusion of ^{3}H-thymidine throughout the previous 24 h. All the large lymphocytes were labelled but only 1% of small lymphocytes (none in this field).

continuously for 24 h before isolating lymphocytes. This labels almost all large lymphocytes but only a minority of small lymphocytes (Fig. 57.4).

Thus different populations can be labelled by varying the regime of ^{3}H-thymidine administration but homogeneous labelling of lymphocytes with ^{3}H-thymidine is not possible.

5-^{125}I-iodo-2-deoxyuridine

This compound can be used for labelling DNA synthesizing cells by injection into intact animals. It has the same two advantages over ^{3}H-thymidine and the same serious disadvantage of radiation toxicity as were described for *in vitro* labelling. Lance & Cooper used a dose of 4 μCi/mouse to label lymph node cells responding to a skin allograft [70]. The uptake can be increased by the administration of fluorodeoxyuridine (FUdR) which inhibits thymidylate synthetase and so reduces competition from endogenous DNA precursors [62].

The detection of radioactive lymphocytes

Autoradiography

Smears of lymphocytes for autoradiography are fixed in methanol and washed in water to remove low

molecular weight compounds. Tissue specimens are fixed, processed, and embedded by routine methods. Paraffin sections, 5 μm thick, are cut and mounted in the usual way. After de-waxing they are ready for autoradiography. Alternatively, epoxy resin embedded sections may be cut at 1.0 μm and etched in saturated alcoholic NaOH for 15 min.

Techniques of autoradiography have been described fully by Rogers [71]. No special modifications are necessary when dealing with lymphoid cells or tissues. In Manchester, a dipping technique using Ilford nuclear research emulsion G5 or K5 is used. The emulsion is diluted 2 parts to 1 part distilled water and is warmed to 42 °C before dipping. Exposure times are long enough to produce a satisfactory intensity of grains, but usually the amount of radioactive label is such that exposure for 2 weeks is sufficient. After the film is developed, smears are stained with Giemsa and sections with methyl green and pyronin (paraffin) or 1% toluidine blue (epoxy resin).

When assessing autoradiographs of ^{3}H-labelled cells it is vital to remember that the penetration of the weak β-emission of ^{3}H is only 1–3 μm, and that considerable self-absorption occurs in 5 μm sections and in the average smear. Special techniques have been described for the autoradiography of haemolytic plaque-forming cells [72]. It is possible to score ^{3}H-labelled and ^{14}C-labelled cells separately on smears provided that the emulsion is > 5 μm thick and the cells are well separated [71].

Organ counting

Rat or mouse recipients of labelled lymphocytes are anaesthetized with ether to take a large sample of blood from the abdominal vena cava into a heparinized syringe. Then the aorta is severed to exsanguinate the animal. The lymph nodes, spleen and other organs are dissected out, cleaned and weighed after insertion into pre-weighed counting vials.

The measurement of ^{51}Cr, ^{111}In or ^{125}I in tissues requires a gamma counter but no sample preparation apart from aliquotting material that is too large to fit into the counting tubes. By contrast measurement of the weak β-emissions of ^{3}H and ^{14}C in tissue samples requires a liquid scintillation counter and fairly elaborate sample preparation. In the previous edition of this handbook, one of the many methods available for preparing samples for liquid scintillation counting was described in detail [14].

Sample experiment: to measure lymphocyte influx and blood flow to the antigenically stimulated popliteal lymph node of the rat [22]

Equipment

Bollman restraining cages, continuous infusion pump, and instruments for thoracic duct cannulation as described in the third edition of this book [14].
Gamma counter capable of counting ^{51}Cr and ^{86}Rb in dual labelled samples.
Bench centrifuge and 37 °C water bath.

Materials

Sodium-^{51}Cr-chromate (CJS.IP) and ^{86}Rb-rubidium chloride (RGS.2), Amersham International.

Procedure

Day 1   To study lymph nodes three days after antigenic stimulation inject 0.1 ml of 10% washed sheep erythrocytes into right footpads of anaesthetized rats to stimulate the right popliteal lymph nodes. Inject antigen-free carrier solution into left feet.
Day 2   Thoracic duct cannulation of 4–5 donor rats [14]. Collect lymph in Erlenmayer flasks in ice buckets from about 6 p.m. until about 12 noon the following day.
Day 3   Centrifuge cells from lymph (or alternatively start the experiment with a lymph node cell suspension). Label cells *in vitro* with ^{51}Cr as described earlier.

Inject late in the afternoon i.v. into 2–3 recipients with well established thoracic duct cannulae (usually some of the donors can be used in this role.) Discard overnight collection.
Day 4   Take 2–3 collections for periods of not more than 4 h at room temperature of lymph from intermediates [20]. Centrifuge cells out of lymph, resuspend at a known concentration, take three injection samples of 0.1 ml and inject 2.0 ml i.v. into each of a series of recipients.

Kill recipients one hour after the injection of lymphocytes: Anaesthetize with ether 10 min before killing and insert needle (G23) into tail vein attached to flexible plastic tubing; inject ^{86}RbCl (10 μCi) in 0.5 ml of PBS quickly and flush with 1.0 ml of physiological saline; at 45 s after ^{86}Rb inject 0.5 ml of saturated KCl via the tail vein cannula to stop the heart abruptly.

The right and left popliteal lymph nodes, the superficial cervical lymph nodes, the spleen and the kidneys are removed, cleaned, weighed to within 0.1 mg, and put into vials for counting ^{86}Rb separately from ^{51}Cr. Lymphocyte influx is represented by the ^{51}Cr activity per g of lymph node expressed as % of the dose of ^{51}Cr injected in association with lymphocytes. Relative blood flow to the lymph nodes is represented by the ^{86}Rb activity per gram of lymph node (or per organ) expressed relative to the ^{86}Rb activity in the kidney as a 'standard' organ [73].

Non-radioactive methods of cell tracing

Methods of cell labelling with radioactive markers lend themselves to automated counting of large numbers of cells, but in general are less technically satisfactory when applied to small cell numbers, and are of no use for some purposes because labelled cells cannot be individually identified while viable. By contrast, stable fluorescent labels or alloantigenic markers permit simultaneous identification and phenotypic analysis of individual marked cells, yet also allow rapid examination of large cell numbers through flow cytofluorometry, and even permit re-isolation of viable marked cells by fluorescence activated cell sorting. This section describes a simple method of direct cell labelling by stable conjugation with fluorescein or tetramethylrhodamine isothiocyanate (FITC or TRITC), and the section on page 57.17 outlines the use of cell surface alloantigenic determinants as cell markers.

Incubation of cells with free fluorescein or tetramethylrhodamine isothiocyanate (FITC or TRITC) near physiologic pH in normal media results in stable conjugation of fluorescein or rhodamine to intracellular and cell surface proteins [74,75]. Fluorescence

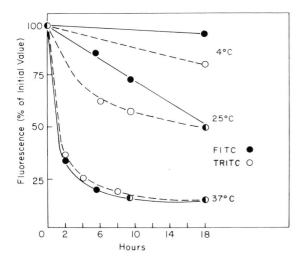

Fig. 57.5. Fading of fluorescence of viable FITC- or TRITC-labelled lymphocytes. Labelled lymphocytes were thoroughly washed and incubated *in vitro* in medium containing fetal calf serum. At various times, the median fluorescence of viable cells was determined on the FACS. From ref. 74, with permission.

microscopy of labelled cells reveals fluorescence throughout the cell, although chromatin appears to be relatively spared. Cellular fluorescence is fairly stable at 4 and 25 °C, decays rapidly at 37 °C, but is nonetheless visible for several days even at this temperature (Fig. 57.5). Although excessive labelling is possible, intense cellular fluorescence can be obtained without affecting cell viability, and without altering lymphocyte migratory properties [75] or immune responsiveness in a graft vs. host assay [74].

Preparation of stock solutions of FITC and TRITC

Equipment

Centrifuge.
Spectrophotometer.
Millipore filters, 0.45 μm pore size.

Materials and reagents

FITC (isomer I, Sigma Chemical Company, St. Louis, MO).
TRITC (isomer R, BBL, Cockeysville, MD).
Phosphate-buffered saline, pH 7.4.

Procedure (FITC)

1   Add 100 mg dry FITC to 100 ml PBS.
2   Stir at room temperature for 3–5 h in the dark.

3   Centrifuge at 1500 rev./min or more for 15–30 min to remove large crystals.
4   Filter supernatant through 0.45 μm Millipore filter.
5   Determine O.D. of the FITC solution at 495 nm, diluting in PBS for measuring the O.D.
6   Adjust FITC solution with PBS to 500 μg/ml (53 O.D. units based on an extinction coefficient of 68 000 at 495 nm, and a Mr of FITC of 389).
7   Freeze 1 ml aliquots in tightly capped tubes at -35 °C until use.

Procedure (TRITC)

1   Add 10 mg TRITC to 100 ml PBS.
2   Stir at room temperature for 3–5 h in the dark.
3   Centrifuge at 1500 rev./min or more for 15–30 min to remove large crystals.
4   Filter supernatant through 0.45 μm Millipore filter.
5   Determine O.D. at 550 nm, diluting TRITC solution in 70% ethanol for O.D. reading.
6   Adjust with PBS to 30 μg/ml (4.7 O.D. units, based on an estimated extinction coefficient of 70 000 at 500 nm in 70% ETOH, and a Mr of TRITC of 444.).
7   Freeze 0.5 ml aliquots at -35 °C until use.

Alternatively, FITC or TRITC can be dissolved at high concentration in dimethyl sulphoxide (DMSO) and diluted with PBS for use; in this case, one must of course control for possible effects of the low concentration of DMSO present during cell labelling.

Cell labelling

Equipment

Centrifuge.
37 °C incubator or water bath.

Materials and reagents

Stock solutions of FITC (about 500 μg/ml) or TRITC (about 30 μg/ml) in PBS (see above), thawed.
Cells to be labelled, suspended at 5×10^7 cells per ml in Hanks' balanced salt solution, pH 7.4, containing 5.0% serum and 20 mM-HEPES.
New-born or fetal calf serum.

Procedure (FITC)

1   Pre-warm cell suspension to 37 °C.
2   Add FITC stock solution to a final concentration of 10–40 μg FITC per ml; pipette to mix.
3   Incubate for 15 min at 37 °C.

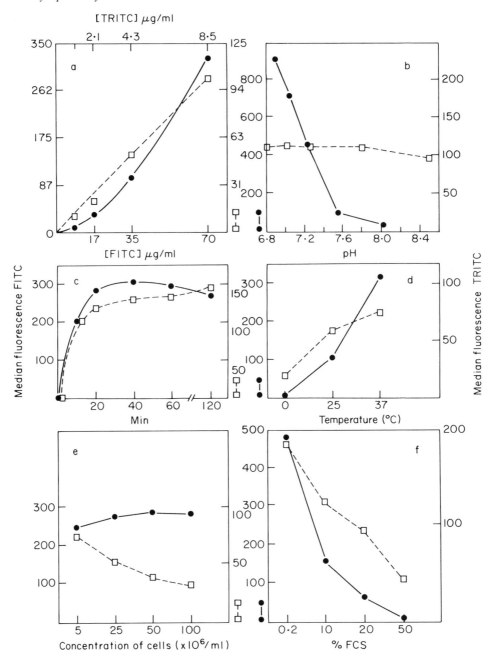

Fig. 57.6. The effect of various factors on cell labelling with FITC (●) and TRITC (□). Each of the important elements of the incubation were varied individually under otherwise standard labelling conditions. Standard conditions of incubation were 2.5×10^7 cells per ml in medium composed of 5% fetal calf serum in an equal mixture of medium 199 and PBS, pH 7.4, for 20 min at 37 °C with 69 μg/ml FITC, or for 15 min at room temperature with 3.4 μg/ml TRITC. Figures show the effect on mean cellular fluorescence of variation in: (a) concentration of reactive fluorochrome; (b) pH (adjusted with 1 M-acetic acid or sodium hydroxide); (c) time of incubation; (d) temperature; (e) concentration of cells; (f) concentration of protein (fetal calf serum) in the medium. From ref. 74, with permission.

4 Layer cell suspension on a 5 ml cushion of serum in 15 ml centrifuge tube.

5 Centrifuge at 1200 rev./min for 10–15 min.

6 Aspirate FITC-containing supernatant, then the serum layer.

7 Resuspend labelled cells for use.

The importance of each of the conditions of incubation is illustrated in Fig. 57.6. Note that the level of cellular fluorescence obtained is not strictly linear with FITC concentration, and is highly sensitive to both the concentration of serum in the labelling medium and to alterations in pH. An alteration of 0.1 pH unit can cause a two- to threefold difference in cellular fluorescence, and thus could determine the difference between functional versus toxic levels of cell labelling. The exquisite sensitivity of cellular labelling to pH may be related to the charge of FITC: lower pH would increase the proportion of singly ionic and neutral FITC molecules, thus allowing more FITC to penetrate the cell membrane to label internal proteins. At pH 7.4 concentrations of FITC over about 60 μg/ml are required before any alteration in short-term lymphocyte migration can be detected, although this may vary with the lot of FITC.

FITC labels all cell types examined, but to different extents. Erythrocytes are poorly stained compared with lymphocytes, and surprisingly B cells stain more heavily than T cells [74].

Procedure (TRITC)

1 Warm cell suspension to room temperature.

2 Add TRITC stock solution to a final concentration of 0.4–4.0 μg TRITC per ml.

3 Incubate 15 min at room temperature.

4–7 As for FITC labelling.

Labelling with TRITC differs in many respects from that with FITC. Labelling with TRITC varies with temperature of incubation and serum concentration, but less so than with FITC. Whereas cell concentration has only a slight effect on labelling with FITC, the amount of TRITC per cell declines significantly with increasing cell concentrations. Finally, in striking contrast to the marked pH dependence of labelling with FITC, the level of cellular fluorescence obtained with TRITC is essentially independent of pH over the range examined (6.8–8.0); this may reflect the fact that TRITC is a neutral molecule within this pH range. Unlike FITC, TRITC labels B and T lymphocytes equally, with cellular fluorescence increasing with cell size.

A significant amount of apparently unreacted TRITC may remain associated with labelled cells after simple washing, and this label can be transferred to subsequently admixed unlabelled lymphocytes.

Transfer of fluorescence (per unlabelled cell) increases with the concentration of labelled cells, the ratio of labelled to unlabelled cells, and the time of co-incubation. Such transfer of fluorescence is insignificant for most *in vivo* applications (see below), but can be a nuisance for experiments *in vitro*. In this case, it is advisable to use the lowest level of TRITC labelling possible, and to pre-incubate the washed labelled cells at 37 °C in protein-containing medium for several hours or overnight to reduce the level of unreacted fluorochrome prior to mixing with unlabelled cells.

Application to studies of lymphocyte migration: (1) *identification and phenotyping of transfused lymphocytes*

The use of fluorescence as a cell marker allows identification of donor lymphocytes in cell suspension of recipient lymphoid organs or lymph, and permits counterstaining with immunologic reagents to determine the surface phenotype of the localized cells. As illustrated in the following sample experiments, the approach allows rapid and quantitative comparisons of the ability of defined lymphocyte subsets to localize in particular lymphoid sites.

Sample experiment: differences in *in vivo* localization of B versus T lymphocytes

TRITC-labelled spleen cells (5×10^7) were injected intravenously into a syngeneic recipient. Four hours later, cell suspensions were made from recipient Peyer's patches, spleen, and peripheral lymph nodes. Each of these cell suspensions was counterstained with FITC conjugated rabbit anti-mouse immunoglobulin. Donor lymphocytes were identified by fluorescence microscopy using filter combinations for rhodamine, and were scored as B (surface Ig$^+$) or T (surface Ig$^-$) by switching to fluorescein filters. The fraction of TRITC-labelled cells bearing surface Ig was 29% (116/400) among cells in recipient axillary and brachial lymph nodes, 62% (248/400) in the spleen, and 55% (220/400) in Peyer's patches. Thus B lymphocytes localized preferentially in Peyer's patches and spleen, whereas T lymphocytes localized better than B cells at this time point in peripheral lymph nodes.

This general approach has already found application in studies of the differential migration of B versus T lymphocytes [76], and of the migratory capabilities of germinal centre lymphocytes [77] and thymocyte subsets [78]. It should allow characterization of *in vivo* migratory characteristics of any lymphocyte or leucocyte population for which cell surface antigenic markers exist.

Although both FITC- and TRITC-labelled cells can

be easily identified in recipient cell suspensions, TRITC may be the label of choice for this type of *in vivo* investigation because (1) it labels B and T lymphocytes more uniformly than FITC, and (2) it produces useful fluorescence, visible for days, even at levels of fluorescence ten times less than those affecting lymphocyte migratory behaviour [74,75].

(2) *Immunohistologic localization of injected lymphocytes*

In order to determine the micro-environmental localization of an injected population within a given tissue or lymphoid organ, it is desirable to be able to identify marked cells within tissue sections. Traditionally, sample lymphocytes are labelled with a radioactive isotope, injected, and identified within recipient tissues by performing autoradiography on routine histologic sections. While autoradiography is still the method of choice for many such experiments, FITC labelling can be employed to follow the histological localization of cells for up to 1–2 days *in vivo* [75, and see Fig. 57.7]. Labelled cells are readily identified by fluorescence microscopy in frozen sections of recipient tissues. The main advantages of FITC over radioactive labels are simplicity and the rapidity of results. The principal disadvantages are decreased sensitivity after 1–2 days, and impermanence of the tissue sections. Both of these disadvantages can be overcome at least partially by using an immunoperoxidase method of staining for FITC: frozen sections are fixed for 10 min in cold dry acetone, incubated with affinity-purified rabbit anti-FITC antibodies followed after washing by horse-radish peroxidase-conjugated swine anti-rabbit immunoglobulin (DAKO Products, Accurate Scientific Company, Westbury, New York) (see Chapter 116) by Rouse & Warnke, for details of immunohistologic staining procedures). Detection of bound antibody with diaminobenzidine and hydrogen peroxide identifies the FITC labelled cells, creating a permanent slide that can be counterstained with methylene blue to allow histologic assessment of the relation of localized cells to tissue architectural components.

TRITC-labelled cells are difficult to visualize in frozen sections even at early times after injection, but TRITC or FITC-labelled cells can be easily visualized in, unstained routine histologic sections of fixed tissues: organs are fixed in 10% buffered formalin, processed routinely for paraffin embedding, and untreated sections are examined under fluorescence microscopy.

(3) In situ *labelling with FITC*

Although much can be learned by following transfused sample lymphocyte populations, in some cases it

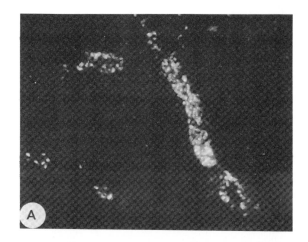

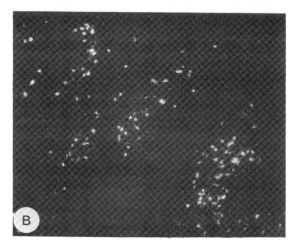

Fig. 57.7. Short-term localization of labelled lymphocytes visualized by fluorescence microscopy in frozen sections of lymph nodes. A: localization in post-capillary high endothelial venules within minutes after i.v. injection. B: subsequent migration into the lymph node parenchyma; 30 min after injection. Approx. × 200. From ref. 75, with permission.

is desirable or essential to examine the behaviour of cells without first removing them from their natural micro-environment. Injection of small volumes of reactive fluorochrome into lymphoid organs results in the labelling of cells around the local site of injection, and thus allows the experimenter to mark and determine the fate of cells under reasonably physiological circumstances [75,79]. FITC has several advantages over metabolically incorporated radiolabels for this type of experiment. FITC labels all cell types randomly, whereas metabolic labelling varies with the status of cells. Cells leaving the site of FITC labelling can be rapidly identified in cell suspensions or tissue sections of organs to which they migrate. Their phenotype can be determined by counterstaining with immunologic reagents, and they can even be purified as viable cells by fluorescence activated cell sorting. Since FITC reacts extremely rapidly with most proteins, FITC labels all cell types at the site of injection, but FITC leaking away from the local site is rapidly inactivated and thus does not significantly label cells elsewhere [79]. An alternative method to micro-injection of label has been described by Pabst *et al.* [80], who labelled the pig spleen and mesenteric node by perfusing them with an FITC solution in isolation from the systemic vasculature, and then re-anastomosed the splenic vessels.

A significant problem with labelling cells by *in situ* injection of FITC is the difficulty of determining whether the levels of labelling achieved are toxic. Possibly the best way to rule this out is to compare the fluorescence of cells labelled *in situ* with the fluorescence of similar cells labelled *in vitro* at high FITC concentrations, approaching those known to interfere with lymphocyte migration (i.e. 60–80 μg/ml).

In situ labelling with FITC has been used to examine the frequency and phenotype of cells emigrating from thymus to peripheral lymphoid organs [79, and see below]. As far as the authors know, the suitability of TRITC for *in situ* labelling has not been tested yet.

Sample experiment: phenotypic analysis of thymus migrants

Ten microlitres of FITC stock solution (500 mg/ml in PBS) were injected into each lobe of the thymus of a young mouse. Three hours later, cell suspensions were made of the thymus and of peripheral lymph nodes. 30% of the thymocytes were labelled detectably (under fluorescence microscopy) with FITC, and flow cytofluorometric analysis revealed that only about 5% of the labelled cells were excessively labelled, i.e. exhibited levels of fluorescence brighter than that of thymocytes incubated at 37 °C for 3 h after *in vitro* labelling with 80 μg/ml FITC, a concentration known to depress the ability of lymphocytes to enter lymph nodes. Thymic migrants were identified microscopically as FITC-labelled cells in a suspension of recipient lymph node cells at a frequency of about 10^{-4}. Control experiments in which FITC was injected intravenously or subcutaneously yielded no labelled lymph node cells, demonstrating clearly that the visualized cells were derived from labelled thymocytes. The accumulation of labelled cells in the periphery was roughly linear with time after labelling, indicating that the migrants were not randomly spilled or flushed from the thymus by the injection procedure but were leaving

at a controlled rate [79]. Counterstaining of the FITC-labelled cells in lymph nodes with TRITC demonstrated that thymus migrants are phenotypically mature—PNA^{lo}, Thy-1^{lo}, H-2K^{hi}—and already divided into Lyt-2$^+$ and Lyt-2$^-$ subsets [81,82,83]. As is consistent with their localization in lymph nodes, the migrants also were found to bear high levels of an antigenic determinant (defined by a monoclonal antibody, MEL-14) thought to be associated with a lymphocyte surface molecule involved in lymphocyte emigration the blood into lymph nodes through post-capillary high endothelial venules [22,103].

Intrinsic markers for cell tracing

Alloantigens

Two disadvantages of any artificial method of cell labelling—whether by radioactivity or fluorescence—are the potential toxicity, and the limited lifespan of the label, especially in metabolically active or dividing cells. The use of actively synthesized cell surface antigens as cell markers avoids these problems, and offers the potential not only to study the relatively short-term migration and differentiation of selected cells, but also to follow their maturational sequence over extended periods. In this approach, one is constrained to use alloantigens that are well represented on the cell surface, for which well defined reagents (preferably monoclonal antibodies) are available, and for which congenic mouse or rat strains have been developed. Several immunoglobulin heavy chain allotype congenic mouse strains are available [84], and monoclonal antibodies against Igh-5a or b (IgD allotypes) [85] or Igh-6a (IgM allotype) (M. Loken, Becton-Dickinson, Monoclonal Antibodies Division, Mountain View, CA, personal communication) would allow tracing of IgD$^+$ of IgM$^+$ cells in congenic recipients. Surface IgD and IgM are not universal markers of B cells, however, and in fact IgD may be lost by regulation or heavy chain class switching from the surface of B cells activated by antigen [e.g. 86,87]. Monoclonal antibodies to rat κ light chain allotype determinants [88], used in conjunction with κ allotype congenic rats [89], might be more generally useful for following B cell differentiation, but even the expression of immunoglobulin light chains is modulated during B lymphocyte development and differentiation [90,91]. In addition to these immunoglobulin allotype systems for tracing B cells, there are two other very powerful marker systems in the mouse, one suitable for following T cells, and the other of more general applicability.

1   The *Thy-1* antigen is expressed on all or nearly all mouse T cells. Monoclonal antibodies have been produced against the two Thy-1 allotypes, Thy-1.1 and Thy-1.2, and such antibodies are available from several commercial sources. Essentially congenic mouse strains are also available: AKR/J (Thy-1.1) and AKR/Cum (Thy-1.2); C57BL/Ka (Thy-1.2) and C57BL/Ka Thy-1.1 mice (M. Lieberman, Stanford University) [92].

2 The *T200* (Ly-5) family of molecules is expressed on almost all haematopoietically derived cells except erythrocytes. Monoclonal antibodies against Ly-5.1 and 5.2 are available commercially as ascites fluid suitable for biotinylation (New England Nuclear, Boston, Massachusetts), and Ly-5.2 congenic mice on the C57BL/6 background are available from Drs F.W. Shen and E.A. Boyse (Memorial Sloan-Kettering Cancer Center, New York, [93]).

Both Ly-5 and Thy-1 are highly represented surface antigens, and positive cells are brightly labelled in cell suspensions or immunohistologic studies, either by direct or indirect immunofluorescence or by indirect immunoperoxidase staining with the relevant monoclonal antibodies. Numerous other lymphocyte surface alloantigens have been described in the recent literature, and in the future many of these may also prove suitable for cell marker studies.

Alloantigens are suitable for tracing cells in short and long term studies of lymphocyte migration and histologic localization, and also for examination of lymphocyte maturation sequences.

Sample experiment: detection of minor differences in the localization of T cell subsets in Peyer's patches vs. peripheral lymph nodes

Lymph node lymphocytes (5×10^7) from AKR/J (Thy-1.1) donors were injected i.v. into AKR/Cum (Thy-1.2) recipients. Twenty-four hours later suspensions of recipient axillary and brachial lymph nodes and of Peyer's patches were made. These suspensions, as well as an aliquot of the originally injected population, were stained with an anti-Thy-1 monoclonal antibody (used as a biotin conjugate with Texas red conjugated avidin as second stage—see Chapter 40, by R. Hardy) and with a fluorescein-indicated monoclonal antibody against Lyt-2. Stained cells were examined under fluorescence microscopy, and the proportion of Thy-1.1$^+$ cells bearing Lyt-2 was determined in each sample population. The ratio of Lyt-2$^-$, Thy-1.1$^+$ cells to Lyt-2$^+$, Thy-1.1$^+$ in recipient lymph nodes was about 2, similar to that in the injected population. By contrast there were nearly six times as many Lyt-2$^-$ as Lyt-2$^+$ donor T cells in recipient Peyer's patches, indicating that Lyt-2$^-$ T cells localize more efficiently than Lyt-2$^+$ T cells in Peyer's patches, whereas both T

cell subsets localize roughly as well in lymph nodes [See also reference 94].

Non-antigenic markers

Several other intrinsic cell markers have been used to follow sample populations for more specialized applications. Use of the chromosomal translocation marker T6 allows identification of donor-derived T6/T6 homozygous cells among host populations, but identification requires examination of mitotic spreads and thus is restricted to mitotically active cell fractions. Allelic variants in enzymes, notably the X-linked enzyme phosphoglycerate kinase, have also been used to follow the contribution of donor derived cells to particular cellular compartments in the host. These systems are discussed in more detail in Chapter 53, by H.S. Micklem.

In vitro assay of lymphocyte binding to post-capillary high endothelial venules

During the process of recirculating, lymphocytes leave the blood and enter lymph nodes and Peyer's patches by binding to the endothelial cells of specialized post-capillary high endothelial venules (HEV) in these organs, and then migrating through the HEV walls into the lymphoid parenchyma [17]. The ability of lymphocytes to recognize and bind to HEV appears to be carefully regulated during lymphocyte development and antigen-induced differentiation, and is of central importance in controlling the migratory characteristics and tissue distribution of different lymphocyte classes and virgin and effector cell subsets [reviewed in 95].

A major advance in our ability to examine this aspect of lymphocyte circulation was the development by Stamper & Woodruff of an *in vitro* assay for measuring lymphocyte-HEV interaction [96]. The assay has since been employed with various modifications by several groups; one version is described below [97]. When quantified using an internal standard population as described below, the binding of lymphocytes to HEV in this *in vitro* system accurately reflects their ability to bind to HEV under more physiologic conditions (i.e. either *in vivo*, or during perfusion at 37 °C through the vasculature of lymphatic tissues [97]). This *in vitro* assay system has been used to demonstrate: (1) that HEV in peripheral lymph nodes and mucosa-associated Peyer's patches express distinct determinants for lymphocyte recognition; (2) that many lymphocytes (including most mature but unstimulated B and T cells, although not their bone marrow and thymocyte precursors) can apparently bind to both lymph node and Peyer's patch HEV, but do so with quantitative preferences for one or the other HEV type as a function of lymphocyte class; (3) that upon stimulation by antigen or mitogen many lymphocytes go through a local, presumably transient period of differentiation during which they fail to express the functional ability to interact with HEV; and (4) that some lymphocytes (including various murine lymphomas, and some memory cells or effector cells or their precursors) can express surface recognition molecules specific for lymph node or for Peyer's patch HEV determinants, thus presumably directing their traffic selectively through mucosal vs. non-mucosal lymphoid tissues [reviewed in 95]. The *in vitro* frozen section assay has also permitted study of the molecular basis of this cell–cell interaction: lymphocyte surface glycoproteins with an apparent relative molecular mass of 80 000–90 000 appear to mediate recognition of lymph node HEV in the mouse [22] and human (Jalkanen, Bargatze, Herron & Butcher, submitted), and monoclonals against rat lymphocyte adhesion molecules for HEV have been recently isolated as well [98; Y.H. Chin & J. Woodruff, personal communication].

Frozen section assay of lymphocyte-HEV binding

Equipment

Cryostat.
Marktex Tech-pen (Scientific Products).
Microshaker II microcytotoxicity shaker (Dynatech products, Division of Cooke, New Jersey) or a rotating platform, $\frac{3}{4}''$ radius of rotation (Tekpro Tektator V variable speed rotator, Scientific Products, or equivalent).
Bull's-eye level.
Flat board or tray suitable for placing on the rotating platform or shaker.
Glass slide staining tray.
Absorbent paper towels.
Cold room, 5–10 °C.

Materials and reagents

Sample lymphocytes, suspended at $1–2 \times 10^7$ viable cells per ml in Hanks' BSS or HEPES-buffered RPMI. (Ca^{2+} is required for binding, so that calcium-free PBS or saline are not suitable media; 5% serum or 0.1–1.0% BSA may be added; pH is not critical in the range of 6.7–7.9.)
Lymph nodes and/or Peyer's patches from several 5–10 week old mice, mounted in a tight cluster for frozen section cutting in Tissue Tek II OCT compound (Lab Tech Products, Naperville, Illinois). (See Chapter 116, by Rouse & Warnke for section cutting procedure.) C57BL mice have small Peyer's patches,

so that other strains such as BALB/c or AKR should be employed when testing binding to Peyer's patch HEV. The mounted organs can be stored in an airtight container at −70 °C until used.
Glass slides (3″ × 1″), pre-cleaned (Scientific Products No. M6132 or equivalent).
Glutaraldehyde (Baker grade, J.T. Baker, Philipsburg, New Jersey) or equivalent.
Slightly hypertonic (1.25 ×) PBS.

Procedure

1   Prepare sample cell suspensions, described above.
2   Cut 10 μm thick frozen sections of mouse lymph nodes and/or Peyer's patches, usually 6–8 sections for each sample population. Use within 2–3 h of cutting.
3   Ring each section with a circle of water-repellent (Tech-pen) ink. The tissue sections should be centred in the circle, and the resulting 'wells' should have a defined inside diameter (see below).
4   Place sides on the flat, levelled board or tray on the shaker or rotator in the cold room at 5–10 °C, and distribute 100 μl of cell suspension in each well while agitating.
5   Incubate for 30 min with continual agitation. The shear forces experienced by the cells appear to be critical, and a proper balance must be achieved between the elements that determine them—the diameter of the wells, the volume of medium applied, and the character and rate of agitation. The authors recommend 100 μl of cells in wells of 1.9 cm internal diameter, agitating either at 170 rev./min on the microcytotoxicity shaker, or at 70 rev./min on the rotating platform. It is advisable to allow the rate of rotation of the shaker or rotator to stabilize in the cold room prior to beginning the assay.
6   Gently decant the medium by tipping the slides on edge on a paper towel.
7   Place slides gently and individually on edge into recently prepared 1% glutaraldehyde in cold 1.25 × PBS in the slide staining tray.
8   After 15 min or longer, the slides can be examined microscopically and they can be gently and individually flooded with PBS to rinse off non-adherent cells if necessary.

Recently, Braaten *et al.* [101] have reported the important observation that the *in vitro* HEV assay can be performed at 25 or 37 °C, as well as at 7 °C, if the lymphoid tissues used for frozen sections are mounted in 35% BSA: OCT compound is apparently cytotoxic at elevated temperatures.

Adherent cells are easily visualized bound to HEV under dry dark-field illumination; the HEV in the glutaraldehyde-fixed sections can be identified as round-to-elongate, plump vessels that are less refrac-

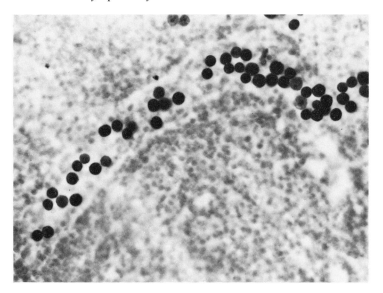

Fig. 57.8. Mouse lymphoid cells (round, dark cells) bound to HEV in a frozen section of a peripheral lymph node. Thionine stain. The adherent, whole cells (from an AKR lymphoma, TK-37) stain more darkly than the fragmented lymphocytes in the tissue section and are further accentuated because they lie in a higher plane of focus. The HEV is identified by its large diameter, plump or 'high' endothelium, and delimiting poorly stained basement membrane.

tile than the surrounding paracortical parenchyma and are fringed by a dark basement membrane. Alternatively slides may be stained with thionine [96] or toluidine blue [99], basophilic dyes that stain intact HEV-bound cells more intensely than the fragmented lymphocytes in the tissue section (see Fig. 57.8).

Two methods of quantifying the HEV-binding ability of lymphocytes have been employed. In one method, the number of lymphocytes bound per HEV, or the proportion of HEV to which more than a certain number of lymphocytes are bound are used as indications of binding ability [96,99,100]. This approach has the advantage of simplicity and general applicability, but suffers to some extent from the significant variability in lymphocyte binding observed from well to well, and even from one area to another within a well. The second approach is to employ a constant internal standard population [3,26]: FITC-labelled lymph node cells (the internal standard) are mixed 1:1 with each unlabelled sample population, and the sample/standard mixtures are incubated on frozen sections. HEV adherent cells are identified under dark field illumination, and the ratio of sample (non-fluorescent cells visualized only under dark field illumination) to standard (FITC-labelled) cells on HEV is determined for each sample population. The contribution of the standard population can be cancelled mathematically to yield direct comparison of the relative binding ability of the sample populations. The assay results are reproducible, and accurately reflect lymphocyte binding to HEV under more physiologic conditions [97].

More detailed descriptions of particular modifications of the assay, and of the methods of data reduction and analysis, may be found in refs. 76, 96, 99–102. Of particular importance are recent demonstrations that lymphocyte–HEV interaction can be studied in non-murine species, including rabbits and guinea-pigs [101] and man [102]. The method has also proved useful for studying neutrophil–endothelial cell interactions [104], and modified section assays have been developed to study the interaction of metastasizing tumour variants with particular organ sites of metastasis [105]. This type of assay may be applicable to the study of a wide variety of cellular interactions.

References

1 GOWANS J.L. & MCGREGOR D.D. (1965) The immunological activities of lymphocytes. *Prog. Allergy*, **9**, 1.

2 HERMAN P.G., UTSONOMIYA R. & HESSEL S.J. (1979) Arteriovenous shunting in the lymph node before and after antigenic stimulus. *Immunology*, **36**, 793.

3 HERMAN P.G., LYONNET D., FINGERHUT R. & TUTTLE R.N. (1976) Regional blood flow to the lymph-node during the immune response. *Lymphology*, **9**, 101.

4 HERMAN P.G. (1980) Microcirculation of organized lymphoid tissues. *Monogr. Allergy*, **16**, 126. *Essays on the Anatomy and Physiology of Lymphoid Tissues*, (eds. Trnka Z. & Cahill R.N.P.). Karger, Basel.

5 ANDERSON N.D., ANDERSON A.O. & WYLLIE R.G. (1976) Specialized structure and metabolic activities of high endothelial venules in rat lymphatic tissues. *Immunology*, **31**, 455.

6 NIEUWENHUIS P. & FORD W.L. (1976) Comparative migration of B and T lymphocytes in the rat spleen and lymph nodes. *Cell. Immunol.* **23**, 254.

7 FORD W.L. (1980) The lymphocyte—its transformation from a frustrating enigma to a model of cellular

function. In *Blood Pure and Eloquent*, (ed. Wintrobe M.M.). McGraw-Hill, New York.

8 LASCELLES A.K. & MORRIS B. (1961) Surgical techniques for the collection of lymph from unanaesthetised sheep. *Quart. J. exp. Physiol.* **46**, 199.

9 HALL J.G. & MORRIS B. (1963) The lymph-borne cells of the immune response. *Quart. J. exp. Physiol.* **48**, 235.

10 HECKER J.F. (1974) *Experimental Surgery on small ruminants.* Butterworth, London.

11 SMITH J.B., McINTOSH G.H. & MORRIS B. (1970) The traffic of cells through tissues: a study of peripheral lymph in sheep. *J. Anat.* **107**, 87.

12 DREXHAGE H.A., MULLINK H., DE GROOT J., CLARKE J. & BALFOUR B.M. (1979) A study of cells present in peripheral lymph of pigs with special reference to a type of cell resembling the Langerhans cell. *Cell Tissue Res.* **202**, 407.

13 ENGESET A., HAGER B., NESHEIM A. & KOLBENSTVEDT A. (1973) Studies on human peripheral lymph I. Sampling method. *Lymphology*, **6**, 1.

14 FORD W.L. (1977) The preparation and labelling of lymphocytes. In *Handbook of Experimental Immunology*, 3rd edn., Ch. 23, (ed. Weir D.M.). Blackwell Scientific Publications, Oxford.

15 BOAK J.L. & WOODRUFF M.F.A. (1965) Modified technique for collecting mouse thoracic duct lymph. *Nature*, **205**, 396.

16 SMITH M.E. & FORD W.L. (1983) The recirculating lymphocyte pool of the rat: a systematic description of the migratory behaviour of recirculating lymphocytes. *Immunology*, **49**, 83.

17 GOWANS J.L. & KNIGHT E.J. (1964) The route of recirculation of lymphocytes in the rat. *Proc. R. Soc.* Series B, **159**, 257.

18 BØYUM A. (1968) Separation of leucocytes from blood and bone marrow. *Scand. J. clin. Lab. Invest.* **21** (suppl. 97), 77.

19 WAGSTAFF J., GIBSON C., THATCHER N., FORD W.L., SHARMA H., BENSON W. & CROWTHER D. (1981) A method for following human lymphocyte traffic using indium-111 oxine labelling. *Clin. exp. Immunol.* **43**, 435.

20 SMITH M.E. & FORD W.L. (1983) The migration of lymphocytes across specialized vascular endothelium. (VI) The migratory behaviour of thoracic duct lymphocytes retransferred from the lymph nodes, spleen, blood or lymph of a primary recipient. *Cell. Immunol.* **78**, 161.

21 DE SOUSA M.A.B. (1981) *Lymphocyte circulation. Experimental and clinical aspects.* Wiley (John) & Sons Ltd.

22 GALLATIN W.M., WEISSMAN I.L. & BUTCHER E.C. (1983) A cell-surface molecule involved in organ-specific homing of lymphocytes. *Nature*, **303**, 30.

23 BAINBRIDGE D.R. & GOWLAND G. (1966) Detection of homograft sensitivity in mice by the elimination of chromium-51 labelled lymph node cells. *Ann. N.Y. Acad. Sci.* **129**, 257.

24 ROLSTAD B. & FORD W.L. (1983) The rapid elimination of allogeneic lymphocytes: relationship to established mechanisms of immunity and to lymphocyte traffic. *Immunol. Revs.* **73**, 87.

25 SMITH M.E., MARTIN A.F. & FORD W.L. (1980) Migra-
tion of lymphoblasts in the rat. Preferential localization of DNA-synthesizing lymphocytes in particular lymph nodes and other sites. *Monogr. Allergy*, **16**, 203. *Essays in the Anatomy and Physiology of Lymphoid Tissues* (eds. Trnka Z. & Cahill R.N.P.). Karger, Basel.

26 OTTAWAY C.A. & PARROTT D.M.V. (1979) Regional blood flow and its relationship to lymphocyte & lymphoblast traffic during a primary immune response. *J. exp. Med.* **150**, 218.

27 DRAYSON M.T., SMITH M.E. & FORD W.L. (1981) The sequence of changes in blood flow and lymphocyte influx to stimulated rat lymph nodes. *Immunology*, **44**, 125.

28 SCAIFE J.F. & VITTORIO P.V. (1964) The use of ^{51}Cr as a sensitive quantitative criterion of early radiation damage to rat thymocytes. *Canad. J. Biochem.* **42**, 503.

29 RONAI P.M. (1969) The elution of ^{51}chromium from labelled leukocytes—a new theory. *Blood*, **33**, 408.

30 RONAI P.M. (1969) High resolution autoradiography with ^{51}Cr. *Int. J. appl. Radiat. Isot.* **20**, 471.

31 BAINBRIDGE D.R., BRENT L. & GOWLAND G. (1966) Distribution of allogeneic ^{51}Cr-labelled lymph-node cells in mice. *Transplantation*, **4**, 138.

32 ZATZ M.M. & LANCE E.M. (1970) The distribution of chromium-51 labelled lymphoid cells in the mouse. *Cell. Immunol.* **1**, 3.

33 ROLSTAD B. & TOOGOOD E. (1978) Toxicity of Na$_2$ ^{51}Cr O$_4$ when used to label rat lymphocytes. *J. immunol. Meth.* **21**, 271.

34 HOWARD J.C., HUNT S.V. & GOWANS J.L. (1972) Identification of marrow-derived and thymus-derived small lymphocytes in the lymphoid tissue and thoracic duct of normal rats. *J. exp. Med.* **135**, 200.

35 RANNIE G.H. & DONALD K.J. (1977) The migration of thoracic duct lymphocytes to non-lymphoid tissues. A comparison of the distribution of radioactivity at intervals following i.v. transfusion of cells labelled with ^{3}H, ^{14}C, ^{75}Se, ^{99m}Tc, ^{125}I and ^{51}Cr in the rat. *Cell Tissue Kinet.* **10**, 523.

36 McAFEE J.G. & THAKUR M.L. (1976) Survey of radioactive agents for *in vitro* labelling of phagocytic leukocytes I. Soluble agents. *J. nucl. Med.* **17**, 480.

37 RANNIE G.H., THAKUR M.L. & FORD W.L. (1977) An experimental comparison of radioactive labels with potential application to lymphocyte migration studies in patients. *Clin. exp. Immunol.* **29**, 509.

38 CHISHOLM P.M., DANPURE H.J., HEALEY G. & OSMAN S. (1979) Cell damage resulting from the labelling of rat lymphocytes and Hela S3 cells with In-111 oxine. *J. nucl. Med.* **20**, 1308.

39 ISSEKUTZ T., CHIN W. & HAY J.B. (1980) Measurement of lymphocyte traffic with indium-111. *Clin. exp. Immunol.* **39**, 215.

40 FROST P., WILTROUT R., MACIOROWSKI Z. & ROSE N.R. (1977) An isotope release cytotoxicity assay applicable to human tumours: the use of ^{111}Indium. *Oncology*, **34**, 102.

41 SPARSHOTT S.M., SHARMA M., KELLY J.I. & FORD W.L. (1981) Factors influencing the fate of ^{111}Indium-labelled lymphocytes after transfer to syngeneic rats. *J. immunol. Meth.* **41**, 303.

42 WAGSTAFF J., GIBSON C., THATCHER N. & CROWTHER D. (1982) A method for studying the dynamics of the primary migration of human lymphocytes using indium-111 oxine cell labelling. *Adv. exp. Med. Biol.* **149**, 153.

43 FROST H., FROST P., WILCOX C. & THRALL J. (1979) Lymph node scanning in sheep with Indium-111-labelled lymphocytes. *Int. J. Nucl. Med. Biol.* **6**, 60.

44 ISSEKUTZ T.B., CHIN G.W. & MAY J.B. (1981) Lymphocyte traffic through chronic inflammatory lesions: differential migration versus differential retention. *Clin. exp. Immunol.* **45**, 604.

45 DANPURE M.J., OSMAN S. & BRADY F. (1982) The labelling of blood cells in plasma with ^{111}In-tropolonate. *Br. J. Radiol.* **55**, 247.

46 HAYHOE F.G.J. & QUAGLINO D. (1965) Autoradiographic investigations of RNA and DNA metabolism of human leucocytes altered with phytohaemagglutinin; uridine-5-^{3}H as a specific precursor of RNA. *Nature*, **205**, 151.

47 COMINGS D.E. (1966) Incorporation of tritium of ^{3}H-5-uridine into DNA. *Expl Cell. Res.* **41**, 677.

48 GUTMAN G. & WEISSMAN I. (1975) Evidence that uridine incorporation is not a selective marker for mouse lymphocyte subclasses. *J. Immunol.* **115**, 739.

49 SCOTT D.W. & JOSEPHS S.H. (1975) Uridine labelling of human lymphocytes: Differential uptake by T and B cells. *Cell. Immunol.* **20**, 64.

50 THURSH D.R. & EMESON E.E. (1973) Selective DNA synthesis by cells specifically localising in response to xenogeneic erythrocytes. *J. exp. Med.* **138**, 659.

51 FORD W.L. & SIMMONDS S.J. (1972) The tempo of lymphocyte recirculation from blood to lymph in the rat. *Cell Tissue Kinet.* **5**, 185.

52 ATKINS R.C. & FORD W.L. (1975) Early cellular events in a systemic graft vs. host reaction. (1) The migration of responding and non-responding donor lymphocytes. *J. exp. Med.* **141**, 664.

53 GOLDSCHNEIDER I. & McGREGOR D.D. (1968) Migration of lymphocytes and thymocytes in the rat. (II) Circulation of lymphocytes and thymocytes from blood to lymph. *Lab. Invest.* **18**, 397.

54 WAGNER H.P., COTTIER H., CRONKITE E.P., CUNNINGHAM L., JANSEN C.R. & RAI K.R. (1967) Studies on lymphocytes. (V) Short *in vivo* DNA synthesis and generation time of lymphoid cells in the calf thoracic duct after simulated or effective extracorporeal irradiation of circulating blood. *Expl Cell Res.* **46**, 441.

55 HALL J.G. & SMITH M.E. (1970) Homing of lymph-borne immunoblasts to the gut. *Nature*, **226**, 262.

56 FEINENDEGEN L.E., BOND V.P. & HUGHES W.L. (1966) Physiological thymidine reutilisation in rat bone marrow. *Proc. Soc. exp. Biol. (NY)*, **122**, 448.

57 MITCHELL J., McDONALD W. & NOSSAL G.J.V. (1963) Autoradiographic studies on the immune response. (3) Differential lymphopoiesis in various organs. *Aust. J. exp. Biol. Med. Sci.* **41**, 411.

58 ROBINSON S.H., BRECHER G., LOURIE S.I. & HALEY J.E. (1965) Leukocyte labelling in rats during and after continuous infusion of tritiated thymidine: implications for lymphocyte longevity and DNA reutilisation. *Blood*, **26**, 281.

59 McGREGOR D.D. (1969) Effect of tritiated thymidine and 5-bromodeoxyuridine on development of immunologically competent lymphocytes. *Immunology*, **16**, 83.

60 HOFER K.G. & HUGHES W.L. (1971) Radiotoxicity of intranuclear tritium, ^{125}iodine and ^{131}iodine. *Radiat. Res.* **47**, 94.

61 DETHLEFSEN L.A. (1970) Reutilization of ^{131}I-5-iodo-2′-desoxyuridine as compared to ^{3}H-thymidine in mouse duodenum and mammary tumour. *J. Nat. Canc. Inst.* **44**, 827.

62 CLIFTON K.H. & COOPER J.M. (1973) Reutilization of thymidine and iododeoxyuridine by mouse mammary carcinoma strain MTG-B. *Proc. Soc. exp. Biol.* **142**, 145.

63 OLDMAN R.K. & HERBERMAN R.B. (1973) Evaluation of cell-mediated cytotoxic reactivity against tumour associated antigens with ^{125}I-iododeoxyuridine labelled target cells. *J. Immunol.* **111**, 1862.

64 PORTEUS D.D. & MUNRO T.R. (1972) The kinetics of the killing of mouse tumour cells *in vivo* by immune response. *Int. J. Cancer* **10**, 112.

65 SPRENT J. (1976) Fate of H-2-activated T lymphocytes in syngeneic host. I. Fate in lymphoid tissues and intestines traced with ^{3}H-thymidine, ^{125}I-deoxyuridine and ^{51}chromium. *Cell. Immunol.* **21**, 278.

66 HALL J.G., PARRY D.M. & SMITH M.E. (1972) The distribution and differentiation of lymph-borne immunoblasts after intravenous injection into syngeneic recipients. *Cell Tissue Kinet.* **5**, 269.

67 ROSE M.L., PARROT D.M.V. & BRUCE R.G. (1976) Migration of lymphoblasts to the small intestine. *Immunology*, **31**, 723.

68 EVERETT N.B. & TYLER R.W. (1967) Lymphopoiesis in the thymus and other tissues: functional implications. *Int. Rev. Cytol.* **22**, 205.

69 EMESON E.E. & THURSH D.R. (1971) Immunologically specific retention of long-lived lymphoid cells in antigenically stimulated lymph nodes. *J. Immunol.* **106**, 635.

70 LANCE E.M. & COOPER S. (1972) Homing of specifically sensitized lymphocytes to allografts of skin. *Cell. Immunol.* **5**, 66.

71 ROGERS A.W. (1973) *Techniques of autoradiography*, 2nd edn. Elsevier, Amsterdam.

72 KOROS A.M.S., MAZUR J.M. & MOWERY M.J. (1968) Radioautographic studies of plaque-forming cells. (1) Antigen-stimulated proliferation of plaque-forming cells. *J. exp. Med.* **128**, 235.

73 SAPIRSTEIN L.A. (1958) Regional blood flow by fractional distribution of indicators. *J. appl. Physiol.* **193**, 161.

74 BUTCHER E.C. & WEISSMAN I.L. (1980) Direct fluorescent labelling of cells with fluorescein or rhodamine isothiocyanate: (I) Technical aspects. *J. immunol. Meth.* **37**, 97.

75 BUTCHER E.C., SCOLLAY R.G. & WEISSMAN I.L. (1980) Direct fluorescent labelling of cells with fluorescein or rhodamine isothiocyanate. (II) Potential application to studies of lymphocyte migration and maturation. *J. immunol. Meth.* **37**, 109.

76 STEVENS S.K., WEISSMAN I.L. & BUTCHER E.C. (1982)

Differences in the migration of B and T lymphocytes: organ-selective localization *in vivo* and the role of lymphocyte-endothelial cell recognition. *J. Immunol.* **128**, 844.

77 REICHERT R.A., GALLATIN W.F., WEISSMAN I.L. & BUTCHER E.C. (1983) Germinal center B cells lack homing receptors necessary for normal lymphocyte recirculation. *J. exp. Med.* **157**, 813.

78 KRAAL G., BODEN D. & KORS N. (1981) Localization of PNA binding and non-binding thymus cells in peripheral lymphoid organs. *Cell. Immunol.* **60**, 228.

79 SCOLLAY R., BUTCHER E.C. & WEISSMAN I.L. (1980) Thymus cell migration: quantitative aspects of cellular traffic from the thymus to the periphery in mice. *Eur. J. Immunol.* **10**, 210.

80 PABST R. & BINNS R.M. (1981) *In vivo* labelling of the spleen and mesenteric lymph nodes with fluorescein isothiocyanate for lymphocyte migration studies. *Immunology*, **44**, 321.

81 SCOLLAY R. & WEISSMAN I.L. (1980) T cell maturation: thymocytes and thymus migrant subpopulations defined with monoclonal antibodies to the antigens Lyt-1, Lyt-2 and ThB. *J. Immunol.* **124**, 2841.

82 SCOLLAY R., JACOBS S., JERABEK L., BUTCHER E.C. & WEISSMAN I. (1980) T cell maturation: thymocyte and thymus cell migrant subpopulations defined with monoclonal antibodies to MHC region antigens. *J. Immunol.* **124**, 2845.

83 SCOLLAY R. (1982) Thymus cell migration; cells migrating from the thymus to the peripheral lymphoid organs have a mature phenotype. *J. Immunol.* **128**, 1566.

84 ALTMAN P.L. & KATZ D.D. (1979) Inbred and genetically defined strains of laboratory animals. *FASEB*, Bethesda, Md., p. 111.

85 OI V.T., JONES P.P., GODING J.W., HERZENBERG L.A. & HERZENBERG L.A. (1978) Properties of monoclonal antibodies to mouse Ig allotypes, H-2 and Ia antigens. *Curr. Top. Microbiol. Immunol.* **81**, 115.

86 KRAAL G., WEISSMAN I.L. & BUTCHER E.C. (1982) Germinal center B cells: antigen specificity and changes in heavy chain class expression. *Nature*, **298**, 377.

87 PREUD'HOMME J.-L. (1977) Loss of surface IgD by human B lymphocytes during polyclonal activation. *Eur. J. Immunol.* **7**, 191.

88 LANIER L.L., GUTMAN G.A., LEWIS D.F., GRISWOLD S.T. & WARNER N.L. (1982) Monoclonal antibodies against rat Ig kappa chains. **1**, 125.

89 ROZING J., JERABEK L., GUTMAN G. & WEISSMAN I.L. (1979) The derivation of the LEW RI-Ia(DA)/STA rat line. *Rat News Letter*, **5**.

90 BUTCHER E.C., ROUSE R.V., COFFMAN R.L., NOTTENBURG C.N., HARDY R.R. & WEISSMAN I.L. (1982) Surface phenotype of Peyer's patch germinal center cells: implications for the role of germinal centers in B cell differentiation. *J. Immunol.* **129**, 6.

91 COFFMAN R.L. (1982) Surface antigen expression and Ig gene rearrangement during mouse pre-B cell development. *Immunol. Revs.* **69**, 5.

92 BONVIER J., DECLÉVE A., LIEBERMAN M., HONSI K.C., TRAVIS M. & KAPLAN H.S. (1981) Marrow-thymus interactions during radiation leukemogenesis in C57BL/Ka mice. *Cancer Res.* **41**, 390.

93 YAKURA H., SHEN F.-W., BOURCET E. & BOYSE E.A. (1983) On the function of Ly-5 in the regulation of antigen-driven B cell differentiation. *J. exp. Med.* **157**, 1077.

94 KRAAL G., WEISSMAN I.L. & BUTCHER E.C. (1983) Differences in *in vivo* distribution and homing of T cell subsets to mucosal vs. non-mucosal lymphoid organs. *J. Immunol.* **130**, 1097.

95 BUTCHER E.C. (1985) The regulation of lymphocytic traffic. Curr. Top. Microbiol. Immunol. (in press).

96 STAMPER H.B. JUN. & WOODRUFF J.J. (1976) Lymphocyte homing into lymph nodes: *in vitro* demonstration of the selective affinity of recirculating lymphocytes for high endothelial venules. *J. exp. Med.* **144**, 828.

97 BUTCHER E.C., SCOLLAY R.G. & WEISSMAN I.L. (1979) Lymphocyte adherence to high endothelial venules: characterization of a modified *in vitro* assay, and examination of the binding of syngeneic and allogeneic lymphocyte populations. *J. Immunol.* **123**, 1996.

98 RASMUSSEN R.A., CHIN Y.-H., WOODRUFF J.J. & EASTON J.G. (1985) Lymphocyte recognition of lymph node high endothelium. (VII) Cell surface proteins involved in adhesion defined by monoclonal anti-HEBF$_{LN}$ (A.11) antibody. *J. Immunol.* **135**, 19.

99 BUTCHER E.C., SCOLLAY R.G. & WEISSMAN I.L. (1980) Organ specific lymphocyte migration: mediation by highly selective lymphocyte interaction with organ-specific determinants on high endothelial venules. *Eur. J. Immunol.* **10**, 556.

100 STOOLMAN L.M. & ROSEN S.D. (1983) A possible role for cell surface carbohydrate binding molecules in lymphocyte recirculation. *J. Cell Biol.* **96**, 722.

101 BRAATEN B.A., SPANGRUDE G.J. & DAYNES R.A. (1985) Molecular mechanisms of lymphocyte extravasation: II. Studies of *in vitro* lymphocyte adherence to high endothelial venules. J. Immunol. (in press).

102 JALKANEN S.T., BUTCHER E.C. (1985) *In vitro* analysis of the homing properties of human lymphocytes: Developmental regulation of functional receptors for high endothelial venules. Blood, (in press)

103 REICHERT R.A., GALLATIN W.M., BUTCHER E.C. & WEISSMAN I.L. (1984) A homing receptor-bearing cortical thymocyte population: Implications for thymus cell migration and the nature of cortisone-resistant thymocytes. *Cell*, **38**, 89.

104 BUTCHER E.C., LEWINSOHN D., DUIJVESTIJN A., BARGATZE R., WU NB. & JALKANEN S.T. (1985) Interactions between endothelial cells and leukocytes. J. cell. Biochem. (in press).

105 NETLAND P.A. & ZETTER B.R. (1984) Organ-specific adhesion of metastatic tumour cells *in vitro*. *Science*, **224**, 1113.

Chapter 58
Human leucocyte subpopulations

P. BEVERLEY

Techniques for identification and
separation of leucocyte subsets,
58.1

Assays of function of leucocyte
subsets, 58.9
Media, 58.13

Understanding of human leucocyte function has progressed rapidly in recent years, in part because experimental rodent models have provided a great deal of information which can be applied to man, but also because recent technical advances have provided tools for studying more effectively the function of human cells. Thus experiments in mice (and to a lesser extent, rats) have demonstrated that in all immune responses a complex series of cellular interactions are required for the generation of effector cells and that the participating cells can be identified by their expression of distinctive phenotypic markers. In rodents the most widely used means of identifying and separating lymphocyte subsets have been conventional alloantisera [1] or, more recently, monoclonal antibodies [2].

In man, improvements in methods for *in vitro* culture of lymphocytes have made it possible to study specific immune responses to antigens as well as the traditional polyclonal mitogen responses. The development of monoclonal antibodies to lymphocyte differentiation antigens has provided reagents for identifying reproducibly different leucocyte subsets. Indeed, perhaps because of the great phylogenetic disparity between men and mice, it has proved possible to produce monoclonal antibodies to important human lymphocyte surface antigens [3], such as T3 and T4, whose homologues either have not yet been recognized in mice (T3) or have only very recently been identified (T4) [2].

Methods for separating phenotypically distinct subsets of cells and assaying their function allow correlation of phenotype and function. A further stage of analysis is to identify the function of the molecules expressed on a subset of cells. However, even if a molecule is expressed on a relatively small subset of cells with a well defined function, this may often prove difficult and at present the true function of most lymphocyte differentiation antigens is unknown.

Nevertheless, examination of the distribution of a phenotypic marker and correlation of its expression with cell function remains an important initial step in understanding molecular function. This chapter provides some basic tools for examining the cellular distribution of human lymphocyte differentiation antigens, separating subsets of lymphocytes and assaying their function.

Techniques for identification and separation of leucocyte subsets

Method for separation of peripheral blood mononuclear cells (PBM)

Equipment

For separation and characterization of human leucocytes the following are required.

A temperature controlled centrifuge capable of carrying tubes of various sizes up to at least 100 ml capacity.
A laminar down-flow tissue culture hood for maintenance of sterility.
A humidified CO_2 incubator.
Bench microscope and haemocytometer for cell counting.
Fluorescence microscope with epi-illumination.
Minor additional equipment includes sterile glass or plastic pipettes (1–25 ml volumes), both single-channel and 8-channel adjustable volume (5–50 μl and 50–200 μl) micropipettes with autoclavable disposable plastic tips, and sterile flasks and beakers.

Materials

Media

For cell preparation, minimal essential medium containing 2 g/l sodium bicarbonate and 20 mM-HEPES buffer (MEM-H).
Heat-inactivated (56 °C for 30 min) fetal calf serum or human serum.
Preservative-free heparin (Weddel Pharmaceuticals, Wrexham, UK).

Ficoll–Hypaque, density 1.077 g/l.
Trypan blue (0.2%) for cell counts.

Other disposables

Glass or plastic centrifuge tubes, e.g. 50 ml tubes (Falcon 2070), 20 ml universals (Sterilin 128C), 12 ml plastic conical-bottomed centrifuge tubes (Nunc N-1200-4), and small plastic 6×63 mm centrifuge tubes (Luckhams LP-3).
Glass beads, 2 mm diameter (BDH, UK). Disposable syringes and 19- or 21-gauge needles.

Method A: heparinized blood

1 Blood is drawn by sterile venepuncture into a syringe containing sufficient preservative-free heparin to give a concentration of approximately 5 u/ml.
2 The blood is mixed with an equal volume of MEM-H and run gently into a tube one-third filled with Ficoll–Hypaque so that an interface is maintained.
3 The tube is centrifuged at 1500 *g* for 15 min at room temperature. Mononuclear cells can then be recovered from the interface using a pipette.
4 At this point, the cells are suspended in medium still containing some Ficoll–Hypaque which must be diluted with 4 or 5 vols. of medium before a further centrifugation at 300 *g* for 10 min.
5 After decanting the supernatant the PBM are resuspended in MEM-H containing 5% serum (FCS or human serum depending on the experiment to be performed) for a further wash before use.

Method B: defibrinated blood

1 Blood is taken by sterile venepuncture into a heparin-free syringe and placed in a flask containing glass beads (up to 25 ml in a 100 ml conical flask containing fifteen to twenty 2 mm glass beads).
2 The beads are then gently swirled in the flask until the swirling is inaudible and the beads are seen to become enmeshed in a fibrin clot.
3 The blood is then mixed 1:1 with medium and PBM are separated on Ficoll–Hypaque as above (Method A).

Notes and recommendations

Defibrination has the advantage over heparinizing that in the former case platelets are removed while in the latter they may cause some agglutination of the PBM, although the relatively slow centrifugation of the first wash, after recovery of the cells from the density gradient, leaves the bulk of platelets in the supernatant. In contrast, defibrination usually gives a 'clean' PBM preparation but in the author's experience the yield is generally lower and there may be selective loss of monocytes. There are unfortunately few studies comparing the composition and function of PBM isolated by these methods or by centrifugation over Percoll, although the latter is said to give a slightly better yield than standard Ficoll–Hypaque methods [4].

Method for sheep red blood cell (E) rosette formation and separation

Equipment

As for separation of PBM.

Materials

Media

MEM-H, FCS, Dulbecco's phosphate-buffered saline (PBS).
Percoll (PVP coated colloidal silica, Pharmacia, Uppsala, Sweden), 1.080 g/ml.
Fluorescein diacetate 1 μg/ml in PBS.
Haemolytic gelatin Gey's solution.

Other disposables

S-2-aminoethylisothiouronium bromide hydrobromide (AET). Sheep red blood cells (SRBC) in Alsever's solution (Gibco).

Procedure

The procedure is essentially that of Kaplan & Clark [5]. Sterility may be maintained by using Millipore-filtered reagents throughout.
1 Stock SRBC in Alsever's solution are washed three times by centrifugation at 600 *g* in PBS.
2 After the last wash, 1 vol. of SRBC is mixed with 5 vols. of AET (40.2 mg/ml in distilled water, pH 9.0) and incubated at 37 °C for 20 min in a water bath before washing three times again in PBS.
3 SRBC are finally stored at 4% v/v in PBS at 4 °C.
4 For rosette formation, 1 vol. of 4% SRBC is mixed with 1 vol. of mononuclear cells at 10^7 cells/ml and 0.5 vol. of FCS.
5 After centrifugation at 300 *g* for 10 min, the cells are incubated for 1 h on ice and resuspended by gently rotating the tube.
6 For analysis of the percentage of rosetted cells, a drop of the cell suspension is diluted 1:1 with PBS

containing 1 μg/ml fluorescein diacetate and pipetted on to a haemocytometer.

7 Counting is performed using a × 40 objective on a microscope equipped with UV epi-illumination. Addition of fluorescein diacetate facilitates discrimination between rosettes and red cell clumps and allows dead cells, which do not fluoresce, to be excluded from the count. If the fluorescence epi-illumination and a low level of transmitted light are used simultaneously, it is possible to see both the SRBC and the fluorescence of viable lymphocytes. Acridine orange or methylene blue can be used as alternative dyes for detecting rosetted lymphocytes. The latter has the advantage that a fluorescence microscope is not required; however these dyes do not discriminate between dead and live cells [6].

8 For separation of E$^+$ and E$^-$ cells the resuspended mixture is layered on to Percoll (density 1.080 g/ml) in an appropriate tube such that approximately one-third of the volume of the tube contains Percoll and the upper two-thirds the rosetted mixture. The tube is centrifuged at 1500 **g** for 20 min at room temperature.

9 E-cells are harvested from the interface using a pipette. The remaining medium and Percoll are removed by suction without disturbing the pellet containing E$^+$ cells. Both E$^+$ and E$^-$ cells are diluted in MEM-H 5% FCS and centrifuged to remove remaining Percoll. The E$^-$ cells can then be resuspended in appropriate medium for functional assay.

10 SRBC are removed from the E$^+$ cells by resuspending the washed cell pellet in haemolytic gelatin Gey's solution [7] for 3 min (1 ml Gey's/10^7 E$^+$ cells) and then washing the cells once more.

11 Separated cells are finally suspended in appropriate medium for functional assays.

Notes and recommendations

A variety of procedures for E rosetting have been described, including the use of untreated red cells or red cells treated with neuraminidase [8,9]. These methods have the drawback that batches of red cells and enzyme vary whereas AET is a stable chemical reagent and, in the author's experience, different batches of SRBC after AET treatment behave reproducibly. AET SRBC rosetting on ice gives 'maximal' rosette formation, in other words detects lymphocytes with both high- and low-affinity SRBC receptors [10]. The author has not described methods for detecting only higher-affinity E rosetting cells because these procedures do not give consistent results from day to day and because isolation of low-affinity E rosetting population may be possible by other means [11].

Separation of rosettes on Ficoll–Hypaque rather than Percoll is possible but, in the author's experience,

contamination of both E$^+$ and E$^-$ fractions is much less when they are separated on Percoll [12] and comparable to that achieved by two cycles of rosetting on Ficoll–Hypaque.

Method for detection of Fc receptors

Equipment

As for separation of PBM.

Materials

Media

PBS with 0.2% w/v bovine serum albumin (PBS-BSA) (BSA, Fraction V, Sigma).
MEM-H, FCS, PBS fluorescein diacetate, 1 μg/ml in PBS.
Haemolytic gelatin Gey's solution.

Other disposables

Ox red blood cells (ORBC) in Alsever's solution (Gibco).
IgG fraction of hyperimmune rabbit anti-ORBC antiserum [13], IgM fraction of primary rabbit anti-ORBC antiserum [14].

Procedure

For Fcγ receptor detection [15]

1 ORBC are washed three times in PBS, resuspended at 2% v/v in PBS-BSA and mixed with an equal volume of a maximal subagglutinating dilution of IgG rabbit anti-ox antibody, held at room temperature for 90 min, washed three times with PBS-BSA and made up to 0.8% v/v in PBS-BSA.

2 For analysis 100 μl of mononuclear cells at 2 × 10^6 cells/ml in PBS-BSA are mixed with an equal volume of sensitized ORBC and centrifuged at 300 **g** for 2 min.

3 Half the supernatant is removed and an equal volume of PBS-BSA, containing 1 μg/ml of fluorescein diacetate, is added before the cells are gently resuspended and an aliquot transferred to a haemocytometer chamber for counting on a fluorescence microscope in the same manner as for E rosettes.

For Fcμ receptors

1 Three-times-washed ORBC are sensitized by incubation of a 2% v/v suspension in PBS-BSA with an equal volume of a maximal subagglutinating dilution of the IgM fraction of a primary rabbit anti-ox red cell serum for 15 min at 0 °C.

2   The ORBC are washed three times and resuspended to 1% v/v in PBS-BSA.

3   For analysis 100 μl of cells at 2×10^6/ml are mixed with an equal volume of sensitized ox cells and incubated for 15 min at 37 °C centrifuged at 300 g for 2 min and kept on ice for 30 min.

4   Half the supernatant is removed and replaced by 100 μl of PBS-BSA containing fluorescein diacetate before the cells are gently resuspended and counted on a fluorescence microscope.

5   Fcμ receptors are not readily detected on fresh PBM so that it is usual to hold the PBM in medium with low IgM (MEM-H 5% FCS) for 24 h prior to assay [14,16].

Notes and recommendations

The use of Fc rosette formation as a test system for detection of leucocyte subsets has become less fashionable since the advent of monoclonal antibodies. This is because of the simplicity of testing with monoclonal antibodies, because it is clear that Fc receptors can be detected on several different subsets of monoclonal antibody defined cells and because many studies have shown that expression of FcR is readily altered by culture conditions or other stimuli [13,17]. Furthermore, the function of cells can be modulated via Fc receptors [13,17] so that separations based on Fc rosette formation may alter the function of the separated cells. In reality, this does not justify the abandonment of Fc rosetting. There is no a priori reason why subsets of cells are better defined by monoclonal antibodies than Fc receptors, and few surface antigens are stable under all conditions. It is also clear that antibodies to surface antigens can stimulate cells [18], block various functions [19,20] and cause rapid modulation of surface antigens [20,21]. Fc rosetting, therefore, remains a useful method for defining the phenotype of human lymphocyte subsets.

Specific antibody rosettes

Equipment

Vortex mixer.
Other equipment: as for separation of PBM.

Materials

Media

Aged chromic chloride solution 1 mg/ml.
0.9% w/v saline.

MEM-H.
Ficoll–Hypaque, density 1.077 g/ml.
Fluorescein diacetate, 1 μg/ml in PBS.

Other disposables

ORBC in Alsever's solution.

Method

Detection of specific antigens by rosette formation can be carried out as a direct or indirect procedure. In the latter case, the indicator red blood cells are coated with anti-immunoglobulin. For both direct and indirect rosette formation the essential first step is the coupling of antibody to red blood cells. This is performed as follows.

1   An immunoglobulin fraction is prepared of the antibody which it is desired to couple to red cells. With high-titre specific antibodies or monoclonal antibody containing ascites it is usually adequate to prepare an IgG fraction by ammonium sulphate precipitation and ion-exchange chromatography.

2   The antibody containing fraction is dialysed exhaustively against saline and centrifuged to remove any precipitate (10 000 g for 30 min). Protein concentration is measured by spectrophotometry ($E_{1cm/280}$ 1.4 for 1 mg/ml IgG). Aliquots of purified antibody, at least 1 mg/ml, are stored at -20 or -70 °C.

3   ORBC are prepared from ox blood stored in Alsever's solution by repeated washing in saline. Cells are centrifuged at 600 g for 5 min at room temperature and the supernatant and buffy coat removed by suction.

5   After five washes the cells are packed by centrifugation at 600 g for 10 min. The packed cells are diluted $1+9$ with sterile saline.

6   Aliquots of 1 ml of this 10% suspension are pipetted into a 10–15 ml conical centrifuge tube and centrifuged again (600 g, 5 min).

7   After removal of the supernatant an appropriate amount, usually 300 μg, of purified antibody is added and the cells resuspended by vortex mixing.

8   Aged chromic chloride (stock diluted 1:10 in saline) is added in a suitable volume (usually 0.2–0.8 ml; see 'Notes and recommendations') using the vortex to mix the suspension.

9   One millilitre of saline is then used to wash down the walls of the tube and the mixture is left overnight at 4 °C.

10   The following day the cells are washed in MEM-H and stored as a 2.5% r.b.c. suspension in MEM-H $+0.2\%$ FCS at 4 °C.

Direct rosette formation

1 In a plastic tube place 50 μl of lymphocyte suspension at 2×10^6/ml with 50 μl of coated red cell suspension, centrifuge at 200 g for 1 min and incubate on ice for 30 min.

2 Gently resuspend and add 100 μl of fluorescein diacetate in PBS.

3 Pipette cells on to a haemocytometer and count using a fluorescence microscope with both the fluorescent light source and visible light switched on and the visible light dimmed so that the haemocytometer grid lines and the cells are just visible. Viable cells only are stained green.

Indirect rosette formation is performed in an essentially similar fashion except that the lymphocytes are first coated with antibody by a 30 min incubation on ice and then washed three times before mixing, as above, with red cells, in this case coated with an appropriate anti-immunoglobulin antibody.

Antibody rosetting can also be used for separation of cells. In this case up to 15×10^6 cells/ml are rosetted with an equal volume of coated red cells. (With larger volumes it is necessary to centrifuge at 300 g for 5 min before incubation for 30 min on ice.) The rosettes are gently resuspended, layered on to Ficoll–Hypaque and centrifuged for 30 min at room temperature. Unrosetted cells are harvested from the interface and rosetted cells from the pellet by lysis of the red cells (see 'Method for sheep red blood cell (E) rosette formation and separation').

Notes and recommendations

Several points relating to the above methodology require discussion. The source of red cells is important. Ox red cells are variably agglutinable and samples which are relatively agglutinable give greater sensitivity in rosette tests [22]. It is sensible, therefore, if possible always to obtain red cells from the same animal. The amount of antibody coupled is important. It is useful initially to titrate the optimum amount of coupling reagent using constant amounts of antibody. This amount can then be used in future couplings. Coated cells should give an even, clump-free suspension when centrifuged, held on ice and resuspended as for rosetting. Coated cells should also be tested on an appropriate antigen-positive cell type, preferably in parallel with an independent method. An appropriate anti-immunoglobulin reagent should also cause strong agglutination of coated red cells.

In rosette tests, as in any other procedure, appropriate controls must be included. For direct rosettes the extent of Fc rosette formation can be examined by using red cells coated with irrelevant Ig of the same class. In indirect rosette tests an irrelevant antibody of the same class as that under test is used to coat the lymphocytes before rosetting. Anti-immunoglobulins of sheep or goat origin bind less strongly to Fc receptors and are therefore more appropriate for indirect rosetting than are rabbit sera [22].

Method for indirect immunofluorescence and fluorescence activated cell sorting

Equipment

Centrifuge and carriers for spinning 96-well microtitre plates.
Vortex mixer.
Hot-plate.
Microfuge.

Materials

Media

MEM-H 5% FCS.
Isoton II and Zap-oglobin (Coulter Electronics Ltd).

Other disposables

Paraffin wax (BDH).
Monoclonal antibodies.
Anti-mouse immunoglobulin FITC.
Microtitre plates, 96-well round-bottomed (e.g. Titertek 76-013-05).

Procedure

For routine analysis of human leucocytes by indirect immunofluorescence and microscopy or cytofluorometry it is sufficient to stain 2×10^5 cells.

1 This number of cells are pipetted into the wells of a microtitre plate (in any volume up to 200 μl). The plate is centrifuged for 2 min at 400 g and the supernatant dumped out by inverting the plate and jerking downward. The face of the plate should then be wiped clear of traces of medium with a tissue.

2 The cells are resuspended in the residue of medium left in the wells (10–20 μl) by holding the plate firmly on to a vortex mixer for a few seconds.

3 First-layer antibody (50 μl) is added and the plate covered with a lid and incubated for 30 min after pressing the plate into an ice bucket.

4 Three washes are carried out by adding 100 μl of ice-cold MEM-H 5% FCS, centrifuging, dumping and resuspending.

5 Fifty microlitres of FITC-conjugated anti-mouse immunoglobulin antibody is then added and the plate again incubated for 30 min on ice, followed by a further three washes as before.

6   For microscopy after the last wash no further medium is added but 10 μl of the cell suspension is transferred to a slide, a 22 mm square coverslip is applied and the edges are sealed with wax or clear nail varnish.

7   For cytofluorometry 100–200 μl of medium are added to each well and if necessary the cell suspension is then transferred to an appropriate tube for analysis.

In either case the appropriate controls should be included. The author always runs (as a minimum) a negative control, in which the cells are incubated first with medium and then with fluorescent second layer, and a positive control, in which cells are incubated with an antibody known to bind to the target cells.

When cell separation using the FACS is intended it is generally appropriate to stain the cells in tubes since adequate washing of $> 10^6$ cells in plates is difficult to obtain. In other respects the procedure is similar to that described above. After staining, cells should be kept on ice and maintained at 4 °C while sorting so that capping or shedding of antibody is minimized.

Notes and recommendations

If stained cells are to be examined by fluorescence microscopy, red cell contamination presents no problem since these can be distinguished under phase and not counted. If FACS analysis is performed, it may be difficult to separate red cells from white cells on the basis of forward-angle light scattering, particularly if immature red cells are present. Two strategies are possible for dealing with this problem. Either the red cells may be lysed immediately before analysis (add an equal volume of 2 drops of Zap-oglobin in 10 ml Isoton II to the cell suspension [23]), or a control may be included to determine the percentage of leucocytes in the scatter-gated population. The author normally uses an antibody against a leucocyte common antigen, or a non-polymorphic determinant of HLA, or a mixture of the two in order to stain all leucocytes [24]. A more detailed description of procedures for cell sorter analysis and separation is given in Volume 1 of this handbook.

With monoclonal antibodies there is seldom a major problem of non-specific staining, particularly if culture supernatant or purified immunoglobulin is used. It is wise, however, to avoid procedures, e.g. repeated freezing and thawing, which cause aggregation, and as a routine all antisera should be microfuged before use (2 min, 14 000 *g*).

Methods for cell separation by panning with monoclonal antibodies

Equipment

As for separation of PBM.

Materials

Media

MEM-H.
FCS.

Other disposables

Antibodies.
Anti-mouse immunoglobulin antibody.
Fifty millimetre or 90 mm plastic Petric dishes (Nunc, Intermed, Denmark).

Procedure

Panning [25]

This procedure can only be satisfactorily performed with cells which do not adhere significantly to plastic surfaces. It is, therefore, most useful for monocyte-depleted peripheral blood mononuclear cells or T-enriched cells prepared by E-rosette separation (see 'Method for sheep red blood cell (E) rosette formation and separation').

1   Petri dishes are first coated with anti-mouse immunoglobulin (anti-MIg) (affinity-purified and human immunoglobulin absorbed using insolubilized human immunoglobulin). Coating is carried out by incubating with enough anti-MIg to cover the bottom of the Petri dish for 1 h at 4 °C (5 ml/90 mm Petri dish). (The optimum concentration of anti-MIg must be determined by titration for each batch but is in the range of 10–50 μg/ml.)

2   Non-specific binding sites are then saturated by incubating the plate for a further hour with MEM-H containing 10% fetal or newborn calf serum. Immediately before use this is removed by suction.

3   Whilst the plates are being prepared, the cell suspension can be readied.

4   Adherent cells are depleted by incubating cells at 10^7/ml in RPMI-H 10% FCS for 1 h at 37 °C in a Petri dish.

5   Non-adherent cells are recovered by pipetting and then coated with monoclonal antibody by incubating for 30 min on ice and washing three times (see 'Method for indirect immunofluorescence and fluorescence activated cell sorting').

6 Coated cells are introduced into the prepared anti-MIg plates in suspension at 10^7/ml. For 90 mm dishes a maximum of 5 ml is advisable.

7 The cells are allowed to settle while the dish is maintained at 4 °C in a refrigerator for 1 h.

8 Non-adherent cells are recovered with a Pasteur pipette after the dish has been gently 'swirled' to free non-adherent (antigen negative) cells from the plastic surface.

9 The plate is then refilled with medium, swirled gently and the medium discarded three times.

10 Finally, adherent (antigen positive) cells can be recovered by vigorous pipetting of a stream of medium on to the attached cells. The purity of the recovered cells can be readily checked by staining a sample with FITC anti-MIg conjugate and microscopic or FACS counting (see 'Method for indirect immunofluorescence and fluorescence activated cell sorting').

Notes and recommendations

Panning is a useful method for bulk separation of leucocyte subpopulations. The main drawback is the necessity for using non-adherent cells. Surprisingly, even at 4 °C many cells can adhere to plastic and adherent cells include some T lymphocytes. Preadsorption, while it may allow clean separation of the non-adherent population to be carried out, is itself a separation procedure with unpredictable effects.

Bearing in mind this drawback, the method can produce good separations. The author has achieved $>95\%$ purity in bound and $>90\%$ in unbound populations. Good separation depends partly on the antibodies used (antibodies giving bright immunofluorescent staining usually work well) and partly on the properties of the plastic Petri dishes used. Of plastic Petri dishes available locally, Nunc plates give low non-specific adsorption and good separation. It is worth trying several brands when setting up the technique.

Complement mediated cytotoxicity

Equipment

As for separation of PBM.

Materials

Media

Fresh normal rabbit serum.
0.2% Trypan blue.
MEM-H.

Other disposables

Round-bottomed microtitre plates for analytical cytotoxicity.
Centrifuge tubes for preparative cytotoxicity.

Procedure

Antibody-mediated, complement-dependent cytotoxicity can be used either as an analytical method for enumeration of lymphocyte subsets or for elimination of a subpopulation for functional experiments [26].

1 Cells for test or treatment are resuspended at 2.5×10^6/ml.

2 To 8 vols. of cells in medium is added 1 vol. of monoclonal antibody such that a saturating concentration is obtained. (In the author's experience under these conditions most monoclonal antibodies can be used out to a final dilution of 1 μg/ml of Ig).

3 After 5 min incubation at 37 °C 1 vol. of fresh rabbit serum is added, to give a final 1 : 10 dilution, and the incubation continued for a further 45 min at 37 °C.

4 At the end of the incubation a sample of the incubation mixture is withdrawn and added to an equal volume of 0.2% trypan blue.

5 After 5 min at room temperature samples can be scored by counting at least 100 cells in a haemocytometer.

6 Appropriate controls are cells incubated with monoclonal antibody but no complement, cells with no antibody but complement, and cells with neither.

Notes and recommendations

It is the general experience that for lysis with most mouse monoclonal antibodies to human leucocytes, rabbit complement is required [26]. Unfortunately, not all batches of rabbit serum work equally well and some give unacceptably high ($>5\%$) background lysis so that it may be necessary to screen several rabbits. Furthermore, both absorption and freezing and thawing of the rabbit serum render the procedure less reliable. In addition, many existing mouse monoclonal antibodies are of the non-complement fixing IgGl class. Nevertheless, complement-dependent cytotoxicity can be a useful method for experimental [27] or *in vitro* therapeutic purposes [28] although in the former one subpopulation is of course lost to the experimenter. If it is essential to use cytotoxicity to remove a specific subpopulation of lymphocytes it may be possible to produce a specific monoclonal by screening only for cytotoxic murine antibodies, by using the rat hybridoma system [29] or by deriving cytotoxic switch variants of IgG1 antibodies [30].

Methods for separation of cells by adherence

Equipment

As for separation of PBM.

Materials

Media

MEM-H.
FCS.
Versene.
Three millimolar EDTA in PBSA (see 'Media' section).

Other disposables

Nylon fibre (Leucopak, Fenwal).
Nylon mesh (80 μm mesh, J. Stainer and Co., Manchester, England).
Sephadex G-10 (Pharmacia).
Baby hamster kidney cells (Flow Laboratories).
Ten millilitre disposable plastic syringes.

Procedure

By separation on Sephadex G-10 [31]

1 Sephadex G-10 is resuspended in distilled water and autoclaved for 10 min at 69 kPa.
2 The sterile slurry is washed twice in MEM-H by centrifugation and resuspension and stored in MEM-H at 4 °C until used.
3 Columns are prepared in plastic 10 ml syringes. A plug of nylon wool is inserted into the nozzle end of the syringe and overlaid with nylon mesh.
4 The syringes are then packed in a suitable container (e.g. a beaker with silver foil over the top) and autoclaved.
5 Sterile slurry is then poured into the syringe and allowed to sediment until a column volume of about 8 ml is achieved.
6 The columns are then washed with 20–30 ml of MEM-H containing 20% FCS prewarmed to 37 °C. PBM, up to 60×10^6, in 2 ml of MEM-H 20% FCS are added to the top of each column and the column is incubated at 37 °C for 30 min.
7 PBM are eluted with 10–15 ml of prewarmed MEM-H 20% FCS.
8 Cell yields vary from 45% to 55% and in the author's experience effluent cells contain less than 0.5% of monocytes as assessed by staining for non-specific esterase [32].

By adherence to micro-exudate coated plates [33]

1 Baby hamster kidney cells are grown to confluence on 90 mm plastic Petri dishes.
2 The cell layer is then detached by first removing the medium, rinsing with versene and then, after adding 15 ml versene, incubating the plates at 37 °C until the cells detach.
3 The plates are then washed vigorously with versene by pipetting, and stored at 4 °C with enough PBS to cover the bottom. (If sterility is in question they can be sterilized by exposure to a bactericidal UV light source for 5 min.) Up to 60×10^6 PBM can be depleted per plate.
4 Cells are added in 10 ml MEM-H 10% FCS medium and the plate incubated at 37 °C for 45 min.
5 Non-adherent cells are recovered by pipette and the plate is washed with medium.
6 Adherent cells can be recovered by incubating the plate with PBSA containing 3 mM-EDTA for a further 15 min and washing vigorously to detach the cells.

The non-adherent cells usually contain less than 5% and the adherent cells more than 75% non-specific esterase positive monocytes.

Notes and recommendations

Adherence methods are commonly used to remove monocytes but other cell types in peripheral blood are able to adhere to most surfaces. Thus, in using this type of methodology, it is important to decide at the outset what it is intended to achieve by the adherence step. If, for example, it is desired to remove the most 'sticky' monocytes in order to perform serological analyses on the remaining mononuclear cells without the problem of clumping and high backgrounds which monocytes sometimes produce, then a short adherence to a plastic Petri dish may be sufficient [34]. More usually it is intended either to remove monocytes in order to study lymphocyte function in the absence of monocytes or to enrich sufficiently to be able to study monocyte function in the absence of lymphocytes. Neither of these are easy to achieve by single-step adherence procedures. Even the G-10 procedure described above, which suffers from the problem of considerable loss of non-monocytic cells, does not remove all cells bearing monoclonal antibody defined monocytic antigens. G-10 depleted cells do, however, usually fail to respond in an antibody response in flat-bottomed culture vessels, while they may still respond in round-bottomed vessels, suggesting that accessory cell depletion by this method is incomplete [35]. It is in fact hardly surprising that depletion of accessory cell function by adherence is difficult and unreliable since recent data both in man [36] and the mouse [37] have shown that accessory cells are extremely heterogeneous and do not necessarily adhere actively.

Enrichment to homogeneity of monocytes is also difficult. While plastic adherence yields populations contaminated with B and T cells, the use of micro-exudate plates should in theory overcome this by selecting specifically for cells able to adhere to fibronectin. In routine use, however, some contamination with other cells occurs, even if the removal of non-adherent cells is followed by vigorous washing. At present, therefore, no totally satisfactory method for purification of monocytes exists. At least in part this is because the extent of heterogeneity among accessory cells has only recently been fully recognized, while the functional significance of this heterogeneity remains to be resolved.

Gradients

Equipment

As for separation of PBM.

Materials

Media

Percoll (Pharmacia).
PBS, 10 × concentration.

Procedure

For discontinuous Percoll gradients [4]
1   Percoll is made isotonic by addition of 1.5 M-PBS in a ratio of 1 part PBS to 9 parts Percoll. This isotonic solution is usually termed 100% Percoll and has a density of 1.1294 g/ml. For cell separation appropriate densities can be readily made up by dilution with tissue culture medium or PBS (single strength) since dilution and density are linearly related. Commonly used densities are as follows: 70% Percoll 1.090, 60% 1.077, 50% 1.067, 40% 1.056, 30% 1.043 and 20% 1.031 g/ml. PBM, (up to 10^8/gradient) are resuspended in 2 ml of 100% Percoll and placed in 15 ml plastic centrifuge tubes.
2   Aliquots of 2 ml of successively less dense solutions of Percoll are carefully run into the tube so that an interface is retained between each layer.
3   The gradient is then spun in a bench top centrifuge at approximately 500 *g* for 10 min at room temperature.
4   Cells at each interface can be harvested with a Pasteur pipette and are then washed in medium to remove contaminating Percoll.

Notes and recommendations

A variety of procedures for separation of cells on the basis of density have been published utilizing various separation media [38,39]. Percoll has the advantage that it is readily made isosmotic and appears to be non-toxic to human lymphocytes [4]. It can also be used to form continuous gradients when single-density solutions are centrifuged at high speed [4]. Gradient centrifugation methods have been most used for separation of lighter cells from the main (T) small lymphocyte population of peripheral blood. The lighter cell populations include monocytes [12] large granular lymphocytes [40] and blast cells [41]. While in most cases separation into subpopulations identifiable by other properties may not be complete, useful enrichment can often be achieved. Gradient separations are, therefore, often combined with other methods such as adherence, rosetting or separation with antibodies.

Assays of function of leucocyte subsets

Method for lymphoproliferation assays

Equipment

Multiple automatic cell harvester (MASH).
Hamilton repeating syringe (Comlab Ltd., Cambridge, UK) or Stepper (Tridak, Indicon Inc., USA) for dispensing 10 μl volumes.
Other equipment: as for separation of PBM.

Materials

Media

RPMI 1640 medium with 2 g/l sodium bicarbonate and 25 mM-HEPES buffer (Flow or Gibco).
Heat-inactivated FCS or Human AB RH + serum.
^{3}H-methyl thymidine or ^{125}I-iododeoxyuridine at 100 μCi/ml (Amersham International, UK).

Procedure

1   Separate mononuclear cells by Ficoll–Hypaque density gradient centrifugation wash twice and resuspend to 2×10^6 cells/ml.
2   Plate out 100 μl of the cell suspension in each well.
3   Add 100 μl of medium alone or containing mitogen or antigen at twice the intended final concentration.
4   Culture at 37 °C in a humidified atmosphere of 5% CO_2 in air.
5   At an appropriate time add either 1 μCi/well of ^{125}I-iododeoxyuridine (IUDR) or ^{3}H-thymidine in 10 μl.

6 Culture overnight and harvest cells onto filter discs using a cell harvester.

7 If IUDR is used, filter discs can be counted directly in a gamma counter.

8 Thymidine-labelled cells must be appropriately processed for scintillation counting.

Notes and recommendations

The use of microtitre plates, multiple-tip micropipettes and automatic cell harvesters has greatly simplified the assay of proliferative responses to mitogens and soluble antigens. In man, phytohaemagglutinin (PHA), concanavalin A (con A) and pokeweed mitogen (PWM) are the most commonly used mitogens. Optimal doses for stimulation with these agents vary, depending on the purity of the preparation and exact culture conditions, but it is in any case important to use a range of doses in order to obtain an optimal response. The same argument applies to soluble antigens such as tetanus toxoid. The kinetics of responses to mitogens and antigens also vary, depending on plate configuration, cell density, serum supplement and antigen or mitogen concentration. In general, however, peak proliferative responses to mitogens are assayed at 3–4 days (the radioactive DNA precursor is added late on the third day and cultures are harvested the following morning) while antigen-specific responses are pulsed on day 6 or 7 of culture. As in all *in vitro* responses, the source of serum is important. While mitogen responses are robust and background incorporation into unstimulated cultures is usually low at 3–4 days, high backgrounds are frequently seen at 6–7 days. Selection of FCS batch for ability to support a response but not stimulate may be necessary. Alternatively, human serum can be used. Pooled blood group AB serum is preferable to avoid agglutination of contaminating red cells by blood group isoagglutinins. The use of IUDR or thymidine as label is largely a matter of personal preference. In general, thymidine gives higher c.p.m. but IUDR has the advantage that the harvested samples do not need to be processed for scintillation counting.

Pokeweed mitogen driven immunoglobulin synthesis

Equipment

Enzyme immunoassay plate-reader (Titertek Multiskan, Flow Laboratories).
Other equipment: as for separation of PBM.

Materials

Media

RPMI 1640 with 2 g/l sodium bicarbonate.
10 mM-HEPES.
10% Heat-inactivated FCS and 10^{-5} M-hydrocortisone (Sigma).
PBS 1% BSA.
0.004% Orthophenylenediamine (Sigma) in citrate buffer, pH 5.0.
1 M-Sulphuric acid.

Other disposables

Round-bottomed tubes (Falcon 2054) or round-bottomed microtitre plates (Titertek #76-013-05) for culture, and flat-bottomed micro-ELISA plates (Titertek #76-381-04) for enzyme immunoassay.
Pokeweed mitogen (Gibco).
Peroxidase-conjugated anti-human immunoglobulin M, G and A antibodies.

Procedure

1 Mononuclear cells isolated by Ficoll–Hypaque separation from peripheral blood or lymphoid organs are counted and made up to 2×10^6/ml in medium.

2 Aliquots of 1 ml are dispensed into round-bottomed tubes.

3 PWM is added to triplicate cultures in volumes from 0 to 80 μl/ml.

4 The loosely capped tubes are cultured for 7 days at 37 °C in a humidified atmosphere of 5% CO_2 in air and at the end of this period the supernatant fluid is collected for immunoglobulin assay.

5 Flat-bottomed microtitre plates are coated with affinity-purified rabbit anti-human IgG, IgM or IgA antibody by incubation of the plates for 1 h at 37 °C with 100 μl of antibody diluted in PBS (an appropriate concentration must be determined by preliminary experiments but, as a guide, the author uses 2.5 μg/ml).

6 The wells are emptied by dumping out the liquid, and washed by adding PBS-BSA and dumping this out.

7 Non-specific binding sites are blocked by a further 1 h incubation at 37 °C with 200 μl PBS-BSA.

8 At the end of this time the liquid is dumped out and 100 μl of serial dilutions of supernatant or standards of known IgG, M or A concentration are added.

9 After a further 1 h incubation, the plates are washed three times and an appropriate dilution of peroxidase-conjugated anti-human IgG, M or A is added and incubated for a further hour.

10 After a further three washes, 100 μl of freshly

made up 0.004% orthophenylenediamine in citrate buffer is added and the plates incubated for 20–30 min.

11 The reaction is stopped by addition of 50 μl 1 M-sulphuric acid.

12 Optical density at 492 nm is read on an ELISA plate-reader. The Ig concentration of the supernatants is calculated from the log/linear regression curve obtained from the standards.

Notes and recommendations

Very many different procedures for performing PWM-induced immunoglobulin synthesis assays have been published. Many of the variations relate to the method of measurement of immunoglobulin synthesis. It is possible either to measure secreted immunoglobulin, as described above, or to measure numbers of plaque-forming cells by reverse plaque assay [42], or to count numbers of plasma cells by staining for cytoplasmic immunoglobulin [43]. The author prefers to use an ELISA method because it is rapid, quantitative and can handle many samples. Alkaline phosphatase may be used equally as well as peroxidase (see next section). Automatic (Skatron, Norway) or manual (Titertek Handiwash) plate-washing devices make washing steps more rapid and reproducible.

The method described utilizes tube cultures with relatively high numbers of cells (2×10^6) but more economical methods have been published using microtitre plates [42,44]. Such methods make it easier to set up many replicates but may not always work as reliably.

As with all *in vitro* culture systems, many variables affect the magnitude of response but perhaps the most important is the serum source. Not all batches of fetal calf serum support responses equally well and some give unacceptably high stimulation of control cultures. Other heterologous serum sources may work well [45] but again there is batch-to-batch variation; thus the use of serum-free medium has been advocated [42].

Method for specific antibody responses to influenza or varicella zoster viruses

Equipment

Centrifuge for spinning 96-well plates.
Enzyme immunoassay plate-reader.
Other equipment: as for separation of PBM.

Materials

Media

RPMI 1640 with 2 g/l sodium bicarbonate, 25 mM-HEPES, 10% heat-inactivated horse serum and 10^{-5} M-hydrocortisone.
RPMI 1640 with 2 g/l sodium bicarbonate, 20 mM-HEPES and 5% FCS.
PBS 1% BSA.
Bicarbonate buffer, pH 9.6.

Other disposables

Influenza viruses are obtainable from the Bureau of Biologics, National Institute of Health, USA, varicella zoster antigen (VZA) from Flow Laboratories, and *p*-nitrophenylphosphate from Sigma.
Cultures tubes and microtitre plates as for the last method.
Alkaline phosphatase conjugated anti-human immunoglobulin antibody.

Procedure

1 PBM are prepared from heparinized peripheral blood by separation on Ficoll–Hypaque.

2 After three washes in MEM-H 5% FCS, they are resuspended at 2×10^6/ml for culture in complete RPMI with 10% horse serum.

3 Cultures may be carried out in round-bottomed tubes [46] or round-bottomed microtitre plates [47]. For tube culture 1 ml of cells and for microtitre plates 0.2 ml are used.

4 An appropriate concentration of antigen is added in 0.1 ml to tubes or 10 μl to plates and the cells are cultured for 6 days in an atmosphere of 5% CO_2 in air.

5 At the conclusion of the culture the supernatant is removed by suction, and the cells are washed once by addition of the same volume of RPMI 5% FCS, centrifugation (5 min at 300 *g* for tubes, 3 min at 400 *g* for plates) and removal of the supernatant by suction.

6 The medium is replaced by 0.5 ml for tubes or 0.1 ml for plates of RPMI 5% FCS and the cells are cultured for a further 24 h.

7 Supernatants are then harvested and stored at -20 °C until assayed.

ELISA antibody assay

1 Flat-bottomed microtitre plate wells are coated with 60 μl of antigen diluted in saline (100 μg/ml of influenza virus or a 1:5 dilution of VZA) by incubation for 1 h at 37 °C.

2 The plates are washed twice with PBS and once

with PBS 1% BSA before non-specific binding sites are blocked by addition of 100 μl of PBS 1% BSA and a further 1 h incubation.

3   The plates are then washed again twice with PBS and once with PBS 1% BSA.

4   After washing, 50 μl of culture supernatant is added and the plates are incubated for a further 1 h at 37 °C.

5   The plates are washed as before and 50 μl of alkaline phosphatase coupled and immunoabsorbent-purified anti-human Ig added at an appropriate concentration.

6   After incubation as before the plates are washed twice with PBS, once with PBS 1% BSA and three times with bicarbonate buffer, pH 9.6, before addition of 100 μl of freshly made-up *p*-nitrophenylphosphate in bicarbonate buffer (1 mg/ml).

7   The colour is allowed to develop at room temperature for 1–18 h and absorbance at 405 nm measured with an automatic plate-reader.

8   Results can be presented as optical density (OD) of the sample. The author has also used specific antibody to influenza virus purified by absorption and elution from antigen to construct a standard curve of OD against immunoglobulin concentration. Since the relationship between OD and Ig concentration is linear only over a restricted range, logit transformation [48] is applied to the OD readings to produce a straight line when plotted against log antibody concentration [47].

Notes and recommendations

The method described above for generating specific antibody responses from human peripheral blood mononuclear cells was developed to provide a system for studies of the cellular requirements for human immune responses in health and disease. It is, therefore, appropriate to mention a number of problems and shortcomings of this methodology. First, it should be noted that consistent responses to a few antigens only can be obtained with this culture system. The author has studied in particular responses to influenza viruses and herpes zoster and a majority of normal subjects give measurable antibody responses to these viruses. However, the level of response is extremely variable and may not always be sufficiently high above background to provide reproducible results if cell separation and recombination experiments are envisaged. What is the source of this variability and low responsiveness in some individuals? It is clear that subjects without measurable serum antibody to influenza or herpes zoster viruses do not make *in vitro* responses; thus this system measures secondary antibody responses. This implies that in order to detect a response memory cells are required. Data from nor-

mal and Hodgkin's disease patients suggest that whereas T memory cells circulate for long periods of time after exposure to antigen, B memory cells may not [49]. The results of experiments on normal subjects immunized with tetanus toxoid [50] or keyhole limpet haemocyanin [51] also suggest that, while shortly after immunization responses to these soluble antigens are readily obtained, at later dates no specific antibody is produced unless B cells are stimulated with polyclonal activators such as *Staphylococcus* Cowan A [50]. In these experiments it is not clear whether the differences in requirements for activation of B cells are due to changes in the B cells or changes in the balance of different T-helper subsets [50]. It should also be noted that though the *in vitro* response is a secondary one, accessory cells are required [35]. The exact nature of these circulating accessory cells has not been defined, nor how their recirculation is affected by natural or deliberate immunization.

That the *in vitro* response is a secondary one also implies that the same antigen must be used *in vitro* and *in vivo*. With herpes zoster or tetanus toxoid this presents no problem but with influenza virus the situation is less straightforward. In the author's experience responses to Type A and B viruses are non-cross-reacting but the degree of cross-reactivity between various A subtypes is variable. Thus, obtaining an optimal response to influenza viruses *in vitro* will require the use of the same subtype of virus to which the subject has recently been exposed. This may pose problems so that an alternative, if the precise antibody specificity is unimportant, is to use a 'cocktail' of different subtypes of A viruses. The optimal dose of each batch of virus must also be determined by titration. Finally, the author has in recent years noted a decline in responsiveness of normal individuals to influenza virus. A parallel decrease in cytotoxic T cell responses has been documented and has been attributed to the unusually long time which has elapsed since the last major influenza virus epidemic [52]. Antibody responses to influenza virus can be boosted at least for a short time by vaccination.

The original description of the methodology for *in vitro* responses to influenza viruses [53] utilized sucrose density gradient purified virus which was not inactivated but had low infectivity; however, formalin inactivated virus works well in this system [54]. The nature of the serum supplement for the medium may also be important. The author has mainly used horse serum but others have used fetal calf serum. Not all batches support antibody responses equally well but the factor(s) present in the serum which are necessary are not defined. Whether mitogenic factors play a role in B cell activation is not clear [50].

Media

Aged chromic chloride

Aged chromic chloride is prepared as follows: 100 mg of $CrCl_3.6H_2O$ is dissolved in 100 ml of 0.9% saline and left at room temperature for 3 weeks. The solution is adjusted to pH 5.0 by dropwise addition of NaOH and stored at room temperature. It is best used after at least 5 months of storage. During this time it may be necessary to readjust the pH repeatedly to pH 5.0 until it stabilizes.

Substrate for peroxidase enzyme immunoassay

Stock solutions: 0.2 M-Na_2HPO_4 and 0.1 M-citric acid.
Mix 25.7 ml 0.2 M-Na_2HPO_4, 24.3 ml 0.1 M-citric acid and 50 ml distilled H_2O.
Add 40 mg orthophenylenediamine and 60 μl 33% hydrogen peroxide.

Substrate for alkaline phosphatase immunoassay

Bicarbonate buffer, pH 9.6.
Na_2CO_3, 1.59 g.
Dissolve in one litre of distilled H_2O.
Add *p*-nitrophenyl phosphate, 1 mg/ml.

Versene

NaCl, 0.8 g.
KCl, 0.2 g.
Na_2HPO_4, 1.15 g.
KH_2PO_4, 0.2 g.
Ethylenediaminetetraacetic acid (EDTA), 0.2 g.
1% Phenol red, 1.5 ml.
Make up to one litre with distilled water (sterilize if necessary by autoclave).

Dulbecco's PBS

Solution A	*Solution B*
NaCl, 1.0 g.	$CaCl_2.2H_2O$, 1.33 g.
KCl, 0.25 g.	
Na_2HPO_4, 1.44 g.	*Solution C*
KH_2PO_4, 0.25 g.	$MgCl_2.6H_2O$, 1 g.

Make up each solution to one litre with distilled water. For use mix 8 parts A, 1 part B and 1 part C. Sterilize each solution separately by autoclave.

Ficoll–Hypaque for cell separation density 1.077 g/ml

Ficoll, 96 g (Mr 400 000 Pharmacia, Uppsala, Sweden).

Sodium diatrizoate, 56 g (Hypaque, Sterling Research Laboratories, Surbiton, UK).
Make up to one litre and sterilize by autoclave.

Haemolytic gelatin Gey's solution

Solution A	*Solution B*
NH_4Cl, 35.0 g.	$MgCl_2 \cdot 6H_2O$, 4.2 g.
KCl, 1.85 g.	$MgSO_4 \cdot 7H_2O$, 1.4 g.
$Na_2HPO_4 \cdot 12H_2O$, 1.5 g.	$CaCl_2$, 3.4 g.
KH_2PO_4, 0.119 g.	*Solution C*
Glucose, 5 g.	$NaHCO_5$, 22.5 g.
Gelatin (Difco), 25 g.	
1% Phenol red, 1.5 ml.	

Make up each solution to one litre with distilled water. For use, mix 20 ml A, 5 ml B, 5 ml C and 70 ml H_2O. Sterilize each solution separately by autoclave.

Fluorescein diacetate

Dissolve 10 mg in 1 ml of acetone.
Dilute 1 : 10 000 in PBS. Store at 4 °C.

Percoll

One hundred per cent Percoll is prepared as follows. To 900 ml of Percoll add 100 ml of 10 × concentrated PBS (PBS Solution A × 10; see under PBS). Sterilize by autoclaving.

For cell fractionations, 100% Percoll is diluted with MEM-H 5% FCS. To obtain a solution of a chosen density, first measure accurately the density of the 100% Percoll and the MEM-H 5% FCS using density bottles. Then mix Percoll and MEM-H 5% FCS in volumes calculated according to the formula:

$$\text{Vol. of 100\% Percoll} = \frac{\text{desired final density} - \text{density of MEM-H 5\% FCS}}{\text{density of 100\% Percoll} - \text{density of MEM-H 5\% FCS}} \times 1000 \text{ ml}$$

Vol. of MEM-H 5% FCS = 1000 − vol. of 100% Percoll

References

1 SIMPSON E. & BEVERLEY P.C.L. (1977) T lymphocyte heterogeneity. In *Progress in Immunology III*, (eds. Mandel T.E., Cheers C., Hosking C.S., McKenzie I.F.C. & Nossal G.J.V.), p. 206. Elsevier/North–Holland, New York.

2 SWAIN S.L. (1983) T cell subsets and the recognition of MHC class. *Immunol. Revs.* **74**, 129.

3 REINHERZ E.L. & SCHLOSSMAN S.F. (1980) The differentiation and function of human T lymphocytes. *Cell*, **19**, 821.

4 KURNICK J.T., OSTBERG L., STEGAGNO M., KIMURA A.K., ORN A. & SJOBERG O. (1979) A rapid method for the separation of functional lymphoid cell populations of human and animal origin on PVP-silica (Percoll) density gradients. *Scand. J. Immunol.* **10**, 563.

5 KAPLAN M.E. & CLARK C. (1974) An improved rosetting assay for detection of human T lymphocytes. *J. immunol. Meth.* **5**, 131.

6 JANOSSY G. (1981) Membrane markers in leukaemia. In *The Leukemic Cell*, Chapter 5, (ed. Catovsky D.), p. 167. Churchill Livingstone, Edinburgh.

7 DRESSER D.W. (1978) Assays for immunoglobulin-secreting cells. In *Handbook of Experimental Immunology*, 3rd edn., Chapter 28, (ed. Weir D.M.), p. 28.22. Blackwell Scientific Publications, Oxford.

8 WHO/IARC Workshop (1974) Identification, enumeration and isolation of B and T lymphocytes from human peripheral blood. *Scand. J. Immunol.* **3**, 521.

9 WEINER M.S., BIANCO C. & NUSSENZWEIG V. (1973) Enhanced binding of neuraminidase treated sheep erythrocytes to human T lymphocytes. *Blood*, **42**, 939.

10 WEST W.H., BOOZER R.B. & HERBERMAN R.B. (1978) Low affinity E rosette formation by the human K cell. *J. Immunol.* **120**, 90.

11 BEVERLEY P.C.L. & CALLARD R.E. (1981) Distinctive functional properties of 'T' lymphocytes defined by E rosetting or a monoclonal anti T cell antibody. *Eur. J. Immunol.* **11**, 329.

12 CALLARD R.E. & SMITH C.M. (1981) Histocompatibility requirements for T cell help in specific *in vitro* antibody responses to influenza virus by human blood lymphocytes. *Eur. J. Immunol.* **11**, 206.

13 SAMARUT C. & REVILLARD J.-P. (1980) Active and passive re-expression of Fcγ receptors on human lymphocytes. *Eur. J. Immunol.* **10**, 352.

14 BURNS G.F., CAWLEY J.C., BARKER C.R., GOLDSTONE A.H. & HAYHOE F.G.J. (1977) New evidence relating to the nature and origin of the hairy cell of leukaemic reticuloendotheliosis. *Br. J. Haematol.* **36**, 71.

15 HALLBERG T., GURNER B.W. & COOMBS R.R.A. (1973) Opsonic adherence of sensitized ox red cells to human lymphocytes as measured by rosette formation. *Int. Archs Allergy appl. Immunol.* **44**, 500.

16 MORETTA L., FERRARINI M., DURANTE M.L. & MINGARI M.C. (1975) Expression of a receptor for IgM by human T cells *in vitro*. *Eur. J. Immunol.* **5**, 565.

17 PICHLER W.J., LUM L. & BRODER S. (1978) Fc-receptors on human T-lymphocytes. (1) Transition of T_G cells to T_M cells. *J. Immunol.* **121**, 1540.

18 VAN WAUWE J.P., DEMEY J. & GOOSSENS J. (1980) OKT3: a monoclonal antibody with potent mitogenic properties. *J. Immunol.* **124**, 2708.

19 LANDEGREN U., RAMSTEDT U., AXEBERG I., ULLBERG M., JONDAL M. & WIGZELL H. (1982) Selective inhibition of human T cell cytotoxicity at levels of target recognition or initiation of lysis by monoclonal OKT3 and Leu 2a antibodies. *J. exp. Med.* **155**, 1579.

20 ZANDERS E.D., LAMB J.R., FELDMANN M., GREEN N. &

BEVERLEY P.C.L. (1983) Tolerance of T cell clones is associated with membrane antigen changes. *Nature*, **303**, 625.

21 REINHERZ E.L., MEUER S.C. & SCHLOSSMAN S.F. (1983) The human T cell receptor: analysis with cytotoxic T cell clones. *Immunol. Revs.* **74**, 83.

22 LING N.R. & RICHARDSON P.R. (1981) A critical appraisal of the direct antibody-rosette test for the detection of cell surface antigens. *J. immunol. Meth.* **47**, 265.

23 LINCH D.C., BEVERLEY P.C.L., LEVINSKY R. & RODECK C.H. (1982) Phenotypic analysis of foetal blood leucocytes: potential for antenatal diagnosis of immunodeficiency disorders. *Prenatal Diagn.* **2**, 211.

24 BEVERLEY P.C.L. (1982) The use of the fluorescence activated cell sorter for the identification and analysis of function of cell population. In *Monoclonal Antibodies in Clinical Medicine*, (eds. McMichael A.J. & Fabre J.W.), p. 557. Academic Press, London.

25 WYSOCKI L.J. & SATO V.L. (1978) Panning for lymphocytes: a method for cell selection. *Proc. natn. Acad. Sci. U.S.A.* **75**, 2844.

26 VAN WAUWE J. & GOOSSENS J. (1981) Monoclonal anti-human T-lymphocyte antibodies: enumeration and characterization of T-cell subsets. *Immunology*, **42**, 157.

27 REINHERZ E.L., MORIMOTO C., FITZGERALD K.A., HUSSEY R.E., DALEY J.F. & SCHLOSSMAN S.F. (1982) Heterogeneity of human T4$^+$ inducer cells defined by a monoclonal antibody that delineates two functional subpopulations. *J. Immunol.* **128**, 463.

28 PRENTICE H.G., BLACKLOCK H.A., JANOSSY G., GILMORE M.J., PRICE-JONES L., TREJDOSIEWICZ L.K., SKEGGS D.B.L., PANJUVANI D., BALL S., GRAPHAKOS S., PATTERSON J., IVORY K. & HOFFBRAND A.V. (1984) Depletion of T lymphocytes in donor marrow prevents significant graft-versus-host disease in matched allogeneic leukaemic marrow transplant recipients. *Lancet*, **i**, 472.

29 HALE G., BRIGHT S., CHUMBLEY G., HOANG T., METCALF D., MUNRO A.J. & WALDMANN H. (1983) Removal of T cells from bone marrow for transplantation: A monoclonal anti-lymphocyte antibody that fixes human complement. *Blood*, **62**, 873.

30 DANGL J.L. & HERZENBERG L.A. (1982) Selection of hybridomas and hybridoma variants using the fluorescence activated cell sorter. *J. immunol. Meth.* **52**, 1.

31 LY I.A. & MISHELL R.I. (1974) Separation of mouse spleen cells by passage through columns of Sephadex G10. *J. immunol. Meth.* **5**, 239.

32 KOSKI I.R., POPLACK D.G. & BLAESE R.M. (1976) In In Vitro *Methods in Cell Mediated and Tumour Immunity*, (eds. Bloom B.R. & David J.R.), p. 359. Academic Press, New York.

33 ACKERMAN S.K. & DOUGLAS S.D. (1978) Purification of human monocytes on microexudate-coated surfaces. *J. Immunol.* **120**, 1372.

34 KUMAGAI K.K., ITOH S., HINUMA S. & TADA M. (1979) Pretreatment of plastic Petri dishes with foetal calf serum. A simple method for macrophage isolation. *J. immunol. Meth.* **29**, 17.

35 MITCHELL D.M., BEVERLEY P.C.L., BOYLE D., WINGER L. & CALLARD R.E. (1983) Accessory cell and HLA compatibility requirements for the generation of specific *in*

vitro antibody responses to influenza virus by human blood lymphocytes. *Immunology*, **50**, 239.

36 POULTER L.W. (1983) Antigen presenting cells *in situ*: their identification and involvement in immunopathology. *Clin. exp. Immunol.* **53**, 513.

37 STEINMAN R.M. & COHN Z.A. (1974) Macrophages dendritic cells and reticular cells. In *Mononuclear Phagocytes*, (ed. Van Furth R.), p. 237. Blackwell Scientific Publications, Oxford.

38 BOYUM A. (1976) Isolation of lymphocytes, granulocytes and macrophages. In *Lymphocytes. Isolation, Fractionation and Characterisation*, (eds. Natvig J.B., Perlmann P. & Wigzell H.), p. 9. *Scand. J. Immunol.* **5**, (suppl. 5).

39 GORCZYNSKI R.M., MILLER R.G. & PHILLIPS R.A. (1970) Homogeneity of antibody-producing cells as analysed by their buoyant density in gradients of ficoll. *Immunology*, **19**, 817.

40 TIMONEN T., ORTALDO J.R. & HERBERMAN R.B. (1981) Characteristics of human large granular lymphocytes and relationship to natural killer and K cell. *J. exp. Med.* **153**, 569.

41 LAMB J.R., ECKELS D.D., LAKE P., JOHNSON A.H., HARTZMAN R.J. & WOODY J.N. (1982) Antigen-specific human T lymphocyte clones: induction, antigen specificity and MHC restriction of influenza virus-immune clones. *J. Immunol.* **128**, 233.

42 TANNO Y., ARAI S. & TAKISHIMA T. (1982) Induction of immunoglobulin-producing human peripheral blood lymphocytes in serum-free medium. *J. immunol. Meth.* **52**, 255.

43 JANOSSY G. & GREAVES M. (1975) Functional analysis of murine and human B lymphocyte subsets. *Transplant. Rev.* **24**, 177.

44 MORETTA L., WEBB S.R., GROSSI C.E., LYDYARD P.M. & COOPER M.D. (1977) Functional analysis of two human subpopulations: Help and suppression of B cell responses by T cells bearing receptors for IgM or IgG. *J. exp. Med.* **146**, 184.

45 CALLARD R.E., SMITH C.M., WORMAN C., LINCH D., CAWLEY J.C. & BEVERLEY P.C.L. (1981) Unusual phenotype and function of an expanded subpopulation of T cells in patients with haemopoietic disorders. *Clin. exp. Immunol.* **43**, 497.

46 SOUHAMI R.L., BABBAGE J. & CALLARD R.E. (1981) Specific *in vitro* antibody response to varicella zoster. *Clin. exp. Immunol.* **46**, 98.

47 ZANDERS E.D., SMITH C.M. & CALLARD R.E. (1981) A micromethod for the induction and assay of specific *in vitro* antibody responses by human lymphocytes. *J. immunol. Meth.* **47**, 333.

48 ARMITAGE P. (1971) *Statistical Methods in Medical Research.* Blackwell Scientific Publications, Oxford.

49 SOUHAMI R.L., BABBAGE J. & SIGFUSSON A. (1983) Defective antibody production to varicella zoster and other virus antigens in patients with Hodgkin's disease. *Clin. exp. Immunol.* **53**, 297.

50 BRENNER M.K., NEWTON C.A., NORTH M.E., WEYMAN C. & FARRANT J. (1983) The interaction of specific T cell help and non-specific B-cell growth factors in the production of anti-tetanus antibody by human B cells grown in serum-free microcultures. *Immunology*, **50**, 377.

51 LANE H.C., VOLKMAN D.J., WHALEN G. & FAUCI A.S. (1982) *In vitro* antigen-induced, antigen-specific antibody production in man. Specific and polyclonal components, kinetics and cellular requirements. *J. exp. Med.* **154**, 1043.

52 MCMICHAEL A.J., GOTCH F.M., DONGWORTH D.W., CLARK A. & POTTER C.W. (1983) Declining T-cell immunity to influenza 1977–82. *Lancet*, **ii**, 762.

53 CALLARD R.E. (1979) Specific *in vitro* antibody response to influenza virus by human blood lymphocytes. *Nature*, **282**, 734.

54 LAMB J.R., WOODY J.N., HARTZMAN R.J. & ECKELS D.D. (1982) *In vitro* influenza virus specific antibody production in man: antigen specific and HLA restricted induction of helper activity mediated by cloned human T lymphocytes. *J. Immunol.* **129**, 1465.

Chapter 59
Lymphokines

J. KAPPLER & PHILIPPA MARRACK

Methods for the production of
  lymphokines, 59.2

Methods for assaying
  lymphokines, 59.4

Purification of lymphokines, 59.6

Lymphokines are non-antigen-specific, hormone-like polypeptides produced by cells of the immune system. Traditionally, as the name suggests, these molecules were defined as products of lymphocytes, particularly of T cells, but in practice mediators produced by other leucocytes, such as macrophages, have been included in this group. Recently, the name 'interleukins' has been suggested to reflect this heterogeneity of the source of these factors. The cells most often identified as the targets of the hormone-like action of lymphokines are other leucocytes, especially T cells, B cells, and macrophages, although there are a number of cases where non-leucocyte targets for these mediators have also been observed.

Lymphokine activities may be broadly grouped into four categories: growth factors, activation or differentiation factors, lymphotoxins, and chemotactic factors. The first two categories account for the great bulk of the published research. Lymphokine growth factors have been reported for T cells (Interleukin-2—IL-2), B cells (B cell growth factors—BCGFs), macrophages and granulocytes (colony stimulating factor—CSF), and mast cells (Interleukin-3—IL-3). The star of this group and of lymphokine research in general has been IL-2. This lymphokine has been fully purified and cloned [1–3]. Moreover, its receptor has now been identified [4,5]. Activation or differentiation lymphokines have also been reported for many different cell types. For example, interferon-γ was the first lymphokine to be molecularly cloned and expressed [6]. In addition to its induction of protection from viral infection in many cell types [6], this mediator has been identified as a powerful inducer of the expression of MHC-products in various cell types [7,8], an activator of macrophages, and a differentiation factor for B cells. Another pleiotropic lymphokine is macrophage-derived Interleukin-1 (IL-1), which has been implicated in both T cell and B cell activation [13,15]. In addition, evidence has suggested that IL-1 can be a growth factor for fibroblasts and is a pyrogen [16,17]. Most recently, a number of additional lymphokine activities have been described which appear to play a role in the activation and differentiation of T cells and B cells [18–22].

Non-lymphokine chemotactic factors for various types of leucocytes have been widely reported and characterized. Such activities among the lymphokines have been reported [23], but are much less well-documented. Lymphotoxins were originally reported a number of years ago as a complex set of proteins produced by activated T cells capable of killing off susceptible cell types, especially fibroblasts [24,25]. Their complexity has hampered their purification.

In a few cases the purification of a particular lymphokine has allowed experiments to establish their credentials as hormones. For example, using purified radiolabelled IL-2 Robb *et al.* have established that proliferating T cells have about 15 000 receptors for IL-2 with a binding constant of about 10^{-11} M [1]. As the availability of purified lymphokines increases, undoubtedly more experiments of this type will be performed.

At present the cell biology of lymphokines is an area of research only in its infancy, because of the preoccupation with the identification and purification of the molecules themselves. In a few cases, cellular receptors for particular lymphokines have been identified, most notably for IL-2 [4,5], but our knowledge of the intracellular messages involved in the action of these mediators is minimal. However, if the recent progress in the purification and cloning of lymphokines continues, we can expect that this type of research will expand rapidly in the next few years.

For many years investigators have entered the field of lymphokine research with some well-warranted trepidation. Since the early discovery of macrophage inhibition factor (MIF), a formidable list of lymphokine acronyms has accumulated in the literature. Until recently, progress in the study of these activities has been painfully slow. There were at least two reasons for this lack of progress. The first had to do with the source of lymphokines for research. Lymphokines were prepared from supernatants of stimulated cultures of mixed lymphoid cells. It became apparent that these supernatants contained many activities which were not separable by simple techniques, such as gel filtration. When these mixtures were tested for particular biological activities, one could never be sure how many activities contributed to the effect seen. Therefore new lymphokines were inevitably named on the basis of an assay which measured the synergy of several activities, some of which were already known. Problems of this type are well illustrated by studies of factors which are active in B cell responses [12,15–21]. A second problem had to do with the lack of purity of the target cells. IL-2, for example, is a very potent stimulator of activated T cells [26]. If an IL-2-containing lymphokine preparation is added to cultures contaminated with but a very small proportion of T cells, any activity observed may not be due to the action of the added lymphokines directly on the target cell, but rather due to the production of additional activities by IL-2 stimulated bystander T cells.

Although these problems still haunt many experiments, since the last edition of this book recent technical advances both in lymphokine sources and purification, and in target cell preparation, have led to remarkably rapid progress in the study of some lymphokines and have resurrected interest in this field. It is, of course, impossible to catalogue here all the techniques currently in use in lymphokine research. Rather, an attempt is made to discuss some of the technical points and pitfalls in order to help investigators design or adapt lymphokine assays for their own use.

Methods for the production of lymphokines

Equipment

Sterile dissecting instruments.
Sterile plastic Petri dishes.
Sterile Pasteur pipettes.
Sterile centrifuge tubes.
Incubator at 37 °C.
Centrifuge.
Microscope.
Haemocytometer chamber.
Rocking platform.

Materials

An activating agent for the cells, e.g. concanavalin A, phytohaemagglutinin, lipolysaccharide, phorbol myristic acetate.
Tissue culture medium.

Procedure

The example given below is for the preparation of supernatants containing (amongst other lymphokines) IL-2 from mouse spleen.

1 Mouse spleens are placed in sterile saline or balanced salt solution, in sterile 3.5 cm diameter Petri dishes, and teased into a single cell suspension with toothed forceps.

2 The cell suspension is transferred into a sterile tube and left to stand on ice for about 4 min. During this time clumps and debris sink to the bottom of the tube.

3 The cell suspension is then removed from the sediment and transferred to a sterile centrifuge tube.

4 A small sample is set aside for use in counting the nucleated cells using a microscope or a cell counter. Red blood cells should be lysed prior to counting using either dilute acetic acid and Giemsa stain or the detergent provided for this purpose by the manufacturers of the automated cell counter.

5 The remaining cells are sedimented by centrifugation at 500 g for 10 min.

6 They are resuspended at 10^7 mediated cells per ml in a suitable medium (RPMI 1640, modified Eagle's medium or Dulbecco's medium) containing 5×10^{-5} M-2-mercaptoethanol, 5% fetal bovine serum and 4 μg/ml concanavalin A.

7 Four millilitres of this suspension is added to each 3.5 cm sterile Petri dish, and the suspension rocked at 37 °C in a suitably gassed environment, usually 95% air, 5% CO_2 or 90% air, 10% CO_2, depending on the medium, for 24 h.

8 Supernatants are then harvested by centrifugation (see above), sterilized by passage through a 0.22 μm filter and stored in aliquots at -20 °C.

Notes and recommendations

Producing lymphokines from unfractionated cells

Techniques for culturing normal lymphoid cells from mouse, man, and other species have become standardized and are in widespread use. In mouse, the original techniques of Mishell & Dutton [27] have been improved by Click *et al.* [28] and most recently by Iscove & Melchers [29]. In general, more complex media have reduced or eliminated the requirement for serum supplementation, a consideration when large scale production, concentration and purification of lymphokines are required.

In man, either tonsil or peripheral blood can be used as the source of lymphoid cells. In mouse and most other species, spleen and lymph node cells are generally used. Single cell suspensions containing T cells, B cells, and adherent cells are cultured by standard techniques and stimulated with a T cell mitogen. Phytohaemagglutinin (PHA) has most often been used with human cells and concanavalin A (con A) with murine cells. Cell concentrations can vary from 1×10^6 to 10×10^6 per ml. Optimal mitogen concentration varies with the source, cell dose, and serum concentration but is generally in the order of 1–5 μg/ml.

Extensive experiments have shown a similar kinetics of production of many different types of lymphokines following stimulation of T cells with mitogens. Most lymphokine activities begin to appear in the extracellular supernatant after about 4 h. Peak levels are usually reached within 12–24 h, at which time synthesis stops. Surprisingly, many lymphokine activities are quite stable at 37 °C and persist at high levels for several days in cultures of stimulated, proliferating T cells. An exception is IL-2, or T cell growth factor (TCGF) which, although quite stable at 37 °C, is rapidly utilized by the proliferating T cells such that its activity can drop to undetectable levels within four days of culture. Since IL-2 can often be a confusing activity in many lymphocyte assays, this method can sometimes be used to prepare a lymphokine preparation selectively depleted of IL-2.

Lymphokine production cultures are harvested at some time between one and four days and the cell-free supernatant is prepared by centrifugation and filtration through a 0.2 μm filter. As with many biological active molecules, storage may be critical at this point. Most lymphokine activities survive freeze-thawing and can be stored at -20 °C. Some may require more careful handling by storage at -70 °C and avoiding multiple freeze-thawing. Rapid loss of IL-2 activity at -20 °C has ben observed in preparations made without serum. Similar preparations made with as little as 0.5% serum have been stable at -20 °C for many months. Whether this loss of activity is due to denaturation in the absence of stabilizing protein or to serum-inhibitable, contaminating proteases is not known, but it is a good idea to purify lymphokines produced in serum-free medium as soon as possible and to consider the use of protease inhibitors or stabilizing protein in these preparations.

Preparing lymphokines from cloned T cell lines

Methodology has been developed over the past few years for the routine production of T cell clones [30]. There are numerous reports of the use of these clones for the production of lymphokines [11]. The methods are similar to those used to produce lymphokines from heterogenous populations described above except that in this case specific antigen as well as mitogens can be used to stimulate high levels of lymphokine production. In general, T cell clones are grown by periodic restimulation with specific antigen presented by MHC-compatible accessory cells with or without supplementation with additional IL-2. Typically, restimulation is performed at weekly to biweekly intervals. As with uncloned T cells, peak lymphokine levels are obtained in these cultures within about 24 h of antigen restimulation. Similar results are seen using mitogen restimulation.

It was originally suggested that the range of lymphokines produced by individual T cell clones would be more restricted than that produced by T cells as a whole reflecting the different functions of T cell subsets. Although the results reported thus far indicate that individual T cell clones produce a wide variety of lymphokine activities, it has been possible to identify clones and subclones which produce a more limited set of activities [31]. Whether these clones reflect the inherent production of the T cell from which they were derived or arose as variants during cloning is not always clear. Nevertheless, these clones can make the task of purifying a particular activity easier.

Preparing lymphokines from T cell tumours and hybridomas

A number of T cell tumours in mouse and man have been identified which are capable of lymphokine production [20]. These cells have the advantage that they make large scale lymphokine production possible and often produce higher levels of lymphokines than normal T cells. Interestingly, nearly all these cells fail to secrete lymphokines constitutively, but rather must be stimulated with mitogen with or without phorbol myristate acetate (PMA). Kinetics of production are similar to that seen with normal T cells. The best characterized of these tumour cells is a subline of the C57BL/6 tumour, EL-4 [20]. When stimulated with con A and PMA this line produces a wide variety of lymphokines (IL-2, BCGF, thymus replacing factor). Care must be taken in utilizing PMA as a stimulus for lymphokine production. PMA can have dramatic effects on the functions of many different cell types and can bind tightly to various proteins. Procedures for removing PMA from supernatants, such as passage over activated charcoal, may not always lower its concentration sufficiently to be without effect in all lymphokine assays. Binding of PMA to proteins may result in its co-purification with particular proteins. Furthermore, even though PMA itself may have no effect in a particular lymphokine assay, it may synergize with a lymphokine, obscuring the mode of action of the lymphokine. These considerations lead us to suggest that if possible PMA be avoided as a stimulus for lymphokine production. The lower lymphokine production seen without PMA may be offset by fewer artifacts to deal with during purification.

Techniques are now widely available for the production of T cell hybridomas in both mouse [32] and man [21]. T cell tumour cells carrying the appropriate drug resistance markers can be fused to normal T cells with the same techniques used to produce monoclonal antibody secreting B cell hybridomas. The resulting T cell hybridomas are often capable of high levels of lymphokine production. Again, as with normal and tumour T cells, these hybridomas nearly always require a stimulus to secrete lymphokines. Mitogens such as con A and PHA can be used. Alternatively when the normal T cell partner in the fusion is a population of enriched or cloned antigen-specific T cells, T cell hybrids can be identified which secrete lymphokines when stimulated with specific antigen presented by MHC-compatible cells. With either type of stimulation, kinetics of lymphokine production are similar to that of normal T cells such that supernatants are harvested at about 24 h.

T cell hybridomas offer the same advantage as T cell tumours in that they make large scale lymphokine production possible. They have the disadvantage that even after cloning they may not be as stable as T cell tumours. This problem can usually be circumvented by establishing a large frozen stock of a functional hybridoma immediately after cloning. Production runs can then be made with a freshly thawed aliquot of cells expanded rapidly in culture just prior to stimulation. Alternatively, as with B cell hybridomas, particularly unstable hybridomas can usually be stabilized by multiple cloning. The authors have recently shown that T cell hybrid instability can be used to advantage in lymphokine purification, since during cloning and recloning it is sometimes possible to segregate the production of particular lymphokines to individual subclones [12].

Producing lymphokines from other cell types

Some lymphokines, most notably IL-1 are not produced by T cells. In these cases a number of approaches toward lymphokine production have been used. Interleukin 1, for example, may be made from normal macrophages by activating them with bacterial lipopolysaccaride with or without PMA, or by other means [15]. Interleukin-1 may also be prepared from the culture supernatants of macrophage tumours [33,34].

Methods for assaying lymphokines

It is impossible to discuss all of the various assays for different lymphokines. The authors instead discuss some general considerations in developing lymphokine assays.

Target cells

The vast majority of bioassays for lymphokines involve either the stimulation of the growth of a particular cell type or the induction of a particular function in the appropriate target cell. The most successful and reliable of these assays are those which use a clonal cell line as the target cell. Clonal cells are, of course, more likely to respond uniformly to the lymphokine. Moreover, the presence of more than one cell type in the target cell population always leaves the actual target of the lymphokine in doubt. Clonal targets for a number of the growth promoting lymphokines are available. Most notably the HT-2 [35] and CTLL [36] T cell lines are widely distributed for use in measuring the TCGF activity of IL-2. These cell lines are absolutely dependent on IL-2 for their growth and viability and have been used to develop dependable, reproducible assays of IL-2. Recently cloned cell lines similarly dependent on IL-3 have been reported [37].

In a number of cases where it has not been possible to establish clones of normal cells which respond to particular lymphokines, tumour cell lines of the appropriate cell type have been identified. For example, in mouse the macrophage tumour cell lines P388D1 and WEHI 3 have been shown to respond to the IaIF activity of IFN$_\gamma$ in a similar way to normal macrophages with increased surface expression of Ia antigens [12,38–40]. Similarly, both in mouse [41,42] and man [21] B cell tumour cell lines have been identified which respond to certain B cell growth and differentiation lymphokines. Obviously, care must be taken in using tumour cell lines as targets for lymphokines, since there is no guarantee that these transformed cells will exactly reflect their normal cell counterpart. Therefore, although tumour cell targets may be useful in the purification and initial characterization of a lymphokine, it is wise to confirm its activity on normal cell targets for critical findings and at periodic points in its purification.

Since it is not always possible to identify cloned normal or tumour cell targets, many lymphokine assays require preparation of primary cultures of target cells. Heterogeneity in this population may lead to confusion about the actual target of the lymphokine. Therefore it is worth the effort to purify the target cell as much as possible for the assay. The additional work pays off in sharper, more reproducible, less ambiguous results. Some of the most commonly used target cells are T cells and B cells. There have been some recent improvements in the purification of these populations. For example, T cell partially purified using nylon wool fibre columns [43] can be further purified by treatment with anti-Ia or anti-Ig antibody and complement [44]. The traditional purification of B cells with anti-Thy-1 and complement [45] can be improved by *in vivo* pre-treatment of donor mice with anti-thymocyte serum, passage of cells over G-10 Sephadex, and treatment with other anti-T cell and anti-null cell antibodies and complement [46]. Furthermore, size fractionation can be used to separate B cells in various states of activation, which respond differently to various lymphokines [47,48].

How pure a target cell must be clearly depends on the particular lymphokine and its state of purity. For example, contaminating T cells in either B cell or macrophage preparations can confuse assays for B cell or macrophage stimulating lymphokines if IL-2 is present as well in the lymphokine preparation. These T cells can respond to IL-2 with the production of other lymphokines. Contaminating T cells may be less of a problem when a more purified lymphokine preparation is used.

Proliferative assays

Many assays measure the ability of lymphokines either directly or in synergy with other factors to stimulate target cell growth. Usually the incorporation of radioactive DNA precursors into DNA is used to estimate the rate of growth. Tritiated thymidine is the most commonly used precursor. There are a number of important considerations in using this type of assay. In order to be confident that the amount of incorporation of label is a measure of the rate of DNA synthesis and, therefore, a measure of cell growth, it is important that incorporation be linear during the period of labelling. An important factor controlling the linearity of incorporation is the extracellular concentration of the DNA precursor. For example, most mammalian cells can synthesize thymidine *de novo* and maintain a relatively small, but measurable internal pool. Although externally added thymidine can enter the cell very rapidly, unless the external concentration is high enough significant dilution of the specific activity by the internal cold pool can occur, resulting in variable and non-linear incorporation. In general, this problem can be kept to a minimum by keeping the concentration of thymidine at or above 5 μM in the medium.

A second factor influencing the linearity of incorporation is the total radioactivity incorporated during the label. Exponentially growing cells, especially lymphocytes, can incorporate radiolabelled thymidine rapidly enough to be destroyed by the radioactivity. Depending on the cell type, as little as 1 c.p.m./cell may be lethal. During the course of a long labelling period the rate of incorporation levels off and may even drop as the cells die. Therefore, as a general rule, lower rather than higher specific activity DNA precursors and shorter rather than longer incubation periods are best for measuring the rate of DNA synthesis. For example, in growth assays using either T cell or B cell targets for growth factors and ^{3}H-TdR as DNA precursor, specific activities of 2 mCi/μmol or less and pulse label periods of under 4 h are best in order to keep incorporation linear.

Two final considerations in proliferation assays for lymphokine activity are the kinetics of incorporation and the percentage of the total input incorporated. Obviously, it is important that the measurement of growth be done during the exponential phase of cell growth which can be determined in an experiment to establish the kinetics of growth of the target cell. Also, it is a good idea to adjust cell concentrations so that no more than 10% of the added label becomes incorporated during the assay. This precaution will assure that the absolute external concentration of the DNA precursor will not vary appreciably, and dilution of the specific activity by the cell's cold internal pool will thus be constant in all samples.

Most of the points raised above can be dealt with in a few preliminary experiments when setting up a new growth factor assay or adapting one from the literature. This extra effort will pay off in an assay which is more reliable and quantitative.

Induction assays

Many lymphokine assays involve the induction of the synthesis of a known protein by the target cell. This protein may be cytoplasmic, as in MAF induction of lyzosomal enzymes in macrophages [49], secreted, as in BCDF induction of Ig secretion by B cells [22,42], or membrane associated, as in IFNγ induction of Ia antigens on macrophages [7,8,12]. In these cases the assay for lymphokine activity can be no better than the assay for the induced protein. Space does not permit a description of the specifics of all the various assays used for measuring induced proteins. Two general types of assays are used. First are those that measure the function of the induced protein, such as the catalytic activity of enzymes [49] or, in the cases of B cell targets, binding activity of specific antibody [27]. Second are assays that use specific antiprotein antibodies to quantify the induced protein, e.g. the use of anti-Ia monoclonal antibodies to follow the induction of I-region encoded molecule on the cell surface [12]. Both methods can be extremely sensitive and quantitative.

Titration curves and the definition of a unit of activity

One of the most important but often ignored aspects of lymphokine research is the requirement that lymphokine activity be titrated in quantifying any biological effect. This is particularly important in lymphokine measurements for several reasons. First of all, it is unusual for lymphokines to have linear dose–response curves, i.e. seldom does doubling the concentration of the lymphokine double the biological effect. Therefore, without a knowledge of the shape of the dose–response curve, it is impossible to use changes in effect to calculate changes in lymphokine levels. Second, the shape of a dose–response curve may be very revealing about the nature of the lymphokine activity or assay. For example, shallow titration curves that become steeper during the purification of a lymphokine may point to the presence of an inhibitor in the initial preparation which was separated during purification. Alternatively, progressively shallower titration curves during a purification may indicate an assay that depends on two lymphokine activities which separate during purification.

Seldom is it possible or desirable in a publication to include the complete titration data for all lymphokine measurements. Rather, one needs a method of reducing the titration data to units of lymphokine activity. A good general method is to use a plot of the titration data to define and measure units of lymphokine activity. Scale becomes important in the usefulness of these plots. In general, a log dose scale on the abscissa is most helpful in analysis, both because many lymphokine assays utilize serial twofold dilutions of the lymphokine and because with such a scale the shape of the titration curve should be the same for all samples. Only the position of the titration curve should change in proportion to the concentration of the lymphokine in the various samples. Changes in the shape of the titration curve are, therefore, easy to spot with such a plot.

The scales of the effect-ordinate axis can be somewhat aribitrary. Depending on the assay one may use a linear scale or transform the data to log, logit, or probit, or perhaps some more complicated function. There are two considerations. First, it is helpful to use a scale that distributes the data evenly along the titration curve so as to avoid weighting the data too heavily toward either end of the titration. Second, it is desirable to use a scale which gives a curve with a shape which is easy to approximate with a simple equation, so that simple curve-fitting equations can be used to approximate the curve. Of course, the simplest curves to fit are straight lines, so that often transformations are used which yield linear titration curves.

In the vast majority of lymphokine assays a unit of lymphokine activity is defined as the amount required to achieve a half maximal effect above background. The amount of each lymphokine preparation required to achieve this effect can be estimated from the titration curves of each sample and the relative lymphokine concentration estimated as the reciprocal of this value. Often within a group of samples some will be found with no detectable activity and some others will be found that are so active that they yield the maximal effect at all concentrations tested. The titration curves of the other samples may be used to extrapolate these other curves to assign a maximal or minimal activity to them. The sample curves of idealized data shown in Fig. 59.1 illustrate some of these points.

Purification of lymphokines

Purification of lymphokines has always been a very difficult problem. However, it has become clear that the use of impure lymphokines has often clouded the interpretation of experimental results, making the work involved in purification worth the effort. Recent advances in purification of lymphokines have involved the application of standard biochemical methods as well as the production of pure lymphokines via recombinant DNA methods.

Most of the techniques currently in use to purify proteins in general have been applied to lymphokines. These include gel, ion-exchange and reverse-phase chromatography, preparative isoelectric focussing and chromatofocussing, and gel electrophoresis. In many instances the chromatography techniques lend themselves to high-performance liquid chromatography (HPLC). A typical scheme entails the production of several litres of lymphokine containing culture supernatant in low serum or serum-free medium using one of the sources described above. This supernatant is concentrated either by ammonium sulphate precipitation or by one of the membrane filtration techniques. Very often gel filtration is used at this point to isolate a molecular weight fraction containing the activity, which is then further purified using one or more of the techniques listed above. As with the purification of any protein, it is essential to quantify recovery at each step in the purification.

Much to everyone's surprise, many lymphokines have proved to be remarkably stable, surviving very harsh treatments. For example, in some cases activity has been recovered from SDS-PAGE gels. One should, therefore, keep in mind that losses in activity at particular steps in purification may be an indication of the separation of two synergizing activities rather than of the denaturation or destruction of the lymphokine. This possibility can be easily tested by recombin-

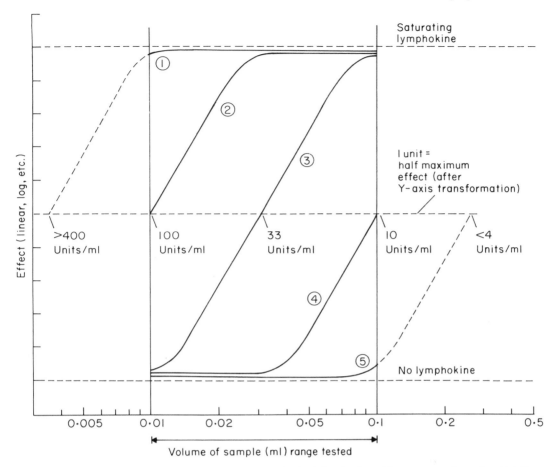

Fig. 60.1. Idealized titration curves for lymphokine activity. Idealized data is plotted from an experiment in which five samples were titrated in a lymphokine assay. A number of volumes of each sample between 0.01 and 0.1 ml were tested. The measured effect on the target cell was plotted (perhaps after transformation to log or some other function) vs. the volume of sample. Samples 2, 3, and 4 contained a concentration of lymphokine such that within some part of the range of volumes tested the lymphokine activity was limiting. Within this limiting range there was a roughly linear relationship between the log volume and effect (or transformed effect). A unit of activity was defined as the amount of lymphokine required to achieve the half maximum stimulatable effect. This was defined as the difference between the maximum effect (or transformed effect) and the background effect (or transformed effect) with no lymphokine divided by two. For samples 2, 3, and 4 this corresponded to 0.01, 0.03, and 0.10 ml of each sample respectively. Taking the reciprocal of these volumes, these samples were calculated to contain 100, 33, and 10 units/ml of the lymphokine activity.

Sample 1 contained a high enough concentration of lymphokine such that a maximal effect was seen at all volumes tested. By extrapolating this curve parallel to curves for samples 2, 3, and 4 it could be estimated that this sample had at least 400 units/ml of the lymphokine. Sample 5 showed no activity at any volume tested. By a similar extrapolation of this curve it could be estimated that this sample had not more than 4 units/ml of lymphokine activity.

ing a portion of each fraction to see if the activity is restored.

One technique which as yet has not been exploited fully is the use of monoclonal antibodies to purify lymphokines by affinity chromatography. Although a few monoclonal antibodies to particular lymphokines have been reported, their routine use in purification has not. Given the discriminating power of these antibodies it seems likely that eventually, as they become more widely distributed, they will become incorporated into purification schemes. Techniques for the production of monoclonal antibodies make possible the use of impure lymphokines as immunogens, since the specificities of the antibodies are sorted out at the clonal level. By far the easiest screening technique is to test the antibodies for inhibition of the activity of the lymphokine, even though one pays the price of missing those antibodies whose binding to the lymphokine fails to interfere with function.

The effectiveness of these purification schemes pales in the light of recently developed recombinant DNA methods. Expression in *E. coli* of cDNA clones encoding lymphokine mRNAs can lead to preparations many thousand times more active than those obtained conventionally and, of course, biologically pure from the start. One must still be cautious about bacterial products that might contaminate the preparation, such as lipopolysaccharide, which may interfere in some lymphokine assays; however, purification at this point is much simpler than from lymphocyte culture supernatants.

One of the commonly used recombinant DNA techniques is to probe cDNA libraries with oligonucleotides prepared to match some portion of the amino acid sequence of the protein. This, of course, requires that the protein has already been purified and at least partially sequenced. For many lymphokines this is a formidable, if not impossible, task. Other techniques sometimes allow the circumvention of the need for protein sequence. One commonly used method is to isolate mRNA from the appropriate source and to translate this mRNA in either *Xenopus* oocytes or *in vitro* translation systems. If one can detect the translated protein, either with an antibody or by its biological activity, then a cDNA library can be screened by the ability of cDNA clones to hybridize with the translatable message. The property of lymphokines which makes them particularly amenable to this approach is their inducibility. In general, as discussed above, normal, tumour, and hybridoma T cells produce no lymphokines unless induced. All evidence suggests that mRNA synthesis is essential during induction, i.e. that T cells do not have a store of inactive mRNA prior to induction. Therefore one of the major mRNA differences between induced and non-induced T cells is the group of lymphokine mRNAs. Using subtraction hybridization techniques it is possible to enrich for these mRNAs during the construction of a cDNA library, thus making the job of identifying the correct cDNA clone easier. Once a clone containing a full length cDNA insert is identified, there are a number of vectors which allow cDNA expression in *E. coli* as protein. Since all of the factors controlling expression of eukaryotic genes in bacteria are not fully understood, expression of the cDNA can vary tremendously for individual clones; however, high level expression of at least three different lymphokines (IFNγ IL-2, and IL-3) has been reported and it seems likely that this will be an extremely valuable technique in the future.

References

1 ROBB R.J., MUNCK A. & SMITH K.A. (1981) T cell growth factor receptors: quantitation, specificity and biological relevance. *J. exp. Med.* **154,** 1455.

2 TANIGUCHI T., MATSUI H., FUJITA T., TAKAOKA C., KASHIMA N., YOSHIMOTO R. & HAMURO J. (1983) Structure and expression of a cloned cDNA for human interleukin-2. *Nature,* **302,** 305.

3 ROSENBERG S.A., GRIMM E.A., McGROGEN M., DOYLE M., KAWASOKI E., KOTHS K. & MARK D.F. (1984) Biological activity of recombinant human interleukin 2 produced in *E. coli. Science,* **223,** 1412.

4 LEONARD W.J., DEPPER J.M., UCHIYAMA T., SMITH K.A., WALDMANN T.A. & GREENE W.C. (1982) Monoclonal antibody that appears to recognize the receptor for human T-cell growth factor; partial characterization of the receptor. *Nature,* **300,** 267.

5 MALEK T.R., ROBB R.J. & SHEVACH E.M. (1983) Identification and initial characterization of a rat monoclonal antibody reactive with the murine interleukin 2 receptor–ligand complex. *Proc. natn. Acad. Sci. U.S.A.* **80,** 5694.

6 GOEDDEL D.V., YELVERTON E., ULLRICH E., HEYNEKER H.L., MIOZZARI G., HOLMES W., ICEBURG P.H., DULL T., MAY L., STEBBING N., CREA R., MAEDA S., McCANDLESS R., SLOMA A., TABOR J.M., GROSS M., FAMILLETTI P.C. & PESTKA S. (1980) Human leukocyte interferon produced by *E. coli* is biologically active. *Nature,* **387,** 411.

7 STEEG P.S., MOORE R.N., JOHNSON H.M. & OPPENHEIM J.J. (1982) Regulation of murine Ia antigen expression by a lymphokine with immune interferon activity. *J. exp. Med.* **156,** 1780.

8 WONG G.H.W., CLARK-LEWIS I., McKIMM-BRESCHKIN J.L., HARRIS A.W. & SCHRADER J.W. (1983) Interferon-γ induces enhanced expression of Ia and H-2 antigen on B lymphoid, macrophage and myeloid cell lines. *J. Immunol.* **131,** 788.

9 PACE J.L., RUSSELL S.W., TORRES B.A., JOHNSON H.M. & GRAY P.W. (1983) Recombinant mouse gamma interferon induces the priming step in macrophage activation for tumor cell killing. *J. Immunol.* **130,** 2011.

10 ROBERTS W.K. & VASIL A. (1982) Evidence for the identity of murine gamma interferon and macrophage activating factor. *J. Interferon Res.* **2,** 519.

11 KELSO A., GLASEBROOK A.L., KANAGAWA O. & BRUNNER K.T. (1982) Production of macrophage activating factor by T cell clones and correlation with other lymphokine activities. *J. Immunol.* **129,** 550.

12 ZLOTNIK A., ROBERTS W.K., VASIL A., BLUMENTHAL E., LARISA F., LEIBSON H.J., ENDRES R.O., GRAHAM S.D. jun., WHITE J., HILL J., HENSON P., KLEIN J.R., BEVAN M.J., MARRACK P. & KAPPLER J.W. (1983) Coordinate production by a T cell hybridoma of gamma interferon and three other lymphokine activities. Multiple activities of a single lymphokine? *J. Immunol.* **131,** 794.

13 LARSSON E., ISCOVE N.N. & COUTINHO A. (1980) Two distinct factors are required for T cell growth. *Nature,* **283,** 664.

14 SMITH K.A., LACHMAN L.B., OPPENHEIM J.J. & FAVATA M.F. (1980) The functional relationship of the interleukins. *J. exp. Med.* **151,** 1551.

15 HOFFMANN M.K. & WATSON J. (1979) Helper T cell-replacing factors secreted by thymus-derived cells and macrophages: cellular requirements for B cell activation and synergistic properties. *J. Immunol.* **122,** 1371.

16 WAHL S.M., WAHL L.M., McCARTHY J.B., CHEDID L. & MERGENHAGEN S.E. (1979) Macrophage activation by mycobacterium water soluble compounds and synthetic muramyl dipeptide. *J. Immunol.* **122,** 2226.

17 ROSENWASSER L.J., DINARELLO C.A. & ROSENTHAL A.S. (1979) Adherent cell function in murine T-lymphocyte antigen recognition. (IV) Enhancement of murine T-cell antigen recognition by human leukocyte program. *J. exp. Med.* **150,** 709.

18 SWAIN S.L., DENNERT G., WARNER J.F. & DUTTON R.W. (1981) Culture supernatants of a stimulated T-cell line have helper activity that acts synergistically with interleukin 2 in the response of B cells to antigen. *Proc. natn. Acad. Sci. U.S.A.* **78,** 2517.

19 TAKATSU K., TANAKA K., TOMINAGA A., KUMAHARA Y. & HAMAOKA T. (1980) Antigen-induced T cell-replacing factor (TRF). (III) Establishment of a T cell hybrid clone continuously producing TRF and functional analysis of released TRF. *J. Immunol.* **125,** 2646.

20 HOWARD M., FARRAR J., HILFIKER M., JOHNSON B., TAKATSU K., HAMAOKA T. & PAUL W.E. (1982) Identification of a T cell-derived B cell growth factor distinct from interleukin 2. *J. exp. Med.* **155,** 914.

21 OKAWA M., SAKAGUCHI N., YOSHIMWA N., HARA H., SHIMIMIEU K., YOSHIDA N., YOSHIZAKI K., KISHIMOTO S., YAMAMURA Y. & KISHIMOTO T. (1983) B cell growth factors and B cell differentiation factor from human T hybridomas. Two distinct kinds of B cell growth factor and their synergism in B cell proliferation. *J. exp. Med.* **157,** 583.

22 ISAKSON P.C., PURÉ E., VITETTA E.S. & KRAMMER P.H. (1982) T cell-derived B cell differentiation factor(s). Effect on the isotype switch of murine B cells. *J. exp. Med.* **155,** 734.

23 ROCKLIN R.E., BENDITZEN K. & GREINEDER D. (1980) Mediators of immunity—lymphokines and monokines. *Adv. Immunol.* **29,** 55.

24 RUDDLE N.H. & WAKSMAN B.H. (1967) Cytotoxic effect of lymphocyte–antigen interaction in delayed type hypersensitivity. *Science,* **157,** 1060.

25 GRANGER G.A. & WILLIAMS T.W. (1968) Lymphocyte cytotoxicity *in vitro*: activation and release of a cytotoxic factor. *Nature,* **218,** 1253.

26 HOWARD M., MATIS L., MALEK T.R., SHEVACH E., KELL W., COHEN D., NAKAMISHI K. & PAUL W.E. (1983) Interleukin 2 induces antigen-reactive T cell lines to secrete BCGF-1. *J. exp. Med.* **158,** 2024.

27 MISHELL R.I. & DUTTON R.W. (1967) Immunization of dissociated spleen cell cultures from normal mice. *J. exp. Med.* **126,** 423.

28 CLICK R.E., BENCK L. & ALTER B.J. (1972) Enhancement of antibody synthesis *in vitro* by mercaptoethanol. *Cell. Immunol.* **3,** 156.

29 ISCOVE N.N. & MELCHERS F. (1978) Complete replacement of serum by albumin, transferrin and soybean lipid in cultures of lipopolysaccharide reactive B lymphocytes. *J. exp. Med.* **147,** 923.

30 MOLLER G. (ed.) (1981) T cell clones. *Immunol. Revs.* **54.** Munksgaard, Copenhagen.

31 ELY J.M., PRYSTOWSKY M.B., EISENBERG I., QUINTANS J., GOLDWASSER E., GLASEBROOK A.L. & FITCH F.W. (1981) Alloreactive cloned T cell lines. (V) Differential kinetics of IL-2, CSF and BCSF release by a cloned and amplifier cell and its variant. *J. Immunol.* **127,** 2345.

32 HARWELL L., SKIDMORE B., MARRACK P. & KAPPLER J. (1980) Concanavalin A inducible, interleukin 2 producing T cell hybridoma. *J. exp. Med.* **152,** 893.

33 MIZEL S., OPPENHEIM J. & ROSENTREICH D. (1978) Characterization of lymphocyte-activating factor (LAF) produced by the macrophage cell line, P388D1. (I) Enhancement of LAF production by activated T lymphocytes. *J. Immunol.* **120,** 1497.

34 LEIBSON H.J., MARRACK P. & KAPPLER J. (1982) B cell helper factors. (II) Synergy among three helper factors in the response of T cell- and macrophage-depleted B cells. *J. Immunol.* **129,** 1398.

35 KAPPLER J.W., SKIDMORE B., WHITE J. & MARRACK P. (1981) Antigen-inducible, H-2-restricted interleukin-2 producing T cell hybridomas. Lack of independent antigen and H-2 recognition. *J. exp. Med.* **153,** 1198.

36 SMITH K.A. (1980) T cell growth factor. *Immunol. Revs.* **51,** 337.

37 IHLE J.N. (1982) Phenotypic characteristics of cell lines requiring interleukin 3 for growth. *J. Immunol.* **129,** 1377.

38 WALKER E.B., LANIER L.L. & WARNER N.L. (1982) Concomitant induction of the cell surface expression of Ia determinants and accessory cell function by a murine tumor cell line. *J. exp. Med.* **155,** 629.

39 KING D.P. & JONES P.P. (1983) Induction of Ia and H-2 antigens on a macrophage cell line by immune interferon. *J. Immunol.* **131,** 135.

40 ZLOTNIK A., SHIMONKEVITZ R.P., GEFTER M.L., KAPPLER J. & MARRACK P. (1983) Characterization of the γ-interferon-mediated induction of antigen-presenting ability in P388D cells. *J. Immunol.* **131,** 2814.

41 SWAIN S.L. & DUTTON R.W. (1982) Production of a B cell growth-promoting activity, (DL) BCGF, from a cloned T cell line and its assay on the BCL₁ B cell tumor. *J. exp. Med.* **156,** 1821.

42 PURÉ E., ISAKSON P.C., KAPPLER J.W., MARRACK P., KRAMMER P.H. & VITETTA E.S. (1983) T cell-derived B cell growth and differentiation factors. Dichotomy between the responsiveness of B cells from adult and neonatal mice. *J. exp. Med.* **157,** 600.

43 JULIUS M.F., SIMPSON E. & HERZENBERG L.A. (1973) A rapid method for the isolation of functional thymus-derived murine lymphocytes. *Eur. J. Immunol.* **3,** 645.

44 MISHELL B.B. & SHIIGI S.M. (1980) *Selected Methods in Cellular Immunology.* W.H. Freeman & Co., San Francisco.

45 RAFF M.C. (1970) Role of thymus derived lymphocytes in the secondary humoral immune response in mice. *Nature,* **226,** 1257.

46 LEIBSON H.J., MARRACK P. & KAPPLER J.W. (1981) B cell helper factors. (I) Requirement for both interleukin 2 and another 40 000 molecular weight factor. *J. exp. Med.* **154,** 1681.

47 RATCLIFFE M.J.H. & JULIUS M.H. (1982) H-2 restricted

T-B interactions involved in polyspecific B cell responses mediated by soluble antigens. *Eur. J. Immunol.* **12,** 634.

48 RATCLIFFE M.J.H. & JULIUS M.H. (1983) Two classes of bystander B cell response: activation requirements reflect those of B cells in general. *J. Immunol.* **131,** 581.

49 SCHNYDER J. & BAGGICHINI M. (1978) Secretion of lysosomal hydrolases by stimulated and nonstimulated macrophages. *J. exp. Med.* **148,** 435.

50 JERNE N.K., NORDIN A.A. & HENRY C. (1963) In *Cell Bound Antibodies*, (ed. Amos B. & Koprowski H.), p. 109. The Wistar Institute Press, Philadelphia.

Chapter 60
Natural killer cells

H. WIGZELL & U. RAMSTEDT

Preparation of cell suspensions, 60.2

Lysis of red blood cells (RBC) using water, 60.3

Subfraction of NK cells, 60.3

Measurement of NK cell activity: *in vitro* assays, 60.4

Measurement of NK cell activity: *in vivo* assays, 60.5

Augmentation of NK activity by biological substances, 60.7

Morphology of NK cells, 60.7

Specificity of NK cells, 60.7

Growth of NK cells *in vitro*, 60.8

Summary, 60.9

Media, 60.9

Studies of cell-mediated reactions *in vitro* may sometimes reveal the existence of normally occurring cytotoxic cells, existing in the absence of any known immunity. There are several explanations for the presence of such killer cells. The actual cell type involved as effector cells may also vary. It became apparent in 1975 that a specific cell type exists amongst such cytotoxic cells, expressing private features of a kind justifying its classification as a cell type of its own [1,2]. This cell type was called natural killer or NK. The particular interest in NK cells stems primarily from the demonstration that they display a certain preference for malignant cells as targets. Yet, certain normal cell types can also serve as susceptible target cells for NK cytolysis. NK cells can also participate in the defence against infectious agents, in part directly and in part through the production of interferons. Likewise, interferons are known to be potent regulators of NK activity [3,4]. Classification of NK cells includes specificity studies as to target types, analysis of their ability to function *in vivo* as well as *in vitro*, and surface marker analysis to classify the cells in relation to other potential cytotoxic cell types. No single unique marker has been found for NK cells. A battery of tests is therefore sometimes required to safely classify killer cells as being of NK type.

Definition of NK cells

Natural killer cells have the ability to lyse their targets in the absence of any prior sensitization towards structures present on the target cells. They exert their lytic capacity in a rapid way via contact, and within each species the majority of NK cells have a characteristic specificity profile with regard to their targets. They are bone marrow derived cells and exist in normal numbers in individuals lacking B and/or T

lymphocytes. Within the body the NK cells have a typical distribution profile, with high NK cell activity being present in peripheral blood and spleen, low to intermediate levels in bone marrow and lymph nodes, and virtually none in the thymus.

In several species the NK activity can be shown to be physically associated with a large, granular lymphocyte (LGL) with characteristic physical and serological features. Cells sharing with NK cells one or several of the above features may arise upon activation of other cell types, notably T cells. The problem of NK heterogeneity in relation to such cells will be discussed separately in this chapter.

Handling of NK cells in short-term studies

Some general recommendations for studies of NK cells should be considered. It is generally agreed amongst scientists studying NK cells that the lytic activity of such cells upon harvesting from *in vivo* conditions may rapidly wane initially if not kept on ice [5]. The actual underlying mechanism for this is unknown and may be indirectly caused by other cells and/or their products. One should keep the temperature around 0 °C, if convenient, when handling the cells in order to ensure retention of lytic power of the NK cells.

Several reports exist indicating that increase of the pH intracellularly in natural killer cells may temporarily inactivate the lytic capacity of the cells [6,7]. Such consequences may be produced when using ammonium chloride to induce red cell lysis in blood or spleen cell samples [7]. It is therefore recommended that lysis of erythrocytes should be carried out using distilled water protocols (see below).

The donor of NK cells

NK cell activity is regulated by many factors. An investigator who would like to use NK cells for a particular experiment but who would not be interested in NK cells in general may benefit from some advice.

Human NK cells are most easily obtained from peripheral blood. The age of the donor does not play any major role in regulating NK activity in the human. However, certain individuals may have a lower NK level than normal and the level of each individual tends to maintain itself at a characteristic level.

Murine NK cells, on the other hand, display a striking variation according to age, with very low NK activities being found before 3 weeks of age; a decay in NK activity will also start around 3 months of age. With the availability of inbred strains of mice, it is now also well established that there exist high and low NK cell strains [1,2]. Table 60.1 summarizes this information. With regard to variations of NK activities in other species the reader is referred to other studies [8].

In their early phases infections do normally induce an increase in NK activity due to interferon production, but may at a later stage be followed by suppressed NK levels. It is thus wise not to use donors with known infections or to use recently received animals within two weeks after arrival.

Preparation of cell suspensions

Equipment

Water bath, ordinary type.
Microperistaltic pump with a constant and steady flow rate at 0.5 ml/min.
Osmometer (Advanced Instrument Inc., Needham Heights, Mass. USA).
Centrifuge, swing-out rotor, capacity 300–700 g.
Fifteen or fifty millilitre tube capacity.
Microscope, ordinary light.

Materials

Plastic Petri dishes.
96-well microtitre plates.
Centrifuge tubes, 15 and 50 ml.

Table 60.1. Grouping of mouse strains according to their levels of NK activity

High-reactive strains	CBA/J	C3H/J	C57Bl/6	C57Bl/10	DBA/2
Low-reactive strains	A/Sn	A/J	AKR	SJL	Balb/c

Nylon wool (Fenwal Laboratories, Deerfield, Ill. USA).
Pipettes, ordinary and Pasteur.
Trypan blue (Fluka AG, Buchs, Switzerland).
Ficoll-Isopaque (Pharmacia, Uppsala, Sweden).
Percoll (Pharmacia, Uppsala, Sweden).
CPD-sagman solution (Travenol).

Procedure

Splenic NK cells

1   Mice and rats are killed by cervical dislocation. Their spleens are removed and transferred to a Petri dish containing 3 ml of tissue culture medium or PBS with HEPES and antibiotics. The cells are then teased from the capsule by injecting medium into the spleen with a syringe or a Pasteur pipette, while pressing the organ with a pair of forceps with broad, blunt ends. Clumps are further dispersed by pipetting up and down with a Pasteur pipette.
2   The suspension is transferred to a centrifuge tube where the remaining clumps are allowed to settle for 2–3 min. The cells are then decanted into another centrifuge tube.
3   The cells are centrifuged at 300 g for 5–10 min and washed twice before they are resuspended in medium and counted in trypan blue solution. The viability is consistently above 95%.

Peripheral blood NK cells

Buffy coats prepared in many blood centres in hospitals producing leucocyte-deprived erythrocytes constitute a convenient source for human NK cells. If freshly obtained on the same day of collection of the blood, using citrate as anticoagulant, such white-cell preparations are normally excellent sources for NK cells. Alternatively, peripheral blood can be obtained by venous puncture with either citrate in a CPD solution or heparin. In the authors' opinion, heparin may sometimes be less suitable than citrate in this regard, perhaps because citrate is more efficient in blocking possible activation of the complement system *in vitro* [9]. The authors will here consider citrate in the CPD solution as an anticoagulant.
1   Blood is collected into CPD solutions using a ratio of 7 vols. of blood to 1 vol. of CPD.
2   Blood is then centrifuged at 700 g for 10 min. The plasma is removed with a pipette without disturbing the cell pellet.
3   A pipette of suitable volume is used to remove the upper half of the cell pellet in a single suction step; this contains the leucocyte-enriched cells.
4   The cells are diluted threefold with PBS. Three

millilitres of Ficoll–Isopaque are added to the bottom of a 15 ml centrifuge tube, followed by addition of 10 ml of the cell suspension, taking care not to mix the two phases. The tubes are centrifuged at 400 *g* for 20 min.

5 The interface band containing the white blood cells is collected with a Pasteur pipette and the cells are washed twice in medium. When the cells are collected from the interface band, care must be taken to suspend the collected cells in the washing medium before centrifugation to avoid formation of a concentration gradient of Ficoll–Isopaque.

Lysis of red blood cells (RBC) using water

Erythrocytes are often found after the initial steps of preparation. If a pure leucocyte preparation without any RBC contamination is needed when the effector cells are to be used, the method preferred is H_2O lysis of the RBCs.

1 Centrifuge the leucocyte–RBC cell suspension in a V-shaped centrifuge tube, to obtain a distinct pellet of cells (400 *g*, 10 min).

2 During this centrifugation, prepare two syringes, one with 4.5 ml distilled water and one with $10\times$ concentrated PBS.

3 Discard the supernatant in the tube and shake up the pellet. Water is added by fast and firm resuspension with a Pasteur pipette.

4 After this has been done (in about 5 s), 0.5 ml $10\times$ concentration PBS is added and resuspended to restore isotonicity.

5 Dead cells are allowed to sediment for 3 min and then the cell suspension is transferred to a new tube. After centrifugation the cells are resuspended in medium.

Subfractionation of NK cells

Enrichment of NK cells from a mixed leucocyte population can be achieved by various features distinguishing the majority of NK cells from the other white blood cells. Some of the most commonly used methods to obtain such a subfractionation will be described. For alternative protocols, consult refs. 10 and 11.

Adherence

Plastic adherence

1 Effector cells depleted of adherent cells can be prepared by incubating 10^8 cells in 10 ml medium in plastic dishes (0.9 cm) for 60 min at 37 °C.

2 Non-adherent (NA) cells are collected via two gentle washes with a Pasteur pipette. If required, the

remaining adherent cells can be scraped off with a rubber policeman, washed with cold Ca^{2+}- and Mg^{2+}-free PBS and kept at 4 °C.

Nylon wool column

1 Plastic NA cells or unseparated leucocytes are incubated at a concentration of 1×10^8 cells per 1.5 g of nylon wool in a 20 ml plastic disposable syringe. The syringe containing the nylon wool should be pre-incubated with medium for 30 min at 37 °C before adding the cells. The cells are incubated in the cotton wool for 45 min at 37 °C, 5% CO_2.

2 The non-adherent cells are eluted using 4 column vols. of medium warmed to 37 °C.

Notes and recommendations

The NA cell yield after plastic adherence and passage through a nylon wool column will normally range between 45% and 53% of the initial unseparated leucocytes.

Density

Discontinuous Percoll density gradient centrifugation

1 Percoll is adjusted to 285 mosmol/kg H_2O for human and mouse and 290 mosmol/kg H_2O for rat NK effector cells by addition of $10\times$ concentrated PBS at pH 7.2. The medium is adjusted by addition of sterile water. If an osmometer is unavailable, a close approximation to the proper osmolarity (285–290 mosmol/kg H_2O) is reached by the addition of 8 vols. of $10\times$ concentrated PBS to 92 vols. undiluted Percoll. Here, however, each cell fraction after the centrifugation has to be checked for cytotoxicity, since the enriched NK-cell fraction may be present in fractions other than the expected fractions 2 and 3.

2 For human and rat, seven different concentrations of osmotically correct Percoll are then prepared, ranging from 40% to 57.5% of Percoll in medium. Each concentration should vary from the next by 2.5% Percoll. For mouse NK cells, five concentrations are prepared, ranging from 38.6% to 56.6% with 4.5% concentration steps.

3 Gradients are then layered in a 15 ml test tube with a micro-peristaltic pump using a rate of 0.5 ml/min. Between 0.5×10^8 and 1.0×10^8 cells in 1 ml medium are placed on the top and the tubes spun at 550 *g* for 30 min at room temperature, except for mouse NK separation which is spun at 300 *g* for 45 min.

4 The cells are then collected from the top using a Pasteur pipette, washed twice and resuspended in medium. The top fraction between medium and the first Percoll layer is designated fraction 1.

5 Percoll separation of mouse effector cells can be further improved by running a second gradient with collected fraction 2 and 3 cells on a similar gradient as for human or rat, but ranging from 37.5% Percoll to 50%.

Notes and recommendations

The recovery of cells should always be >85% and the viability >95%. The human NK–LGL fractions (fractions 2 and 3) were enriched to approximately 80%, as defined by morphology (see 'Morphology of NK cells'). From fraction 2 and 3 of the second mouse gradient the enrichment is 30–45% LGL. Rat LGL enrichment is 70–85%. Table 60.2 gives typical results using gradient centrifugations.

Table 60.2. Distribution of human peripheral blood mononuclear cells in discontinuous Percoll gradient centrifugation

Fraction	Input	1	2	3	4	5
Percoll concentration (%)	—	40.0	42.5	45.0	47.5	50.0
Cell recovery (%)	100	1.6	3.5	8.5	28.5	21.5
LGL (%)	12	5	82	74	7	2
LU/10^7 cells*	42	16	192	143	4	1

* Lytic unit (LU) is defined as the number of effector cells required to induce 30% specific lysis of 5×10^3 target cells (K 562)

SRBC high-affinity rosettes

For further enrichment of human LGLs, cells from fraction 2 and 3 are depleted of high-affinity sheep red blood cell (SRBC) rosette forming cells with no cytotoxic potential.
1 Effector cells (5×10^6/ml) are mixed with 2 ml of fetal calf serum (FCS) and 2 ml of SRBC at 1×10^8/ml in a round-bottomed test tube.
2 The tube is centrifuged for 5 min at 100 *g* and incubated at 29 °C for 1 h in a water bath.
3 The cells are then gently resuspended with a Pasteur pipette, layered on 3 ml Ficoll–Isopaque, and centrifuged for 30 min at 400 *g* and room temperature.
4 The interface cells are washed twice in medium (the rosette-forming cells can be washed and the SRBC lysed by sterile water). The purity of cells that did not bind SRBC was >90% LGL determined by Giemsa staining.

Other surface markers usable for fractionation of NK cells

Using conventional techniques for cell separation, it is

Table 60.3. Surface markers on NK cells of murine or human cells

	Human NK	Murine NK	References
Fc receptors, IgG	+ + +	+	[55]
Asialo-GM$_1$*	±	+ + +	[56,24]
Differentiation antigen	—	NK-1 NK-2	[58,57]
Differentiation antigen	HNK-1/Leu-11	—	[60,59]

* As defined using cytotoxic antibodies with complement.

possible to take advantage of other surface markers characterizing either non-NK cells (negative selection) or NK cells (positive selection) to further purify NK cells from a mixed population. The markers for NK cells are not precise. Table 60.3 gives a summary of some markers shown to be suitable in the studies of murine or human NK cells. This list is rapidly expanding and may soon contain truly unique markers for NK features. A problem in designing such a table is the relative heterogeneity of NK cells in relation to their stage of activation. Table 60.3 is conservative, containing the classical NK cells normally obtained from *in vivo* situations using normal donors.

Measurement of NK cell activity: *in vitro* assays

Like all systems measuring selective cell-mediated lysis, the cytotoxicity of NK cells can be divided into discrete steps: binding to target, triggering and mediation of lysis. Several analyses of each discrete step have been published [12–15] but the precise mechanisms of this lytic reaction are still unknown. Two methods for measuring NK activity are presented: the ^{51}Cr-release assay functioning in a batch assay, and the target-conjugate assay, where individual effector–target conjugates can be isolated and observed during their potentially lytic interactions.

Equipment

Centrifuge for microplates and 15 ml tubes. Whirl-mixer.
Water bath for 37 °C and 42 °C.
Isotope counter for gamma-rays.

Materials

Na$_2$^{51}CrO$_4$, ≥10 mCi/ml (Amersham, England).
96-Well, V-shaped microtitre plates of any brand.
Trypan blue (Fluka Ag, Buchs, Switzerland).
Formic or glutaric aldehyde.

Nonidet P-40 (Sigma, St. Louis, Mo., USA). Agarose, high quality of any brand.

^{51}Cr-release assay

A common problem in NK assays is the rather low cytolytic activity per unit cell number. Thus care to reduce non-specific background problems is important to obtain a satisfactory signal: noise ratio. Effector cells are prepared according to protocols indicated above.

1 Target cells of high viability (> 95%) at a concentration of $2–10 \times 10^6/0.1$ ml RPMI-1640 are incubated with 100 μCi Na$_2$^{51}CrO$_4$ (using 10 μl from a 10 mCi/ml stock solution) for 1–1.5 h at 37 °C in 5% CO$_2$.

2 The cells are then washed three times and resuspended in medium before use. If the cells are incubated for another hour and washed once again, the spontaneous release will be significantly reduced.

3 The lytic assay is carried out in 96-well, V-bottomed microtitre plates. Effector cells are first titrated into the plates aiming at effector:target ratios ranging from 200:1 to 1:1 depending on the system. Target cells are about $0.5–1 \times 10^4$ per well. The total reaction volume should be 0.2 ml.

4 Controls include target cells with medium alone for spontaneous release and with 0.05% Nonidet P-40 for maximum release figures. Each titration is done in triplicate to reduce variation.

5 The effector target cells are then incubated for 4 h at 37 °C in 5% CO$_2$. The plates are spun at 200 **g** for 5–10 min and 100 μl of the supernatant removed for counting in a gamma-counter.

Table 60.4. Natural killer effect of human blood lymphocytes against K 562 tumour cell line

	Specific ^{51}Cr-release (%)*				
	50:1	25:1	12:1	6:1	3:1
Nylon wool separated lymphocytes	68.5	50.3	36.2	29.0	18.2

* Four hour cytotoxic assay at the indicated effector cell:target cell ratio.

A typical experiment is shown in Table 60.4. The following formula is used to calculate percent specific lysis:

% Specific lysis =

$$\frac{\text{c.p.m. in experiment} - \text{c.p.m. spontaneous release}}{\text{c.p.m. maximum release} - \text{c.p.m. spontaneous release}} \times 100$$

Lysis can also be presented as lytic units per cell [16]. A lytic unit is defined as the number of effector cells required to induce a defined percentage of specific lysis. (see Table 60.2)

Conjugate cytotoxic assay

The principle here is to incubate effector and target cells in free solution to allow contact, whereafter the cells are suspended in a solid phase for further analysis [12,17]. The following protocol has been found useful in such NK-target studies.

1 A 0.5% agarose solution in RPMI-1640 is prepared with HEPES in a boiling water and kept in a 42 °C water bath.

2 An equal number of effector and target cells (2×10^5) is mixed in a total volume of 0.2 ml of RPMI-1640 containing 15% FCS in a centrifuge tube.

3 The mixture is centrifuged at 400 **g** for 2 min and incubated for 10 min at 37 °C. The pellet is resuspended with a whirl-mixer (10 min) or by five gentle suctions up and down using a Pasteur pipette.

4 The cells are then added to 0.5 ml of agarose precooled to around 37 °C by holding the pipette with agarose solution for some 20 s at room temperature before mixing with the cells.

5 The mixture in a Pasteur pipette is then dropped from a height of 30 cm on to a plastic Petri dish (diameter around 3 cm). A thin layer of cells in agarose is formed and allowed to solidify. After this, 1 ml of RPMI-1640 with 15% FCS is added.

6 Control dishes, with target or effector cells only, are also normally included.

7 The dishes are incubated for 4 h at 37 °C in 5% CO$_2$.

8 The medium is removed and 2 ml of a 0.1% trypan blue solution is added and left for 10 min.

9 The solution is removed and the plates washed three times for 5 min with PBS, whereafter 1% formic aldehyde is added for final fixation. Alternatively, 0.5% glutaraldehyde can be used a fixative. The Petri dishes can be kept at 4 °C for several months, provided humidity is maintained to prevent drying.

10 After fixation the cells are ready for reading with an ordinary light microscope. Killed cells are clearly blue. The percentage of target binding cells and percentage of targets killed is then determined. An experiment is shown in Table 60.5.

Measurement of NK cell activity: *in vivo* assays

Evidence that NK cells can function *in vivo* against relevant targets has accumulated in a large number of experimental systems [18–22]. The most convincing results have come from short-term *in vivo* reactions

Table 60.5. Target-binding cells and cytotoxic fraction therein

	Target	% Bound to targets*	% Bound targets lysed†
Human non-enriched lymphocytes	K 562	15.3	26.3
	Molt-4	17.0	31.7
	Raji	14.7	1.0

Each value represents a triplicate, with 150 lymphocytes for each value.

$$* \% \text{ bound to targets} = \frac{\text{number bound to targets}}{\text{total (free} + \text{bound) number of lymphocytes}} \times 100$$

$$† \% \text{ bound targets lysed} = \frac{\text{number of conjugates with dead targets}}{\text{total (live} + \text{dead) targets}} \times 100$$

where presence or absence of NK cells has been linked to a rapid elimination and death of the NK-susceptible target cells. Selective depletion of NK cells *in vivo* can be obtained by treatment with radioactive strontium [23] or antisera with comparatively selective action on NK cells [24]. Genetic defects may sometimes result in a more significant impact on NK cells than on most other cell types [25,26]. A useful technique when trying to assess *in vivo* elimination of NK targets *in vivo* has been to have the potential target cells pre-labelled with a marker before inoculation.

The elimination of IUDR-labelled target cells **in vivo**

Equipment

Centrifuge for 15 ml tubes.
Light microscope.
Gamma-counter.

Materials

^{125}I-5-2'-deoxyuridine (sp.act. 36 Ci/mmol); Radio-chemical Centre, Amersham, England).
5-Fluoro-2'-deoxyuridine (Sigma, St. Louis, Mo., USA)

Procedure

1 The target cells are first labelled using ^{125}I-deoxy-uridine *in vitro* or *in vivo*. *In vivo* labelling is done in the mouse by the injection of 50 μCi of ^{125}I-IUDS i.p. to mice which have received tumour cells for passage, at a concentration of 10^7 cells, 3 days before. The cells are harvested 6 h later [22].
2 *In vitro* labelling is accomplished by incubating 3×10^7 cells in 50 ml RPMI-1640 in 20% FCS for 18 h at 37 °C, 5% CO_2 in the presence of 5–10 μg of

5-fluoro-2'deoxyuridine and 20 μCi of ^{125}I-IUDR using a suitable tissue culture bottle.
3 Both labelling procedures are followed by four washes of the cell suspension in medium (0.5–1 × 10^6 cells).
4 Around 500 000 c.p.m. are injected i.v. into the recipient mouse. After 4–18 h the animal is killed and the spleen, liver and lungs are removed.
5 The amounts of radioactivity in the whole body and organ are determined with a gamma-counter.
6 Results are calculated as total c.p.m. or percentage of injected c.p.m. retained.

Notes and recommendations

Viability of labelled cells should be > 95% and the rate of release of ^{125}I-UDR less than 1% per hour. The rate of elimination of ^{125}I-UDR from the lung and spleen would give an indication of the target cell susceptibility to NK attack *in vivo* [20,22].
Table 60.6 exemplifies this method.

Table 60.6. *In vivo* clearance of radiolabelled tumour cells

Strain	Tumour	% Cytotoxicity *in vitro**	Recovery of radioactivity (%)†		
			Spleen	Liver	Lung
CBA/J	YAC-1	69.2	0.5	2.1	0.5
SJL	YAC-1	5.2	1.1	5.2	7.8

* Percentage cytotoxicity of spleen cells against ^{51}Cr-labelled target cells at an effector cell:target cell ratio of 100:1.
† Percentage ^{125}I-UDR retained in different organs 4 h after injection of 10^6 labelled tumour cells.

Augmentation of NK activity by biological substances

It is well established that the lytic activity of NK cells can be regulated *in vivo* and *in vitro* by several biological substances. A major family of proteins shown to enhance NK activity contains the interferons [3,4,27–29]. All three types of interferon (IFN) can function as enhancers of NK activity by an inductive process requiring both RNA and protein synthesis [30,31]. At the same time, the IFN can act at the level of the target cell surface, making that cell resistant to attack by NK cells [27]. If possible, it is thus wise to activate NK cells separately from the target cells with IFN or IFN-inducers, when optimal NK activities are wanted at the level of lysis.

Inoculation of anti-IFN antibodies *in vivo* does also tend to reduce background NK levels [32,33]. The consequences of IFN treatment with regard to NK activity can be shown to reside at several levels. Pre-NK cells may be recruited into active NK cells via differentiation [34,35,61]. Binding to NK target cells is frequently improved by IFN treatment of NK cells. Their capacity to recycle, i.e. to kill more than one target, is improved [12,36,61].

Induction of NK activities may also be regulated by other proteins, such as interleukin-2 [37–39], but the major pathway of NK activation *in vivo* would seem to be through IFN.

Equipment

There is no special equipment besides that required for preparation and testing of NK cells.

Materials

Poly(I:C), poly(inosinic:cytidylic) acid, (Sigma, St. Louis, Mo., USA).
Tilorone (Sigma; see above).
Statolone (Sigma; see above).
IFN (from various sources).

Procedure

In vivo augmentation

If interferon inducers are used, 24 h is required to obtain induction of maximal IFN release, which is then secondarily inducing an increase in NK activity. In the mouse, the following doses and tests for NK activity are recommended: poly(I:C), 100 μg/mouse i.p., 24–48 h before test; Tilorone, 2 mg orally, 24 h before test; Statolone, 2 mg i.v., 24 h before test; IFN, > 1000 I.U. i.p., 12–24 h before test.

In vitro augmentation

Poly(I:C), 25–100 μg/ml, is pre-incubated with cells 4 h before testing. IFN, 100–1000 I.U./ml, is pre-incubated with cells 2 h before test.

Morphology of NK cells

Cells with a distinct morphology called large granular lymphocytes (LGL) are responsible for NK activity in cells freshly obtained from humans [40], rats [41] and, at least in part, mice [42,62]. Percoll fractionation, as indicated above, allows purification of NK cells and their subsequent morphological studies [31,43].

Equipment

Cytocentrifuge.
Light microscope.

Materials

Giemsa stain (Sigma, St. Lousi Mo., USA).
Methanol.

Procedure

1 Cells are prepared using Percoll gradients, as described above; see 'Density'. Using ordinary glass slides, 1.5×10^5 cells, in medium with 10% FCS, are centrifuged in a cytocentrifuge for 5 min at 35 **g**.
2 The slides are air dried and fixed for 5 min in methanol and dried again. The cells can then be stained with Giemsa solution diluted 10% in water for 5–10 min.
3 LGL are identified by their comparatively high ratio of cytoplasma to nucleus with several azurophilic granules in a weak basophilic cytoplasm. The nuclear shape is that of a kidney. Cell size is around 10–15 μm, and the LGL differ from macrophages by the larger size and vacuolar cytoplasm of the latter. Murine LGL have a nucleus typically more kidney shaped than NK cells of human origin.

Specificity of NK cells

This question is intimately linked to that of the possible heterogeneity of NK cells. There is little doubt, however, that the 'average' NK cell obtained from *in vivo* situations has a typical specificity pattern shared by most NK cells of the same species. The binding features of NK cells to their targets do express one of the necessary requirements for NK lysis to occur, i.e. cellular contact. Data exist, however, indicating that several sets of bone marrow derived cells may have the capacity to express binding specificities similar or identical to conventional NK cells without expressing lytic abilities [44]. This would suggest the possibility that the selectiveness of NK cells may be linked to the expression of certain differentiation- or activation-linked stages of several cell types. Support for such a view comes from data in which cloned T cells can be found to express both T cell specificity *and* NK specificity; this feature may be permanently expressed [45] or induced at will with lymphokines [46]. The simultaneous linkage between such 'NK specificity structures' and lytic capacity in a single cell may be the reason that NK activity *in vivo* is normally associated with classical NK cells and only to a minor degree with other cells of lytic potential, such as T cells and monocytes or macrophages. Some typical cell lines used around the world in the studies of NK cells are listed in Table 60.7. It is recommended that the investigator try to grow some 'resistant' and 'susceptible' cell lines in the laboratory, as relative comparison of target susceptibilities still serves as the best marker when defining NK cells. It may be particularly advantageous to use target cells with little or no MHC antigens on their surface to reduce possible problems with more conventional killer T cells.

Cold target inhibition is one assay used when studying cell-mediated lysis as to specificity [47]. It is done using a radiolabelled target and unlabelled competitor cells. It is a useful but complex technique when it comes to interpretations and does require extensive controls. Passively coated IgG antibodies may also add to specificity problems, in particular in human NK studies, as the Fc receptor on human NK cells has a high enough affinity for antibodies to allow a relatively firm coating. This endows the NK cells with additional specificity because NK cells are potent effector cells in antibody-dependent, cell-mediated cytolysis [48,49]. Inhibition of human ADCC activities in the NK cell population can normally be achieved, if necessary using F(ab) fragments of antibodies directed against human IgG [50].

Growth of NK cells *in vitro*

Several studies report the outgrowth *in vitro* of cell lines with more or less striking similarities to NK cells [51–53]. Frequently, however, discrepancies also exist, making it very difficult to compare them with NK cells obtained *in vivo*. In essence, the same protocols described in this book for the maintenance of T cell clones can also be applied to the growing of NK cells or NK-like cells *in vitro*. The reader is referred to these protocols [75, 110].

Leukaemias with NK-like features have also been reported and in some situations it has been possible to establish these tumour lines *in vitro* and maintain cytolytic ability, especially of the rat NK leukaemia type [54,63]. Growth conditions cannot be standardized and have to be varied according to the species and type of cells.

Table 60.7 Tissue culture lines used as targets using NK cells from the same species

Human targets

*Sensitive to lysis**		*Insensitive to lysis**	
Molt-4	Acute T-lymphatic leukaemia	Daudi	Burkitt lymphoma
K 562	Myeloid leukaemia	Raji	Burkitt lymphoma
Jurkat	Acute T lymphatic leukaemia	1301	Acute lymphatic leukemia
U-937	Histocytoma		

Mouse targets

*Sensitive to lysis**		*Insensitive to lysis**	
Yac-1	Moloney virus induced T lymphoma A/Sn mice	L 1210	Methylcholanthrene induced lymphoma DBA/2
MPC-11	Mineral oil induced plasmocytoma Balb/c	EL-4	Benzpyrene induced lymphoma C57Bl/6
X-63	Mineral oil induced plasmocytoma Balb/c	P 815	Methylcholanthrene induced mastocytoma DBA/2
RLol	Radiation induced leukaemia Balb/c	RBL-5	Rauscher virus induced lymphoma C57Bl/6
Nulli-SCCl	Mouse teratocarcinoma lacking MHC	PYS-2	Mouse yolk-sac carcinoma lacking MHC

---

* Sensitive and insensitive should not be considered absolute terms.

Summary

NK cells were originally defined as cells with natural cytotoxicity and a typical physiology, morphology and regulatory properties. Cells with similar specificity can also be found amongst more conventional cell types, if such cells are activated to express cytolytic activities. At present, the most relevant problems to be solved in the NK area include questions of cellular lineage, structures containing NK specificity and triggering capacity, and the actual relevance of NK cells in health and disease.

Media

CPD solution (Travenol)

One hundred millilitres of solution contains: 327 mg citrate monohydrate acid, 2.63 g sodium citrate dihydrate, 222 mg monosodium phosphate monohydrate, 2.55 g glucose monohydrate.

Phosphate-buffered saline (Dulbecco), PBS (Flow Laboratories, England)

Component	mg/dm^3
NaCl	8000.0
KCl	200.0
Na$_2$HPO$_4$	1150.0
KH$_2$PO$_4$	200.0
CaCl$_2$ (anhyd.)	100.0
MgCl$_2$·6H$_2$O	100.0
Calibrated to pH 7.2	

RPMI-1640, (Flow Laboratories, England)

Component	mg/dm^3
L-Arginine	200.0
L-Asparagine H$_2$O	56.82
L-Aspartic acid	20.00
L-Cystine, disodium salt	59.15
L-Glutamic acid	20.00
L-Glutamine	300.0
Glutathione	1.00
Glycine	10.00
L-Histidine	15.00
L-Hydroxyproline	20.00
L-Isoleucine	50.00
L-Leucine	50.00
L-Lysine HCl	40.00
L-Methionine	15.00
L-Phenylalanine	15.00
L-Proline	20.00
L-Serine	30.00
L-Threonine	20.00
L-Tryptophane	5.00
L-Tyrosine	20.00
L-Valine	20.00
Biotin	0.20
D-Calcium pantothenate	0.25
Choline chloride	3.00
Folic acid	1.00
i-Inositol	35.00
Nicotinamide	1.00
p-Aminobenzoic acid	1.00
Pyridoxine HCl	1.00
Riboflavin	0.20
Thiamin HCl	1.00
Vitamin B12	0.005
Ca(NO$_3$)$_2$	69.49
KCl	400.0
MgSO$_4$·7H$_2$O	100.0
NaCl	6000
NaHCO$_3$	2000
Na$_2$HPO$_4$	800.7
Glucose	2000
Sodium phenol red	5.00

RPMI-1640 supplemented with:

Buffer: HEPES (N-2-hydroxyethyl-piperazine N'-2-ethanesulphonic acid; Sigma, St. Louis, Mo., USA) at a concentration of 10 mM.
Antibiotics: benzylpenicillin (Sigma, St. Louis, Mo., USA) at a concentration of 120 mg/dm^3; streptomycin (Sigma, St. Louis, Mo., USA) at a concentration of 100 mg/dm^3.

Trypan blue solution

0.18% trypan blue in PBS or 0.9% NaCl in H$_2$O.

References

1 HERBERMAN R.B., NUNN M.E. & LAVRIN D.H. (1975) Natural cytotoxic reactivity of mouse lymphoid cells against syngeneic and allogeneic tumors. (I) Distribution of reactivity and specificity. *Int. J. Cancer*, **15**, 216.

2 KIESSLING R., KLEIN E. & WIGZELL H. (1975) Natural killer cells with specificity for mouse Moloney leukemia cells. Specificity and distribution according to genotype. *Eur. J. Immunol.* **5**, 112.

3 GIDLUND M., ÖRN A., WIGZELL H., SENIK A. & GRESSER I. (1978) Enhanced NK cell activity in mice injected with interferon and interferon inducers. *Nature*, **223**, 259.

4 HERBERMAN R.B., ORTALDO J.R. & BONNARD G.D. (1979) Augmentation by interferon of human natural and antibody-dependent cell mediated cytotoxicity. *Nature*, **277**, 221.

5 HERBERMAN R.B., NUNN M.E., HOLDEN H.T. & LAVRIN D.H. (1975) Natural cytotoxic reactivity of mouse lym-

phoid cells against syngeneic and allogeneic tumors. (II) Characterization of effector cells. *Int. J. Cancer*, **16**, 230.

6 RODER J.C., ARGOV S., KLEIN M., PETERSSON C., KIESSLING R., ANDERSSON K. & HANSSON M. (1980) Target–effector cell interaction in the natural killer cell system. (V) Energy requirements, membrane integrity, and the possible involvement of lysosomal enzymes. *Immunology*, **40**, 107.

7 EREMIN E. & PLUMB D. (1978) Antibody-dependent cellular cytotoxicity and natural cytotoxicity: Effect of pre-treatment of human lymphocytes with deionised water and ammonium chloride. *J. immunol. Meth.* **24**, 257.

8 LEIBOLD W., JANOTTE G. & PETER H.H. (1980) Spontaneous cell-mediated cytotoxicity (SCMC) in various mammalian species and chickens: selective reaction pattern and different mechanisms. *Scand. J. Immunol.* **11**, 203.

9 CHARRIAUT C., SENIK A., KOLB J.P., BAREL M. & FRADE R. (1982) Inhibition of *in vitro* natural killer activity by the third component of complement: Role for the C3a fragment. *Proc. natn. Acad. Sci. U.S.A.* **79**, 6003.

10 SERROU B., ROSENFELD C., & HEBERMAN R.B. (1982) *Human Cancer Immunology*, Vol. 4, *Natural Killer Cells*, Elsevier Biomedical Press, Amsterdam.

11 HERBERMAN R.B. (1982) *NK Cells and Other Natural Effector Cells*. Academic Press, New York.

12 ULLBERG M., MERRIL J. & JONDAL M. (1981) Interferon-induced NK augmentation in humans. An analysis of target recognition, effector cell recruitment and effector cell recycling. *Scand. J. Immunol.* **14**, 285.

13 HISERODT J.C., BRITVAN L.J. & TARGAN S.R. (1982) Characterization of the cytolytic reaction mechanism of the human natural killer (NK) lymphocyte: resolution into binding, programming and killer cell-independent steps. *J. Immunol.* **129**, 1782.

14 QUAN P.C., ISHIZAKA T. & BLOOM B.R. (1982) Studies of the mechanism of NK cell lysis. *J. Immunol.* **128**, 1786.

15 WRIGHT S.C. & BONAVIDA B. (1982) Studies on the mechanism of natural killer (NK) cell mediated cytotoxicity (CMC). (I) Release of cytotoxic factors specific for NK-sensitive target cells (NKCF) during co-culture of NK effector cells with NK target cells. *J. Immunol.* **129**, 433.

16 BRUNNER K.T. & CEROTTINI J.-C. (1974) Cell-mediated cytotoxicity, allograft rejection and tumor immunity. *Adv. Immunol.* **18**, 67.

17 GRIMM E. & BONAVIDA B. (1979) Mechanism of cell-mediated cytotoxicity at the single cell level. (I) Estimation of cytotoxic T-lymphocyte frequency and relative lytic efficiency. *J. Immunol.* **123**, 2861.

18 HALLER O., HANSSON M., KIESSLING R. & WIGZELL H. (1977) Nonconventional natural killer cells may play a decisive role in providing resistance against syngenic tumor cells *in vivo*. *Nature*, **270**, 609.

19 KIESSLING R., PETRÁNYI G., KLEIN G. & WIGZELL H. (1976) Non-T-cell resistance against a mouse Molonyy lymphoma. *Int. J. Cancer*, **17**, 1.

20 RICCARDI C., PUCETTI P., SANTONI A. & HERBERMAN R.B. (1979) Rapid *in vivo* assay of mouse natural killer (NK) cell activity. *J. Nat. Cancer Inst.* **63**, 1041.

21 RIESENFELD I., ÖRN A., GIDLUND M., AXBERG I., ALM G. & WIGZELL H. (1980) Positive correlation between *in vitro* NK activity and *in vivo* resistance towards AKR lymphoma cells. *Int. J. Cancer*, **25**, 399.

22 CARLSON G.A. & WEGMAN T.G. (1977) Rapid *in vivo* destruction of semi-syngeneic and allogeneic cells by nonimmunized mice as a consequence of non-identity at H-2. *J. Immunol.* **118**, 2130.

23 HALLER O. & WIGZELL H. (1977) Suppression of natural killer cell activity with radioactive strontium: effector cells are marrow-dependent. *J. Immunol.* **118**, 1503.

24 KASAI M., YONEDA T., HABU S., MARUYAMA Y., OKUMURA K. & TOKUNAGA T. (1981) *In vivo* effect of anti-asialo GM 1 antibody on natural killer activity. *Nature*, **291**, 334.

25 RODER J.C. & DUWE A.K. (1979) The beige mutation in the mouse selectively impairs NK cell function. *Nature*, **278**, 451.

26 ÖRN A., HÅKANSSON E.M., GIDLUND M., RAMSTEDT U., AXBERG I., WIGZELL H. & LUNDIN L.-G. (1982) Pigment mutations in the mouse which also affect lysosomal functions lead to suppressed natural killer cell activity. *Scand. J. Immunol.* **15**, 305.

27 WALLACH D. (1982) Interferon induced resistance to the killing by NK cells: A preferential effect of IFN-gamma. *Cell. Immunol.* **75**, 390.

28 EINHORN S., BLOMGREN H. & STRANDER H. (1978) Interferon and spontaneous cytotoxicity in man. (I) Enhancement of spontaneous cytotoxicity of peripheral lymphocytes by human leukocyte interferon. *Int. J. Cancer*, **22**, 405.

29 TRINCHERI G., SANTOLI D. & KOPROWSKI H. (1978) Spontaneous cell-mediated cytotoxicity in humans: role of interferon and immunoglobulins. *J. Immunol.* **120**, 1849.

30 ORTALDO J.R., HERBERMAN R.B. & DIEU J.Y. (1980) Characteristics of augmentation by interferon of cell-mediated cytotoxicity. In *Natural Cell-mediated Immunity Against Tumors*, (ed. Herberman R.B.), p. 593. Academic Press, New York.

31 SENIK A., KOLB J., ÖRN A. & GIDLUND M. (1980) Study of the mechanism of *in vitro* activation of mouse NK cells by interferon. *Scand. J. Immunol.* **12**, 51.

32 CLARK E.A., RUSSEL P.H., EGGHART M. & HORTON M.A. (1979) Characteristics and genetic control of NK cell mediated cytotoxicity activated by natural acquired infection in the mouse. *Int. J. Cancer*, **24**, 688.

33 ÖRN A., GIDLUND M., OJO E., GRÖNVIK K.-O., ANDERSSON J., WIGZELL H., MURGITA R.A., SENIK A. & GRESSER I. (1980) Factors controlling the augmentation of natural killer cells. In *Natural Cell-mediated Immunity Against Tumors*, (ed. Herberman R.B.), p. 581. Academic Press, New York.

34 SAKSELA E., TIMONEN T. & CANTELL K. (1979) Human natural killer cell activity is augmented by interferon via recruitment of 'pre-NK' cells. *Scand. J. Immunol.* **10**, 257.

35 TIMONEN T., ORTALDO J.R. & HERBERMAN R.B. (1982) Analysis by a single cell cytotoxicity assay of natural killer (NK) cell frequencies among human large granular lymphocytes and of the effect of interferon on their activity. *J. Immunol.* **128**, 2514.

36 TARGAN S. & DOREY F. (1980) Interferon activation of 'pre-spontaneous killer' (pre-SK) cells and alternations in kinetics of lysis of both 'pre-SK' and active SK cells. *J. Immunol.* **124**, 2157.

37 HENNEY C.S., KURIBAYASHI K., KERN D.E. & GILLIS S. (1981) Interleukin-2 augments natural killer cell activity. *Nature*, **291**, 335.

38 SUZUKI R., HANDA K., ITOH K. & KUMAGAI K. (1983) Natural killer (NK) cells as responder to interleukin-2 (IL-2). (I) Proliferative response and establishment of cloned cells. *J. Immunol.* **130**, 981.

39 DEMPSEY R.A., DINARELLO C.A., MEIR J.W., ROSEN-WASSER L.J., ALLEGRETTA M., BROWN T.E. & PARKINSON D.R. (1982) The differential effect of human leukocytic pyrogen/lymphocyte activating factor, T cell growth factor, and interferon on human natural killer cell activity. *J. Immunol.* **129**, 2504.

40 TIMONEN T., SAKSELA E., RANKI A. & HÄYRY P. (1979) Fractionation, morphological and functional characterization of effector cells responsible for human natural killer activity against cell line targets. *Cell. Immunol.* **48**, 133.

41 REYNOLDS C.W., TIMONEN T. & HERBERMAN R.B. (1981) Natural killer (NK) cell activity in the rat. (I) Isolation and characterization of the effector cell. *J. Immunol.* **127**, 282.

42 KUMAGI K., ITHO K., SUZUKI R., HINUMA S. & SAITOH F. (1982) Studies of murine large granular lymphocytes. (I) Identification as effector cells in NK and K cytotoxicities. *J. Immunol.* **129**, 388.

43 TIMONEN T., REYNOLDS C.W., ORTALDO J.R. & HERBERMAN R.B. (1982) Isolation of human and rat natural killer cells. *J. Immunol. Meth.* **51**, 269.

44 PIONTEK G.E., GRÖNBERG A., AEHRLUND-RICHTER L., KIESSLING R. & HENGARTNER H. (1982) NK-patterned binding expressed by non-NK mouse leukocytes. *Int. J. Cancer*, **30**, 225.

45 BINZ H., FENNER M., FREI D. & WIGZELL H. (1983) Two independent receptors allow selective target lysis by T cell clones. *J. exp. Med.* **157**, 1252.

46 BROOKS C. (1983) Reversible induction of natural killer cell activity in cloned murine cytotoxic T lymphocytes. *Nature*, **305**, 155.

47 HANSSON M., KÄRRE K., BAKACS T., KIESSLING R. & KLEIN G. (1978) Intra- and interspecies reactivity of human and mouse natural killer (NK) cells. *J Immunol.* **121**, 6.

48 TIMONEN T., ORTALDO J.R. & HERBERMAN R.B. (1981) Characteristics of human large granular lymphocytes and relationship to natural killer and K cells. *J. exp. Med.* **153**, 569.

49 PERLMAN H.P., PERLMAN G.R. & HALLDEN G. (1976) Purification, fractionation and assay of antibody-dependent lymphocyte effector cells (K-cells) in human blood. *Scand. J. Immunol.* **5** (suppl. 5), 57.

50 TROYE M., PERLMAN P., PAPE G.R., SPEIGELBERG H.L., NÄSLUND I. & GIDLÖF A. (1977) The use of Fab fragments of anti-human immunoglobulin in the spontaneous cytotoxicity to cultured tumor cells by lymphocytes from patients with bladder carcinoma and from healthy donors. *J. Immunol.* **119**, 1061.

51 DENNERT G. (1980) Cloned lines of natural killer cells. *Nature*, **287**, 47.

52 NABEL G., BUCALO L.R., ALLARD J., WIGZELL H. & CANTOR H. (1981) Multiple activities of a cloned cell line mediating natural killer cell function. J. exp. Med. **153**, 1582.

53 BROOKS C.G., KURIBAYASHI K., SALE G.E. & HENNEY C. (1982) Characterization of five cloned murine cell lines showing high cytotoxic activity against YAC-1 cells. *J. Immunol.* **128**, 2326.

54 WARD J.M. & REYNOLDS C.W. (1983) Large granular leukemia. A heterogenous lymphocytic leukemia in F 344 rats. *Am J. Path.* **111**, 1.

55 WEST W., CANNON G.B., KAY H.D., BONNARD G.D. & HERBERMAN R.B. (1977) Natural cytotoxic reactivity of human lymphocytes against a myeloid cell line: characterization of effector cells. *J. Immunol.* **118**, 355.

56 KASAI M., IWAMORI M., NAGAI Y., OKUMURA K. & TADA T. (1980) A glycolipid on the surface of mouse natural killer cells. *Eur. J. Immunol.* **10**, 175.

57 GLIMCHER L., SHEN F.W. & CANTOR H. (1977) Identification of a cell-surface antigen selectively expressed on the natural killer cell. *J. exp. Med.* **145**, 1.

58 POLLACK S.B. & EMMONS S.L. (1982) NK-2.1: An NK-associated antigen detected with NZB Anti-Balb/c serum. *J. Immunol.* **5**, 2277.

59 ABO T. & BALCH C.M. (1981) A differentiation antigen of human and NK and K cells identified by a monoclonal antibody (HNK-1). *J. Immunol.* **127**, 1024.

60 LANIER L.L., LE A.M., PHILLIPS J.H., WARNER N.L. & BABCOCK G.F. (1983) Subpopulations of human natural killer cells defined by expression of the Leu-7 (HNK-1) and Leu-11 (NK-15) antigens. *J. Immunol.* **131**, 1789.

61 HURME M., SILVENNOINEN O. & RENKONEN R. (1984) Highly increased natural killer cell number and lytic activity in the murine peripheral blood and lungs after interferon induction *in vivo*. *Scand. J. Immunol.* **20**, 371.

62 PATEL M.R. & LINNA T.J. (1984) Enrichment of mouse splenic natural killer cells using discontinuous polyvinyl-pyrrolidone silica (PercollR) gradients. *Immunology*, **53**, 721.

63 BLUMENTHAL P., MILLARD P.J. HENKART M.P., REYNOLDS C.W., HENKART P.A. (1984) Liposomes as targets for granule cytolysin from cytotoxic large granular lymphocyte tumors. *Proc. natn. Acad. Sci. U.S.A.* **81**, 5551.

Chapter 61
Genetics and cell distributions of mouse cell surface alloantigens

LORRAINE FLAHERTY & J. FORMAN

Classification, 61.1
Methods of detection, 61.4

Analysis, 61.4
Perspective, 61.5

There are over fifty known lymphocyte cell surface alloantigens in the mouse. The alloantigens are important because they serve as useful genetic markers and because they seem to distinguish functionally distinct subpopulations of lymphocytes. The purpose of this review is to catalogue these markers according to their genetic, serologic, biochemical, and tissue distribution characteristics. This discussion will be limited to serologically defined alloantigens and to those which do not belong to the H-2, Ig or Ia class of molecules determined by the major histocompatibility complex (MHC). It will, however, include the Qa and TL series of alloantigens determined by the MHC.

Classification

Various systems have been used to categorize these alloantigens. One such system proposed by Snell [1] involves the use of letter prefixes to indicate the tissue representation of a particular alloantigen: Ea for erythrocyte antigen, Ly for lymphocyte antigen, Thy for thymocyte antigen, Pca for plasma cell antigen, and Sk for skin antigen. These symbols do not necessarily mean that the antigen resides solely on the tissue in question; rather, the antigen is detectable (or was first detectable) on that tissue. In general, these classifications are still being used today.

Boyse et al. [2] introduced an additional terminology to distinguish lymphocyte alloantigens which reside exclusively on T cells ('Lyt') or B cells ('Lyb'). In certain cases these classifications have been useful, but some presumed Lyt or Lyb antigens have been shown to appear on both T and B cells. Thus some investigators have reverted to the practice of naming a lymphocyte alloantigen simply Ly and have dropped the T and B cell designations.

Since the advent of monoclonal antibodies, many new alloantigens are being identified and characterized with these reagents. In such cases, an 'm' (standing for monoclonal) usually follows the letter designation.

To distinguish one molecule bearing an alloantigen from another, three criteria are generally used: the genetic map position, the biochemical characterization, and the tissue distribution. Even with these three criteria, however, it is often difficult to distinguish between alloantigens. There are three major reasons for this difficulty.

1 The genes which determine alloantigens are often clustered in short stretches of the chromosome. In particular, several main clusters are evident on chromosomes 1, 2, 4, and 17. Since crossing over is rare in these regions, the distinctions cannot always be based on chromosomal mapping studies. More precise linkage relationships are needed.

2 Molecules determined by a single cluster often have striking biochemical similarities, making biochemical distinctions more difficult to define.

3 If two alloantigens have different tissue distributions, they are often considered unique. However, two uncertainties must be considered in this type of analysis. First, different detection systems are often more sensitive on a particular tissue type. Thus different tissue distributions may simply reflect our inability to measure the alloantigen's expression on certain tissues with a particular antiserum. Second, the expression of molecules bearing alloantigens is sometimes altered in a given cell type (e.g. by glycosylation). If these alterations are genetically determined, it may be difficult to compare the alloantigenic tissue distribution characterized in one mouse strain with that of another.

All known murine alloantigens which are expressed on lymphoid cells are listed in Table 61.1. In some cases their predominant expression occurs on an unrelated tissue. Wherever possible, synonyms are given for these alloantigens. Where distinctions between alloantigens have been questioned in the literature, similar alloantigens are indicated in column 3. The detection systems used for these antigens, as well as their genetic and relative molecular mass characteristics and their tissue distributions, are indi-

Table 61.1. Murine lymphocyte alloantigens

Allo-antigen	Synonym	Similar or identical molecule[a]	Chromosome	Number of alleles	Mono-clonal?	Tissue distribution[b]	Relative molecular mass	Functional marker[c]	References
Ly1	LyA,Mu, Lyt-1		19	2	Yes	T,LN,S	67000	T helper, T cytotoxic, B cell subset	[3-7]
Ly2	LyB,Lyt-2		6	2	Yes	T,LN,S	34000, 38000	T cytotoxic/suppressor	[3,4,8-10]
Ly3	LyC,Lyt-3		6	2	Yes	T,LN,S	30000	T cytotoxic/suppressor	[3,4,8-11]
Ly4	Lyb-1	H-3,β2m, Lym11	2	2		E?,T?,LN, S,O?			[12-14]
Ly5	Lyt-4	T200,B220	1	2	Yes	T,LN,S,O	200000, 205000, 220000	Haematopoietic cells	[15-21]
Ly6		Ala-1,Ly8,DAG	2 or 9[d]	2	Yes	T,LN,S,O	33500	Some T, some B	[22-29]
Ly7				3	Yes	T,LN,S			[30-32]
Ly8		Ly6,Ala-1, DAG	2 or 9	2		T,LN,S,O			[25,26]
Ly9	T100,Lgp100		1	2	Yes	T,LN,S	100000	Some T, some B	[33-36]
Lym10			19	2	Yes	T,LN,S,O		Prothymocytes, NK	[37]
Ly11(a)	Ly10		2	2		T,LN,S			[38-40]
Lym11(b)	β2m	H-3,Ly4	2	2	Yes	E?,T,LN, S,O	12000		[14,41]
Ly11(c)				2		T,LN,S,O	18000-22000?		[42]
Ly12				2		T,LN,S			[42]
Ly13				2		E,T,LN,S,O			[42]
Ly14				2		T,LN,S,O			[42]
Ly15			7	2	Yes	T,LN,S,O			[43]
Ly17	Lym20					T,LN,S,O			[44]
Ly18(a)			1	2		LN[e]	73000?	T cytotoxic	[45]
Lym18(b)			12	2	Yes	T,LN,S,O			[46]
Ly19(a)			12	2	Yes	T,LN,S			[47]
Lym19(b)			4	2	Yes	T,LN,S			[48]
Lym20	Ly17,LyM-1 Mls		1	2	Yes	T,LN,S,O		B cells?	[49]
Lym-21			7	2	Yes	T,LN,S,O			[50]
Ly-22(a)			4	2		T,LN,S		T cells	[51]
Lym-22(b)			1	2	Yes	T,LN,S			[52]
Lyb-2	Lyb-4,Lyb-6		4	3		T?,LN,S	40000-50000	B cells?	[53-55]
Lyb-3	Lyb-5		X[f]	2		LN,S	68000	B cells	[56,57]
Lyb-4	Lyb-2,Lyb-6		4	2		LN,S	44000	B cells?	[58,59]
Lyb-5	Lyb-3		X[f]	2		LN,S		B cells	[60]
Lyb-6	Lyb-2,Lyb-4		4	2		LN,S	44000?	B cells	[59]
Lyb-7			12	2		LN,S		B cells	[61]
Lyb-8			7	2	Yes	LN,S	95000	B cells	[62]
Ea-1			8	3		E			[63,64]

Table 61.1 (*cont.*)

Allo-antigen	Synonym	Similar or identical molecule[a]	Chromosome	Number of alleles	Mono-clonal?	Tissue distribution[b]	Relative molecular mass	Functional marker[c]	References
Ea-2	R,Z,ρ,H-14			2		E,T,LN,S,O			[64,65]
Ea-3				2		E			[64,66]
Ea-4	BL,D			2		E,T,LN,S,O			[64,67]
Ea-5	α,H-5.A			2		E,T,LN,S,O			[64,68]
Ea-6	δ,H-6.A		2	2		E,LN,S,O			[64,68]
Ea-7	T	Ea-5		2		E,T			[64,69]
Thy-1	θ		9	2	Yes	T,LN,S,O	25 000	T cells	[70,71]
Thy-2			17	2		T,LN,S,O	150 000		[72]
TL			17	6	Yes	T	44 000 + β2m	Immature thymocytes	[73,74]
Qa-1		Qed-1,H-2T	17	4?		T,LN,S,O	45 000 + β2m	Haematopoietic cells	[75–78]
Qa-2			17	2	Yes	T,LN,S,O	40 000 + β2m	Haematopoietic cells	[78–81]
Qa-3		Qa-2	17	2		LN,S			[78,82]
Qa-4		Qa-2	17	2	Yes	LN,S,O?			[78,81,83]
Qa-5		Qa-2	17	2	Yes	LN,S			[78,81,83]
Qa-6			17	2		LN,S			[84]
Lq			17	2		LN,S	41 000 + β2m		[85]
Ala-1		Ly6,Ly8,DAG	2 or 9	2	Yes	T,LN,S			[22–29]
H-Y			Y[g]	1?	Yes	E,T,LN,S,O		Male cells	[86]
H9/25		ThB	2 or 9	2	Yes	T,LN,S	12 000–16 000		[29,87,88]
Lna-1			2	2		LN		Lymph node lymphocytes	[89]
LyM-1		Mls	1	3?		LN,S		B cells?	[90,91]
NK-1				2		LN,S		NK cells	[92]
NK-2			2?	2		S		NK cells	[93]
Pc-1				2		LN,S,O	2 × 110 000		[94–96]
Pgp-1			2	2	Yes	T,LN,S,O	95 000	Haematopoietic cells	[97–99]
Tind[d]			12	2	Yes	T?,LN,S		T cell subset	[100–102]
Tsu[d]			12	2	Yes	LN,S		T cell	[101–103]
Tthy[d]			12	2	Yes	T,LN,S		T cell subset	[100–102]
Tpre			12	2	Yes	T,S,O		Fetal cells	[104]

a Molecules or alloantigens which have similar genetic and/or biochemical properties.

b Symbols: erythrocytes, E; thymus, T; lymph nodes, LN; spleen and/or bone marrow, S; other, O.

c Only alloantigens which have been used to separate functionally distinct subpopulations of haematopoietic cells are indicated. Separation could be based either on selective elimination by use of complement, or on cell sorting.

d There is currently some debate in the literature on the chromosomal position of the Ly6 family of alloantigens, including Ly6, Ly8, DAG, Ala-1, H9/25, and ThB [100,101]. They are tightly linked on either chromosome 2 or chromosome 9.

e On activated spleen cells only.

f Lyb-3 and Lyb-5 are missing in CBA/N mice with a defective X-linked gene. The structural gene controlling these antigens has not been mapped.

g Only males express H-Y. However, it is still unclear whether the serologically defined H-Y antigen is determined by the Y chromosome or is simply sex-limited.

cated. Finally, when these alloantigens are frequently used to isolate functionally distinct subpopulations of cells, the subpopulations are also indicated.

Methods of detection

Reagents

Three basic types of reagents are used to detect mouse alloantigens: xenogeneic antisera, allogeneic antisera, and monoclonal antibodies. In the case of antisera, particularly xenogeneic antisera, caution must be observed, since these reagents often contain auto-antibodies and anti-viral components and may react against multiple alloantigenic specificities. Absorption tests as well as negative controls are often necessary to clarify their reactivity. Moreover, different batches or pools of antisera may have different contaminants or activities. Antisera do have the advantage, however, of being polyvalent and thus are more strongly reactive to the target molecule.

Monoclonal reagents have the advantages of being specific and easily produced in large quantities. Since the same antibody can be made in multiple laboratories, these reagents are useful for standardization of many immunologic assays. However, it is important to remember that cross-reactions also occur with monoclonal reagents (i.e. one monoclonal antibody may react with more than one molecule; see Chapter 107). Moreover, when ascites fluid from mice is used to raise the monoclonals, the possibility of contamination with auto-antibodies and anti-viral antibodies should be considered.

Test procedures

Several assays can be used to detect the binding of antibodies to cell surface alloantigens. These assays are listed in Table 61.2 with their advantages and disadvantages. Because combinations of certain classes of antibodies with particular assays are more sensitive than others, one technique may be superior to another for a given purpose. Therefore the selection of an appropriate technique is critical and dependent on the experimental design. This choice is especially important when the alloantigen varies quantitatively on different subpopulations. For example, immuno-fluorescent techniques and fluorescence-activated cell sorter (FACS) analysis have shown that the Ly1 antigen is present on all T cells but in different quantities [107], yet in some experiments cytotoxicity assays show only helper T cells [4]. No definitive conclusions should be drawn from results obtained with any single assay.

Analysis

Genetic

As previously stated, genetic analysis of an alloantigen is essential to distinguish it from other alloantigens. Several useful genetic tools are available in the murine system for this purpose. First, a preliminary strain distribution should be performed. In general, strains with different origins should be screened to determine the prevalance of this alloantigen in the general mouse population. In particular, it would be judicious to

Table 61.2. Detection systems

Detection system	Main variations	Usage	Advantages	Disadvantages
Haemagglutination	Polyvinylpyrrolidone method Dextran-fetal calf serum (FCS) method Capillary method	Detection of allo-antigens on red blood cells	Sensitive for red blood cells	Only certain classes of antibodies are haemagglutinating
Complement-dependent cytotoxicity	^{51}Cr release Trypan blue method	Detection of alloantigens on viable cell suspensions	Sensitive for thymo-cytes and lymphocytes	Dependent on complement-binding antibodies and sensitivity of cells to lysis by complement
Binding procedures	Immunofluorescence Radioimmunoassays ELISA techniques	Detection of allo-antigens on cell suspensions or on tissue slices Allows for the detection of antigen at the single cell level	Sensitive for thymocytes and lymphocytes Easily quantified	Fixation procedures for tissue sections sometimes destroy antigenicity Non-specific binding of anti-Ig conjugates to Fc-receptor-bearing cells

screen the inbred parents of commonly available recombinant inbred (RI) lines since this approach avoids the use of extensive back-cross typings. Next, either RI lines or back-crosses employing multiple markers should be performed to locate the chromosome which contains the alloantigen-determining locus. Finally, this location should be confirmed by the use of congenic strains or by back-cross experiments employing suitable markers.

One of the most serious considerations in these genetic studies is the effect of genetic background on the expression of the alloantigen in question. Modifier genes in the genetic background can often change the expression of an alloantigen. For example, the level of expression of Ly4 (β_2m?) is dependent on the expression of MHC genes [11]. Another obstacle may be the occurrence of clusters of alloantigen-determining loci which often make it difficult to distinguish one alloantigen from another. If an alloantigen-determining locus maps to one of these clusters, extensive back-cross analyses may be needed to show the individuality of the alloantigen.

Tissue distribution

Because many alloantigens are now being used as tools to dissect out functionally distinct subpopulations of lymphocytes, a careful examination of the tissue distributions of these markers is necessary.

The first step in this procedure is to ascertain whether the marker in question is limited to the lymphoid cells. Such a limitation is unusual; most of the antigens listed in Table 61.1 are also represented on other somatic tissues. Some markers, however, are even more narrowly restricted to subsets within the lymphoid population; a case in point is Ly2.

Functional analysis

The first marker found to be represented on a functionally distinct population of lymphoid cells was Thy-1 [66]. This marker is frequently used to separate T cells from B cells. Several markers also seem to separate T cell subclasses and are specific for T-helper cells, T-suppressor cells, and/or T-cytotoxic cells. Here, however, the method of detection and separation is critical, since this distinction may depend on a quantitative difference rather than a qualitative one (e.g. Ly1).

Several separation techniques are employed in this type of analysis. These include selective elimination of antigen-positive cells by use of antibody and complement, panning techniques, and cell sorting analysis.

Perspective

Even though certain of these alloantigens appear to distinguish functional subpopulations of lymphocytes and a great deal is known about their genetics and biochemistry, it is remarkable how little we know about their actual function. In fact, not one of the alloantigens listed in Table 61.1 has yet been identified with a clearly defined function associated with them.

At the very least, however, these alloantigens are important tools for analysis of the immune system and for biomedical studies. Since a variety of immune-related diseases are characterized in part by altered ratios of functionally distinct T and/or B cell subpopulations, alloantigens are now being used to diagnose those diseases.

References

1 SNELL G. (1971) The Histocompatibility Systems. *Transplant. Proc.* **3**, 1133.
2 BOYSE E.A., CANTOR H., SHEN F.-W. & McKENZIE I.F.C. (1977) Nomenclature for antigens demonstrable on lymphocytes. *Immunogenetics*, **5**, 189.
3 BOYSE E.A., MIYAZAWA M., AOKI T. & OLD L.J. (1968) Ly-A and Ly-B: two systems of lymphocyte isoantigens in the mouse. *Proc. R. Soc.* Series B, **170**, 175.
4 CANTOR H. & BOYSE E.A. (1975) Functional subclasses of T lymphocytes bearing different Ly antigens. (I) The generation of functionally distinct T-cell subclasses is a differentiative process independent of antigen. *J. exp. Med.* **141**, 1376.
5 ITAKURA K., HUTTON J., BOYSE E. & OLD L.J. (1971) Linkage groups of the θ and LyA loci. *Nature New Biol.* **230**, 126.
6 DURDA P.J., SHAPIRO C. & GOTTLIEB P.D. (1978) Partial molecular characterization of the Ly-1 alloantigen on mouse thymocytes. *J. Immunol.* **120**, 53.
7 LANIER L.L., WARNER N.L., LEDBETTER J.A. & HERZENBERG L. (1981) Expression of Lyt-1 antigen on certain murine B cell lymphomas. *J. exp. Med.* **153**, 998.
8 DURDA P.J. & GOTTLIEB P.D. (1978) Sequential precipitation of mouse thymocyte extract with anti-Lyt-2 and anti-Lyt-3 sera. (I) Lyt-2.1 and Lyt-3.1 antigenic determinants reside on separable molecular species. *J. Immunol.* **121**, 983.
9 REILLY B.B., AUDITORE-HARGREAVES K., HAMMERLING U. & GOTTLIEB P.D. (1980) Lyt-2 and Lyt-3 alloantigens: precipitation with monoclonal and conventional antibodies and analysis on one- and two-dimensional polyacrylamide gels. *J. Immunol.* **125**, 2245.
10 LEDBETTER J.A., SEAMAN W.E., TSU T.T. & HERZENBERG L.A. (1982) Lyt-2 and Lyt-3 antigens are on two different polypeptides linked by disulfide bonds: relationship of subunits to T cell cytotoxic activity. *J. exp. Med.* **153**, 1503.
11 BOYSE E.A., ITAKURA K., STOCKERT E., IRITANI C. & MIURA M. (1971) Ly C, a third locus specifying alloantigens expressed only on thymocytes and lymphocytes. *Transplantation*, **11**, 351.

12 SNELL G., CHERRY C., MCKENZIE I. & BAILEY D. (1973) Ly4, a new locus determining a lymphocyte cell surface alloantigen in mice. *Proc. natn. Acad. Sci. U.S.A.* **70**, 1108.

13 MICHAELSON J., ROTHENBERG E. & BOYSE E.A. (1980) Genetic polymorphism of murine β_2-microglobulin detected biochemically. *Immunogenetics*, **11**, 93.

14 TADA N., KIMURA S., HATZFELD A. & HAMMERLING U. (1980) Ly-m11: the H-3 region of mouse chromosome 2 controls a new cell surface alloantigen. *Immunogenetics*, **11**, 441.

15 KOMURO K., ITAKURA E., BOYSE E.A. & JOHN M. (1975) Ly-5: a new lymphocyte antigen system. *Immunogenetics*, **1**, 452.

16 SCHEID M.P. & TRIGLIA D. (1979) Further description of the Ly-5 system. *Immunogenetics*, **9**, 423.

17 MICHAELSON J., SCHEID M.P. & BOYSE E.A. (1979) Biochemical features of Ly-5 alloantigen. *Immunogenetics*, **9**, 193.

18 SIADAK A.W. & NOWINSKI R.C. (1980) Identification of Ly-5 and T200 antigens on identical cell surface proteins. *J. Immunol.* **125**, 1400.

19 OMARY M.B., TROWBRIDGE I.S. & SCHEID M.P. (1980) The T200 cell surface glycoprotein of the mouse: polymorphism defined by the Ly-5 system of alloantigens. *J. exp. Med.* **151**, 1311.

20 COFFMAN R.L. & WEISSMAN I.L. (1981) B220: a B cell-specific member of the T200 glycoprotein family. *Nature*, **289**, 681.

21 SHEN F.-W. (1981) Monoclonal antibodies to mouse lymphocyte differentiation alloantigens. In *Monoclonal Antibodies and T-Cell Hybridomas*, (eds. Hammerling G.J., Hammerling U. & Kearney J.F.), p. 25. Elsevier/North–Holland Biomedical Press.

22 MCKENZIE I.F.C., CHERRY M. & SNELL G.D. (1977) Ly-6.2: a new lymphocyte specificity of peripheral T-cells. *Immunogenetics*, **5**, 25.

23 FEENEY A.J. & HAMMERLING U. (1976) Ala-1: a murine alloantigen of activated lymphocytes. *Immunogenetics*, **3**, 369.

24 FEENEY A.J. (1978) Expression of Ly-6 on activated T and B cells: possible identity to Ala-1. *Immunogenetics*, **7**, 537.

25 FRELINGER J.A. & MURPHY D.B. (1976) A new alloantigen, Ly-8, recognized by C3H anti-AKR serum. *Immunogenetics*, **3**, 481.

26 HORTON M.A. & SACHS J.A. (1979) Identity of murine lymphocyte alloantigens DAG, Ala-1, Ly-8, and Ly-6. *Immunogenetics*, **9**, 273.

27 TAKEI F., GALFRE G., ALDERSON T., LENNOX E.S. & MILSTEIN C. (1980) H9/25 monoclonal antibody recognizes a new allospecificity of mouse lymphocyte subpopulations: strain and tissue distribution. *Eur. J. Immunol.* **10**, 241.

28 AUCHINCLOS H., OZATO K. & SACHS D.H. (1981) Two distinct murine differentiation antigens determined by genes linked to the Ly-6 locus. *J. Immunol.* **127**, 1839.

29 MATOSSIAN-ROGERS A., ROGERS P., LEDBETTER J.A. & HERZENBERG L.A. (1982) Molecular weight determination of two genetically linked cell surface murine antigens: ThB and Ly6. *Immunogenetics*, **15**, 591.

30 MCKENZIE I.F.C., GARDINER J., CHERRY M. & SNELL G.D. (1977) Lymphocyte antigens: Ly-4, Ly-6, and Ly-7. *Transplant. Proc.* **9**, 667.

31 LANIER L.L. & WARNER N.L. (1982) Lym 7.2—monoclonal antibody defining an alloantigen similar or identical to Ly 7.2. *Hybridoma*, **1**, 227.

32 LANIER L.L. & WARNER N.L. (1983) Lym 7.3—a new murine specificity defining a third allele of the Ly7 locus. *Hybridoma*, **2**, 177.

33 MATHIESON B.J., SHARROW S.O., BOTTOMLY K. & FOWLKES B.J. (1980) Ly9, an alloantigenic marker of lymphocyte differentiation. *J. Immunol.* **125**, 2127.

34 HOGARTH P.M., CRAIG J. & MCKENZIE I.F.C. (1980) A monoclonal antibody detecting the Ly-9.2 (Lgp 100) cell-membrane antigen. *Immunogenetics*, **11**, 65.

35 DURDA P.J., BOOS S.C. & GOTTLIEB P.D. (1979) T100: a new murine cell surface glycoprotein detected by anti-Lyt-2.1 serum. *J. Immunol.* **122**, 1407.

36 LEDBETTER J.A., GODING J.W., TSU T.T. & HERZENBERG L.A. (1979) A new mouse lymphoid alloantigen (Lgp100) recognized by a monoclonal rat antibody. *Immunogenetics*, **8**, 347.

37 KIMURA S., TADA N. & HAMMERLING U. (1980) A new lymphocyte alloantigen (Ly-10) controlled by a gene linked to the Lyt-1 locus. *Immunogenetics*, **10**, 363.

38 MERUELO D., PAOLINO A., FLIEGER N. & OFFER M. (1980) Definition of a new T lymphocyte cell surface antigen, Ly 11.2. *J. Immunol.* **125**, 2713.

39 MERUELO D., PAOLINO A., FLIEGER N., DWORKIN J., OFFER M., HIRAYOMA N. & OVARY Z. (1980) Functional properties of Ly 11.2 lymphocytes: a role for these cells in leukemia? *J. Immunol.* **125**, 2719.

40 MERUELO D., PAOLINO A., FLIEGER N. & DWORKIN J. (1980) Definition of a new T lymphocyte cell surface antigen, Ly 10.2. *Fedn Proc.* **39**, 798.

41 TOMONARI K., TADA N., KIMURA S., HAMMERLING U. & WEKSLER E. (1982) Inhibition of killer-target cell interaction by monoclonal anti-Ly-m11 antibody. *Immunogenetics*, **15**, 605.

42 POTTER T.A. & MCKENZIE I.F.C. (1981) Identification of new murine lymphocyte alloantigens: antisera prepared between C57L, 129 and related strains define new loci. *Immunogenetics*, **12**, 351.

43 POTTER T.A., HOGARTH P.M. & MCKENZIE I.F.C. (1981) Ly15: a new murine lymphocyte alloantigenic locus. *Transplantation*, **31**, 339.

44 SHEN F.-W. & BOYSE E.A. (1980) An alloantigen for B cells: Ly-17.1. *Immunogenetics*, **11**, 315.

45 FINNEGAN A. & OWEN F.L. (1981) Ly-18, a new alloantigen present on cytotoxic T cells and controlled by a gene(s) linked to the Igh-V locus. *J. Immunol.* **127**, 1947.

46 KIMURA S., TADA N., LIU Y. & HAMMERLING U. (1981) A new mouse cell surface antigen (Ly-m18) defined by a monoclonal antibody. *Immunogenetics*, **12**, 547.

47 FINNEGAN A. & OWEN F.L. (1981) *ICN-UCLA Symposium on Immunoglobulin Idiotypes and Their Expression*, p. 51 (Abstract).

48 TADA N., KIMURA S., LIU Y., TAYLOR B. & HAMMERLING U. (1981) Ly-m19: the Lyb-2 region of mouse chromo-

some 4 controls a new surface alloantigen. *Immunogenetics*, **13**, 539.

49 KIMURA S., TADA N., NAKAYAMA E., LIU Y. & HAMMERLING U. (1981) A new mouse cell-surface antigen (Ly-m20) controlled by a gene linked to *Mls* locus and defined by monoclonal antibodies. *Immunogenetics*, **14**, 3.

50 KINNARD J. & MERUELO D. (1982) A new murine lymphocyte alloantigen, Ly-21.2, mapping to the seventh chromosome. *Immunogenetics*, **15**, 239.

51 MERUELO D., OFFER M. & FLIEGER N. (1983) A new lymphocyte cell surface antigen, Ly-22.2, controlled by a locus on chromosome 4 and a second unlinked locus. *J. Immunol.* **130**, 946.

52 TADA N., KIMURA S., LIU-LAM L. & HAMMERLING U. (1983) Mouse alloantigen system Lym-22 predominantly expressed on T lymphocytes and controlled by a gene linked to Mls region of chromosome 1. *Hybridoma*, **2**, 29.

53 SATO H. & BOYSE E.A. (1976) A new alloantigen expressed selectively on B cells: the Lyb-2 system. *Immunogenetics*, **3**, 565.

54 TUNG J.S., MICHAELSON J., SATO H., VITETTA E. & BOYSE E.A. (1977) Properties of the Lyb-2 molecule. *Immunogenetics*, **5**, 485.

55 SHEN F.-W., SPANONDIS M. & BOYSE E.A. (1977) Multiple alleles of the Lyb-2 locus. *Immunogenetics*, **5**, 481.

56 HUBER B., GERSHON R.K. & CANTOR H. (1977) Identification of a B-cell surface structure involved in antigen-dependent triggering: absence of this structure on B cells from CBA/N mutant mice. *J. exp. Med.* **145**, 10.

57 CONE R.E., HUBER B., CANTOR H. & GERSHON R.K. (1978) Molecular identification of a surface structure on B cells (Lyb-3) and its relationship to B cell triggering. *J. Immunol.* **120**, 1733.

58 FREUND J.G., AHMED A., BUDD R.E., DORF M.E., SELL K.W., VANNIER W.E. & HUMPHREYS R.E. (1976) The L1210 leukemia cell bears a B lymphocyte specific, non H-2 linked alloantigen. *J. Immunol.* **117**, 1903.

59 KESSLER S., AHMED A. & SCHER I. (1979) Identification and partial molecular and genetic characterization of an alloantigen expressed on murine B cells. In *B Lymphocytes in the Immune Response*, (eds. Cooper M., Mosier D.E., Sher I., Vitetta E.), p. 47. Elsevier/North–Holland Biomedical Press.

60 AHMED A., SCHER I., SHARROW S.O., SMITH A.H., PAUL W.E., SACHS D.H. & SELL K.W. (1977) B-Lymphocyte heterogeneity: development and characterization of an alloantiserum which distinguishes B-Lymphocyte differentiation alloantigens. *J. exp. Med.* **145**, 101.

61 SUBBARAO B., AHMED A., PAUL W.E., SCHER I., LIEBERMAN R. & MOSIER D.E. (1979) Lyb-7, a new B cell alloantigen controlled by genes linked to the IgG4 locus. *J. Immunol.* **122**, 2279.

62 SYMINGTON F.W., SUBBARAO B., MOSIER D.E. & SPRENT J. (1982) Lyb-8.2: a new B cell antigen defined and characterized with a monoclonal antibody. *Immunogenetics*, **16**, 381.

63 SINGER M., FOSTER F.M., PETRAS M.L., TOMLIN P. &

SLOANE R.W. (1964) A new case of blood group inheritance in the house mouse. *Genetics*, **50**, 285.

64 KLEIN J. (1975) *Biology of the Mouse Histocompatibility-2 Complex*. Springer Verlag, Berlin.

65 HOECKER G., PIZARRO O. & RAMOS A. (1959) Some new antigens and histocompatibility factors in the mouse. *Transplant. Bull.* **6**, 407.

66 EGOROV I.K. (1965) A new isoantigen of mouse erythrocytes. *Genetika*, **6**, 80.

67 SHREFFLER D.C. (1966) A new erythrocytic antigen in the house mouse. *Genetics*, **54**, 362.

68 AMOS D.B., ZUMPFT M. & ARMSTRONG P. (1963) H-5.A and H-6.A, two mouse isoantigens on red cells and tissues detected serologically. *Transplantation*, **1**, 270.

69 AMOS D.B. (1959) Some iso-antigenic systems of the mouse. *Proc. Can. Cancer Res. Conf.* **3**, 241.

70 REIF A.E. & ALLEN J.M. (1963) Specificity of isoantisera against leukemic and thymic lymphocytes. *Nature*, **200**, 1332.

71 TROWBRIDGE I.S. & MAZAUSKAS C. (1976) Immunological properties of murine thymus-dependent lymphocyte surface glycoproteins. *Eur. J. Immunol.* **6**, 557.

72 SIADAK A.W. & NOWINSKI R.C. (1981) Thy-2: a murine thymocyte brain alloantigen controlled by a gene linked to the major histocompatibility complex. *Immunogenetics*, **12**, 45.

73 OLD L.J., BOYSE E.A. & STOCKERT E. (1963) Antigenic properties of experimental leukemias. (I) Serological studies *in vitro* with spontaneous and radiation-induced leukemias. *J. Nat. Cancer Inst.* **31**, 977.

74 SHEN F.-W., CHORNEY M. & BOYSE E.A. (1982) Further polymorphism of the *Tla* locus defined by monoclonal TL antibodies. *Immunogenetics*, **15**, 573.

75 STANTON T.H. & BOYSE E.A. (1976) A new serologically defined locus, Qa-1, in the *Tla* region of the mouse. *Immunogenetics*, **3**, 525.

76 STANTON T. & HOOD L. (1980) Biochemical identification of the Qa-1 alloantigen. *Immunogenetics*, **11**, 309.

77 FLAHERTY L., RINCHIK E. & DIBIASE K. (1981) New complexities at the Qa-1 locus. *Immunogenetics*, **13**, 339.

78 FLAHERTY L. (1981) The Tla region antigens. In *Role of the Major Histocompatibility Complex in Immunobiology*, (ed. Dorf M.) p. 33. Garland Press.

79 FLAHERTY L. (1976) The Tla region of the mouse: identification of a new serologically defined locus, Qa-2. *Immunogenetics*, **3**, 533.

80 LYNES M.A., TONKONOGY S. & FLAHERTY L. (1982) Qa-1 and Qa-2 expression on CFU-s. *J. Immunol.* **129**, 928.

81 FORMAN J., TRIAL J., TONKONOGY S. & FLAHERTY L. (1982) The *Qa-2* subregion controls the expression of two antigens recognized by H-2 unrestricted cytotoxic T cells. *J. exp. Med.* **155**, 749.

82 FLAHERTY L., ZIMMERMAN D. & HANSEN T.H. (1978) Further serological analysis of the Qa antigens. Analysis of an anti-H-2.28 serum. *Immunogenetics*, **6**, 245.

83 HAMMERLING G., HAMMERLING U. & FLAHERTY L. (1979) Qat-4 and Qat-5, new murine T-cell antigens governed by the Tla region and identified by monoclonal antibodies. *J. exp. Med.* **150**, 108.

84 FLAHERTY L., KARL M. & REINISCH C.L. (1982) Syn-

geneic tumor immunizations produce Qa antibodies. Discovery of a new Qa antigen, Qa-6. *Immunogenetics*, **16**, 329.

85 DEMANT P. & ROOS M.H. (1982) Molecular heterogeneity of D-end products detected by anti-H-2.28 sera. (I) A molecule similar to Qa-2, detected in the BALB/cBy but not in the BALB/c-H-2^{dm2} mutant. *Immunogenetics*, **15**, 461.

86 GOLDBERG E., BOYSE E., BENNETT D., SCHEID M. & CARSWELL E. (1971) Serological demonstration of H-Y (male) antigen on mouse sperm. *Nature*, **232**, 478.

87 TAKEI F., GALFRE G., ALDERSON T., LENNOX E.S. & MILSTEIN C. (1980) H9/25 monoclonal antibody recognizes a new allospecificity of mouse lymphocyte subpopulations: strain and tissue distribution. *Eur. J. Immunol.* **10**, 241.

88 TAKEI F. (1982) Biochemical characterization of H9/25, an allospecificity encoded by the Ly-6 region. *Immunogenetics*, **16**, 201.

89 SHEN F.-W., VIAMONTES G. & BOYSE E.A. (1982) A system of alloantigens that selectively identified lymphnode lymphocytes. *Immunogenetics*, **15**, 17.

90 TONKONOGY S.L. & WINN H.J. (1977) Further genetic and serological analysis of the LyM-1 alloantigenic system. *Immunogenetics*, **5**, 57.

91 SATO H., KIMURA S. & ITAKURA K. (1981) Genetic and serologic re-evaluation of the LyM-1 antigen specified by a gene closely linked to Mls. Establishment of LyM-1 antigen of the mouse. *J. Immunol.* **8**, 27.

92 GLIMCHER L., SHEN F.-W. & CANTOR H. (1977) Identification of a cell-surface antigen selectively expressed on the natural killer cell. *J. exp. Med.* **145**, 1.

93 POLLACK S.B. & EMMONS S.L. (1982) NK-2.1: an NK-associated antigen detected with NZB anti-BALB/c serum. *J. Immunol.* **129**, 2277.

94 TAKAHASHI T., OLD L.J. & BOYSE E.A. (1970) Surface alloantigens of plasma cells. *J. exp. Med.* **131**, 1325.

95 TUNG J.-S., SHEN F.-W., BOYSE E.A. & FLEISSNER E. (1978) Properties of the PC-1 molecule. *Immunogenetics*, **6**, 101.

96 GODING J. & SHEN F.-W. (1982) Structure of the murine plasma cell alloantigen, PC.1: comparison with the receptor for transferrin. *J. Immunol.* **129**, 2636.

97 COLOMBATTI A., HUGHES L.N., TAYLOR B.A. & AUGUST J.T. (1981) The gene for a major cell surface glycoprotein of mouse macrophages and other phagocytic cells is located on chromosome 2. *Proc. natn. Acad. Sci. U.S.A.* **79**, 1926.

98 TROWBRIDGE I.S., LESLEY J., SCHULTE R., HYMAN R. & TROTTER J. (1982) Biochemical characterization and cellular distribution of a polymorphic, murine cell-surface glycoprotein expressed on lymphoid tissues. *Immunogenetics*, **15**, 299.

99 LESLEY J. & TROWBRIDGE I.S. (1982) Genetic characterization of a polymorphic murine cell-surface glycoprotein. *Immunogenetics*, **15**, 313.

100 SPURLL G.M. & OWEN F.L. (1981) A family of T-cell alloantigens linked to Igh-1. *Nature*, **293**, 742.

101 OWEN F.L., SPURLL G.M. & PANAGEAS E. (1982) Tthy^d, a new thymocyte alloantigen linked to Igh-1. Implications for a switch mechanism for T cell antigen receptors. *J. exp. Med.* **155**, 52.

102 OWEN F.L. (1982) Products of the IgT-C region of chromosome 12 are maturational markers for T cells. Sequence of appearance in immunocompetent T cells parallels ontogenetic appearance of Tthy^d, Tind^d, and Tsu^d. *J. exp. Med.* **156**, 703.

103 OWEN F.L., RIBLET R. & TAYLOR B.L. (1981) The T suppressor cell alloantigen Tsu^d maps near immunoglobulin allotype genes and may be a heavy chain constant-region marker on a T cell receptor. *J. exp. Med.* **153**, 801.

104 OWEN F.L. (1983) Tpre, a new alloantigen encoding in the IgT-C region of chromosome 12, is expressed on bone marrow of nude mice, fetal T cell hybrids, and fetal thymus. *J. exp. Med.* **157**, 419.

105 HORTON M.A. & HETHERINGTON C.M. (1980) Genetic linkage of Ly-6 and Thy-1 loci in the mouse. *Immunogenetics*, **11**, 521.

106 MERUELO D., OFFER M. & ROSSOMANDO A. (1982) Evidence for a major cluster of lymphocyte differentiation antigens on murine chromosome 2. *Proc. natn. Acad. Sci. U.S.A.* **79**, 7460.

107 MCKENZIE I.F.C. & POTTER T. (1979) Murine lymphocyte surface antigens. *Adv. Immunol.* **27**, 179.

Chapter 62
Overview: Lymphocyte responses

G. J. V. NOSSAL

The anatomical-
  descriptive era, 62.1
The era of lymphocyte
  biology, 62.2

The era of lymphocyte
  interaction: T cells
  regulate immune
  responses, 62.2

The molecular era of
  lymphocyte research, 62.3
Conclusions, 62.5

It is an exciting challenge to attempt an overview of the history and current directions of research dealing with lymphocyte responses, particularly as molecular genetics and protein chemistry are at last revealing the mysteries of the T lymphocyte receptor for antigen. One can discern four eras in lymphocyte research, each punctuated by major advances in knowledge, but illuminated by quite different perspectives.

The anatomical-descriptive era

The first era occupies approximately the first half of the twentieth century and is here termed the anatomical-descriptive era. The early giants of immunology, following Pasteur's work on immunization, all held firm theories about how immune protection was achieved by the body. The sometimes quite heated debates between proponents of the cellular and humoral theories are amusing in retrospect, but the theorizing that has best stood the test of time is undoubtedly Paul Ehrlich's, whose side-chain theory [1] to explain antibody production was the forerunner of the clonal selection hypothesis. Interestingly, the anatomic location of antibody production appeared not to interest Ehrlich a great deal, although as early as 1898, Pfeiffer & Marx [2] elegantly showed that the spleen was a major site of production of antibodies protective against cholera, and that lymph nodes and bone marrow also made significant contributions. Carrel & Ingebrigtsen [3] drove the notion that lymphoid tissues are important in antibody production a great deal further when they showed that spleens from immunized animals could form antibody in tissue culture. The special importance of lymph nodes draining the site of a subcutaneous injection was documented by McMaster & Hudack [4] in 1935. Up to this time, relatively little attention had been given to the question of which cell in these lymphoid organs actually made the antibodies. As the monocytes and macrophages were active in taking up antigens, many

workers came naturally to the view that they would subsequently make antibody, particularly after the direct template hypothesis of antibody production became popular.

Serious attempts to understand the histological changes accompanying immune responses were made on both sides of the Atlantic about the time of World War II. In the United States, a group in Philadelphia headed first by W.E. Ehrich and later by T.N. Harris contributed significantly. They showed that particulate antigens engendered a series of hypertrophic changes in lymph nodes, which included a marked outpouring of small lymphocytes into the efferent lymph, as well as enlargement of the lymphoid follicles [5]. When later experiments [6] showed that the cells of efferent lymph could form antibody *in vitro*, it was concluded that the lymphocyte was the antibody-producing cell. In Europe, in the meantime, the chief focus of interest was the plasma cell. Bing & Plum [7] showed that patients with hyperglobulinaemia had excessive numbers of plasma cells in their tissues, and Bjorneboe & Gormsen [8] drew attention to a marked and widespread increase in plasma cells in heavily immunized animals. A particularly influential study was that of Fagraeus [9]. She noted a developmental sequence occurring in the red pulp of the spleen following immunization, in which a large lymphoid blast cell was seen as giving rise to immature and then mature plasma cells. Splenic fragments derived from the red pulp formed far more antibody *in vitro* than did white pulp fragments. Fagraeus proposed that plasma cells, not lymphocytes, made antibody. Using differential centrifugation to enrich for splenic plasma cells, Thorbecke & Keuning confirmed this view [10].

The anatomical-descriptive era drew to a close with the development of the fluorescent antibody technique by Coons' group [11]. The ingenious 'sandwich' variant of this method, in which frozen sections of tissues from immunized animals were treated first with antigen and then with fluorescein-labelled antibody to that antigen, sheeted home the importance of the plasma cell series as the chief formers of antibody [12]. While the origin of plasma cells was highly controversial, Harris & Harris [13] came close to the truth in placing emphasis on lymphocytes as the best cells for adoptive transfer of immune responses to sublethally irradiated animals and, therefore, as the ancestors of the antibody-forming cells.

The era of lymphocyte biology

Cellular immunology became an independent discipline in the mid-1950s, and knowledge of lymphocyte biology grew rapidly over the next fifteen years. In 1955, Jerne [14] published his natural selection theory of antibody formation which Burnet [15] and Talmage [16] soon developed into the clonal selection theory. This saw the small lymphocyte as bearing cell surface recptors for antigen, the receptors themselves being antibody molecules, with each lymphocyte having only one receptor specificity. Lederberg and the author [17] were able to show that when an animal was immunized with two or three antigens, a single cell from the draining lymph node always formed only one antibody, and this 'one cell–one antibody' rule seemed consistent with clonal selection, though certainly not proving it. The idea of the small lymphocyte as an immunocompetent cell, capable of being activated by antigen, received a major boost from the work of Gowans [18], who showed that recirculating small lymphocytes from thoracic duct lymph could transform themselves into large, rapidly-dividing lymphoid blast cells upon stimulation with alloantigens. However, the demonstration of unique receptors on the lymphocyte surface had to wait quite a few years, until Naor & Sulitzeanu's [19] discovery that a tiny minority of lymphocytes from an unimmunized animal could bind a given radioactively-labelled antigen to their surface. It was soon discovered [20,21] that when such antigen-binding lymphocytes were removed or inactivated, immune responses to that antigen were selectively ablated. By the end of the 1960s, clonal selection was virtually universally accepted, although formal proof at the single cell level [22] only came in 1976.

It was certainly clear that lymphocyte responses fell into two broad groups, namely humoral responses leading to antibody production, and cell-mediated responses leading to a cellular immunity, of which delayed-type hypersensitivity was the prototype example. A major achievement of the lymphocyte biology era was the recognition that these two kinds of responses reflect the existence of two broad families of lymphocytes, namely B cells and T cells. But this insight did not come in one fell swoop; it evolved over nearly a decade. The drastic effects of neonatal thymectomy on later immune response capacity [23,24] focussed interest on the thymus as a source of immunocompetent cells. In the chicken, early removal of the bursa of Fabricius impeded later antibody formation [25], suggesting that the bursa was important in lymphocyte ontogeny; Szenberg & Warner [26] investigated the differential effects of ablation of the thymus and the bursa in the chick embryo. They found that there was a dissociation of responsiveness, with bursectomy impeding later antibody formation and thymectomy abolishing cellular responses. So each primary lymphoid organ produced a morphologically similar but functionally distinct lymphocyte population. Even though Möller [27] had introduced good immunofluorescent methods to identify cell membrane antigens in 1961, it was only at the end of the decade that Raff [28] demonstrated that B cells were characterized by possessing cell surface immunoglobulin, whereas T cells lacked this but possessed readily-demonstrable theta (Thy-1) antigen.

Many important methods were developed during this lymphocyte biology era. The haemolytic plaque technique for the study of antibody formation by single cells [29] made the study of antibody formation a much more quantitative science, and the ^{51}Cr-release method for the assay of cytotoxic T lymphocytes [30] had a parallel effect on cell-mediated immunity. The development of a reliable method for the initiation of a primary antibody response in tissue culture [31] also had a pivotal influence on the field. By the mid-1960s, lymphocyte biology was ready for the next paradigm shift.

The era of lymphocyte interaction: T cells regulate immune responses

No sooner had it become clear that lymphocytes fell into two major populations than the *interdependence* of the two lineages became manifest. Claman *et al.* [32] demonstrated that a given number of bone marrow cells gave only a low adoptive immune response. Thymus cells did not produce antibody on transfer. When the two populations were mixed and transferred, substantial antibody formation resulted. It soon became clear that, while B cells made antibody, T cells were required to exert a 'helper' effect [33,34]. Moreover, the helper T cell and the B cell being stimulated to antibody production recognized different portions of the same antigen molecule [35]. Interacting T cells and B cells by themselves were not enough to initiate immune responses; macrophages first had to 'present' antigen to the T cell to initiate the immunoproliferative cascade [36]. Furthermore, the regulatory effects of T cells were not only amplifying. In fact, a separate subset of suppressor T lymphocytes

[37] was shown to be at least equally important. These cells can powerfully down-regulate both humoral and cellular immune responses and are responsible for some forms of immunologic tolerance.

While the period 1966–1973 was chiefly devoted to sorting out the details of these regulatory cell interactions, a subtlety of the interaction process of an altogether different nature occupied cellular immunologists for the rest of the 1970s. This was the progressive unfolding of the role of the major histocompatibility complex (MHC) in lymphocyte interactions, crystallizing in the concept of MHC gene products as restriction elements and of the T cell somehow recognizing foreign antigen and 'self' MHC antigen in a combinatorial fashion. Several strands of research had to come together before the issue came into full focus. It was noted that antigen on macrophages will only stimulate T lymphocytes of the same MHC genotype [38]. Moreover, T cell–B cell collaboration requires the interacting cells to share MHC molecules [39,40]. Finally, cytotoxic T lymphocytes will kill antigen-bearing target cells only if killer and target share MHC determinants [41,42]. All of these findings are interpretable if one postulates that T lymphocytes effectively only 'see' antigen in combination with a 'self' MHC determinant. This requires either that the T cell receptor for antigen is so designed as to be able to recognize only foreign antigen in molecular association with an MHC antigen; or that T cells have two receptors, one for foreign antigen and one for self-MHC, both of which have to be engaged for effective recognition.

This era of research on regulatory mechanisms saw increasing emphasis placed on subsets of lymphocytes within the two great families. However, apart from the major subdivision of T cells into helper-inducer versus cytotoxic-suppressor categories, consensus has been difficult to reach. Efforts to sub-classify various categories of suppressor cells are ongoing, as are ways to divide B cells into sets, e.g. 'T-dependent' versus 'T-independent'. On the whole, the differentiation antigens available to characterize B cell subsets lag well behind those for T cell subsets, and monoclonal antibody reagents against the former are badly required.

Many aspects of immunoregulation are dealt with in much greater detail in the next major section of this volume. This will also amplify the immense value of cloned lines of T cells in lymphocyte research, addressed in some chapters of the present section.

The molecular era of lymphocyte research

During the 1980s, the recombinant DNA revolution struck lymphocyte biology with full force. We have now entered the molecular era of lymphocyte research, and are able to approach many of the key issues with new and sharper tools. Of the many exciting vistas opening up, three deserve special mention as particularly relevant to lymphocyte responses.

The T cell receptor

First, the T cell receptor for antigen is at last emerging from the fog. Several groups [e.g. 43–46] have identified a molecule of Mr ~ 80 000 with characteristics that make it an excellent candidate, namely: (1) it is clonally distributed, like the Ig receptors on B cells; (2) attaching specific ligands to the molecule can, depending on circumstances, block the capacity of antigen to activate the T cell, or activate the cell—this is akin to the various effects of anti-μ-immunoglobulin chain antibodies on B cells; (3) the molecule is electrophoretically heterogeneous, more so when derived from pooled T cell sources than from a monoclonal source; (4) the molecule consists of two disulphide-bonded subunits, i.e. two families of chains of Mr ~ 40 000, differing slightly from each other in pI and relative molecular mass.

Perhaps even more excitingly, in an unscheduled oral presentation to the Fifth International Congress of Immunology, which is in press at the time of writing, Dr. Mark Davis [47] presented evidence suggesting that the cDNA from messenger RNA of one of the two chains of the T cell receptor has been cloned through recombinant DNA technology. Three cDNA clones from a thymocyte library of this putative receptor chain showed that 600 nucleotides at the 3′ end were all the same in the three clones, whereas the 5′ regions were quite different. The imputed amino acid sequence implies intrachain disulphide bonds not unlike in position to those of Ig domains, though homology with Ig is only distant. Most importantly, the gene seems to be rearranging systematically and specifically in T cells, being in a different context there than in liver DNA. All of eight T cell hybridomas showed rearrangement whereas no B lymphoma did so. This is highly reminiscent of V-C joining in Ig genes.

All this progress suggests that knowledge of the T cell receptor, so crucial to an understanding of T cell responses, will now move very rapidly. However, substantial conceptual problems remain. Why is the receptor for the OKT3 monoclonal antibody a 'triggering' receptor and loosely associated (co-capping) with the clonotypic 'receptor' [48]? Why does anti-

Ly-2 antibody block the killer action of T cells? How does the Mr $\sim 80\,000$ clonotypic receptor relate to suppressor and helper factors alleged to possess I region *and* antigen-binding determinants? Above all, how does the new knowledge about the T cell receptor accommodate the phenomena of MHC restriction? These are enormous challenges for the student of T lymphocyte responses.

The enzymology and ontogeny of Ig gene rearrangement

While one generation of lymphocyte biologists gloats over the extraordinary discovery of the VDJC gene rearrangements inherent in clonal individuation of B cells and isotype switching, another generation is coming up fast and posing deep questions about how it all happens! It is clear that special enzymes are required to break the gene in such a specific manner and to re-anneal the join, and the enzymology is beginning to be addressed as a problem in its own right. This is important not only for an understanding of the generation of antibody diversity, but also of B lymphocyte malignancy. The consistent finding of a chromosomal translocation of the c-myc gene to the Ig gene in B lymphocyte malignancy (reviewed in ref. 49) indicates that the switch regions of Ig C genes represent a vulnerable point, at which things can at times go gravely wrong. The other question that will require to be fitted in is the ontogenetic organization of the whole process. On the other hand, it is now clear that VDJC joining for the μ heavy chain antedates both VJC joining for κ and λ light chains at the single cell level, and that these primary choices precede the appearance of cell surface receptors in the development of the pre-B cell clone. The antigenic universe, including self antigens, cannot influence the primary processes at work. Obviously, a receptorless repertoire cannot be influenced by antigen. What, then, assures a moderately even expression of the germ line v genes? If it is an entirely random process, must we not postulate a good deal of redundancy? If p = the total number of v-heavy genes and q = the total number of v $\kappa + \lambda$ genes, the number of B cells in which the primary rearrangement takes place must be considerably greater than pq for each v gene pair to be expressed combinatorially even once, and this does not take into account the further problems of multiple D and J genes. There are doubtless very important regulatory rules governing these processes during B lymphocyte ontogeny still waiting to be discovered.

Growth and differentiation factors for lymphocytes and the question of lymphocyte subsets

One of the most rapidly moving areas of research to be addressed later in this section, by Dr. M. Howard, is that of growth and differentiation factors for lymphocytes. The reason that this field is so crucial is that it stands at the crossroads of so many branches of immunobiology. We now know that growth and differentiation of tissues is under the control of complex families of hormone-like regulators and in the case of lymphocytes we face an interesting specialized issue. There are in fact two cascades of proliferation to be considered. First, there are the processes in primary lymphoid organs which generate the 'virgin' lymphocytes that then seed out to populate the secondary lymphoid organs. While these processes are similar in concept to those generating other formed elements of the blood, e.g. polymorphs or erythrocytes, they may nevertheless not be entirely antigen-independent, as encounters with self antigens are possible, and processes of repertoire purging or suppressor cell generation may well occur within this primary lymphoid compartment (reviewed in ref. 50). It is a pity to have to admit that we know virtually nothing about the molecular regulators of lymphoneogenesis, despite the enormous effort that has gone into the 'thymus hormone' field. Taking a line from molecular haematology, however, it seems certain that glycoprotein regulators of lymphoneogenesis do exist and are waiting to be discovered. The second cascade of immunoproliferation takes place when lymphocytes encounter antigens to which they must respond. Here we know much more, and are beginning to address both the MHC-restricted, antigen-specific cell interactions concerned, and the MHC-independent, antigen non-specific T cell- and accessory cell-derived molecular factors which are operative. The challenge here is threefold: to devise assay systems which genuinely define the cellular mechanisms and target cell populations operative for each factor of interest; to purify the various factors; and to generate large amounts of them by recombinant DNA technology, so that the cell biology and pharmacology could be more fully investigated.

T cell-derived factors will also help in the progressive definition of lymphocyte subsets. The author does not believe the question of the separate existence of 'T-dependent' versus 'T-independent' B cell lineages has been settled, and controversy continues to surround the question of whether 'T-independent' antigens can signal the B cell in the complete absence of accessory factors [51]. There do not yet exist the battery of monoclonal antibodies for B cell surface differentiation antigens corresponding to these which have materially increased our understanding of T cell subsets.

Finally, the field of lymphocyte growth factors requires to be integrated with that of haemopoietic malignancies. On the one hand, there is the possibility that cellular oncogenes are related to growth-regulatory molecules or to receptors for them; on the other, it could turn out that a crucial event in oncogenesis is the transcription and translation within a cell of the gene for its own growth factor [52]. From that point of view, we need to increase our knowledge not only of the factors, but also of specific receptors for them.

Conclusions

One of the most appealing things about science is that all of our most beautiful symphonies are unfinished ones. None of the eras described in this overview has ended. In the anatomical-descriptive area, we have to admit the depth of our ignorance concerning the functional meaning of much of the beautiful micro-anatomic architecture of lymphatic tissues. What do germinal centre B cells *really* do? What *is* a Hassal's corpuscle? What *does* control lymphocyte traffic flows within and amongst lymphoid organs? As we examine the other eras in turn, each will be found to bristle equally with challenges.

The *Handbook of Experimental Immunology* is much more than a collection of experimental recipes. It is also much more than a compendium of scholarly essays. In fact, it represents an attempt to link the world of experimental technologies in immunology with the world of biological concepts at the very margin of advancing knowledge. In the field of lymphocyte responses, this is very much what is needed, because there has been somewhat of a tendency for ideas and speculations to be based on methodology that is at best incomplete and at worst, sloppy. Cellular immunology is a field in which it is easy to publish papers, but difficult to prove a novel point with the finality that is required for it to enter definitively into the corpus of established knowledge. For this reason, most of the chapters in this section on lymphocyte responses have assay methods as a central concern. We are indebted to the authors who have themselves contributed to the methodological revolution and have summarized the 'state of the art' in nine overlapping areas. The challenge now is to do even better—to make the methods more and more precise so that cellular immunology gradually moves from its present status of an exciting, soft-edged field to one which compares favourably with biochemistry in its rigour and discipline.

Acknowledgements

The author's own contributions as summarized in this overview have been supported by the National Health and Medical Research Council, Canberra, Australia, and by Grant No. AI-03958 from the National Institute of Allergy and Infectious Diseases, U.S. Public Health Service. The help of many able colleagues and technicians at the Walter and Eliza Hall Institute is gratefully acknowledged.

References

1 EHRLICH P. (1900) On immunity with special reference to cell life (Croonian Lecture). *Proc. R. Soc.* Series B: Biological Sciences, **66**, 424.

2 PFEIFFER R. & MARX E. (1898) Die Bildungsstätte der Choleraschjutzstoffe. *Z. Hyg.* **27**, 272.

3 CARREL A. & INGEBRIGTSEN R. (1912) The production of antibodies by tissues living outside of the organism. *J. exp. Med.* **15**, 287.

4 MCMASTER P.D. & HUDACK S.S. (1935) The formation of agglutinins within lymph nodes. *J. exp. Med.* **61**, 783.

5 EHRICH W.E. & HARRIS T.N. (1942) The formation of antibodies in the popliteal lymph node in rabbits. *J. exp. Med.* **76**, 335.

6 HARRIS T.N., GRIMM E., MERTENS E. & EHRICH W.E. (1945) The role of the lymphocyte in antibody formation. *J. exp. Med.* **81**, 73.

7 BING J. & PLUM P. (1937) Serum proteins in leucopenia. *Acta med. scand.* **92**, 415.

8 BJORNEBOE M. & GORMSEN H. (1943) Experimental studies on the role of plasma cells as antibody producers. *Acta path. microbiol. scand.* **20**, 649.

9 FAGRAEUS A. (1948) The plasma cellular reaction and its relation to the formation of antibodies *in vitro*. *J. Immunol.* **58**, 1.

10 THORBECKE G.J. & KEUNING F.J. (1953) Antibody formation *in vitro* by haemopoietic organs after subcutaneous and intravenous immunization. *J. Immunol.* **70**, 129.

11 KAPLAN M.H., COONS A.H. & DEANE H.W. (1950) Localization of antigen in tissue cells, (III) Cellular distribution of pneumococcal polysaccharides Types II and III in the mouse. *J. exp. Med.* **91**, 15.

12 COONS A.H., LEDUC E.H. & CONNOLLY J.M. (1955) Studies on antibody production, (I) A method for the histochemical demonstration of specific antibody and its application to the study of the hyperimmune rabbit. *J. exp. Med.* **102**, 49.

13 HARRIS S. & HARRIS T.N. (1955) Studies on the transfer of lymph node cells (V) Transfer of cells incubated *in vitro* with suspensions of *Shigella paradysenteriae*. *J. Immunol.* **74**, 318.

14 JERNE N.K. (1955) The natural-selection theory of antibody formation. *Proc. natn. Acad. Sci. U.S.A.* **41**, 849.

15 BURNET F.M. (1957) A modification of Jerne's theory of antibody production using the concept of clonal selection. *Aust. J. Sci.* **20**, 67.

16 TALMAGE D.W. (1957) Allergy and immunology. *Ann. Rev. Med.* **8**, 239.

17 NOSSAL G.J.V. & LEDERBERG J. (1958) Antibody production by single cells. *Nature*, **181**, 1419.

18 GOWANS J.L. (1962) The fate of parental strain small lymphocytes in F_1 hybrid rats. *Ann. N.Y. Acad. Sci.* **99**, 432.

19 NAOR D. & SULITZEANU D. (1967) Binding of radioio-

dinated bovine serum albumin to mouse spleen cells. *Nature*, **214**, 687.

20 ADA G.L. & BYRT P. (1969) Specific inactivation of antigen-reactive cells with ^{125}I-labelled antigen. *Nature*, **222**, 1291.

21 WIGZELL H. & ANDERSSON B. (1969) Cell separation on antigen-coated columns. Elimination of high rate antibody-forming cells and immunological memory cells. *J. exp. Med.* **129**, 23.

22 NOSSAL G.J.V. & PIKE B.L. (1976) Single cell studies on the antibody-forming potential of fractionated, hapten-specific B lymphocytes. *Immunology*, **30**, 189.

23 MILLER J.F.A.P. (1961) Immunological function of the thymus. *Lancet*, **ii**, 748.

24 JANKOVIC B.D., WAKSMAN B.H. & ARNASON B.G. (1962) Role of the thymus in immune reactions in rats, (I) The immunologic response to bovine serum albumin in rats thymectomized or splenectomized at various times after birth. *J. exp. Med.* **116**, 159.

25 GLICK B., CHANG T.S. & JAAP R.G. (1956) The bursa of Fabricius and antibody production. *Poult. Sci.* **35**, 224.

26 SZENBERG A. & WARNER N.L. (1962) Dissociation of immunological responsiveness in fowls with a hormonally arrested development of lymphoid tissues. *Nature*, **194**, 146.

27 MÖLLER G. (1961) Demonstration of mouse isoantigens at the cellular level by the fluorescent antibody technique. *J. exp. Med.* **114**, 415.

28 RAFF M.C. (1970) Two distinct populations of peripheral lymphocytes in mice distinguishable by immunofluorescence. *Immunology*, **19**, 637.

29 JERNE N.K. & NORDIN A.A. (1963) Plaque formation in agar by single antibody-producing cells. *Science*, **140**, 405.

30 BRUNNER K.T. & CEROTTINI J.C. (1971) Cytotoxic lymphocytes as effector cells of cell-mediated immunity. *Prog. Immunol.* **1**, 385.

31 MISHELL R.I. & DUTTON R.W. (1967) Immunization of dissociated spleen cell cultures from normal mice. *J. exp. Med.* **126**, 423.

32 CLAMAN H.N., CHAPERON E.A. & TRIPLETT R.F. (1966) Thymus-marrow cell combination. Synergism in antibody production. *Proc. Soc. exp. Biol. Med.* **122**, 1167.

33 MILLER J.F.A.P. & MITCHELL G.F. (1968) Cell to cell interaction in the immune response, (I) Hemolysin-forming cells in neonatally thymectomized mice reconstituted with thymus or thoracic duct lymphocytes. *J. exp. Med.* **128**, 801.

34 NOSSAL G.J.V., CUNNINGHAM A., MITCHELL G.F. & MILLER J.F.A.P. (1968) Cell to cell interaction in the immune response, (III) Chromosomal marker analysis of single antibody-forming cells in reconstituted, irradiated or thymectomized mice. *J. exp. Med.* **128**, 839.

35 RAJEWSKY K., SCHIRRMACHER V., NASE S. & JERNE N.K. (1969) The requirement of more than one antigenic determinant for immunogenicity. *J. exp. Med.* **129**, 1131.

36 CHUSED T.M., KASSAN S.S. & MOSIER D.E. (1976) Macrophage requirement for the *in vitro* response to TNP Ficoll: a thymic independent antigen. *J. Immunol.* **116**, 1579.

37 GERSHON R.K. & KONDO K. (1971) Infectious immunological tolerance. *Immunology*, **21**, 903.

38 ROSENTHAL A.S. & SHEVACH E.M. (1973) Function of macrophages in antigen recognition by guinea pig T lymphocytes, (I) Requirement for histocompatible macrophages and lymphocytes. *J. exp. Med.* **138**, 1194.

39 KINDRED B. & LOOR F. (1974) Activity of host-derived T cells which differentiate in nude mice grafted with co-isogenic or allogeneic thymuses. *J. exp. Med.* **139**, 1215.

40 KATZ D.H., HAMAOKA T. & BENACERRAF B. (1973) Cell interactions between histoincompatible T and B lymphocytes, (II) Failure of physiologic cooperative interactions between T and B lymphocytes from allogeneic donor strains in humoral response to hapten–protein conjugates. *J. exp. Med.* **137**, 1405.

41 ZINKERNAGAL R.M. & DOHERTY P.C. (1974) Restriction of *in vitro* T cell-mediated cytotoxicity in lymphocytic choriomeningitis within a syngeneic or semiallogeneic system. *Nature*, **248**, 701.

42 SHEARER G.M. (1974) Cell-mediated cytotoxicity to trinitrophenyl-modified syngeneic lymphocytes. *Eur. J. Immunol.* **4**, 527.

43 ACUTO O., HUSSEY R.E., FITZGERALD K.A., PROTENTIS J.P., MEUER S.C., SCHLOSSMAN S.F. & REINHERZ E.L. (1983) The human T cell receptor: appearance in ontogeny and biochemical relationship of α and β subunits on IL-2 dependent clones and T cell tumors. *Cell*, **34**, 717.

44 KAPPLER J., KUBO R., HASKINS K., WHITE J. & MARRACK P. (1983) The mouse T cell receptor: comparison of MHC-restricted receptors on two T cell hybridomas. *Cell*, **34**, 727.

45 MCINTYRE B.W. & ALLISON J.P. (1983) The mouse T cell receptor: structural heterogeneity of molecules of normal T cells defined by xenoantiserum. *Cell*, **34**, 739.

46 WILDE D.B., MARRACK P., KAPPLER J., DIALYNAS D.P. & FITCH F.W. (1983) Evidence implicating L3T4 in class II MHC antigen reactivity: monoclonal antibody GK1.5 (Anti-L3T4a) blocks class II MHC antigen-specific proliferation, release of lymphokines, and binding by cloned murine helper T lymphocyte lines. *J. Immunol.* **131**, 2178.

47 DAVIS M. (1983) Unscheduled oral presentation to the Fifth International Congress of Immunology, Kyoto, Japan, August 1983.

48 MEUER S.C., HODGDON J.C., HUSSEY R.E., PROTENTIS J.P., SCHLOSSMAN S.F. & REINHERZ E.L. (1983) Antigen-like effects of monoclonal antibodies directed at receptors on human T cell clones. *J. exp. Med.* **158**, 988.

49 CORY S. (1983) Oncogenes and B lymphocyte neoplasia. *Immunology Today*, **4**, 205.

50 NOSSAL G.J.V. (1983) Cellular mechanisms of immunological tolerance. *Ann. Rev. Immunol.* **1**, 33.

51 PIKE B.L. & NOSSAL G.J.V. (1984) A reappraisal of 'T-independent' antigens, (I) Effect of lymphokines on the response of single adult hapten-specific B lymphocytes. *J. Immunol.* **132**.

52 SCHRADER J.W. & CRAPPER R.M. (1983) Autogenous production of a hemopoietic growth factor, persisting-cell-stimulating factor, as a mechanism for transformation of bone marrow-derived cells. *Proc. natn. Acad. Sci. U.S.A.* **80**, 6892.

Chapter 63
Lymphocyte responses to polyclonal B and T cell activators

EVA SEVERINSON & EVA-LOTTA LARSSON

Polyclonal B cell activators, 63.1   Polyclonal T cell activators, 63.8   Media, 63.15

Polyclonal activators (PA) are widely used as agents to activate T and B lymphocytes [1–3]. When it was established that lymphocytes could be separated into T and B cells, it was discovered that phytohaemagglutinin (PHA) and concanavalin A (con A) stimulated T cells [4,5], whereas lipopolysaccharide (LPS) stimulated B cells [5]. At that time, proliferation was primarily studied and measured by induction of DNA synthesis. An important finding was that LPS, con A, and PHA also induced effector functions [6–9]. The discovery that the cellular requirements for mitogen-induced responses were similar to those of antigen-specific induction [10,11] and the later identification of various lymphokines [11,12] led a step further and reinforced the notion that PA are appropriate model systems to study lymphocyte function.

Today, polyclonal activation is one of the most important systems used to study the mechanisms of activation, growth, and maturation of lymphocytes. The reason for this is mainly that it is easier to study activation of a large lymphocyte population than that of rare antigen specific cells. Most likely, the cellular mechanisms of lymphocyte stimulation are the same in specific and polyclonal responses. Furthermore, culture techniques have improved with time, and they are now simple and reproducible. Finally, the development of assays which measure effector functions non-specifically have further advanced the field.

By definition, PA stimulate B or T cells of many different specificities [13]. PA normally induce both proliferation and maturation to effector function, but there are exceptions to this rule. For example, anti-Ig have been reported to induce DNA synthesis, without inducing Ig secretion in B cells [14].

Some years ago, it was thought that PA stimulated lymphocytes independent of cell co-operation. This opinion has now been modified. Con A, for example, induces secretion of lymphokines, which in turn activate other cells [15]. Lymphokines can be called PA, although unlike classical PA, most of them do not activate uncommitted lymphocytes, but act on already PA- or antigen-experienced cells. Whether or not lymphokines are PA is in essence a question of semantics.

In this chapter, the authors describe methods for lymphocyte activation by PA. They deal with the most current and widely used methods, and only briefly comment on older methods; they deal separately with T and B cell activators, and focus on the most commonly used activators. As the authors' experience is mainly confined to murine systems, they make only brief mention of the experimental use of PA in man.

Polyclonal B cell activators

A list of widely used polyclonal B cell activators (PBA) is given in Table 63.1. The PBA are grouped into three categories depending on whether they activate murine lymphocytes, at high or low cell density, or human peripheral blood lymphocytes. For each PBA, the standard concentration range and references are also indicated.

The question of cell density deserves a comment, because it is decisive on what type of response will be achieved. Most cell types which proliferate in culture stop dividing at a particular cell density. A number of factors dictate when saturation density is reached, such as the amount of fetal calf serum (FCS) in the culture medium. Furthermore, different cell types may also have inherent differences regarding their saturation density. During activation, B cells gradually differentiate and eventually start to secrete IgM; and thereafter, they switch to other Ig classes. These events are highly dependent on proliferation.

The high cell density cultures ($2{-}10 \times 10^6$ cells/ml) only permit limited cell proliferation, because the cells are cultured at concentrations above the saturation density. Therefore this culture system will give results that differ from those obtained with the low cell density cultures exposed to the same PBA. For example, the responses reach their maxima early, and activation leads to secretion of IgM only.

Table 63.1. Common polyclonal B cell activators

PBA	Source	Recommended concentration (μg/ml)	References
	High cell density cultures of murine lymphocytes		
Lipopolysaccharide (LPS)	*Escherichia coli, Salmonella*	10–100	[5,6,16]
Lipoprotein (LP)	*E. coli*	1–50	[17]
Dextran sulphate (DxS)	*Leuconostoc mesenteroides*	50–250	[18,19]
Purified protein derivative (PPD)	*Mycobacterium tuberculosis*	100–200	[20,21]
Dextran	*L. mesenteroides*	1000–2000	[19]
Anti-Ig	Rabbit, goat		[22,23]
Nocardia water-soluble mitogen (NWSM)	*Nocardia opaca*	1–100	[24]
	Low cell density cultures of murine lymphocytes		
LPS	*E. coli*	10–100	[25]
LP	*E. coli*	1–50	[26]
NWSM	*N. opaca*	50	[27]
T helper cells	Mouse	—	[28]
	Cultures of human peripheral blood lymphocytes		
Pokeweed mitogen (PWM)	*Phytolacca americana*	1–80	[29]
Epstein-Barr virus (EBV)	Marmoset EBV-infected cell line	—	[30]
Cowan strain I bacteria	*Staphylococcus aureus*	$1–20 \times 10^{6}$*	[31]
NWSM	*N. opaca*	10–100	[32]

* Number of organisms.

The low cell density culture system (i.e. 5×10^5 cells/ml or lower) is the most often employed system for activation with PBA, because it closely resembles *in vivo* activation with antigen, in the sense that cells proliferate extensively, secrete IgM and switch to IgG secretion. As opposed to the high cell density system, this system requires the presence of 2-mercaptoethanol (2-ME) and high concentrations of FCS.

Some PBA will activate murine B cells only in high cell density cultures, for unknown reasons. Among these are PPD (purified protein derivative of *Mycobacterium tuberculosis*) and dextran of high relative molecular mass from *Leuconostoc mesenteroides*. The PBA activity of dextran is poor unless added at high concentrations (more than 1 mg/ml). Dextran sulphate (DxS) is normally a good mitogen in high cell density cultures, i.e. it induces DNA synthesis, but it activates IgM secretion poorly [21]. In many respects, DxS is different from the other PBA. For example, it has a much more marked dependence on adherent cells than the other PBA [33]. Furthermore, the optimal concentration of DxS is related to the cell concentration in culture, whereas this is not the case with other PBA (Eva Severinson, unpublished observation). Moreover, it can act synergistically with both PBA and polyclonal T cell activators [18,34]. There are a number of polyanions with similar properties as DxS

[18]. However, since they are used rarely, they are not included in Table 63.1.

The prototype PBA in low cell density cultures is LPS. Lipoprotein (LP) from *Escherichia coli* or *Nocardia* water-soluble mitogen (NWSM) both act as LPS in low cell density cultures, except that they can also activate B cells from the LPS low responder mouse strains, C3H/HeJ and C57BL.10/ScCr. Although DxS alone is only weakly active at low cell density, it gives a strong synergistic effect together with LPS or LP [35]. Soluble, purified goat anti-mouse IgM, or Sepharose-bound anti-Ig are mitogens with little or no ability to induce Ig secretion. Cultures of enriched T cells or cloned T cell lines, which react specifically with cell surface antigens on the responding B cells and adherent cells, can activate B cells to proliferation, and IgM and IgG secretion, to a level comparable with activation caused by LPS.

The authors will not discuss high cell density cultures further. The interested reader will find references in Table 64.1. They will concentrate instead on the basic method for activation of mouse spleen cells with lipopolysaccharide (LPS) in low cell density cultures.

Method for activation of mouse spleen cells with LPS in low cell density cultures

Equipment

Sterile hood.
Incubator with 100% humidity, set at 5% CO_2 and 37 °C.
Light microscope.
Inverted microscope.
Centrifuge.
Tools (sterilized scissors and forceps).
Sterile pipettes and Pasteur pipettes (cotton plugged).
Hamilton syringe for 10–20 μl aliquots.
Multichannel pipette with sterile tips (Flow Laboratories Ltd., PO Box 17, Irvine, Scotland KA12 8NB, UK).
Sterile tubes, Petri dishes and flasks.
Microculture plates.

A good incubator is important and should keep constant temperature and CO_2 level. Furthermore, it should re-equilibrate quickly after the doors have been opened. The humidity should be as close to saturation as possible. This is very important when microculture plates or other vessels with small culture volumes are used.

The kind of culture vessels to be used depends on how many cells are needed for the experiment. Microcultures plates are suitable for measuring DNA synthesis or plaque forming cells. Alternative culture vessels are Terasaki plates for 10–20 μl volumes, Linbro cultures for 1–2 ml cultures, tissue culture flasks for 5–10 ml, 30–100 ml or 200–300 ml, respectively, of culture fluid. Flasks should be incubated flat, with the tops loose to permit CO_2 entry. Activation of cell with PBA can be done with all these vessels, provided the cell number/ml of culture fluid and the density of cells per cm^2 of the bottom of the culture vessel is kept constant. Tissue culture plastics can be bought from many different producers. The brands tried all work equally well for cultures with PA.

Materials

Balanced salt solution (BSS).
Trypan blue.
RPMI 1640 + L-gln, penicillin/streptomycin, and 2ME.
FCS.
LPS (Difco Laboratories, Detroit, MI, U.S.A.), stock solution at 0.2–10 mg/ml in BSS.
Mouse spleens.

The stock concentration of LPS (or other PBA to be tested) depends on the concentration to be used in the assay. A number of different mouse strains can be used, e.g. C57BL.10, C3H/Tif or CBA. These and many other strains are high responders to LPS. However, C3H/HeJ, C57BL.10/ScCr, CBA/N, SJL or SJA should not be used. The first two are non-responders to LPS [20,36], and cells from CBA/N respond poorly to all PBA in low cell density cultures (Eva Severinson & Carmen Fernandez, unpublished observation). SJL and SJA respond poorly to LPS in low cell density cultures (Eva Severinson, unpublished observation).

Culture procedure

A single cell suspension of the spleens is made, clumps are allowed to sediment in a 10 ml tube and the remaining suspension transferred to a 50 ml tube. During this procedure, the cells should be kept on ice. Thereafter, the cells are washed 2–4 times in BSS in the cold. Extensive washing often improves the results, but cells are lost in each centrifugation. After the last centrifugation, the cells are resuspended in 5–10 ml BSS, and the viable nucleated cells counted by trypan blue exclusion. The cells should be kept on ice in BSS until they are ready for culturing.

Aliquot the PBA or the same amount of BSS to control cultures. The PBA should preferably be added in not higher than one-tenth of the total culture volume. Thus, in microcultures with 0.2 ml of total volume per well, the PBA should be added in 10–20 μl aliquots. Hamilton pipettes are suitable and can be kept sterile by storing and rinsing them in 70% ethyl alcohol. Before and after use, they should be washed extensively in sterile BSS. For culture vessels which contain 1 ml or more, normal pipettes can be used to aliquot the PBA. When Terasaki cultures are used, it is advisable to dilute the PBA directly into the complete medium together with the cells. For each test-group and test-day, 3–5 cultures should be set up. When several concentrations of PBA are used, the lowest concentration should be added first. Generally, the amount of PBA used is expressed as weight per volume in the cultures, independent of the volumes of the vessels or the cell density. It is concentration rather than the total amount of PBA that determines the response. If the incubator has a low humidity, it is advisable not to use the outer wells of the microplates for cell cultures, but rather to fill them with sterile water or BSS.

The medium is prepared as indicated in the media section and the FCS (5–15% depending on the experiment, see below) is added. It is essential that the medium has a proper pH when the cells are added. Therefore it should be kept in a bottle with a closed lid. If the pH has increased, due to contact with air, place the medium in a 5% CO_2 environment until the desired pH has been reached. For the same reason, the cells should be kept in a non-carbonate-buffered solution like BSS, until they are ready to be distributed into the cultures. The cells are diluted in the complete medium to $3–4 \times 10^5$ cells/ml, for LPS-induced responses, or other cell concentrations depending on the PBA used. When a new PBA is tested, it is advisable to culture several different concentrations of the cells, diluted two- to threefold between each step. Aliquot 0.2 ml of the cell suspension into each microculture well. A normal 1 ml pipette can be used, but it is faster with a multichannel pipette with sterile tips. Quick handling of the cells diluted in medium is essential since cell death is very rapid at low cell concentrations. Place the culture plates in the incubator as soon as possible.

Notes and recommendations

The inverted microscope is very useful for screening cultures. If this is done routinely, the experimenter gets a fair impression of the cultures' comfort and infected or otherwise poor cultures can be discarded, without having to test them. Since there is inevitably a certain variability in lymphocyte responses, microscopic screening may tell for example when the peak of proliferation has occurred (or will occur) and thus, at what day it is best to test the cultures.

The typical morphological events that can be detected by daily screenings of standard LPS-induced cultures are the following. After one day of culture, the first blast cells appear, and there are signs of cells dividing, i.e. pairs of cells close together. The numbers of cells have also decreased after the first day. By day two, the blasts are more numerous and there is a tendency for big clumps of cells to form. Between days 2 and 5 there is a marked increase in the total number of cells and huge clumps of cells have developed. By now, the majority of the cells are blasts. Later, cell death becomes obvious, unless the cells are subcultured (see below).

The percentage of FCS to be used depends on the type of response and the day of assay. High cell density cultures are less dependent of fetal calf serum [13] than low cell density cultures. In the latter system, 5–10% FCS is sufficient when assaying DNA synthesis or IgM secretion measured on or before day 4. For measurements of IgG responses on day 5 or later, 15% or more is required [26].

As mentioned previously, the optimal cell density may vary considerably, depending on the PBA used. Among other things this depends on the proportion of cells which can be activated by the particular PA used. Thus when only a small fraction of the cells can be activated, the cell density should be higher. Contrariwise, when a large part of the cells are stimulated, the cell density should be lower. The higher the cell density, the earlier is the maximum response achieved [26]. Some PBA act synergistically, e.g. LPS and DxS, and together they can activate about 80% of the splenic B cells, whereas LPS or DxS alone activate less than 25% or 5%, respectively, in the same system [37]. Thus with LPS plus DxS at least a fourfold lower cell concentration can be used as compared to LPS alone. The optimal cell density is generally the one where the response is highest per number of input cells and which allows cell proliferation for a longer time. At suboptimal cell concentrations, the response may rapidly drop to zero [38].

In many systems, it is necessary to work with purified B cells. Suitable purification methods are described in detail elsewhere in this book. We recommend procedures where both positive and negative selections for B cells are performed. For example, as a first step, macrophage-like cells are removed by adherence to glass or plastic, or by filtering the cell suspension through Sephadex G-10 beads [39]. This is followed by a positive selection like 'panning' to enrich for B cells, i.e. adherence of Ig positive cells to anti-Ig coated Petri dishes [40]. This method works well provided the anti-Ig does not inhibit PBA responses. The best source of anti-Ig is a monoclonal antibody of the IgM class. After selection of B cells through panning, the remaining contaminating T cells are removed by antibody- (anti-Thy-1 or anti-Lyt-1 and anti-Lyt-2) and complement-mediated killing. This three-step procedure may result in a partial or complete loss of the response, depending on which PBA is used. For example, both anti-Ig- and LPS-induced responses are considerably reduced when using extensively purified B cells [41,42].

Thus this system can be used to asses whether a PBA response depends on accessory cells. This is done by comparing the responses of purified B cells and whole spleen cells at several different cell concentrations. If the response is lost more rapidly with decreasing concentration of pure B cells as compared to unseparated spleen cells, the system is likely to be accessory cell-dependent. Restoration of the response can then be tested by addition of various accessory cells and/or lymphokines [41,42].

Activation of mouse cells with PBA have been used in a number of systems, which in essence are based on the same principles as the low cell density system described above. A summary of these methods indicating references and applications is given in Table 63.2.

Table 63.2. Different culture methods for PBA induced responses

Method	PBA	Application	References
Limiting dilutions using thymocytes as filler cells	LPS	Frequency of responding cells	[43]
Limiting dilutions using tumour cells as filler cells	LPS + anti-Ig + T cell supernatants	Frequency of responding cells	[44]
Single cell cultures	LPS + DxS	Frequency of responding cells	[37]
Colony formation in agar	LPS	Frequency of responding cells	[45,46]
Repeated subculture	LPS, LPS + DxS	Study of activation for a prolonged time	[35,47]
Polyclonal activation with T-helper cells	T cells, T cells + anti-Ig	Study of the mechanism of thymus-dependent responses	[28,48,49]
Activation with PBA + antigen	LPS LPS + T cell supernatants	Study of the mechanism of antigen induced responses	[50,51]
B cell growth factor assays	LPS, anti-Ig	Study of induction of B cell proliferation	[41,52]
B cell maturation factor assays	LPS	Study of induction to IgM secretion	[52]
B cell differentiation factor assays	LPS	Study of induction to IgG secretion	[53]

Measuring the response: proliferation

^{3}H-thymidine uptake

The degree of proliferation can be determined in a number of different ways. The most common is measurement of ^{3}H-thymidine uptake (for the detailed method, see below under polyclonal T cell activators). It is a reliable and rapid method. Short pulses with ^{3}H-thymidine should be avoided, since there is a risk of measuring the uptake in the cytoplasm and equilibration of the nuclear pool of thymidine may take several hours. Twelve-to 24-hour pulses are normally used. It is essential to determine that sufficient thymidine is present during the pulse. Usually, the tritiated thymidine is mixed with cold thymidine for this purpose. The stock solution is prepared as follows. One bottle of methyl-^{3}H-thymidine (The Radiochemical Centre, Amersham, England; TRA 120; specific activity 5 Ci/mmol), with 5 mCi in 5 ml, is mixed with 7.5 ml cold thymidine at 50 μg/ml and 50 ml BSS. This mixture is aliquoted and kept at -20 °C. For the assay, the stock solution is diluted four-fold in BSS and 20 μl added per microculture. The specific activity is thus 2 Ci/mmol, and 0.4 μCi is added per culture.

Cell counts

Another method of determining the rate of proliferation is simply to count the cells at different times after culture and to record the increase in cell numbers. In Fig. 63.1, a proliferation curve for the LPS response is shown. During the first two days there is a drop in cell number, which is normally seen with low cell density cultures. Thereafter, the numbers of cells steadily increase up to day 5. In control cultures without PBA, there is no increase in cell numbers and the cultured

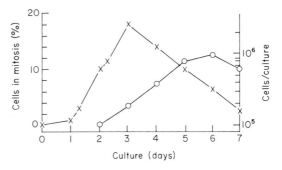

Fig. 63.1. Mitotic activity of LPS-activated cells cultured at 4×10^5 cells/ml with 1.5 ml/culture. Cultures were pulsed with 0.1 μg/ml of colcemid for 2 h at different times and the relative percentage of cells in mitosis was estimated ($\times$). The values represent the mean of duplicate slides. The number of viable cells were determined by trypan blue exclusion ($\bigcirc$). The values represent the mean of four experiments. Reprinted from ref. 54, with permission from the editor of *Journal of Immunology*.

cells die rapidly. To compare the numbers of cells in cultures containing PBA with unstimulated cultures can thus be a good measurement of the PBA-induced proliferation.

Mitotic index

Fig. 63.1 also shows the mitotic index, i.e. the percentage of cells which enter mitosis after a two-hour pulse with the mitosis-inhibiting drug, colcemid. This method shows the proliferative capacity of the individual cells. As shown in Fig. 63.1, the proliferation capacity was highest on day 3, when (by extrapolation) close to 100% of the cells were actively proliferating. Although an increase in cell numbers was observed later than day 3, the cells were dividing at a slower rate or fewer cells were dividing at this time.

Prolonged proliferation after subculture

The cells stop dividing at the end of the culture period because they lack nutrients in the medium and/or they reach saturation density. Longer time periods can be studied if the cells are recultured at lower cell concentrations in fresh medium and PBA [35]. An example of this is shown in Fig. 63.2 in which the proliferation induced by LPS + DxS was studied. The cells were allowed to grow until they reached saturation density, which in this experiment usually occurred 2–4 days after initiation of the cultures. At this time the cells were washed and recultured in new medium containing the PBA. As shown in Fig. 63.2, the cells responded by vigorous growth the first time they were cultured and also after the two subsequent times. After the third

reculturing, there was a rapid cell loss the first day of culture, but the remaining cells could continue growing. At the fourth reculturing, the cells were unable to proliferate further. Such prolonged proliferation can also be obtained when cells are activated by LPS only [47] and probably also other PBA which induce a response in low cell density cultures. It is important to subculture the cells at the time they reach saturation density. When this occurs has to be determined in each case, since it depends on the PBA and the initial cell concentration.

Measuring the response: Ig secretion

Cells secreting Ig *in vitro* can be detected by measuring Ig in the supernatants, as cells containing Ig as determined by fluorescence techniques or as plaque forming cells. The methods will not be described in detail, since they are dealt with elsewhere in this book; the authors will only give their view on the possibilities of using them in the context of PBA activation.

Ig in culture supernatants

Suitable methods for detecting Ig in supernatants are radioimmunoassays and enzyme-linked immunosorbent assays (ELISA) (see Chapters 26 and 27). These two techniques are sensitive and can be used to detect even the small amounts of Ig present in the culture supernatants. In cloning or limiting dilution assays, this may be a superior method, since one can measure Ig accumulated over a long period of time, whereas another method, like the plaque assay, would demand that the cultures were assayed on the optimal day of

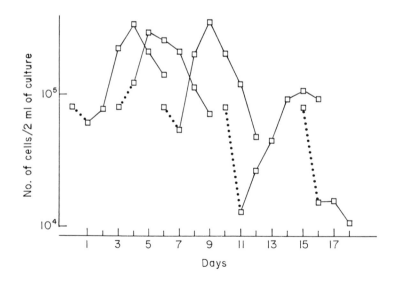

Fig. 63.2. The proliferative activity of cells activated by LPS + DxS. Eight × 10^5 spleen cells were cultured with PBA in 2 ml of medium. On days 3, 6, 10, and 15, the cells were washed and recultured at 8 × 10^5 cells/2 ml in newly prepared medium and PBA. On each day of culture, cells were washed and viable cells counted by trypan blue exclusion.

the response. A disadvantage with the radioimmunoassay and ELISA is that it can be difficult to achieve the low background levels which are required for successful interpretation of the test. However, the use of monoclonal antibodies may avoid these problems.

Intracytoplasmic staining

The method for detecting intracellular Ig, using fluorochrome conjugated antisera, is normally used to determine secreting cells, although non-secreting Ig-containing cells (i.e. B cell precursors) can also be detected. This method has a lower threshold of sensitivity than the plaque assay, but the background fluorescence may sometimes be disturbing and can make it difficult to distinguish a negative from a weakly positive cell. A clear advantage with this technique, as opposed to plaque assays, is that all sources of antisera can be used, e.g. monoclonal antibodies, provided they can be coupled to the fluorochrome. Furthermore, the technique allows detection of cells producing two different isotypes, by the use of two fluorochromes with different emission spectra.

Plaque assays

There are two non-specific plaque assays: the reverse plaque assay using anti-Ig coated red cells as targets [55], and the protein A plaque assay employing staphylococcal protein A coupled to erythrocytes [56] (see also Chapter 64). Both these methods need developing antisera to detect plaques. The antisera should be complement-fixing and in the latter method they should also be able to bind protein A. The assays seem to be equally sensitive.

When cultured cells are to be assayed in a plaque assay, they have to be washed in BSS to remove Ig present in the culture supernatants, which otherwise will be inhibitory. The cells should be diluted so that there will be 50–200 plaques per sample. Since there is often quite a high number of secreting cells in cultures activated by PBA, extensive dilution may be necessary. This dilution step should be done immediately before plaquing, since the cells tend to die very fast at these extreme dilutions.

Fig. 63.3 shows the kinetics of the LPS-induced IgM and IgG response as measured in the protein A plaque assay. The IgM response generally appears earlier than the IgG response. Furthermore, the kinetics for induction of IgM- and IgG-secreting cells are often different from each other, in that the IgM response increase at a slower rate than the IgG response. The rapid kinetics is a characteristic of the IgG response.

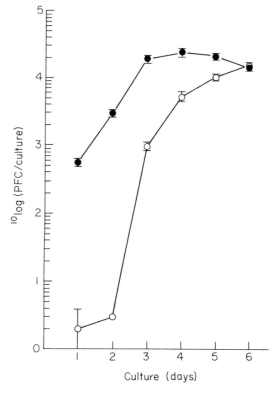

Fig. 63.3. IgM and IgG secreting cells induced by LPS. Three $\times 10^5$ cells/ml/culture were stimulated by LPS. Each day, cultures were assayed for the numbers of IgM- and IgG-secreting cells, using the protein A plaque assay. Each point represents the geometrical mean $\pm$ S.D. of triplicates. ● IgM PFC; ○ IgG PFC. Reprinted from ref. 57, with permission from the editor of *Journal of Immunology*.

Ig responses are not induced in cultures without PBA, unless a fetal calf serum which in itself has PBA activity is used (see media section). Furthermore, the Ig secreting cells present in the normal spleen tend to die rapidly after culturing.

Two major subclasses of IgG appear after *in vitro* activation of murine cells with LPS, i.e. IgG2b and IgG3. LP, NWSM, and the combination LPS plus DxS, give similar subclass patterns [27,28,35]. Polyclonal activation of B cells with helper T cells, on the other hand, gives rise to an IgG response consisting mostly of the IgG1 subclass, while little or no IgG3 is formed [28].

How to express the results

As already mentioned, the low cell density culture system allows for exponential growth over a limited period of time. The responses are logarithmic and not linear, and whenever possible, logarithmic scales should be used. Likewise, the results should not be represented by the stimulation index (i.e. the ratio of the activity in cultures with PBS over the activity in the background cultures). The background activity, e.g. spontaneous DNA synthesis, is generally not related to the activity induced by a stimulant. When the background activity is disturbing for the reader, net responses (i.e. backgrounds subtracted) can be shown instead.

When studying PBA-induced responses it is important to first perform complete kinetics experiments, in order to be able to determine the time of exponential rise and the peak of the response. When that has been done, one can choose to assay on one or two points during the exponential phase of the response. In general, it is more important to determine an increased response over time than to record the response at the peak of activity.

Activation of B cells from human

PBA can stimulate B cells from a number of species other than mouse, e.g. monkey, rabbit, rat, guinea-pig, and human. The same basic principles as used for activation of mouse cells are valid here, although little work has been published on activation of cells from other species, with the exception of human peripheral blood lymphocytes.

Most PBA seem to be more T cell dependent in man as compared to mouse, with the sole exception of Epstein-Barr virus (EBV). The most commonly used PBA in man are pokeweed mitogen (PWM, which is primarily a polyclonal T cell activator), protein A or whole *Staphylococcus aureus* bacteria, and EBV. LPS is normally not a particularly active PBA, although it has been found to induce a high response in adherent cell depleted peripheral blood lymphocytes. Addition of adherent cells suppressed this response [58].

Activation of human peripheral blood lymphocytes by PBA has mostly been performed with a relatively high density of cells, i.e. 1×10^6 cell/ml or more. Human AB serum of FCS are both common serum sources. 2-ME is often not included in the medium, at least when AB serum is used. It may not be necessary, since a relatively high cell density is used. Alternatively, the human AB serum may contain molecules which perform the same function as 2-ME. It has been found that adherent cell depleted peripheral blood lymphocytes respond better to LPS when 2-ME is present in FCS containing medium [58]. Thus 2-ME can at least sometimes potentiate the response of human lymphocytes.

As opposed to the murine system, the IgM and the IgG responses of human cells seem to appear with similar kinetics and, furthermore, IgA responses are also obtained [59].

A more extensive description of PBA activation of human cells can be found in a review article by Waldner & Broder [59], and in the book *Human B-Lymphocyte Function. Activation and Immunoregulation* (eds. Fauci A.S. & Ballieux R.E.), [60].

Polyclonal T cell activators

Lectin-induced T lymphocyte responses have been extensively studied during the last few years. This experimental approach is largely responsible for the rapid progress in the understanding of the mechanisms underlying T lymphocyte activation and subsequent responses [15].

Lectins are non-enzymatic, non-antibody, sugar-binding proteins (or glycoproteins) isolated from several plant genera and some invertebrates, with variable cell agglutinating properties. A limited number of lectins are mitogenic for T cells of which some of the most commonly used are listed in Table 63.3 [61]. The most extensively characterized lectin is concanavalin A (con A) which has high specificity for the sugar α-methyl-D-mannoside (α-MM).

It was believed at first that lectins would exert a direct activating effect on T lymphocytes by merely binding to cell surface glycoproteins [62]. However, the demonstration that lectin-induced T cell activation required the participation of specialized accessory cells [11], as well as the finding that soluble mediators with growth promoting activity were released in lectin stimulated cultures lead to the notion, and later the conviction, that these responses involved complex cellular interactions, similar to those required for antigen-specific responses. The biological significance of growth factors was given relevance when it became evident that such factors, and *not* the lectins themselves, were the 'physiological mitogens' for lymphocytes [12,63]. On the other hand, the discovery that T cell growth factors (TCGF) had no effect on resting, non-induced T cells demonstrated that mitogenic lectins not only induce production of TCGF but also render resting T cells susceptible to the growth promoting activity of TCGF produced *in situ* [64,65]. It is now established that lectin-induced proliferation reflects TCGF-dependent expansion of TCGF reactive T cells. Although T cell mitogenic lectins bind to specific sugar residues that are more or less equally represented on *all* T lymphocytes membranes (and on non-T cells for that matter), they appear to activate exclusively T cells and to exert different effects depending on the T cell subset.

The methods used to analyse the different events comprising lectin-induced T cell activation will be presented herein. The various assays described are restricted to the analysis of lectin-induced T cell activation in the mouse, mainly using con A as the inducing ligand. The principles are, however, applicable to other T cell lectins and other species.

Methods for preparation of various cell populations and description of assay systems

Equipment

Same as listed above.

Materials

Balanced salt solution (BSS pH 7.2).
RPMI 1640 + HEPES, 2-ME, L-gln, penicillin-streptomycin.
FCS.
Concanavalin A (con A; Pharmacia Fine Chemicals, Uppsala, Sweden).
Phytohaemagglutinin (PHA; Difco).
Leukoagglutinin (LA; Pharmacia).
α-Methyl-D-mannoside (α-MM; Sigma Chemical Co., P.O. Box 14508, St. Louis, MO 63178, U.S.A.).
Phorbol myristic acid (PMA; Sigma).
Sephadex G-10 (Pharmacia).
Ficoll-Isopaque (Pharmacia).
Nylon wool.
Rabbit complement (C′).
^{3}H-thymidine (Amersham Radiochemical Centre 2 Ci/mmol).
^{14}C-thymidine (Amersham Radiochemical Centre 56 mCi/mmol).
^{51}Cr (Na$_2$CrO$_4$ specific activity 362 mCi/mg; CEA Laboratoire de Produits Biomedicaux B.P. 21, 91190 Gif sur Yvette, France).

Normal and T cell enriched spleen cells

Single cell suspensions from spleens are prepared by gentle teasing of the tissue fragments with forceps and then collecting the cells in BSS. Cell aggregates are removed by a 3-min, 1-g sedimentation and the non-sedimented cells are pelleted and washed twice in BSS. The cells are subsequently resuspended in culture medium and viable cells are counted by trypan blue exclusion. Such spleen cells are then enriched for T cells by passage over nylon wool columns [66]. Three grams of sterile nylon wool is lightly packed in a 10 ml

syringe, after which culture medium is added and the flow-rate adjusted to around one drop per second. The columns are incubated for 45 min at 37 °C. Subsequently, 100×10^6 spleen cells in 1 ml are applied and the column incubated for 45 min at 37 °C before they are eluted with 10 ml of pre-warmed (37 °C) medium. The average yield is around 50–60% of the input T cells.

Macrophages

Macrophage-rich populations are obtained from peritoneal cells (PC), by injecting 8–10 ml of cold (4 °C) medium into the peritoneal cavity of mice sacrificed by cervical dislocation immediately prior to the injection. Five minutes later the peritoneal cavity is punctured, the cells collected and resuspended in culture medium. Macrophage populations devoid of T cells are obtained by treatment with monoclonal anti-θ antibodies and complement.

Macrophage-depleted populations

Normal spleen cells are resuspended in culture medium (1 ml per spleen equivalent) and applied to Sephadex G-10 columns for depletion of macrophages. Normally around 100×10^6 spleen cells are applied on a 5 ml column. The columns are pre-incubated in culture medium at 37 °C for 45 min prior to addition of cells. After adding the cells, the columns are re-incubated at 37 °C for another 15 min before dropwise elution of the cells with warm (37 °C) culture medium. The average recovery of non-bound cells is around 40% of the input.

Preparation of TCGF-reactive T cell blasts

T cell blasts are prepared by culturing $1-2 \times 10^6$ spleen cells per ml in culture medium and 5 μg/ml con A. After 48–72 h of culture, the cells are harvested and washed in BSS containing 10 mg/ml α-MM in order to dissociate agglutinated cells and displace cell-bound con A. Blast cells are purified by centrifugation on a cushion of Ficoll-Isopaque for 20 min at 1500 rev./min at room temperature. The blasts can be used either directly or after prolonged periods of culture in TCGF-supplemented medium (see below).

Production and assay of TCGF

Mouse spleen cells are incubated at 5×10^6/ml for 24 h in the presence of 5 μg/ml con A in culture medium. The TCGF-containing supernatants are harvested, supplemented with 20 mg/ml α-MM, filtered through 0.45 μm Nalgene filters and stored at −20 °C until used. TCGF is also readily obtained from con A-induced rat spleen cell cultures using the same protocol as above. Large quantities of TCGF are preferentially obtained from the EL-4 lymphoma cell line [67]. EL-4 cells are cultured for 36 h at 1×10^6/ml in serum free medium in the presence of 1–10 ng/ml phorbol-myristic acid (PMA) and 5 μg/ml con A. A two-step procedure for obtaining partially purified TCGF has been described [68] which involves ammonium sulphate precipitation followed by hydrophobic chromatography. This method gives a PMA- and con A-free TCGF preparation.

TCGF-activity is assayed and quantified by using long-term cultured cytotoxic T lymphocyte (CTL) lines which are strictly TCGF-dependent for their growth. If CTL lines are not available, TCGF-activity can be readily assayed on short-term, con A-induced, TCGF-reactive T cell blasts (prepared as described above). Both types of target cells give the same activity profiles.

TCGF-activity is quantified by titrating the TCGF-rich supernatants, into microtitre wells containing 5×10^4–1×10^5/ml of TCGF-reactive T cell blasts (CTL or con A-induced), from 1:2 to 1:1000 (v/v). Con A-containing TCGF-supernatants are supplemented with α-MM prior to assay in order to avoid possible non-specific stimulation (or inhibition) by the lectin. The proliferative response is measured by ^{3}H-thymidine incorporation (see below).

The amount of TCGF present in an unknown sample can be determined by the reciprocal of the sample dilution that results in a value that is 50% of a standard TCGF preparation [69]. In other words, if the standard TCGF preparation gives 50% maximum activity at a final dilution of 1:10 (assigned 1 unit per ml) and the unknown sample gives 50% activity at a dilution of 1:20, then the test sample has a TCGF-activity of 2 units per ml.

Production and assay of LAF

LAF (lymphocyte activating factor) is a macrophage product. LAF production by normal macrophages is obtained by stimulating 1–2×10^6/ml peritoneal cells with 1–10 μg/ml LPS for 36 h in culture medium.

To obtain large quantities of LAF, macrophage tumour cell lines are to be preferred. A good source for LAF is the macrophage cell line P388D$_1$ which, upon induction, elaborates large amounts of this factor, as described in detail elsewhere [70].

LAF activity is assayed by titrating the LAF-rich supernatants on 2–3×10^5/ml G-10 passed spleen cells, in the presence of 5 μg/ml con A. Such macrophage-depleted cell populations do not respond to con A, but will do so upon addition of macrophages or of LAF.

Thus the LAF-assay is an indirect assay which reflects reconstitution of the LAF-dependent induction of TCGF-production and the proliferation induced in TCGF-reactive T cell blasts [71]. When LAF is obtained from LPS-induced macrophages, the LAF activity is assayed as above but using a LPS-nonresponder strain like C3H/HeJ.

Proliferation assay

Proliferation is determined by incorporation of ^{3}H-thymidine (1 μCi/well) which is added to the cultures 4–6 h before termination. The cultures are collected with a multiple cell harvester on to glass-fibre filters and after washing and lysis with water the filters are dried and counted in a liquid scintillation counter. The results are expressed as mean counts per minute (c.p.m.) of triplicate cultures.

Non-specific killer assay

Normally lectin-induced and TCGF-expanded T cells (effector cells) are assayed for cytolytic activity after 4–5 days. The harvested cells are washed and resuspended to desired concentrations. The non-specific cytolytic activity is revealed by co-culturing a constant number of ^{51}Cr-labelled target cells (48 h con A-activated spleen cells or tumour cells) which have been pre-incubated for 30 min with agglutinating concentrations of con A or PHA (5 μg/ml and 10 μg/ml respectively) prior to the assay [72]. Usually 0.1 ml of the target cells (1×10^5/ml) plus 0.1 ml of at least three dilutions (in steps of 1:3) of the effector cells are distributed in V-shaped microtitre plates. The plates are centrifuged for 5 min at 100 rev./min (20 **g**) and incubated at 37 °C for 3 h, after which 100 μl supernatant is removed from each well. The cytolytic activity is calculated as follows:

$$\% \text{ lysis} = \frac{\text{experimental c.p.m.} - \text{spontaneous c.p.m.}^1}{\text{maximum c.p.m.}^2 - \text{spontaneous c.p.m.}}$$

(1) ^{51}Cr-release of target cells cultured alone.
(2) ^{51}Cr-release of target cells cultured with a detergent.

Limiting dilution assay

The limiting dilution assays are performed in V-bottom microtitre plates. Irradiated (2000R) peritoneal cells are resuspended at 1×10^5/ml in culture medium containing TCGF (50% v/v). Each well receives 100 μl of this mixture. Subsequently, limiting numbers of nylon wool passed spleen cells resuspended in culture medium are added in 50 μl aliquots, using a Hamilton repeating dispenser. For each cell concentration, 24–96 replicate cultures are set up. Finally, optimal doses of the lectin are added in 5 μl (thus 30 times the final desired concentration). After 5–8 days of incubation, proliferation and lectin-dependent cytolytic activity are determined in the same wells in the following way: 14–16 h before the killer assay, all wells receive 0.1 μCi of ^{14}C-thymidine. Before the assay the plates are centrifuged for 5 min at 500 rev./min and the radioactive supernatant discarded. The pellets are resuspended in 100 μl culture medium containing 1000-fold excess of cold thymidine (to prevent incorporation of residual ^{14}C-thymidine by the target cells during the killer assay). To assay for lectin-dependent cytotoxicity, ^{51}Cr-labelled target cells are pre-incubated with lectin (10 μg/ml PHA or 5 μg/ml con A) for 20 min, washed and added to the wells at a final concentration of 1×10^4 in 50 μl. The killer assay is performed as described above. The proliferative responses of the same effector cells, which are left in the pellet in the microtitre wells after the killer assay, are now harvested and ^{14}C-thymidine incorporation measured as described above. The individual cultures are considered positive for proliferation and cytolytic activity when they exceed, by more than 3 standard deviations, the mean activity observed in 24 parallel cultures containing no responder cells. The frequencies are determined by using the zero-order term of the Poisson distribution [for detailed description see ref. 73].

Stepwise analysis of lectin-induced T cell responses

As mentioned above, a T cell mitogenic lectin must be capable of performing two functions in order to induce T cell proliferation [64,65]. First, it must be capable of inducing a resting T cell precursor to become susceptible to TCGF ('step 1'). Second, it must induce the production of such factors ('step 2'). Neither of the two events will *per se* lead to proliferation. Since step 1 and step 2 display different kinetics and cellular requirements, they can readily be studied separately. The procedures used for 'screening' different lectins for step 1 and/or step 2 activity are schematically presented in Fig. 63.4.

The mitogenic property of a lectin, i.e. both step 1 and step 2 activities, is easily assayed by simply titrating the desired lectin on whole spleen cell populations and measuring the proliferative responses. Fig. 63.5 depicts a typical experiment where the optimal con A concentrations for the overall proliferative response is determined in the presence of various amounts of FCS. As shown, the optimal con A-concentrations on day 3, using 1%, 10%, and 20% FCS are 1, 5, and 10 μg/ml respectively.

When measuring proliferative responses, it is fundamental to study kinetics. Fig. 63.6 illustrates the different kinetic profiles over a 6-day period, using three different cell concentrations and 5 μg/ml con A in the presence of 10% FCS. The day of 'peak-response' will of course occur earlier in high cell density cultures

ASSAY FOR 'STEP 1' AND/OR 'STEP 2' ACTIVITY

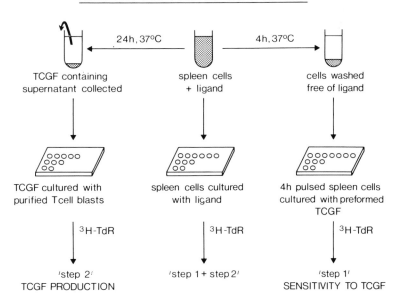

Fig. 63.4. Schematic diagram for dissecting lectin-induced T cell responses.

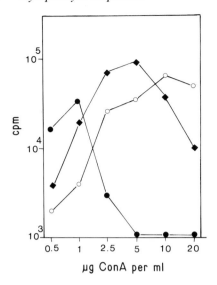

Fig. 63.5. Optimization of con A-induced responses in the presence of various concentrations of FCS. Normal spleen cells were cultured at 3×10^5/ml in the presence of 1% (●); 10% (◆) or 20% (○) FCS and the indicated concentrations of con A. The proliferative response on day 3 of culture was determined by incorporation of ^{3}H-thymidine.

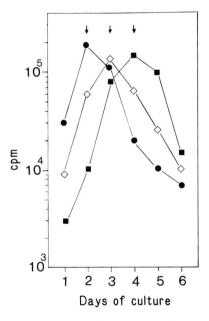

Fig. 63.6. Kinetic profiles of con A-induced responses using different cell concentrations. Normal spleen cells were cultured at 2×10^5/ml (■); 4×10^5/ml (◊) or 8×10^5/ml (●) in RPMI + 10% FCS in the presence of 5 µg/ml of con A. The proliferative response was measured during 6 consecutive days by incorporation of ^{3}H-thymidine.

since more cells are induced to proliferate, thereby causing a more rapid consumption of TCGF and deterioration of the culture conditions.

Step 1 is known to occur during a short pulse (4–5 h) with specific ligands, which results in the expression of functional growth receptors for TCGF. This induction of TCGF-reactivity is a non-mitotic response of resting T cells [74] which most likely constitues a G_0 to G_1 transition. To assay for step 1 activity of a lectin, normal spleen cells are pre-incubated at 37 °C for 4–5 h with the ligand in question, extensively washed and recultured in the presence of TCGF-containing culture medium. Alternatively, the ligand can be present throughout the whole culture period in the presence of preformed TCGF. If the lectin possesses step 1 activity, a proliferative response is observed since the exogenously provided TCGF will substitute for the eventual lack of step 2 activity of the lectin (see below). Figs. 63.7 and 63.8 exemplify such step 1 analysis using con A and LA respectively as inducing ligands. In Fig. 63.7, normal spleen cells are incubated with the indicated concentrations of con A for 4 h, subse-

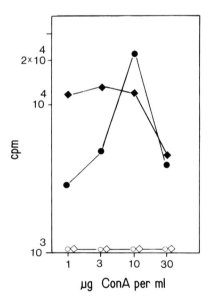

Fig. 63.7. Expression of growth receptors and production of TCGF by con A. Spleen cells (5×10^6/ml) were pre-incubated in various concentrations of con A for 4 h, washed and recultured (2×10^5/ml) with (●) or without (○) TCGF. C.p.m. of spleen cells, pre-incubated in medium and recultured in TCGF, are subtracted. TCGF, produced with the different concentrations of con A for 24 h, were tested on T cell blasts (5×10^4/ml) (◆). T cell blasts were cultured with different concentrations of con A alone (◊). Responses were measured on day 3. Reprinted from ref. 75, with permission.

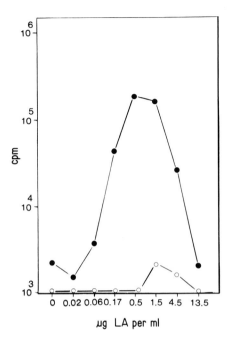

Fig. 63.8. Dose–response curve of spleen cells to LA in the presence or absence of TCGF. Spleen cells (2×10^5/ml) were cultured with different concentrations of LA in TCGF-conditioned medium (●) or in normal medium (○) on day 4 of culture. Reprinted from ref. 75, with permission.

quently washed and recultured in the presence or absence of preformed TCGF. The proliferative response obtained in the secondary cultures supplemented with TCGF reveals that step 1 is induced. Fig. 63.8, on the other hand, demonstrates that LA is a very poor mitogenic lectin for murine T cells. If an excess of TCGF, however, is added to such LA-containing cultures, a good proliferative response is obtained. The concentrations of LA which are totally devoid of mitogenicity on spleen cells by themselves are optimal for inducing sensitivity to TCGF. Thus LA is a potent step 1 lectin and its poor mitogenicity is due to its inability to produce TCGF (step 2).

Production of TCGF requires the presence of both θ-positive cells and macrophages since depletion of either of these two cell types results in lack of TCGF-production [76]. Step 2 activity of a lectin is determined by incubating spleen cells with various concentrations of the ligand for 24 h (as described in detail above). TCGF-activity is subsequently assayed by its capacity to induce growth in T cell blasts. The amount of TCGF produced in the presence of different concentrations of con A is shown in Fig. 63.7. In the case of this lectin, the optimal amount for step 2

activity is quite different from that of step 1 activity. Thus con A is preferentially a good step 2 ligand since TCGF is produced in the presence of low concentrations of con A, while to obtain maximal step 1 activity a tenfold higher concentration is required. The dose–response profiles for the overall con A responses shown in Fig. 63.5 reflect, therefore, the two different dose–response curves presented in Fig. 63.7.

It is well established that TCGF is a T cell product and not a macrophage product, since macrophage-depleted lectin-stimulated cultures will produce TCGF if the cultures are provided with LAF [77,78]. Step 2 activity of a lectin includes its capacity (1) to induce the macrophages to produce LAF, and (2) in conjunction with LAF, to induce the TCGF-producing T-helper cells to elaborate TCGF. Whether or not a lectin is deficient in inducing LAF-production can be revealed by supplemention of 'production cultures' with preformed LAF and subsequent measurements of TCGF-production in such lectin-stimulated cultures on TCGF-reactive T cell blasts.

Frequency analysis of lectin-inducible T cells

The improvements of *in vitro* culture conditions have made it possible to develop sensitive quantitative assay systems which allow estimation of the numbers of specific T cell precursors [79,80]. Such quantitative estimates can be readily performed with polyclonal lectins and the frequency of lectin-inducible T cells that grow in TCGF, as well as their functional properties, can be defined with precision [81,82].

Basically, many replicates of limiting numbers of responder cells are cultured in and assayed as described above. An example of such limiting dilution analysis is presented in Fig. 63.9. In this particular case, the frequency of LA-inducible T cells that grow in TCGF and develop into cytolytic T lymphocytes (CTL) was analysed. Limiting numbers of cells were seeded into microcultures containing irradiated peritoneal cells as fillers, optimal concentrations of LA and TCGF. As shown in Fig. 63.9 (left panel) a fraction of the cultures containing, on the average, a single cell incorporate high amounts of ^{14}C-thymidine after 8 days of culture. The frequency of CTL generated under these conditions can also be determined by using the 'non-specific' killer assay, since, as shown in Fig. 63.9 (right panel), the system allows for detection of single clones of CTL precursors. Since the plot of the logarithm of the fraction of negative wells versus the number of responder cells per well is a straight line, intercepting the y-axis at zero, one can conclude that the growth-inducible responder cells are the only limiting variable in the system. The frequency of cells induced by LA (Fig. 63.9) to grow in TCGF, as

Table 63.3. Properties of some commonly used lectins

Lectin	Source	Main sugar specificity[1]	Relative molecular mass
Concanavalin A (con A)	*Canavalia ensiformis* (jack bean)	α-D-Man α-D-Glc	102 000
Phytohaemagglutinin (PHA)	*Phaseolus vulgaris* (red kidney bean)	(complex)	140 000
Leucoagglutinin (LA)	*Phaseolus vulgaris* (red kidney bean)	(complex)	140 000
Lentil lectin (LL)	*Lens culinaris* (lentil)	α-D-Man α-D-Glc	40 000–60 000
Pokeweed mitogen (PWM)	*Phytolacca americana* (pokeweed)	—	19 000–31 000
Soybean agglutinin (SBA)	*Glycine max* (soybean)	α-D-Gal *N*-Ac α-D-Gal	120 000

[1] Man = mannoside; Glc = glucose; Gal = galactose; D-Gal *N*-Ac = *N*-acetyl-D-galactosamine.

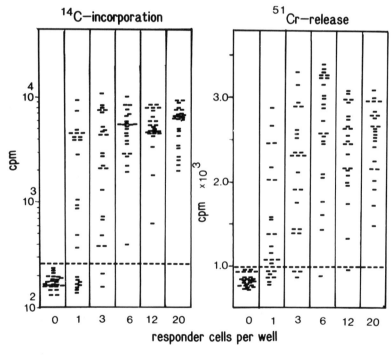

Fig. 63.9. Proliferative and cytolytic responses by limiting numbers of LA-induced, nylon-wool-purified spleen cells in TCGF-conditioned media. Groups of 24 wells containing the indicated numbers of nylon-wool-purified spleen cells and 1×10^4 irradiated peritoneal cells were cultured for 8 days in the presence of 1 μg/ml LA and 50% TCGF-conditioned media. Day 7: 1 μCi of ^{14}C-thymidine was added per well. Day 8: each well was simultaneously assayed for proliferation (left panel) and non-specific cytotoxicity against 1×10^4 ^{51}Cr-labelled target cells (right panel). The dotted line represents 3SD above the mean value of ^{14}C-thymidine incorporation and ^{51}Cr-release observed in the 24 parallel wells containing all supplements except responding cells.

well as the frequency of CTL precursors, can, therefore, be calculated applying Poisson statistics; in this particular experiment, it is 1 in 3.

Media

Balanced salt solution: Earl's BSS $10 \times$ solution (Flow Laboratories Ltd., Victoria Park, Heatherhouse Rd., Irvine Ayrshire, Scotland, UK) without sodium bicarbonate; dilute in sterile water and adjust to pH 7.2 with sodium hydroxide.

Components of tissue culture media:
RPMI 1640 Flow or Gibco (3175 Staley Rd., Grand Island, NY 14072, U.S.A.) $10 \times$ solutions or powder medium without sodium bicarbonate and L-gln;
L-glutamine (200 mM, Flow or Gibco);
penicillin/streptomycin (5000 I.U. of each, Flow or Gibco);
2-mercaptoethanol (2-ME; prepare a 1 M stock solution in H_2O and keep frozen in small (100 μl) aliquots);
fetal calf serum (FCS) or human serum.

L-Glutamine and penicillin/streptomycin can be kept in 1–10 ml aliquots at $-20\,°C$. They are diluted 100-fold in the medium. The 1 M solution of 2-ME is diluted 20-fold in BSS (0.05 M). This solution can be kept at 4 °C for several weeks without losing activity. The 0.05 M solution is diluted 1000-fold in the medium. FCS need not be heat-inactivated, but should be centrifuged or filtered to remove precipitated protein. FCS and human serum is kept in aliquots and frozen.

Prepare $1 \times$ RPMI 1640 medium, add sodium bicarbonate and adjust the pH as described by the manufacturers. Add L-glutamine, penicillin/streptomycin, 2-ME, and the desired amount of serum. This complete medium should be used within one week, if kept at 4 °C.

The most commonly used medium is RPMI 1640, originally adapted to provide growth of human and murine leukaemic cells. Dulbecco's Modified Eagles medium (DMEM) is also a common medium, but it appears to be inadequate for cultures stimulated by PBA, unless it is supplemented with certain components present in RPMI 1640 medium. RPMI 1640 and DMEM have different concentrations of sodium bicarbonate, because they are meant for culturing at 5% and 10% CO_2, respectively. When RPMI 1640 is incubated at 10% CO_2, it becomes more acid. A constant pH is very important for the results and therefore a strong buffering capacity of the medium is desirable. HEPES is extensively used with good results with concentrations up to 20 mM. When the medium is supplemented with serum, HEPES is not necessary, since the serum has strong buffering capacity. The initial pH of the medium should be around 7.2 (for cell cultures stimulated by PBA, pH 7.4 is optimal), but the pH tends to decrease during the time of culturing, when there is a high proliferating activity of the cells.

A new medium has been developed and used in lymphocyte cultures by Iscove & Melchers [83]. It is based on DMEM and supplemented with amino acids and a number of other components. It can support activation, growth and maturation of both T and B lymphocytes in the absence of serum in low cell density cultures. Some constituents are labile, and therefore the medium should be kept frozen. Considerable variability from one batch to another has been observed and this may be the reason why it has sometimes been used supplemented with FCS.

2-Mercaptoethanol (2-ME), or related thiol compounds, are necessary ingredients in many culture systems of haemopoietic cells in particular. Its optimal concentration range is rather narrow, and the peak is around 5×10^{-5} M.

Serum, as mentioned previously, is normally also provided to the cultures. That most commonly used is FCS. Different batches vary in their growth supporting activity and normally several batches should be tested in order to select an optimal one for the system used. Some batches of FCS contain unwanted mitogenic or inhibitory activities. As discussed above, a high concentration of FCS is sometimes required but not all batches can be used at these high concentrations without being inhibitory.

A good strategy for testing different batches of FCS is as follows. To test the mitogenic activity, cells at a high cell density are cultured in medium with different percentages of FCS, and DNA synthesis is measured on days 2 to 4. To test the supporting activity, a low concentration of cells is cultured with the activator(s) and FCS in different concentrations. The pertinent activity is measured, e.g. proliferation, Ig synthesis or cytolytic activity. In this way, one can select a batch of FCS which has low mitogenic activity on non-activated cells and high supporting activity with the activators present.

The widespread use of FCS is in a way unfortunate, since it is costly. When using RPMI 1640 medium, FCS cannot be replaced by human serum, newborn calf serum or horse serum for activation by LPS in low cell density cultures of mouse spleen cells. This is not the case with the proliferative T cell responses to con A, which develop in cultures supplemented with selected batches of human sera.

Acknowledgements

S. Bergstedt-Lindqvist is thanked for providing the data for Fig. 63.2. The authors thank S. Bergstedt-Lindqvist, S. Britton, G. Möller, and C. Wood for reviewing the manuscript.

References

1 NOWELL P.C. (1960) PHA: an initiator of mitosis in cultures of normal human leukocytes. *Cancer Res.* **20**, 562.

2 WECKSLER M., LEVY A. & JAFFÉ W.G. (1968) Acción mitogénica de extractos de *Canavalia ensiformis* y concanavalina A. *Acta cient. venez.* **19**, 154.

3 PEAVY D.L., ADLER W.H. & SMITH R.T. (1970) The mitogenic effects of endotoxin and staphylococcal enterotoxin B on mouse spleen cells and human peripheral lymphocytes. *J. Immunol.* **105**, 1453.

4 STOBO J.D., ROSENTHAL A.S. & PAUL W.E. (1972) Functional heterogeneity of murine lymphoid cells. (I) Responsiveness to and surface binding of Concanavalin A and phytohemagglutinin. *J. Immunol.* **108**, 1.

5 ANDERSSON J., MÖLLER G. & SJÖBERG O. (1972) Selective induction of DNA synthesis in T and B lymphocytes. *Cell. Immunol.* **4**, 381.

6 ANDERSSON J., SJÖBERG O. & MÖLLER G. (1972) Induction of immunoglobulin and antibody synthesis *in vitro* by lipopolysaccharide. *Eur. J. Immunol.* **2**, 349.

7 HOLM G., PERLMANN P. & WERNER B. (1964) Phytohaemagglutinin-induced cytotoxic action of normal lymphoid cells on cells in tissue culture. *Nature*, **203**, 841.

8 STAVY L., TREVES A.J. & FELDMAN M. (1971) Effect of Concanavalin A on lymphocyte-mediated cytotoxicity. *Nature*, **232**, 56.

9 MÖLLER G., SJÖBERG O. & ANDERSSON J. (1972) Mitogen-induced lymphocyte-mediated cytotoxicity *in vitro*: Effects of mitogens selectively activating T or B cells. *Eur. J. Immunol.* **2**, 586.

10 GERY I., GERSHON R.K. & WAKSMAN B.H. (1972) Potentiation of the T-lymphocyte response to mitogens. (I) The responding cell. *J. exp. Med.* **136**, 128.

11 HABU S. & RAFF M.C. (1977) Accessory cell dependence of lectin-induced proliferation of mouse T lymphocytes. *Eur. J. Immunol.* **7**, 451.

12 GILLIS S. & SMITH K.A. (1977) Long-term culture of tumour-specific cytotoxic T-cells. *Nature*, **268**, 154.

13 MÖLLER G. (ed.) (1972) Lymphocyte activation by mitogens. *Transplant. Rev.* **11**.

14 MÖLLER G. (ed.) (1980) Effect of anti-immunoglobulin sera on B lymphocyte function. *Immunol. Revs.* **52**.

15 MÖLLER G. (ed.) (1980) T cell stimulating growth factors. *Immunol. Revs.* **51**.

16 COUTINHO A., MÖLLER G., ANDERSSON J. & BULLOCK W.W. (1973) *In vitro* activation of mouse lymphocytes in serum-free medium: effect of T and B cell mitogens on proliferation and antibody synthesis. *Eur. J. Immunol.* **3**, 299.

17 MELCHERS F., BRAUN V. & GALANOS C. (1975) The lipoprotein of the outer membrane of *Escherichia coli*: a B-lymphocyte mitogen. *J. exp. Med.* **142**, 473.

18 DIAMANTSTEIN T., VOGT W., RÜHL H. & BOCHERT G. (1973) Stimulation of DNA synthesis in mouse lymphoid cells by polyanions *in vitro*. (I) Target cells and possible mode of action. *Eur. J. Immunol.* **3**, 488.

19 COUTINHO A., MÖLLER G. & RICHTER W. (1974) Molecular basis of B-cell activation. (I) Mitogenicity of native and substituted dextrans. *Scand. J. Immunol.* **3**, 321.

20 SULTER B. & NILSSON B. (1972) PPD Tuberculin—a B-cell mitogen. *Nature New Biol.* **240**, 198.

21 GRONOWICZ E. & COUTINHO A. (1974) Selective triggering of B cell subpopulations by mitogens. *Eur. J. Immunol.* **4**, 771.

22 PARKER D.C. (1975) Stimulation of mouse lymphocytes by insoluble anti-mouse immunoglobulin. *Nature*, **258**, 361.

23 SIECKMANN D.G., ASOFSKY R., MOSIER D.E., ZITRON I.M. & PAUL W.E. (1982) Activation of mouse lymphocytes by anti-immunoglobulin. (I) Parameters of the proliferative response. *J. exp. Med.* **147**, 814.

24 BONA C., DAMAIS C. & CHEDID L. (1974) Blastic transformation of mouse spleen lymphocytes by a water-soluble mitogen extracted from *Nocardia*. *Proc. natn. Acad. Sci. U.S.A.* **71**, 1602.

25 KEARNEY J.F. & LAWTON A.R. (1975) B lymphocyte differentiation induced by lipopolysaccharide. (I) Generation of cells synthesizing four major immunoglobulin classes. *J. Immunol.* **115**, 671.

26 ANDERSSON J., COUTINHO A. & MELCHERS F. (1978) Stimulation of B lymphocytes to IgG synthesis and secretion by the mitogens lipopolysaccharide and lipoprotein and its inhibition by anti-immunoglobulin antibodies. *Eur. J. Immunol.* **8**, 336.

27 PRIMI D., MAMI F., LE GUERN C. & CAZENAVE P.-A. (1982) Mitogen-reactive B cell subpopulations selectively express different sets of V regions. *J. exp. Med.* **156**, 181.

28 AUGUSTIN A.A. & COUTINHO A. (1980) Specific T helper cells that activate B cells polyclonally. *In vitro* enrichment and cooperative function. *J. exp. Med.* **151**, 587.

29 GREAVES M. & JANOSSY G. (1972) Elicitation of selective T and B lymphocyte responses by cell surface binding ligands. *Transplant. Rev.* **11**, 87.

30 ROSÉN A., GERGELY P., JONDAL M., KLEIN G. & BRITTON S. (1977) Polyclonal Ig production after Epstein-Barr virus infection of human lymphocytes *in vitro*. *Nature*, **267**, 52.

31 FORSGREN A., SVEDJELUND A. & WIGZELL A. (1976) Lymphocyte stimulation by protein A of *Staphylococcus aureus*. *Eur. J. Immunol.* **6**, 207.

32 BONA C., BRODER S., DIMITRIU A. & WALDMANN T.A. (1979) Polyclonal activation of human B lymphocytes by *Nocardia* water soluble migoen (NWSM). *Immunol. Revs.* **45**, 69.

33 PERSSON U.C.I., HAMMARSTRÖM L.L.G. & SMITH C.I.E. (1977) Macrophages are required for the dextran-sulfate induced activation of B lynphocytes. *J. Immunol.* **119**, 1138.

34 GRONOWICZ E. & COUTINHO A. (1976) Heterogeneity of B cells: direct evidence for selective triggering of distinct subpopulations by polyclonal activators. *Scand. J. Immunol.* **5**, 55.

35 BERGSTEDT-LINDQVIST S., SEVERINSON E. & FERNANDEZ C. (1982) Limited life span of extensively proliferating B cells. No evidence for a continuous class of subclass switch. *J. Immunol.* **129**, 1905.

36 COUTINHO A., FORNI L., MELCHERS F. & WATANABE T. (1977) Genetic defect in responsiveness to the B cell mitogen lipopolysaccharide. *Eur. J. Immunol.* **7**, 325.

37 WETZEL G.D. & KETTMAN J.R. (1981) Activation of

murine B lymphocytes. (III) Stimulation of B lymphocyte clonal growth with lipopolysaccharide and dextran sulphate. *J. Immunol.* **126**, 723.

38 ANDERSSON J., COUTINHO A., LERNHARDT W. & MELCHERS F. (1977) Clonal growth and maturation to immunoglobulin secretion *in vitro* of every growth inducible B lymphocyte. *Cell*, **10**, 27.

39 LY L. & MISHELL R. (1974) Separation of mouse spleen cells by passage through Sephadex G-10. *J. immunol. Meth.* **5**, 239.

40 MAGE M.G., MCHUGH L.L. & ROTHSTEIN T.L. (1977) Mouse lymphocytes with and without surface immunoglobulin: preparative scale separation in polystyrene tissue culture dishes coated with specifically purified anti-immunoglobulin. *J. immunol. Meth.* **15**, 47.

41 HOWARD M., FARRAR J., HILFIKER M., JOHNSON B., TAKATSU K., HAMAOKA T. & PAUL W.E. (1982) Identification of a T cell-derived B cell growth factor distinct from interleukin 2. *J. exp. Med.* **155**, 914.

42 FERNANDEZ C. & SEVERINSON E. (1983) The polyclonal LPS response is accessory cell dependent. *Scand. J. Immunol.* **18**, 279.

43 ANDERSSON J., COUTINHO A. & MELCHERS F. (1977) Frequencies of mitogen-reactive B cells in the mouse. (I) Distribution in different lymphoid organs from different inbred strains of mice at different ages. *J. exp. Med.* **145**, 1511.

44 ZUBLER R.H. (1984) Polyclonal B cell responses in the presence of defined filler cells: Complementary effects of lipopolysaccharide and anti-Ig antibodies. *Eur. J. Immunol.* **14**, 357.

45 METCALF D., NOSSAL G.J.V., WARNER N.L., MILLER J.F.A.P., MANDEL T.E., LAYTON J.E. & GUTMAN G.A. (1975) Growth of B-lymphocyte colonies *in vitro*. *J. exp. Med.* **142**, 1534.

46 KINCADE P.W., RALPH P. & MOORE M.A.S. (1976) Growth of B-lymphocyte clones in semisolid culture is mitogen dependent. *J. exp. Med.* **143**, 1265.

47 MELCHERS F., COUTINHO A., HEINRICH G. & ANDERSSON J. (1975) Continuous growth of mitogen-reactive B lymphocytes. *Scand. J. Immunol.* **4**, 853.

48 MARTINEZ-ALONSO C., COUTINHO A. & AUGUSTIN A.A. (1980) Immunoglobulin C-gene expression. (I) The commitment to IgG subclass of secretory cells is determined by the quality of the nonspecific stimuli. *Eur. J. Immunol.* **10**, 698.

49 JULIUS M.H., VON BOEHMER H. & SIDMAN C.L. (1982) Dissociation of two signals required for activation of resting B cells. *Proc. natn. Acad. Sci. U.S.A.* **79**, 1989.

50 JAWORSKI M.A., SHIOZAWA C. & DIENER E. (1981) Triggering of affinity-enriched B cells. Analysis of B cell stimulation by antigen-specific helper factor or lipopolysaccharide. (I) Dissection into proliferative and differentiative signals. *J. exp. Med.* **155**, 248.

51 ZUBLER R.H. & GLASEBROOK A.L. (1982) Requirement for three signals in 'T-independent' (lipopolysaccharide-induced) as well as in T-dependent B cell responses. *J. exp. Med.* **155**, 666.

52 ANDERSSON J. & MELCHERS F. (1981) T cell dependent activation of resting B cells: requirement for both nonspecific unrestricted and antigen-specific Ia-restricted soluble factors. *Proc. natn. Acad. Sci. U.S.A.* **78**, 2497.

53 ISAKSSON P.C., PURÉ E., VITETTA E.S. & KRAMMER P.H. (1982) T cell-derived B cell differentiation factor(s). Effect of the isotype switch of murine B cells. *J. exp. Med.* **155**, 734.

54 SEVERINSON GRONOWICZ E., DOSS C. & SCHRÖDER J. (1979) Activation to IgG secretion by lipopolysaccharide requires several proliferation cycles. *J. Immunol.* **123**, 2057.

55 MOLINARO G.A. & DRAY S. (1974) Antibody coated erythrocytes as a manifold probe for antigens. *Nature*, **248**, 515.

56 GRONOWICZ E., COUTINHO A. & MELCHERS F. (1976) A plaque assay for all cells secreting Ig of a given type or class. *Eur. J. Immunol.* **6**, 588.

57 VAN DER LOO W., SEVERINSON GRONOWICZ E., STROBER S. & HERZENBERG LA. (1979) Cell differentiation in the presence of cytochalasin B: studies on the 'switch' to IgG secretion after polyclonal B cell activation. *J. Immunol.* **122**, 1203.

58 LAWTON A.R., LUCIVERO G., LEVITT D. & COOPER M.D. (1982) Aspects of mitogen activation of human B cells. In *Human B-Lymphocyte Function. Activation and Immunoregulation*, (eds. Fauci A.S. & Ballieux R.E.), p. 37. Raven Press, New York.

59 WALDMANN T.A. & BRODER S. (1982) Polyclonal B cell activators in the study of the regulation of immunoglobulin synthesis in the human system. *Adv. Immunol.* **32**, 1.

60 FAUCI A.S. & BALLIEUX R.E. (eds.) (1982) *Human B-Lymphocyte Function. Activation and Immunoregulation.* Raven Press, New York.

61 LIS H. & SHARON N. (1977) Lectins: their Chemistry and Application to Immunology. In *The Antigens*, vol. IV, (ed. Sela M.), p. 429. Academic Press, New York.

62 ANDERSSON J., SJÖBERG O. & MÖLLER G. (1972) Selective induction of DNA synthesis in T and B lymphocytes. *Cell. Immunol.* **4**, 381.

63 MORGAN D.A., RUSCETTI F.W. & GALLO R.C. (1976) Selective *in vitro* growth of T lymphocytes from normal human bone marrows. *Science*, **193**, 1007.

64 LARSSON E.-L., ANDERSSON J. & COUTINHO A. (1978) Functional consequences of sheep red blood cell rosetting for human T cells: gain of reactivity to mitogenic factors. *Eur. J. Immunol.* **8**, 693.

65 LARSSON E.-L. & COUTINHO A. (1979) On the role of mitogenic lectins in T cell triggering. *Nature*, **280**, 239.

66 JULIUS M.H., SIMPSON E. & HERZENBERG L.A. (1973) A rapid method for the isolation of functional thymus-derived murine lymphocytes. *Eur. J. Immunol.* **3**, 645.

67 FARRAR J.J., FULLER-FARRAR J., SIMON P.L., HILFIKER M.L. & FARRAR W.L. (1980) Interleukin-2 production by EL-4 thymoma cells. *Behring Institute Mitteilungen*, **67**, 58.

68 CLARK-LEWIS J., SCHRADER J.W. & MCKIMM-BRESCHKIN J.L. (1982) Preparation of T cell growth factor free from interferon and factors stimulating hemopoietic cells and mast cells. *J. immunol. Meth.* **51**, 311.

69 GILLIS S., FERM M.M., OU W. & SMITH, K.A. (1978) T cell growth factor: parameters of production and a quantitative microassay for activity. *J. Immunol.* **120**, 2027.

70 MIZEL S.B. & MIZEL D.J. (1981) Purification to apparent homogeneity of murine Interleukin I. *J. Immunol.* **126,** 834.

71 LARSSON E.-L., GULLBERG M., IVARS F., HOLMBERG D. & COUTINHO A. (1980) T cell producing and responding to TCGF. *Behring Institute Mitteilungen*, **67,** 12.

72 BERETTA A., PERSSON U., RAMOS T. & MÖLLER, G. (1982) Concanavalin A inhibits the effector phase of specific cytotoxicity. *Scand. J. Immunol.* **16,** 181.

73 LANGHORNE J. & FISCHER-LINDAHL K. (1981) Limiting dilution analysis of precursors of cytotoxic T lymphocytes. In *Immunological Methods*, vol. II, (eds. Lefkovits S.I. & Pernis B.), p. 221. Academic Press, New York, San Francisco, London.

74 LARSSON E.-L. (1981) Mechanism of T cell activation. (II) Antigen- and lectin-dependent acquisition of responsiveness to TCGF is a nonmitotic, active response of resting T cells. *J. Immunol.* **126,** 1323.

75 LARSSON E.-L. & COUTINHO A. (1980) Mechanism of T cell activation (I) A screening of 'step one' ligands. *Eur. J. Immunol.* **10,** 93.

76 ANDERSSON J., GRÖNVIK K.-O., LARSSON E.-L. & COUTINHO A. (1979) Studies on T lymphocyte activation (I) Requirements for the mitogen-dependent production of T cell growth factors. *Eur. J. Immunol.* **9,** 581.

77 LARSSON E.-L., ISCOVE N.N. & COUTINHO A. (1980) Two distinct factors are required for induction of T cell growth. *Nature*, **283,** 664.

78 SMITH K.A., GILBRIDGE K.-J. & FAVATA M.F. (1980) Lymphocyte activating factor promotes T cell growth factor production by cloned murine lymphoma cells. *Nature*, **287,** 853.

79 FISCHER-LINDAHL K. & WILSON D.B. (1977) Histocompatibility antigen-activated cytotoxic T lymphocytes. (II) Estimates of the frequency and specificity of precursors. *J. exp. Med.* **145,** 508.

80 MACDONALD H.R., CEROTTINI J.C., RYSER J.E., MARYANSKI J.L., TOSWELL C., WIDMER M.B. & BRUNNER K.T. (1980) Quantitation and cloning of cytolytic T lymphocytes and their precursors. *Immunol. Revs.* **51,** 93.

81 LARSSON E.-L., FISCHER-LINDAHL K., LANGHORNE J. & COUTINHO A. (1981) Quantiative studies on Concanavalin A-induced, TCGF-reactive T cells. (I) Correlation between proliferation and lectin-dependent cytolytic activity. *J. Immunol.* **127,** 1081.

82 LARSSON E.-L. (1982) One third of murine splenic T cells are cytotoxic precursors induced to grow by leucoagglutinin and TCGF. *Scand. J. Immunol.* **15,** 515.

83 ISCOVE N.N. & MELCHERS F. (1978) Complete replacement of serum by albumin, transferrin and soybean lipid in cultures of lipopolysaccharide-reactive B lymphocytes. *J. exp. Med.* **147,** 923.

Chapter 64
Assays for immunoglobulin-secreting cells

D. W. DRESSER

Immunoglobulin-(antibody) secreting cells, 64.1

Localized haemolysis in gel (LHG) (conventional plaque assay), 64.1

Non-erythrocyte antigens, 64.12

Nucleated target cells, 64.16

Immunoglobulin-(antigen) secreting cells (reversed plaque assay), 64.16

Preparation of cell suspensions, 64.17

Anti-immunoglobulin sera, 64.18

Coda, 64.21

Media, 64.22

The analysis of the cellular events underlying the immune response has been helped by the development of sensitive and reliable methods for the enumeration of individual cells producing antibody (immunoglobulin—Ig). Antigen-induced antibody synthesis occurs as a result of a differentiation process in lymphoid cells and it is clear that the precursors of actively secreting cells either secrete minimally or not at all. In addition, many lymphoid cells (particularly those that spend an essential part of their life history in the thymus—T cells) do not undergo a differentiation process leading to antibody secretion. Of the other lymphoid cell types, however, many have reactivity towards antigen and have presumably undergone at least limited antibody production, possibly in the form of antigen-receptor molecules associated with the cell surface. In order to study such cells which are secreting immunoglobulins, a variety of techniques have been developed. In principle (Table 64.1), there are three distinctive approaches to the study of antibody (Ig) producing cells. Although few comparative studies have been reported it is likely that many individual antibody-producing cells give a positive reaction in more than one or even in all three test systems. In this chapter, techniques designed to enumerate immunoglobulin-(*antibody*) *secreting cells* are described.

Immunoglobulin-(antibody) secreting cells

A variety of techniques have been evolved for enumerating Ig-(antibody) secreting cells (Table 64.1). This chapter will describe the localized haemolysis in gel technique which, with its modifications, is one of the more widely used methods.

Localized haemolysis in gel (LHG) (conventional plaque assay)

The LHG assay is analogous to the plaque or colony technique of the microbiologist in that a situation is created in which a visible plaque is formed at a focal point of activity, in this case an individual cell-releasing antibody. For example, a suspension of spleen cells prepared from a mouse immunized with sheep red blood cells (SRBC) is mixed with SRBC *in vitro*, in a suitable semi-solid medium spread into a thin film. During or after incubation at 37 °C, complement (fresh guinea-pig serum) is added to the system, whereupon those SRBC that are close to a spleen cell that secreted a complement-fixing antibody specific for SRBC, and that have bound sufficient of this antibody, will lyse. This will result in a localized area of lysis around the antibody-secreting lymphoid cell, which will appear as a macroscopic 'hole' or plaque in the otherwise continuous layer of target erythrocytes.

The LHG technique as originally described by Jerne *et al.* [58], detected only those cells which produced antibody capable of fixing complement (C) and lysing erythrocytes directly. With certain minor exceptions this antibody is IgM and the cells secreting such antibody are often referred to as *direct* PFC (plaque-forming cells). However, a majority of humoral antibodies belong to other classes (IgG, IgA) which are incapable or inefficient at fixing C; but C will be fixed if this antibody is complexed with an antiglobulin antibody [30,97]. Cells responsible for plaques formed in this manner can be conveniently called *indirect* PFC. The use of specific antiglobulin developing reagents enables the experimenter to enumerate independently PFCs secreting different classes and subclasses of immunoglobulin: in mice, for example, an immune response can be readily measured in terms of IgM, IgA, IgG1, IgG2a, IgG2b and IgG3 or L chain secreting PFC [103].

In the past a degree of confusion has existed in the nomenclature of immunoglobulin classes. This arose on the one hand from the existence of obvious homologies in gross structure and function in the major immunoglobulin classes of different species, and on the other hand from the use of homonyms,

Table 64.1. Enumeration of cells synthesizing immunoglobulin (Ig)

Localization of Ig	Cell	Method
Intracellular	Ig (antibody) containing	Immunofluorescence, enzymatic (histochemical)
Cell surface (mIg)	Antigen binding (mIg + ve B cell)	Immunofluorescence rosettes (E,EA,EAC,EAb)
Secreted	Plaque forming (PFC)	
	Antigen-specific	Bacterial immobilization (microdroplet)
		Autoradiographic
		Localized haemolysis in gel (LHG)
		Conventional plaque (E,EA)
	Non-specific	Autoradiographic
		LHG
		Reversed plaque (EAb)

especially for subclasses, where such homologies do not exist or homology of primary structure has not yet been established. Table 64.2 gives a general nomenclature for the major immunoglobulin classes which is used in this chapter.

LHG assays

There are three commonly used methods of assaying a population of lymphoid cells for haemolytic plaque forming cells. These will be described in the following sections. Many of the principles discussed in section 1 also apply to the other methods described in sections 2 and 3.

1   *Petri-dish (Jerne plaque) assay*

A modified version of the original technique first described by Jerne *et al.* [59] is now described in sufficient detail for an inexperienced person to carry out the assay satisfactorily.

Reagents and equipment

Disposable polystyrene 9 cm Petri dishes, grease-free and with no irregular edges.
Water bath to run at 39–44 °C, with racks to contain sufficient 12×90 mm glass test-tubes.
Hot-plate magnetic stirrer.
Level platform; alternatively, a sheet of glass and three lumps of plasticine, and a spirit level.
Adjustable automatic pipetting device (A. R. Horwell or Becton-Dickinson).
Repeater syringe to deliver 100 μl aliquots (Oxford).
Eppendorf-Marburg Pipetter (or Oxford equivalent)—100 μl and 10 μl.

Agarose A.37 (A.45) (Indubiose) (L'Industrie Biologique: Gennevilliers, Seine, France) or equivalent (Seaplaque) from Marine Colloids (Miles). Difco Noble agar with 0.5 mg/ml DEAE Dextran (Pharmacia can be used as an alternative).
Concentrated balanced salt solutions, e.g. $\times 5$ or $\times 10$.
An incubator set at 37 °C and containing a humid atmosphere; if a bicarbonate buffer is used in the cell suspension medium, the atmosphere would be 95% air and 5% CO_2. A cheap alternative is to make a gas-tight box from a freezer storage container. An inlet and outlet can be made by cutting a hole and fitting a bung with suitable hose fittings and clips. The box can then be gassed with a ready made mixture, sealed, and placed in an ordinary 37 °C incubator.
Dulbecco's PBS, Hanks', Eagle's MEM or 199.
As a source of complement (C), 1 ml of 10% fresh guinea-pig serum in Hanks' solution is necessary for each plate. Undiluted guinea-pig complement can be stored for at least 18 months at −70 °C. Freeze-dried guinea-pig serum, commercially available, is a satisfactory although expensive substitute. It is advisable to absorb the complement with target erythrocytes before use; e.g. 1 ml packed SRBC for 20–30 ml serum, for a few minutes at 0 °C is usually sufficient.

Procedure

Bottom layer. Two layers of gel are required. The bottom layer provides a smooth, level, non-toxic surface for the thin top layer containing the mixture of PFC and target erythrocytes. In addition the bottom layer also prevents the top layer forming a meniscus with a large proportion of its volume.

Five millilitres of 1.2% agarose in Dulbecco's

Table 64.2. Nomenclature of immunoglobulin classes (IgC$_H$ variants)

General	Mouse [40,43,49,51,67]			Rat [7,8,10]			Human [35,102]		
	Isotype	C$_H$ gene**	Allotype locus***	Isotype	C$_H$ gene	Allotype locus***	Isotype	C$_H$ gene	Allotype locus***
IgM	IgM	μ	Igh-6	IgM	μ	–	IgM	μ	–
IgD	IgD	δ	Igh-5	IgD	δ	–	IgD	δ	–
IgG	IgG$_3$	$\gamma3$	–	IgG$_{2c}$	$\gamma2c$	–	IgG$_1$	$\gamma1$	G$_1$m
	IgG$_1$	$\gamma1$	Igh-4	IgG$_1$	$\gamma1$	–	IgG$_2$	$\gamma2$	G$_2$m A$_2$m
	IgG$_{2b}$	$\gamma2b$	Igh-3	IgG$_{2b}$	$\gamma2b$	Igh-2	IgG$_3$	$\gamma3$	G$_3$m
	IgG$_{2a}$	$\gamma2a$	Igh-1	IgG$_{2a}$	$\gamma2a$	–	IgG$_4$	$\gamma4$	–
IgE	IgE	ε	Igh-7 [90a]	IgE	ε	–	IgE	ε	–
IgA	IgA	α	Igh-2	IgA	α	Igh-1	IgA$_1$	$\alpha1$	–
							IgA$_2$	$\alpha2$	–

* The major isotypes of mammals and birds [15,52,82].
** The nomenclature for the 'C$_H$ gene' and 'allotype locus' are operational alternatives.
*** The dash indicates that IghC allotypic variants (or equivalent) have not yet been described for these isotypes.

In the mouse allotype, polymorphisms on Ig are confined to IgC$_H$; the homologies between mouse and rat on the same horizontal line above, are believed to be fairly close, but human isotypes are considerably different. This is emphasized by the genomic order of the IgC$_H$ genes in the germ line of the mouse (5' . . . . μ-δ-$\gamma3$-$\gamma1$-$\gamma2b$-$\gamma2a$-ε-α . . . . 3') [93] and human (5' . . . . μ-δ . . . . $\gamma1$-$\gamma3$-$\psi\varepsilon$-α_1 . . . . $\gamma2$-$\gamma4$-ε-α_2 . . . . 3') [34]. IgC$_H$ pseudogenes (ψ) exist in the human but not the mouse. Human but not mouse IgG$_1$ can fix guinea-pig C.

phosphate-buffered saline (PBS), at about 50 °C is pipetted into a sterile Petri dish using an automatic pipetting device. The lid is quickly replaced and the molten agarose is spread over the dish which is placed on a level surface until set. Dishes containing bottom layers can be stored in a refrigerator for up to 4 days, or if in sealed containers (polythene bags) they can be stored at 2 °C for up to 3 weeks. For example, if 200 bottom layers were to be prepared, 12 g agarose would be placed in 450 ml distilled water in a conical flask; this would be brought to the boil whilst being constantly stirred. It is essential to dissolve the agarose by boiling in this manner prior to sterilization by autoclaving at 103.5 kPa (120 °C) for 15 min. When the agarose is completely dissolved, a further 450 ml of cold (sterile) distilled water can be added with constant stirring. When the temperature is below 60 °C, 80 ml of concentrated ($\times$12.5) PBS solution and 10 ml of Dulbecco's solutions 2 and 3 can be added in order (appropriate amounts of concentrated solutions of other media could be used instead).

Top layer. Two millilitres of top layer are required for each dish. With A.37 Agarose a 0.75% solution (w/v) is recommended (although 0.6% is sufficient). The top layer is prepared in exactly the same way as described above for the bottom layer, although concentrated Hanks' solution (with bicarbonate, HEPES buffer or Eagle's MEM) usually replaces the PBS. Molten top layer can be filtered through a clean, hot (no. 3), sintered glass filter or a coarse fluted filter paper and then dispersed in 2 ml aliquots into 12 $\times$ 90 mm tubes in a water bath at 40–42 °C (for agarose A.45 or agar, this temperature should be 46–48 °C).

If developing antiglobulin reagents are to be used, they can be added at this stage; 0.1 ml of a suitable dilution in balanced salt solution can be quickly added using a repeater syringe.

Preparation of the assay plates. A tube containing top layer is removed from the water bath and quickly wiped dry; 0.1 ml of target cells (20% washed SRBC or 30% horse RBC) are added from a repeater syringe, followed quickly by 0.1 ml of a suitable dilution of a suspension of cells to be assayed for PFC, using an Eppendorf type of dispenser. The contents of the tube are thoroughly mixed on a vortex mixer poured on to a prepared dish (warmed to room temperature), spread evenly by shaking, and left to set on a level surface. (This should take less than 20 s per plate.) It is advisable to check early on in the proceedings that the target cell layer is perfectly homogeneous; a likely cause of trouble is a temporary chilling of the medium leading to the formation of small foci of gel prior to the addition of target cells.

The plates are incubated for 2 h at 37 °C. One

millilitre of C (10% fresh guinea-pig serum diluted in Hanks' solution) is added to each plate, and spread over the surface. The plates are incubated for a further 40–50 min at 37 °C, taking care to ensure that the incubator shelf is level. Plates can be counted at once or later, in which case the cell layer can be fixed by the addition of 6–8 ml of a solution of 0.25% glutaraldehyde in physiological saline (or PBS); this should be done in an appropriate fume hood.

Plaque counts. Plaques can best be counted under low magnification ($\times 2$–4) under dark ground illumination. Conductivity type colony counters are adequate for this purpose.

Although theoretical considerations [86] suggest that means of PFC per organ or PFC per 10^6 lymphocytes should be calculated geometrically from transformed data, practical considerations (occasional non-responders) dictate that arithmetic means should be used.

Developed plaques (conventional assay). The LHG assay relies on antibody mediated complement-dependent lysis of the target erythrocyte (or antigen-coated erythrocyte). It seems that only one IgM antibody molecule can lead to the lysis of an erythrocyte: antibodies of classes other than IgM are either extremely inefficient or incapable of mediating lysis unless complexed with another (antiglobulin) immunoglobulin with the ability to bind C of allo- or xenogeneic origin [54]. Anti-γ,-α-sera develop indirect plaques of IgG, IgA isotype but high levels of anti-μ activity inhibit direct (IgM) plaques. It is essential that every developing serum is exhaustively absorbed and tested to ensure that it is specific within the limits of the available techniques; a further discussion of this point follows on page 64.20. It is assumed for the moment that developing sera will be free of any activity whatsoever against IgM antibody (no anti-μ or anti-Fab activity) and will therefore not reduce the number of direct plaques. Such developing sera may be used at suboptimal concentrations if economy of material is of prime importance and providing that the value of an appropriate correction factor (KD) is known. Nevertheless, it is always best to use a developing serum at a concentration where the KD is as near unity as possible. Within the limits outlined above, the number of developed PFC can be calculated as follows:

$$\text{Dev PFC} = (\text{total PFC} - \text{direct PFC})\ \text{KD}$$

where 'Dev PFC' are specifically developed PFC (or indirect PFC); 'total PFC' are derived from a plate treated with developing serum, and therefore contain both IgM and developed PFC; 'IgM PFC' are from a direct plate, which received no developing antiserum. Dev PFC and IgM PFC should be calculated for each animal (pool of cells) separately before the mean PFC

per organ or PFC per 10^6 lymphocytes is calculated for the group.

Indirect plaques can be estimated without recourse to a calculation of the difference in count between two sets of plates. This is achieved by totally inhibiting direct (IgM) plaques while at the same time allowing development of indirect plaques. For example, most (but not all) goat and sheep anti-(mouse) μ sera added to an assay plate at the start of incubation inhibit IgM plaques and do not interfere with the development of IgG plaques developed by a rabbit antiserum. Inhibitory sera must be tested to show that they are specifically anti-μ (IgM) and, if necessary, absorbed to remove activity against Fab or non-μ determinants. The inhibitory sera should be titrated and used at a concentration giving >99% inhibition and yet having no detectable effect on the activity of admixed developing sera. It has been found that this method is especially effective when there are less indirect than direct plaques: in this situation the 'difference method' usually results in a very high variance.

Titration of KD for a developing serum. The inhibitory effect of sera on IgM plaques can be measured by adding serial dilutions of serum to the gel containing PFC and target cells. Spleen cells from mice immunized 44–48 h earlier with 10^8 SRBC (or 2–4 days after 4×10^6 SRBC), should be used as a source of IgM PFC which contains a minimum number of indirect PFC. Inhibition is seen with sera possessing anti-μ or anti-Fab activity [103]. A serum which is intended for use as a developing reagent for non-IgM PFC, by the 'difference method', should not exhibit any inhibition in this test. The developing capacity of an antiglobulin serum can be tested as described above, but using spleen cells from mice immunized intraperitoneally with 10^8 SRBC 8–12 days previously. Fig. 64.1 illustrates such a titration and shows how the value of KD is obtained.

2   LHG assay on slides

This assay is similar in principle to the Jerne (Petri dish) method described in the previous section with the exception that there is no 'bottom layer'.

Procedure

Glass microscope slides (25×75 mm), frosted for 15–20 mm on one side of one end, should be grease free. Pre-cleaned slides are readily available from most supply houses. Slides should be numbered on the frosting using a soft graphite pencil. Clean dry slides are subbed by being dipped into hot (60–90 °C) 0.5% A.37 or A.45 agarose in distilled water and then allowed to dry. Any slides that show any sign of

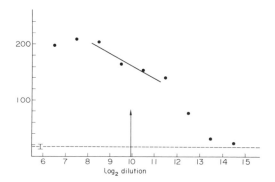

Fig. 64.1. Plot of a KD titration, using spleen cells from CBA males injected 9 days before with 4×10^7 SRBC. The abscissa is the $\log_2$ concentration of antiglobulin serum in the gel medium. The ordinate is the geometric mean number of PFC per plate. The dashed line indicates the mean number of PFC on twelve untreated plates, with one standard deviation indicated. The vertical arrow indicates 0.1% serum, i.e. the concentration of developing serum it was decided to use in subsequent experiments. The KD is calculated as follows:

$$KD_{0.1\%} = \frac{\text{PFC per plate at optimum}}{\text{PFC per plate at 0.1\% serum} - \text{direct PFC}}$$
(concentration of serum) $-$ direct PFC

$$= \frac{210 - 20}{160 - 20}$$

$$= \frac{190}{140}$$

$$= 1.36$$

greasiness must be discarded. Subbed slides may be sterilized by dry heat and can be stored for considerable lengths of time in a dry, dust-free atmosphere. Metal histology racks may be used to hold slides for both subbing and drying. It must be emphasized that patchy or irregular subbing leads to the detachment of the gel medium during the addition of complement or during subsequent washing procedures.

A 0.75% solution of LGT agarose (Miles) in HEPES/Eagle's or Eagle's medium buffered with bicarbonate or phosphate buffers (pH 7.2–7.4), is prepared and kept at 35–37 °C. It has been found when LGT agarose, glass-distilled water and commercially available × 10 concentrated Eagle's medium are used, filtration of the gel medium is not necessary. It should be noted that if for economy reasons A.37 agarose is used in place of the lower melting (and setting) point LGT, the temperature of the water bath should be set to about 41 °C. Subbed slides and Pasteur pipettes are pre-warmed on a thermostatically controlled his-

tology or photographic warming plate with the surface temperature set at 30–37 °C.

In a typical experiment, 0.2 ml aliquots of the gel medium are pipetted, using a pre-warmed pipetting device, into small test-tubes held in a water bath at 35 °C. Ten microlitres of a suitable dilution of developing serum can be added to the appropriate tubes using a suitable pipetting device such as a Hamilton repeater. Ten microlitres of 8–9% (washed) SRBC are added to 0.2 ml of gel medium, which is agitated to thoroughly disperse the target cells. Immediately, 20 µl of an appropriate dilution of lymphoid cells are added (by Eppendorf or Oxford pipette) and mixed with the gel medium, after which the contents of each tube are put on a slide on the warm plate, using a warm Pasteur pipette. The narrow part of the pipette is then used to spread the medium over the full width and about 50 mm of the length of the slide. After about 5 s to allow the layer of molten gel medium to become completely even, the slide is transferred to a cool level surface to allow the gel to set. After about a further 20–40 s has elapsed, the slides are transferred face downwards on to a 'culture tray' (see Fig. 64.2). If LGT agarose is being used in conditions of high ambient tempera-

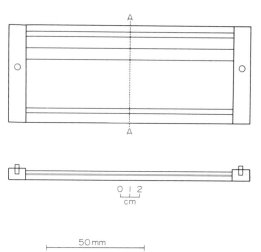

Fig. 64.2. Culture tray for LHG assay on slides. The trays can be milled from perspex (acrylic) and the ends stuck on using a suitable glue. Alternatively, they can be made from a single piece and cut using a horizontal mill. The pins on the end pieces are intended to allow stacking of the trays—to allow for this an appropriately located hole must be cut in the underside of each tray.

tures, it is advisable to use a plate cooled below 15 °C since this form of agarose remains molten down to 28 °C. The medium containing living cells can be kept at 35–37 °C for up to 10 min without there being a significant diminution in the plaque count. Slides should be checked throughout the process. When held up to the light they should appear perfectly homogeneous to the naked eye; if any granularity is apparent, the slides should be discarded, the temperature of the water bath checked and fresh medium or target cells prepared as appropriate.

After 2–4 h incubation at 37 °C in a humid atmosphere, which should contain 5% CO_2 if a bicarbonate buffer is used, complement (5% fresh guinea-pig serum previously absorbed with target cells) is flooded under the slides. After a further 45 min incubation, the plaques on the slides can be counted at once; alternatively, the slides can be fixed in 0.25% glutaraldehyde in physiological saline for 5 min, washed for several minutes in running tap water, rinsed in distilled water and finally dried. The washing procedure can be carried out by placing the slides in a standard 10-slot glass histology tray. They can be dried by being laid face upwards on absorbent paper on the bench.

Notes and recommendations

Apart from a greater sensitivity and convenience than the Jerne technique, the slide assay has two other significant advantages: (1) autoradiographic procedures may be carried out with slides fixed, washed and dried as described above; and (2) reduction and alkylation of IgM (direct) antibody and other such manipulations are possible; the technique as described by Plotz *et al.* [84] has proved to be simple to perform and reliable. For reduction and alkylation, slides are prepared without developing serum and incubated for 1–2 h as described above. One millilitre of dithiothreitol (DTT) or dithioerythritol—McClellan's reagent—(Calbiochem) in 0.1 M-Tris-HCl, pH 8.6, is added to each slide (or flooded between the slide and tray). Plotz *et al.* used 0.01 M-DTT [84]; however, when HEPES buffered Eagle's medium is used it has been found that this must be increased to 0.025 M. After incubation for 30 min at room temperature (20 °C), the excess fluid is removed; 1 ml of 0.02 M-iodacetamide (Koch-Light) (0.05 M if 0·025 M-DTT is used) in 0.1 M-Tris-HCl, pH 7.6, is added to each slide and allowed to remain in contact with the gel for 10 min at room temperature. After a brief rinse in Hanks' solution, the slides are each treated with 1 ml of an optimum concentration of developing serum in Hanks' solution for 45 min at room temperature. Subsequent to a rinse with Hanks' solution, the

reduced and alkylated slides treated with developing serum, plus controls treated with Hanks' solution and further control slides that have neither been reduced and alkylated nor treated with developing serum (IgM-direct PFC), are all exposed to complement as described above.

Monolayer (Cunningham technique)

In this version of the haemolytic plaque assay [18] target cells and PFC as a suspension in liquid medium are introduced into an extremely thin planar chamber, which is placed horizontally to allow the cells to settle down on to the lower face of the chamber, where they form a monolayer. The supporting liquid tissue-culture medium contains a suitable buffering agent for an enclosed chamber, e.g. HEPES (see HEG, page 64.22), or a phosphate-buffered BSS, together with fresh guinea-pig serum (C) at a suitable concentration. Visible plaques can form in 30 min at 37 °C and they are usually optimal after an hour. In a liquid medium, Brownian movements or slight convection currents can lead to the occlusion of small plaques in a few hours; it is therefore necessary to count the plaques within relatively strict time limits.

Procedure

Pre-cleaned plain glass microscope slides (25×75 mm) are used. A row of slides are laid side-by-side on a flat surface and are lined against a straight edge. Three strips of $\frac{1}{4}''$ (about 6 mm) wide, double-sided, self-adhesive tape (Scotch Tape No. 410—Minnesota Mining and Manufacturing Co.) are applied in parallel strips, across the ends and middle of the individual slides, as shown in Fig. 64.3. The backing is peeled off, and another layer of slides are placed exactly on top of the first row and pressed down very firmly using a rubber-faced roller. The tape is trimmed off at the ends of the row of double slides and the individual chambers are separated by breaking them apart.

Each double-chamber has a volume of about 180 μl, so that 200 μl of medium-containing cells should be prepared for each double-chambered slide. For example, 150 μl of a suitable number of spleen cells, in HEPES-buffered Eagle's medium with 0.5% gelatin (HEG), is pipetted into a tube, followed by 20 μl of a suitable dilution of developing (antiglobulin) serum, 20 μl of a 16% suspension of target erythrocytes (SRBC), and 10 μl of fresh target-cell-absorbed guinea-pig serum. For high precision, 160 μl of the mixture can be pipetted into the chamber using an adjustable micropipette and the residual space can be filled with a 'chaser' of target cells in medium. Air

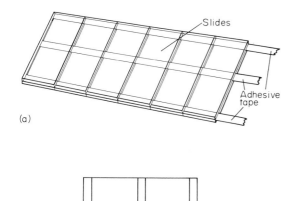

(a)

(b)   Hotplate

Fig. 64.3 Cunningham slide chambers. (a) Making the chambers, and (b) sealing the chamber in molten wax. For details, see text.

Table 64.3. Plaque-forming cells per spleen assayed for a single pool of cells by three variations of the LHG method. Cells prepared 7 days after the intraperitoneal injection of 4×10^7 sheep erythrocytes into male CBA mice. Five samples per point; one standard deviation indicated. Guinea-pig complement absorbed with target cells.

	IgM	IgG$_2$*
Jerne plates	$17\,480 \pm 1560$	$10\,240 \pm 1444$
Slides	$34\,240 \pm 4480$	$15\,680 \pm 3230$
Cunningham chambers	$35\,880 \pm 1098$	$10\,854 \pm 1053$

* Anti-(mouse)-IgG$_2$-globulin was prepared in rabbits. The serum was absorbed and tested for specificity according to the criteria outlined in the text.

bubbles in the chamber lead to movement in the liquid medium with consequent loss of definition of small plaques; this situation can be avoided by ensuring that the slides are absolutely clean and grease-free and that the cell suspension is allowed to warm to room temperature immediately before pipetting into the chamber. The chamber can be most easily sealed after filling by dipping the long edges into a bath of molten paraffin wax–petroleum jelly at 70 °C (Fig. 64.3).

Notes and recommendations

Several workers have shown that the Cunningham assay is more sensitive than the original Jerne assay for the detection of IgM (direct) PFC. In the Cunningham assay the complement has to be added to the system at the start of incubation: unpublished experiments in this laboratory, using the original Jerne method, have shown that the addition of complement at the start of incubation results in the detection of fewer *indirect* plaques than when the complement is added after 2 h of incubation. Table 64.3 shows that, as might be expected, the Cunningham assay is less efficient at detecting indirect PFC than the slide assay where the C has been added after 2 h of incubation (C added after 2 h on the Jerne plates also). In addition, this assay has been found to be unsatisfactory for reversed assays (q.v.) or in assays for RF plaques.

Micromanipulation

It is possible to set up LHG assays in microdrops in such a way that the cell at the centre of a plaque which

is producing the lytic antibody can be micromanipulated and transferred to a new medium. A very simple procedure has been evolved by Cunningham [20].

Procedure

Between 6 and 8 ml of sterile liquid paraffin oil (BP), equilibrated against saline or tissue culture medium, is spread evenly over a clean, grease-free 25×75 mm glass microscope slide. For ease of handling, and to help prevent oil running off the edge, the slide should be supported on a slightly larger piece of glass or Perspex (Acrylic). Medium containing lymphoid cells, target cells and complement (made up exactly as described earlier) is taken up in a Pasteur pipette which has been drawn out into an extremely fine point. Minute drops of medium are placed on the glass surface, beneath the layer of oil. A mouth tube gives better control of the pipetting than a bulb. With a little assistance, the microdrop can be flattened out in contact with the glass, whereupon the cells contained in the liquid will quickly settle to form a monolayer.

The micromanipulator necessary for the removal of a single plaque-forming cell is very simple. A Pasteur pipette drawn out into an exceedingly fine point (20–40 μm i.d.) is fixed firmly in a clamp held on a rack and pinion to allow controlled up and down movement (an old microscope stage can be modified for this). The rack and pinion is attached to a stand with a heavy flat base which rests on a firmly supported level sheet of plate glass; this allows for coarse movement of the pipette point in a horizontal plane; fine movement in this plane is obtained by using the stage of the microscope. The pipetting action is controlled by mouth. A binocular microscope with phase contrast and $\times 40$ high dry lens is suitable.

Notes and recommendations

A somewhat more elaborate method has been described in detail by Nossal *et al.* [76]. They use a medium with a high viscosity derived from its content of carboxymethyl cellulose (CMC) as originally described by Ingraham & Bussard [55]. Despite restrictions on its general usefulness, the CMC-gum technique as described by Nossal *et al.* is very sensitive and may be capable of detecting a 'plaque' formed by the lysis of as 'few as five to seven erythrocytes'.

Special applications

For the micro- or cell biologist, plaque assays provide a selective technique for the identification and enumeration of rare individuals or events. For example, using the LHG assay it is a simple matter to find as few as 10^2 antibody-forming cells in a population of 10^8 spleen cells. However, identification and enumeration are sometimes not enough and the experimenter may want to know the answer to simple questions such as these: (1) does an antibody-forming cell ever make antibodies of more than one specificity? [42]; (2) are antibodies produced by one cell simultaneously of one or more specificities, or of more than one immunoglobulin class?; (3) has a cell, responsible for a particular plaque, incorporated a radiolabelled precursor at some point in its life history?; (4) what is the cellular basis of the humoral response to non-erythrocyte antigens?

Most of these questions can be answered by micro-manipulation experiments (see previous section); however, this is far too cumbersome for many situations. Certain techniques which bypass this limitation are now described.

Replica analysis

This can be made by forming a sandwich of antibody-forming cells between two layers of gel containing target cells. The two layers which contain the target cells can be of different antigenic specificity or of the same specificity, in which case the two layers can be treated differently, e.g. by mild reduction and alkylation of one and not the other or combination of this with different specificities of developing serum.

Experience has shown that it is absolutely essential that the target cell layers are flat, thin and uniform. Any complexity which may enter into the technique is due to the necessity of achieving this end [56].

Procedure

Perfectly flat but thin layers of 1.5% agarose in Dulbecco's phosphate-buffered saline (PBS) are formed on agarose-subbed (25×75 mm) slides in the following manner. Large (15 cm diameter) Petri dishes are placed on a level surface. Thirty-five millilitres of molten 1.5% agarose in 0.9% saline is added to each dish and allowed to set. When set, four subbed slides are carefully placed on the surface of the gel. Twenty-five millilitres of molten 1.5% agarose prepared as described on page 64.3 (bottom layer), is poured over the slides; the Petri dish is then shaken to ensure that the layer of agarose is evenly spread. The lid of the Petri dish is replaced and the gel allowed to set. These prepared slides can be stored in sealed containers for up to a week at 4 °C.

The gel used to suspend the target cells (SRBC) is 0.9% agarose in Eagle's minimal essential medium, plus 10% fetal calf serum. The medium is dispersed in 4 ml aliquots in 75×12 mm test-tubes supported in a water bath at a suitable temperature (37 °C for LGT agarose).

The Petri dishes containing the slides are placed without their lids on a warm plate (60 °C) for 5 min. A volume of 0.2 ml of a washed 25% suspension of target erythrocytes (SRBC) in Hank's solution is added to a 4 ml aliquot of gel-medium, dispersed evenly and the mixture then poured on to a warmed Petri dish. The target erythrocyte suspension is quickly spread and then allowed to set with the covered Petri dish on a level surface. After 10 min at room temperature the slides are cut out and freed of excess gel using a scalpel. Orientation marks consisting of transverse sections of polythene cannula, 0.3–0.4 mm in length can now be added to about half the slides. The prepared slides may be stored in a humid atmosphere for up to 5 h at room temperature.

'Slide-pairs' are formed by first placing a slide with orientation marks face upwards on a suitable surface. A volume of 0.3 ml of a lymphoid cell suspension containing PFC is then pipetted along one of the longer edges. Another slide is then taken face downwards and lowered at such an angle that one of its longer edges is the first part to come into contact with the lymphoid cell suspension: lowering continues, with care being taken to avoid trapping bubbles of air between the two slides. Excess fluid is then removed from the edge by brief contact with absorbent tissue. The slides are then incubated at 37 °C for 2 h in a humid atmosphere; slight pressure is applied by laying a 3 mm thick sheet of glass on top of the slide pairs. After incubation the slides are gently prized apart with a scalpel and placed face upwards in a humid atmosphere: they can then be processed as described on page 64.4 and, where appropriate, different treatments such as reduction-alkylation and use of specific developing sera can be given to the separated slides from each slide pair. A photographic (q.v) record can be kept of the plaques on these slides.

Plaque inhibition

Plaque formation on an assay slide (or plate) can be inhibited by the addition of free soluble antigen or hapten of the same, or cross-reactive, specificity as the target cells. In general, it is clear from experimental observation that the degree of inhibition increases with increasing free antigen concentration [2]. It was once thought that the rate and nature of this increase reflected the distribution of affinities of secreted antibody: the lower the amount of free antigen required to inhibit to an arbitrary level, the higher the affinity of the antibody [58]. However, it is apparent that in practice the situation is very much more complex [75], e.g. an earlier study of Pasanen & Mäkelä showed that high epitope density can be a requirement for the detection of low affinity antibodies [77]. In theoretical studies [21–25,106] it has been concluded that for high epitope density on the sensitized red cells, plaque inhibition curves do indeed reflect the affinity distribution of antibody sites for free hapten. In contrast, where low epitope density allows only monovalent antibody binding, the inhibition curves almost certainly reflect the mean rate of antibody secretion by individual cells.

Since in practice a given situation is likely to be at some ill-defined position between the theoretical limits, it follows that plaque inhibition data cannot be used to give indications of absolute values for either affinity or rate of secretion. Bearing this in mind, it will be clear that accurate control and quantitative monitoring of the coupling of epitopes to target RBC is important.

Photography

Slides produced in the course of a replica experiment, or as described on page 64.5, can be photographed unstained after fixation and drying, by inserting them in the plate (film-negative) carrier of a standard darkroom enlarger; prints can then be made directly on a suitable high contrast photographic paper. Prints of replicate slides can be placed back-to-back, carefully aligning them by the orientation marks: coincident and non-coincident plaques can then be scored by pricking through with a fine needle from one side to another.

Slides or Cunningham chambers can be photographed 'wet' using a suitably constructed illuminator. In principle, the illuminator is based on an inverted enlarger. Light from an enlarger bulb is focussed on to film in a camera using a standard biplanar-convex condenser. The camera lens and film take the place of the enlarger lens and easel, respectively. A 35 mm camera (single lens reflex) and a high contrast fine-

grain film such as 'Microfile' have been found to be ideal. Fig. 64.4 was prepared from photographs made in this way.

Mixed antigens

Target cells of different specificities can be mixed and in certain circumstances it is possible to distinguish the specificity of the plaques which are formed. For example, Petersen & Ingraham coupled a hapten (arsanilazo) to mammalian erythrocytes and mixed this target cell with pigeon erythrocytes to create an experimental situation capable of detecting the specificities of antibodies being released by cells from rabbits immunized by arsanilazo-pigeon-erythrocytes [79]. They were able to distinguish between anti-pigeon and anti-sheep plaques on the grounds of the presence or absence of free nuclei. Incidentally, they ascribed the twenty concentric plaques which they observed (out of a total of 12 665) to a low level of cross-reactivity inherent in the system and not to the presence of 'double-producers': this background 'coincidence' compares with the level of 1–3% with the replica technique.

Cunningham & Sercarz [19] have used mixtures of sheep and bovine erythrocytes as target cells to enumerate cells producing antibody against antigenic determinants common to both species of red cell; Fig. 64.4b illustrates that clear and partial plaques can be distinguished from each other. The same basic methodology was used by Gershon *et al.* in an unsuccessful search for cells producing antibody of more than one specificity [37]; they used both non-cross-reacting erythrocytes and haptens in their experiments.

It is sometimes possible, using fluoresceinated cell-specific antibodies, to visualize antigenic markers on the surface of plaque forming cells detected using the slide method (q.v.) [87]. This technique is greatly simplified in the case of a reversed plaque assay for IgM or IgG producing cells since the high frequency of PFC entails the use of great dilution leading to very few instances of more than one lymphoid cell in each plaque. Fixed and dried slides can also be stained histologically or with radiolabelled reagents for autoradiographic analysis (see next section).

Autoradiography

Slides fixed, washed and dried as described on page 64.6 can be used in autoradiographic experiments. The incorporation of labelled metabolites and other substances into PFC can be followed by this means. For example, Perkins *et al.* have used ^{3}H-thymidine in a study of the role of cell proliferation in the primary immune response of mice to sheep RBC [78]. It is

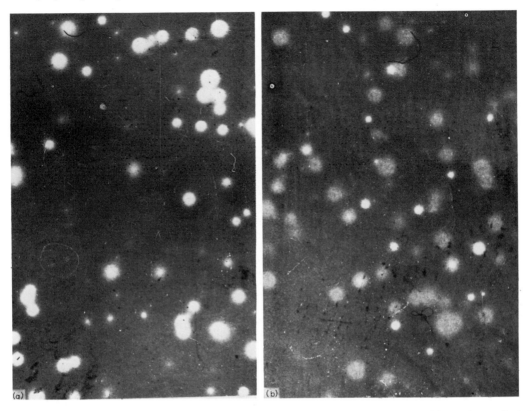

Fig. 64.4. Plaques formed in the Cunningham slide chamber. (a) Normal plaques, and (b) clear and furry plaques (including some sombreros) in a monolayer of mixed sheep and goat erythrocytes (clear plaques indicate cells secreting antibody to determinants common to both target cells).

important to remember that the radiation from ^{3}H and from ^{125}I have a very low penetration, which means that the dried layer of gel must not be thicker than 1 μm. Kennedy & Axelrad have overcome this problem by developing a system where a monolayer of RBC (which are negatively charged) is formed on negatively charged polystyrene (Falcon Petri dish) by means of a positively charged intermediary layer such as poly-L-lysine or 'Polybrene' (Sigma). The plates should be treated with 1% polybrene in water for 10 min at 20 °C, followed by two rinses with PBS and a final treatment with 0·3% BSA (bovine serum albumin) in PBS for 30 min to block non-specific binding. PFC are held in position after the formation of plaques and before autoradiographic procedures by fixation for several hours in glutaraldehyde vapour [62].

It has been found that the standard autoradiographic methodology, as described by Rogers using Ilford K2 or K5 dipping emulsion, is satisfactory [89].

Slice

The microanatomical distribution of groups (clones?) of cells producing antibody can be found by making 50–100 μm sections of quickly frozen lymphoid tissue and laying the sections as they thaw on to a layer of target cells in a gel medium. This method, used originally by Playfair *et al.* [83], is in some respects more convenient than cutting an organ into many small pieces and carrying out a separate plaque assay on each piece. The earlier methodology has been greatly improved by Berenbaum & Stringer, who mount very thin frozen sections on glass slides, cover the sections with a thin layer of gel medium, target erythrocytes and, after addition of complement and suitable incubation, fix, stain and examine the preparation *in toto* [11]. The resolution of their technique is sufficiently good for them to be able to say with confidence that in the primary and secondary response to sheep RBC in the mouse spleen, PFC first appear in the red pulp and are subsequently found in germinal centres.

IEF overlay

Proteins and antibodies which have been isoelectrically focussed in thin polyacrylamide layers, can be visualized by histochemical or autoradiographic staining, as originally described by Awdeh *et al.* [4] An overlay of target erythrocytes followed by complement dependent lysis has also been used to detect bands of focussed antibody [80]. As would be expected by analogy with the cellular LHG, antibody spectrotypes (clonotypes) to erythrocytes or to determinants coupled to erythrocytes [80,81], can be visualized. The method has the advantage that, by using isotype specific developing sera (q.v.), the Ig class of individual spectrotypes can be identified. In practice, it has been found that (1) any target erythrocyte system which is satisfactory in the cellular LHG can be used successfully in the IEF overlay, and (2) IgM antibodies do not *focus* well, unless specially prepared high porosity gels bound covalently to silane-treated glass plates are used [73a,12a].

Procedure

The basic system using riboflavin as a catalyst for UV-activated polymerization (described in Chapter 9 in the 3rd edition of this handbook) is used but modified to give thinner polyacrylamide ampholyte gel layers. Subbed (with 0.1% gelatin, 0.01% chrome alum) 152 × 76 mm glass plates or 38 × 75 mm microscope slides are used. Gels are formed between the glass and a perspex block (not siliconed) using 0.57 mm (or 0.3 mm for microscopic slides) nylon tubing as spacers. For the larger plate, 7.5 ml of solution is pipetted onto the perspex block with nylon tubing spacers already mounted, the glass is then lowered subbed side down, taking care not to trap air. The sandwich is then exposed to UV (365 nm) for several hours. The polymerized gel sticks to the glass but not the perspex.

One to ten microsamples can be loaded on to the polyacrylamide gels [80]. The products of cell clones, or individual cells, or the cells themselves together with their products, can be micromanipulated on to the gels or they can be applied to the gel by the method of Cotton *et al.* [16], who grew microcultures in agarose gel on strips of dialysis membrane; after a period of culture the strips were inverted on to the polyacrylamide-ampholyte gel just prior to focussing.

After focussing for 18 h in the manner described in Chapter 9 in the 3rd edition of this handbook, the polyacrylamide plates are washed for 20–30 min in alkaline Hanks' solution. The plates are then drained free of excess liquid and placed face upwards on a warm plate at 42 °C; 3 ml (for the larger plates) agarose medium containing target erythrocytes and, if necessary, a developing serum (q.v) is spread over the plate. After setting, the plates are put in a humid box for 2 h at about 20 °C. The plates are then inverted on to 1.35 mm diameter nylon tubing on perspex blocks and 10% fresh guinea serum in Hanks' solution is flooded

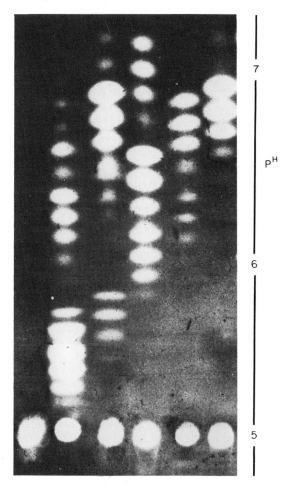

Fig. 64.5. Visualization of anti-sheep RBC spectrotypes in the IEF-overlay method described in the text. Three microlitres of sera from six individual CBA mice injected i.p. 9 days previously with 4×10^6 sheep RBC were applied to the surface of the polyacrylamide gel. The point of application is indicated by a round area of lysis which can be seen at the bottom of the plate: this is due to the presence of IgM which cannot run in the gel. The target cell overlay contained a developing serum for the IgG_{2a} subclass. The pH gradient achieved after 18 h of focussing is indicated. This IEF plate was photographed wet using the apparatus described in an earlier section (q.v.).

between the gel and the perspex. The plates are incubated at 37 °C and are then photographed. Fig. 64.5 is a photograph of a plate of focussed CBA anti-sheep RBC antibodies (3 μl samples of serum) visualized by the complement dependent lysis of sheep RBC in a layer of agarose containing a specific anti-IgG$_{2a}$ developing serum. Spectrotypes (sets of bands) have been visualized on microscope-slide-sized plates with 1 μl samples of serum diluted by a factor of 10^{-3}. Providing suitable controls, such as limiting dilutions, are carried out, a distinct spectrotype can in many situations be used as a 'clonal marker' and in this respect may make a V region marker additional to idiotypic determinants.

Cytotoxicity

A technique to measure cytotoxicity by a reduction in numbers of haemolytic plaques has been described by Ezaki *et al.* [33,107]. Hybridoma cells producing antibody (and hence PFC) to RBC are the target cells for cytotoxicity. The effect, which is measured in terms of a reduction in numbers of PFC against the RBC, is very sensitive since few of the antibody-secreting target cells (PFC) are required.

Non-erythrocyte antigens

Proteins

Segre & Segre measured the response of mice to immunization with rabbit IgG by means of the LHG assay, using as target cells sheep RBC coated with sub-haemolytic amounts or rabbit antibody to sheep RBC [92]. Dresser & Wortis showed that serum albumins could be coupled to tannic acid treated sheep RBC and that these coated erythrocytes could be used as target cells [31]. They also showed that bis-diazo-benzidine (BdB)* is a successful and economical reagent for coating sheep RBC with bovine γ-globulin for use in the LHG assay. Golub *et al.* [38] successfully used 1-ethyl-3(3-dimethyl-aminopropyl) carbodi-imide HCl (ECDI) as a coupling reagent for linking human γ-globulin to goat RBC and used these cells as targets in the LHG assay. Kapp & Ingraham [61] confirmed earlier findings that BdB is more economical of antigen than ECDI in the preparation of passively sensitized target cells.

---

* This method [60] is not described in this chapter, not only because it has been superceded by simpler and perhaps more reliable methods but because benzidine is a powerful carcinogen and its use should be avoided whenever possible.

ECDI method

The methodology described here was originally that used by Dr Eli Sercarz (UCLA) for conjugating lysozymes to erythrocytes and it has not received any notable alteration in the author's laboratory.

Procedure

Goat RBC stored in Alsever's solution for at least 10 days are washed four times in 0.15 M-NaCl (phosphate ions *must* be avoided at all costs). Forty micrograms of lysozyme are dissolved in 6 ml of 0.15 M-NaCl, which is then added to 0.4 ml of packed, washed goat RBC. Meanwhile, 20 mg of ECDI (Ott Chemical Co.) are quickly dissolved in 0.4 ml of 0.15 M-NaCl and the solution is then added immediately, with brisk mixing, to the mixture of protein and goat RBC. The reaction mixture is left at room temperature (20 °C) for 30–60 min and the RBC then washed three times in 1% NRS–0.15 M-NaCl (the NRS should be absorbed with both the goat RBC and an insoluble form of the protein antigen). The coated RBC may be stored for a day at 4 °C before being used as target cells.

Notes and recommendations

The method works well with other proteins, but it has been found that the optimal concentrations differ; e.g. serum albumins should be at a concentration of 50 mg/ml of reaction volume, IgG at 20–30 mg/ml and lysozymes at about 5 mg/ml. HEPES-buffered media should not be used in LHG assays with target cells prepared by the ECDI method.

Chromic chloride method

In an elegant study of the effects of metallic cations on erythrocyte membranes, Jandl & Simmons showed that Cr^{3+} was effective as a coupling reagent for linking certain proteins to red blood cells [57]. Subsequently, Gold & Fudenberg [41] introduced the method for immunological purposes. The simplicity and reliability of the method has been demonstrated by several workers both for 'normal' [26,39,53] and reversed LHG applications [72].

Procedure

The method that has been found in the author's laboratory to be the most reliable and simple, is as follows. Sheep RBC are washed three or four times in saline (0.15 M-NaCl) at 20 °C; it is important to note that (1) the RBC of some sheep tend to agglutinate spontaneously in low concentrations of CrCl$_3$, (2) phosphate ions strongly inhibit the coupling reaction and should therefore be avoided at this stage in the proceedings, and (3) all glassware must be scrupulously clean.

Chromic chloride ($CrCl_3$) is dissolved in 0.15 M-NaCl at a concentration of 10 mg/100 ml ($\sim 4 \times 10^{-5}$ M).

One volume of 50% (packed cell volume) SRBC, plus 10 vols. of a saline solution of protein (1–2 mg/ml for goat IgG; 0.25–0.5 mg/ml for mouse IgG) at 20 °C, are mixed together in a 15 ml graduated plastic centrifuge tube (Falcon 2095). While the tube of RBC–protein is being briskly agitated on a vortex mixer, 10 vols. of the freshly prepared chromic chloride solution is added quickly. The mixture is then incubated at 20 °C for 20 min (10 min for mouse IgG) before the reaction is stopped by the addition of a phosphate containing BSS (Hanks' gelatin-HG). The RBC are washed three or four times in HG and can be stored in HG at 0 °C for several days before use.

Notes and recommendations

An alternative methodology [39] using 'matured' chromic chloride may be very effective for the preparation of stable target cells for rosetting or agglutination tests.

The need to select a 'good' sheep as a source of stable RBC for $CrCl_3$ coupling cannot be over-emphasized. As mentioned above the RBC of some sheep spontaneously agglutinate in dilute $CrCl_3$ solution and of others the coupled RBC are noticeably unstable. The authors selects sheep on the basis of both the suitability of their RBC for $CrCl_3$ coupling and as positive responders in Dutton-Mishell type cultures using mini-Marbrook culture chambers (Hendley Engineering, Loughton, Essex LG10 3TZ) [69]. On two occasions he has found two 'good' sheep in a group of ten or a dozen cross-bred Welsh mountain sheep.

The following general points may be relevant in particular instances. (1) The optimal concentration of protein, which may differ from one type of protein to another, should be determined by experimentation. (2) An optimum for haemolysis may sometimes be suboptimal for agglutination. (3) Economy of protein may be effected by reducing the volumes of $CrCl_3$ and protein solutions used in the recipe, keeping the *concentration* of protein the same and the *absolute amount* of $CrCl_3$ (for a given amount of RBC) constant. (4) The use of piperazine buffer is unnecessary. (5) The chromic chloride method is perfectly satisfactory for coating goat and horse RBC. (6) The method is suitable for some but not all viral antigens [117]

Benzoquinone method

Ternynck & Avrameas [100] have published a method for coupling antigens to enzymes or red blood cells. Professor J. H. Humphrey (personal communication) has successfully used the method to couple arsanylated-bovine γ-globulin (Ars-BGG) to sheep RBC, and used the coated target cells to detect anti-arsanyl antibodies by means of agglutination and haemolytic plaques.

Procedure

Two milligrams of Ars-BGG dissolved in 0.4 ml PBS, is added to 3 mg benzoquinone (*p*-1,4-benzoquinone) in 0.1 ml ethanol. (The benzoquinone (Fluka-AG) can be used without further purification or doubtful preparations can be recrystallized from Ligroin to give brownish-yellow crystals).

The mixture is kept at 20 °C for 20 min in the dark, and then passed down a Sephadex G-25 (fine) column equilibrated against fresh 0.1 M-NaHCO$_3$—two coloured bands form: the first, a clean orange/brown, is retained on elution and the second, a muddy brown colour, is discarded.

The retained material is added to 0.4 ml of packed saline-washed SRBC in 2 ml 0.1 M-NaHCO$_3$. The mixture is gently rotated or stirred for 3 h at 20 °C (or $\frac{1}{2}$ h at 37 °C). The coated SRBC are washed three times in PBS or Hanks' solution.

'Anti-enzyme plaques'

Rotman & Cox [90] have described a method for enumerating lymphoid cells which bind (as an antigen) the enzyme β-D-galactosidase. After binding the enzyme, the cells are washed and then plated in agarose containing riboflavin-β-D-galactopyranoside, streptomycin, riboflavin-deficient medium and a streptomycin-resistant strain of *Streptococcus faecalis* that requires riboflavin. Release of riboflavin occurs around each individual cell binding β-D-galactosidase and initiates the localized growth of bacteria which form a visible colony. The technique is not limited to the detection of enzyme binding cells since haptens and proteins can be coupled to the enzyme.

Certain mutant strains of *E. coli* produce an inactive β-galactosidase which can be activated when bound by an IgG antibody. The substrate 5-bromo-4-chloro-3 indoxy-β-D-galactopyranoside, when split by activated enzyme, produces an insoluble blue-green stain *in situ*. This reagent has been used to detect spectrotypes of anti-β-galactosidase antibodies [63] and at least in principle might be applied to the detection of antibody produced by single cells.

Rheumatoid factor plaques

Rheumatoid factors (RF) are often IgM antibodies with specificity for IgG molecules (M-anti-G) in the same individual or species (homophile) and sometimes cross-reacting with IgG of other species (heterophile). Other combinations have been demonstrated (G-anti-G) [47] or suspected (M-anti-A; G-anti-A, etc.). A direct plaque assay for M-anti-G RF producing cells has been described for human lymphoid cells [27]. In contrast it has been shown that mouse M-anti-G RF plaques are unusual in that they are indirect and must be developed by a C-fixing μ-specific developing serum [29]. These plaques are inhibited by guinea-pig IgG_1 anti-mouse-μ but developed by an IgG_2 with the same specificity and obtained from the same individual guinea-pig [29a].

Recently, Petersen *et al.* [79a] have evaluated a methodology for detecting heterophile human G–anti-G PFC, using as target cells SRBC coated with rabbit IgG. A key step in their procedure seems to be the use of IgG-depleted guinea-pig serum as a source of complement. See reference 121 which suggests RF plaques may be due to cross-linking of effector IgM and contaminating IgM in target IgG preparation by developing serum.

Procedure

The assay for mouse RF-PFC is essentially that described earlier as the 'slide method', but using sheep RBC coated with mouse IgG by the chromic chloride method as the target cells. However, since these target cells are very susceptible to non-specific lysis, the following extra precautions must be taken.
1   The sheep RBC are coated with as little mouse IgG as possible—about 0.25–0.5 mg/ml of protein solution in the recipe given earlier.
2   The mouse IgG is prepared by passage through a column of DEAE cellulose (DE52) in 0.01 M-Tris-HCl, (pH 8.1)–0.02 M-NaCl. The 'performance' of mouse (and rat) IgG is improved by one or both of the following procedures. The first is precipitation in 25% v/v ethanol (in 0.075 M-acetate buffer, pH 6.7) by putting one volume of protein solution in an ice/salt bath until ice crystals start to form, whereupon an equal volume of 50% ethanol at −10 °C, is added slowly so that the temperature of the mixture is lowered progressively to −7 °C. The precipitate is centrifuged down and after removal of the supernatant is dissolved in cold saline. The second procedure is mild acid treatment in which the pH is adjusted to 4.0–4.1 with 0.1 M-acetate buffer, after incubation for 1 h at 37 °C, the pH is returned to 7. Aliquots of mouse IgG treated in this way have been stored satisfactorily for up to 2 years at −70 °C.

3   The guinea-pig complement is carefully absorbed with coated target cells or mouse IgG-Sepharose, before use.

As mentioned above, the experiments of Petersen *et al.* [79a] suggest that in some circumstances the guinea-pig serum used as a source of complement should be depleted of IgG. This can be done by passage down a column of Protein A–Sepharose (Pharmacia) after dialysis of the serum against a suitable buffer at pH 8 (0 °C).
4   Since the numbers of RF-PFC are very high, even in a 'normal' mouse spleen, it is essential to dilute the spleen cell suspension sufficiently (spleen in 100 ml HG—20 μl of suspension per slide), if general lysis due to confluent plaques is to be avoided.

Glycolipid

Several workers have successfully used lipopolysaccharide (LPS) antigens of Gram-negative bacteria in the LHG and rosette assay. Schwarts & Braun described a plaque assay which used intact *E. coli* organisms as the targets [91]. Most other workers have used purified extracts of LPS prepared from such bacteria [13,46,65,73] (see Chapter 3). Sheep RBC are quickly and easily coated by incubating the LPS and RBC at 37 °C. For example, 1 ml of PBS containing 1 mg of LPS prepared from *E. coli* by the method of Westphal & Jann [104] (can be purchased from Difco) is added to 0.5 ml of washed sheep RBC and incubated at 37 °C for 30–60 min. The erythrocytes are then washed before being used in the LHG assay as targets. LPS can be sterilized by boiling for 2 h without affecting its antigenicity [13]: alternatively, it may be sterilized by filtration through a Millipore membrane.

Hämmerling & Westphal have used *O*-stearoylpolysaccharide for the preparation of passively sensitized erythrocytes [48], and in the course of their experiments showed that it is the lipid moiety which is responsible for binding to erythrocyte membranes.

Carbohydrate antigens

Certain antigens, including many carbohydrates—e.g. PVP (polyvinylpyrolidone), SIII (pneumococcal polysaccharide type III and some parasite antigens—are not easily coupled directly to target RBC. An interesting technique has been described recently [5] which avoids this problem by passively binding these antigens to latex beads (1.0–1.5 μm diameter; Dow Diagnostics), which together with uncoated sheep RBC in a ratio of 50:1 are added to the plaquing mixture in a Cunningham chamber (q.v.). Binding of antibody to the antigen on the beads initiates complement fixation and by a 'bystander-effect' leads to lysis of closely adjacent sheep RBC, thereby forming a visible plaque. The method visualizes IgM (direct) plaques and with the use of suitable developing sera can be used to detect IgG PFC.

Haptens

DNP (2,4-dinitrophenyl) is one of the most widely used haptenic determinants. In general, most of the procedures which can be used to coat erythrocytes with DNP can also be used for other haptenic groupings. The hapten or an activated form of the hapten can be (1) chemically linked directly to the erythrocyte membrane or (2) coupled to a protein or carbohydrate intermediate (carrier), which in turn can be linked to the erythrocyte membrane by one of the procedures described in the previous section.

1   DNP comes in two readily available active forms: FDNB (1-fluoro-2,4-dinitrobenzene) or as DNBS (2,4-dinitrobenzene sulphonic acid). Both reagents are regularly used for coupling DNP groups on to protein carriers [32], but FDNB seems to be too active and DNBS not quite active enough for reliable and successful direct coupling to erythrocytes. However, TNP (2,4,6-trinitrophenyl; picryl) can be used as a satisfactory determinant on plaque assay indicator (target) cells in experiments where animals have been immunized by DNP carrier. The active reagent TNBS seems to be ideal for coupling to sheep or horse RBC. The 100% cross-reaction between TNP and DNP is operational for plaque experiments when DNP is the immunogen but is only partial if humoral antibodies are being measured qualitatively.

Procedure

(i) Coupling procedures [88]: sheep or horse RBC are washed three or four times in PBS. Six to sixty milligrams of TNBS (Sigma) is dissolved in 7 ml of PBS which contains phenol red. The pH is adjusted to 7.0–7.4 by the addition of 0.5 M NaOH. Sixty milligrams of TBNS in this recipe gives 'heavy coupling' which favours the detection of PFC producing low affinity antibodies [77]. The RBC of some sheep show spontaneous lysis with this amount of TNBS. It has been found that 40 mg TNBS is sufficient for the optimum detection of low-affinity PFC with these RBC. Ten milligrams is the amount used in the standard procedure.

One millilitre of packed RBC is added to the TNBS solution, and gently stirred for 20 min at 20 °C, after which triglycine (1.1 mg for every 1 mg TNBS) dissolved in PBS is added to the mixture to stop the reaction.

The coated RBC are washed in Hanks' gelatin or PBS until there is no free colour (four or five times).

After each centrifugation (1700 *g*) the RBC should be resuspended using a Pasteur pipette.

It is essential that complement (fresh guinea-pig serum) is absorbed with hapten-lys-Sepharose 4B and RBC before use in assays employing hapten-RBC target cells.

(ii) NIP (3-iodo-5-nitro-4-hydroxyphenyl acetic acid) (or NP: 3-nitro-4-hydroxyphenyl acetic acid) can be coupled to erythrocyte membranes using the azide forms. NIP-azide prepared by the method of Brownstone *et al.* [14] is stored dry at −70 °C.

To 0.1–1(5) mg of NIP azide is added 1 ml of 10% saline washed sheep RBC (three times). After 10 min at 20 °C with occasional stirring, the RBC are washed four or five times in Hanks' gelatin. Complement should be absorbed with coupled RBC or NIP-Sepharose. The exact amount of a particular preparation of NIP azide required for a particular purpose should be determined experimentally: the quality of preparations can vary considerably. Sometimes, higher epitope densities are required when low affinity antibodies are to be detected [78].

2   (i) Proteins conjugated with DNP by the method of Eisen [32] or with NIP by the method of Brownstone *et al.* [14], may be coupled to RBC by one of the methods for 'protein coupling' described earlier.

(ii) DNP (or NIP) can be linked by stearo-amino-ethyl-polyvinylalcohol to form a synthetic hapten-'LPS' [96] which can then be coupled to RBC by the method described above under the heading 'Glycolipid antigens'.

(iii) The following method has proved to be both easy to perform and reliable. It is essentially an extension of the technique of Segre & Segre [92] and is similar to the methodology described by Strausbauch *et al.* [98]. The principle involved is to conjugate antigenic determinants (haptens) to erythrocytes via Fab monomers of anti-erythrocyte antibodies.

A rabbit is hyperimmunized with sheep RBC by injecting it three or four times intravenously at 2–3 day intervals with 10^8 sheep RBC. Eight to twelve days after the last injection of antigen, the rabbit is bled and IgG is prepared from the antiserum by the method outlined on page 64.18. As an example of the procedure now adopted, 10 mg of the IgG in 1.0 ml of saline is mixed with an equal volume of acetate buffer pH 4.5 (43 ml 0.3 M-NaAc plus 57 ml 0.2 M HAc). To this mixture is added 1 mg of *pepsin* (Worthington) in the same acetate buffer. A single drop of toluene is added to inhibit bacterial growth and the mixture is incubated at 37 °C overnight. Next morning sufficient of a molar solution of Tris is added to raise the pH to 7.0. The digested protein is reduced by adding sufficient dithiothreitol (DTT: Calbiochem or Koch Light) to make the solution $5(-50) \times 10^{-4}$ M, for 1 h at 20 °C, pH 7.0. The reduced protein is alkylated by adding α-iodoacetyl ε-N-DNP-lysine (IDNPL) [12,44] allowing a 10% molar excess over the active sites of the DTT added to the mixture. This procedure couples a DNP group to the C-terminal end of the Fab monomer. Providing the original rabbit anti-sheep RBC serum had a reasonably high titre, about 0.02 mg of DNP-Fab added to 1 ml 10% washed sheep RBC, followed by further centrifugal washes, results in passively sensitized DNP-RBC for use in the LHG assay.

Alternatively, DNP and NIP can be coupled to Fab (from rabbit (anti-SRBC) IgG) using the general methods for coupling these haptens to proteins, which are described by Iverson in Chapter 69. Sheep RBC sensitized passively in these ways can be used in the LHG assay but are not quite as efficient as the method detailed above. Each batch must be tested carefully before being used in a routine assay.

Whole fowl antibody directed against mammalian target erythrocytes can be used as a vehicle for attaching haptens to the RBC [94]. The Fc portion of chicken IgG does not fix guinea-pig complement, so there is no problem with a general spontaneous lysis. It has, however, been observed in the author's laboratory that this method using IgG prepared from fowl anti-sheep RBC serum is less sensitive than the use of the best preparations of Fab from the IgG of rabbit antisera to sheep RBC. It seems that the substitution ratio of hapten to fowl globulin is critical, with only a narrow optimum range.

Nucleated target cells

In 1971, Fuji, Zaleski & Milgrom [36] and Nordin, Cerottini & Brunner [74] published papers describing plaque assays for enumerating cells secreting antibody against nucleated allogeneic mouse cells. Both groups made monolayers of target cells, added antibody secreting cells and after a period of incubation added rabbit complement. Plaques were visualized by fixing and staining the unlysed cells in the target cell layer. Fuji *et al.* who used thymus (Thy-1) and lymphoblast (H-2) target cells incubated for 1 h in complement before fixing and staining, whereas Nordin *et al.*, using the DBA/2 mastocytoma (P815Y) cell line (H-2^d), found it necessary to wash the monolayer 1 h after complement addition and incubate it in medium plus antibiotic for a further 24 h before fixation and staining.

Intact bacteria may be used as target cells in a plaque methodology described by Schwartz & Braun [91].

Zones of inhibited phage plaques

'Plaques' may be visualized as opaque discs (colonies of growing bacteria) surrounding cells secreting antibody against bacteriophages [99]. Antibody-secreting cells are incubated at 37 °C in a thin layer of agarose containing tissue culture medium and a target bacteriophage such as φX174 or Fd. This gel is then overlaid by a thin layer of suspension of an appropriate strain of bacteria in nutrient agar. After a short incubation at a temperature optimal for bacteria, the active lysis of bacteria in the indicator lawn is stopped by the addition of an excess of hyperimmune antiphage antibody. The slides are then washed and dried before the ZIPPs (zones of inhibited phage plaques) are enumerated.

The technique, which is basically a 'reversed plaque' method, is fairly difficult to carry out successfully. The optimal concentration of phage, the various incubation times and the concentration of the 'stopping antiserum' must be determined experimentally. An assay of this difficulty and complexity should never be used if a simpler method can be used, such as, for example, conventional phage inactivation assay for humoral antibody [1].

The principle of the ZIPP assay has been extended to the visualization of antiphage antibody bands (spectrotypes) on IEF plates by an overlay procedure analogous to that described earlier (Dr Jan Obel, personal communication).

Immunoglobulin-(antigen) secreting cells
(reversed plaque assay)

At the beginning of this chapter, a description was given for using the LHG methodology for detecting cells synthesizing antibody against antigenic determinants (epitopes) on target erythrocytes: these epitopes can be either native to the erythrocytes or coupled to them by one of the methods described earlier. It is possible to turn this system inside out, coat the target erythrocytes with antibody (EAb), and thus be able to detect cells secreting antigen. The method was first described by Dray *et al.* [70–72] who used a chromic chloride method to couple either IgG from hyperimmune (rabbit) sera or 'pure antibody' eluted from affinity columns, to sheep erythrocytes. These target cells (EAb) were used to detect cells synthesizing human IgG in one series of experiments and, in another, rabbit lymphoid cells secreting Ig bearing a particular allotypic marker (b locus).

The methodology has been used to enumerate mouse cells secreting IgM, using target cells coated with goat anti-(mouse)-μ by the chromic method described earlier. It has been found that it is unnecessary to make affinity preparations from the goat IgG providing that the goat has been hyperimmunized. The IgG is prepared by precipitation in half-saturated ammonium sulphate (4 °C) followed by elution from DEAE cellulose (DE52—Whatman) in 0.01 M-Tris-HCl, pH 8.1, containing 0.04 M-NaCl. General lysis of target cells when complement is added to the assay slides has not been observed in this system.

Problems with lysis of target cells have been experienced when sheep RBC have been coated with rabbit IgG, human IgG, and canine IgG. In the 'reversed plaque' assay, such general lysis can be avoided either (1) by using 'pure antibody' prepared by affinity chromatography, thus leading to a reduction to sub-lytic levels of IgG on the target erythrocytes, or (2) by blocking the complement binding site on the IgG molecules through fluoresceination [101].

Dr J. M. Phillips has shown (in unpublished experiments) that the reversed LHG procedure of Dray et al. can be used successfully in the IEF-overlay methodology described on page 64.11. Allotypically marked rabbit IgG spectrotypes have been visualized using sheep RBC coated with rabbit (anti-allotype) IgG by the chromic chloride method.

False or pseudoplaques can be formed by aggregations of platelets or damaged lymphoid cells or by the presence of microcolonies of haemolytic bacteria. These hazards of the LHG assay can be avoided by differential centrifugation, and by using a medium containing protein, sterile solutions and thoroughly clean glassware.

Universal method

An elegant modification of the methodology of 'reversed plaquing' has been described by Gronowicz, Coutinho & Melchers [45]. The method has been confirmed as being both practical and simple although not giving plaque counts as high as some of the goat IgG preparations used in the direct coupling method described above. As originally described [45], the modified assay makes use of the fact that protein A from *Staphylococcus aureus* (Cowan 1) binds to Fc portions of IgG molecules. Three versions of the reversed assay have been compared recently [120]: an agarose in Petri dish, agar under coverslip and the Cunningham assay. While the Cunningham version was the most efficient of the methods used in this comparison, the 'slide' method using LGT agarose (p. 64.4) was not included in that study. It is the author's experience that the 'slide' method is more efficient than the Cunningham assay for the detection of rheumatoid plaques and is of about equal efficiency for reverse plaques.

Procedure

Protein-A coated (CrCl$_3$ method q.v.) (sheep) RBC are plated in a Cunningham chamber together with Ig-secreting cells, complement and the IgG fraction of (rabbit) antisera specific for the various types and classes of Ig. If the slide method is used, the C can be added after 2–3 h incubation. Complexes of the secreted Ig and IgG antibodies specific for the secreted Ig, bound to protein A on the red cell surface, activate sufficient amounts of complement to lyse the protein A-coated red cells. As a result of a prozone phenomenon, the effectiveness of developing serum-IgG has a pronounced concentration maximum and optimum values must be determined by experimentation.

Notes and recommendations

It is clear that SRBC coated with protein A will make a universal reversed-plaque target cell whose versatility depends only on the availability and specificity of (rabbit) sera specific for various secreted proteins. There are many obvious clinical and experimental applications [108,116,118,119].

An interesting variant of the reversed plaque assay designed for the detection of red blood cells carrying abnormal or mutant haemoglobins, has been described recently [6]. For example, sheep RBC are coated (using CrCl$_3$ with or without protein A intermediary) with a monospecific anti-(DBA/2 mouse) haemoglobulin; these target cells are mixed with a polyspecific anti-mouse haemoglobin developing serum together with a mixture of say DBA/2 and C57B1 RBC in a ratio of 1:100, in an agarose gel on a slide or in a Cunningham chamber. An antiserum specific for mouse RBC (absorbed with sheep RBC) is added with C to lyse all the mouse RBC, the target (coated) sheep RBC surrounding each lysed DBA/2 will lyse to form a visible plaque. In principle, this is a powerful method for searching for rare mutants providing the appropriate monospecific (hybridoma) antisera are available. The technique, which is at least as sensitive as immunofluorescence for detecting Ig-producing cells [113], can have its sensitivity increased further by lowering the threshold for lysis by the controlled addition of antigen (Ig) to the target cells [112]

Preparation of cell suspensions

Harvesting cells from lymphoid organs

For example, a mouse is killed by cervical dislocation, thoroughly wetted with 70% alcohol, opened with the aid of clean (sterile) dissecting instruments and the spleen removed. The pellicle of the spleen should then be cut as the spleen is dropped into 1–2 ml of HG in a 15 ml round-bottomed centrifuge tube. The spleen is then gently homogenized using a very loose-fitting PTFE (polytetrafluoroethylene; Teflon) pestle. The homogenizer pestles which may be purchased from most large supply houses can be turned down on a lathe so that they have about a 1 mm clearance in the centrifuge tube, and in addition the surface of the pestle can be finished with a fine screw thread. The cell suspension is sieved through a 30–35 hole/cm stainless steel mesh into a 15 ml graduated centrifuge tube to remove connective tissue. The suspension is then immediately made up to 15 ml with HG (20 °C) and centrifuged at 600 g for 5 min in a refrigerated centrifuge at 4 °C. The supernatant which contains platelets and cell debris is discarded and the cells are resuspended in 1–2 ml of cold HG. The prepared cell suspensions can be stored at 0 °C for up to 3 h without any detectable deterioration taking place: in many instances mouse spleen cells have been kept for 24 h with only very marginal reduction in the number of detected plaques. It should not take longer than 30 min from killing the animal to putting the tube containing the prepared cell suspension into an ice water bath.

The following points may be of interest in certain circumstances.

1   Very high viable cell counts can be obtained if a spleen is gently teased in tissue culture medium, although the total number of cells obtained is lower.

2   Large numbers of spleens in a 'pool' experiment can be homogenized by gently pressing them through a fine-meshed nylon strainer.

3   Individual lymph nodes can be easily homogenized with minimal cell damage providing the pellicle of the node is first cut two or three times with scissors.

4   Thymus and to a lesser extent mesenteric lymph nodes contain cells which are very sensitive to adverse conditions in that they lyse, releasing DNA which agglutinates the lymphoid cells. Although the condition can be treated with DNAase (1 mg/ml) it is better to prevent lysis by using scrupulously clean glassware and Hanks' solution containing 15–20% fetal calf serum or 0.5% gelatin (HG).

5   RBC in a spleen cell suspension can be removed by centrifugally washing the cells in haemolytic HG (NaCl is replaced by an equimolar amount of NH_4Cl) followed by suspension of the lymphoid cells in HG. It has been observed that two washes in haemolytic HG, involving the spleen cells being in contact with ammonium chloride for up to 20 min, has no measurable effect on the five main classes of CBA mouse PFC to sheep RBC. Use of Tris-buffered NH_4Cl was found to be detrimental in this experiment.

6   Very convenient sieves can be made by pressing small pieces of mesh into a shape like a bowler hat which when inverted fits neatly into the top of a 15 ml graduated centrifuge tube.

Harvesting cells from blood

Peripheral blood leucocytes (PBL) may be prepared from whole blood using the method of Crispens [17]. The procedure used in the author's laboratory for mouse PBL is now described. A heparinized 1 ml tuberculin syringe fitted with a 27-gauge, $\frac{5}{8}''$ needle is used to obtain 0.4 ml blood from the heart of chloroform-anaesthetized mice. Immediately after collection the blood is diluted in an equal volume of 0.15 M-NaCl at ambient temperature (20–22 °C). After not more than 1 h, 0.4 ml of the diluted blood is layered on top of 1 ml of Ficoll-Paque (Pharmacia) at ambient temperature in a round-bottomed 75×11 mm (i.d.) glass tube—these dimensions are important. Following centrifugation at 200 g for 25 min at 20–22 °C, the white cell layer at the interface is removed and transferred to standard centrifuge tubes for three centrifugal washes in HG. This number of washes is necessary to remove free serum Ig which can have serious detrimental effects on the target cells in reversed plaque assays. The prepared PBL can be stored in HG at 0 °C for up to 24 h.

Anti-immunoglobulin sera

Anti-immunoglobulin sera can be used *inter alia* for the development and inhibition of plaques. When using such serum it is essential that its specificity and optimal working concentration is known. Fig. 12.1 (Chapter 12) is a highly simplified diagram of an archetypal mouse immunoglobulin unit and from this it can be deduced that if class-specific antisera are required the best immunizing antigen preparation (immunogen) would be the Fc of a homogeneous globulin of the desired class. The most practical source of such material lies in myeloma or hybridoma protein, produced in inbred strains of mice by lines of transplantable plasmacytomas or hybridomas. There are many such lines which are readily available and can be used for this purpose. General methods for immunizing animals to raise such anti-Ig sera are described and discussed in Chapter 8.

Preparing immunogen

1   Many plasmacytoma (myeloma) lines are grown as solid tumours, although some may be grown for a limited number of generations as ascites. Cell lines may be obtained from American Type Culture Collec-

tion, 12301 Parklawn Drive, Rockville, Md 20852, U.S.A. or from Litton Bionetics, 5516 Nicholson Lane, Kensington, Md. Both organizations produce useful catalogues.

A small lump of tumour, about 1–2 mm³, is taken up in a trochar and is implanted subcutaneously either in the flank or the back of a mouse of the appropriate strain. The tumour will grow to optimum size in 10–20 days; allowing the tumour to grow too long will result in the formation of large areas of necrosis in the tumour itself. During the growth of the tumour the mouse can be bled so that myeloma protein can be separated from the serum.

Hybridoma and myeloma lines can be propagated by serial transplantation. The sera of potential donors must be tested by a simple electrophoretic run in agar gel, so that a selective procedure can ensure that the property of high protein production is retained by the line. Myelomas and hybridoma lines have been stored successfully for many years in a liquid nitrogen refrigerator.

When preparing such tissue for preservation, the author chops solid tissue into small lumps (1–2 mm³) in Hanks' solution containing 10% fetal calf serum and 10% dimethyl sulphoxide (DMSO-BDH); alternatively he makes up a cell suspension in the same medium. The material is then dispensed in 1 ml ampoules (NUNC) which are sealed and then frozen down at 1 °C/min from zero to −15 °C and at up to 4 °C/min thereafter [3]. These freezing rates can be obtained precisely by using a programmed machine [3,95], but it has been found that the rates obtained using the cheap adaptor made by Linde and BOC to fit the neck of their liquid nitrogen refrigerators are satisfactory. Frozen material should be thawed rapidly to 37 °C and implanted immediately or injected into pristane primed mice; 2,6,10,14-tetra-methylpentadecane, 0.5 ml i.p. into BALB/c mice a few days before injection of cells.

2 Ascitic fluid or serum from mice bearing a myeloma or hybridoma can be purified as follows. An equal volume of ammonium sulphate, saturated at 4 °C (pH 6.5), is added dropwise with constant stirring to the protein solution. The mixture is left for several hours at 4 °C before the precipitate is centrifuged down and washed in half-saturated ammonium sulphate (10 000 *g* for 15 min). It is finally dissolved in a small volume of physiological saline. If the protein is to be further purified by ion-exchange chromatography on DEAE-cellulose, it should be exhaustively dialysed against several changes of 0.01 M-Tris-HCl, pH 8.1, for at least 36 h. Because of their homogeneity, myeloma proteins can, if the appropriate conditions are known, be eluted from a DEAE column (DE-52; Whatman) by a stepwise procedure; e.g. 5563 protein

can be eluted by 0.01 M-Tris-HCl, pH 8.1, 0.06 M-NaCl but not at any lesser concentration of salt. However, if the *exact* conditions for elution are not known, elution should be made using a shallow gradient of NaCl (0–0.1 M) in 0.01 M-Tris-HCl, pH 8.1. Peaks should be concentrated by pressure dialysis and then tested as described on page 64.21.

IgM should not be precipitated in ammonium sulphate but should be partially purified by gel filtration on, for example, Ultrogel (ACA22-LKB). α₂-Macroglobulin can be separated from IgM by preparative electrophoresis or by the method of Bazin *et al.* [9].

3 The following simplified method has been found to be adequate for the preparation of Fc and Fab fragments of mouse IgG by Dr G. M. Iverson.

An equal volume of 0.2 M Sørensen phosphate buffer, pH 7.2, containing 0.008 M-EDTA is added to a 0.5–5% solution of protein in saline. To this is added 10 mg of Mercuripapain suspension (Worthington) for every gram of protein to be digested. The reaction mixture is then made 0.01 M with 2-mercaptoethanol (Koch-Light) and incubated for 4 h at 37 °C; the optimum incubation time varies with different species of IgG—4 h is about right for mouse IgG. The digestion is stopped by adding 1/33 the volume of the reaction mixture of 0.5 M-iodoacetamide in 1 M-Tris, after which the protein mixture is dialysed exhaustively against 0.01 M-Tris-HCl, pH 8.1, prior to ion-exchange chromatography (DE-52) using a gradient of NaCl from 0 to 0.2 M. The order of elution is Fab, then undigested protein, followed closely by IgG2-Fc and IgG1-Fc. All peaks should be concentrated and tested by immunoelectrophoresis.

4 Since most hybridomas and some myelomas have antibody activity, it is possible to prepare highly purified immunoglobulins from antigen affinity columns. The reliability of this method depends on rigorous control (frequent screening and cloning) of the cell lines concerned, to prevent accumulation of revertant or mutant sub-clones. Ascitic fluid or serum from mice bearing myelomas such as MOPC 315 (αλ₂) and MOPC 460 (ακ), both with anti-DNP activity, or from mice bearing one of hundreds of hybridoma lines now available, is used as the source of immunoglobulin. Many hybridomas have the additional advantage of growing well *in vitro* and secreting their antibody into the culture fluid, from which it can be readily recovered. Appropriate techniques for screening, re-cloning and growing hybridoma lines are described in Chapters 108 and 111.

An example of a usable procedure with anti-DNP hybridomas and myelomas, is now given. Fluid (pH 7) containing immunoglobulin with anti-DNP activity is passed slowly down a column of DNP-BSA-Sepharose 4B. The DNP_{10-20}-BSA is made as described earlier (page 64.15) and is coupled to cyanogen bromide (CNBr) activated Sepharose 4B (Pharmacia) using the manufacturers instructions. The column is washed until the effluent is free of protein ($OD_{280}^{1cm} < 0.01$). The antibody is now eluted by lowering the pH to 2.5–3.0. Suitable acid buffers are 0.1 M-acetate-acetic acid with or without 1 M-NaCl; 0.2 M-glycine-HCl or 1 M-propionic acid. Alternatively, a chaotropic agent such as 1 M potassium thiocyanate (pH 7) can be used. Not generally recommended since it leads to a measurable degree of elution of antigen from the column, is a combination of extreme alkalinity (pH 11) and chaotropic agent (1 M-KSCN plus 0.5 M-NH$_4$OH): this should only be used if the Ig (antibody) binds so tightly to the antigen that the other elutants do not work.

An interesting and possibly useful alternative to the above is a column of DNP-cysteinyl-Sepharose, prepared according to the method of Klaus [64]. After adsorption to the column and subsequent washing, elution of antibody is carried out in reducing conditions maintained for 30 min with 2×10^{-2} M-cysteine in 0.15 M-phosphate buffer, pH 7. Excess, but not all, hapten can be removed from the eluted antibody by

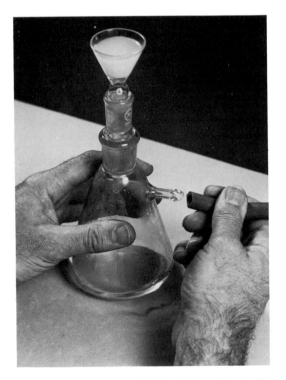

Fig. 64.6. The fast antibody elution technique. For details, see text.

dialysis against PBS. This elution method, which is independent of the affinity of the antibody, gives a very high yield, although high affinity antibodies will tend to retain a high proportion of hapten in their specific sites.

Fast elution

Since some antigens and antibodies of some species (mouse, goats) are extremely labile in acid conditions, a simple and rapid elution method has been devised [66]. Antibodies are absorbed on to an antigen column, which is then thoroughly washed as described above. The Sepharose–antigen–antibody complex is now gently blown from the column into a small sintered glass filter funnel set on a side-arm flask (Fig. 64.6). An appropriate volume of acid is used, e.g. for 3–4 ml of Sepharose, 10 ml of 1 M-propionic acid would be suitable. An equivalent volume of Tris buffer (10 ml 1 M-Tris-HCl, pH 8) is placed in the side-arm flask. About one-third of the acid is now placed on the Sepharose, and after stirring is sucked through, the process being controlled by manipulation of the tube from the vacuum pump (see Fig. 64.6). This is repeated twice more. The total time of exposure to acid is about 90 s. Finally, the Sepharose is quickly rinsed twice on the filter with 2 or 3 ml saline before being removed to a beaker of borate-buffered saline (pH 8.5). The eluted antibody is concentrated by pressure dialysis against PBS (pH 7, 4 °C). This method has been found to be very effective indeed when antibody stability and activity is of prime importance, although protein yields (OD units) are somewhat less than by more conventional methods.

Reducing non-specificity of antisera

Absorption of antisera

If indirect plaques are to be meaningful in a quantitative sense, the antiglobulin sera must be specific for a particular class of immunoglobulin. For example, a polyspecific developing serum which reacts against Fab will react to some extent with immunoglobulins of all isotypes including IgM and thus will inhibit direct plaques. Such inhibition can be measured and allowed for but its existence leads to an enormous increase in the variance of indirect plaque counts [31].

Several methods exist for preparing insoluble immunoabsorbents but only the one which was originally described by Porath *et al.* [85] is described here. This method is used routinely in a wide range of experimental situations, both for negative absorption (removal of unwanted antibodies) and positive absorption (elution of specific antibody).

Procedure

About 200 mg of Sepharose 4B (Pharmacia) (approximately 14 ml of the slurry which is supplied) is added to 10 ml of distilled water in a small beaker and a small PTFE-covered magnet is added. Ten millilitres of a freshly prepared solution of 50 mg/ml cyanogen bromide (weigh out in a fume hood) in water is added; then the beaker is put on a magnetic stirrer and monitored with a pH meter while 2 M NaOH is added dropwise to maintain the pH at 11.0–11.5 for 5 min (20 °C). The Sepharose is then washed on a small sintered glass filter with cold (4 °C) distilled water followed by cold borate buffer (0.15 M, pH 8.3). The Sepharose is then placed in a small beaker or bottle with 5 ml or less of protein in borate buffer (say 100–135 mg of IgG for 200 mg of Sepharose). The mixture is then left overnight at 4 °C without stirring if the protein was 5 ml; if in a greater volume the mixture should be mixed by the bottle being turned end-over-end (3–6 times/min). Three or four hours at 20 °C will also be sufficient. Residual activity is then inactivated in 0.05 M-ethanolamine (pH 8.0–9.0) for 5 min. The Sepharose–protein conjugate is then washed with borate buffer; then with 0.15 M-NaCl:0.1 M acetic acid—twice, 1 min each; then with saline until all acetic acid is removed, and finally in borate buffer. The preparation can be stored in borate buffer or phosphate-buffered saline (pH 7.2) containing 0.02% w/v sodium azide. For negative absorption, Sepharose containing at least 1 mg antigen for each mg of antibody to be removed, is made up into a column and then the serum is allowed to trickle slowly through the column. The absorbent is regenerated (unwanted antibody eluted) by washing it on a small sintered glass filter with saline; three quick washes with 1 M-propionic acid or 0.1 M-acetic acid, followed by saline and borate buffer as before. Pharmacia supply various pre-activated Sepharose preparations, including CNBr-activated Sepharose 4B. Each preparation is supplied by the manufacturer with excellent instructions.

In addition, all sera should be absorbed with one-fifth volume packed mouse/sheep RBC for 40 min.

When coated RBC are used as target cells, developing sera and complement should be absorbed for a few minutes with an insoluble form of the target antigen such as a protein–Sepharose conjugate. Complement absorption should be carried out at 0 °C. In certain circumstances [79a] IgG is removed from the guinea-pig serum used as a source of complement by passage down a column of Sepharose–Protein A (see page 64.14). Further absorptions with thymocytes or liver cells may be necessary for certain applications.

Notes and recommendations

It has been shown using the IEF overlay assay described earlier, that anti-allotype antisera, even when used in a reciprocal context, may not be operationally specific [28]. For example, CBA (IgG$_{2a}$) anti-sheep RBC spectrotypes can be developed both by an anti-*j* serum raised in C57B1/6 mice, as would be expected, and by an anti-*b* serum raised in CBA mice, which was unexpected. This phenomenon is not clearly seen when anti-sheep RBC plaques are developed. However, when hapten-coated erythrocytes (e.g. NIP-azide) were used to detect cells secreting anti-hapten antibody, the phenomenon was sufficiently pronounced to invalidate attempts to use allotype markers in adoptive immunization experiments.

The non-specific activity is confined to a macroglobulin fraction and has been shown to be a M-anti-G RF. It can be removed by gel filtration on Ultrogel ACA22 or removed by standard reduction and alkylation procedures [61a] (see page 64.6). The M-anti-G activity can be induced in SPF animals by injecting them with *B. pertussis* or LPS, or by keeping them for a time in 'dirty' (non-SPF) conditions. The IgG fractions of several gel-filtrated anti-allotype sera have been shown to be allotype specific.

Testing specificity of antisera

Antiglobulin sera should be tested in the following ways:

1   Double diffusion in gel (Ouchterlony) using specific test antigens (Chapter 19).
2   Immunoelectrophoresis (Chapter 19).
3   Quantitative micro-precipitin test described in detail by Herzenberg *et al.* [50]. RIA (radioimmune assay) and ELISA (enzyme linked immunosorbent assay) using standard isotype specific reagents, may also be used (see Chapters 26 and 27). The Mancini radial immunodiffusion technique [68] provided a simple method for making quantitative assessments of antisera.
4   An antiglobulin serum to be used for the development of plaques should be tested at a range of concentrations in a LHG assay, using spleen cells from mice immunized 2 days before with 10^8 sheep RBC i.p., or 3 or 4 days before with 4×10^6 sheep RBC (85% direct PFC), or 8–10 days before with 10^8 sheep RBC i.p. (85% indirect). A serum which inhibits direct PFC at the optimal concentration for development of indirect PFC should be reabsorbed with Sepharose-Fab or Sepharose-IgM and if still inhibitory it should be discarded for use in the LHG assay [103]. A correction factor (KD) can be calculated for develop-

ing sera which for reasons of economy must be used at sub-optimal concentrations (see Fig. 64.1).

Coda

Immunological techniques are evolving very rapidly at the present, and specific advice in a chapter such as this can rapidly be superceded by new advances in immuno-technology. It follows, therefore, that a research worker about to expend time and energy on a project should use this chapter only as a guide and should consult the appropriate technical literature for details of new methodologies or useful modifications to old ones. In this context the *Journal of Immunological Methods* is especially useful and it is well worth skimming through the contents pages (also published in *Current Contents*) before starting. Careful controls and checks on specificity of antisera, etc., should be carried out whatever the technique finally chosen: there can be considerable variation in conditions from one laboratory or reagent to another. For example, commercial anti-immunoglobulin sera sold as being isotype specific almost always appear so in IEP or Ouchterlony tests, but some may be effectively non-specific when used as developing sera in a haemolytic plaque assay.

Media

Balanced salt solutions

Dulbecco's PBS (PBS)

		Mass (g)
1	NaCl	40.45
	KCl	1.45
	KH_2PO_4	1.45
	$Na_2HPO_4 \cdot 12H_2O$	21.90
	Water to 400 ml	
2	$CaCl_2$	0.95
	Water to 50 ml	
3	$MgCl_2 \cdot 6H_2O$	0.95
	Water to 50 ml	

Sterilize all components by autoclaving (120 °C).
To use: 80 ml (1); 900 ml water; 10 ml (2); 10 ml (3).

Phosphate-buffered (BSS)

(For use in situations where bicarbonate or HEPES-buffered solutions cannot be used.)

		Mass (g)
1	Glucose	10.0
	KH_2PO_4	0.6
	$Na_2HPO_4 \cdot 12H_2O$	7.6

	Phenol red	0.1
	Water to one litre	
2	$CaCl_2 \cdot 2H_2O$	1.86
	KCl	4.0
	NaCl	80.0
	$MgCl_2 \cdot 6H_2O$	2.0
	$MgSO_4 \cdot 7H_2O$	2.0
	Water to one litre	

Autoclave (120 °C) both solutions. It is best to add the phenol red after autoclaving as a sterile (filtered) solution.
To use: add 100 ml (1) to about half a litre water, mix, add 100 ml (2), mix, and make up to one litre.

Bicarbonate-buffered (BSS)

Hanks' gelatin (HG).

		Mass (g)
1	NaCl*	40.0
	KCl	2.0
	$Na_2HPO_4 \cdot 12H_2O$	0.9
	KH_2PO_4	0.3
	Glucose	5.0
	Phenol Red	0.085
	Gelatin	25.0
	$MgSO_4 \cdot 7H_2O$	1.0
	$CaCl_2 \cdot 2H_2O$	0.925

Water to one litre Autoclave (120 °C)

2	$NaHCO_3$	0.7

Water to 100 ml Autoclave (120 °C)
To use: 20 ml(1); 75 ml water; 5 ml(2); adjust to pH 7.2 with CO_2.

N.B. Stock solutions containing phenol red if stored for long periods should be kept in the dark. Concentrated solutions containing (2.5%) gelatin may have to be warmed before dilution. Working strength (0.5%) gelatin solutions do not gel at normal room temperature but may over a period of several days at 0 °C.

Bicarbonate may be omitted and HEPES (23.35 g) added to stock solution (1).

It is convenient to make up Hanks' solution (minus bicarbonate) at working strength and autoclave at this stage. For use in the laboratory, sufficient bicarbonate is added to raise the pH to 7.2. This avoids the need for gassing the solution with CO_2 to adjust the pH. Hanks' made up with bicarbonate in this way is not suitable for use in a CO_2-gassed incubator.

---

* For haemolytic Hanks', NaCl may be replaced by an equal weight of NH_4Cl.

HEPES Eagle's gelatin (HEG)

10 ml × 10 concentrated Eagle's MEM (with phenol red).
70 ml water.
10 ml HEPES (0.467 g) in water.
10 ml gelatin (5% w/v) in water.
pH to 7.3 with 0.5 M NaOH.
Autoclave at 120 °C for 15 min.

Standard solutions such as MEM and Hanks' are available from several commercial sources as ready-to-use solutions or concentrates.

Note added in proof

Since this chapter was written there have been few if any major adances in the haemolytic plaque technique. However, one trend of some practical importance has been the modification of the micro-plaque assay of Kappler [109,111,114,116]. This assay is carried out *in situ* in the flat-bottomed wells of a 96-well micro-tissue culture plate. Cells to be assayed are centrifuged (300–400 g; 3–5 min) on to the bottom of the plate, the supernatant is shaken off in a single careful movement and an aliquot of a mixture of target cells, developing serum and complement, similar to that used in the Cunningham assay (p. 64.6), is added to each well. The plate is shaken to mix the contents of the wells and is again centrifuged prior to being incubated at 37 °C for 1–2 h to allow for the development of visible plaques which can be counted using a binocular microscope. Since this method can be semi-automated using, for example, standard micro-titre multi-channel pipetting devices, the technique is ideal for limiting dilution assays which require a large number of replicate analyses [107,110] and for routine clinical applications [108,116] where it is necessary to enumerate cells producing, for example, immunoglobulins, components of complement [105], enzymes [115] or hormones [108].

References

1 ADAMS M.H. (1959) *Bacteriophages*. Interscience Publishers, New York.
2 ANDERSSON B. (1970) Studies on the regulation of avidity at the level of the single antibody-forming cell. *J. exp. Med.* **132**, 77.
3 ASHWOOD-SMITH M.J. (1964) Low temperature preservation of mouse lymphocytes with dimethyl sulphoxide. *Blood*, **23**, 494.
4 AWDEH Z.L., WILLIAMSON A.R. & ASKONAS B.A. (1970) One cell–one immunoglobulin. *Biochem. J.* **116**, 241.
5 BAGASRA O. & DAMJANOV I. (1982) Detection of plaque-forming cells by a latex bead technique. *J. immunol. Meth.* **49**, 283.

6 BAIG M.A., ANSARI A.A. & MALLING H.V. (1982) A hemolytic plaque assay for the detection of red blood cells carrying abnormal or mutant hemoglobin. *J. immunol. Meth.* **55**, 43.
7 BAZIN H., BECKERS A. & QUERINJEAN P. (1974) Three classes and four (sub)classes of rat immunoglobulins: IgM, IgA, IgE and IgG₁, IgG₂ₐ, IgG₂ᵦ, IgG₂ᵨ. *Eur. J. Immunol.* **4**, 44.
8 BAZIN H., BECKERS A., VAERMAN J.-P. & HEREMANS J.F. (1974) Allotypes of rat immunoglobulins. (I) An allotype at the α-chain locus. *J. Immunol.* **112**, 1035.
9 BAZIN, H., SAVIN M.-C. & MICKLEM H.S. (1968) Separation of mouse immunoglobulins on the basis of water solubility on Sephadex G-25 *J. Chromatog.* **34**, 180.
10 BECKERS A. & BAZIN H. (1975) Allotypes of rat immunoglobulins. (III) An allotype of the γ₂ᵦ chain locus. *Immunochemistry*, **12**, 671.
11 BERENBAUM M.C. & STRINGER I.M. (1970) The localization of haemolytic antibody in sections of lymphoid organs: an improved method. *Immunology*, **18**, 85.
12 BRENNEMAN L. & SINGER J.T. (1970) On homogeneous antigens and antibodies. (III) The preparation and properties of the univalent hapten–protein conjugate papain-DNPL. *Ann. N.Y. Acad. Sci.* **169**, 72.
12a BRITTLE M.P., BRADLEY N.J., GOMER K.J., PLAYFAIR J.H.L. & DAVIES A.J.S. (1984) The control of antibody diversity during IgM and IgG anti-sheep red cell responses in mice. *Immunology*, **52**, 97.
13 BRITTON S. (1969) Regulation of antibody synthesis against *Escherichia coli* endotoxin. *Immunology*, **16**, 513.
14 BROWNSTONE A., MITCHISON N.A. & PITT-RIVERS R. (1966) Chemical and serological studies with an iodine-containing synthetic immunological determinant 4-hydroxy-3-iodo-5-nitrophenylacetic acid (NIP) and related compounds. *Immunology*, **10**, 465.
15 CHEN C.-L.H., LEHMEYER J.E. & COOPER M.D. (1982) Evidence for an IgD homologue on chicken lymphocytes. *J. Immunol.* **129**, 2580.
16 COTTON R.G.H., SECHER D.S. & MILSTEIN C. (1973) Somatic mutation and the origin of antibody diversity. Clonal variability of the immunoglobulin produced by MOPC21 cells in culture. *Eur. J. Immunol.* **3**, 135.
17 CRISPENS C.G. (1979) Preparation of lymphocytes from small volumes of peripheral mouse blood. *Experientia*, **35**, 833.
18 CUNNINGHAM A.J. & SZENBERG A. (1968) Further improvements in the plaque technique for detecting single antibody-forming cells. *Immunology*, **14**, 599.
19 CUNNINGHAM A.J. & SERCARZ E.E. (1971) The asynchronous development of immunological memory in helper (T) and precursor (B) cell lines. *Eur. J. Immunol.* **1**, 413.
20 CUNNINGHAM A.J., SMITH J.B. & MERCER E.H. (1966) Antibody formation by single cells from lymph nodes and efferent lymph nodes of sheep. *J. exp. Med.* **124**, 701.
21 DELISI C. (1975) The kinetics of hemolytic plaque formation. (III) Inhibition of plaques by antigens. *J. theor. Biol.* **51**, 337.
22 DELISI C. (1975) The kinetics of hemolytic plaque

formation. (IV) IgM plaque inhibition. *J. theor. Biol.* **52**, 419.

23 DELISI C.P. & BELL G.I. (1974) The kinetics of hemolytic plaque formation. *Proc. natn. Acad. Sci. U.S.A.* **71**, 16.

24 DELISI C.P. & GOLDSTEIN B. (1974) On the mechanism of hemolytic plaque inhibition. *Immunochemistry*, **11**, 661.

25 DELISI C. & GOLDSTEIN B. (1975) The kinetics of hemolytic plaque formation. (II) Inhibition of plaques by haptens. *J. theor. Biol.* **51**, 313.

26 DRESSER D.W. (1974) Factors influencing the rate of induction of tolerance by bovine gamma globulin. In *Immunological Tolerance: mechanisms and potential therapeutic applications*, (eds. Katz D.H. & Benacerraf B.), pp. 3–24. Academic Press, New York.

27 DRESSER D.W. (1978) Most IgM producing cells in the mouse secrete autoantibodies (rheumatoid factor). *Nature*, **274**, 480.

28 DRESSER D.W., KEELER K.D. & PHILLIPS J.M. (1976) Immunoglobulin allotypes of the mouse. *Biochem. Soc. Trans.* **4**, 34.

29 DRESSER D.W. & POPHAM A.M. (1976) Induction of an IgM anti-(bovine)-IgG response in mice by bacterial lipopolysaccharide. *Nature*, **264**, 552.

29a DRESSER D.W. & POPHAM A.M. (1980) Rheumatoid factors in mice: plaque assay for homophile and heterophile rheumatoid factors. *Immunology*, **41**, 569.

30 DRESSER D.W. & WORTIS H.H. (1965) Use of an antiglobulin serum to detect cells producing antibody with low haemolytic efficiency. *Nature*, **208**, 859.

31 DRESSER D.W. & WORTIS H.H. (1967) Localized haemolysis in gel. In *Handbook of Experimental Immunology*, 1st edn. (ed. Weir D.M.), p. 1054. Blackwell Scientific Publications, Oxford.

32 EISEN H. (1964) Preparation of purified anti-2,4-dinitrophenyl antibodies. *Meth. med. Res.* **10**, 94.

33 EZAKI T. & MARBROOK J. (1982) The hemolytic plaque reduction technique to measure cytotoxicity with hybridoma cells as a target. *J. immunol. Meth.* **54**, 281.

34 FLANAGAN J.G. & RABBITTS T.H. (1982) Arrangement of human immunoglobulin heavy chain constant region genes implies evolutionary duplication of a segment containing γ, ε and α genes. *Nature*, **300**, 709.

35 FRANGIONE B. (1975) Structure of human immunoglobulins and their variants. In *Immunogenetics and immunodeficiency*, (ed. Benacerraf B.), pp. 1–53, MTP, Lancaster.

36 FUJI H., ZALESKI M. & MILGROM F. (1971) Allogeneic nucleated cells as immunogen and target for plaque-forming cells in mice. *Transplant. Proc.* **3**, 852.

37 GERSHON H., BAUMINGER S., SELA M. & FELDMAN M. (1968) Studies on the competence of single cells to produce antibodies of two specificities. *J. exp. Med.* **128**, 223.

38 GOLUB E.S., MISHELL R.I., WEIGLE W.O. & DUTTON R.W. (1968) A modification of the hemolytic plaque assay for use with protein antigens. *J. Immunol.* **100**, 133.

39 GODING J.W. (1976) The chromic chloride method of coupling antigens to erythrocytes: definition of some important parameters. *J. immunol. Meth.* **10**, 61.

40 GODING J.W., WARR G.W. & WARNER N.L. (1976) Genetic polymorphism of IgD-like cell surface immuno-globulin in the mouse. *Proc. natn. Acad. Sci. U.S.A.* **73**, 1305.

41 GOLD E.R. & FUDENBERG H.H. (1967) Chromic chloride: a coupling reagent for passive hemagglutination reaction. *J. Immunol.* **99**, 859.

42 GREEN I., VASSALI P., NUSSENZWEIG V. & BENACERRAF B. (1967) Specificity of antibodies by single cells following immunisation with antigen bearing two types of antigenic determinants. *J. exp. Med.* **125**, 311.

43 GREEN M.C. (1979) Genetic nomenclature for the immunoglobulin loci of the mouse. *Immunogenetics*, **8**, 89.

44 GREEN N.M. (1978) (quoted by D.W. Dresser) Assays for immunoglobulin secreting cells. In *Handbook of Experimental Immunology*, 3rd edn., (ed. Weir D.M.), p. 28.16. Blackwell Scientific Publications, Oxford.

45 GRONOWICZ E., COUTINHO A. & MELCHERS F. (1976) A plaque assay for cells secreting Ig of a given type or class. *Eur. J. Immunol.* **6**, 588.

46 HALLIDAY W.J. & WEBB M. (1965) A plaque technique for counting cells which produce antibacterial antibody. *Austr. J. exp. Biol. Med. Sci.* **43**, 163.

47 HAY F.C., NINEHAM L.J. & ROITT I.M. (1975) Routine assay for the detection of IgG and IgM antiglobulins in seronegative and seropositive rheumatoid arthritis. *Br. med. J.* **3**, 203.

48 HÄMMERLING U. & WESTPHAL O. (1967) Synthesis and use of O-stearoyl polysaccharides in passive hemagglutination and hemolysis. *Eur. J. Biochem.* **1**, 46.

49 HERZENBERG L.A., McDEVITT H.O. & HERZENBERG L.A. (1969) Genetics of antibodies. *Ann. Rev. Genet.* **2**, 209.

50 HERZENBERG L.A. & WARNER N.L. (1968) Genetic control of mouse immunoglobulin. In *Regulation of the Antibody Response*, (ed. Cinader B.), p. 322. Charles C. Thomas, Illinois.

51 HERZENBERG L.A., HERZENBERG L.A., BLACK S.J., LOKEN M.R., OKUMURA K., VAN DER LOO W., OSBOURNE B.A., HEWGILL D., GODING J.W., GUTMANN G. & WARNER N.L. (1977) Surface markers and functional relationships of cells involved in murine B-lymphocyte differentiation. *Cold Spring Harb. Symp. quant. Biol.* **41**, 33.

52 HIGGINS D.A. (1975) Physical and chemical properties of fowl immunoglobulins. *Vet. Bull.* **45**, 139.

53 HOSONO M. & MURAMATSU S. (1972) Use of 2-mercaptoethanol for distinguishing between IgM and IgG antibody-producing cells of mice immunized with bovine globulin. *J. Immunol.* **109**, 857.

54 HUMPHREY J.H. & DOURMASHKIN R.R. (1969) The lesions in cell membranes caused by complement. *Adv. Immunol.* **11**, 75.

55 INGRAHAM J.S. & BUSSARD A. (1964) Application of a localised haemolysin reaction for specific detection of individual antibody forming cells. *J. exp. Med.* **119**, 667.

56 IVANYI J. & DRESSER D.W. (1970) Replica analysis of the class of antibodies produced by single cells. *Immunology*, **6**, 493.

57 JANDL J.H. & SIMMONS R.L. (1957) The agglutination and sensitization of red cells by metallic cations: interac-

tions between multivalent metals and the red-cell membrane. *Br. J. Haematol.* **3**, 19.

58 JERNE N.K., HENRY C., NORDIN A.A., FUJI H., KOROS A.M.C. & LEFKOVITS I. (1974) Plaque forming cells: methodology and theory. *Transplant. Rev.* **19**, 130.

59 JERNE N.K., NORDIN A.A. & HENRY C. (1963) The agar plaque technique for recognizing antibody producing cells. In *Cell-bound Antibody*, (eds Amos B. & Koprowski H.), p. 109. Wistar Institute Press, Philadelphia.

60 KABAT E. & MEYER M.M. (1962) *Experimental Immunochemistry*. Charles C. Thomas, Illinois.

61 KAPP J.A. & INGRAHAM J.S. (1970) Anti-protein plaque-forming cells detected with high efficiency by the use of red cells coupled to bovine serum globulin through bis-diazo-benzidine. *J. Immunol.* **104**, 1039.

61a KEELER K.D., PHILLIPS J.M. & DRESSER D.W. (1979) IgM rheumatoid factor as a source of non-specificity in murine anti-allotype sera. *Immunology*, **37**, 263.

62 KENNEDY J.C. & AXELRAD M.A. (1971) An improved assay for haemolytic plaque-forming cells. *Immunology*, **29**, 253.

63 KOHLER G. & MELCHERS F. (1972) Isoelectric focusing spectra of antibodies which activate mutant β-galactosidases. *Eur. J. Immunol.* **2**, 453.

64 KUNKL A. & KLAUS G.G.B. (1981) The generation of memory cells. (V) Preferential priming of IgG₁ B memory cells by immunization with antigen-IgG₂ antibody complexes. *Immunology*, **44**, 163.

65 LANDY M., SANDERSON R.P. & JACKSON A.L. (1965) Humoral and cellular aspects of the immune response to the somatic antigen of *Salmonella enteritidis*. *J. exp. Med.* **122**, 483.

66 LEE S-K. & DRESSER D.W. (1981) Allotype suppression of the responsiveness of adoptively transferred adult spleen cells induced by affinity prepared anti-allotype antibody. *Immunology*, **42**, 601.

67 LIEBERMAN R. (1978) Genetics of IgCH (allotype) locus in the mouse. *Springer Semin. Immunopath.* **1**, 7.

68 MANCINI G., CARBONARA A.O. & HEREMANS J.F. (1965) Immunochemical quantitation of antisera by single radial immunodiffusion. *Immunochemistry*, **2**, 235.

69 MAIZELS R.M. & DRESSER D.W. (1977) Conditions for the development of IgM- and IgG-antibody-secreting cells from primed mouse splenocytes *in vitro*. *Immunology*, **32**, 793.

70 MOLINARO G.A. & DRAY S. (1974) Antibody coated erythrocytes as a manifold probe for antigens. *Nature*, **248**, 515.

71 MOLINARO G.A., BESSINGER B.A., GILMAN-SACHS A. & DRAY S. (1975) Sensitive detection of immunoglobulin light and heavy chains on rabbit lymphocytes by antibody-coated erythrocytes. *J. Immunol.* **114**, 908.

72 MOLINARO G.A., MARON E. & DRAY S. (1974) Antigen-secreting cells: enumeration of immunoglobulin allotype-secreting cells in non-immunized rabbits by means of hybrid-antibody-coated erythrocytes in a reverse hemolytic plaque assay. *Proc. natn. Acad. Sci. U.S.A.* **71**, 1229.

73 MÖLLER G. (1965) 19S antibody production against soluble lipopolysaccharide antigens by individual lymphoid cells *in vitro*. *Nature*, **207**, 1166.

73a NICOLOTTI R.A., BRILES D.E., SCHROER J.A. & DAVIE J.M. (1980) Isoelectric focusing of immunoglobulins: improved methodology. *J. Immunol. Meth.* **33**, 101.

74 NORDIN A.A., CEROTTINI J.-C. & BRUNNER K.T. (1971) The antibody response of mice to allografts as determined by a plaque assay with allogeneic target cells. *Eur. J. Immunol.* **1**, 55.

75 NORTH J.R. & ASKONAS B.A. (1974) Analysis of affinity of monoclonal antibody response by inhibition of plaque-forming cells. *Eur. J. Immunol.* **4**, 361.

76 NOSSAL G.J.V., BUSSARD A.E., LEWIS H. & MAZIE J.C. (1970) *In vitro* stimulation of antibody formation by peritoneal cells. (I) Plaque technique of high sensitivity enabling access to the cells. *J. exp. Med.* **131**, 894.

77 PASANEN V.J. & MÄKELÄ O. (1969) Effect of the number of haptens coupled to each erythrocyte on haemolytic plaque formation. *Immunology*, **16**, 399.

78 PERKINS E.H., SADO T. & MAKINODAN T. (1969) Recruitment and proliferation of immunocompetent cells during the log phase of the primary antibody response. *J. Immunol.* **103**, 669.

79 PETERSEN B.H. & INGRAHAM J.S. (1969) The limitation of individual cells to the production of a single specificity of antibody in response to a coupled hapten–antigen complex. *Immunochemistry*, **6**, 379.

79a PETERSEN J., HEILMANN C., BJERRUM O.J., INGEMANN-HANSEN T. & HALJKAER-KRISTENSEN J. (1983) IgG rheumatoid factor-secreting lymphocytes in rheumatoid arthritis: evaluation of a haemolytic plaque-forming cell technique. *Scand. J. Immunol.* **17**, 471.

80 PHILLIPS J.M. & DRESSER D.W. (1973) Isoelectric spectra of different classes of anti-erythrocyte antibodies. *Eur. J. Immunol.* **3**, 524.

81 PHILLIPS J.M. & DRESSER D.W. (1973) Antibody isoelectric spectra visualized by antigen coated erythrocytes. *Eur. J. Immunol.* **3**, 738.

82 PINK J.R.L. & IVANYI J. (1975) Close linkage between genes coding for allotypic markers in chicken IgG and IgM. *Eur. J. Immunol.* **5**, 506.

83 PLAYFAIR J.H.L., PAPERMASTER B.W. & COLE L.J. (1965) Focal antibody production by transferred spleen cells in irradiated mice. *Science*, **149**, 998.

84 PLOTZ P.H., TALAL N. & ASOFSKY R. (1968) Assignment of direct and facilitated hemolytic plaques in mice to specific immunoglobulin classes. *J. Immunol.* **100**, 744.

85 PORATH J., AXEN R. & ERNBACH S. (1967) Chemical coupling of protein to agarose. *Nature*, **215**, 1491.

86 QUENOUILLE M.H. (1950) Transformation and non-normal distributions. In *Introductory Statistics*. Butterworth-Springer, London.

87 REPKE H.H. (1977) The fluorescence-plaque test—a new sensitive technique for the detection of antigens on antibody plaque-forming cells. *J. immunol. Meth.* **16**, 263.

88 RITTENBERG M.B. & PRATT K.L. (1969) Antitrinitrophenyl (TNP) plaque assay. Primary response of BALB/c mice to soluble and particulate immunogens. *Proc. Soc. exp. Biol. (NY)* **132**, 575.

89 ROGERS A.W. (1967) *Techniques of autoradiography.* Elsevier Publishing Co., Amsterdam.

90 ROTMAN B. & COX D.R. (1971) Specific detection of antigen-binding cells by localised growth of bacteria. *Proc. natn. Acad. Sci. U.S.A.* **68**, 2377.

90a RUDOLPH A.K., BURROWS P.D. & WABLE M.R. (1981) Thirteen hybridomas secreting hapten-specific immunoglobulin E from mice with Ig^a or Ig^b heavy chain haplotype. *Eur. J. Immunol.* **11**, 527.

91 SCHWARTZ S.A. & BRAUN W. (1965) Bacteria as an indicator of formation of antibodies by single spleen cells in agar. *Science*, **159**, 200.

92 SEGRE D. & SEGRE M. (1968) Hemolytic plaque formation by mouse spleen cells producing antibodies to ovalbumin. *Immunochemistry*, **5**, 206.

93 SHIMIZU A., TAKAHASHI N., YAOITA Y. & HONJO T. (1982) Organization of the constant-region gene family of the mouse immunoglobulin heavy chain. *Cell*, **28**, 499.

94 SILVER H., MILLER J.F.A.P. & WARNER N.L. (1971) A simple hemolytic plaque technique for the enumeration of anti-hapten antibody forming cells. *Int. Archs Allergy*, **40**, 540.

95 SMITH A.U. (1965) Survival of frozen chondrocytes isolated from cartilage of adult mammals. *Nature*, **205**, 782.

96 SORG C., HIMMELSPACH K., RÜDE E. & WESTPHAL O. (1969) Synthesis of stearo-aminoethyl-polyvinyl-alcohol and its use for preparation of agents for specific adsorptive sensitization of erythrocytes. *Israel J. Med. Sci.* **5**, 253.

97 STERZL J. & RIHA I. (1965) Detection of cells producing 7S antibodies by the plaque technique. *Nature*, **208**, 857.

98 STRAUSBAUCH P., SULICA A. & GIVOL D. (1970) General method for the detection of cells producing antibodies against haptens and proteins. *Nature*, **277**, 68.

99 TAO T.-W. & DRESSER D.W. (1972) The Zipp assay: a method for enumerating cells producing antiphage antibody. *Eur. J. Immunol.* **2**, 262.

100 TERNYNCK T. & AVRAMEAS S. (1976) A new method using benzoquinone for coupling antigens and antibodies to marker substances. *Ann. Immunol. (Paris)*, **127C**, 197.

101 THRASHER S.G., BIGAZZI P.E., YOSHIDA T. & COHEN S. (1975) The effect of fluorescein conjugation on Fc-dependent properties of rabbit antibody. *J. Immunol.* **114**, 762.

102 TURNER M.W. (1977) Structure and function of immunoglobulins. In *Immunochemistry: An Advanced Textbook*, (ed. Glynn L.E. & Steward M.W.), pp. 1–57. Wiley (John) & Sons Ltd.

103 WORTIS H.H., DRESSER D.W. & ANDERSON H.R. (1969) Antibody production studied by means of the localized haemolysis in gel (LGH) assay. (III) Mouse cells producing five different classes of antibody. *Immunology*, **17**, 93.

104 WESTPHAL O. & JANN K. (1965) Bacterial lipoplysaccharides: extraction with phenol-water and further applications of the procedure. In *Methods in Carbohydrate Chemistry*, Vol V, (ed. Whistler R.L.) p. 83. Academic Press, New York.

105 ALPERT S.E., AUERBACH H.S., COLE S. & COLTEN H.R. (1983) Macrophage maturation: differences in complement secretion by marrow, monocyte and tissue macrophages detected with an improved hemolytic plaque assay. *J. Immunol.* **130**, 102.

106 CRONKHITE R., CERNY J. & DELISI C. (1984) Inhibition of plaque-forming cells with anti-idiotype or hapten: variation due to hapten density on indicator red cells. *J. Immunol.* **68**, 109.

107 EZAKI T., CHRISTENSEN N.D., SKINNER M.A. & MARBROOK J. (1984) The adaptation of the plaque reduction assay for measuring specific cytotoxic cells in limiting dilution cultures. *J. immunol. Meth.* **66**, 357.

108 FRAWLEY L.S. & NEILL J.D. (1984) A reverse hemolytic plaque assay for microscopic visualization of growth hormone release from individual cells: evidence for somatotrope heterogeneity. *Neuroendocrinology*, **39**, 484.

109 KAPPLER J.W. (1974) A micro-technique for hemolytic plaque assays. *J. Immunol.* **112**, 1271.

110 LEFKOVITS I. & WALDMAN H. (1979) *Limiting dilution analysis of cells in the immune system.* Cambridge University Press.

111 LIBRACH C.L. & MACKAY I.R. (1982) Rapid replicate reverse hemolytic plaque assay directly in microwells used for tissue culture. *J. immunol. Meth.* **52**, 43.

112 MAKONKAWKEYOON S. & VITHAYASAI V. (1983) A preamplified reverse hemolytic plaque assay. *J. immunol. Meth.* **62**, 365.

113 VAN OUDENAREN A., HAAIJMAN J.J. & BENNER R. (1983) Comparison of the sensitivity of the Protein A plaque assay and the immunofluorescence assay for detection of immunoglobulin producing cells. *J. immunol. Meth.* **56**, 117.

114 PIKE B.L., JENNINGS G. & SHORTMAN K. (1982) A simple semi-automated plaque method for the detection of antibody-forming cell clones in microcultures. *J. immunol. Meth.* **52**, 25.

115 RICHTER J., OLOFSSON T., BRITTON S. & OLSSON I. (1984) Detection of lactoferrin and myeloperoxidase release from single neutrophils by a protein A plaque assay. *Scand. J. Immunol.* **20**, 349.

116 ROW V.V. & VOLOE R. (1984) A micro reverse haemolytic plaque technique for the detection of antithyroglobulin antibody producing-lymphocytes in Hashimoto's thyroiditis. *J. Clin. Lab. Immunol.* **15**, 219.

117 STEINMANN J. & MARZOCK H.-J. (1983) Chemical linkage of erythrocytes and viral antigen in the hemolysis-ingel (HIG) test for viral antibodies. *J. immunol. Meth.* **59**, 221.

118 TAURIS P. (1983) Plaque-forming cells in man I. Basic technical results obtained with the Protein A technique. *Scand. J. Immunol.* **18**, 241.

119 TAURIS P. (1983) Plaque-forming cell in man II. Evidence of the existence of active suppressor cells in peripheral blood of normal plaque-forming cell non-responders. *Scand. J. Immunol.* **18**, 249.

120 WANGEL A.G., POIKONEN H.K. & ESKOLA J. (1984) A comparison of three reverse haemolytic plaque assays. *Immunobiology*, **116**, 403.

121 DZIARSKI R. (1984) Anti-immunoglobulin autoantibodies are not preferentially induced in polyclonal activation of human and mouse lymphocytes and more anti-DNA and anti-erythrocyte autoantibodies and induced in polyclonal activation of mouse than human lymphocytes. *J. Immunol.* **133**, 2537.

Chapter 65
Limiting dilution analysis of effector cells and their precursors *in vitro*

M. ZAUDERER

Probability distributions, 65.1
Limiting dilution analysis, 65.2
Frequency analysis for a specific helper T cell, 65.2

Functional properties of a limiting cell type, 65.3
Isolation and expansion of clonal precursors *in vitro*, 65.4

Assays for specific antibody secretion, 65.6
Conclusion, 65.7

The antigenic and regulatory specificity of immune responses derives from the properties and interactions of a heterogenous population of immunocompetent cells. Recognition of this cellular complexity and the development of methods for the analysis of lymphocyte subpopulations and clones has made possible the remarkable advances of cellular immunology in recent years. Limiting dilution analysis offers a means to determine the relative frequency within a population of effector cells with defined specificity and function. If culture conditions can be defined that will permit the expansion of precursors to effector cells *in vitro*, then limiting dilution methods can be applied to enumerate and isolate such precursors. This is useful both for obtaining clones of a particular cell type for intensive characterization and for studies of regulation at the level of precursors. This article will focus on limiting dilution analysis of helper T cells and their precursors *in vitro*. The methods are, however, equally applicable to other effector cells. Lefkovits & Waldmann [1] have recently published an excellent volume with detailed treatment of many aspects of limiting dilution analysis. Miller *et al.* [2] have described conditions for limiting dilution assays of precursors to cytotoxic T lymphocytes.

Probability distributions

Suppose an identifiable cell type T occurs in a population with frequency p. Cells that are not of that type must then occur with frequency $q = 1 - p$. If cells are randomly and independently sampled from this population, then over many samples of size n the mean number, μ, of cells of type T is the product np. A probability, P_r, can be assigned for finding in any sample of size n a number r $(0 \leq r \leq n)$ of cells of type T. It will be apparent that for the extreme values $r = 0$, $P_0 = q^n$ and $r = n$, $P_n = p^n$. In general the probability

of finding any number r of cells of type T is given by the successive terms in the expansion of the binomial $(p+q)^n$. If, for example, $n = 3$, $(p+q)^3 = p^3 + 3p^2q + 3pq^2 + q^3$, and the probability of finding $r = 1$ is $3pq^2$. Note that $p+q = 1$ and, therefore, the sum of all terms of the binomial distribution $(p+q)^n = 1$. For large values of n it is useful to have a general formula for individual terms of the distribution:

$$P_r = \frac{n!}{r!(n-r)!} p^r q^{n-r}$$

It can be shown that when n is relatively large and p is relatively small the binomial distribution is closely approximated by the Poisson distribution:

$$P_r = \frac{(np)^r}{r!} e^{-np} = \frac{\mu^r}{r!} e^{-\mu}$$

The probability then of observing $r = 0, 1, 2, 3, \ldots$ in samples with a mean number, μ, of cells of type T is $P_r = e^{-\mu}, \mu e^{-\mu}, \mu^2/2! \, e^{-\mu}, \mu^3/3! \, e^{-\mu} \ldots$. A distinctive property of the Poisson distribution is that the mean is equal to the variance. Knowledge of the variance, a measure of the spread of a distribution, makes it possible to draw conclusions from a sample concerning the properties of the parent population at any desired level of confidence (usually 95%). Perhaps more relevant for experimental purposes, it makes it possible to determine whether two independent samples are likely to derive from the same unaltered parent population. This is normally expressed in the statement that measurements on two samples are or are not significantly different. Circumstances in which there is a need to make such determinations and some specific statistical tests that can be applied will be identified below.

Limiting dilution analysis

It will be readily appreciated that just as known values of the mean lead to predictions of P_r, experimentally determined values of P_r (termed F_r below) permit an estimate of the mean. In practice, this requires that an assay system be established in which the ability to induce a specific response is limited only by the presence of the cell type of interest. All other accessory and target cells necessary for a readout should be introduced in excess from an independent source. In the case of assays for helper T cells that co-operate in the induction of specific antibody secretion, both B cells and antigen-presenting cells are required. These can derive from a population of primed spleen cells depleted of endogenous T cells by treatment with anti-Thy1 and complement. Multiple sets of cultures are then established, each of which receives a standard number of T-depleted spleen cells sufficient to support a specific response. In the absence of any further cellular additions, antigen stimulation would induce either no response or perhaps a low background response that defines the T-independent threshold. Upon addition of some large number of cells, N, from a population known to include helper T cells, it should be confirmed that a specific response can be induced in every culture. To the extent that the T cell donor population is depleted of B cells and/or accessory cells, this demonstrates that these cells have been introduced in adequate numbers from the independent source. As decreasing numbers of cells from the T cell donor population are added to different sets of cultures, the mean number of helper T cells introduced per culture becomes limiting. This is reflected in both a reduced level and frequency of response. It may, in principle, be possible over some range of the absolute level of response to estimate the number, r, of limiting cells introduced into a particular culture. In theory this would determine F_r at several values of r and permit an estimate of the mean number, μ, of limiting cells per culture from the corresponding terms of the Poisson distribution. In practice this is likely to require more precise measurements than are convenient for the large number of cultures that need to be assayed in such experiments. Many simple assays, however, readily distinguish between the presence or absence of a response. It is convenient, therefore, to focus on those cultures that fail to give rise to a response (r = 0) and to estimate μ from the zero term of the Poisson distribution, $F_0 = e^{-\mu}$. Estimates of μ are most reliable in the range $0.1 < F_0 < 0.37$. If several estimates of μ are obtained for different numbers of cells (N) added per culture, then since $\mu = -\ln F_0$, a semi-log plot of F_0 vs. N should give a straight line passing through the origin (see Fig. 65.1). The larger the number of

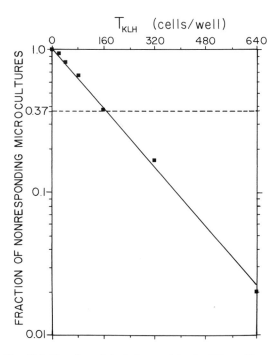

Fig. 65.1. Titration of the helper activity for PC-specific responses of a population of KLH-primed lymph node cells enriched *in vitro* (T_{KLH}).

cultures assayed at any number of cells, N, the more reliable the estimate of μ (see remarks on data analysis below).

Frequency analysis for a specific helper T cell

Helper T cells are greatly enriched in populations of KLH-primed lymph node cells selected during 18 days *in vitro* culture with 40 μg/ml KLH [3]. A titration of the helper activity recovered in one such population for secondary phosphorylcholine-(PC) specific responses *in vitro* is shown in Fig. 65.1. Sets of sixty 10 μl test cultures, including $3 \times 10^4 B_{PC}$ per culture, were assayed for responses to PC_2KLH. Each point represents the fraction of test cultures in a set of sixty that fail to respond at a particular concentration of *in vitro* selected T cells. Antibody-secreting cells induced in each culture were assayed on day 5. At higher T cell concentrations (3×10^3 per culture) every culture gives rise to a PC-specific response, indicating that PC-specific B precursors and any accessory cells required are present in excess. When either no T cells or no antigen was added, the mean number of plaque forming cells (PFC) per 10 μl test culture was less than one. This background contrasts with and is readily distinguished from a mean of 53 PFC per positive culture induced with PC_2KLH at a limiting T cell concentration (160 T_{KLH} per culture). From the Poisson relationship, $F_0 = e^{-\mu}$, when the mean number of helper events per culture, μ, equals 1, $F_0 = 0.37$. This intercept occurs at 160 viable T cells per culture for this KLH selected population.

In this analysis what is actually detected is the response induced by each helper event. If a single limiting T cell of a single type gives rise to a helper event, then the number of such T cells will be equal to the number of helper events. The data should then fit a single hit model and as indicated above a plot of log F_0 vs. N would give a straight line passing through the origin. If, however, a detectable helper event requires more than one cell of the limiting type (multi-hit) or more than one type of limiting cell (multi-target), then a more complex relationship between log F_0 and N is predicted. It may be useful to recognize that in the case of a multi-target model the fraction of cultures that are lacking more than one of m different required cell types is a higher order function of $e^{-\mu}$ (where for simplicity it is assumed that each of m cell types is represented at equal frequency, μ). As the number of cells added per culture increases, these terms become negligible and F_0 becomes a function of $m\, e^{-\mu}$. A plot of log F_0 vs. μ, therefore, takes on a defined slope whose extrapolation back to $\mu = 0$ gives a y axis intercept equal to m. Clearly $F_0 > 1$ is not possible and a line drawn through experimental points at low values of μ will in this case curve towards the origin ($F_0 = 1$).

The best estimate of μ from assays of replicate cultures at a single limiting T cell concentration is given by $\mu = -\ln F_0$. There are several ways to estimate μ from a set of values of F_0 determined at a number of different limiting T cell concentrations. When a substantial number of cultures (≥ 60) are assayed at each cell concentration, then for most purposes fitting a line that passes through the origin to these points by the method of least squares will prove satisfactory [1]. The significance of any deviation in the observed values of F_0 from those predicted by this line can then be evaluated by the chi-square test for goodness of fit. This will determine whether the experimental points are consistent with a single hit Poisson model. When a smaller number of cultures (≥ 20) are assayed at each limiting cell dilution, the method of maximum likelihood may give a more precise estimate of the frequency [4,5]. A program for carrying out the necessary calculations has been published [4].

Functional properties of a limiting cell type

Limiting dilution analysis can be applied to determine the frequency of a limiting cell and to test whether the relationship between F_0, the fraction of cultures in which a response fails to be induced, and N, the number of cells added per culture, is consistent with a single hit model. It is also possible to derive information concerning functional properties of the limiting cell type. This is not, however, entirely straightforward. Suppose, for example, it is determined that a population of helper T cells induces a positive response only with MHC-syngeneic B cells. This could be a property of either the limiting helper cell or of a second required cell type. If the second cell is not limiting at the cell concentrations being assayed, it would not affect the titration curve although its functional properties influence the ability to detect a response. In this example of MHC-restricted function it might be possible to assign this property to the limiting cell if it could be shown that in a population derived from an $(A \times B)F_1$ hybrid donor some limiting cells are restricted to parent A and others to parent B. Multiple assays of each limiting cell would be required to determine specificity. This is not usually possible for an effector cell but could be carried out at the level of limiting precursors that are induced to clonal expansion *in vitro*. An example of such an analysis will be presented in the next section. Here the author presents an example of functional analysis for a limiting effector cell.

In a study of helper T cell heterogeneity, it was of interest to determine whether the limiting T cells in two different populations selected under different *in vitro* conditions co-operate with hapten-specific B cells via similar or distinct mechanisms. It had been previously suggested that MHC-restricted carrier-specific T cells are limited to participate in only one helper event *in vitro* [8]. This limitation is consistent with a co-operation mechanism that proceeds through direct cell–cell interaction but would not be expected for T cells whose helper function is mediated by readily diffusible factors. In order to assay for this property, the author determined whether independent B precursors compete *in vitro* for a limiting helper T cell. Enriched populations of dinitrophenol (DNP)-specific and phosphorylcholine (PC)-specific B cells were obtained from independent primed donors. The DNP-specific response to DNP-KLH and the PC-specific response to PC-KLH are T-dependent and do not cross-react on hapten-conjugated red blood cells. The number of T cells per culture at which help is limiting was determined for a population specifically enriched in MHC-restricted, carrier-specific T cells. At a single limiting concentration of these T cells, the fraction of cultures in which a DNP-specific or PC-specific response can be induced was determined in three sets of 60 cultures each, that received either B_{DNP}, B_{PC} or both B_{DNP} and B_{PC}. The results in Table 65.1 demonstrate

Table 65.1. B$_{PC}$ and B$_{DNP}$ compete for helper T cells selected in limiting dilution cultures

Precursors added to each culture		Fraction of microcultures in which a hapten specific response is detected		
B$_{DNP}$	B$_{PC}$	DNP	PC	PC or DNP
+	+	0.30	0.32	0.58
+	−	0.55	−	0.55
−	+	−	0.55	0.55
		$P < 0.01$	$P < 0.01$	

All test cultures received both PC$_2$KLH and DNP$_4$ KLH. Reproduced from *The Journal of Immunology* (1982) **129**, 1845, by copyright permission of the American Association of Immunologists.

that in the presence of the two types of B cells the frequency of both DNP-specific and PC-specific responses is substantially reduced relative to that observed when only homologous B cells are present. The total amount of help (i.e., total number of positive cultures) remains constant. The statistical significance of the observed difference between the fraction of cultures in which a DNP-specific or PC-specific response is detected when both B$_{DNP}$ and B$_{PC}$ or only homologous B cells are present was determined by the test for a difference between two proportions. These results demonstrate that B$_{DNP}$ and B$_{PC}$ compete for limiting carrier-specific helper T cells. By carrying out a similar analysis of T cell populations selected under different conditions, it was possible to identify a second type of helper T cell for which B cell competition could not be demonstrated. The helper activity of these latter T cells was subsequently shown to be mediated by soluble factors freely available to multiple B cells. Although the same populations of primed B cells could be used to assay both types of helper T cell, it was shown that different B cells within that population are responsive to the different helper signals. The details of this analysis have been presented elsewhere [3].

To ensure that only helper T cells are limiting *in vitro* it is necessary to confirm that indicator B cells have been provided in excess. If helper T cells are titrated in the presence of a fixed but limiting concentration of B cells, then the titration curve takes on a more shallow initial slope and levels off at an F$_0$ that corresponds to the fraction of cultures that fail to receive an inducible B cell. In the course of the experiments described above, the author encountered an unexpectedly complex situation in which it could be shown that because of heterogeneity in the T cell population being titrated, different B cells were activated when T cells were present in excess and when T cells were limiting. To ensure that all relevant *in vitro* inducible B cells are present in excess, it was necessary to titrate T cells in 0.1 ml test cultures with 3×10^5 B cells from hyperimmune donors.

Limiting dilution experiments can also be applied to determine whether two events are independent. If, for example, a single T cell limits the ability to give rise to two different responses, then at a limiting concentration the presence or absence of the two responses should correlate. The analysis of helper T cell function described above demonstrates, however, that although a single cell may in principle be able to co-operate in two different responses, in practice its participation in one response may preclude participation in another. If sufficient information is available to exclude this possibility, then the independence of two responses in a single set of cultures can be tested in 2×2 contingency tables. Lefkovits & Waldmann [1] provide a useful set of tables for evaluating the probability of obtaining various numbers of double positives in a set of 60 cultures if two events are independent.

Isolation and expansion of clonal precursors *in vitro*

Limiting dilution analysis may reveal the presence of multiple interacting cell types. Definitive identification of such cells, however, requires that they be isolated on the basis of unique surface markers or as cloned lines *in vitro*. The most widely used method for isolating clonal precursors is limiting dilution in the presence of supporting cells and factors. Although precursors will normally be present in the initial population at relatively low frequency, they may be recloned through successive cycles of enrichment. Provided a high cloning efficiency can be achieved, this serves to ensure that each clone has a high probability of deriving from a single precursor. The requirement for repeated cloning is, however, laborious and limits the number of clones that can be characterized in this way. When the information desired is limited to the distribution of specificities within a population, a short-term cloning procedure permits characterization of a larger number of clonal precursors. The author has taken this approach to determine MHC-restriction specificities in an F$_1$ hybrid population of precursors to KLH-specific helper T cells [6,7].

Procedure

1 (BALB/c × BALB.B)F$_1$ KLH-primed lymph node cells are cultured at between 2×10^3 and 30×10^3 viable cells per 100 μl culture and supplemented to a final concentration of 35×10^3 cells per well with anti-Thy1.2, and C'- and mitomycin C-treated normal F_1 spleen cells. After 21 days, the cellular contents of 30–50 cultures at each initial input concentration are individually transferred in equal aliquots to six 10 μl test wells. Cells are washed in the new culture plates and helper activity is assayed by addition of 3×10^4 DNP-FGG-primed, anti-Thy-1.2, anti-Lyt-2.2, and C'-treated spleen cells (B_{DNP}), and DNP-KLH (0.1 μg/ml) to each well. In each set of six test cultures, three receive B_{DNP} of BALB/c origin and three of BALB.B origin.

2 A titration curve for precursors to helper T cells in one primed lymph node cell population is plotted in

Fig. 65.2. At 30×10^3 F_1 hybrid lymph node cells per culture, T cell precursors are in excess and virtually every culture transfers helper activity on day 21 to test wells of both parental types. As decreasing numbers of lymph node cells are added per culture, a required cell type becomes limiting and an increasing number of cultures fail to transfer helper activity to test wells of either parental type. In this particular primed lymph node population, the limiting cell occurs at an initial frequency of ~ 1 in 10^4 cells. The linear relationship between log F_0 and the number of lymph node cells added per culture indicates that, in the presence of mitomycin C-treated splenic filler cells, only one cell in the F_1 population limits the ability of a lymph node culture to transfer helper activity.

3 The results of two independent experiments in which MHC-restriction specificity of clonal progeny was determined are presented in Table 65.2. For each experiment, data are shown for those initial lymph node cell concentrations at which a significant proportion of cultures failed to transfer helper activity to any of the six corresponding test wells. Under these conditions, the majority of F_1 lymph node cultures transfer helper activity to recipient wells of only one parental type. As discussed below, this is not due to a limitation in the number of helper T cells present in a single culture on day 21 because when helper activity is transferred to test wells of one parental type it is most often transferred to all three test wells of that type. These results indicate that F_1 hybrid precursors to helper T cells restricted to co-operation with one or the other parental haplotype, segregate in the limiting dilution. The predicted frequency of lymph node cultures that include precursors for both H-2 specificities is the product of the individual frequencies and could, in fact, account for all of the cultures that were observed to transfer helper activity to recipient wells of both parental types.

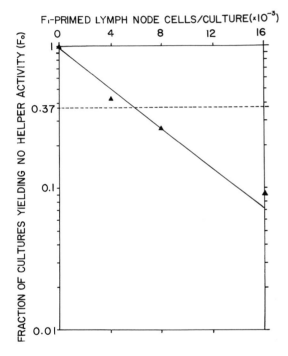

FRACTION OF CULTURES YIELDING NO HELPER ACTIVITY (F_0)

F_1-PRIMED LYMPH NODE CELLS/CULTURE($\times 10^{-3}$)

Fig. 65.2. Semi-log plot of the fraction of a set of lymph node cultures that fail to transfer any helper activity for a DNP-specific response vs. the number of (BALB/c × BALB.B) F_1 KLH-primed lymph node cells added to each 100 μl culture. Each culture was supplemented with syngeneic filler cells to 35×10^3 cells/well. This is the same experiment as experiment 1 of Table 65.2 but with additional data points. Helper activity was assayed as described in the legend to Table 65.2. If a DNP-specific response was induced in any test culture of either BALB/c or BALB.B origin, the donor F_1 lymph node culture was scored positive for helper activity. The points conform to a straight line determined by least squares analysis with correlation coefficient > 0.95. Reproduced from *The Journal of Experimental Medicine* (1980), **152**, 924, by copyright permission of the Rockefeller University Press.

Notes and recommendations

It is most important for these experiments that each clonal precursor give rise to an adequate number of helper T cells so that their specificity may be characterized by assay of helper function in independent test cultures with B_{DNP} of diverse origin. A minimal estimate for the mean number of helper cells present on day 21 in lymph node cultures that receive a limiting precursor can be derived from a Poisson analysis of the distribution of responses in test cultures to which progeny of such precursors have been transferred. For this purpose, data are pooled from all sets of three test wells for which a DNP-specific response is detected in at least one well. The fraction of test cultures in which a DNP-specific response is not

Table 65.2. Isolation of (BALB/c × BALB.B)F$_1$ helper T cells restricted to parental MHC haplotypes

Experiment	(BALB/c × BALB.B)F$_1$-primed lymph node cells per culture ($\times 10^3$)	Number of cultures assayed	Helper activity (number of cultures)			
			BALB/c only	BALB.B only	BALB/c and BALB.B	None
1	7.5	30	5	10	2	13
	15.0	30	5	8	9	8
2	7.5	50	7	16	10	17

(BALB/c × BALB.B)F$_1$ KLH-primed lymph node cultures were initiated at the indicated number of cells in 100 μl round-bottomed wells and supplemented with anti-Thy-1.2 and C′- and mitomycin C-treated F$_1$ filler cells. The helper activity in 30 or 50 identical lymph node cultures was assayed on day 21 by transfer to triplicate 10 μl microculture wells with DNP$_7$FGG-primed B cells and macrophage of either BALB/c or BALB.B origin. If a DNP-specific response was induced in at least one test well in a set of three, the donor lymph node culture was scored positive for helper activity restricted to that haplotype. In control plates that received the same number of B$_{DNP}$, but to which T cells were added in excess, a DNP-specific response was detected in every culture indicating that B$_{DNP}$ are also in excess. DNP-specific responses were detected as PFC on day 5 of secondary culture. The mean PFC per positive well for each B cell donor in both experiments was ≥ 100. Reproduced from *The Journal of Experimental Medicine* (1980) **152**, 925, by copyright permission of the Rockefeller University Press.

detected (F$_0$) then represents the fraction that did not receive a helper T cell. The mean number of helper T cells transferred to each test culture at that concentration of lymph node cells is determined from the Poisson relationship, F$_0$ = e$^{-\mu}$, and the mean number of helper T cells derived from one positive 100 μl lymph node culture can be calculated (6 × μ). In many experiments this value, after limited expansion *in vitro*, is greater than twenty functional progeny per precursor. If necessary higher levels of expansion can be obtained in lymph node cultures by repeated cycles of weekly stimulation with fresh filler cells and antigen prior to assay of helper activity.

Assays for specific antibody secretion

The more cultures are assayed at informative dilutions, the more precise and reliable are the conclusions of limiting dilution experiments. Since it is often not possible to predict what will be an informative dilution, it is necessary to set up many cultures at each of a number of different T cell concentrations. A useful assay for specific antibody secretion must, therefore, be simple as well as reliably discriminate background from positive responses. The author has found haemagglutination assays with haptenated red blood cells well-suited for this purpose. The following procedure has been used in our laboratory to detect a variety of hapten-specific responses when helper T cells derive

from the expanded progeny of an isolated clonal precursor.

Procedure

1 3×10^5 primed B cells and antigen are introduced in 0.1 ml cultures of 96-well round-bottomed tissue culture plates in complete RPMI 1640 medium with 20% FCS.
2   One set of test cultures is set up without T cells to determine the T-independent background and define a threshold level of response. A second set of test cultures receives helper T cells in excess from a bulk population to confirm that B cells and accessory cells are present in excess. The remaining test cultures receive cellular aliquots from day 21 limiting dilution lymph node cultures that may have included a clonal precursor to helper T cells.
3   On day 4 culture supernatants are removed and replaced with fresh medium. This step removes any background antibody derived from early secretion by residual antibody-producing cells in hyperimmune B cell donors. It is not necessary at this stage to add back antigen.
4   Antibody produced in a 24 h pulse through day 5 is assayed by transfer of 10 μl of the final culture supernatant to assay wells containing 60 μl HBSS, 10 μl 2.5% haptenated-horse red blood cells, and 10 μl polyvalent rabbit anti-mouse Ig serum. The final 1:8

dilution of culture supernatant was selected to avoid inhibitory pro-zone effects of high titre supernatants that are induced when multiple T cell progeny of a single isolated lymph node precursor are transferred to a B cell test well. Equivalent high titre supernatants are not induced by individual helper T cells isolated in limiting dilutions of effector cells. In this case, supernatants should not be diluted with buffer.

5 The contents of assay wells are mixed and red cells allowed to settle at room temperature for 1 h. Unagglutinated red cells will form a tight button and indicate the absence of specific antibody. In the presence of enhancing serum the haemagglutination pattern is stable for at least 3 h.

Conclusion

Limiting dilution analysis can provide information concerning the frequency within a population of effector cells with defined specificity and function. Because of the possibility of repeated sampling, these methods are uniquely powerful when applied at the level of clonal precursors that can be induced to expand and differentiate *in vitro*. The identification of tissue-specific growth factors greatly facilitates this application of limiting dilution analysis.

References

1 LEFKOVITS I. & WALDMANN H. (1979) *Limiting Dilution Analysis of Cells in the Immune System.* Cambridge University Press.
2 MILLER R.G., TEH H.-S., HARLEY E. & PHILLIPS R.A. (1977) Quantitative studies of the activation of cytotoxic lymphocyte precursor cells. *Immunol. Revs.* **35**, 38.
3 IMPERIALE M.J., FAHERTY D.A., SPROVIERO J.F. & ZAUDERER M. (1982) Functionally distinct helper T cells enriched under different culture conditions cooperate with different B cells. *J. Immunol.* **129**, 1843.
4 FAZEKAS DE ST. GROTH S. (1982) The Evaluation of Limiting Dilution Assays. *J. immunol. Meth.* **49**, R11.
5 TASWELL C. (1981) Limiting dilution assays for the determination of immunocompetent cell frequencies. (I) Data analysis. *J. Immunol.* **126**, 1614.
6 SPROVIERO J.F., IMPERIALE M.J. & ZAUDERER M. (1980) Clonal analysis of F_1 hybrid helper T cells restricted to parental or F_1 hybrid major histocompatibility determinants. *J. exp. Med.* **152**, 920.
7 SPROVIERO J.F., IMPERIALE M.J. & ZAUDERER M. (1981) Clonal analysis of F_1 hybrid helper T cells. I-A subregion-encoded hybrid determinants restrict the activity of KLH-specific helper T cells. *J. exp. Med.* **154**, 1255.
8 PHILLIPS J.M. & WALDMAN H. (1977) Monogamous helper T cell. *Nature,* **268**, 641.

Chapter 66
In vitro evaluation of human lymphocyte function

H. C. LANE, GAIL WHALEN & A. S. FAUCI

Methods for obtaining human lymphoid cell populations, 66.1
Methods for identifying lymphocyte surface markers, 66.3

Methods for evaluating *in vitro* lymphocyte blast transformation, 66.5

Methods for *in vitro* evaluation of B cell effector function (Ig production), 66.6
Methods for *in vitro* evaluation of T cell effector function, 66.10

The human immune system is one of the most difficult organ systems in human physiology to assess accurately *in vitro* [1–2]. The complexity of this organ, which is comprised of peripheral blood, bone marrow, lymph node, thoracic duct, and splenic lymphocytes and accessory cells, makes it virtually impossible to develop *in vitro* systems that accurately take into account the totality of the intricate interplay of cells which is occurring *in vivo*. The survival of the host is dependent upon the presence of a functioning immune system. Thus attempts to develop ways to at least in part provide a quantification of immune system function are of considerable importance.

The human immune system is a dynamic organ and constantly changes to meet the antigenic challenges of the environment. Any *in vitro* measurements of *in vivo* immune function will be influenced by the degree of activation of the immune system at the time a specimen is obtained for assay. For example, the percentage of peripheral blood lymphocytes from a normal subject bearing certain cell surface antigens will fluctuate as a function of the length of time since the last viral infection experienced by the individual [3–4]. In attempting to dissect out the mechanisms of abnormal immune function in diseases, it is often difficult to distinguish between aberrations of immune function due to the immunologic disease itself and changes in immune function due to other diseases occurring as a complication of the abnormal immune status of the host. This is particularly true in the study of immunodeficiency diseases in which the patients are often prone to recurrent severe infections and neoplasms, which may result in profound changes in the immune profile.

In the sections which follow, the authors outline some of the *in vitro* tests of human immune function which have been established as being valuable in delineating the mechanisms of human immune function in normal and disease states (see Chapter 26).

Methods for obtaining human lymphoid cell populations

General considerations

Human lymphoid cell populations may be obtained from peripheral blood, bone marrow, lymph nodes or spleen. As a result of its easy accessibility, as compared to the other lymphoid organs, the most commonly utilized source of lymphocytes is peripheral blood. It should be pointed out, however, that peripheral blood only reflects immunocompetent cells present in the bloodstream at the time the sample is taken and may not accurately reflect the overall immune status of the host. It is quite clear that human peripheral blood is not as immunocompetent an organ as is mouse spleen; therefore it may be difficult to correlate studies in these two systems. A pertinent fact is that while it is quite simple to induce a primary antigen-specific immune response utilizing lymphocytes obtained from a mouse spleen [5], it is quite difficult, and some feel perhaps impossible, to do so utilizing lymphocytes from human peripheral blood [6]. Despite these limitations, lymphocytes obtained from human peripheral blood have greatly increased our understanding of the workings of the human immune system in normal and disease states.

Equipment

Room temperature centrifuge and carriers.
Cytocentrifuge.
Phase-contrast microscope.

Materials

Hypaque-Ficoll (Ficoll-paque, Pharmacia Fine Chemicals, Piscataway, NJ).
18-gauge Spinal needle.
Pipettes.

Pipette-aid.
Thirty-five millilitre syringes.
Haemocytometer.
Wright's stain.
Erlenmeyer flask.
Fifty millilitre sterile conical tubes.
Microscope slides.
Heparin.
Sucrose.

Procedures

Separation of peripheral blood mononuclear cells from whole blood [7]

1   Blood is collected by phlebotomy into a syringe containing approximately 1000 units of heparin per 50 ml of blood.
2   Heparinized blood thus obtained is diluted 1:1 with phosphate-buffered saline (PBS) in an Erlenmeyer flask, mixed well, and poured in 35 ml aliquots into 50 ml conical tubes.
3   Using the spinal needle attached to a syringe, 12 ml of Hypaque-Ficoll are layered underneath the diluted blood in each tube.
4   The tubes are then balanced and placed in a room temperature centrifuge to spin at 400 *g* for 35 min.
5   Following centrifugation, the mononuclear cell layer will appear as a white band, underneath the plasma layer and above the red blood cell and granulocyte pellet (Fig. 66.1). This layer may be removed by gentle aspiration, utilizing a 10 ml pipette and a pipette-aid. Aspirated layers are transferred to a clean 50 ml conical tube (no more than two layers per tube). The tubes are then filled to 50 ml with media and centrifuged at 800 *g* for 5 min.
6   Following centrifugation, the tubes are decanted, and the pellets (which contain the peripheral blood mononuclear cells) are resuspended in approximately 5–10 ml of media and combined in one tube. This tube is filled to 50 ml with media and centrifuged at 600 *g* for 5 min.
7   Following centrifugation, the tube is decanted, the cells are resuspended in 10.1 ml of media, and a 0.1 ml aliquot is removed for counting cells and preparing a cytoprep. The tube is again filled with 50 ml media and centrifuged at 600 *g* for 5 min. A portion of the aliquoted cells are placed in the cytocentrifuge and then fixed and stained in order to determine the cell types present in the population. The number of cells in the aliquot is determined, and the number of cells/ml in the aliquot multiplied by 10 to obtain the total number of peripheral blood mononuclear cells collected.
8   Following this last centrifugation, the tubes are

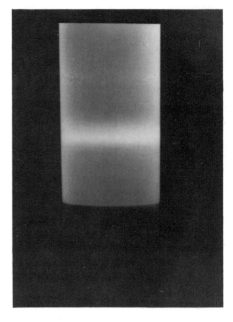

Fig. 66.1. Diluted human peripheral blood immediately following centrifugation over Hypaque-Ficoll density gradient. The mononuclear cells appear as a layer at the plasma-Ficoll interface. The red blood cells and granulocytes form a pellet at the bottom of the tube.

decanted and the cells resuspended in media at 10^7 cells per ml. Cell suspensions thus obtained are placed on ice until needed.

Separation of mononuclear cells from bone marrow aspirates [8]

1   Aspirate 2.5–3.0 ml of bone marrow aspirate into a syringe containing 0.5 ml of acid citrate.
2   Mix syringe contents with 10 ml of ammonium chloride solution to lyse red blood cells in a 50 ml conical tube. Pipette contents of tube up and down several times over a period of 2 min to ensure lysis of the red cells. Bring contents of tube to 50 ml with media, and centrifuge at 600 *g* for 5 min.
3   Decant the supernatant, resuspend the button in 50 ml of media, and centrifuge at 600 *g* for 5 min.
4   Decant the supernatant, resuspend the button in 2 ml of media, and carefully layer on a sucrose density gradient in a 12 ml test-tube (2 ml layers of 35, 30, 25, 20, and 15% sucrose in Hanks' balanced salt solution [HBSS] containing 20% fetal calf serum [FCS]).
5   Centrifuge at 200 *g* for 7 min.
6   Aspirate with a pipette the top half of the gradient, and place in a 50 ml conical tube. Bring contents of the

tube to 50 ml with culture media, and centrifuge at 600 *g* for 5 min.

7 Resuspend the button in 10.1 ml, and take a 0.1 ml aliquot for cell count and preparation of cytoprep as outlined above. Bring the remainder of the tube to 50 ml with media, and centrifuge at 600 *g* for 5 min.

8 Decant or aspirate the supernatant, and resuspend the cells at 10^7 per ml.

Separation of mononuclear cells from spleen, lymph node or tonsil

1 Place tissue to be processed in a sterile Petri dish containing enough media to completely cover the bottom of the dish. Tease the tissue apart, utilizing two pairs of forceps. An optional step at this point involves passage of the cell suspension through a fine wire mesh.

2 Transfer the cell suspension from the Petri dish to a 50 ml sterile conical tube, using a 10 ml pipette. Fill the tube to 50 ml with media and allow to sit on ice for 5 min.

3 Aspirate the cell suspension from the tube and place in a clean 50 ml conical tube. Be careful not to disturb the debris which has settled out.

4 Bring the contents of the tube containing the cell suspension to 50 ml with media and centrifuge at 600 *g* for 5 min.

5 Decant the supernatant, resuspend the button in 50 ml of media, and centrifuge at 600 *g* for 5 min.

6 Decant the supernatant, resuspend the button in 10.1 ml of media, and remove 0.1 ml for cell count and cytoprep. Bring the tube to 50 ml, centrifuge for 5 min at 600 *g*, decant the supernatant, and resuspend the button to give a cell density of 10^7 per ml.

Notes

Care must be taken to maintain sterility if cells are to be used for culture conditions. Peripheral blood may be separated undiluted if one desires plasma from the donor.

Methods for identifying lymphocyte surface markers

Since the earliest observations that the lymphocyte was not a uniform cell type, investigators have been developing ways to identify and enumerate distinct subpopulations of lymphocytes. The development of monoclonal antibody technology has resulted in the production of a large number of murine monoclonal antibodies which can identify unique human cell surface antigens [9–10]. Despite this degree of complexity, the investigator wishing to classify a given immune system as grossly normal or abnormal can

often do so simply by enumerating the number of T cells and B cells present in the peripheral blood by either the classic method of sheep red blood cell (SRBC) rosetting or through the binding of appropriate polyclonal or monoclonal antibodies tagged with a fluorescent probe. For the individual wishing to probe subset identification more precisely, a wide panel of commercial monoclonal antibodies are available for this purpose.

Equipment

Rotator.
37 °C Incubator.
Fluorescent microscope or fluorescence-activated cell sorter (FACS) analyser.
Phase-contrast microscope.

Materials

Washed sheep red blood cells (SRBC).
Fluorescein isothiocyanate (FITC)-conjugated F(ab')$_2$ fragment goat anti-human immunoglobulins (Ig).
FITC-conjugated F(ab')$_2$ fragment goat anti-mouse IgG (γ- and light-chain specific).
Latex beads.
Mononuclear cells obtained from Hypaque-Ficoll separation.
12×75 mm. 5 ml test-tubes.
1-*n*-Propyl glycolate.
Appropriate monoclonal antibodies.

Procedures

Enumeration of the total T cell number by SRBC rosetting [11]

1 Add 0.1 ml (1×10^6) unfractionated peripheral blood mononuclear cells to 0.15 ml of media and 0.25 ml of 0.5% SRBC in a 5 ml test-tube.

2 Centrifuge at 400 *g* for 5 min at 4 °C.

3 Gently aspirate media and carefully layer 0.5 ml of 5% albumin of FCS over the cells. Be careful not to disturb the button.

4 Incubate for 2 h or overnight at 4 °C.

5 Gently resuspend the button completely by slowly turning the test-tube until all cells are resuspended.

6 Place one drop of the cell suspension on a slide, cover with a coverslip, and read under phase-contrast microscopy.

7 Count 100–200 cells and score them as rosette-positive or rosette-negative. A rosette-positive cell is one that has bound 3 or more SRBC (Fig. 66.2).

8 The percentage of rosette-positive cells × the total

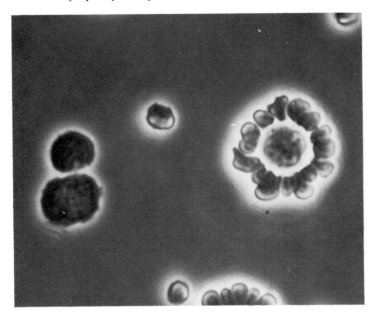

Fig. 66.2. Phase-contrast microscopy of erythrocyte rosette-positive and rosette-negative cells.

number of monocytes and lymphocytes in the peripheral blood (determined from the total white blood count and differential) yields the total number of T lymphocytes. The normal range for this value will vary depending upon the laboratory. It is usually in the range of 1000–2000/mm³.

Determination of total T cell number utilizing monoclonal antibodies [9]

1   Place 0.1 ml (1 × 10⁶) unfractionated peripheral blood mononuclear cells in a 5 ml test-tube.
2   Add 5 μl (this value may vary, depending upon the monoclonal antibody) monoclonal antibody to the suspension.
3   Incubate for 45 min on ice.
4   Wash twice with 4 ml of FACS buffer.
5   Aspirate the last wash fluid and add 5 μl of FITC-conjugated goat anti-mouse IgG to the cell button.
6   Incubate for 45 min on ice.
7   Wash twice with 4 ml of FACS buffer.
8   Resuspend the final cell button in 1 ml of FACS buffer if sample is to be analysed by a FACS analyser, or in 0.2 ml of FACS buffer if the sample is to be counted manually utilizing a fluorescence microscope.
9   The total number of T cells equals [the percentage of cells binding the monoclonal antibody multiplied by the total number of lymphocytes and monocytes (obtained from the white blood cells and differential)] minus the total number of monocytes. If the mono-

cytes have been gated out by the FACS, the total number of T cells equals the percentage of cells binding the monoclonal multiplied by the total lymphocyte count.

Determination of total number of B lymphocytes by staining for surface Ig [12]

1   Place 0.1 ml (1 × 10⁶) unfractionated peripheral blood mononuclear cells in a 5 ml test-tube.
2   Add 2 ml of serum-free media, 5 μl of a 1% suspension of latex beads and incubate on rotator for 30 min at 37 °C (removal of cytophilic antibody from B cells and latex bead ingestion by monocytes).
3   Fill tube with media, spin at 600 *g* for 5 min.
4   Decant supernatant, add 5 μl of fluorescein-conjugated goat F(ab′)₂ fragment polyvalent anti-human Ig.
5   Incubate at 4 °C for 45 min or overnight.
6   Wash three times with cold PBS.
7   Add a drop of *n*-propyl glycolate [13]; resuspend cells. Keep sample at 4 °C to prevent capping of surface Ig on B cells.
8   Place a drop on a slide and cover, read with phase contrast on fluorescence microscope.
9   The total number of B cells equals (the percentage of fluorescent cells minus the percentage of fluorescent cells containing latex beads—monocytes) multiplied by the total number of lymphocytes.

Notes

Lymphocyte subsets defined by monoclonal antibodies can be enumerated by modifications of the methods in the section on pages 66.3 and 66.4.

Methods for evaluating *in vitro* lymphocyte blast transformation

The *in vivo* function of lymphocytes is felt to involve a complex series of cellular interactions among immunocompetent cells and antigen [14]. The ability to assess lymphocyte function on a qualitative as well as a quantitative level is hampered because it is currently impossible to precisely duplicate *in vivo* conditions *in vitro*. The *in vitro* evaluation of lymphocyte function is greatly influenced by the precise conditions of the individual experimental method. Variables such as cell density, culture vessel geometry, and length of culture may greatly influence the end result (Fig. 66.3). Accordingly, it is important in such measurements that lymphocytes from control subjects be processed along with lymphocytes from patients. In addition, it is virtually impossible to establish absolute normal ranges for these values as they will fluctuate substantially from laboratory to laboratory and even within a given laboratory from time to time.

The main *in vitro* measurements of lymphocyte function take advantage of the fact that certain plant lectins as well as some microbial products have the ability to activate human peripheral blood lymphocytes. This activation, which involves a G_0 to S transition of lymphocytes, results in the synthesis of DNA. This DNA synthesis can be easily quantified by the use of radioisotope labelling, generally employing tritiated thymidine.

While plant lectins induce a non-specific triggering

of peripheral blood lymphocytes, the ability of the immune system to undergo blast transformation following a specific signal can be assessed with the use of an antigen such as tetanus toxoid. This soluble protein makes an ideal *in vitro* test due to the fact that most individuals have been immunized with it at some point in their lives. However, the use of a test which is dependent upon prior immunization results in the introduction of a new variable, namely the interval since the last antigenic exposure. In addition to the ability to respond to a soluble recall antigen, the specific recognition capabilities of peripheral blood lymphocytes can be assessed through the measurement of alloreactivity.

Equipment

CO_2 incubator.
Scintillation counter.
Skatron cell harvester (Skatron, Inc., Sterling, VA).

Materials

Phytohaemagglutinin (PHA, Burroughs-Wellcome Laboratories, Research Triangle Park, NC) at a concentration of 40 µg/ml.
Tetanus toxoid (TT) at a concentration of 100 µg/ml (Lederle Laboratories, Pearle River, NY).
Concanavalin A (Con A) at concentrations of 1000 µg/ml and 2000 µg/ml.
Whole formalinized *Staphylococcus aureus* Cowan strain 1 (SAC, Bethesda Research Laboratories, Gaithersburg, MD) at a 1:625 dilution.
Pokeweed mitogen (PWM, GIBCO Laboratories, Grand Island, NY) at a 1:10 dilution.

a

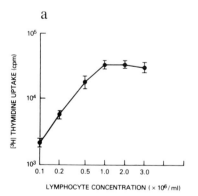

b

Culture Tube	Cell Count	Unstimulated	Stimulated
Round bottom	0.5×10^6	9	6,700
Round bottom	1.0×10^6	54	10,100
Round bottom	2.0×10^6	25	18,000
Round bottom	4.0×10^6	27	5,400
Flat bottom	0.5×10^6	7	3,500
Flat bottom	1.0×10^6	26	4,400
Flat bottom	2.0×10^6	15	2,900
Flat bottom	4.0×10^6	22	310

(column headers: Culture Tube | Cell Count | ^{3}H/TdR Incorporation into DNA (dpm) — Unstimulated / Stimulated)

c

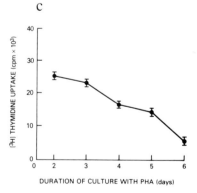

Fig. 66.3. Influence of lymphocyte concentration, culture vessel geometry, and duration of culture on phytohaemagglutinin-induced incorporation of ^{3}H-thymidine. In a, cultures were performed in a total volume of 0.2 ml; thus 0.5×10^6 lymphocytes per ml corresponds to 1×10^5 lymphocytes per culture. (a) and (c) from ref. 15; (b) from ref. 17.

Tritiated thymidine, specific activity 6.7 Ci/mmol, diluted 1:50.

96-Well tissue culture plates.

All dilutions are performed in RPMI 1640.

Procedures

In vitro *measurement of lymphocyte blast transformation to T cell mitogens PHA or con A* [15–17]

1 Place 0.05 ml (5.0×10^5) unfractionated peripheral blood mononuclear cells in a 5 ml test tube containing 0.15 ml of human serum, 0.75 ml of RPMI 1640, and 0.05 ml of mitogen or additional media (control).

2 Gently vortex the contents of the tube and pipette in triplicate 200 μl of the contents into the wells of a 96-well microtitre plate.

3 Allow the tissue culture plate to incubate for 3 days at 37 °C in a 5% CO_2 atmosphere.

4 Add 20 μl of the tritiated-thymidine mixture to each well.

5 Return the plate to the incubator for an additional 4 h.

6 Harvest the contents of the plate, utilizing any of the automated cell harvesters (SKATRON), and count the amount of tritium incorporated during the pulse.

7 The amount of tritiated thymidine incorporation induced by the mitogen can be determined by subtracting the mean of the control points from the mean of the mitogen stimulated points.

In vitro *measurement of lymphocyte blast transformation to the pure B cell mitogen SAC* [18,19]

1 Place 0.05 ml (5.0×10^5) peripheral blood mononuclear cells into a 5 ml test-tube containing 0.10 ml of FCA, 0.80 ml of RPMI 1640, and 0.05 ml of SAC suspension or media (control).

2–6 Same at outlined above.

In vitro *measurement of lymphocyte blast transformation to the T and B cell mitogen PWM or the soluble protein antigen TT*

1 Place 0.05 ml (5.0×10^5) peripheral blood mononuclear cells into a 5 ml test-tube containing 0.15 ml of human serum, 0.75 ml of RPMI 1640, and 0.05 ml of mitogen, antigen or media (control).

2–6 Same as outlined above, with the exception that the plate is pulsed and harvested on day 5 rather than day 3.

In vitro *measurement of alloreactivity*

1 Place 0.025 ml (2.5×10^5) peripheral blood mononuclear cells into a 5 ml test-tube containing 0.15 ml human serum, 0.8 ml RPMI 1640, and 0.025 ml (2.5×10^5) irradiated (3000 R) peripheral blood mononuclear cells from either the same individual (control) or from the individual to be used as the stimulator.

2–6 Same as outlined above, with the plate pulsed and harvested on day 5 or 6.

Notes

Pooled human A sera is used to maintain a low background of proliferation during a 3- or 5-day incubation. SAC will not induce proliferation of B cells in human A sera because of the binding of human Ig to the protein A component of the SAC; therefore FCS must be used in the SAC assay. FCS has mitogenic properties in itself; therefore different lots should be pre-screened before use in order to avoid lots with substantial stimulatory activity. The authors have chosen concentrations of mitogens or antigens that give maximal proliferation in their laboratory. Dose–response curves should be set up for each of the mitogens where initially used since there is some variability among the reagents.

Methods for *in vitro* evaluation of B cell effector function (Ig production)

While measurements of blast transformation give an indication of the ability of peripheral blood lymphocytes to respond to an activation signal, they provide little insight into the ability of these cells to differentiate into mature effector cells. One of the easiest effector cell functions to measure is that of the B lymphocyte, namely Ig production. Ig secretion may be measured at the single cell level in the PFC assay or as a soluble product in culture supernatants. In addition, one may measure spontaneous antibody secretion, mitogen-induced antibody secretion, or antigen-induced antibody secretion. The former measurement provides an excellent indicator of *in vivo* polyclonal B cell activation, while the latter two reveal the ability of the B lymphocyte repertoire to respond to non-specific or specific stimulation. As in the case of antigen-induced blast transformation, the character of antigen-induced antibody production is greatly influenced by the exposure history of the particular subject to the antigens in question.

Method for PFC assay [20,21]

Equipment

CO_2 incubator.
Dissecting microscope.
30 °C and 56 °C water baths.
Heating block.

Materials

SRBC washed three times in 0.85% NaCl and spun at 250 *g* for all washes.
Chromic chloride stock solution (10 mg in 10 ml 0.85% NaCl).
Staphylococcal protein A [SPA, Pharmacia Fine Chemicals]—5 mg vial brought up in 1 ml 0.85% NaCl diluted to 0.5 mg/ml for use in preparation of SPA-coated SRBC.
IgG fraction polyvalent rabbit anti-human Ig (Cappel Laboratories, West Chester, PA).
French agarose gel at 45 °C.
60 × 15 mm Petri dishes.

Procedures

Preparation of reagents

1   SPA-coated SRBC. Add 1 ml of chromic chloride stock solution to a 15 ml test-tube containing 9 ml 0.85% NaCl. To this tube add 1 ml of the diluted SPA solution, followed by 1 ml of packed SRBC. Gently mix the contents of the tube and incubate at 30 °C in a shaker water bath for 40 min.

Pellet contents of tube by centrifugation at 800 *g* for 5 min at 4 °C. Wash once with normal saline. Supernatant should appear fairly clear at this point. If there is gross haemolysis present, protein has probably not been attached to the red cell; discard and attempt again. If no gross hemolysis, resuspend pellet in 3 ml HBSS (25% solution) for use in PFC assay.

2   Agarose mixture. Mix 1400 mg agarose with 100 ml distilled water in a small Wheaton bottle. Boil mixture until agarose dissolves completely. Once agarose is dissolved, add 100 ml of 2 × RPMI which has been preheated to 56 °C. Mix contents of bottle and keep in water bath at 56 °C.

3   Guinea-pig serum adsorbed to remove antibodies directed against SRBC. Add 2 ml packed SRBC to 25 ml of freshly thawed guinea-pig serum. Mix and incubate on ice for 10 min. Centrifuge at 3000 rev./min at 4 °C for 10 min. Pipette off serum; discard packed cell button.

Repeat above procedure for second absorption. Pipette off serum, filter through a 0.45 μm Millipore filter, aliquot in 1 ml aliquots, and freeze at −70 °C until ready for use.

Performing the assay

Add 4 ml of agarose mixture to 60 × 15 mm plastic Petri dishes, swirl the contents quickly to cover the bottom of the plate, and cool to room temperature. These plates may be used the same day or stored at 4 °C for several weeks.

Prepare the suspension of lymphoid cells to be tested such that the desired number of cells are contained in 0.10 ml of RPMI 1640. This concentration should be adjusted such that 0.10 ml will contain approximately 100–200 PFC. If one is unsure of the number of PFC in a cell population, several different concentrations should be assayed.

Place 0.85 ml of agarose mixture, 0.06 ml of SPA-coated SRBC and 0.10 ml of cells to be tested into a 5 ml test tube pre-warmed to 47 °C in a heating block. For each cell suspension to be tested, three plates should be set up in order to allow for three different concentrations of developing antisera (0, 1 : 50, and 1 : 100).

Vortex the contents of the tube, and quickly pour its contents into an agarose-coated Petri dish. Swirl the dish to distribute the cell mixture evenly.

Allow the contents of the dish to cool with the lid ajar, then close the lid and place the dish in a 37 °C incubator for 2 h. Following this incubation, add to the triplicate plates either 1 ml of RPMI 1640, 1 ml of rabbit anti-human Ig (IgG, IgM and IgA) diluted 1 : 50 or 1 ml of anti-human Ig diluted 1 : 100 (all dilutions done in RPMI 1640).

Incubate plates for 2 h at 37 °C. Aspirate the antibody and add 1 ml of SRBC-absorbed guinea-pig serum (a source of complement) diluted 1 : 40 in RPMI 1640. Return the plates to the 37 °C incubator for 1 h. Remove the complement and count the number of plaques under a dissecting microscope (10 ×) (Fig. 66.4). Data are usully expressed as PFC/10^6 total cells.

Method for measurement of supernatant Ig production by enzyme-linked immunosorbent assay (ELISA) (Fig. 66.5) [22–25].

Equipment

Immulon I flat-bottomed plates.
96-Well ELISA plate (Dynatech Laboratories, Alexandria, VA).
Microelisa auto-reader (Dynatech).
Multichannel pipette with tips (Flow Laboratories, Inc., McLean, VA).

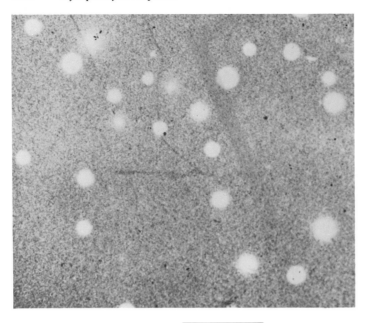

Fig. 66.4. Photomicrograph of haemolysis-in-gel plaque-forming cell assay. Each clear spot in the gel corresponds to an individual immunoglobulin-secreting cell.

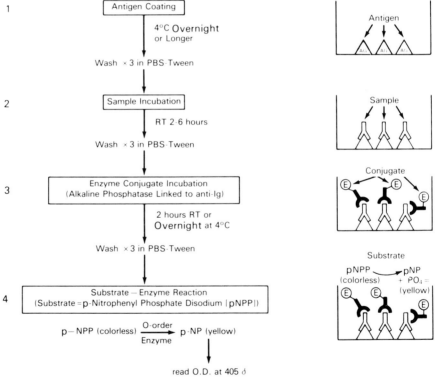

Fig. 66.5. Enzyme-linked immunosorbent assay for quantification of supernatant immunoglobulin (Ig) production. The antigen (which may be anti-human Ig) is bound to the solid phase. The plate is then incubated with sample, washed, incubated with enzyme-(alkaline phosphatase) linked anti-human Ig, washed, and incubated with substrate (e.g., *p*-nitrophyenyl phosphate). The degree of enzymatic conversion of colourless substrate to coloured product is proportional to the amount of enzyme present, which is proportional to the amount of sample bound. Graphic provided by Drs Thomas R. Cupps and David J. Volkman.

Materials

Coating antibodies: IgG fraction goat anti-human IgM μ-chain specific; IgG fraction goat anti-human IgG F(ab')$_2$ fragment specific (N.L. Cappel Laboratories, Cochranville, PA).

Conjugates: goat anti-human IgM (μ-chain specific) alkaline phosphatase conjugate; goat anti-human IgG (γ-chain specific) alkaline phosphatase conjugate; goat anti-human IgA (α-chain specific) alkaline phosphatase conjugate.

Standards of defined concentrations of human Ig.

p-Nitrophenyl phosphate (Sigma Chemical Co., St. Louis, MO) at 1 μg/ml in substrate buffer.

3 M NaOH.

PBS containing 0.05% Tween-20.

Coating buffer.

Procedures

1   Culture supernatants from peripheral blood lymphocyte cultures established as described below are harvested and stored at 4 °C until assay. Cultures for measurement of spontaneous Ig production usually need to be diluted 1:50, and cultures stimulated with PWM diluted 1:200 prior to assay. PBS-Tween is a good diluent.

2   ELISA plates for assaying IgG or IgA are prepared by coating 96-well, flat-bottomed microtitre ELISA plates with 200 μl carbonate-bicarbonate coating buffer, pH 9.6, containing 10 μg/ml of goat anti-human F(ab')$_2$. ELISA plates for assaying IgM are prepared by coating 96-well, flat-bottomed microtitre ELISA plates with 200 μl of a carbonate-bicarbonate coating buffer, pH 9.6, containing 10 μg/ml of goat anti-human IgM.

3   Plates with anti-Ig coating buffer solution (200 μl per well) are allowed to incubate overnight at 4 °C.

4   Plates are washed three times with 200 μl PBS-Tween per well per wash. The final amount of fluid in each well is aspirated with suction or a sharp blow on an absorbent pad.

5   In duplicate, 200 μl of sample or standard (generally four concentrations in the 10–100 ng range) are applied to the plate.

6   The plate is allowed to incubate for 2 h at room temperature.

7   The samples are then removed and the plate again washed three times with PBS-Tween.

8   Depending upon the particular assay, the wells are then filled with 200 μl diluted in 1:1000 PBS-Tween: goat anti-IgG conjugated to alkaline phosphatase, or goat anti-IgA conjugated to alkaline phosphatase, or goat anti-IgM conjugated to alkaline phosphatase.

9   The plates are allowed to sit for 2 h at room temperature or overnight at 4 °C.

10   Plates are then washed four times with PBS-Tween and 200 μl of substrate solution added.

11   The plates are allowed to sit at room temperature until sufficient substrate conversion has occurred to allow for the development of a yellow colour among all four standards, generally ranging from an OD_{402} of 0.1 to 1.0. At this point, the reaction is stopped by the addition of 25 μl of NaOH solution to the wells.

12   The optical density of each well is determined with the use of an ELISA reader (Titertek multiscan; Dynatech ELISA reader), a standard curve created from the standard values, and the experimental points interpolated on the curve.

Method for measurement of spontaneous Ig secretion [26]

1   The cell population to be studied is harvested as outlined on page 66.2 and adjusted to a concentration of 10^7 cells per ml.

2   3×10^6 cells (0.3 ml) are placed in a 5 ml test-tube containing 3 ml of RPMI 1640. The cell mixture is placed on a rotator in a 37°C incubator for 45 min to remove cytophilic antibody.

3   The cells are then washed three times in RPMI 1640 and recounted.

4   For determination of spontaneous PFC, the cells are resuspended at 10^7 per ml and used as outlined above for PFC assay.

5   For determination of spontaneous supernatant Ig production, the cells are resuspended at 5×10^5 per ml in 1 ml cultures of RPMI 1640 containing 10% FCS in triplicate and allowed to incubate for 10 days. Supernatants are harvested and assayed by ELISA. Cultures may be performed in 5 ml test-tubes or 24-well Costar plates. Cultures are performed in 37°C incubators in 5% CO_2.

Method for measurement of PWM-induced Ig production [6,21,27]

1   Place 5×10^5 cells (0.5 ml), 0.10 ml FCS, 0.05 ml of a 1:10 dilution of PWM, and 0.800 ml of RPMI 1640 into either triplicate 5 ml test-tubes or the wells of a 24-well Costar plate.

2   Cultures for PFC assay are incubated 5 or 6 days in a 5% CO_2, 37 °C incubator, then washed and resuspended at 2×10^6 and 2×10^5 cells per ml. Cell suspensions thus obtained are used as outlined above for the PFC assay.

3   Cultures for supernatant Ig production are incu-

bated for 10 days and supernatants harvested and assayed by ELISA.

Measurement of antigen-induced Ig production

Many systems currently exist for the *in vitro* measurement of antigen-induced, antigen-specific antibody production [6,25,28–32]. Currently, there is no uniform agreement on which are the most appropriate for the study of human antigen-specific B cell responses *in vitro*. These systems vary considerably, with some independent [28,29,32] and some dependent [6,25,30,31] upon prior *in vivo* immunization of the subject. All of these systems are similar, however, in that culture vessel geometry, cell density in culture, and kinetics of the response are critical variables that must be clearly understood in order to generate reproducible results. Optimal conditions for antigen-induced, antigen-specific antibody production may vary considerably from those which give optimal results in a PWM-driven system (Fig. 66.6). The references noted above provide the experimental details of these various systems.

Notes

SPA-PFC: the preparation of coating of SPA to SRBC must always be done in 0.85% NaCl. PBS cannot be used as an alternative for diluting or washing cells.

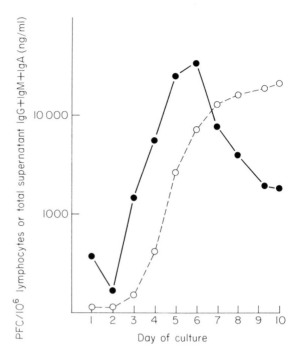

Fig. 66.7. Differential kinetics of plaque-forming cell response and supernatant immunoglobulin production.

ELISA: the coating antibodies must be tested to obtain maximal binding. Each lot will vary between 1 μg and 15 μg/ml. The optimum concentration for each lot of reagents needs to be tested for specificity as well. PWM-induced PFC responses peak at day 5–6, while 10 days of culture are required for maximal supernatant Ig production (Fig. 66.7).

Methods for *in vitro* evaluation of T cell effector function

In addition to measurements of lymphocyte blast transformation and DNA synthesis, final T cell effector function can be assessed *in vitro* as well. This includes the ability to mount a cytotoxic T cell response, the ability to help or suppress Ig production by B lymphocytes, and the ability to produce soluble mediators of the immune response such as interleukin-2 and B cell growth factor. As the *in vitro* assays of human immune function become more complex, however, the precise *in vivo* significance of the *in vitro* observations becomes more difficult to assess. It is of critical importance that measurements of this sort are always done in parallel with an age-matched control.

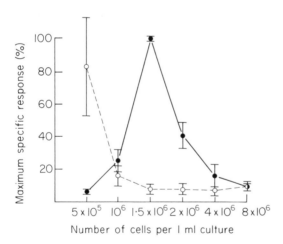

Fig. 66.6. Effect of cell concentration on antigen-induced (●) and pokeweed mitogen-induced (○) antigen-specific antibody production. The concentration of cells yielding peak antigen-induced, antigen-specific antibody production is several times higher than that required for peak mitogen-induced specific antibody production. Taken from ref. 6.

Equipment

Scintillation counter.

Materials

^{51}Cr, PHA, PWM.

2-Aminoethylisothiouronium (AET)-treated SRBC: 0.5 g AET (Sigma Chemical Co., St. Louis, MO) is dissolved in 12.5 ml distilled water adjusted to pH 9 with 4 M NaOH. Washed, packed SRBC (3 ml) are added to this solution and the resulting suspension is incubated at 37 °C for 15 min. The cells are then washed three times in cold PBS and finally brought up in RPMI 1640 to make a 2% suspension [33].

Procedures

Evaluation of cytotoxic T cell function [34,35]

Preparation of ^{51}Cr-labelled target cells (PHA-blasts) from the donor of stimulator cells

1   Peripheral blood mononuclear cells (20×10^6) are placed in 10 ml of RPMI 1640 containing 15% human serum and 20 μg of PHA and incubated in a 25 cm^2 tissue culture flask for 3 days.
2   At the end of 3 days, the cultures are harvested and the viable lymphocytes obtained by passage over a Hypaque-Ficoll gradient as outlined on page 66.2 and irradiated with 5000 rad.
3   Following washing, the lymphocytes are resuspended at 10^7 per ml in RPMI 1640 with 15% human serum.
4   Then 0.3 ml of washed cells and 500 μCi of buffered ^{51}Cr are added to a 5 ml test-tube.
5   The contents of the tube are incubated at 37 °C for 1 h in a shaking water bath.
6   The cells are then washed 3 times and resuspended at 1×10^5 cells per ml.

Performing the assay

1   Peripheral blood mononuclear cells (1×10^6) from the test subject (responder) are placed in 1 ml of RPMI 1640 with 15% human serum and 1×10^6 irradiated (5000 rad) peripheral blood mononuclear cells from an unrelated individual (stimulator) in at least 10 wells of a 24-well Costar plate.
2   The one-way mixed lymphocyte cultures thus established are incubated at 37 °C and 5% CO$_2$ for 7 days.
3   After 7 days, the cells are harvested from the culture and live cells obtained via purification over a Hypaque-Ficoll density gradient.

4   The cells are then resuspended at 8×10^6 per ml, 4×10^6 per ml, 2×10^6 per ml, 1×10^6 per ml, and 1×10^5 per ml.
5   The assay is then set up employing quadruplicate wells of a 96-V-shaped-well microtitre plate. To each well are added: 50 μl of ^{51}Cr PHA blasts, 50 μl of one of the concentrations of mixed lymphocyte culture-stimulated test cells, and 100 μl of RPMI 1640 containing 15% human serum.

To one set of quadruplicate wells (maximal release), 150 μl of distilled water is substituted for the test cells and RPMI 1640.

To another set of quadruplicate wells (spontaneous release), 50 μl of RPMI 1640 with 15% human serum is substituted for the test cells.

Centrifuge the plate at 100 **g** for 5 min. Incubate the plate at 37 °C, 5% CO$_2$ for 4 h. Centrifuge the plate at 200 **g** for 5 min. Aspirate 100 μl of supernatant from each well, place in 2 ml of scintillation fluid, and count in a gamma counter.

The percentage of specific lysis may be obtained from the following formula:

$$\text{Percentage specific lysis} = (E-S)/(M-S) \times 100$$
$$E = \text{experimental counts per minute}$$
$$S = \text{spontaneous counts per minute}$$
$$M = \text{maximum counts per minute}$$

One may then plot percentage specific lysis as a function of lymphocyte to target cell ratio. For the concentrations of lymphocytes chosen above, one would have set up lymphocyte to target cell ratios of 80:1, 40:1, 20:1, 10:1, and 1:1. By definition, the lymphocyte to target cell ratio required for 33% lysis is called 1 lytic unit (Fig. 66.8) [34].

Evaluation of T cell help or suppression of Ig production

Preparation of an indicator population of B cells + T cells + monocytes [36]

1   To two 50 ml conical tubes add 4×10^7 peripheral blood lymphocytes (4 ml) cells, 18 ml of a 2% suspension of washed AET-treated SRBC, 6 ml of a 5% human albumin RPMI 1640 solution, and 8 ml of RPMI.
2   Incubate the mixture for 15 min at 37 °C in a water bath.
3   Centrifuge into a pellet by spinning for 5 min at 800 **g** in a 4 °C centrifuge.
4   Incubate the tubes on ice for 45 min.
5   Gently resuspend the buttons by rocking the tubes. Layer 12 ml of Hypaque-Ficoll solution under the resuspended cells and centrifuge the tubes at 400 **g** for 35 min in a 10 °C centrifuge.

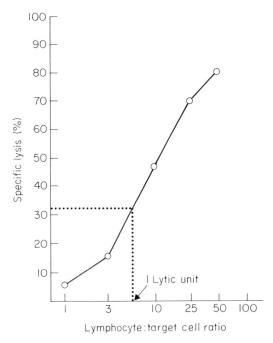

Fig. 66.8. Relationship between effector cell concentration and target cell lysis. The number of lymphocytes corresponding to an effector-target ratio yielding 33% lysis is arbitrarily defined as 1 lytic unit. Adapted from ref. 34.

6 Aspirate the interfaces and combine into one tube. These are the rosette-negative cells and will consist of B cells, monocytes, and a small number of T cells.
7 Aspirate the fluid remaining in the two 50 ml conical tubes and discard. The resulting buttons contain the rosette-positive cells and consist primarily of T cells. The red cells in the rosette-positive fractions can be lysed by the addition of 10 ml of the ammonium

chloride buffer. The ammonium chloride buffer should be pipetted up and down for approximately 2 min or until complete lysis is observed. The contents of the two tubes are then washed with RPMI 1640.
8 Both rosette-positive and rosette-negative cells are washed three times with RPMI 1640, counted, and resuspended at 10^7 cells per ml.
9 An erythrocyte (E) rosette determination as outlined on page 66.3 is then performed on the rosette-negative fraction to determine the number of T cells present. Since the PWM-induced production of Ig is a T cell-dependent event, at least 2% E rosette-positive cells must be in the indicator population to obtain a response. If less than 2% rosette-positive cells are present, an appropriate number of cells from the rosette-positive fraction are added to bring the percentage of rosette-positive cells to approximately 2%.

Assay for helper or suppressor cell function [9,37]

1 Triplicate cultures are set up in a volume of 1 ml containing 250 000 indicator population cells, a 1:200 final dilution of PWM, 10% FCS, and graded numbers of the cell population to be tested. One standard procedure is to add serial dilutions of the test cells from 160 000 to 20 000. Cultures may be performed in either 5 ml test-tubes or 24-well Costar plates.
2 The cultures are allowed to incubate for 5 or 10 days depending upon whether the assay for B cell function is to be a PFC assay or a measurement of supernatant Ig production.
3 Assays are performed at the end of culture as outlined on pages 66.6 and 66.7.
4 The helper or suppressor capabilities of the test population is measured by the degree to which B cell function in the suboptimal indicator population is enhanced or suppressed (Fig. 66.9).

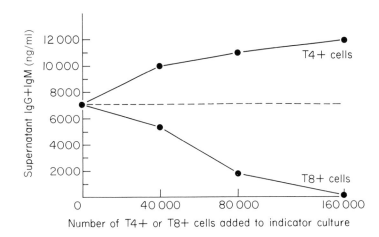

Fig. 66.9. Help or suppression in a pokeweed mitogen-driven system of immunoglobulin production. The addition of T4+ cells results in increased immunoglobulin production; the addition of T8+ cells results in decreased Ig production.

Evaluation of soluble mediator production

Generation of mediator-containing supernatants
1 Replicate cultures containing 2×10^6 peripheral blood mononuclear cells and 10 μg of PHA are established in 24-well Costar plates containing 1 ml of RPMI 1640 with 10% FCS and incubated at 37 °C in a 5% CO_2 atmosphere for 48 h.
2 Supernatants are then harvested and stored in 0.5 ml aliquots until ready for assay.

Assays for mediator production

Many different lymphokines have been described, along with the assays for their presence in culture supernatants [38–42]. The majority of these assays are described in detail elsewhere in the handbook (chapters 59, 77, 78, 80).

Media

RPMI 1640 with glutamine (M.A. Bioproducts, Walkersville, MD) with 10 μg/ml gentamicin (GIBCO Laboratories, Grand Island, NY).
Phosphate-buffered saline (PBS, M.A. Bioproducts, Walkersville, MD).
Fetal calf serum (FCS, Dutchland Laboratories, Denver, PA). Heat-inactivate at 57 °C for 30 min.
Hanks' Balanced Salt Solution (HBSS, Biofluids, Rockville, MD).
Acid citrate: 2.92 g citric acid, 9.16 g sodium citrate, 400 ml distilled water.
Fluorescein-activated cell sorter (FACS) buffer: 1 g bovine serum albumin, 0.1 g sodium azide, 1000 ml PBS.
Substrate buffer for enzyme-linked immunosorbent assay (ELISA): 1.3 g $NaHCO_3$, 1.27 g $NaCO_3$, 0.95 g $MgCl_2$, 1000 ml distilled water.
Coating buffer for ELISA: 1.59 g Na_2CO_3, 2.93 g $NaHCO_3$, 0.2 g NaN_3, 1000 ml distilled water.
Human A serum (Dutchland Laboratories).
Ammonium chloride lysing buffer: 8.29 g NH_4Cl, 1.00 g $KHCO_3$, 0.0372 g EDTA disodium salt, 1000 ml distilled water.

Acknowledgements

The authors wish to acknowledge the work of Dr David J. Volkman in developing the ELISA assay used in their laboratory and the expert editorial assistance of Ms Ann C. London.

References

1 STILES D.P. (1980) Clinical laboratory methods of detecting cellular immune function. In *Basic and Clinical Immunology*, 3rd edn., (eds. FUDENBERG H.H., SITES D.P., CALDWELL J.L. & WELLS F.J.), p. 382. Lange Medical Publications, California.
2 ROSE N.R. & FRIEDMAN H. (1980) *Manual of Clinical Immunology*, 2nd edn. American Society for Microbiology, Washington D.C.
3 REINHERZ E.L., O'BRIEN C., ROSENTHAL P. & SCHLOSSMAN S.F. (1980) The cellular basis for viral-induced immunodeficiency: analysis by monoclonal antibodies. *J. Immunol.* **125**, 1269.
4 RAMEY W.P., RUBIN R.H., HOFFMAN R.A., HANSEN W.P., HEALEY K. & HIRSH M.J. (1981) Analysis of T lymphocyte subsets in cytomegalovirus mononucleosis. *J. Immunol.* **126**, 2116.
5 MISHELL R.I. & DUTTON R.W. (1967) Immunization of dissociated spleen cell cultures from normal mice. *J. exp. Med.* **126**, 423.
6 LANE H.C., VOLKMAN D.J., WHALEN G. & FAUCI, A.S. (1981) *In vitro* antigen-induced, antigen-specific antibody production in man. *J. exp. Med.* **154**, 1043.
7 BOYUM A. (1968) Isolation of mononuclear cells and granulocytes from human blood. *Scand. J. clin. Lab. Invest.* **21**, 77.
8 OSMOND P.G. (1967) The separation of lymphocytes from bone marrow by centrifugation in a density gradient. *Anat. Rec.* **157**, 295.
9 REINHERZ E.L., KUNG P.C., GOLDSTEIN G. & SCHLOSSMAN S.F. (1979) Separation of functional subsets of human T cells by a monoclonal antibody. *Proc. natn. Acad. Sci. U.S.A.* **76**, 4061.
10 HAYNES B.F. (1981) Human T cell antigens as defined by monoclonal antibodies. *Immunol. Revs.* **57**, 1.
11 LAY W.H., MENDES N.F., BIANCO C. & NUSSENZWEIG V. (1971) Binding of sheep red blood cells to a large population of human lymphocytes. *Nature*, **230**, 531.
12 WINCHESTER R.J. & FU S.M. (1976) Lymphocyte surface membrane immunoglobulin. *Scand. J. Immunol.* **5**, 77.
13 GILOH H. & SEDAT J.W. (1982) Fluorescence microscopy. Reduced photobleaching of rhodamine and fluorescein protein conjugates by *n*-propyl gallate. *Science*, **217**, 1252.
14 PAUL W.E. (1984) *Fundamental Immunology*, 1st edn. Raven Press, New York.
15 PENHALE W.J., FARMER A., MACCUISH A.C. & IRVINE W.J. (1974) A rapid micromethod for the phytohemagglutinin-induced lymphocyte transformation test. *Clin. exp. Immunol.* **18**, 155.
16 OPPENHEIM J.J. & SCHECTOR B. (1980) Lymphocyte transformation. In *Manual of Clinical Immunology*, 2nd edn., (eds. ROSE N.R. & FRIEDMAN H.), p. 233. American Society for Microbiology, Washington D.C.
17 LING N.R. & KAY J.E. (1974) Lymphocyte Stimulation, 2nd edn. American Elsevier Publishing Company, New York.
18 FORSGREN A., SVEDLJELUND A. & WIGZELL H. (1976) Lymphocyte stimulation by protein A of *Staphylococcus aureus*. *Eur. J. Immunol.* **6**, 207.
19 FALKOFF R.J.M., ZHU L.P. & FAUCI A.S. (1982) Separate

signals for human B cell proliferation and differentiation in response to *Staphylococcus aureus*: evidence for a two-signal model of B cell activation. *J. Immunol.* **129**, 97.

20 GRONOWICZ E.A., COUTINHO A. & MELCHERS F. (1976) A plaque assay for all cells secreting immunoglobulin of a given type of class. *Eur. J. Immunol.* **6**, 558.

21 FAUCI A.S., WHALEN G. & BURCH C. (1980) Activation of human B lymphocytes. (XVI) Cellular requirements, interactions, and immunoregulation of pokeweed mitogen-induced total immunoglobulin producing plaque-forming cells in peripheral blood. *Cell Immunol.* **54**, 230.

22 ENGVALL E., JONSSON K. & PERLMAN P. (1971) Enzyme-linked immunosorbent assay. (II) Quantitative assay of protein antigen, immunoglobulin G, by means of enzyme-labelled antigen and antibody-coated tubes. *Biochem. biophys. Acta*, **251**, 427.

23 ENGVALL E. & PERLMAN P. (1972) Enzyme-linked immunosorbent assay, ELISA. (III) Quantitation of specific antibodies by enzyme-labelled anti-immunoglobulin in antigen-coated tubes. *J. Immunol.* **109**, 129.

24 KELLY B.S., LEVY J.G. & SIKOVA L. (1979) The use of the enzyme-linked immunosorbent assay (ELISA) for the detection and quantification of specific antibody from cell cultures. *Immunology*, **37**, 45.

25 VOLKMAN D.J., LANE H.C. & FAUCI A.S. (1981) Antigen-induced *in vitro* antibody production by humans: a model for B cell activation and immunoregulation. *Proc. natn. Acad. Sci. U.S.A.* **78**, 2528.

26 FAUCI A.S., WHALEN G. & BURCH C. (1980) Activation of human B lymphocytes. (XV) Spontaneously occurring and mitogen-induced indirect anti-sheep red blood cell plaque-forming cells in normal human peripheral blood. *J. Immunol.* **124**, 2410.

27 KEIGHTLY R.G., COOPER M.D. & LAWTON A.R. (1976) The T cell dependence of B cell differentiation induced by pokeweed mitogen. *J. Immunol.* **117**, 1538.

28 DOSCH H.M. & GELFAND E.W. (1977) Generation of human plaque-forming cells in culture: tissue distribution, antigenic and cellular requirements. *J. Immunol.* **118**, 302.

29 HEIJNEN C.J., UYTDE HAAG F., GMELIG-MEYLING F. & BALLIEUX R.E. (1979) Localization of antigen-specific helper and suppressor function in distinct T cell subpopulations. *Cell. Immunol.* **43**, 282.

30 CALLARD R.E. (1979) Specific *in vitro* antibody responses to influenza virus by human blood lymphocytes. *Nature*, **282**, 734.

31 YARCHOAN R., MURPHY B.R., STROBER W., SCHNEIDER H.S. & NELSON D.L. (1981) Specific anti-influenza virus antibody production *in vitro* by human peripheral blood mononuclear cells. *J. Immunol.* **127**, 2588.

32 MISITI J. & WALDMANN T.A. (1981) *In vitro* generation of antigen-specific hemolytic plaque-forming cells from human peripheral blood mononuclear cells. *J. exp. Med.* **154**, 1069.

33 PELLEGRINO M.A., FERRONE S., DIERICH M.P. & REISFIELD R.A. (1975) Enhancement of sheep red blood cell human lymphocyte rosette formation by the sulfhydryl compound 2-aminoethylisothiouronium bromide. *Clin. Immunol. Immunopath.* **3**, 324.

34 CERROTINI J.C. & BRUNNER K.T. (1974) Cell mediated cytotoxicity, allograft rejection, and tumor immunity. *Adv. Immunol.* **18**, 67.

35 MORETTA A., MINGARI M.C., HAYNES B.F., SEKALY R.P., MORETTA L. & FAUCI, A.S. (1981) Phenotypic characterization of human cytolytic T lymphocytes in mixed lymphocyte culture. *J. exp. Med.* **153**, 213.

36 FALKOFF R.M., PETERS M. & FAUCI A.S. (1982) T cell enrichment and depletion of human peripheral blood mononuclear cell preparations. Unexpected findings in the study of the functional activities of the separated populations. *J. immunol. Meth.* **50**, 39.

37 THOMAS Y., SOSMAN J., IRIGOYEN O., FRIEDMAN S.M., KUNG P.C., GOLDSTEIN G. & CHESS L. (1980) Functional analysis of human T cell subsets defined by monoclonal antibodies. (I) Collaborative T-T interactions in the immunoregulation of B cell differentiation. *J. Immunol.* **125**, 2402.

38 GILLIS S., FERM M.M., OU W. & SMITH K.A. (1978) T cell growth factor: parameters of production and a quantitative microassay for activity. *J. Immunol.* **120**, 2027.

39 LACHMAN L.B., HACKER M.P. & HANDSHUMACHER R.E. (1977) Partial purification of human lymphocyte-activating factor (LAF) by ultrafiltration and electrophoretic techniques. *J. Immunol.* **119**, 2019.

40 MURAGUCHI A., KISHIMOTO T., MIKI Y., KURITANI T., KAIEDA T., YOSHIYAKI K. & YAMAMURA Y. (1981) T cell-replacing factor (TRF)-induced IgG secretion in a human B blastoid cell line and demonstration of acceptors for TRF. *J. Immunol.* **127**, 412.

41 MURAGUCHI A. & FAUCI A.S. (1982) Proliferative responses of normal human B lymphocytes. Development of an assay system for human B cell growth factor (BCGF). *J. Immunol.* **129**, 1104.

42 SCHWARTING R., LANE C., RINNOOY KAN E.A., CHIORAZZI N. & WANG C.Y. (1984) Human B-cell stimulatory-factor production in both T4$^+$ and T8$^+$ lymphocytes. *Cell. Immunol.* **88**, 41.

Chapter 67
Assay for *in vivo* adoptive immune response

G. M. IVERSON

Method for the preparation of immunogens, 67.2

Method for the primary immunization of donor mice, 67.3
Method of cell transfer, 67.5

Methods for assaying the immune response in the adoptive hosts, 67.6
Media, 67.8

Immunity against both hapten and carrier protein is required to elicit a maximum secondary anti-hapten response (carrier effect) [1]. An animal that has been immunized with hapten–protein A will not respond with a maximum secondary anti-hapten response when boosted with hapten–protein B. Yet the anti-hapten antibody produced by immunization and boosting with the same hapten–protein conjugate (homologous carrier) will bind almost equally well to both conjugates. Therefore the secondary anti-hapten response is dependent, to a large degree, upon carrier specificity. It is assumed that antigen must act through specific immunoglobulin-like receptors on the surface of lymphocytes. Carrier specificity must, therefore, reside with these specific immunoglobulin-like receptors. Yet specific anti-hapten immunoglobulins secreted by the lymphocytes do not recognize this carrier specificity. Either (1) the immunoglobulin-like receptors on the surface of lymphocytes are different, with regard to their specificity, from the immunoglobulin they secrete, or (2) than one cell type is involved in the secondary anti-hapten humoral immune response [2,3].

An important technique that has been used in the experimental approach to the above problems is the adoptive transfer, via lymphoid cells, of the secondary humoral immune response [4]. Spleens were harvested from primed mice, single cell suspensions made and then injected into X-irradiated syngeneic recipients. When these recipients were injected with the priming immunogen, a secondary humoral immune response was detected. This procedure has been slightly altered to study the carrier effect in the secondary anti-hapten humoral immune response [5]. Mice are immunized against a carrier protein, say protein A. Other syngeneic mice are immunized against a hapten on a different non-cross-reacting carrier, say hapten–protein B. Some time later, lymphoid organs are harvested separately from each group of mice, single cell suspensions made and injected into X-irradiated syngeneic

hosts. These recipients are then challenged with hapten–protein A. An appropriate time later, the mice are bled and the sera serologically tested for anti-hapten antibody (Fig. 67.1).

This biological assay system allows experimental manipulations to be applied to the two different lymphoid populations independently. For example, both populations of cells, from an experiment like the one described above, have been treated *in vitro*, prior to the cell transfer into X-irradiated syngeneic hosts, with different antisera (plus a source of complement) specific for surface antigens on the thymus-derived lymphocyte (anti-θ) or the bone-marrow-derived lymphocyte antigen (anti-MBLA). The results clearly indicated that the carrier-primed cells were sensitive to treatment with anti-θ whereas the hapten-primed cells were not [6]. On the other hand, it has been shown that the hapten-primed cells are sensitive to anti-MBLA and not to the carrier-primed cells [7,8].

In this way the carrier effect in mice has been shown to be the result of an act of antigen-mediated cellular co-operation between at least two types of lymphocytes. One is derived from the thymus and the other from the bone marrow. The thymus-derived or T lymphocytes require an intact thymus for maturation [9,10] and are found in varying proportions in the peripheral lymphoid tissue (see Table 67.1 for organ distribution) [7,11]. The thymus-derived lymphocyte does not secrete any detectable antibody [12] but is involved in both the humoral and cell-mediated immune responses [9]. It is a helper cell. The bone-marrow-derived or B lymphocyte develops independently of the thymus. The B lymphocyte is the antibody-forming cell precursor (AFCP) [13]. The thymus-derived lymphocyte binds antigen by means of a carrier determinant and presents the hapten determinant to a bone-marrow-derived lymphocyte, AFCP, which is then somehow triggered to produce antibody.

This implies that for a molecule to be immunogenic it must possess at least two antigenic determinants

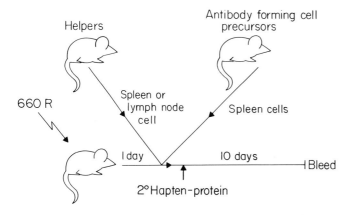

Fig. 67.1. Diagram of the cell transfer system.

Table 67.1. Tissue distribution of thymus-derived and bone-marrow-derived lymphocytes in the mouse

Tissue	Thymus-derived (%)	Bone-marrow-derived (%)
Thymus	100	0
Thoracic duct lymphocytes	80–90	10–20
Lymph node	60–85	25–35
Spleen	25–45	50–60
Bone marrow	0	20

The above values are estimates derived from data published by Raff [26] and Niederhuber & Moller [7], using anti-θ and anti-MBLA antisera.

[14]. One determinant acts as the carrier and the other determinant then acts as the 'hapten equivalent'.

The advantages of this type of assay are obvious. The combination of interactions of sets and subsets of lymphocytes are almost limitless. The advantages of this type of assay over *in vitro* assays are numerous: (1) one need not have all of the equipment required for sterile tissue culture; (2) it obviates the need for having different batches of 'screened' fetal calf serum for each kind of assay; (3) probably most important is the reliability of the assay system—it works every time!

The limitations of this type of assay are not always so obvious. One can only study the interactions of populations of cells. It does not lend itself to studies at the single cell level. Also, one must remember that the observed interactions are influenced by the immunological history of both the donor and the recipient.

Method for the preparation of immunogens

Equipment

Magnetic stirrer.
pH meter.
Spectrophotometer.

Materials

Proteins

CGG: chicken γ-globulin, prepared from fresh chicken serum by fractionation with 45% saturated ammonium sulphate.
BSA: bovine serum albumin, Cohn fraction V.
HSA: human serum albumin.
OA: egg albumin.
MGG: mouse γ-globulin.
KLH: keyhole limpet haemocyanin.

Haptens

DNP: 2,4-dinitrophenyl.
NIP: 4-hydroxy-3-nitrophenacetyl, prepared according to the method of Brownstone *et al.* [15].
OX: 4-ethoxymethylene-2-phenyloxazolone.

Heterologous red blood cells

RBC: red blood cells obtained from whole blood that contains Alsever's solution as an anticoagulant.

All of the above reagents are available commercially. A good source of the various suppliers, including addresses, is *Linscott's Directory of Immunological and Biological Reagents*, (from 40 Glen Drive, Mill Valley, CA 94941, U.S.A.).

Table 67.2. Physico-chemical data of haptens used in the adoptive transfer of the secondary humoral immune response

Hapten	λ_{max}	$E^{M, 1\ cm}$	Correction factor (%)	Molar coupling efficiency (%)	Solvents used
NIP	430	4.95×10^3	67.5	60	DMSO, ethoxy-ethanol
DNP	360	1.74×10^4	38.5	50	Dioxane, acetone
OX	360	2.63×10^4	25.0	60	Ethanol, ethoxy-ethanol

Procedures

Conjugation of haptens to proteins

1 Dissolve protein in 0.5 M-NaHCO₃.
2 An appropriate amount of NIP-azide, prepared according to the method of Brownstone *et al.* [15], 1-fluoro-2-4-dinitrobenzene (FDNB), or 4-ethoxy-methylene-2-phenyloxazolone (Ox), is added to the protein and stirred for 2–3 h at room temperature. The amount of hapten to add is calculated using the molar percentage coupling efficiencies for the different haptens given in Table 67.2. The volume of hapten added should never exceed 5% of the volume of protein.
3 The mixture is then exhaustively dialysed for 48 h with at least two changes of buffer. The pH of the buffer should be below 8.0. Phosphate-buffered saline is ideal.

Determination of hapten:protein ratios

1 The average molar coupling ratio is calculated by dividing the molar concentration of hapten by the molar concentration of the protein. All of the haptens listed here do absorb monochromatic light at 280 nm. Therefore the OD_{280} reading, after coupling, will be increased according to the degree of coupling and the hapten used. The protein concentration is estimated by lowering the observed OD_{280} reading by the appropriate correction factor given in Table 67.2. For example, one wants to couple four DNP groups per molecule of mouse γ-globulin; they have 111 mg of protein; from Table 67.3 the relative molecular mass of MGG is assumed to be 150 000.

$$111/1.5 \times 10^8 = 74 \times 10^{-8} \text{ mol protein} \quad (1)$$

From Table 67.2 assume 50% coupling efficiency for FDNB. Therefore add

$$8 \times 74 \times 10^{-8} = 592 \times 10^{-8} \text{ mol FDNB} \quad (2)$$

After dialysis the volume is 8.5 ml. The observed $OD_{280} = 20$ and the $OD_{360} = 4.7$.

$$38.5\% \text{ of } 4.7 = 1.8 \quad (3)$$
$$20 - 1.8 = 18.2 \quad (4)$$

$$\frac{18.2/1.4}{1.5 \times 10^8} \times 8.5 = 7.4 \times 10^{-7} \text{ mol MGG} \quad (5)$$

in the 8.5 ml.

$$\frac{4.7}{1.74 \times 10^4} \times 8.5 \times 10^{-3} = 22.9 \times 10^{-7} \text{ mol DNP} \quad (6)$$

in the 8.5 ml.

$$\frac{22.9 \times 10^{-7}}{7.4 \times 10^{-7}} = 3.1 \quad (7)$$

Therefore there are, on the average, 3.1 DNP groups per molecule of MGG, i.e. DNP₃.₁MGG.

Method for the primary immunization of donor mice

When protein antigens are used, the donors of helper cells and AFCPs are primed by an intraperitoneal injection of alum-precipitated protein (or hapten–protein conjugate), along with *B. pertussis* as an adjuvant. Alum precipitation is after the method of Proom [16].

Helper cell activity develops earlier than AFCP activity in response to immunization. Helper cell activity is optimal as early as 7 days post-immunization, whereas AFCP activity is optimal at about 21 days [17]. Both helper cell activity and AFCP activity remain in the primed animal for at least 5 months. Therefore, in the adoptive transfer system, the donors of helper cells need to be primed as little as 1 week or as long as 5 months before the cell transfer. The donors of the AFCPs need to be primed at least 3 weeks or as long as 5 months prior to the cell transfer.

It has also been shown that haptens can act as the carrier determinant [18,19]. One can engender a population of helper cells specific for the hapten by direct immunization with hapten–protein conjugates, as explained in the previous section. An alternative method is by skin painting the mice with the appropriate form of the hapten [18,19].

The helper cell activity of 20×10^6 lymph node cells

Table 67.3. Physico-chemical value for various proteins used in the adoptive secondary humoral immune responses

Protein	λ_{max}	$E^{1mg/ml\ 1cm}$ λ_{max}	Mol. wt.	Optimal amount of alum-precipitated protein for primary (μg)	Optimal amount of protein for secondary (μg) Homologous*	Heterologous†
BSA	280	0.68	69 000	800	100	800
OA	280	0.735	45 000	800	0.25	1500
CGG	280	1.4	150 000	10	0.1	30
BGG	280	1.4	150 000	100	0.1	ND
MGG	280	1.4	150 000	100	1.0	ND
KLH	280	1.12	100 000	10	1.0	ND

* The same protein as used in the initial hapten–protein priming primary.
† A protein non-cross-reacting with the primary protein. These values represent the amount of carrier protein required to override the carrier effect and give an anti-hapten response equal to that achieved when the values of column '*' are used.

from mice skin painted once is as effective a helper population as 40×10^6 spleen cells from either the same skin painted animal or conventionally immunized mice in the adoptive secondary immune response to DNP-protein. The helper-cell activity of 20×10^6 lymph node cells from mice skin painted five times (at weekly intervals) is significantly better than 40×10^6 spleen cells from mice immunized conventionally [20]. Even so, as can be seen from Table 67.4, it is more economical to use spleen cells. For every donor, three recipients can be used if spleen cells are transferred whereas only one recipient per donor is available if lymph node cells are transferred.

Table 67.4. Approximate cell yields from adult, primed, CBA mice

Organ	No. of cells ($\times 10^6$) per organ
Thymus*	200
Thoracic duct (24 h drainage)	50–100
Spleen	120
Bone marrow	20
Lymph nodes Superficial cervicals Axillary Brachial Inguinal	20

* The value given is for young (4-week-old), normal CBA mice.

The hapten carrier system generally requires priming for AFCP specific for a protein determinant. This is done as described earlier (for helper cells) but is complicated by the fact that helper cells specific for the protein are also generated. Spleens of such mice can be effectively depleted of helper cells by *in vivo* treatment with heterologous anti-thymocyte serum (ATS) prior to harvesting the spleens [21]. See Levey & Medawar [22] for the production of ALS(ATS). Mice donating the spleens for AFCP are given 0.25 ml of ATS on days -6, -4, -2, and the spleens are harvested on day 0. Alternatively, helper cells can be eliminated by an *in vitro* treatment of the spleen cells with anti-thy-1 plus complement.

The same general principles are applied when heterologous red cells are used as the immunogen. Heterologous red cells have at least two antigenic determinants. One determinant acts as the carrier and the other determinant then acts as the 'hapten equivalent'. For a maximum, secondary, anti-heterologous red cell immune response there must be both primed helper cells for the carrier determinant and primed AFCPs for the 'hapten equivalent' determinant(s) on the red cells. A major difference is that priming for helper cells and AFCPs is not only temporally distinct but is accomplished with different antigen doses [23]. Priming for helper cells is derived with low doses of antigen and early harvesting. Priming for AFCPs results from immunization with high doses of antigen and late harvesting. Fig. 67.2 gives the number of plaque-forming cells (per 10^6 recipient spleen cells) obtained in adoptive hosts receiving $5–10 \times 10^6$ spleen cells from donor mice primed with varying doses of

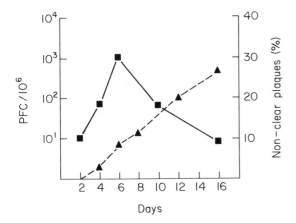

Fig. 67.2. Helper cell and AFPC activity of SRBC primed spleen cell populations as a function of antigen dose and days between priming and harvesting for cell transfer. The irradiated syngeneic hosts received 5×10^6 primed spleen cells, were boosted with 2×10^8 SRBC and the spleens harvested for plaquing 7 days later. ■, mice primed with a low dose of antigen, 2×10^5 SRBC, and plaqued with SRBC. This represents the helper cell activity. ▲, mice primed with a high dose of antigen, 2×10^9 SRBC and plaqued with a cross-reacting red blood cell. This represents the AFCP activity.

sheep red blood cells and transferred to irradiated syngeneic hosts at various times after priming. The hosts were boosted with 2×10^8 SRBC and the spleens harvested for plaquing 7 days later.

Another problem that arises is that both helper cells and AFCPs are engendered against the same antigenic determinants. A unique way of measuring the helper cell or AFCP activity of such a cell population is to use slightly cross-reacting red cells as the different antigens used in priming and challenging. The antibody-forming cells are then plaqued against a mixture of both kinds of red cells. Clear plaques indicate that cells are producing antibody detecting antigens on both red cells, thus detecting helper activity. Non-clear plaques indicate that the antibody is detecting antigens on only one kind of red cell, thus detecting the AFCP activity of the transferred spleen population [23].

Materials

9% (w/v) Potassium aluminum sulphate (alum).
5 M NaOH.
Saline.
pH paper.
Table-top centrifuge.
B. pertussis vaccine. The best source of *B. pertussis* vaccine as an adjuvant is: Dept. of Public Health,

Division of Biologic Laboratories, Commonwealth of Massachusetts, Boston, Mass., U.S.A.

Procedures

Protein and/or hapten–protein conjugates

1 Alum precipitation: equal volumes of 2% (2 g/ml) protein, or conjugate, and 9% alum are mixed. The pH is adjusted to 6.5 by adding 5 M NaOH dropwise. The precipitate is centrifuged at 600 **g** for 5 min and washed twice with saline. 100% recovery of protein, or conjugate, in the precipitate is assumed.
2 Donor mice are primed by an i.p. injection of 0.2 ml suspension of alum-precipitated protein plus adjuvant. Each donor receives 2×10^9 *B. pertussis* organisms as an adjuvant. The volume of the alum precipitate is adjusted such that after adding the concentrated *B. pertussis* there will be the correct amount of protein and adjuvant in 0.2 ml. Table 67.3 is a list of the amounts of various proteins, or conjugates, needed for optimal priming.

Hapten as the carrier determinant

1 One can engender a population of helper cells specific for hapten by direct immunization with hapten–protein conjugates as described above.
2 An alternative method is by painting the mice with the appropriate form of the hapten. Table 67.2 is a list of haptens used in sensitizing mice by skin painting. The hapten sensitizing agent is applied to the clipped abdomen of each mouse. Seven to ten days later, both the spleen and lymph nodes can be used as a source of hapten-sensitive helper cells.

Heterologous red cells as the immunogen

Mice are primed with heterologous red cells by a single, intraperitoneal, injection of the appropriate dose of red blood cells. The appropriate dose, depending on whether one wants to engender helper cells or AFCPs is either 2×10^5 RBC per mouse or 2×10^9 RBC per mouse respectively. The best time to harvest the primed cells for adoptive transfer can be determined from Fig. 67.2.

Method of cell transfer

Equipment

Access to an X-ray machine or other suitable way to irradiate recipient mice.
Centrifuge.
Microscope for cell counting.

Materials

Salt solution for cell suspension.
Screen sieve or microscope slides with ground-glass ends.
Needle and syringe.

Procedures

Irradiation of the adoptive hosts

The adoptive syngeneic hosts are irradiated 4–24 h before the cell transfer. Table 67.5 lists the different dosages of irradiation that have been reported for different strains of mice. This list is by no means exhaustive. It is merely a list gathered from various sources of systems that are being used in various laboratories. Older mice tend to be healthier adoptive hosts after irradiation than do younger mice. A good source of older animals are the 'retired breeder' mice from the local source of animals.

Table 67.5. Doses of irradiation for adoptive hosts

Strain	Amount of whole body irradiation (rad)
CBA	600–800
(CBA × C57BL)F$_1$	600–800
Balb/c	600
C3H/snhz	600–800
C57BL/10	600
CWB/8	600–800

These values are intended only as a guide. They vary between laboratories probably depending upon the general state of health of the mice. The amount of irradiation used for mice from any given source should be determined empirically.

Cell suspensions

If the cell suspensions have to be kept for some time prior to transfer, such as when treatment of the cells *in vitro* is part of the experimental design, then it is suggested that balanced salt solution be used to make the cell suspensions. Gey's solution, being bicarbonate buffered, tends to change pH (becoming alkaline) more rapidly than the phosphate-buffered BSS (see page 67.8).
1 Single cell suspensions are obtained by gently pressing the tissue (spleen, lymph nodes or thymus) in a few drops of salt solution through a screen sieve. The screen sieve can be as simple or elaborate as you choose. Some workers use elaborate stainless-steel screen sieves with 10 wires per cm soldered to sturdy steel holders. A simple and inexpensive sieve is a plastic tea-strainer obtained at most household goods stores. Some workers prefer to grind the tissue between the ground-glass ends of two microscope slides. Both techniques have been used successfully.
2 Bone marrow cells are obtained from the femur and tibia. After cutting off the epiphyses, the marrow is extruded by forcing cold salt solution through with a small needle and syringe. Cell clumps are broken up by repeated gentle aspiration through a 15-gauge hypodermic needle. Care must be taken to avoid causing excess air bubbles in the cell suspension. The cell suspension is allowed to stand, at 4 °C, for 2–3 min, allowing large fragments to settle. The supernatant is carefully removed and centrifuged, in the cold, at 600 **g** for 5 min. The supernatant is aspirated off and enough fresh, cold salt solution is added to give the desired cell concentration. As a guide, the approximate cell yield per organ in adult primed CBA mice is given in Table 67.4.

Cell transfer

With two exceptions, cells are injected i.p. into the irradiated syngeneic hosts. Volumes of 0.5–1.0 ml are generally used. The two exceptions are: (1) thymocytes, in all cases, and (2) all cell suspensions when the secondary immune response will be assayed by plaquing the spleen cells. In both of these situations, the cells are injected intravenously into the tail vein. In the case of thymocytes, additional precautions are necessary: (1) lower cell concentrations should be used—10^7 thymocytes per ml is the upper limit; (2) the cells should be injected slowly, i.e. 0.7 ml in about 0.5–1 min; and (3) the recipient mice should be given 10 units of heparin i.p. 10–60 min prior to the cells. This will greatly reduce the mortality caused by small clumps of thymocytes in the cell suspension.

Methods for assaying the immune response in the adoptive hosts

A modification of the Farr assay is used to detect antibodies to haptens and albumins. Readings from the salt precipitations are converted to antigen binding capacity (ABC) as described in detail by Mitchison [5]. The ABC is linear to the percentage of radioactive antigen bound, up to 35% binding. For bindings greater than 35%, the log of ABC is proportional to the log of the percentage bound and is equal to $2 \times 1/10$ antilog(% binding/35 × log 3.5)/dilution. The ABC is not dependent on titre when the capacities are measured on a log scale. Thus all measurements are expressed as log ABC.

   A co-precipitation assay is used to measure the antibody titre to protein antigens that are precipitated with 50% saturated ammonium sulphate. The $\log_2$ of the dilution of antisera that binds 50% of the maximum precipitable radioactive antigen is calculated.

Anti-heterologous red cell immune responses are measured by the haemolytic plaque assay. The PFC per unit number of cells harvested is generally calculated.

Equipment

Centrifuge.
Gamma counter.

Materials

Radioiodinated antigens.
Saturated (at 4 °C) $(NH_4)_2SO_4$.
Borate buffer (see page 67.8).
Normal rabbit serum.

Procedures

Radiolabelled antigen preparations

Haptens

DNP: for serology, radio-iodine-labelled preparations of the haptens are used. 4-Hydroxyphenacetyl-ε-amino-lysine-ε-amino-2-4-dinitrophenyl (HOP-Lys-DNP), prepared by the method of Meyer-Delius *et al.* [24] is iodinated with ^{125}I, according to the chloramine-T method of Hunter & Greenwood [25]. The iodinated product, 4-hydroxy-3,5-diiodophenactyl-amino-lys-amino-2-4-dinitrophenyl ($D^{125}IP$-lys-DNP) is separated from non-bound ^{125}I by fractionation on a Sephadex G-25 column. The free ^{125}I is contained in the first peak of radioactivity and $D^{125}IP$-lys-DNP in the second. $D^{125}IP$-lys-DNP is stored in borate buffer, pH 8.4, at a concentration of about 3×10^{-7} M. NIP: 4-Hydroxy-3-nitrophenacetyl-ε-amino-n-caproic acid (NP-CAP, prepared according to the method of Brownstone *et al.* [15]) is also iodinated with ^{125}I by the method of Hunter & Greenwood [16], yielding 4-hydroxy-5-iodo-3-nitrophenacetyl-O-amino caproic acid ($N^{125}IP$-CAP). Unbound ^{125}I is separated from $N^{125}IP$-CAP by differential elution from an ion-exchange resin. The radioactive mixture is applied to a small column (2–3 mm in a tuberculin syringe) of Dowex, 1×8, 200–400 mesh Cl form, washed with distilled water and the $N^{125}IP$-CAP differentially eluted with 2 ml of 50% (v/v) glacial acetic acid. The pH of the acid eluate is quickly adjusted to 7.0 with 5 M NaOH. $N^{125}IP$-CAP is stored in borate buffer, pH 8.4, at a concentration of about 2×10^{-6} M.

Proteins

The proteins are iodinated with ^{125}I according to the

chloramine-T method of Hunter & Greenwood [25]. The iodinated proteins can be easily separated from the free ^{125}I by either fractionation on a Sephadex G-25 column or dialysis. The removal of free ^{125}I from the sample, by dialysis, is facilitated by adding 200 mg/l of KI to the dialysis buffer.

Serological assay for anti-hapten and anti-albumin antibodies

Each individual serum sample is tested at a dilution of 1/6 in borate buffer and at further dilutions of 1/36 and 1/180 in 10% normal rabbit serum diluted in borate buffer. To 0.25 ml of diluted serum in a 9×50 mm test-tube is added 0.25 ml of the radioactive hapten or protein antigen. The concentration of the radioactive antigen is 2×10^{-8} M. The tubes are mixed and left to stand for a few minutes; 0.5 ml of saturated ammonium sulphate is then added and quickly mixed. The tubes are centrifuged (3000 **g** for 30 min at 4 °C) and the supernatants decanted. The precipitates are then counted in a well-type gamma-scintillation counter, together with one set of controls containing either 0.25 ml of the radioactive hapten originally added or a TCA (trichloroacetic acid) precipitate in the case of protein antigens (high controls) and with another set containing the ammonium sulphate precipitate of the radioactive hapten or protein (low controls).

Serological assay for anti-γ-globulin antibodies

A co-precipitation assay is used to measure the antibody titre to protein antigens that are precipitated with 50% saturated ammonium sulphate. Ten millilitres of radioactive antigen, at a concentration of 6×10^{-8} M, is added to 50 μl of antiseru, diluted in 1 : 24 normal mouse serum, diluted in borate buffer. The antigen–antiserum mixture is incubated for 30 min at room temperature; then 50 μl of rabbit anti-mouse immunoglobulin serum is added to each tube, mixed and incubated for a further 30 min at 4 °C. It is clear that rabbit anti-mouse immunoglobulin serum must not precipitate the radioactive antigen. This is ensured by absorbing the serum with the antigen made insoluble by conjugation to Sepharose 2B (or some other suitable insoluble absorbent), the absorption being repeated until no precipitation of the radioactive antigen occurs. After incubation, 250 μl of borate buffer is added and the tubes are centrifuged at 2000 **g** for 30 min. The supernatant is removed and the radioactivity of the precipitate measured in a well-type gamma-scintillation counter.

Assay for the immune response to heterologous red cells

Anti-heterologous red cell immune responses are measured by the haemolytic plaque assay.

Media

Borate buffer

6.18 g Boric acid.
9.54 g Sodium tetraborate.
4.38 g Sodium chloride.
Make up to one litre with double-distilled water.
Adjust pH to 8.6 with concentrated NaOH.

Balanced salt solution (BSS)

Stock I

10.00 g Dextrose.
0.60 g KH_2PO_4.
1.89 g Na_2HPO_4 (or 3.58 g $Na_2HPO_4\cdot7H_2O$).
0.10 g Phenol red.
Make up to one litre with double-distilled water.

Stock II

1.86 g $CaCl_2$ (or 2.46 g $CaCl_2\cdot H_2O$).
4.00 g KCl.
80.00 g $MgCl_2\cdot6H_2O$.
2.00 g $MgSO_4\cdot7H_2O$.
Make up to one litre with double-distilled water.
Dilute 100 ml of stock I to about 800 ml with double-distilled water; then add 100 ml of stock II and bring the volume up to one litre.
A commercial source of the above balanced salt solution is available from Irvine Scientific, 2511 Daimler St., Santa Ana, CA 92705, as a powdered medium. Its called 'Cantor's Balanced Salts'. The catalogue number is 9617.

References

1 OVARY X. & BENACERRAF B. (1963) Immunological specificity of the secondary response with dinitrophenylated proteins. *Proc. Soc. exp. Biol. (NY)* **114**, 72.
2 MITCHISON N.A. (1967) Antigen recognition responsible for the induction *in vitro* of the secondary response. *Cold Spring Harb. Symp. quant. Biol.* **32**, 431.
3 RAJEWSKY K. & ROTTLANDER E. (1967) Tolerance specificity and the immune response to lactic dehydrogenase isoenzymes. *Cold Spring Harb. Symp. quant. Biol.* **32**, 547.
4 MITCHISON N.A. (1957) Adoptive transfer of immune reactions by cells. *J. cell. Comp. Physiol.* **50**, 247.
5 MITCHISON N.A. (1971) The carrier effect in the secondary response to hapten–protein conjugates. (I) Measurement of the effect and objections to the local environment hypothesis. *Eur. J. Immunol.* **1**, 10.
6 RAFF M.C. (1970) Role of thymus-derived lymphocytes in the secondary humoral immune response in mice. *Nature*, **226**, 1257.
7 NIEDERHUBER J.E. & MÖLLER E. (1972) Antigenic markers on mouse lymphoid cells: the presence of MBLA on antibody forming cells and antigen binding cells. *Cell. Immunol.* **3**, 559.
8 RAFF M.C., NASE S. & MITCHISON N.A. (1971) Mouse-specific bone marrow-derived lymphocyte antigen (MBLA): a marker for thymus independent lymphocytes. *Nature*, **230**, 50.
9 MILLER J.F.A.P. (1961) Immunological function of the thymus. *Lancet*, **ii**, 748.
10 RAFF M.C. & WORTIS H.H. (1970) Thymus dependence of 0-bearing cells in the peripheral lymphoid tissues of mice. *Immunology*, **18**, 931.
11 RAFF M.C. (1969) Theta isoantigen as a marker of thymus-derived lymphocytes in mice. *Nature*, **224**, 378.
12 HARRIS T.N., RHOADS J. & STOKES J.A. (1948) A study of the role of the thymus and spleen in the formation of antibodies in the rabbit. *J. Immunol.* **58**, 27.
13 MILLER J.F.A.P. & MITCHELL G.F. (1969) Thymus and antigen-reactive cells. *Transplant Rev.* **1**, 3.
14 RAJEWSKY K., SCHIRRMACHER V., NASE S. & JERNE N.K. (1969) The requirement of more than one antigenic determinant for immunogenicity. *J. exp. Med.* **129**, 1131.
15 BROWNSTONE A., MITCHISON N.A. & PITT-RIVERS R. (1966) Chemical and serological studies with a synthetic immunological determinant 4-hydroxy-3-iodo-5-nitrophenylacetic acid (NIP) and related compounds. *Immunology*, **10**, 465.
16 PROOM H. (1943) The preparation of precipitating sera for the identification of animal species. *J. Path. Bacteriol.* **55**, 419.
17 MITCHISON N.A. (1971) The carrier effect in the secondary response to hapten–protein conjugates. (II) Cellular cooperation. *Eur. J. Immunol.* **1**, 18.
18 IVERSON G.M. (1970) Ability of CBA mice to produce anti-idiotypic sera to 5563 myeloma protein. *Nature*, **227**, 273.
19 MITCHISON N.A. (1971) The carrier effect in the secondary response to hapten–protein conjugates. (V) Use of antilymphocyte serum to deplete animals of helper cells. *Eur. J. Immunol.* **1**, 68.
20 TAYLOR R.B. & IVERSON G.M. (1971) Hapten competition and the nature of cell-cooperation in the antibody response. *Proc. R. Soc.* Series B, **176**, 393.
21 MITCHISON N.A. (1970) Mechanism of action of antilymphocyte serum. *Fedn Proc.* **29**, 222.
22 LEVEY R.H. & MEDAWAR P.B. (1966) Nature and mode of action of anti-lymphocytic antiserum. *Proc. natn. Acad. Sci. U.S.A.* **56**, 1130.
23 CUNNINGHAM A.J. & SERCARZ E. (1971) The asynchronous development of immunological memory helper (T) and precursor (B) cell lines. *Eur. J. Immunol.* **1**, 413.
24 MEYER-DELIUS M., MITCHISON N.A., PITT-RIVERS R. & RUDE E. (1971) Synthesis of a radioiodine-labelled 2,4-dinitrophenyl-hapten and its use for binding assays. *Eur. J. Immunol.* **1**, 267.
25 HUNTER W.M. & GREENWOOD F.C. (1962) Preparation of iodine-131 labelled human growth hormone of high specific activity. *Nature*, **194**, 495.
26 RAFF M.C. (1971) Surface antigenic markers for distinguishing T and B lymphocytes in mice. *Transplant. Rev.* **6**, 52.

Chapter 68
Analysis of cytotoxic T cell responses

ELIZABETH SIMPSON & P. CHANDLER

Introduction, 68.1
Cell interactions in generating cytotoxic responses: role of MHC antigens, 68.1
Cytotoxic responses to non-MHC antigens, 68.2
T cell clones: generation and uses, 68.2
The biological role of Tc, 68.3

Methods, 68.3
In vitro mixed lymphocyte culture, 68.3
^{51}Cr release assay of cytotoxic T cells from a mixed lymphocyte culture, 68.5
In vivo generation of cytotoxic T cell responses and assay, 68.8

Separation of subpopulations involved in generating cytotoxic T cell responses, 68.9
Limiting dilution analysis of Tc and Th, 68.9
Cloning Tc, 68.12
Analysis of transfectants with cytotoxic T cells, 68.13
Appendix, 68.14

Introduction

Cell interactions in generating cytotoxic responses: role of MHC antigens

Cytotoxic T cells are perhaps the best defined sub-population of T lymphocytes, in terms of their activation pathway, cell surface phenotype and target cell specificity. Cytotoxic T cell effectors (Tc) are derived from precursors (pTc) that require for their differentiation not only antigen but also a second 'helper' signal, which is provided by helper T cells (Th) but can be substituted by soluble factors. These soluble factors are present in culture supernatants of T cells activated by lectins (concanavalin A, PHA). The necessary factors include interleukin 2 (IL-2) a well defined growth factor, but also less well defined differentiation factors [1–3].

The antigen against which the cytotoxic T cell is capable of responding has to be presented in an appropriate form and by appropriate antigen presenting cells. Cytotoxic T cells, like other T cells, have receptors which recognize not extrinsic antigen (X) alone, but X in association with self major histocompatibility complex (MHC) antigens (H-2 in mouse, HLA in man) [4–10]. Cytotoxic T cells with specificity against viruses and haptens are directed against the virus or hapten in association with class I MHC antigens (H-2K and D in mouse, HLA, HLB and HLC in man) [4,5,10]. Cytotoxic T cells can also be generated against allogeneic MHC antigens and minor histocompatibility (H) antigens. Cytotoxic responses to minor H antigens are MHC restricted in the same way as those directed against viruses and haptens [6,7,9]. When the specificity of individual T cell clones directed against viruses, haptens and minor H antigens

is examined, it is often found that despite the H-2 restriction with respect to recognition of the antigen X, certain non-self MHC target cells will also be killed, i.e. there is cross-reactivity between self plus X and allogeneic MHC (e.g. ref. 11 but see ref. 1 for review). It is possible that the high frequency of pTc found against allogeneic MHC determinants is a reflection of this cross-reactivity, and that the conformation of allogeneic MHC antigens mimics that of self MHC plus X antigens [12].

Whilst cytotoxic T cells are directed at class I MHC determinants (either allogeneic or self plus X), T helper cells are in general similarly directed against class II MHC determinants, H-2I in mouse, HL-D in man [8,13]. Tc and Th are also distinguished by their cell surface phenotypes. In mice, Tc are generally Ly1$^+$2$^+$ and Th are Ly1$^+$2$^-$ [14]. In man, Tc directed against class I MHC alloantigens are T3$^+$4$^-$8$^+$ whilst Th are T3$^+$4$^+$8$^-$ [15]. The biological role of these cell surface markers is not altogether understood but there is evidence for Ly2 in mouse and T3, T4 and T8 in man being involved in antigen recognition [15,16].

The observation that pTc responding to class I MHC determinants need interaction with Th responding to class II MHC antigens was originally established from two lines of evidence obtained from *in vitro* mixed lymphocyte cultures (MLC). The first line of evidence is genetic [13]. When spleen, lymph node or peripheral blood lymphocyte (PBL) cells from one individual (the responder cells) are placed in culture with irradiated lymphoid cells from another (the stimulator cells irradiated to prevent them actively participating in the response), whether a cytotoxic response is generated depends on genetic disparity between the two individuals. If there are both class I and class II MHC differences, the first response to be seen will be a proliferative one between days 2 to 4, and this is followed on days 5 or 6 by a cytotoxic response. The proliferative response is predominantly that of the Th specific for class II MHC alloantigens, whilst the cytotoxic response is that of Tc directed against class I MHC alloantigens. If class I differences only are present, a poor or negligible Tc response and a weak proliferative response will be obtained. If class II differences only are present, there will be little or no Tc developed but strong proliferation will be seen. If an MLC is constructed to include a responder cell type together with two different stimulator cell types, one differing at class I and the other at class II MHC antigens from the responder, then a synergistic effect is seen, and a Tc response towards the stimulating class I antigens is generated [13].

The second line of evidence that two interacting cell populations are involved in generating cytotoxic T cell responses comes from cell separation experiments in which cells of the pTc phenotype (in mouse Ly1$^+$2$^+$) were separated from those of the Th phenotype (in mouse Ly1$^+$2$^-$) and tested both separately and together for their ability to generate a cytotoxic response to cells which carried stimulatory class I and II MHC antigens. Neither population alone generated an effective response, whereas together synergy was observed, with the cytotoxic response from the mixed Tc and Th cells being comparable with that of the original unseparated spleen cell population [17,18].

Initially these observations on synergy between Th and Tc in MLC were made for responses to allogeneic MHC antigens, but it has subsequently been found that similar interactions are necessary for the generation of MHC restricted cytotoxic responses. In such cases Th respond to self class II MHC+X whilst Tc respond to self MHC class I+X [19,20].

Cytotoxic responses to non-MHC antigens

The cytotoxic T cell response to minor histocompatibility antigens is not seen in primary MLC. This probably reflects the low pTc frequency to such antigens [21]. This can be overcome if a responder animal is first immunized *in vivo* before the MLC is set up *in vitro*. The interval between *in vivo* priming and *in vitro* restimulation can be as short as 1 or 2 weeks, and the memory so generated lasts virtually the lifetime of the responder animal (certainly over 1 year in the mouse) [6,7]. The stimulator cells for both the *in vivo* immunization and the *in vitro* MLC must bear the minor histocompatibility antigen(s) against which the anti minor H Tc response is to be generated. MHC matching of responder and stimulator in MLC is essential, otherwise anti-allogeneic MHC responses

will dominate. However, the initial *in vivo* immunization can be done with MHC disparate cells, since antigen processing occurs *in vivo* such that the minor H antigens are re-presented to responder Tc and Th in association with responder type MHC determinants [22,23]. However, in certain circumstances re-presentation of this kind is not as efficient as direct presentation of minor H antigens on MHC matched cells for the initial immunization.

Anti-viral Tc responses can either be generated *in vivo* (6 days after immunizing with virus) or *in vitro* in secondary MLC, using virus infected irradiated syngeneic cells as stimulators [4,24]. Spleen, lymph node or PBL cells from unimmunized individuals make little or no primary *in vitro* MLC cytotoxic T cell response to most viruses, although some, such as Sendai virus, can elicit a primary *in vitro* response [25].

Anti-hapten responses can be generated in primary MLC, using as stimulator cells haptenated syngeneic spleen cells [5]. However, a quantitatively larger response is seen from T cells of animals which have been previously immunized *in vivo* with the hapten [26].

T cell clones: generation and uses

Since the discovery of T cell growth factors (TCGF) it has been possible to grow both cytotoxic T cells and helper cells *in vitro* independently for short or prolonged periods, and such T cell cultures can be cloned. This approach has allowed more accurate estimation of precursor frequencies of both Tc and Th, for the further analysis of the activation pathways and for an examination of target cell specificity [see 1] at the clonal level.

The initial pTc→Tc step requires antigen and a second signal normally produced by Th. This second signal can be bypassed by using medium containing TCGF. An important component of TCGF is the growth factor, IL-2, a product of Th, but TCGF also contains differentiation factors which are less well defined functionally and biochemically. These, together with IL-2, are necessary in order to obtain the initial pTc→Tc differentiation. The use of TCGF with limiting dilution of pTc allows the assessment of pTc frequencies. Once functional Tc are established they can be maintained, cloned and expanded in medium supplemented with purified IL-2. However, the most stable Tc lines and clones are those which are also periodically restimulated with cells carrying the specific antigen against which they are directed. Such clones are karyotypically and functionally much more stable than those which are grown in IL-2 containing medium in the absence of stimulating antigen [1]. The majority of Tc clones are IL-2 dependent: the growth and functions of a small minority are apparently independent of the addition of extrinsic IL-2—they may make their own [27].

The ability to make T cell clones provides homogeneous populations that can be studied with respect to growth and functional characteristics, antigen specificity, cell surface phenotype and receptor composition. An approach to the T cell receptor using cloned T cells has now provided answers to this difficult and tantalizing question [46,47,49,50].

Tc clones may also provide further information about another long vexed question, namely the manner in which target cell killing is achieved. It is known that lysis is dependent on close contact between target and attacker cell, energy (glucose), Mg^{2+} ions and Ca^{2+} ions, but is independent of DNA, RNA or protein synthesis [28]. A complement-type pathway to lysis appears unlikely but the exact mechanism remains obscure.

Cytotoxic T cells, both Tc clones and more heterogeneous populations from primary MLC, have also been used to probe the genetic organization of class I MHC antigens [29–31]. Class I MHC genes have been cloned from cosmid libraries of mouse and human genomic DNA [29,30]. Cosmids containing DNA sequences of interest have been inserted into mouse L cells (H-2 type $H-2^k$) that have been examined for expression of known class I gene products using antibodies and cytotoxic T cells. The detection of expression of the product of an inserted gene is an important part of identifying that gene. These studies have established in the mouse that there are relatively few genes coding the highly polymorphic class I antigens, H-2K, D and L but many coding the less polymorphic class I products of the Qa and Tla region, telomeric to H-2L. These studies also show that both antibody and cytotoxic T cells recognize epitopes (not necessarily the same) on the same molecule.

The biological role of Tc

The biological role of Tc cells *in vivo* lies mainly in defence against invading intracellular organisms such as viruses. Very strong Tc responses against viruses are generated *in vivo* and many of these can be demonstrated to be protective using cell transfer either from immunized mice, or with Tc or Tc clones generated *in vitro* [32,33]. The only tumours which unequivocally stimulate protective Tc responses are those caused by oncogenic viruses such as murine sarcoma virus (MSV). Such tumours regress spontaneously in immunocompetent hosts, and subsequently such animals show high levels of MHC-restricted, virus-specific cytotoxic cells [34].

It is unlikely that the cytotoxic T cell response to

either MHC antigens or minor histocompatibility antigens is the principal mediator of graft rejection. Delayed type hypersensitivity cells (Tdh), which have the same phenotype as Th cells, and are directed against allogeneic class II MHC antigens and self class II restricted minor H antigens, are more likely candidates than Tc cells for the primary role in graft rejection [12,35,37]. This is indicated from genetic studies using the male specific minor H antigen, H-Y, against which the graft rejection and cytotoxic T cell responses are under the control of separate H-2 Ir genes. Mouse strains that can reject H-Y incompatible grafts, although incapable of generating cytotoxic T cell responses, are found, as well as strains which make the reciprocal response, i.e. cytotoxicity but no graft rejection [37]. The separation of Tc and graft rejection responses has also been shown for MHC antigens in mice by cell transfer of either $Ly1^+2^-$ cells (Th/Tdh phenotype) or $Ly1^+2^+$ cells (Tc phenotype) into immunoincompetent recipients. The $Ly1^+2^-$ cells alone were able to transfer ability of the recipients to reject MHC incompatible skin grafts [35,36]. These findings have also been confirmed in rats using a similar experimental approach [38].

In vivo immunization with either MHC or minor H antigen incompatible cells is an efficient way to sensitize the hosts for delayed type hypersensitivity responses (elicited *in vivo*) [36,39], but a poor way to generate cytotoxic T cells when lymphoid organs are removed directly from the animal and tested immediately for Tc function. This may be a reflection of the Th/Tdh response against such antigens predominating (see above) and/or cell migration of the Tc away from the organs usually tested for Tc (spleen, lymph node, peritoneal exudate). The easiest way to obtain cytotoxic T cell responses against MHC and minor H antigens is from *in vitro* mixed lymphocyte culture following *in vivo* sensitization in the case of minor H antigens. Therefore techniques for performing MLC will be described first, followed by a simple quantitative assay for Tc so generated. Details will be given for handling murine cells, but some references will be given for human work.

Methods

In vitro mixed lymphocyte culture

Equipment

(1) A humidified CO_2 incubator at 37 °C and maintaining 5–7% CO_2 in air.
(2) A tissue culture hood—the simplest clean air cabinet will suffice for mouse work, since its function is

merely to protect the cell cultures from contamination from the air or the operator. For human work a laminar flow hood protective of the operator is essential for safety reasons since human cells to be cultured may contain human pathogens.

(3) A microscope for cell counting, a haemocytometer.

(4) A small bench centrifuge.

(5) A water bath.

(6) Sterile instruments: scissors, forceps (rat-toothed or curved).

(7) Access to an irradiation source (or use mitomycin C).

(8) Micropipettes and sterile tips. A single-channel variable 50–200 μl (Fin pipette H40/26/26 Jencons) for sampling for cell counts and an 8-channel multichannel variable 50–200 μl (Cat. no. 77.859.00 Flow) for cell dilutions.

Materials

Media

(1) Preparative: a phosphate-buffered balanced salt solution (BSS) containing 5% fetal calf serum (FCS). FCS must be a tested non-toxic batch.

(2) A culture medium such as bicarbonate-buffered RPMI 1640 or Eagle's MEM(EMEM) containing 5% FCS, 5×10^{-5} M-2-mercaptoethanol, 2 mM-glutamine, 100 i.u./ml penicillin, 100 μg/ml streptomycin and 10 mM-HEPES.

(3) Mitomycin C.

(4) 0.1% Eosin or 0.2% trypan blue for viable cell counts.

Plasticware

Petri dishes; universals (20 ml), 128C (Sterilin) or 50 ml tubes (2070 F, Falcon); culture flasks for 10 ml or 20 ml culture volumes, (1–52094, 1–63371 Nunc) or plates with 12 or 24 wells (76–053–05, 76–063–05, 76–033–05 Flow); 5 and 10 ml pipettes; 1 ml syringes; 19-gauge needles.

Nylon mesh (80 μm, J. Stainer & Co., Manchester) in sterile squares of suitable size.

Mice—one each of 2 MHC disparate strains (e.g. C57BL/10 and BALB/c).

70% Alcohol.

Procedure

1   General

Thaw out additives to be included in preparative (BSS) and culture (EMEM or RPMI) media. Make up media

in the hood and keep at room temperature or at 37 °C. Under sterile conditions dispense 10–20 ml aliquots of BSS/FCS into each of two Petri dishes.

2   Removal of spleen

Kill the two mice (cervical dislocation or CO_2) and swab the left-hand side of the abdominal fur with 70% alcohol. Tent the skin just below the rib-cage on the left side of the abdomen and cut with non-sterile scissors. Pull back skin from the incision, both cranially and caudally exposing abdominal wall musculature. Using sterile scissors and forceps, tent the abdominal wall over the spleen, cut and open abdomen. Grasp spleen gently with the forceps and draw it out of the abdomen cutting through the omental connections. Place each spleen in a separate Petri dish containing the sterile BSS/FCS.

3   Making spleen cell suspensions

Place 19-gauge needles on two 1 ml syringes. Use the syringes as handles and the tips of the needles to tease apart the spleen. Place a square of sterile nylon mesh over the mouth of a universal (20 ml) or 50 ml tube. Using a 5 or 10 ml pipette draw the spleen cell suspension up and down a few times to break up any clumps and then transfer the suspension on to the mesh and let it run through slowly. The mesh will filter out any remaining cell clumps. Cap the universal or 50 ml tube and centrifuge at 1000 rev./min for 5 min at room temperature. Discard supernatant and resuspend cells in 10 ml culture medium (EMEM or RPMI with all additives). Under sterile conditions remove an aliquot from each cell suspension and count viable lymphoid cells after diluting with an equal volume of dye (eosin or Trypan blue). Adjust the concentration of viable spleen cell suspensions to 4 or 5×10^6/ml.

4   Setting up cultures

Irradiate (2000 R) the spleen cell suspension to be used as stimulator cells, or alternatively treat with mitomycin C at 25 mg/ml, with cells at 5×10^7/ml at 37 °C for 10 min followed by three washes in medium. Add the responder and stimulator cell suspensions in equal volumes either into tissue culture flasks, total volume of 10 ml in Nunc 1–52094 or 20 ml in Nunc 1–63371, (incubate standing upright) or into the wells of multiwell plates, 2 ml per well in 76–063–05 and 76–033–05, or 5 ml in 76–053–05 Flow.

5   Incubate at 37 °C in a 5–7% CO_2 atmosphere in air for 5 days. Aliquots of cells can be removed at 3 days for proliferative assays if this is required.

Notes and recommendations

During the preparation and handling of cell suspensions from which cytotoxic responses are to be obtained, never use chilled medium. Prior to *in vitro* incubation at 37 °C keep preparative and culture medium either at room temperature or at 37 °C.

The use of phosphate-buffered BSS/FCS to make the initial cell suspensions enables this procedure to be carried out in the normal atmosphere without the medium becoming too alkaline.

For mouse cultures, it is unwise to use HEPES concentrations over 10 mM (30 mM-HEPES is used for human cultures). Media containing 30 mM-HEPES are better buffered to withstand normal atmospheric concentrations of CO_2 during cell manipulations but such a concentration can be toxic for mouse cells.

Making cell suspensions: the method given works well for spleen or lymph node, but many other methods described in the literature are equally as good. To obtain peripheral blood lymphocytes from small samples of blood from individual mice, see the method of Chandler *et al.* [40].

Human MLC are usually set up using peripheral blood lymphocytes from MHC incompatible donors for responder and stimulator cells [1].

^{51}Cr release assay of cytotoxic T cells from a mixed lymphocyte culture

Equipment

(1–6) As in (1–5) and (8) of previous method (page 68.3).
(7) A centrifuge in which 96-well microplates on appropriate carriers can be spun.
(8) Shaker for water bath, or rocking platform (optional).
(9) Access to hot room (optional).
(10) A gamma counter.

Materials

Media

(1 and 2) As above, page 68.4.
(3) Concanavalin A, stock at 40 μg/ml or LPS, stock at 400 μg/ml.
(4) 10 × Concentrated BSS.
(5) Sterile distilled water.

Plasticware

As in previous method (page 68.4) plus 96-well round-bottomed microtitre plates with lids (M24A Sterilin). These do not need to be sterile. 96-Well Flexiplates (1–222–24 Dynatech) or LP-2 tubes (Luckhams) for harvesting the assay.
^{51}Cr sodium chromate at 1 mCi/ml in isotonic saline.
Mice—one of each of the 2 MHC disparate strains used in setting up the MLC.
70% Alcohol.
Paraffin wax (BDH: congealing point 49 °C).
Wax bath at 52 °C.

Procedure

1   *Preparation of target cells*

Con A blast cultures

These can be set up 24–72 h before the assay. Aseptically remove the spleens from the mice and make each into a cell suspension as described above on page 68.4. Red blood cells (RBC) need to be removed or they will absorb ^{51}Cr and 'leak it' during the assay, giving high levels for spontaneous release. Removal of RBC can be done before culture by adding 4.5 ml sterile distilled water from a syringe to the cell pellet and immediately adding 0.5 ml 10 × concentrated BSS, to bring back the cells to isotonic conditions. Then add 15 ml BSS/FCS and spin the cells. Alternatively, RBC can be removed by lysis in Tris-buffered 0.83% (w/v) ammonium chloride [41]. The pellet will be obviously free of red cell contamination and can be resuspended at 4×10^6/ml in culture medium, to which concanavalin A is added to a final concentration of 4 μg/ml. The cells are incubated at 37 °C in a 5–7% CO_2 humidified atmosphere for 24, 48 or 72 h in tissue culture flasks either in a 10 ml volume (Nunc 1–63371) or in a 20 ml volume (Nunc 52094), or in 4 ml wells of a 12-well cluster plate (76–053–05 Flow).

Alternatively, target cells can be set up at the time of the original MLC, and thus used after 5 days incubation. For this, place $1–2 \times 10^6$ freshly prepared RBC-free spleen cells in 12.5 ml RPMI culture medium containing 10% FCS and 1 μg/ml con A to which 25% rat con A supernatant has been added (for IL-2 preparation see page 68.11). Incubate in a 20 ml tissue culture flask (1-63371 Nunc) standing upright.

At the end of the culture period harvest the target cells into 20 ml universals or 50 ml tubes, spin down and discard the supernatant. To the pellet add 50 or 100 μCi ^{51}Cr sodium chromate, mix, and incubate for 90 min at 37 °C, either on a rocking platform, or with occasional shaking by hand. Wash three times in a large volume (20 or 50 ml depending on the tube used for labelling) of BSS/FCS, count, and make a suspension of the appropriate concentration in culture medium for use in the assay. This concentration usually lies between 5×10^4/ml and 1×10^6 ml.

Alternative sources of target cells

LPS blast cultures: culture spleen cells for 72 h, substituting 40 μg/ml final concentration LPS for the 4 g/ml con A as described above.

Fresh spleen cells, from which RBC have been removed, can be used but these uncultured, unblasted cells are considerably less sensitive to cytotoxic T cell lysis and are not recommended.

Tumour cells: lymphoreticular tumours such as EL-4 (H-2^b) and P815 (H-2^d) either grown *in vivo* or *in vitro* are an excellent source of target cells for cytotoxic cells directed against class I antigens of their H-2 haplotypes. Fibroblast and other attached tumour cell lines are much less sensitive to cytotoxic T cell killing, and their use sometimes requires more prolonged assay periods.

Macrophages from the peritoneal cavity, either washed out of an unstimulated mouse, or from a mouse stimulated by the intraperitoneal injection of thioglycollate broth 3–4 days previously are often good targets for cytotoxic T cells, although they may be somewhat less sensitive than con A blasts and lymphoreticular tumours.

If any of the above alternative target cells are used, it is necessary to make a single cell suspension of them, and then label a pellet of between 10^6 and 10^7 cells with ^{51}Cr sodium chromate as described for con A blasts. In general, it is better to label a number of target cells not much greater than needed for the assay, since with fewer cells, more ^{51}Cr sodium chromate will be incorporated per cell.

2   *Preparation of the attacking cells*

While the target cells are labelling with ^{51}Cr sodium chromate, the MLC cells should be harvested into 20 ml universals or 50 ml tubes. Pipette the cells from the culture flask or wells, making sure to get all cells which can be loosened from the plastic by gentle pipetting. Spin down and resuspend in a volume of culture medium (RPMI or MEM with 5% FCS and 10 mm-HEPES added) convenient for counting and appropriate for the assay. A minimum volume would be 0.6 ml per target to be tested. Count the cells and if necessary adjust the volume to give the desired concentration. For anti-MHC class I cytotoxic cells, generated in primary MLC between class I plus class II disparate responder/stimulator pairs, a starting ratio of 10:1 attacking cells per target cell is appropriate. This ratio would be achieved using attacking cells at 10^6/ml and target cells at 10^5/ml—suitable concentrations for assaying in 200 μl wells of microtitre plates. However, successful assays in microtitre wells can be performed with target cells as few as 5×10^3/well

(5×10^4/ml) or even 1×10^3/well if tumour targets such as P815 or EL-4 are used. Concentrations of attacking cells up to 5×10^6/ml (5×10^5/well) are possible before overcrowding in assay wells is seen.

3   *Plating the attacking cells*

Place 200 μl of the chosen concentration of attacking cells in the first three wells of a 12-well row of a round-bottomed microtitre plate. Using the 8-channel variable micropipette set at 100 μl, place 100 μl culture medium in each of the wells of the rest of the row. Again using the multichannel micropipette, remove 100 μl of the cell suspension from the first three wells, add to the medium in the next three wells, mix gently (no bubbles) then remove 100 μl to the next three wells, repeat the mixing step and transfer 100 μl of this suspension to the end three wells of the row. After mixing, discard 100 μl from each of the end three wells. In this way triplicate doubling dilutions of each attacking cell population will be in a 12-well row of the microtitre plate. If several attacking cell populations are to be assayed, they can be similarly titrated on the same plate, but one row, usually the first, should be left free of attacking cells, for the maximum and spontaneous release values for target cells alone.

4   *Addition of the target cells*

The target cells at the chosen concentrations are added in 100 μl volumes to each well containing attacking cells. In addition, one row of 12 wells should have target cells alone added. To 6 of these wells add 100 μl 5% Triton X-100 (for maximum release) and to the other 6 add 100 μl culture medium (for medium or spontaneous release). The plates can now be centrifuged gently (500 rev./min) for 5 min to co-sediment the attacker and target cells, to facilitate the start of the killing. After centrifugation, place the assay plates for 3 h in a humidified 5–7% CO$_2$ incubator.

5   *Harvesting the assay*

Target cells lysed by the attacking cytotoxic T cells will release their ^{51}Cr into the culture medium. Samples of the supernatants are removed, therefore, and counted for released gamma counts, which give a measure of the level of target cell killing. Using the multichannel micro-pipette set at 100 μl, remove 100 μl supernatant from each well. Transfer the samples into 96-well flexiplates or into LP-2 tubes (Luckhams) set up in 12×8 racks of the same dimension as the microtitre plate. If transferred into flexiplate wells, it will be necessary to leave the samples overnight in a hot room for the liquid to evaporate. Then the plate can be cut up with scissors and each well gamma-counted. If LP-2 tubes are used, they can be sealed by addition of ~100 μl molten paraffin wax to each tube. When the wax has solidified, the tubes can be assessed for gamma counts; 10–60 s per sample should suffice. In general, the lowest counts (medium only) should be at least five times that of the machine background. If 1000 counts are obtained from the maximum, this usually gives 200–300 counts for medium which is adequate for 60 s counts in most machines (having background of <30 counts/min).

6 Calculation of the percentage of specific lysis

The percentage of specific lysis at each attacker:target (A:T) ratio is given by the following formula:

$$\% \text{ specific lysis} = \frac{\text{c.p.m. targets incubated with attacker cells} - \text{c.p.m. in medium}}{\text{c.p.m. targets incubated in 5\% Triton (maximum)} - \text{c.p.m. in medium}}$$

Machine background should be subtracted from each c.p.m. in the above formula.

Thus a figure for percentage of specific lysis will be obtained for each A:T ratio. Four such figures are obtained for each population of cytotoxic T cell attackers tested. These figures can be plotted directly on graph paper, and/or can be subjected to regression analysis, with the curve being solved at a chosen A:T ratio for each attacking cytotoxic T cell population. In this way the relative activity of each population can be compared (see Fig. 68.1). Using a sophisticated computer, it is possible to program the analysis and to obtain (1) a computer printout of the % specific lysis for each point, (2) a graphical representation of this, and (3) a computation of the regression analysis at a chosen A:T ratio, with r^2 value, which is a measure of how well the titrated data fit the semi-logarithmic plot.

Notes and recommendations

Some laboratories do not count the viable cells recovered after an MLC but merely resuspend the harvested cells in a predetermined volume and assay serial dilutions of this. The results are expressed as a percentage specific lysis of the appropriate fraction of the starting culture. Such figures are a measure of the cytotoxic activity developed per culture. This is a perfectly valid way of comparing activities of parallel cultures, but such a manner of doing the assay does not give information about the lytic activity per viable recovered cell. The lytic activity per culture can easily be calculated from the assay as performed in the procedure above, by multiplying the % specific lysis at

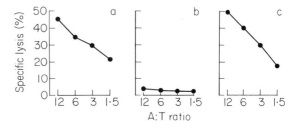

Fig. 68.1. Titration of anti-H-Y and anti-H-2 cytotoxic T cells.
(a) & (b). Attacker cells were C57BL/10 female spleen cells from mice immunized *in vivo* with 10^7 syngeneic male cells i.p., then after three weeks boosted *in vitro* in MLC for 5 days with irradiated syngeneic male cells as described on page 68.9. Assay of anti-H-Y cytotoxic cells was carried out as described on pages 68.5–68.8—against ^{51}Cr labelled C57BL/10 male (a) and female (b) 48 h con A blasts at the attacker to target (A:T) ratios shown.
c. Attacker cells were from a primary C57BL/10 anti-BALB/c MLC, assayed on the 5th day of culture on ^{51}Cr-labelled BALB/c 48 h Con A blasts at the A:T shown.

the chosen A:T ratio by the viable cell recovery per culture.

When comparing the lytic activities of attacking cells assayed on the same target cells, it is not necessary to use exactly the same A:T ratios for each attacking cell population, providing they are roughly within the same range (no more than a twofold difference) and are subjected to regression analysis, since this method of computation calculates from the experimental values a curve from which the solution is taken. It is, however, not desirable to take as values for comparison figures obtained by extrapolating curves beyond the experimental data.

When a wider range of A:T ratios is required, tripling rather than doubling dilutions of the attackers can be made. This is achieved by placing 150 μl rather than 200 μl of the highest concentration of attacking cells in the first three wells of a row and serially transferring 50 μl rather than 100 μl when making he dilutions. The results of such a titration are shown in Fig. 68.4.

An alternative control to the medium release is that of using a population of unsensitized spleen cells (fresh or cultured) as 'attackers': these are titrated at the same A:T ratios as the cytotoxic population(s) under test. This method certainly controls for cell crowding effects but in general most laboratories find that the values for spontaneous release obtained in this way are indistinguishable from target cells incubated in medium alone.

Length of assay incubation: using cytotoxic T cells

from MLC, directed at MHC antigens (for a primary MLC) or minor H antigens (from a secondary MLC) and con A blasts as target cells, a 3 h incubation is certainly long enough. If the assay is prolonged further this may lead to such high spontaneous release of ^{51}Cr that the assay is invalidated (spontaneous release of above 30% is undesirable: if above 40%, the titrations are often poor and the results unreliable). However, attached tumour cell lines such as L929 (of C3H, H-2^k origin) give very little specific release during a 3 h assay and the incubation period if such cells are used needs to be extended to 5 or 6 h. During this time L cells give an acceptably low spontaneous release. It is possible to let such assays incubate for 18 h but then there is a danger of non-specific killing, e.g. C3H attackers raised against H-2^b targets will produce 'self' lysis on L929 cells, of C3H, H-2^k origin.

The reason for using targets such as L929 cells is that they are good for assaying certain H-2 restricted virus cytotoxic T cells (where con A blasts are poor) and that to date these cells have been the only ones that have been successfully transfected with foreign class I MHC DNA in gene transfer experiments.

Other methods for assaying cytotoxicity: in the past laborious methods for counting residual cells after incubation with cytotoxic cells were devised. The methods that relied on visual counting have passed into oblivion as being too time consuming and subjective. Methods which rely on post-labelling with radionucleotides, such as ^{125}I-UdR and ^{3}H-proline, are still in use in some laboratories but produce poor quantification.

Another method of assessing numbers of residual cells at the end of the assay has recently been introduced. It depends on the use of a dye, which is taken up by target cells and then released from them by cell rupture, followed by a spectroscopic measurement. One limitation is that it can only be used on target cells such as macrophages that attach firmly to plastic, so that the potentially confusing attacking cells can be washed away before dye is added. However, quantification and sensitivity of this method appears good [42].

Methods for assessing cytotoxicity of very few cytotoxic cells, such as those clonally derived from a single precursor cell (pTc) during the course of a 6 day limiting dilution MLC will be given when limiting dilution is discussed (page 68.9).

In vivo generation of cytotoxic T cell responses and assay

Equipment for assay, as for the previous method (page 68.5).

Materials

For immunizations

(1) Preparative medium—balanced salt solution (BSS).
(2) Plasticware, syringes, 25-gauge needles.
(3) Tumour cells—grown *in vitro* or *in vivo*, e.g. P815, EL-4 or spleen cells—fresh, prepared as described on page 68.4.

For assay

As in previous method (page 68.6).

Mice

MHC incompatible with the immunizing cells, e.g. C57BL/10 (H-2^b) (for P815); BALB/c (H-2^d) (for EL-4). P815 was derived from a DBA/2 mouse (H-2^d) and EL-4 from a C57BL/6 mouse (H-2^b).

Procedure

1 Harvest the cells to be used for immunization, wash and suspend in BSS without added FCS. Inject $2-5 \times 10^7$ cells i.p. into the recipient mice.

2 Approximately 10 days after immunization, harvest the sensitized cells from the recipient mice. These can be obtained from the spleen or peritoneal cavity. The spleen should be teased (see page 68.4) and counted, and viable counts adjusted to the desired concentration. Cells can be washed from the peritoneal cavity by flushing with 5 ml BSS. Centrifuge cell suspension, resuspend pellet, count, and adjust cell concentration.

3 The cytotoxic assay using *in vivo* primed T cells is performed exactly as for the assay of MLC-induced cytotoxic T cells (pages 68.5–68.7). However, in general rather higher A:T ratios will be needed to obtain lysis of target cells. In the case of mice immunized with allogeneic spleen cells, their spleen cell population will only show activity if A:T ratios starting at 100:1 or 50:1 are used. However, peritoneal cells from mice given allogeneic tumour will have much higher activity, and A:T ratios can start at 20:1 or lower.

Notes and recommendations

Anti-viral cytotoxic T cell responses against many viruses can be readily generated *in vivo* by injecting virus (e.g. vaccinia, LCM, influenza) [see ref. 24] and using the splenic lymphocytes for assay 6 days later. The assay is performed on H-2 matched target cells (usually tumours) and targets should always include infected target cells and control uninfected target cells. The virus-specific kill is that seen on virus infected cells alone. A:T ratios used are generally rather high, starting at about 50:1. Much lower A:T ratios can be used if spleen cells from such immunized mice are placed *in vitro* together with virus infected syngeneic cells for 5 or 6 days before the assay.

It is not possible to generate cytotoxic T cell responses against minor transplantation antigens or haptens following a single *in vivo* immunization. However, if mice are immunized in the footpad and the draining popliteal lymph nodes placed in culture for 3 days in the absence of further stimulating antigen, minor H-specific or hapten-specific cytotoxicity can be generated against the immunogen [43,44]. This is assayed on appropriate target cells as described on pages 68.5–68.7. In the case of haptens, target cells must include syngeneic haptenated cells and as negative control non-haptenated syngeneic cells. In the case of minor transplantation antigens, targets must be H-2 matched and include one bearing the minor H antigen(s) in question, and if possible, one without: in the case of responses to multiple minors, the only negative H-2 matched control will be cells of the responder type.

Very strong anti-hapten and anti-minor H responses can be obtained if spleen cells are taken from *in vivo* immunized mice (immunized 2 weeks to several months previously by the i.p. or s.c. route) and cultured *in vitro* in MLC for 5 days with appropriate irradiated antigen bearing cells. Such *in vivo* primed, *in vitro* boosted attacker cells are assayed, as described on pages 68.5–68.7, and target cell specificity is assessed by using targets as described in the above paragraph. A:T ratios used in the assay of such H-2 restricted secondary MLC cells should start at 20:1 or 10:1, i.e. these attackers will be as active as primary anti-H-2 MLC.

Separation of subpopulations involved in generating cytotoxic T cell responses

Equipment and materials

For cell separation

As described in Chapter 29, on FACS and in Chapter 55, on immunoselection of lymphocyte subpopulations.

For in vitro *MLC and assay of cytotoxicity*

As described for the first two methods (see pages 68.4–68.8).

Procedure

Responder cell populations containing both Tc and Th can be separated into each component using appropriate cell surface markers (e.g. Lyt1, Lyt2) by positive and/or negative selection methods, as described in the chapters cited above. Set these cells up in MLC, as described on page 68.3, using each population alone as responder, and equal numbers of both added together. Add irradiated spleen cells carrying the appropriate stimulating alloantigen to each responder type and mix. If the cell separation procedure yields low cell numbers (as in FACS sorting) micro-MLC can be set up in 200 μl round-bottomed wells of 96-well microtitre plates (1–63320 Nunc), using 1 or 2×10^5 responder cells per well, plus 5×10^5 irradiated spleen cells as antigen per well. Six replicate wells of each type should be set up. At the end of a 5 or 6 day incubation period, harvest and pool cells from replicate wells as described on page 68.6.

Notes and recommendations

Experiments of the type described above, using Lyt1 and/or Lyt2 markers for mouse cells, require a combination of positive and negative selection or sequential positive selection methods, since Tc are $Lyt1^+2^+$ and Th are $Lyt1^+2^-$. Thus using Lyt2-positive selection, Tc can be obtained, leaving Th in the unselected population. Using Lyt2-negative selection, $Lyt2^+$ Tc are removed, leaving $Lyt1^+$ Th cells. Lyt1-negative selection, if appropriately manipulated, can be used to remove $Lyt1^+$ Th cells but leave at least a proportion of $Lyt1^+2^+$ Tc cells, since these generally have quantitatively less Lyt1 on their surface than Th cells. In man, Th cells are $T4^+T8^-$, whilst Tc are $T4^-T8^+$, thus greatly facilitating separation by positive selection from the same starting population.

Recently, a mouse T cell marker, L3T4, has been described which is eqivalent to T4 in man, thus marking class II MHC reactive Th cells and facilitating their separation [48].

The results of such experiments have shown that Tc cultured alone with stimulating antigen in MLC generate little or no cytotoxicity, whilst co-culture in the presence of Th enables the cytotoxic response to develop [19]. However, Th can be substituted for *in vitro* by culture supernatants containing IL-2 and other factors, and this approach has been employed in the limiting dilution analysis described below.

Limiting dilution analysis of Tc and Th

Equipment and materials

As for first method (page 68.3).

Additional materials

Plasticware: 96-well, V-bottomed microtitre plates (Greiner M220-25ARTL Dynatech).

An IL-2 containing source—either (1) con A supernatant taken 24 h after setting up mouse or rat spleen cells at 5×10^6/ml with 4 μg/ml con A or (2) secondary MLC supernatant, prepared from mouse spleen cells at 5×10^6/ml, co-cultured with an equal concentration of Mls and/or H-2 disparate irradiated spleen cells for 14 days, then harvested, resuspended in growth medium at 2×10^6/ml, and restimulated for 2 days in the presence of 5×10^6/ml of the same stimulating cells. After 2 days restimulation, the supernatants contain high concentrations of IL-2 and other growth/differentiation factors or (3) supernatant from the Farrar subline of EL-4 stimulated for 24 h with 1 μg/ml phenorbital acid. Assays for the biological activity of IL-2 containing supernatants are given in Chapter 59 of this handbook. These supernatants can also be tested for their ability to support the end-stage growth and functional activity of cytotoxic effectors by titrating the supernatants into limiting numbers of cells (1×10^4 cells per microwell) of IL-2 dependent secondary MLC cells (see page 68.11) [45]. In general, optimal concentrations for supporting Tc differentiation will be found on inclusion in the range 5–15% by volume of the IL-2 containing culture supernatants described above.

Procedure

For limiting dilution analysis of Tc

1   Remove spleens of responder and stimulator mouse strains, make cell suspensions, as described on page 68.4.

2   Remove RBC from stimulator cells by water lysis, as described on page 68.5. Resuspend at 5×10^6/ml in culture medium supplemented with IL-2 containing supernatant at twice the concentration of IL-2 finally needed. Irradiate (2000 R) as on page 68.4. If mitomycin C is used instead of irradiation, treat before making up at 5×10^6/ml in culture medium supplemented with IL-2.

3   Resuspend responder cells at, for example, 4×10^5/ml in culture medium. Place 200 μl of this suspension in 24 wells (rows 1–3 in lines A–H) of a V-bottomed microtitre plate. Place 100 μl of culture medium in the remaining wells of this plate, and in all 96 wells of a second plate. Using an 8-channel micropipette set at 100 μl, remove 100 μl suspension from the first row (1, A–H) of the first plate, and transfer to the 4th row (4, A–H): mix gently (no bubbles), remove 100 μl to row 7 (7, A–H), repeat the

mixing, and transfer to row 10 of the first plate and subsequently to rows 1, 4, 7 and 10 of the second plate. Repeat this doubling dilution manoeuvre, taking cells from row 2 (A–H) plate 1 to rows 5, 8, 11 of the first plate then on to rows 2, 5, 8 and 11 of the second plate, and again repeat using rows 3, 6, 9 and 12 of both plates. In this way, eight doubling dilutions will have been performed, leaving 4×10^4, 2×10^4, 1×10^4, 0.5×10^4, 0.25×10^4, 0.12×10^4, 0.06×10^4 and 0.03×10^4 cells per well, in replicates of 24. The greater the number of replicates made, the more accurate is the analysis. Twenty-four wells is an acceptable number, and is practical to handle if several responders are to be analysed in one experiment.

4   Add irradiated antigen in IL-2 supplemented medium, 100 μl/well (5×10^5 cells). Twenty-four wells of a third plate should be filled with 100 μl antigen plus 100 μl medium.

5   Culture in a humidified CO_2 incubator (5–7% CO_2) for 6 days, preferably with the plates in a moist container to prevent excessive dehydration.

6   Assay for cytotoxicity: label target cells, either P815 or EL-4, or con A blasts, as described on page 68.5. After washing, resuspend the targets in culture medium at 2.5×10^4/ml. Spin the V-bottomed plates containing the responder cells at 500 rev./min for 5 min. Flick off the supernatants. Add 200 μl labelled targets (i.e. 5×10^3) to each well. Mix responders and attackers gently, starting with wells in which antigen only was placed, then those containing the lowest numbers of responders plus antigen and so on, up to the highest concentration. Place 100 μl target cells at 5×10^4/ml in eight empty wells (i.e. 5×10^3/well), and add 100 μl Triton. These are for the maximum release. Incubate the plates for 4 h after spinning for 5 min at 500 rev./min. Harvest 100 μl supernatant from each well, as described on page 68.6. Count for gamma counts: this will need 30–100 s/sample, depending on how efficiently the targets were labelled.

7   Assessment of results: the manner of calculating the number of positive wells for the 24 wells containing each concentration of responders is to determine the mean c.p.m. plus three standard errors of the 24 wells used for medium release. These were the 24 wells set up initially with 5×10^5/well antigen plus 100 μl medium. Wells showing counts greater than this mean plus 3S.E.s are taken as positive (Fig. 68.2). The percentage of negative wells at each concentration of responders is then plotted against the number of responders per well on a semi-log plot. Providing these points fall on a straight line passing through 0 (one-hit kinetics, so only one cell is limiting, i.e. the Tc) the reciprocal of the number of responder cells giving a 37% negative response is the Tc precursor frequency. This is illustrated in Fig. 68.3. A more detailed analysis of Poisson

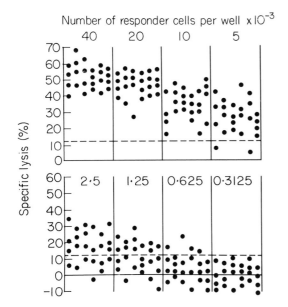

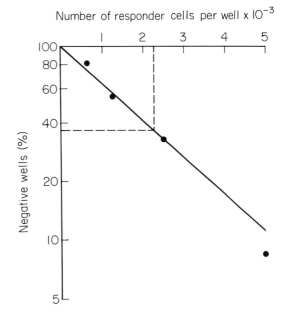

Figs. 68.2 and 68.3. Limiting dilution analysis of cytotoxic T cell precursor frequency in spleen cells from a BALB/c mouse stimulated with irradiated C57BL/6 spleen cells as antigen. BALB/c splenic responder cells were set up in 24 replicates at each concentration tested, according to the method described on pages 68.9–68.10. The assay was carried out using a 5×10^3 ^{51}Cr-labelled EL-4 tumour cells per well.

In Fig. 68.2, the points show the percentage of specific lysis of individual wells. The dotted line indicates 3 standard deviations above the medium release control, and each point above that line is counted as positive for cytotoxicity.

In Fig. 68.3, the data are replotted in terms of the percentage of negative wells at each concentration of responder cells over the range in which the data titrated (5×10^3/well to 0.625×10^3/well). The dotted line is drawn at 37% negative wells and this intersects the regression line to give a precursor (pTc) frequency of 1 in 2327 responder cells. The regression line has an r^2 value of 1.00 in this experiment.

distribution and limiting dilution analysis and assessment of results is given in Chapter 65 of this handbook, by Zaunderer.

For limiting dilution analysis of Th

1–4 Procedure is identical with 1–4 above, except that *no* IL-2 is added to the medium. In fact, the production of IL-2 by limiting numbers of cells is used as a measure of help.
5 The initial incubation period is for 7 days.
6 The plates are then spun and 'flicked' but this step must be done aseptically. A source of sterile tissues on which to blot off the plates after flicking is necessary.
7 Add 150 μl medium containing 5×10^5/well freshly prepared and irradiated spleen cells, genetically identical with those used as antigen in the initial culture.
8 Incubate the plates for a further 2 days.
9 Aseptically remove 100 μl/well supernatants, placing them in round-bottomed wells of microtitre plates

using the same plate plan as the initial plates. At this stage the plates can be taped closed and frozen.
10 Assay for helper activity: a source of secondary MLC cells, dependent on IL-2 for the maintenance of growth and functional cytotoxic activity is required. For this, 7 days before the helper activity is to be assayed, set up a standard bulk culture MLC, using 1×10^7 responder spleen cells and 1×10^7 H-2 disparate irradiated spleen cells as antigen (CBA [H-2^k] responders and BALB/c [H-2^d] as antigen are ideal), in 5 ml volumes of culture medium per well in 12 well cluster plates (76–053–05 Flow). After 5 days incubation, harvest aseptically, count, and resuspend at an appropriate concentration to give 2×10^6 responders per well; add 5×10^6 freshly prepared, irradiated spleen cells as antigen per well, in a total volume of 5 ml culture medium per well in 12-well cluster plates. Incubate for 2 more days, then harvest and resuspend at 1×10^5/ml in culture medium. These are the secondary MLC cells and at this concentration their further

growth in the absence of antigen is IL-2 dependent. Thus their growth and differentiation to Tc is a measure of the presence of IL-2 in the supernatant (page 68.11) above to be tested. Add 100 μl secondary MLC cell suspension, i.e. 1×10^4 cells, to each of the wells to be assessed for helper activity (page 68.11). Incubate for 2–3 days.

The final step in the assay is to determine which of the wells has generated cytotoxic activity. This is done as described on page 68.10, using P815 targets if the CBA anti BALB/c combination was set up as a source of secondary MLC.

11   Assessment of results: this is essentially the same as described on page 68.10. The mean $\pm$ 3S.E. against which positives are to be measured, are taken from those wells of secondary MLC which received no supernatants containing helper factors, i.e. supernatants taken from wells of the original cultures set up with stimulator cells alone. The results are plotted semi-logarithmically with the percentage of negative cultures plotted against the number of cells set up as responders in the original cultures (see page 68.11). The helper frequency (i.e. the frequency of cells capable of making IL-2 which subsequently supports the test secondary MLC) is the reciprocal of the number of responder cells giving a 37% negative response.

Notes and recommendations

The Tc and Th precursor frequencies vary considerably, depending on the many factors of which the genotype of responder and stimulator are the most important: as expected, H-2 differences show the highest precursor frequencies, and minor H antigen specific precursor frequencies of Th and Tc are virtually unmeasurable unless the responder mice have been previously immunized *in vivo*. Other important factors are the general state of health of the mice used and, for Tc precursor frequency, the quality of the IL-2 used. Whenever comparisons between individuals and/or genotypes of responder or stimulator pairs are to be compared, it is necessary to make those comparisons within a single experiment, or always to include reference responders within each experiment to be compared. Another source of variation of the results is the varying sensitivity of target cells—particular targets may be more sensitive to cytotoxic killing one day than the next, again giving variation between experiments.

Cloning Tc

Equipment and materials

As for the first method, on page 68.3.

Additional materials

IL-2 containing supernatants (as described on page 68.10) or purified IL-2 (see Chapter 6 of this handbook).

Procedure

Tc clones against class I MHC alloantigens are perhaps the easiest to obtain, although Tc clones specific for minor H antigens [11,51] and viruses [33] have been obtained.

The starting point for all Tc cloning is a primary or secondary MLC. Responder and stimulator spleen cells of H-2 or minor H disparate strains are bulk-cultured for 12–14 days, using equal numbers of responder and stimulator cells. Convenient plastic vessels in which to set up the initial cultures are 24-well cluster plates (76–063–05 or 76–033–05 Flow), holding a volume of 2 ml (cells usually at concentrations of 4×10^6 responders and 4×10^6 stimulators). When left for 12–14 days, such cultures have passed through the stage of active blasts and most of the viable recovered cells are small, round lymphocytes.

Further stimulation with antigen can either be done in similar bulk cultures, for 2–4 cycles of restimulation, each 12–14 days apart, or cloning can be done immediately after the initial bulk culture. In some cases, best results have been obtained if the bulk culture restimulation is carried through many cycles, with later ones (after the 3rd or 4th) having IL-2 added to them and the number of responders reduced to 5×10^4/well. The timing of cloning is to a certain extent a matter of experience in handling cells making the particular response in question. Restimulation of bulk cultures should be continued anyway until clones are safely established.

Cloning can be done by limiting dilution, setting up 96 microtitre wells (round- or flat-bottomed) with 0.3 cells per well and a further 96 wells with 1 cell per well. To this, antigen at 5×10^5/well should be added, together with a source of IL-2 at a concentration known to support differentiation of Tc (see page 68.11). Growth of individual clones will appear in 8–14 days and wells from plating concentrations yielding <30% wells containing growing cells are likely to contain progeny of single cells, i.e. clones. These can be transferred to 2 ml wells of cluster plates, together with fresh antigen and IL-2. They must be inspected carefully for growth, and transferred to new wells at $\sim 5 \times 10^4$/well with new antigen and IL-2 if they overgrow. Once established, it should be possible to maintain cytotoxic clones so that the cultures need to be split, restimulated and given IL-2 every ~ 14 days. They should be tested for function regularly, and also regularly recloned (1) to increase the chances of their being true clones, and (2) to eliminate somatic variation.

Notes and recommendations

It is now well established that the most stable cytotoxic T cell clones, both karyotypically and functionally, are those which are maintained in the presence of stimulating antigen and IL-2 [1]. Purified IL-2 is all that is necessary to maintain T cell clones once established, i.e. they appear not to require other factors that seem necessary for the pTc→Tc differentiation step. Mouse T cell clones can be maintained in the presence of IL-2 from mouse, rat, gibbon, and human. Human T cell clones will grow in human and gibbon IL-2, but not in IL-2 from rat or mouse.

An excellent account incorporating the experience of many laboratories on the cloning of Tc and Th of man and mouse is given in ref. 1.

Analysis of transfectants with cytotoxic T cells

Equipment and materials

As for method on page 68.5.

Additional materials

Cloned HAT-sensitive L929 cells, transfected with cosmids containing the Tk gene and a class I MHC gene. As a control, L929 (H-2^k) are transfected with cosmids containing the Tk gene only. These cell lines can be obtained from laboratories where workers have developed them and published results using them [29–31]. Alternatively they can be developed, using the appropriate recombinant DNA technology (see also Chapters 91 and 92 of this handbook).

Procedure

1 Generation of cytotoxic T cells

This should be done in primary 5 day bulk MLC. A positive control is needed, i.e. anti-H-2^k Tc, which should kill all L929 (H-2^k) cell clones, regardless of whether they have incorporated foreign DNA. This is a control for the lysability of such cells by Tc. The experimental Tc will depend on the source of the DNA

used in the transfections. C57BL/10 (H-2^b) and BALB/c (H-2^d) mice have been used by two different laboratories. To explore the expression of the K^b gene, of the C57BL/10 strain, anti-H-2K^b Tc can be generated using the mutant strain C57BL/6^{bm-1}, which has a mutant K^{bm-1} gene and can recognize as foreign the K^b gene of the parental of 'wild-type' H-2^b mouse.

Since cells carrying third party H-2 alloantigens are frequently lysed by bulk culture MLC, whilst auto-killing by such cultures is rarer, the most informative way to make Tc to examine an L cell transfectant carrying the K^b gene is to generate
(1) C57BL/10 anti-C3H (H-2^b anti-H 2^k)
(2) C57BL/6^{bm-1} anti-B6 (H-2^{bm-1} anti-H 2^b).
One mouse of each of the genotypes above should be killed, and the spleen removed and teased. The cells should be set up in MLC in 12-well cluster plates with 1×10^7 responder cells and 1×10^7 stimulator cells per well, and a culture medium volume of 5 ml/well (as on pages 68.3–68.5). These MLC should be cultured for 5 days in a humidified CO$_2$ incubator (page 68.4).

2 Preparation of target cells

The L cell transformants grow attached. They must be resuspended by incubation with versene-trypsin for 2–4 min, washed twice in BSS/FCS and counted; $1–2 \times 10^6$ cells should be labelled with 100 μCi ^{51}Cr sodium chromate for 60 min.

Positive control targets, C57BL/10 and C3H 24–72 h con A blasts, should also be labelled (as described on page 68.5) for 60–90 min. After washing all targets two to three times, their counts should be adjusted to a concentration appropriate for the assay, i.e. within the range $1–5 \times 10^5$/ml.

3 Preparation of the attacking Tc cells

As described on page 68.6.

4 Plating of attacking Tc cells and target cells

As described on page 68.6. Concentrations of both attacking Tc cells and target cells should be adjusted so that the highest A:T ratio is approximately 30:1.

5 Incubation and harvesting

Plates with the positive control con A blast target cells should be harvested after 3 h, as on page 68.6, or the background lysis figure will rise too high.

Plates with the L cell transfectants as target cells should be harvested after 5–6 h incubation (as on page 68.6) because the levels of killing at 3 h are too low.

The results of such an experiment are shown in Fig.

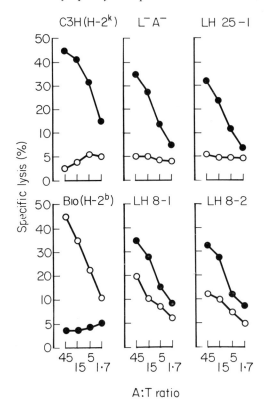

Fig. 68.4. Analysis of L cell transformants by cytotoxic T cells. Attacker cells were generated in 5 day MLC: C3H anti-C57BL/10 (H-2^k anti-H-2^b)○——○; and C57BL/10 anti-C3H (H-2^b anti-H-2^k) ●——●. They were used at the A:T ratio shown, against the ^{51}Cr-labelled target cells indicated at the top of each panel. C3H and B10 were 48 h Con A blast spleen cells, and the assay against them was run for 3 h. The other targets, L$^-$A$^-$, LH25–1, LH8–1 and LH8–2, were L929 cells (L$^-$A$^-$) or L cells transformed with cloned cosmid DNA of H-2 origin. LH8–1 and LH8–2 were subclones of the same transformation using the K^b gene to transfect. LH25–1 was derived from transfection with a cloned gene which did not map to K^b or D^b: the assay against the L cells and their transformants was run for 6 h before harvesting. Reprinted from ref. 30.

68.4, where three transfectants were examined for H-2^b class I expression. Two cloned lines, LH8–1 and LH8–2 expressed the gene whereas the one, LH25–1 did not.

Notes and recommendations

Since the attached L cell lines are trypsin treated to make them into a suspension and this might remove some cell surface H-2 molecules, they must always be checked for endogeneous class I gene expression, to establish whether (1) they are expressing class I genes and (2) they are lysable by Tc cells. The incubation time of 5–6 h appears necessary to obtain lysis under these conditions.

Acknowledgements

The authors would like to thank Bruce Loveland, Brigitte Stockinger, Kyuhei Tomonari, and Gerard Farmer for reading the manuscript and for making helpful suggestions.

Appendix

Names and addresses of suppliers of minor equipment.

Dynatech Laboratory Ltd.,
Daux Road, Billingshurst,
West Sussex RH14 9SJ.

Falcon,
Becton Dickinson (UK) Ltd.,
York House,
Empire Way,
Wembley, Middlesex HA9 0PS.

Flow Laboratories,
PO Box 17,
Second Avenue, Industrial Estate,
Irvine, Ayrshire KA12 8NB,
Scotland.

Jencons Science Ltd.,
Mark Road,
Hemel Hempstead,
Hertfordshire.

Luckhams Ltd.,
Labroworks,
Victoria Gardens,
Burgess Hill,
Sussex RH15 9ON.

Nunc: Gibco-Europe Ltd.,
PO Box 35,
Paisley PA3 4EP.

Sterilin,
43–45 Broad Street,
Teddington,
Middlesex TW11 8QZ.

References

1 FATHMAN C.G. & FITCH F.W. (1982) *Isolation, Characterization, and Utilization of T lymphocyte clones.* Academic Press Inc.

2 MÖLLER G. (ed.) (1980) T cell stimulating growth factors. *Immunol. Revs.* **51.**

3 MÖLLER G. (ed.) (1981) T cell clones. *Immunol. Revs.* **54.**

4 ZINKERNAGEL R.M. & DOHERTY P.C. (1974) Restriction of *in vitro* T cell-mediated cytotoxicity in lymphocytic choriomeningitis within a syngeneic or semiallogeneic system. *Nature,* **248,** 701.

5 SHEARER G.M. (1974) Cell-mediated cytotoxicity to trinitrophenyl-modified syngeneic lymphocytes. *Eur. J. Immunol.* **4,** 527.

6 BEVAN M.J. (1975) The major histocompatibility complex determines susceptibility to cytotoxic T cells directed against minor histocompatibility antigens. *J. exp. Med.* **142,** 1349.

7 GORDON R.D., SIMPSON E. & SAMELSON L.E. (1975) *In vitro* cell-mediated immune responses to the male specific (H-Y) antigen in mice. *J. exp. Med.* **142,** 1108.

8 SCHWARTZ R.H., DAVID C.S., DORF M.E., BENACERRAF B. & PAUL M.E. (1978) Inhibition of dual Ir gene-controlled T-lymphocyte proliferative responses to poly (Glu^{56} Lys^{39} Phe^9)$_n$ with anti-Ia antisera directed against products of either I–A or I–C subregion. *Proc. natn. Acad. Sci. U.S.A.* **75,** 2387.

9 GOULMY E., TERMIJTELEN A., BRADLEY B.A. & VAN ROOD J.J. (1977) Y antigen killing by T cells of women is restricted by HLA. *Nature,* **266,** 544.

10 McMICHAEL A. (1978) HLA restriction of human cytotoxic T lymphocytes specific for influenza virus. Poor recognition of virus associated with HLA A2. *J. exp. Med.* **148,** 1458.

11 VON BOEHMER H., HENGARTNER H., NABHOLZ M., LERHARDT W., SCHREIER M.H. & HASS W. (1979) Fine specificity of a continuously growing killer cell clone specific for H-Y antigen. *Eur. J. Immunol.* **9,** 592.

12 SIMPSON E. (1983) MHC antigens and the genetic control of immune responses. *Transplant. Proc.* **15,** 186.

13 SCHENDEL D.J., ALTER B.J. & BACH F.H. (1973) The involvement of LD- and SD-region differences in MLC and CML: a three cell experiment. *Transplant. Proc.* **5,** 1651.

14 SIMON M.M. & EICHMANN K. (1980) T cell subsets participating in the generation of cytotoxic T cells. *Springer Semin. Immunopath.* **3,** 39.

15 REINHERZ E.L., MEUER S.C. & SCHLOSSMAN S.F. (1983) The delineation of antigen receptors on human T lymphocytes. *Immunology Today,* **4,** 5.

16 NAKAYAMA E., DIPPOLD W., SHIKU H., OETTGEN H.F. & OLD L.J. (1980) Alloantigen-induced T-cell proliferation: Lyt phenotype of responding cells and blocking of proliferation by Lyt antisera. *Proc. natn. Acad. Sci. U.S.A.* **77,** 2890.

17 CANTOR H., SIMPSON E., SATO V.L., FATHMAN C.G. & HERZENBERG L.A. (1975) Characterization of subpopulation of T lymphocytes. (1) Separation and functional studies of peripheral T-cells binding different amounts of fluorescent anti-Thy 1.2 (Theta) antibody using a fluorescence-activated cell sorter (FACS). *Cell. Immunol.* **15,** 180.

18 CANTOR H. & BOYSE E.A. (1975) Functional subclasses of T lymphocytes bearing different Ly antigens. (1) The generation of functionally distinct T-cell subclasses is a differentiative process independent of antigen. *J. exp. Med.* **141,** 1376.

19 SIMON M.M., EDWARDS A.J., HÄMMERLING U., McKENZIE I.F.C., EICHMANN K. & SIMPSON E. (1981) Generation of effector cells from T cell subsets: (III) Synergy between Lyt-1 and Lyt-123/23 lymphocytes in the generation of H-2 restricted and alloreactive cytotoxic T cells. *Eur. J. Immunol.* **11,** 246.

20 PETTINELLI C.B., SCHMITT-VERHULST A.M. & SHEARER G.M. (1979) Cell types required for H-2 restricted cytotoxic responses generated by TNP-modified syngeneic cells or proteins. *J. Immunol.* **122,** 847.

21 MACDONALD H.R., CEROTTINI J.-C., RYSER J.-E., MARYANSKI J.L., TASWELL C., WIDMER M.B. & BRUNNER K.T. (1980) Quantitation and cloning of cytolytic T lymphocytes and their precursors. *Immunol. Revs.* **51,** 93.

22 GORDON R.D., MATHIESON B.J., SAMELSON L.E., BOYSE E.A. & SIMPSON E. (1976) The effect of allogeneic presensitization on H-Y graft survival and *in vitro* cell mediated responses to H-Y antigen. *J. exp. Med.* **144,** 810.

23 BEVAN M.J. (1976) Cross priming for a secondary cytotoxic response to minor H antigens with H-2 congenic cells which do not crossreact in the cytotoxic assay. *J. exp. Med.* **143,** 1283.

24 ZINKERNAGEL R.M. & DOHERTY P.C. (1979) MHC-restricted cytotoxic T cells: studies on the biological role of polymorphic major transplantation antigens determining T-cell restriction-specificity, function and responsiveness. *Adv. Immunol.* **27,** 51.

25 KURRIE R., RÖLLINGHOFF M. & WAGNER H. (1978) H-2-linked murine cytotoxic T cell responses specific for Sendai virus-infected cells. *Eur. J. Immunol.* **8,** 910.

26 COOLEY M.A. & SCHMITT-VERHULST A.M. (1979) Specific helper T cells permit differentiation of thymic anti-self TNP cytotoxic precursor cells. *J. Immunol.* **123,** 2328.

27 WIDMER M.B. & BACH F.H. (1981) Antigen-driven helper cell—independent cloned cytolytic T lymphocytes. *Nature,* **294,** 750.

28 HENNEY C.S. (1980) The mechanism of T-cell-mediated lysis. *Immunology Today,* **1,** 36.

29 GOODENOW R.S., McMILLAN M., ORN A., NICHOLSON M., DAVIDSSON N., FRELINGER J.H. & HOOD L. (1982) Identification of a BALB/c H-2L^d gene by DNA-mediated gene transfer. *Science,* **215,** 677.

30 MELLOR A.L., GOLDEN L., WEISS E., BULLMAN H., SIMPSON E., JAMES R., TOWNSEND A.R.M., TAYLOR P.M., SCHMIDT W., FERLUGA J., LEBEN L., SANTAMARIA M., ATFIELD G., FESTENSTEIN H. & FLAVELL R.A. (1982) Expression of the murine H-2K^b histocompatibility antigen in cells transformed with cloned H-2 genes. *Nature,* **298,** 529.

31 WEISS E.H., MELLOR A., GOLDEN L., FAHRNER K., SIMPSON E., HURST J. & FLAVELL R.A. (1983) Structure of a mutant H-2 gene: generation of polymorphism in H-2 genes by gene conversion-like events. *Nature,* **301,** 671.

32 KEES U. & BLANDEN R.V. (1977) Protective activity of

secondary effector T cells generated *in vitro* against ectromelia virus infection *in vivo*. *Clin. exp. Immunol.* **30**, 338.

33 LIN Y.-L. & ASKONAS B.A. (1981) Biological properties of an influenza A virus-specific killer T cell clone. Inhibition of virus replication *in vivo* and induction of delayed-type hypersensitivity reactions. *J. exp. Med.* **154**, 225.

34 GOMARD E., LEVY J.P., PLATA F., HENIN Y., DUPREZ V., BISMUTH A., REME T. (1978) Studies on the nature of the cell surface antigen reacting with cytotoxic T lymphocytes in murine oncogenic virus induced tumours. *Eur. J. Immunol.* **8**, 228.

35 LOVELAND B.E., HOGARTH P.M., CEREDIG R.H. & MCKENZIE I.F.C. (1981) Cells mediating graft rejection in the mouse. (I) Lyt-1 cells mediate skin graft rejection. *J. exp. Med.* **153**, 1044.

36 LOVELAND B.E. & MCKENZIE I.F.C. (1982) Delayed type hypersensitivity responses and the correlation with graft rejection. *Immunology*, **46**, 313.

37 HÜRME M., CHANDLER P.R., HETHERINGTON C.M. & SIMPSON E. (1978) Cytotoxic T cell responses to H-Y: correlation with the rejection of syngeneic male skin grafts. *J. exp. Med.* **147**, 768.

38 DALLMAN M.J., MASON D.W. & WEBB M. (1982) The role of host and donor cells in the rejection of skin allografts by T-cell-deprived rats injected with syngeneic T cells. *Eur. J. Immunol.* **12**, 511.

39 LIEW F.Y. & SIMPSON E. (1980) Delayed-type hypersensitivity responses to H-Y: characterization and mapping of Ir genes. *Immunogenetics*, **11**, 255.

40 CHANDLER P.R., MATSUNAGA T., BENJAMIN D. & SIMPSON E. (1979) Use and functional properties of peripheral blood lymphocytes in mice. *J. immunol. Meth.* **31**, 341.

41 BOYLE W. (1968) An extension of the ^{51}Cr-release assay for the estimation of mouse cytotoxins. *Transplantation*, **6**, 761.

42 PARISH C.R. & MÜLLBACHER A. (1983) Automated colorimetric assay for T cell cytotoxicity. *J. immunol. Meth.* **58**, 225.

43 STARZINSKI-POWITZ A., PFIZENMAIER K., RÖLLINGHOFF M. & WAGNER H. (1976) *In vivo* sensitization of T cells to hapten-conjugated syngeneic structures of major histocompatibility complex. (I) Effect of *in vitro* culture upon generation of cytotoxic T lymphocytes. *Eur. J. Immunol.* **6**, 799.

44 CZITRON A.A. & GASGOYNE N.R.J. (1983) Primary T cell responses to minor alloantigens. (I) Characterization of cytotoxic effector cells generated from regional lymph nodes after immunization in the footpad. *Immunology*, **50**, 121.

45 WAGNER H. & RÖLLINGHOFF M. (1978) T–T-cell interactions during *in vitro* cytotoxic allograft responses. (1) Soluble products from activated Ly1$^+$ T cells trigger autonomously antigen-primed Ly 23$^+$ T cells to cell proliferation and cytolytic activity. *J. exp. Med.* **148**, 1523.

46 HEDRICK S., COHEN D., NIELSEN E. & DAVIS M.M. (1984) Isolation of cDNS clones encoding T cell specific membrane associated proteins. *Nature*, **308**, 149.

47 YANAGI Y., YOSHIKAI Y., LEGGETT K., CLARK S.P., ALEKSANDER I. & MAK T.W. (1984) A human T cell specific cDNA clone encodes a protein having extensive homology to immunoglobulin chains. *Nature*, **308**, 145.

48 SWAIN S.L., DIALYNAS D.P., FITCH E.W. & ENGLISH M. (1984) Monoclonal antibody to L3T4 blocks the function of T cells specific for class 2 MHC antigens. *J. Immunol.* **132**, 1118.

49 MEUER S.C., ACUTO O., HERCEND T., SCHLOSSMAN S.F. & REINHERZ E.L. (1984) The human T cell receptor. *Ann. Rev. Immunol.* **2**, 23.

50 HOOD L., KRONENBERG M. & HUNKAPILLER T. (1985) T cell antigen receptors and the Immunoglobulin supergene family. *Cell*, **40**, 225.

51 SIMPSON E., MCLAREN A., CHANDLER P. & TOMONARI K. (1984) Expression of H-Y antigen by female mice carrying *Sxr*. *Transplantation*, **37**, 19.

Chapter 69
T cell lines and hybrids in mouse and man

C. G. FATHMAN & E. G. ENGLEMAN

Method for production of culture supernatants containing rat IL-2, 69.2

Method for IL-2 microassay, 69.3

Methods for cloning non-cytolytic, alloreactive murine T cells, 69.3

Cloning of alloreactive cytolytic murine T cells, 69.4

Methods for cloning murine T cells reactive with soluble antigen, 69.5

Cloning of human T cells, 69.6

Production of culture supernatants containing human IL-2, 69.7

Cloning of human T cells by limiting dilution, 69.7

Production of functional human T–T hybridomas, 69.8

Production of murine T–T hybrids, 69.10

Analysis of the molecular basis for cellular interactions and of regulatory and effector functions of lymphocytes has been greatly facilitated by the availability of homogeneous cell populations. Neoplastic myelomas and B cell hybridomas have been particularly useful for determining the structure of antibody molecules and the genetic basis for immunoglobulin formation. Three different approaches have been used to obtain functional monoclonal T cells. Naturally occurring (neoplastic) T lymphomas have been useful for certain purposes such as the production of lymphokines [1,2]. However, relatively few different types of functional T lymphomas exist, and the availability of cells depends largely on the chance occurrence of tumours. Some attempts to induce T lymphomas with specific functions have been successful [3,4]. This technique will not be described in this chapter and interested readers are referred to the publications referenced above. The production of T cell hybridomas has been useful for several purposes, e.g. obtaining a variety of lymphokines, especially suppressor factors [5–12]. In addition, T hybridomas have also been used in attempts to define conditions for activation of T cells by antigen [9]. Methods for obtaining T cell hybridomas will be described in detail below, but it should be recognized that interpretation of results obtained with T lymphomas and T hybridomas are complicated by a possible unrecognized contribution of tumour cell products to the effects observed.

Another approach for obtaining large numbers of identical, functional cells is the derivation of clones of normal T cells using medium containing T cell growth factor (TCGF). Using TCGF (supernate of con A activated splenocytes), long-term lines of mouse cytolytic cells were described [13]. At about the same time, non-cytolytic T cell clones were obtained, utilizing soft agar for cloning in the absence of added TCGF (possibly as a result of endogenous production of T cell growth factor) [14]. Cytolytic T cell clones were developed a few months later [15]. Within a few years, TCGF was renamed interleukin-2 following deliberations at an International Lymphokine Workshop attempting to rationalize lymphokine nomenclature [16]. This designation was given because extensive biochemical and biological data indicated that a single, rather well defined molecule accounted for T cell growth factor activity [17,18].

Most methods now used to obtain cloned T cells depend on the presence of growth factors. In practice, most investigators use crude conditioned medium (CM) or only partially purified material to derive and maintain T cell clones. CM containing IL-2 can be obtained by stimulation of murine lymphoid cells in MLC, by stimulation of rat [17], mouse [18,19], or human [20–22] lymphoid cells with a mitogen, or by appropriate stimulation of selected murine [1,2] or human [23] lymphoma cells. In all of these different CM, IL-2 seems to be (one of) the factor(s) essential for growth of T cells. However, other lymphokines are usually present as well and may account for some of the biological effects observed. It should be noted that unless purified preparations of IL-2 are used, it is hazardous to assume that IL-2 accounts for all of the effects observed when T cells are cultured in the presence of CM. For convenience, the term CM will be used in subsequent discussions to describe the essential T cell growth-promoting material used to support proliferation of cloned T cells, and the above warnings should be remembered.

Two rather distinct approaches have been used to derive and maintain T cell clones. The first employs

CM alone as the stimulus for T cell growth following T cell activation. Responding lymphoid cells, sometimes collected after initial stimulation with antigen *in vivo*, are placed in culture with the appropriate antigen. The cultured cells are then fed (exposed repetitively) only with CM. Usually, with this approach, it is necessary to passage cells in bulk cultures for several weeks before it is possible to isolate clones with a reasonable success rate, since the frequency of T cells capable of growing in CM alone seems to be low [24]. Cloned cells grown with CM alone have a distinct advantage in that the population grows rapidly to large numbers of cells and contains no other type of cell. On the other hand, cloned T cells derived and maintained by culture in CM alone may exhibit fluctuating patterns of antigen reactivity and specificity [15] and frequent karyotypic abnormalities [25].

The second approach for deriving and maintaining T cell clones employs stimulating antigen and 'filler cells' in addition to CM added as a growth 'tonic'. Alloreactive clones can be derived from primary MLC using this approach, and cloning efficiency from secondary cultures may approach 100% [26,27]. In the case of cloned T cells reactive with 'conventional' soluble antigens, the filler cells provide a source of Ia-positive antigen-presenting cells which are required for T cell stimulation [28]. Alloreactive cloned T cells can be stimulated by adherent irradiated allogeneic cells which include macrophages. Although the presence of filler cells may complicate functional studies of T cells cloned with this approach, cloned cells grown with antigen and filler cells appear to be phenotypically and karyotypically more stable than clones grown in CM alone.

The actual clones may be derived by limit dilution [26,29], culture in soft agar [14], or micromanipulation [29]. With repetitive cloning, one can be reasonably confident that cultured cells are clonal descendants if they display uniform and expected phenotypic characteristics. It is possible to obtain a statistical estimate of the likelihood of clonal distribution with both limit dilution and soft agar culture methods, but it may be impossible to be certain that a given 'clone' derived by either of these methods may not consist of descendants of two or more cells. Cloning by micromanipulation, especially if repeated several times, gives the greatest assurance of true clonal derivation.

Method for production of culture supernatants containing rat IL-2

Equipment

CO_2 incubator.
Tissue culture hood.

Materials

Sterile transfer pipettes.
Sterile tissue culture flasks.
Test-tubes.
Adult rats (Sprague-Dawley or other commercially available inbred lines).
Concanavalin A (conA).
Complete culture medium routinely used in the authors' laboratory consists of RPMI 1640 supplemented with 100 units/ml penicillin, 100 μg/ml streptomycin, fetal calf serum at concentrations ranging from 2% to 10%, and 5×10^{-5} M-2-mercaptoethanol. HEPES (12 mM) can be used to buffer the medium. L-glutamine is added at a final concentration of 2×10^{-3} M before use.

Procedure

1 Spleens of 10–40 rats are removed and single cell suspensions are prepared by conventional methodologies. These cells are cultured for 24–48 h at 5×10^6 cells per ml in 70–100 ml portions of complete media and 5 μg per ml con A in 5% CO_2 at 37 °C.
2 Supernates containing T cell growth factors are collected by centrifugation at 1500 rev./min, filtered and stored under sterile conditions at 4 °C until use.

Notes and recommendations

A variety of similar culture conditions have been utilized elsewhere and details of the procedure do not seem to be important [17,18]. Such cultured supernatant can be assayed for T cell growth factor activity in the IL-2 microassay described below. In addition to utilizing rat spleen cells as a source of conditioned medium containing T cell growth factor, secondary mixed lymphocyte culture (MLC) supernates are also a convenient source of conditioned medium. In addition to this source of conditioned medium, there are several murine lymphoma lines which can serve as a source of T cell growth factors. Appropriate sublines of EL-4 tumour cells can be stimulated by phorbol myristate acetate (PMA) and are found to contain high levels of T cell growth factors [2]. For this technique, 1 μg of PMA is added to 100 ml of complete medium in which are cultured 10^8 of the appropriate EL-4 subline. After incubation for 48 h, the supernate is collected by centrifugation and PMA is removed by absorption with charcoal. Briefly activated charcoal (2 g), dextran T-10 (0.5 g), and 165 ml of complete medium are mixed and centrifuged at 9000 **g** in a 200 ml plastic centrifuge tube in a Sorval centrifuge at room temperature for 5 min. The supernate is decanted and the charcoal pellet washed again only with complete medium. After the second wash and decanting, the charcoal pellet is mixed with 165 ml of crude EL-4 TCGF containing supernatant produced by stimulation with PMA. This solution is quickly centrifuged again at 9000 **g**. After 5 min, the supernate is collected as soon as possible and can be stored at 4 °C for use as IL-2 containing conditioned medium without PMA. There are recent reports which suggest that the IL-2 gene has been cloned and expressed by recombinant DNA technology (David Mark, personal communication). The commercial production of IL-2 from such cloned sources may provide a simple and inexpensive method for obtaining large quantities of purified material.

Method for IL-2 microassay

Equipment

CO_2 incubator.
Tissue culture hood.
Microtitre tissue culture plate harvester.
Liquid scintillation counter.

Materials

Complete culture medium.
Tritiated thymidine.
Microtitre plates (Falcon #3072).
Glass fibre filter strips for the automatic harvesting machine.
An IL-2 dependent T cell line such as HT-2.

Procedure

Serial ($\log_2$) dilutions of the sample are plated (100 μl volume) in replicate microtitre culture wells. Dilutions of the sample are made using complete culture medium. Any IL-2 dependent T cell line can serve as an indicator line. Between 3000 and 10 000 T cells harvested from cultures of the IL-2 dependent T cell line are added in 100 μl aliquots of medium to each microplate well. The cells are cultured overnight at 37 °C in an atmosphere of 5% CO_2 in air. After 18 h, each microwell culture is pulsed for an additional 4 h with 1 μCi of tritiated thymidine. The cultures are harvested on the glass fibre filter strips and thymidine incorporation is measured as an index of cellular proliferation. Units per millilitre of IL-2 activity can be standardized. Roughly speaking, a one unit per millilitre of IL-2 sample will induce 50% of the maximum proliferation observed where IL-2 is saturating at a dilution of 1:4 or greater.

Notes and recommendations

In addition to scoring IL-2 activity in serial dilution based upon thymidine incorporation, it is also possible simply to look for viability of cells after 24 h. In the absence of IL-2, IL-2 addicted cell lines die within 24 h. Several laboratories simply use dye exclusion or fluorescein diacetate uptake as a measure of cell viability and as a method for titrating activity of IL-2 in conditioned medium. The IL-2 addicted line, HT-2, as well as the PMA-inducible subline of EL-4, can be obtained from the author.

Methods for cloning non-cytolytic, alloreactive murine T cells

Equipment

CO_2 incubator.
Liquid scintillation counter.
Tissue culture hood.
Microtitre tissue culture plate harvester.
Inverted binocular microscope with phase contrast.
Fluorescence microscope.

Materials

Complete culture medium.
Single cell suspensions of appropriate mouse spleen and/or lymph node cells.
Bacto agar (Difco Laboratories).
10 cm Petri dish (Falcon Plastics, #1001).
Microtitre plates (Falcon #3072).
Costar trays (Costar #3524).
Tissue culture flasks (Falcon #3024).

Procedure

Primary mixed lymphocyte culture

Responder lymph node cells (40×10^6) are co-cultured with $80–100 \times 10^6$ X-irradiated (3300 rads) stimulator cells from the allogeneic spleen. These cells are cultured in Falcon #3024 flasks in complete medium upright at 37 °C, in a water saturated atmosphere of 5% CO_2 in air for 14 days. Recovery of viable cells from a primary MLR using these conditions ranges from 10–50% of the initial responder cell input. Such recovered cells are referred to as primed responder cells (PRC).

Secondary mixed lymphocyte culture

For assay, PRC are recultured at $1–2.5 \times 10^4$ cells in 0.2 ml of fresh complete media in flat-bottom microtitre wells (Falcon #3040) in the presence of 1×10^6 irradiated stimulator spleen cells (these are either syngeneic as control or allogeneic to the PRC). Such cultures are set up in triplicate and harvested at 2 and/or 3 days following initiation of culture. Proliferation is measured in terms of thymidine incorporation of an overnight pulse of 1 μCi of tritiated thymidine.

Soft agar cloning of PRC

PRC obtained after several serial restimulations (more than four) are restimulated with the priming stimulator cell at a cell density of 2×10^6 PRC and 5×10^7 irradiated allogeneic spleen cells in 15 ml of complete medium. Twenty-four hours after initiation of this MLR, cells are centrifuged and aliquots of cells are plated in soft agar. Generally, concentrations of cells ranging from 3×10^4 to 1×10^6 input-primed responder cells are resuspended in 1 ml of their own supernate. Each of these cell suspensions is then mixed with 2 ml of 0.5% Bacto agar in complete medium which has been warmed to 45 °C. This mixture is then spread evenly in a 10 cm Petri dish (Falcon #1001) containing a 15 ml feeder layer of 0.5% Bacto agar made in complete medium. Four to ten days later, colonies can be observed in the soft agar predominantly near the top of the soft agar. These colonies, which consist of 8–100 cells, are picked under an inverted microscope using a drawn out Pasteur pipette and transferred to 0.2 ml of fresh complete medium containing 1×10^6 X-irradiated stimulator spleen cells in microtitre plates (Falcon #3040). After an additional 10–14 days of culture, these cells are transferred into Costar trays (Costar #3524) in 2 ml of complete medium containing 1×10^7 X-irradiated allogeneic spleen cells. After this second transfer, cells are allowed to grow for another 9–14 days, after which time the expanded cells can be transferred into tissue culture flasks containing 5 ml of complete media and 4×10^7 irradiated allogeneic stimulator spleen cells. Such cultures are maintained upright in a water saturated atmosphere of 5% CO_2 in air at 37 °C. Following this expansion, the cells can be assayed for reactivity as described above, further expanded, or, 24 h after restimulation, can be frozen and stored as described below.

Cloning by limit dilution

PRC are diluted in complete media to give a final concentration of 3 cells per ml. Replicate 100 λ aliquots of this cell suspension are then plated into microtitre plates containing 100 μl of complete medium in which 1×10^6 irradiated allogeneic spleen cells and 10% volume per volume rat con A supernate have been added. This gives an average of one cell in every three to four wells. These cells are cultured under the same conditions described above at 37 °C until growth is observed by visual inspection using an inverted microscope. Once cells are growing, they can be transferred to Costar wells in 2 ml of complete medium, in the presence of 1×10^7 irradiated allogeneic stimulator spleen cells. At this second step, it is possible to exclude the addition of exogenous conditioned medium although it can be added as a 'tonic' to ensure a more prompt and reproducible growth of these cells.

Freezing and storage of alloreactive non-cytolytic T cell clones

PRCs or cloned cells may be frozen 24 h after they have been restimulated in culture. The cell mixture is centrifuged; the supernate is discarded; and the cells are resuspended in 1 ml of complete medium containing 10% dimethyl sulphoxide (DMSO) at 4 °C. The cells are frozen by placing them in storage vials within a styrofoam pad in a −70 °C freezer overnight. Under these conditions, freezing occurs at the rate of approximately 1 °C per minute. The cells can then be transferred to liquid nitrogen for storage. Retrieval of these cells can be accomplished by thawing them in a 37 °C water bath, with shaking. At the moment the last ice crystal disappears, the cell suspension is diluted with 10 vols. of fresh complete medium that has been cooled to 4 °C. The cells are then centrifuged and resuspended in 15 ml of complete medium containing 6×10^7 (approximately one-half mouse spleen) irradiated stimulator spleen cells in tissue culture flasks under conditions described above.

Cloning of alloreactive cytolytic murine T cells

Procedure

Conditions for cloning cytolytic T cells are very similar to those outlined above for limit dilution cloning of non-cytolytic T cells. The differences concern the fact that cytolytic murine T cells may be cloned shortly after generation of primary activity *in vitro*; i.e. they are cloned after the initial 14 day primary MLR culture. Such cells are taken 48 h after initiation of the secondary MLC, as described above. Between 0.1 and 1 cell suspended in conditioned medium (see above) is added to a 100 μl aliquot of a microtitre well in a tissue culture plate containing 1×10^6 irradiated (3300 rads) allogeneic spleen cells. The cloning plate is then incubated at 37 °C and fed after 4 days of incubation with an additional 100 λ of a 1:1 mixture of complete medium and conditioned medium. Clusters of cells will begin to appear in the cloning wells approximately 6–9 days after incubation. Screening for cytolytic activity, utilizing a sensitive chromium release microassay, can be performed directly with an aliquot of cells from those wells that contain proliferating cells [30]. Cells that are selected following the microcytotoxicity assay are expanded and maintained routinely by passage at 7 day intervals on irradiated allogeneic stimulator cells in the presence of conditioned medium. For these passages, $1–3 \times 10^4$ cloned T cells in 100 μl are added to Costar wells (Costar #3524) which contain 0.5 ml of CM and 6×10^6 irradiated (3300 rads) stimulator spleen cells in 1 ml of complete medium. Such cloned cells are passaged at 7 day intervals utilizing the same conditions.

Notes and recommendations

Clones of alloreactive T cells can be established from unstimulated spleen or lymph node cells, but the frequency of responding cells is much higher if the responding cells are first stimulated by alloantigen in mixed lymphocyte culture (MLC) [29]. Limit dilution is a convenient method for deriving both cytolytic and non-cytolytic cloned T cells. If unstimulated cells are used, several hundred cells must be added to each microwell.

To develop cloned cells capable of growing in CM alone, it is necessary to maintain bulk cultures for two or more months before cloning is attempted [14,28]. For example, to obtain cytolytic T cells reactive with haptenated cells, mice are immunized by i.p. injection of densely haptenated syngeneic spleen cells. Ten days later, spleen cells from immunized mice are cultured together with hapten-coupled irradiated syngeneic spleen cells. Surviving cells obtained 10 days after initiation of primary culture are cultured at a density of 10^5 cells per ml in rat con A CM, and new cells are established at 4–6 day intervals in fresh rat con A CM. Cell density is maintained between 2×10^4 and 5×10^5 cells per ml. After two months in culture, cells are cloned at limit dilution into microwells containing 10^5 irradiated peritoneal cells in rat con A CM. The frequency of clones capable of indefinite growth in IL-2 containing medium is much greater if cloning is delayed until after several months of bulk culture. Specificity analysis of cytolytic activity of cloned cells derived in this way often indicates that the population has 'cloned' itself [24].

Cellular debris can be removed by centrifugation over a Ficoll-Hypaque gradient [31]. Generally, more than 95% of cells remaining after culture for 7–9 days are cloned T cells. It is possible to maintain cloned T cells for several passages using syngeneic spleen cells and conditioned medium if it is necessary to avoid the presence of alloantigen. It has been possible to use conditioned medium alone to support the short-term growth of such T cell clones, but the yield of cells is significantly lower than if they are maintained on either syngeneic or allogeneic filler cells.

Methods for cloning murine T cells reactive with soluble antigen

Equipment

CO_2 incubator.
Liquid scintillation counter.
Tissue culture hood.
Microtitre tissue culture plate harvester.
Inverted binocular microscope with phase contrast.
Fluorescence microscope.

Materials

Complete culture medium.
Single cell suspensions of appropriate mouse spleen and/or lymph node cells.
Fluorescein diacetate (FDA) (5 mg per ml in acetone stored at -20 °C).
Bacto agar (Difco Laboratories).
10 cm Petri dish (Falcon Plastics, #1001).
Microtitre plates (Falcon #3040).
Costar trays (Costar #3524).
Tissue culture flasks (Falcon #3024).

Procedure

Mice of the haplotype selected for responsiveness (4–5 per group) are immunized with appropriate amounts of soluble antigen (generally around 100 μg of protein) emulsified in complete Freund's adjuvant and injected subcutaneously at the base of the tail, according to the method of Corradin *et al.* [32]. Seven days later, draining lymph nodes are removed and single cell suspensions are made and cultured in Costar trays (Costar #3524) with appropriate amounts of soluble antigen (approximately 10–50 μg per ml) at a cell number of 5×10^6 cells per well in 2 ml of complete medium. Four days later, the cells are harvested and blast cells are selected by layering on Ficoll-Hypaque followed by centrifugation at 2000 rev./min for 20 min. Cells from the interface are collected, washed twice with complete medium, and recultured in Costar wells (#3524) with 5×10^6 irradiated (3300 rads) syngeneic spleen cells as filler cells at a concentration of 1×10^5 primed T cells per ml in 2 ml of complete medium. After 7–14 days, cells are harvested and viability assayed utilizing FDA; 2×10^5 viable recovered cells are restimulated with appropriate amounts of antigen in the presence of 5×10^6 syngeneic irradiated filler cells in 2 ml of complete medium. If recultured after 4 days, the cells are harvested, blast cells are selected by Ficoll-Hypaque centrifugation, and recultured with syngeneic irradiated filler cells in the absence of antigen at a concentration of 1×10^5 blast cells and 2.5×10^6 filler cells per ml in 2 ml of complete medium for an additional 7–14 days. Cells can be assayed 7–14 days after reculture by taking aliquots of viable recovered cells and restimulating them in the presence of appropriate antigen. Generally, we assay 2×10^4 antigen-reactive T cells and 1×10^6 irradiated syngeneic spleen filler cells in 200 μl of complete medium, in the presence of appropriate amounts of antigen. These cells are co-cultured in microtitre plates, in triplicate samples for 48–72 h prior to the addition of tritiated thymidine, and harvested.

Notes and recommendations

This technology has been extremely useful in the generation of antigen-specific helper murine T cell clones. Such cells have been assayed in a variety of *in vitro* and *in vivo* models of help [33–35]. The long-term stability of the helper phenotype has yet to be proved with such cells. It is quite clear from work in the authors' laboratory that a period of rest in the absence of antigen is required only if the ultimate use of the cells is an assay of antigen-specific B cell help. If these antigen-specific T cell clones are simply to be recultured and/or assayed for proliferation, the step of washing away excess antigen may be omitted and the cells may be simply left in the presence of residual antigen. The authors have been able to maintain antigen-reactive T cells by this cyclical restimulation for culture periods of greater than three years. In experiments where large numbers of cells are required, such cells can be restimulated and recultured in an upright position in tissue culture flasks (Falcon #3024) in a total volume of 15 ml complete medium with the appropriate concentration of antigen-reactive T cells, antigen and filler cells. In addition to assays of antigen-specific help, such inducer T cells produce a variety of lymphokines and their production can serve as a separate assay of antigen-specific reactivity of such inducer T cell clones. In fact, the array of lymphokines produced by inducer T cell clones varies. Some secrete a large number of different factors while others release a more restricted variety [36,37]. To date, there appears to be no correlation between the types of lymphokine produced and the antigenic reactivities of cloned T cells. Modifications of this cloning procedure have been utilized to derive cloned

suppressor cells in other laboratories (Richard Hodes and Yoshi Asano, personal communication).

Cloning of human T cells

Introduction

The requirements and techniques for propagation of human T cells are similar in most respects to those described for murine T cells. Although human IL-2 supports the growth of murine T cells, the reverse is not the case and, therefore, human IL-2 is required for the propagation of human T cells. For investigators that have access to large numbers of human lymphoid cells provided by apheresis of a normal blood donor, or pooled buffy coats from several donors, or from spleens removed at surgery, production of CM using mitogen stimulation is not difficult [20]. Alternative sources include T leukaemia cell lines or hybrids that secrete IL-2 either constitutively or on exposure to mitogens and/or phorbal esters. Finally, human IL-2 produced by recombinant DNA technology has already been shown to propagate human T cells for periods of several weeks, and highly purified recombinant IL-2 should soon be generally available for *in vitro* research purposes.

Two problems in the cloning of antigen-specific human T cells are the inability to deliberately immunize humans with any but ethical antigens, and limited access to cells from lymphoid organs, i.e. dependence on peripheral blood lymphocytes (PBL). To date, long term human T cell lines and clones have been limited primarily to those responsive to alloantigens, infectious agents (e.g. influenza and herpes viruses) and protein vaccines (e.g. tetanus and diphtheria toxoids). Primary immunization, *in vitro*, is under study by a number of investigators, but the general experience to date is that sensitization *in vivo* is a prerequisite for production of stable, long term, antigen-specific clones.

Another problem in the propagation of human T cells is the availability of suitable feeder and/or antigen presenting cells, which may be required for maintenance and expansion of antigen-specific clones. For example, it is difficult to obtain blood from the same subject by repeated venipuncture at 7–10 day intervals for more than a few weeks; unless several HLA identical relatives are accessible, the authors generally obtain 10^9–10^{10} lymphoid cells from a consenting subject by leukopheresis, and then cryopreserve aliquots of 10^7 cells per vial so that individual vials can be thawed as necessary for use as feeders. In the case of alloreactive cytotoxic or helper clones, a single cell source can be used as feeder and antigen, and it appears that Epstein-Barr virus transformed lymphoblastoid lines may sometimes be adequate for these purposes. Finally, spleen or lymph nodes removed surgically from tumour bearing hosts may provide all three necessary cell components for the generation of tumour reactive T cell clones: tumour sensitized T cells, tumour antigen, and normal accessory cells.

Production of culture supernatants containing human IL-2

Equipment

Centrifuge.
CO_2 incubator.
Tissue culture hood.
137-Cesium irradiator (J.L. Shepherd, Glendale, CA).

Materials

Sterile transfer pipettes.
Sterile tissue culture flasks.
Ficoll-Hypaque.
Modified Iscove's DMEM medium (Gibco) supplemented with 10% fetal calf serum or human male AB serum.
5×10^{-5} M-2-mercaptoethanol.
25 mM-HEPES and 2 mM-glutamine (basic growth medium).
Phytohaemagglutinin (PHA-P, Burroughs-Wellcome).

Procedure (for production of 100 ml)

1 Isolate peripheral blood mononuclear cells (PBL) from each of two donors by Ficoll-Hypaque gradient centrifugation of either anticoagulated peripheral blood or buffy coats freshly prepared from donated whole blood units. A typical buffy coat contains $2-4 \times 10^8$ PBL, whereas $1-2 \times 10^6$ PBL can usually be obtained from each millilitre of whole blood. Anticoagulation with preservative-free heparin or acid-citrate-dextrose (ACD) is acceptable. For smaller volumes, the authors prefer to defibrinate blood with sterilized glass beads in order to reduce platelet contamination.
2 5×10^7 PBL from each donor are suspended in 10 ml of basic growth medium and irradiated with 1 500 rads.
3 Pool approximately 3.33×10^7 Epstein-Barr virus (EBV) transformed lymphoblastoid cells (in log growth phase) from each of three unrelated donors (representing different HLA-DR allotypes) in a total of 50 ml basic growth medium and irradiate with 10 000 rads.
4 Mix 1×10^8 irradiated PBL and 1×10^8 irradiated EBV cell lines in 70 ml basic growth medium.

By first removing adherent cells from the 50×10^6 PBL mixture and then irradiating the non-adherent cells (1000 rads), the yield of IL-2 can be substantially increased by admixture of the irradiated non-adherent cells with an equal number of EBV transformed B lymphoblastoid cells (i.e. 2×10^6 cells/ml added back to the adherent-cell-containing flasks).
5 Add 1 μg/ml PHA-P, adjust volume to 100 ml, and incubate in 150 cm² flasks at 37 °C in an incubator containing 6–8% CO_2.
6 After 48 h, the supernatant containing IL-2 is harvested by centrifugation at 1 500 **g** for 10 min, followed by filtration through a 0.22 μm filter to ensure sterility. It can be stored at −70 °C.
7 To determine the IL-2 titre, carry out the assay using an IL-2 dependent cell line as described previously for determination of rat IL-2. Murine or human IL-2 dependent cell lines can be used for this purpose; in either case, a rapidly growing line is preferred.

Notes and recommendations

Occasionally, an excess of monocytes will inhibit IL-2 production. This problem can be obviated by removing adherent cells from PBL prior to culture by incubating PBL on plastic Petri dishes for 1–2 h at 37 °C followed by removal of the non-adherent cells.

Cloning of human T cells by limiting dilution

Equipment

CO_2 incubator.
Tissue culture hood.
^{137}Cs irradiator (J.L. Shepherd, Glendale, CA).

Materials

Modified Iscove's DMEM (Gibco) supplemented with 10% fetal calf serum or male AB serum.
5×10^{-5} M-mercaptoethanol and 2 mM-glutamine (basic growth medium).
IL-2 containing growth medium.
Acridine orange–ethidium bromide for determining cell viability.
96-, 24-, and 12-well tissue culture plates (Costar).
Percoll (Pharmacia).

Procedure

1 Prior to propagation in IL-2-containing medium, 10^6 T cells per ml are primed in basic growth medium with 10^6 irradiated (3 000 rads) non-T accessory cells, and an optimal concentration of antigen. Following

7–10 days of culture at 37 °C in 5–8% CO_2, T blasts are isolated over discontinuous Percoll gradients and cloned by the method of limiting dilution.

2   The cloning medium consists of basic growth medium supplemented with 10^7 autologous irradiated (3 000 rads) PBL per ml and IL-2 containing medium, at a concentration found to be optimal in assays on IL-2 dependent lines. The objective is to plate 36 wells of a 96-well tissue culture plate with an average of five cells per well, 36 wells with an average of one cell per well, and the remaining 24 wells with an average of 0.5 cell per well. One of these plating conditions should yield wells with monoclonal growth. The dilutions are carried out by removing samples from the 1 ml cultures and determining the concentration of viable cells by staining with acridine orange–ethidium bromide.

3   A sample of the cells to be cloned should be diluted such that 230 live cells are suspended in 4.6 ml of the PBL-containing cloning medium. Thirty-six wells are plated with 0.1 ml of this mixture, leaving 1 ml of cell suspension. An additional 4 ml of the PBL-containing medium are added to the remaining 1 ml and another 36 wells are plated with 0.1 ml. Finally, 1.4 ml of the PBL containing medium are added to the remaining cell suspension and plated into the last 24 wells [43].

4   At day 5, and again at day 12, the cloning plate is fed by adding two drops of medium with a Pasteur pipette. By days 14–20, the clones should be large enough to expand into 4 replicate wells.

5   Following an additional week of growth in these wells, the cells are pooled and mixed with 1×10^6 autologous PBL, irradiated to 3 000 rads, and transferred in 2 ml to 1 well of a 12-well tissue culture plate for continued growth.

6   Thereafter, the wells are fed every other day in the same medium without antigen. One millilitre of spent medium is removed and 1 ml of fresh medium added, and the proliferating colonies are dispersed.

7   When a well becomes confluent with viable cells, the cells are split into 2 wells. Feeders consisting of 1×10^6 irradiated PBL per well in addition to antigen are usually required every 2 weeks. The growing cells are frozen as often as possible at $5–10 \times 10^6$ cells per ml in 10% dimethyl sulphoxide and 25% fetal calf serum in basic growth medium and stored in liquid nitrogen.

Production of functional human T–T hybridomas

Introduction

The use of T–T hybridomas, produced by the fusion of an activated T cell with a malignant T cell line, offers an alternative source of enriched T cell derived products with the advantage of continuous growth in the absence of exogenous growth promoters. Hybridoma technology, originally developed by Kohler & Milstein for the production of monoclonal antibody secreting B cell hybrids, involves fusion of the two cell types with a fusogen such as polyethylene glycol (PEG), expansion of the hybridomas in a selective medium that allows hybrids but not unfused parent cells to grow, and identification and propagation of hybrids with a desired function or product (see Chapter 108). To produce antigen-reactive hybridomas, it is essential to use antigen sensitized T cells, and such cells can be enriched by secondary stimulation *in vitro* or by longer term propagation, utilizing T cell growth factor and the techniques described in the previous section. Following the growth of hybrids in selective medium for a period of one to a few weeks, hybridomas should be transferred to and expanded in medium free of aminopterin or azaserine because the latter are inhibitory of proliferative assays. The procedures described below for production of mutant T cell lines, fusion with activated T cells, and assay for functional products have worked in the authors' hands [38], but the reader is referred to alternative approaches described by other investigators [39–43].

Equipment

Centrifuge.
Tissue culture hood.
CO_2 and temperature regulated incubator.
Inverted binocular microscope with phase contrast.
Fluorescence microscope.

Materials

RPMI 1640 (Gibco)/25 mM-HEPES/2 mM-L-glutamine/10% fetal calf serum.
6-Thioguanine (SIGMA).
Polyethylene glycol (Mr 1500, BDH Chemicals, Poole, England).
NCTC 109 medium (Microbiological Associates, Walkersville, Maryland).
Hypoxanthine (SIGMA).
Azaserine (SIGMA).
Vinblastine (Lilly).
Methanol/glacial acetic acid, 3:1.
Giemsa stain (SIGMA).
96- and 24-well microtitre trays and 25 cm² tissue culture flasks (Flow Laboratories, McLean, Virginia).

Procedures

Derivation of a 6-thioguanine-resistant T leukaemia line

6-Thioguanine-resistant T cell lines can be derived from human T leukaemia lines (e.g. the Jurkat line) by placing the line in RPMI 1640 medium supplemented with 25 mM-HEPES, 2 mM-glutamine, 10% fetal calf serum, and 1 μM-6-thioguanine. Prior to this step, the line may be optionally exposed to a mutagenic agent in order to increase the frequency of mutants. After one week of growth in humidified 95% air/5% CO_2 at 37 °C, the viable cells should be separated by Ficoll-Hypaque gradient centrifugation and placed in the same nutrient medium with a higher concentration of 6-thioguanine. Over a 6 week period, the levels of 6-thioguanine should be increased to approximately 0.2 mM. A rapidly growing clone can be derived by the method of limit dilution and used in hybridization experiments. One such clone, designated J3R7, has been used in fusion experiments in the authors' laboratory and is available from the authors on request.

Cell isolation and activation

Normal T lymphocytes from a variety of tissue sources may be used in the fusion; peripheral blood mononuclear leukocytes (PBL), spleen cells, thoracic duct cells, lymph node cells, bone marrow cells, and tonsil cells are examples. For convenience, PBL are usually preferred. PBL prepared from normal donor blood by Ficoll-Hypaque gradient centrifugation can be stimulated with antigens or mitogens in bulk culture or propagated and cloned using T cell growth factor as described earlier. Peripheral blood monocytes are enriched by adherence to plastic or glass Petri dishes at 37 °C for 1 h and harvested by pipetting with calcium-free medium containing 0.1% EDTA. Such cells are used as feeders after irradiation with 8000 rads from a ^{137}Cs source.

Fusion procedure

4×10^7 T cells and 4×10^7 mutant tumour cells are mixed in 1 ml of 50% (v/v) polyethylene glycol (Mr 1500; BDH Chemicals, Poole, England) in RPMI 1640 over one minute. The suspension is centrifuged for 3 min at 500 **g**. After 8 min, the cell pellet is suspended in 1 ml of RPMI 1640 with slow mixing over a period of 1 min, followed by addition of 6 ml of RPMI 1640/10% fetal calf serum. The cells are then pelleted at 250 **g** for 10 min and the pellet washed twice in RPMI 1640/10% fetal calf serum. Thereafter, the cells are suspended in RPMI 1640/25 mM-HEPES/2 mM-glutamine/15%

fetal calf serum/100 mM-hypoxanthine/azaserine (1 mg per ml) (SIGMA) (AH medium). The cells are cultured in 24-well trays at a concentration of 10^6 tumour cells per well in a 1 ml volume with a feeder layer of 2×10^5 adherent cells per well. The cultures are maintained in 37 °C in humidified 95% air/5% CO_2. After 10 days, the medium should be altered by removing azaserine. In general, the medium should be changed approximately every 3 days.

Confirmation of hybridization by analysis of chromosomes and cell surface markers

Chromosome preparations are produced according to standard techniques. Approximately 10^6 cells per ml are placed in basic growth medium containing vinblastine at 0.5 mg/ml. After 3 h of incubation, the cells are harvested by centrifugation at 250 **g** for 10 min. The cell pellet is then suspended in 5 ml of hypotonic solution (growth medium/distilled water, 1:2) for 10 min. The cells are then pelleted, washed twice in fixative (methanol/glacial acetic acid, 3:1), suspended in a few drops of fixative, air dried on microscope slides, stained with Giemsa and examined microscopically. Hybrids produced in the manner described should contain substantially more than 46 chromosomes (the number in each fusion partner) and in the authors' hands tend to vary between 70 and 92 immediately after fusion. Over time, the number of chromosomes in individual hybrid clones often declines.

Confirmation of hybridization should also be carried out by detection of cell surface markers on hybrids that are absent from the mutant leukaemia line used as the fusion partner. For example, the J3R7 line expresses the Leu 1 and Leu 4 'pan T' markers but lacks the Leu 2a and Leu 3a subset specific markers, and hybrids of this line and activated Leu 3a⁺ (helper) T cells were shown to express the Leu 3a marker based upon staining with monoclonal anti-Leu 3a antibody and analysis in a cell sorter [38]. The HLA A or B antigens of the normal T cell partner may be expressed on the hybridoma in addition to the A and B antigens of the T cell line, and such antigens can be detected in standard microcytotoxicity assays using defined alloantisera.

Functional assays

T cell hybrids derived from the fusion of activated T cells and a T leukaemia line may produce soluble immunoregulatory factors either constitutively or on exposure to the antigen responsible for the initial sensitization of the normal T cell partner. To identify constitutively produced factors, assays for such factors need only be carried out on spent supernatant (after removal of azaserine). To identify factors produced by antigen reactive hybrids, hybrids must be exposed to the antigen presented by an appropriate accessory cell prior to factor assay. A convenient method for identifying antigen specific helper hybrids is to expose the hybrid to antigen and, thereafter, to measure the production of IL-2 by the hybridoma. Assays for the measurement of IL-2 have been described previously. This technique has been used by Lakow *et al.* [42] to identify antigen reactive human T cell hybrids.

Notes and recommendations

In the authors' experience (which is described in detail in ref. 38), avoidance of thymidine and aminopterin in selection medium is of critical importance in the growth of T–T hybrids. In fact, the observation that thymidine and aminopterin (standard components of HAT selective medium, which has been used extensively in the production of B–B hybrids) were inhibitory of T–T hybrid growth provided the basis of the authors' search for an alternative selective medium. Azaserine was chosen because its main action is irreversible binding of various L-glutamine aminotransferases that are necessary in *de novo* purine synthesis, but it has little or no effect on pyrimidine biosynthesis. Therefore, in selection medium containing azaserine, hypoxanthine is necessary for DNA synthesis but exogenous thymidine is not.

A persistent problem in the production of functional T cell hybrids is their instability over time, due apparently to the loss of chromosomes. To some extent, this problem can be obviated by the frequent cloning of hybrids, and it is possible that as newly derived mutant T cell lines become available their resultant hybrids will be more stable.

Production of murine T–T hybrids

Equipment

CO_2 incubator.
Liquid scintillation counter.
Tissue culture hood.
Microtitre tissue culture plate harvester.
Inverted binocular microscope with phase contrast.
Fluorescence microscope.

Materials

Polyethylene glycol (PEG), Mr 1500, BW5147, an HGPRT-negative AKR thymoma line obtained originally from Dr. R. Hyman (available from the author).
Dulbecco's Modified Eagle's Medium (DMEM).
Hypoxanthine, thymidine, and aminopterin.

Procedure

Approximately 10^8 antigen-primed T cells (having either helper or suppressor function) are admixed with 10^7 BW5147 cells, which are HGPRT-negative, and washed twice in serum-free balanced salt solution (BSS). The cells are then centrifuged at 400 **g** and the supernate is poured off. One-half millilitre of PEG, Mr 1500, 50% in BSS, pH 7.8, is added dropwise over 2 min as the cells are gently shaken into suspension. One-half millilitre of serum-free BSS is then added dropwise at the same rate. An additional 5 ml of BSS is then slowly added before finally filling the tube to 20 ml with BSS. The cells are then spun at 400 **g** and the supernate is discarded. The cells are subsequently resuspended in 100 ml DMEM with 20% FCS and dispensed into 2 ml aliquots in Costar trays.

Approximately 24 h after this fusion procedure, 1 ml of the culture supernate is removed and replaced by 1 ml of HAT medium (DMEM plus 20% FCS containing 1.1×10^{-4} M-hypoxanthine, 1.6×10^{-3} M-thymidine, and 4×10^{-7} M-aminopterin). This procedure is repeated for the next 2 days. On days 6, 8, and 10, HT medium is used (DMEM plus 20% FCS containing 1.1×10^{-4} M-hypoxanthine and 1.6×10^{-5} M-thymidine). Thereafter, starting on days 12 or 13, the medium is slowly changed to DMEM plus 10% FCS by removing 1 ml of the old supernate and replacing it with 1 ml of fresh DMEM with 10% FCS at 3 day intervals. The contents of each Costar well, which begin to grow within the next one to three weeks, can be subcultured in Costar wells and transferred to small tissue culture flasks in this supporting medium. Aliquots of the supernate cultures can then be tested for the function that characterized the cells prior to fusion with BW5147.

References

1 GILLIS S., SCHEID M. & WATSON J. (1980) The biochemical and biological characterization of lymphocyte regulatory molecules. (III) The isolation and phenotypic characterization of Interleukin 2 producing T cell lymphomas. *J. Immunol.* **125,** 2570.

2 FARRAR J.J., FULLER-FARRAR J., SIMON P.L., HILFIKER M.L., STADLER B.M. & FARRAR W.L. (1980) Thymoma production of T cell growth factor (Interleukin 2). *J. Immunol.* **125,** 2555.

3 FINN O.J., BONIVER J. & KAPLAN H.S. (1979) Induction, establishment *in vitro* and characterization of functional

antigen-specific, carrier-primed murine T-cell lymphomas. *Proc. natn. Acad. Sci. U.S.A.* **76**, 4033.

4 RICCIARDI-CASTAGNOLI P., DORIA G. & ADORINI L. (1981) Production of antigen-specific suppressive T cell factor by radiation leukemia virus-transformed suppressor T cells. *Proc. natn. Acad. Sci. U.S.A.* **78**, 3804.

5 HARWELL L., SKIDMORE B., MARRACK P. & KAPPLER J.W. (1980) Concanavalin A-inducible interleukin-2-producing T cell hybridomas. *J. exp. Med.* **153**, 893.

6 TAUSSIG M.J., CORVALAN J.R.F., BINNS R.M. & HOLLIMAN A. (1979) Production of an H-2 related suppressor factor by a hybrid T-cell line. *Nature*, **277**, 305.

7 TANIGUCHI M. & MILLER J.F.A.P. (1978) Specific suppressive factors produced by hybridomas derived from the fusion of enriched suppressor T-cells and a T lymphoma cell line. *J. exp. Med.* **148**, 373.

8 KONTIAINEN S., SIMPSON E., BOHRER E., BEVERLEY P.C.L., HERZENBERG L.A., FITZPATRICK W.C., VOGT P., TORANO A., MCKENZIE I.F.C. & FELDMANN M. (1978) T-cell lines producing antigen-specific suppressor factor. *Nature*, **274**, 477.

9 KAPPLER J.W., SKIDMORE B., WHITE J. & MARRACK P. (1981) Antigen-inducible H-2 restricted, interleukin-2-producing T cell hybridomas. Lack of independent antigen and *H-2* recognition. *J. exp. Med.* **153**, 1198.

10 PACIFICO A. & CAPRA J.D. (1980) T cell hybrids with arsonate specificity. (I) Initial characterization of antigen-specific T cell products that bear a cross-reactive idiotype and determinants encoded by the murine major histocompatibility complex. *J. exp. Med.* **152**, 1289.

11 CLARK A.F. & CAPRA J.D. (1982) Ubiquitous nonimmunoglobulin *p*-azobenzene-arsonate-binding molecules from lymphoid cells. *J. exp. Med.* **155**, 611.

12 TAUSSIG M., HOLLIMAN A. & WRIGHT L.J. (1980) Hybridization between T and B lymphoma cell lines. *Immunology*, **39**, 57.

13 GILLIS S. & SMITH K.A. (1977) Long-term culture of tumour-specific cytotoxic T cells. *Nature*, **268**, 154.

14 FATHMAN C.G. & HENGARTNER H. (1978) Clones of alloreactive T-cells. *Nature*, **272**, 617.

15 NABHOLZ M., ENGERS H.D., COLLAVO D. & NORTH M. (1978) Cloned T cell lines with specific cytolytic activity. *Curr. Top. Microbiol. Immunol.* **81**, 176.

16 AARDEN L.A. *et al.* (1979) Revised nomenclature for antigen non-specific T-cell proliferation and helper factors. *J. Immunol.* **123**, 2928.

17 GILLIS S., SMITH K.A. & WATSON J.D. (1980) Biochemical and biological characterization of lymphocyte regulatory molecules. (II) Purification of a class of rat and human lymphokines. *J. Immunol.* **124**, 1954.

18 WATSON J., GILLIS S., MARBROOK J., MOCHIZUKI D. & SMITH K.A. (1979) Biochemical and biological characterization of lymphocyte regulatory molecules. (I) Purification of a class of murine lymphokines. *J. exp. Med.* **150**, 849.

19 ROSENBERG S.A., SPIESS P.J. & SCHWARZ S. (1978) *In vitro* growth of murine T cells. (I) Production of factors necessary for T cell growth. *J. Immunol.* **121**, 1946.

20 MIER J.W. & GALLO R.C. (1980) Purification and some characteristics of human T-cell growth factor (TCGF) from PHA-stimulated lymphocyte conditioned media. *Proc. natn. Acad. Sci. U.S.A.* **77**, 6134.

21 STRAUSSER J.L. & ROSENBERG S.A. (1978) *In vitro* growth of cytotoxic human lymphocytes. (I) Growth of cells sensitized *in vitro* to alloantigens. *J. Immunol.* **121**, 1491.

22 INOUYE H., HANK J.A., ALTER B.J. & BACH F.H. (1980b) TCGF production for cloning and growth of functional human T lymphocytes. *Scand. J. Immunol.* **12**, 149.

23 GILLIS S. & WATSON J. (1980) Biochemical and biological characterization of lymphocyte regulatory molecules. (V) Identification of an Interleukin 2 producer human leukemia T cell line. *J. exp. Med.* **152**, 1709.

24 HAAS W., MATHUR-ROCHAT J., POHLIT H., NABHOLZ M. & VON BOEHMER H. (1980) Cytotoxic T cell responses to haptenated cells. (III) Isolation and specificity analysis of continuously growing clones. *Eur. J. Immunol.* **10**, 828.

25 JOHNSON J.P., CIANFRIGLIA M., GLASEBROOK A.L. & NABHOLZ M. (1982) Karyotype evolution of cytolytic T cell lines. In *Isolation, Characterization and Utilization of T Lymphocyte Clones*, (eds. Fathman C.G. & Fitch F.W.), p. 183. Academic Press Inc.

26 HENGARTNER H. & FATHMAN C.G. (1980) Clones of alloreactive T cells. (I) A unique homozygous MLR stimulating determinant present on B6 stimulators. *Immunogenetics*, **10**, 175.

27 GLASEBROOK A.L. & FITCH F.W. (1979) T cell lines which cooperate in generation of specific cytolytic activity. *Nature*, **278**, 171.

28 KIMOTO M. & FATHMAN C.G. (1980) Antigen reactive T cell clones. (I) Transcomplementing hybrid I–A region gene products function effectively in antigen presentation. *J. exp. Med.* **152**, 759.

29 MACDONALD H.R., CEROTTINI J.-C., RYSER J.-E., MARYANSKI J.L., TASWELL C., WIDMER M.B. & BRUNNER K.T. (1980a) Quantitation and cloning of cytolytic T lymphocytes and their precursors. *Immunol. Revs.* **51**, 93.

30 ENGERS H.D. & FITCH F.W. (1979) An estimate of the minimal frequency of cytolytic T lymphocyte effector cells generated in allogeneic reactions. *J. immunol. Meth.* **25**, 13.

31 DAVIDSON W. & PARISH C.R. (1975) A procedure for removing red cells and dead cells from lymphoid cell suspension. *J. immunol. Meth.* **7**, 291.

32 CORRADIN G.H., ETLINGER M. & CHILLER J.M. (1977) Lymphocyte specificity to protein antigens. (I) Characterization of the antigen-induced *in vitro* T cell-dependent proliferative response with lymph node cells from primed mice. *J. Immunol.* **119**, 1048.

33 HODES R.J., KIMOTO M., HATHCOCK K.S., FATHMAN C.G. & SINGER A. (1981) Functional helper activity of monoclonal T cell populations: antigen-specific and H-2 restricted cloned T cells provide help for *in vitro* antibody responses to trinitrophenyl-poly(1Try,Glu)-poly(DLAla)--poly(LLys). *Proc. natn. Acad. Sci. U.S.A.* **78**, 6431.

34 HODES R.J., SHIGETA M., HATHCOCK K.S., FATHMAN C.G., SINGER A. (1982) Role of the major histocompatibility complex in T cell activation of B cell subpopulations: antigen-specific and H-2 restricted monoclonal T_H cells activate Lyb-5+ B cells through an antigen-nonspecific and H-2-unrestricted effector pathway. *J. Immunol.* **129**, 267.

35 ASANO Y., SHIGETA M., FATHMAN C.G., SINGER A. & HODES R.J. (1982) Role of the major histocompatibility complex in T cell activation of B cell subpopulations. A single monoclonal T helper cell population activates different B cell subpopulations by distinct pathways. *J. exp. Med.* **156,** 350.

36 GLASEBROOK A.L., KELSO A., ZUBLER R.H., ELY J.M., PRYSTOWSKY M.C. & FITCH F.W. (1982) Lymphokine production by cytolytic and noncytolytic alloreactive T cell clones. In *Isolation, Characterization and Utilization of T Lymphocyte Clones*, (eds. Fathman C.G. & Fitch F.W.), p. 341. Academic Press Inc.

37 PRYSTOWSKY M.B., ELY J.M., BELLER D.I., EISENBERG L., GOLDMAN J., GOLDMAN M., GOLDWASSER E., IHLE J., QUINTANS J., REMOLD H., VOGEL S. & FITCH F.W. (1982) Alloreactive cloned T cell lines. (VI) Multiple lymphokine activities secreted by helper and cytolytic cloned T lymphocytes. *J. Immunol.* **129,** 2337.

38 FOUNG S.K.H., SASAKI D.T., GRUMET F.C. & ENGLEMAN E.G. (1982) Production of functional human T-T hybridomas in selection medium lacking aminopterin and thymidine. *Proc. natn. Acad. Sci. U.S.A.* **79,** 7494.

39 GRILLOT-COURVALINE C., BROUET J.C., BERGER R. & BERNHEIM A. (1981) Establishment of a human T cell hybrid line with suppressive activity. *Nature,* **292,** 844.

40 KOBAYASHI Y., ASADA M., HIGUCHI M. & OSAWA T. (1982) Human T cell hybridomas producing lymphokines. *J. Immunol.* **128,** 2714.

41 LE J., VILCEK J., SAXINGER C. & PRENSKY W. (1982) Human T cell hybridomas secreting immune interferon. *Proc. natn. Acad. Sci. U.S.A.* **79,** 7857.

42 LAKOW E., TSOUKAS C.D., VAUGHAN J.H., ALTMAN A. & CARSON D.A. (1983) Human T cell hybridomas for Epstein-Barr virus infected B lymphocytes. *J. Immunol.* **130,** 169.

43 ENGLEMAN E.G., FOUNG S.K.H., LARRICK J.A. & RAUBITSCHEK A. (eds.) (1985) *Human Hybridomas and Monoclonal Antibodies.* Plenum Press, New York.

Chapter 70
B cell growth factors

MAUREEN HOWARD

Types of B cell growth factors,
  70.1

Assay for mouse BCGF-I, 70.4
Sources of mouse BCGF-I, 70.5

Biochemical characteristics of
  mouse BCGF-I, 70.5
Long-term B cell lines, 70.7

Despite a detailed knowledge of the antigen-specific receptor expressed on the membrane of B lymphocytes, the precise mechanism by which B lymphocytes are activated during antigenic encounter has remained an area of controversy. Contending viewpoints originally attributed induction of B cell proliferation to the delivery of signals at membrane-bound immunoglobulin itself (Ig), at membrane-bound Ia molecules, or at uncharacterized membrane-bound 'mitogen receptors'. However, the recent discovery of soluble factors specifically involved in B cell proliferation has undermined such simplistic models. Now a more tenable hypothesis would seem to be that occupancy of membrane Ig (or mitogen receptors) by antigen and/or cognate T cell interactions involving the Ia antigens of resting B cells results in functional expression of receptors for soluble proliferation co-factors, and that it is these factors which in turn stimulate B cells to replicate. This chapter will discuss the biological and biochemical nature of such B cell specific proliferation co-factors (B cell growth factors) and consider the technical and conceptual advances that their manipulation potentially offers us.

Types of B cell growth factors

For the purpose of this review, the general term B cell growth factor (BCGF) is used to denote a soluble-cell-derived product that is involved functionally in B cell proliferation. Several distinct products of this type have thus far been described. To distinguish these products throughout this chapter, the following system of nomenclature will be adopted.

Mouse BCGF-I (18k BCGF)

The term B cell growth factor was initially used to designate the T-cell-derived B cell co-stimulator that synergizes with affinity-purified anti-IgM antibodies to induce polyclonal B cell proliferation [1]. This factor, a glycoprotein of approximate Mr 18 000 by gel

filtration analysis, will henceforth be referred to as mouse BCGF-I, to distinguish it from the other B cell growth factors discussed in this review. Mouse BCGF-I was identified using a short-term B cell co-stimulator assay where highly purified B cells were cultured with affinity purified goat anti-mouse IgM antibodies for 3 days, with a final 16 h pulse of ^{3}H-thymidine to assess proliferation. As shown in Fig. 70.1, when B cells were cultured at high cell density ($\geqslant 10^5$/microtitre well) and in the presence of doses of anti-IgM which were far in excess of what would be required to saturate membrane Ig receptors (i.e. 50 μg/ml), excellent proliferation was obtained in the absence of exogenously added factor. However, when lower cell densities and/or lower doses of anti-IgM were used, proliferation was dependent upon exogenously added mouse BCGF-I. For the experiments illustrated in Fig. 70.1, this was provided by supplementing cultures with PMA-induced supernatant from a subline of the cloned murine thymoma EL4. On the basis of these data, the routine assay developed for mouse BCGF-I was 5×10^4 purified splenic B cells per microtitre well, plus anti-IgM at a final concentration of 5 μg/ml, plus the factor source under test.

In addition to PMA-induced EL4 supernatant, mouse BCGF-I is found in antigen-induced supernatants from normal T cell helper lines [2] propagated in long-term culture as described by Kimoto & Fathman [3]. Recently, murine B cell growth factors with similar physical and biological properties to BCGF-I have also been detected in constitutive or con A-induced supernatants from two T cell hybridomas [4,5] and in con A-induced supernatants from two alloreactive T cell clones [6]. Mouse BCGF-I is not readily detected in supernatants of spleen cells cultured for 24 h with concanavalin A (con A) or phytohaemagglutinin (PHA). It has little or no apparent action on resting B cells and its effect on anti-IgM-activated B cells is polyclonal, not MHC-restricted, and seemingly limited to DNA synthesis without the production of antibody-forming cells [1]. The fact that exogenously

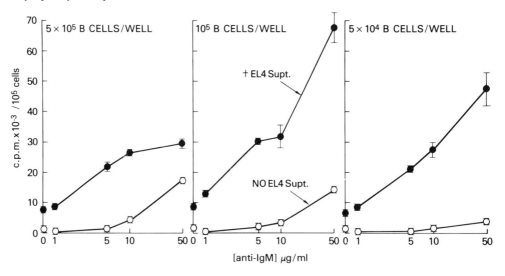

Fig. 70.1. Murine BCGF-I activity in EL4 supernatant: enhancement of anti-IgM induced B cell proliferation. Purified B cells were cultured with various concentrations of affinity purified anti-IgM antibodies, with (●) or without (○) EL4 supernatant added at 5% final concentration. Proliferation was assessed at day 3 via the uptake of ^{3}H-thymidine. Reproduced from ref. 1.

added mouse BCGF-I is not required by anti-Ig-activated B cells cultured at high cell density presumably reflects accessory cell contamination and endogenous factor production under such conditions. Mouse BCGF-I acts as a proliferation co-stimulant for some, but possibly not all, B cells activated with lipopolysaccharide (LPS). When cultures are supplemented with additional differentiation co-factors, mouse BCGF-I is found to be an essential component of both antigen-specific [1] and polyclonal anti-Ig-induced [7] AFC responses. Preliminary experiments indicate that mouse BCGF-I is required for antigen-specific proliferation of affinity-purified, hapten-specific B cells stimulated by hapten conjugated to the semi-synthetic polysaccharide Ficoll (Howard, Pillai, Scott & Paul, work in progress). The proportion of B cells responsive to mouse BCGF-I has not yet been established. However, the levels of proliferation obtained in B cell co-stimulator experiments are consistent with involvement of the entire anti-IgM responsive B cell pool, a pool recently shown to consist of approximately 50% of normal B cells [8]. Splenic B cells from xid mice fail to synthesize DNA in response to the combination of anti-IgM and mouse BCGF-I [2].

Substantial data now suggest mouse BCGF-I is a novel factor distinguishable from all previously described lymphokines. Extensive biochemical details on mouse BCGF-I are summarized below (page 70.5). It does not cause proliferation of IL2-dependent T cell clones, nor is it absorbed by such cells [1]. It can be further distinguished from IL2, the growth factor for

T cells, by several biochemical procedures [1,9,10]. Mouse BCGF-I can also be distinguished both functionally and biochemically from the following T-cell-derived factors: classical TRF [11,14]; colony-stimulating factor [15]; interferon [16]; interleukin-3 [17]; B cell replication and maturation factor [18]; B cell differentiation factor for IgM [6]; B15-TRF and EL-TRF [7]; and B cell maturation factors [20]. It does not cause proliferation of PHA stimulated thymocytes, indicating that it is also distinct from IL-1 [21].

Mouse BCGF-II (B15-TRF, DL-BCGF, BGDF)

As mentioned above, the action of mouse BCGF-I is restricted to B cell proliferation, a fact which readily distinguishes the molecule from those soluble factors which drive proliferating cells into Ig-synthesizing cells. The historical designation for the latter factor(s) is T-cell-replacing factor(s) or TRF [11,12]. Recently, however, the discovery of numerous T cell products involved in different aspects of B cell development (see review, ref. 22) has led to an increased complexity and confusion in nomenclature. Resolution of this confusion is beyond the scope of this chapter. However, it is important to appreciate the existence of several distinct types of molecules which fit the TRF classification: at least two involved in a primary IgM response [7], and probably several more which influence the class of isotype expressed [19,23]. Of particular interest for this discussion is whether any or all of these differentiation molecules are additionally involved in B cell proliferation and thus qualify as B cell growth factors. Several lines of evidence in favour of this notion have been reported. Two groups have shown that certain TRF-containing supernatants (e.g. B15K12 supernatant [7] and DL supernatant [24]), which are mouse BCGF-I-free [7,25], produce significant levels of proliferation in unstimulated, purified B cells [7,24]; they substantially enhance the proliferation obtained with anti-IgM and mouse BCGF-I [7]; they enhance final cell yields in an *in vitro* B cell assay [7]; and they increase the frequency of B cells that undergo clonal expansion in a mitogen dependent cloning assay [24]. Both groups distinguish these bifunctional proliferation/differentiation factors from a second component of the supernatant (i.e. B15-TRF vs. EL-TRF [7]; and DL-BCGF vs. DL-TRF [24]), which behaves as a differentiation factor only.

The notion of such a bifunctional maturation and replication factor is further supported by the recent studies of Pike *et al.* [26] who have identified a component (BGDF) in con-A-induced spleen cell supernatants and various T cell line supernatants capable of driving single-antigen-activated, hapten-specific B cells into both clonal expansion and antibody-forming cell development. The active moiety has an approximate relative molecular mass of 25–60 000 and thus appears to be distinct from BCGF-I. While further evidence is required to exclude the possible co-purification of mouse BCGF-I and a separate differentiation-only factor in these studies, the data is consistent with the existence of a second class of helper factor exhibiting both proliferative and maturational properties.

Recently, a concerted effort to test this proposal has been made by comparing the activities of a variety of B cell growth factor containing supernatants in a number of proliferation bioassays [25]. The data obtained indeed warranted classification of a second mouse BCGF (mouse BCGF-II). As the detailed characteristics of and relationships between B15-TRF, DL-BCGF, and BGDF have not yet been elucidated, it is currently unclear whether mouse BCGF-II represents one or more factors. In view of the limited knowledge of mouse BCGF-II, it will not be discussed further in this chapter.

Interleukin-1

Using either a low-cell-density B cell co-stimulator assay, or a higher-cell-density B cell co-stimulator assay performed in mercaptoethanol-free culture media, it is possible to demonstrate a role for the monokine interleukin-1 (IL-1) in B cell proliferation [27]. Under either of these experimental conditions,

induced supernatants from either the cloned murine monocytic cell line P388D$_1$ or human monocytic leukaemia cells are required for polyclonal proliferation of purified mouse B cells treated with anti-IgM and mouse BCGF-I. Identification of the macrophage product involved as IL-1 is based on correlation of B cell and thymocyte co-stimulating activities following a series of biochemical purification procedures. Both murine IL-1 purified to apparent homogeneity, and human IL-1 purified to high specific activity, show excellent B cell co-stimulating activity in this anti-Ig induced, mouse BCGF-I dependent, B cell co-stimulator assay. Mouse BCGF-I and IL-1 act synergistically in cultures of anti-IgM activated B cells, suggesting that both co-factors operate on the same B cell population.

Human BCGF-I (17k BCGF)

Three groups have reported a human B cell growth factor of approximate Mr 17 000 [28–30]. The experimental systems used in these laboratories vary, and it is not totally clear whether the same factor is being investigated by each of the groups, nor whether this human BCGF is analogous to the biochemically similar mouse BCGF-I. Nevertheless, some uniform conclusions regarding the nature of this human BCGF(s) (designated for the purposes of this review as human BCGF-I) have emerged. Human BCGF-I is currently used to designate *either* a material which co-stimulates with anti-Ig or other polyclonal B cell activators to cause DNA synthesis by normal or leukaemic human B cells [28,30], *or* a material which maintains the proliferation of activated purified human B lymphocytes in suspension culture [29]. Obviously, these two functions may well be mediated by different moieties. Human BCGF-I defined by both assays can be found in supernatants of lectin-activated normal T lymphocytes [28–30] and also in T cell hybridoma supernatants [31,32]. Direct binding of human BCGF-I to B cell blasts has been demonstrated via its depletion following absorption on human leukaemic B cells activated with anti-Ig or anti-idiotypic antibodies [28].

Human BCGF-II (50k BCGF)

Recently, Kishimoto *et al.* have reported a second distinct human B cell growth factor produced by an IL-2-dependent allospecific helper T cell clone upon stimulation with cells bearing the alloantigen for which the T cells are specific [28,31]. This factor (designated for the purposes of this review as human BCGF-II) stimulates proliferation of normal B cells cultured with anti-Ig or of leukaemic B cells cultured with anti-idiotype antibody. It has a Mr of 50 000 by gel filtration. Normal T cells stimulated with the combination of PHA and PMA produced both the 17 000 and 50 000 BCGFs, i.e. human BCGF-I and II. Most interestingly, these two BCGFs showed a synergistic effect on the proliferation of anti-Ig stimulated B cells. This suggests that the larger BCGF is not simply an aggregated form of the smaller, and that both co-factors act on the same population of B cells. Just as in the case of human and mouse BCGF-Is, it is tempting to speculate that human and mouse BCGF-IIs are analogous. While some biological characteristics of the latter two components seem disparate, both synergize with an Mr 18 000 BCGF to cause extensive proliferation of activated B cells.

Assay for mouse BCGF-I

The presence of mouse BCGF-I in a test supernatant can be detected using a B cell co-stimulator assay involving co-culture of purified mouse B lymphocytes, either anti-Ig or LPS as a polyclonal B cell activator, and the supernatant under study [1]. The standard protocol for this assay is illustrated in Fig. 70.2. Precise experimental details are as follows.

Mice

No genetic polymorphism of mouse BCGF-I or of the receptor for this factor has yet been observed, and all mouse strains tested to date (e.g. BALB/c, B10.A, CBA/CaH, DBA/2, DBA/2 × CBA/N), with the exception of mice bearing the xid defect (i.e. CBA/N), are suitable for use in the mouse BCGF-I assay.

B cell purification

B lymphocytes used for mouse BCGF-I co-stimulator assays are highly purified prior to culture in order to remove contaminating T and accessory cells which may either lead to endogenous mouse BCGF-I production (thus obscuring dependency for this factor) or proliferate themselves in response to other factors in the test supernatant. A commonly used B cell purification method is one of negative selection, originally described by Leibson *et al.* [33].

Procedure

Mice are treated with 0.40 ml anti-thymocyte serum (Microbiological Associates, Walkersville, MD), and spleen cells harvested 2 days later are depleted of macrophages, activated lymphocytes, and other adherent cells by passage over Sephadex G-10 as described by Ly & Mishell [34]. T cells and null cells are

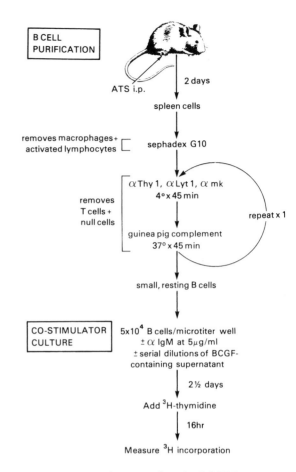

Fig. 70.2. Protocol for assay of murine BCGF-I.

subsequently removed by two treatments with a battery of monoclonal antibodies (4 °C, 45 min), followed by guinea-pig complement at a 1:4 dilution (37 °C, 45 min). The antibodies comprise a monoclonal mouse anti-Thy-1.2 antibody (New England Nuclear, Boston, MA), a non-cytotoxic monoclonal rat anti-Lyt-1 antibody (provided by J. Ledbetter, Stanford University, Palo Alto, CA) combined with a cytotoxic monoclonal mouse anti-rat κ antibody (MAR 18.5, provided by L. Lanier, University of New Mexico, Albuquerque, NM), and a monoclonal mouse cell antibody specific for certain splenic null cells (MK 2.2, provided by P. Marrack, National Jewish Hospital, Denver, CO). The cells obtained by this method comprise 20–30% of the initial B cell population, are all small lymphocytes by density gradient analysis (i.e. are largely free of activated B lymphocytes), are approximately 98% Ig-positive by immunofluorescence, and show the normal range of B cell immunocompetence in a variety of filler-supplemented assay systems (unpublished data).

Anti-IgM

Highly purified resting B lymphocytes are themselves unresponsive to mouse BCGF-I, but can be rendered responsive by exposure to a resting B cell activator such as antigen, anti-IgM, or LPS. For this purpose, the author has most commonly used affinity column-purified goat anti-mouse Ig specific for μ heavy chains (anti-μ), prepared according to the method of Sieckmann [35]. Recent data suggests that some but not all monoclonal rat anti-mouse μ chain antibodies are also suitable. Alternatively, others have successfully utilized the polyclonal B cell activator lipopolysaccharide to replace anti-IgM in sensitizing B cells to mouse BCGF-I [4,5].

Culture conditions

Purified B cells are cultured at a density of 5×10^4/well in 200 μl of medium in flat-bottomed 96-well microtitre plates (3596, Costar, Data Packaging, Cambridge, MA). Cells are cultured with and without anti-IgM antibodies at a final concentration of 5 μg/ml, together with various dilutions of BCGF-containing supernatants. Standard serum-containing culture media (e.g. RPMI supplemented with 10% fetal calf serum, penicillin at 50 μg/ml, streptomycin at 50 μg/ml, gentamicin at 100 μg/ml, L-glutamine at 200 mM, and 2-mercaptoethanol at 5×10^{-5} M), and serum-free modified Iscove's medium [36], both support BCGF-I assays. Cultures are incubated at 37 °C in a humidified atmosphere of air containing 7.5% CO_2 for 3 days. The proliferative response of these cultures is determined by adding ^{3}H-thymidine for the last 16 h of culture and measuring ^{3}H-thymidine incorporation.

Mouse BCGF-I units

Data from mouse BCGF-I assays can be expressed as counts per minute, e.g. Figs. 70.1 and 70.3, or more ideally in terms of units of mouse BCGF-I activity, e.g. Fig. 70.4. A relative unit of activity is generally defined as the amount of material required to produce 50% of the proliferation caused by a saturating amount of EL4 supernatant. Thus, to determine the number of units of mouse BCGF-I in a test supernatant, the supernatant and a control standard, e.g. induced EL4 supernatant, must be assayed at several dilutions. The inverse of the dilution that produces 50% of the proliferation obtained with a saturating level of EL4 supernatant then defines the number of relative units per millilitre in the test supernatant.

Sources of mouse BCGF-I

To date, the most commonly used source of mouse BCGF-I has been an induced supernatant obtained from a cloned subline of the murine thymoma EL4 following stimulation with phorbol myristate acetate (PMA). EL4 cells are harvested in log phase growth when their viability exceeds 90%. They are then recultured at 2×10^6/ml in either serum-supplemented or serum-free standard culture medium containing phorbol myristic acetate (PMA) at 10 ng/ml. Cell-free supernatants are collected after 48 h, aliquoted, and frozen. The PMA content in such supernatants may be reduced by a procedure of adsorption on activated charcoal, as described elsewhere [37]. Fig. 70.3 shows an example of BCGF-I activity in PMA induced EL4 supernatant, assayed as described above.

An alternative source of mouse BCGF-I is provided by the supernatants of antigen-activated, long-term, cultured helper T cell lines [2]. Antigen-reactive T cell lines can be generated by serial restimulation of antigen-primed T cells with irradiated spleen cells plus antigen, followed by antigen-free periods when the cells are maintained on irradiated spleen cells alone [3]. These lines are capable of supporting a variety of *in vitro* B cell responses, and thus were obvious candidates for potential BCGF-producers. When such long-term antigen-reactive T cells are stimulated with antigen in the context of syngeneic antigen-presenting cells, they produce a factor which is indistinguishable biochemically and functionally from the B cell co-stimulating factor found in induced EL4 supernatants, i.e. mouse BCGF-I [2]. The amount of mouse BCGF-I produced within 24 h of stimulating 2×10^5 antigen-reactive T cells is comparable to that produced by ten times as many EL4 cells stimulated for 48 h with PMA (Fig. 70.3). Compared to EL4 supernatants, this source of mouse BCGF-I offers the advantage of being free of PMA; it suffers from the disadvantage of including macrophage-derived products, e.g. IL1.

Finally, two groups have recently developed T cell hybridomas which release mouse BCGF-I either constitutively or in response to con A [4,5].

Biochemical characteristics of mouse BCGF-I

General properties

Farrar *et al.* [1,9,10] have studied the physico-chemical properties of mouse BCGF-I. They have shown that mouse BCGF-I is a glycoprotein by virtue of its trypsin and neuraminadase sensitivity. When produced by PMA-induced EL4 cells in serum-containing media, it is readily separated from the bulk of proteins in such culture supernatants by ammonium sulphate

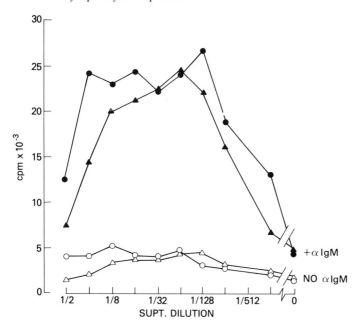

Fig. 70.3. Relative BCGF-I activity in PMA-induced EL4 supernatant (●) and in antigen-activated long-term helper T cell line supernatant (▲). BCGF-I was assayed as in Fig. 70.2.

precipitation. More than 90% of the mouse BCGF-I activity is precipitated between 80% and 100% saturated ammonium sulphate; only 5–9% of the total protein is found in this fraction. By conventional gel filtration on ACA 54 in neutral solution, mouse BCGF-I elutes as a broad peak between 13 000 and 20 000. Analysis of mouse BCGF-I by SDS-PAGE reveals two components which exhibit biological activity after extraction from the gels and dialysis. One has a monomeric Mr of 11 000, the other 14 000. A degree of microheterogeneity is also observed when mouse BCGF-I is examined by electrofocussing. Two peaks of mouse BCGF-I activity are observed migrating with isoelectric points of 6.4–6.7 and 7.4–7.6, respectively. These resolve to one peak of pI 9.3 following neuraminidase treatment. Mouse BCGF-I can be completely separated from the growth factor for T cells, interleukin-2 (IL-2), by a combination of ammonium sulphate precipitation, phenylsepharose column chromatography, and Tris-glycine gel electrophoresis [10]. Surprisingly, mouse BCGF-I displays a lower electrophoretic mobility than IL-2 on Tris glycine gels, despite its lower relative molecular mass; this is probably due to the alkaline isoelectric points of mouse BCGF-Is. Although mouse BCGF-I has not been purified to homogeneity, it has been brought to high specific activity by a sequential purification procedure involving ammonium sulphate precipitation, phenylsepharose chromatography, Tris-glycinate PAGE and SDS-PAGE [10]. In this sequential purification procedure, significant mouse BCGF-I

activity could be recovered from the final SDS-polyacrylamide gel. Surprisingly, no band of appropriate size could be revealed when this final gel was stained using the highly sensitive silver nitrate procedure [38]. As this staining procedure is capable of detecting nanogram amounts of protein, this implies that a unit of BCGF-I activity corresponds to less than nanogram amounts of protein.

Routine purification

The most commonly used source of mouse BCGF-I, i.e. PMA-induced EL4 supernatant, contains numerous other lymphokines (see review, ref. 9) including EL-TRF [7], IL-2 and CSF [9] and BCGF-II [25]. For many biological experiments, it is desirable to use semi-purified mouse BCGF-I which is functionally free of these other lymphokines. A one-step purification method which achieves this purpose is phenyl sepharose chromatography, as described by Farrar *et al.* [10].

Procedure

Approximately 100 ml of PMA-induced EL4 supernatant containing 1% FCS, or up to two litres of serum-free PMA-induced EL4 supernatant, is concentrated to approximately 20 ml by amicon filtration using PM10 or YM5 membranes respectively. This material is then dialysed to 0.8 M $(NH_4)_2SO_4$ in 0.02 M phosphate-buffered saline (PBS), pH 7.2, and applied

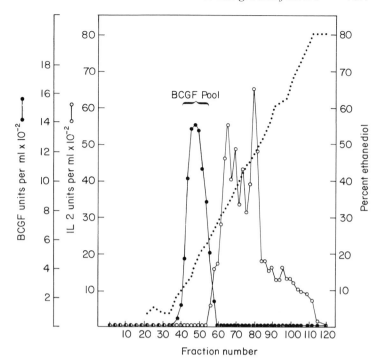

Fig. 70.4. Phenyl sepharose hydrophobic chromatography of PMA-induced EL4 supernatant, showing separation of BCGF-I (●) and IL-2 (○) activities. BCGF-I was assayed as in Fig. 70.2. IL-2 was assayed via proliferation of an IL-2-dependent T cell clone. Units of activity were calculated as described in text. (Courtesy of Dr J. Farrar.) Reproduced from ref. 10.

to a 15 ml bed volume phenyl sepharose CL-4B column previously equilibrated with the same buffer (starting buffer). The column is washed with ≥4 column volumes of starting buffer and then a 200 ml gradient of 1:1 starting buffer to 60% ethanediol in 0.02 M PBS is initiated. The column is run at a flow rate of 20 ml/h, and fractions (2.0 ml volume) are collected, dialysed extensively (at least six changes) against PBS and finally against culture medium, prior to their assay for mouse BCGF-I content. The ethanediol gradient is estimated by reading the conductivity of each fraction and comparing these values to a standard curve constructed using various standard dilutions of ethanediol in starting buffer. As illustrated in Fig. 70.4, mouse BCGF-I activity routinely elutes at between 10% and 25% ethandiol. When 1.5 l of serum-free EL4 supernatant is fractionated in this way, this region of the chromatography contains less than 5% of the total protein (unpublished data). Due to a small and variable amount of overlap in mouse BCGF-I and IL-2 activities recovered from phenyl sepharose chromatography, it is advisable to routinely assay the fractions for IL-2 activity, e.g. via proliferation of an IL-2 dependent T cell clone, (e.g. Fig. 70.4). Only those fractions totally free of IL-2 activity are then taken to make a BCGF-I pool. As shown elsewhere, this BCGF-I pool is additionally free of CSF [9], EL-TRF [7], and BCGF-II [25].

Long-term B cell lines

B cell lymphomas, myelomas, and hybridomas have provided invaluable resources for the study of antibody diversity, idiotypy, and immunoglobulin gene rearrangement and expression [39–41]. The limitation of such tumour lines is that they have relatively little immunocompetence, so they do not allow the analysis of many of the cellular and biochemical mechanisms related to B cell activation, isotype switching, idiotype selection, and immunoregulation. The recent development of long-term cultures of antigen-specific immunocompetent T cell clones [42–46] has raised hopes that the same technology might be possible for B lymphocytes. Indeed, much of the impetus for defining B cell proliferation co-factors as outlined above has been to obtain a growth factor(s) capable of maintaining continuous *in vitro* growth of normal B cells, just as IL-2 maintains continuous *in vitro* growth of some normal T cells. In many respects, the development of B cell clones would seem an easier endeavour than that of T cell clones. The technologies for marked enrichment of antigen-specific B lymphocytes [47] and for isolation of individual, immunocompetent, antigen-specific clones [48] have been established for some years. The one remaining difficulty in producing long-term cloned lines of antigen-specific, immunocompetent B lymphocytes lies in the continuous

Table 70.1. Current status of technology for continuous cultivation of normal B lymphocytes

Starting B cell population	Growth dependence	Evidence of B cell phenotype	Survival of lines (months)	Cloned?	Ref.
1 *Factor dependent lines*					
Mouse, LPS-stimulated, splenic B cells	PMA-induced EL4 or P388D$_1$ supernatant	mIgM; activation to Ig synthesis	>12	No	[52]
Human-T-cell-depleted, PHA-stimulated, peripheral blood B cells	PHA-induced peripheral blood supernatant	mIgM; activation to Ig synthesis	>12	Unclear	[54]
Mouse, LPS-stimulated, DNP-binding, splenic B cells	PHA- or con A-induced spleen supernatant; or LPS-induced EL4 + PEC supernatant	mIg; DNP-binding; activation to Ig synthesis	>9	Unclear	[53]
Human-T-cell-depleted, anti-Ig stimulated, peripheral blood B cells	PHA-induced peripheral blood supernatant	mIg; BCGF absorption	>8	No	[55]
2 *Adherent-cell dependent lines*					
Mouse bone marrow cells	Adherent feeder cell layer derived from bone marrow population	Ig synthesis	>12	Yes†	[56,57]

† B cell lines grown by the adherent-cell-dependent procedure can be cloned by limit dilution on previously prepared adherent layers; the origin of the outgrowing clone is established by using allotypically differentiated feeder cells and B cell lines; evidence of clonality is provided by demonstrating the expression of a single idiotype (O. Witte, personal communication).

propagation of these cells. Although it has been possible to propagate individual B cell clones *in vivo* for periods of up to 10 months [49,50], early attempts to culture B lymphocytes for periods longer than 4 weeks were unsuccessful [51].

Recently activity in the area of continuous cultivation of B lymphocytes has flourished with the emergence of two types of successful procedures. The current status of this field is summarized in Table 70.1. The first procedure to be developed involved repeated feeding of mitogen-activated B cells with crude supernatants rich in B cell growth factors. This approach has yielded lines of both mouse [52,53] and human [54,55] B cells which have been propagated for periods of 12 or more months. Cloning of such growth factor dependent long-term lines has not yet been demonstrated convincingly. Some success at driving these proliferating lines into Ig-synthesizing cells, by providing helper T cells or their products, has been reported [52–54]. The second method of long term B cell cultivation involves growth of bone marrow B cells on adherent layers derived from the same source [56,57].

Such lines have also been maintained for periods greater than one year. These lines appear to grow more rapidly than growth factor dependent lines. Furthermore, using allotypically marked feeder layers to monitor possible adherent layer outgrowth, such cell lines have been cloned by limit dilution to yield cloned lines which express a single idiotype. While both types of procedures are clearly tedious and still difficult to perform on a reproducible and routine basis, it is hoped that they represent a foundation for greater successes ahead.

References

1 HOWARD M., FARRAR J., HILFIKER M., JOHNSON B., TAKATSU K., HAMAOKA T. & PAUL W.E. (1982) Identification of a T-cell derived B-cell growth factor distinct from Interleukin 2. *J. exp. Med.* **155**, 914.
2 HOWARD M., MALEK T., KELL W., COHEN D., ANSEL J., NAKANISHI K., JOHNSON B. & PAUL W.E. (1983) Interleukin 2 induces an antigen-reactive T cell line to secrete BCGF-I. *J. exp. Med.*, **158**, 2024.

3 KIMOTO M. & FATHMAN C.G. (1980) Antigen-reactive T cell clones. (I) Transcomplementing hybrid I-A region gene products function effectively in antigen presentation. *J. exp. Med.* **152**, 759.

4 LEANDERSON T., LUNDGREN E., RUUTH E., BORG H., PERSSON H. & COUTINHO A. (1982) B cell growth factor (BCGF): distinction from T cell growth factor and B cell maturation factor. *Proc. natn. Acad. Sci. U.S.A.* **79**, 7455.

5 LERNHARDT W., CORBEL C., WALL R. & MELCHERS F. (1982) T cell hybridomas which produce B lymphocyte replication factors only. *Nature*, **300**, 355.

6 PURE E., ISAKSON P., KAPPLER J., MARRACK P., KRAMER P. & VITETTA E. (1983) T cell derived B cell growth and differentiation factors: dichotomy between the responsiveness of B cells from adult and neonatal mice. *J. exp. Med.*, **157**, 583.

7 NAKANISHI K., HOWARD M., MURAGUCHI A., FARRAR J., TAKATSU K., HAMAOKA T. & PAUL W.E. (1983) Soluble factors involved in B cell differentiation: identification of two distinct T cell replacing factors (TRF). *J. Immunol.* **130**, 2219.

8 DEFRANCO A., RAVECHE E., ASOFSKY R. & PAUL W.E. (1982) Frequency of B lymphocytes responsive to anti-immunoglobulin. *J. exp. Med.* **155**, 1523–1536.

9 FARRAR J., BENJAMIN W., HILFIKER M., HOWARD M., FARRAR W. & FULLER-FARRAR J. (1982) The biochemistry, biology, and role of IL-2 in the induction of cytotoxic T cells and antibody-forming B cell responses. *Immunol. Revs.* **63**, 129.

10 FARRAR J., HOWARD M., FULLER-FARRAR J. & PAUL W.E. (1983) Biochemical and physiochemical characterization of mouse B cell growth factor: a lymphokine distinct from interleukin 2. *J. Immunol.* **131**, 1838.

11 DUTTON R.W. (1975) Separate signals for the initiation of proliferation and differentiation in the B cell response to antigen. *Transplant. Rev.* **23**, 66.

12 SCHIMPL A. & WECKER E. (1975) A third signal in B cell activation given by TRF. *Transplant. Rev.* **23**, 176.

13 SCHIMPL A., HUBNER L., WONG C. & WECKER E. (1980) Distribution between T helper cell replacing factor (TCGF) and T cell growth factor (TCGF). *Behring Inst. Mitt.* **67**, 221.

14 WATSON J., GILLIS S., MARBROOK J., MOCHIZUKI D. & SMITH K.A. (1979) Biochemical and biological characterization of lymphocyte regulatory molecules. (I) Purification of a class of murine lymphokines. *J. exp. Med.* **150**, 849.

15 BURGESS A. & METCALF D. (1980) The nature and action of granulocyte-macrophage colony stimulating factors. *Blood*, **56**, 947.

16 SIMON P., FARRAR J. & KIND T. (1979) Biochemical relationship between murine interferon and a killer cell helper factor. *J. Immunol.* **122**, 127.

17 ANDERSSON J. & MELCHERS F. (1981) T cell-dependent activation of resting B cells: requirement for both nonspecific unrestricted and antigen-specific Ia-restricted soluble factors. *Proc. natn. Acad. Sci. U.S.A.* **78**, 2497.

18 HAPEL A., LEE J., FARRAR W. & IHLE J. (1981) Establishment of continuous cultures of Thy1.2$^+$, Lyt1$^+$2$^-$ T cells with purified interleukin 3. *Cell*, **25**, 179.

19 ISAKSON P., PURE E., VITETTA E. & KRAMMER P. (1982) T cell-derived B cell differentiation factor(s). Effect on the isotype switch of murine B cells. *J. exp. Med.* **155**, 734.

20 PETTERSON S., LEANDERSON T. & COUTINHO A. (1985) Identification of a factor inducing high rate secretion of immunoglobulin in B lymphocytes. Not yet published.

21 GERY I., GERSHON R.K. & WAKSMAN B.H. (1972) Potentiation of the T-lymphocyte response to mitogens. (I) The responding cell. *J. exp. Med.* **136**, 128.

22 HOWARD M. & PAUL W.E. (1983) Regulation of B cell growth and differentiation by soluble factors. *Ann. Rev. Immunol.* **1**, 307.

23 KISHIMOTO T. & ISHIZAKA K. (1975) Immunologic and physiochemical properties of enhancing soluble factors for IgG and IgE antibody responses. *J. Immunol.* **114**, 1177.

24 SWAIN S. & DUTTON R. (1982) A B cell growth promoting activity DL(BCGF) from a cloned T cell line and its assay on the BCL, B cell tumor. *J. exp. Med.* **156**, 1821.

25 SWAIN S., HOWARD M., KAPPLER J., MARACK P., WATSON J., BOOTH R., WETZEL M. & DUTTON R. (1983) Evidence for two distinct classes of murine B cell growth factors which have activities in different functional assays. *J. exp. Med.*, **158**, 822.

26 PIKE B., VAUX D., CLARK-LEWIS I., SCHRADER J. & NOSSAL G. (1982) Proliferation and differentiation of single, hapten-specific B lymphocytes promoted by T cell factor(s) distinct from T cell growth factor. *Proc. natn. Acad. Sci. U.S.A.* **79**, 6350.

27 HOWARD M., MIZEL S.D., LACHMAN L., ANSEL J., JOHNSON B. & PAUL W.E. (1983) Role of interleukin 1 in anti-immunoglobulin-induced B cell proliferation. *J. exp. Med.* **157**, 1529.

28 YOSHIZAKI K., NAKAGAWA T., FUKUNAGA K., KAIEDA T., MARUYAMA S., KISHIMOTO S., YAMAMURA Y. & KISHIMOTO T. (1982) Characterization of human B cell growth factor (BCGF) from cloned T cells or mitogen-stimulated T cells. *J. Immunol.* **130**, 1241.

29 MAIZEL A., SAHASRABUDDHE C., MEHTA S., MORGAN C., LACHMAN L. & FORD R. (1982) Isolation of a human B cell mitogenic factor. *Proc. natn. Acad. Sci. U.S.A.* **79**, 5998.

30 MURAGUCHI A., KASAHARA T., OPPENHEIM J. & FAUCI A. (1982) Human BCGF and TCGF are distinct molecules. *J. Immunol.* **129**, 2486.

31 OKADA M., SAKAGUCHI N., YOSHIMURA N., HARA H., SHIMIZU K., YOSHIDA N., YOSHIZAKI K., KISHIMOTO S., YAMAMURA Y. & KISHIMOTO T. (1983) B cell growth factors (BCGF) and B cell differentiation factor (BCDF) from human T hybridomas: two distinct kinds of BCGFs and their synergism in B cell proliferation. *J. exp. Med.* **157**, 583.

32 BUTLER J., MURAGUCHI A., LANE C. & FAUCI A. (1983) Development of a human T–T cell hybridoma secreting B cell growth factor. *J. exp. Med.* **157**, 60.

33 LEIBSON H., MARRACK P. & KAPPLER J. (1981) B cell helper factors (I) Requirement for both Il-2 and another 40 000 Mr factor. *J. exp. Med.* **154**, 1681.

34 LY L. & MISHELL R. (1974) Separation of mouse spleen cells by passage through Sephadex G10. *J. immunol. Meth.* **5**, 239.

35 SIECKMANN D., ASOFSKY R., MOSIER D., ZITRON I. & PAUL W.E. (1978) Activation of mouse lymphocytes by anti-immunoglobulin. (I) Parameters of the proliferative response. *J. exp. Med.* **147,** 814.

36 MOSIER D.E. (1981) Primary *in vitro* antibody responses by purified murine B lymphocytes in serum-free defined medium. *J. Immunol.* **127,** 1490.

37 FULLER-FARRAR J., HILFIKER M., FARRAR W. & FARRAR J. (1981) PMA enhances the production of interleukin 2. *Cell. Immunol.* **58,** 156.

38 SWITZER R., MEML C. & SHIFRIN S. (1979) A highly sensitive silver stain for detecting proteins & peptides in polyacrylamide gels. *Analyt. Biochem.* **98,** 231.

39 POTTER M. (1977) Antigen-binding myeloma proteins of mice. *Adv. Immunol.* **25,** 141.

40 MELCHERS F., POTTER M. & WARNER N. (eds.) (1978) *Curr. Top. Microbiol. Immunol.* **81.**

41 SAKANO H., MAKI R., KUROSAWA Y., REEDER W. & TONEGAWA S. (1980) Two types of somatic recombination are necessary for the generation of complete immunoglobulin heavy-chain genes. *Nature,* **286,** 676.

42 GILLIS S. & SMITH K.A. (1977) Long term culture of tumour-specific cytotoxic T cells. *Nature,* **268,** 154.

43 FATHMAN C.G. & HENGARTNER H. (1978) Clones of alloreactive T cells. *Nature,* **272,** 617.

44 NABHOLZ M., ENGERS H., COLLAVO D. & NORTH M. (1978) Cloned T-cell lines with specific cytolytic activity. *Curr. Top. Microbiol. Immunol.* **81,** 176.

45 AUGUSTIN A.A., JULIUS M.H. & COSENZA H. (1979) Antigen-specific stimulation and trans-stimulation of T cells in long-term culture. *Eur. J. Immunol.* **9,** 665.

46 SREDNI B., TSE H.Y. & SCHWARTZ R.H. (1980) Direct cloning and extended culture of antigen-specific MHC-restricted, proliferating T lymphocytes. *Nature,* **283,** 581.

47 HAAS W. & LAYTON J.E. (1975) Separation of antigen-specific lymphocytes. (I) Enrichment of antigen-binding cells. *J. exp. Med.* **141,** 1004.

48 PILLAI S. & SCOTT D. (1981) Hapten-specific murine colony-forming B cells: *in vitro* response of colonies to fluoresceinated thymus independent antigens. *J. Immunol.* **126,** 1883.

49 WILLIAMSON A. & ASKONAS B. (1972) Senescence of an antibody-forming cell clone. *Nature,* **238,** 337.

50 ASKONAS B.A., WILLIAMSON A.R. & WRIGHT B.E.G. (1970) Selection of a single antibody-forming cell alone and its propagation in syngeneic mice. *Proc. natn. Acad. Sci. U.S.A.* **67,** 1398.

51 MELCHERS F., COUTINHO A., HEINRICH G. & ANDERSSON J. (1975) Continuous growth of mitogen-reactive β lymphocytes. *Scand. J. Immunol.* **4,** 853.

52 HOWARD M., KESSLER S., CHUSED T. & PAUL W.E. (1981) Long-term culture of normal mouse B lymphocytes. *Proc. natn. Acad. Sci. U.S.A.* **78,** 5788.

53 ALDO-BENSON M. & SCHEIDERER L. (1983) Long-term growth of lines of murine dinitrophenol-specific B lymphocytes *in vitro*. *J. exp. Med.* **157,** 342.

54 SREDNI B., SIECKMANN D., KUMAGAI S., HOUSE S., GREEN I. & PAUL W.E. (1981) Long-term culture and cloning of nontransformed human B lymphocytes. *J. exp. Med.* **154,** 1500.

55 MAIZEL A., MORGAN J., MEHTA S., KOUTTAB N., BATOR J. & SAHASRABUDDHE C. (1983) Long-term growth of human B cells and their use in a microassay for BCGF. *Proc. natn. Acad. Sci. U.S.A.* **80,** 5047.

56 WHITLOCK C. & WITTE O. (1982) Long-term culture of B lymphocytes and their precursors from murine bone marrow. *Proc. natn. Acad. Sci. U.S.A.* **79,** 3608.

57 WHITLOCK C., ROBERTSON D. & WITTE O. (1984) Murine B cell lymphopoiesis in long term culture. *J. Immunological Methods,* **67,** 353.

Chapter 71
Overview: helper and suppressor T cells

K. OKUMURA & T. TADA

Family of helper T cells, 71.1
Families of suppressor T cells,
    71.3

Interaction between
    carrier-specific and Ig-specific
    regulatory pathways, 71.4
A synthetic view, 71.4

The authors must start by admitting that the terms helper (Th) and suppressor (Ts) T cells have been only arbitrarily used to designate T cell types that are involved in the induction and suppression of the antibody synthesis by B cells against T cell dependent antigens. However, we are now aware that such terminal inductive and suppressive signals are produced via the complex processes of a series of cellular interactions. Thus it is difficult to define Th and Ts by the simple phenomenological data that was used in the first decade of 'T-ology'. A typical example is found in a model of a regulatory circuit, where a Th is required for the induction of Ts, which suppresses another Th. A circuit model formulated by Herzenberg et al. [1] accommodates two Th and two Ts interconnected in one circular interaction system. In this model, because the temporal locking of the circuit into suppression or help is primarily dependent on the first cell activated, it is not easy to define the true nature of Th and Ts. Largely as a result of the elaborate effort by the late R.K. Gershon, the circuitry of cellular regulation of the antibody response has been greatly elucidated [2,3], and the regulatory mechanisms are no longer in a black box.

It is, however, still a matter of controversy to define Th and Ts by simple phenotypic markers and phenomenological functions. In fact, the definition of Th by Lyt-1 is not always valid, since such a marker is also expressed on cell types in the suppressor pathway. The term inducer T cell has also been proposed, but the multifaceted concept of 'induction' more confuses than compromises. The authors will, therefore, describe in this short chapter some of the known properties of different types of Th and Ts, and try to comprehend the interrelationship between different regulatory T cells in the immune circuit.

Family of helper T cells

Carrier-specific helper T cell (CTh)

Because of the well-known interaction between carrier-specific T cells and hapten-specific B cells in the secondary antibody response [4,5], we designate antigen-specific Th as CTh. They are specific for carrier antigen in terms of interaction with both hapten-specific B cells and antigen-presenting cells (APC), the latter of which is required for the activation of CTh. As a result of this dual-faceted specificity, CTh are divided into two types (CTh1 and CTh2) [6]. Although it is not excluded that a single CTh, especially a cloned CTh, can function in both pathways, they help B cells via the different mechanisms. The successful separation of these two CTh allowed their functional analyses, and several interesting facets have been revealed. They can also be quantitatively discriminated by limiting dilution analysis [7].

CTh1

CTh1 can be defined as the classical CTh originally described by Rajewsky & Rottrander [4] and Mitchison [5], which is involved in the 'cognate interaction' with B cells for the antibody formation by the latter. The term 'cognate interaction' indicates the necessity for two functionally different cells to recognize antigenic determinants on the same single molecule in order for an effective cell communication to occur. This type of cell interaction is often called 'linked recognition', since the regulatory signal of one cell type is conveyed to another via the antigen bridge between two interacting cells.

CTh is probably essential in all the T cell dependent antibody response and is the only legitimate T cell type for true definition of helper activity. The resting B cells lacking Lyb-5 differentiation marker cannot be triggered for antibody formation without CTh1. CTh1 is known to belong to Lyt-1^+2^- subset, and is radioresistant. The most important feature in CTh1–B cell interaction is the requirement of the identity of I region genes (A and/or E genes) between these two cell types for effective co-operation. Thus CTh1 seems to specifically recognize Ia structure together with antigen on partner B cells to interact with. Since this restriction specificity of CTh1 is altered under the chimeric condition where T cells differentiate in an environment with genotypically different Ia antigens, CTh1 seem to acquire the restriction specificity through an adaptive process. It is suggested that CTh1 recognize antigen fragments in the context of class II molecules on B cells. One of the central issues in current cellular immunology is to determine the molecule which imposes this restriction specificity of CTh1. It has been suggested that CTh1 effect is mediated by antigen-specific MHC-restricted helper factor, while the formal proof is still pending. Recently, it became possible to maintain cloned CTh1 cell lines by stimulating the primed T cells with antigen and APC and allowing them to divide in IL-2-containing medium. These cloned CTh1 will enable us to study the molecular basis of CTh1–B cell interactions.

CTh2

CTh2, by the authors' criteria, is the cell type which produces antigen non-specific mediators that induce B cell proliferation and maturation into antibody-synthesizing cells. B cells competent to respond to non-specific factors seem to be limited. Such B cells generally carry the Lyb-5 differentiation marker and are already in a proliferative phase (G_1) by previous exposure to antigen and CTh1. This early step leading to activation may be replaced by certain anti-Ig reagents. Upon stimulation with antigen on APC, CTh2 produce multiple non-specific B cell stimulating factors (BSF), including B cell growth factors and B cell differentiation or maturation factors. One of the B cell differentiation factors is called T cell replacing factor (TRF). CTh2 is, therefore, considered to be a heterogeneous population of T cells producing different mediators, and thus it has to be realized that the effect of CTh2 resulting in antibody synthesis by B cells is the net effect of different CTh2 cells. Various T cell clones and tumour cell lines producing BCFs are now available, and thus the biochemical consequences of B cell activation are rapidly being clarified. CTh2 also belong to Lyt-1^+2^- subset and are probably relatively radiation sensitive. In certain strains of mice, CTh1 and CTh2 can be separated by passage through a tightly packed nylon wool column. CTh2 activity is found enriched in the cells adherent to nylon wool, and is sensitive to treatment with anti-Ia (I-J) and complement (C) [6]. Probably because of the production of

IL-2 by CTh2, the mixture of CTh1 and CTh2 gives a synergistic helper effect rather than an additive one. The activation of CTh2 is dependent on MHC compatible APC. The recognition of antigen on APC is, therefore, MHC-restricted, while the effect on B cells is unrestricted. A number of CTh2 type cell lines and hybridomas have been produced, with which one can analyse the molecules and genes involved in MHC-restricted antigen recognition and production of unrestricted mediators including BCFs and IL-2.

Ig specific helper T cells (IgTh)

There exist T cells that regulate the production of antibody of a particular isotype, allotype or idiotype. Although the mechanisms involved in the regulation of isotype and idiotype seem different, it is probable that this process is due to the presence of a special subset of T cells that can recognize the Ig structure on the B cell surface. This type of helper cell is designated as IgTh. In allotype specific suppression in the mouse, it was found that the target of allotype-specific Ts is not the carrier-specific CTh but, instead, a cell type that preferentially helps the production of one of the allotypes in F_1 mice [8]. This allotype-specific Th has been found to exert a regulatory effect on B cells for the maturation of antibody affinity but not for the development of memory [9]. Thus IgTh may be involved in highly sophisticated regulation of certain processes of B cell differentiation carrying a particular allotype and antibody affinity. Another example is the presence of Ig-restricted Th, which recognizes certain Ig structure, particularly the idiotype in association with antigen [10]. It has been postulated that the induction of IgTh depends on the idiotype expressed on B cells or on circulating Ig, and that IgTh has dual specificities for both the antigen and the antigen-receptor (idiotype). This is in contrast to MHC-restricted CTh. In this context, IgTh recognizes antigen but interacts only with B cells expressing the corresponding Ig structure. The T15 idiotype-specific helper T cell is a well-documented IgTh of this sort where a population of carrier-specific helper T cells also identify T15-positive B cells to help them preferentially [11]. The nature of this dual recognition is presently unknown. Woodland & Cantor [12] demonstrated another type of IgTh which is not antigen specific but is solely specific for idiotype of the antibody produced. They separated carrier-specific and idiotype-specific T cells from carrier-primed mice, the combination of which was required for the production of the idiotype-positive response. This IgTh is anti-idiotypic, does not require antigenic stimulation for its generation, and is therefore probably induced by internal network regulation. Woodland & Cantor postulated that two concurrent signals from CTh and IgTh are required for the production of idiotype-positive antibodies by B cells. In general, IgTh seem to recognize allotype, idiotype or isotype of the B cell receptors. The B cells also have to be co-stimulated by antigen to lead to differentiation towards antibody production.

The authors are, of course, aware of the presence of Fc-receptor-positive T cells that regulate the production of antibodies carrying a given class of Fc (Ig isotype) [13–16]. Especially noteworthy is the regulation of IgE which is conducted by two types of Fc_ε-positive T cells producing IgE-augmenting and suppressor factors. They are triggered by antigen on APC, but the effect is not antigen specific. The non-specific regulatory factors have affinity for the Fc component of IgE. Such regulatory T cells with discriminatory activity for the Fc portion of Ig may play important roles in the class distribution of produced antibodies. It is still unknown whether such T cells are the counterparts of CTh2, which may be designated as antigen non-specific IgTh2.

Carrier-specific augmenting T cell (CTa)

The authors would like to depict CTa cells as important regulatory T cells, because they may be involved in specific augmentation of the antibody response or in the counter-suppressor action of T cells. It has been found that there is an antigen-specific T cell that has no helper activity by itself but augments the helper T cell dependent antibody response. The effect was mediated by a soluble factor designated as TaF [17]. TaF has specific affinity for antigen and acts on MHC-compatible T cells to augment the helper activity. TaF is composed of two polypeptides of mol. wt. 33 000, one with antigen-binding activity and the other with I region controlled determinants [18]. Recently, Asano & Hodes [19] demonstrated that normal unprimed T cells collaborate with cloned CTh1 to augment the antibody response. Their TaF also show MHC genetic restriction.

Although not much is known about the mechanism of augmentation by CTa, the authors expect the presence of a complex regulatory system activated by CTa as the mirror image of the suppressor circuit (see below). It is suggested that the TaF described here is an inducer factor to activate the final effector cell that synergizes with CTh1 or makes CTh1 resistant to the suppressor signal (contrasuppressor; see below).

Families of suppressor T cells

Carrier-specific suppressor T cells (CTs)

Suppressor T cells (Ts) have been envisaged as the counterparts of Th, since their ultimate effect is to suppress the T cell dependent antibody response. However, most Ts do not directly suppress the B cell response, but inhibit Th function, leading to the inability of B cells to make antibodies. Therefore it is not realistic to see Ts as the mirror image of Th. It is more likely that they are the counterparts of Ta cells, as described above. Ts can be divided into several categories which act at different levels in the regulation of the antibody response. Ts having antigen-dependent functions are designated as carrier-specific Ts (CTs) by simple comparison with CTh. There are different types of CTs described in different experimental systems [reviewed in refs. 20 and 21]. The most definitive feature of CTs is their exquisite binding specificity for antigen. MHC restriction is not always apparent in the stimulation of CTs, while in certain cases their *effects* are clearly MHC-restricted.

In a number of experimental systems, different subsets of CTs interact with each other to induce the ultimate suppressor effect. Such interactions among CTs subsets are often mediated by antigen-specific soluble factor (TsF). The general agreement is that antigen, alone or in association with Ia of APC, stimulates the first stage in Ts generation called *inducer Ts* (Tsi or Ts1). Tsi is either Lyt-1$^+$ or Lyt-2$^+$ depending on the experimental systems and derived from a cyclophosphamide-sensitive population. Tsi in many cases are I-J$^+$ and Qa-1$^+$ and produce I-J$^+$ TsiF (inductive suppressor factor). TsiF acts on other T cells (in many cases Lyt-1$^+$2$^+$ acceptor cells) to activate the second order Ts called *effector Ts* (Tse or Ts2) of Lyt-2$^+$ subclass. This inductive stage cell interaction may be a little more complicated, because it has been suggested that the Lyt-1$^+$2$^+$ acceptor T cells that accepted the TsiF do not directly differentiate into Tse but promote the induction of Tse from other precursor sources (transduction). Variable types of genetic restrictions have been reported in the induction of Tse by TsiF [reviewed in ref. 21]. Tse carries the same antigen specificity and produces the effector type TsF designated as TseF. TseF is antigen-specific and acts on CTh1 to stop the essential helper activity. It has been noted that the same TseF probably also act on Tsi to inhibit the inductive signal for Tse (feedback suppression) [22].

Molecular analyses of TsiF and TseF are now being conducted in a number of laboratories. At the moment, ample evidence indicates that TsiF and TseF exhibit considerable differences in their structure, serological determinants and functions. Some of the TsF are two-chain molecules composed of antigen-binding and I region controlled (I-J) polypeptides [23,24] and others consist only of a single polypeptide with full functional activity [25,26]. It is not yet known what the interrelationships are between these different TsF, as no critical comparisons have been made.

There are probably two types of CTs (CTs1 and CTs2), at least at the level of their effector phase. The generation of Tse is dependent on antigen and antigen-specific Tsi, as described above. However, the final suppression of Th1 is either via the antigen bridge between TseF and Th (cognate interaction) or by non-specific suppressor factors.

There are a number of T hybridomas and cloned T cell lines with suppressor function that belong to either Tsi or Tse. The biochemical analysis of TsF and trials to isolate genes coding for these biologically important factors are in progress.

Ig-specific Ts (IgTs)

It is evident that there exist Ts that regulate B cell responses having a particular Ig structure, as one of the earliest descriptions of the suppressor function of T cell was on chronic allotype suppression [27]. Here again, the direct targets of allotype specific IgTs were neither B cells nor CTh, but IgTh [8]. Since the suppressive effect was dominant for certain classes of Ig over others, and the affinity maturation of antibody produced was also suppressed, the effect of IgTs thus seems to be manifested via a highly sophisticated regulatory mechanism that governs B cell differentiation.

Prenatal or postnatal treatment of animals with anti-idiotypic reagents directed at a major cross-reactive idiotype of the strain induces chronic suppression of the idiotype upon stimulation with corresponding antigen [28–30]. At least a part of this idiotype suppression has been shown to be due to induction of idiotype-specific Ts. This idiotype suppression is at first glance very similar to a clonal expression of allotype suppression (see below), while not much is known about the cellular interactions involved in the suppressor mechanism activated by idiotype-specific IgTs. IgTs so far tested are Lyt-2+ and I-J+. Since allotype-specific IgTs can neutralize Lyt-1+ IgTh, it probably corresponds to the effector type of Ts. Since IgTh itself does not carry Ig allotype, it is yet to be determined how IgTs can recognize IgTh having specificity for one allotype. The authors are inclined towards the view that Ig-allotype-linked determinants detected on functional T cells [31,32] are involved in such Ig-restricted cell interactions.

Interaction between carrier-specific and Ig-specific regulatory pathways

Two important observations give clues to enable the comprehension of the relationship between CTs and IgTs. First, the regulatory cascade initiated by CTh proceeding via idiotype–anti-idiotype interactions [33–35]: CTsi is activated by antigens such as 4-hydroxy-3-nitrophenyl acetyl (NP) and p-azobenzenarsonate (PAB) coupled to syngeneic lymphoid cells, and L-glutamic acid^{60}-L-alanine^{30}-L-tyrosine^{10} (GAT), which can induce antibodies carrying cross-reactive idiotypes in certain selected strains. Analysis of the consequence of cellular interactions leading to the suppression of the antibody response and of delayed type hypersensitivity to corresponding antigens indicated that the initial CTs (Ts1) induces the second (Ts2, anti-idiotypic) and third (Ts3, idiotypic and antigen-specific) order suppressor T cells for the final suppression of the response. Since this linear activation of Ts is not dependent on antigen itself but on the idiotype carried by CTsi (Ts1), Ts2 is a type of IgTs rather than a CTs. Ts3 seems to have dual functions similar to IgTs and CTs because the final suppression is not restricted to the given idiotypic response where antigen-specific as well as polyclonal suppression should have taken place.

The second observation is the conversion of the CTs effect into IgTs, as described by Leonore A. Herzenberg elsewhere in this volume (Chapter 74). Thus the CTs circuit is closely linked to the IgTs circuit via the utilization of Ig-related epitopes of effector molecules such as TsiF. The authors' recent observations have also indicated that idiotype-positive TsiF acts on natural anti-idiotypic T cells of Lyt-1+2+ subclass to transduce Lyt-2+ CTse [36]. In this case, CTsi can act on T cells derived from strains with the same Igh allotype but not others showing apparent Ig allotype restriction. This is, however, the manifestation of an internal idiotype–anti-idiotype interaction between CTsi, acceptor T cell and IgTse that finally suppresses the dominant idiotype. Complex and sophisticated interactions between CTh, CTs, IgTh and IgTs and other members of the group are implied in the responses to certain interesting protein antigens carrying particular epitopes specialized in stimulating the separate regulatory T cell subsets referred to above [37,38].

A synthetic view

The complex regulatory principles of help and suppression are of major interest in contemporary basic immunology; at the same time it has to be admitted that definition of helper and suppressor T cells

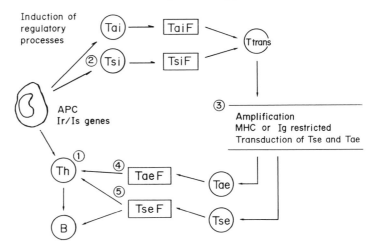

Fig. 71.1. Regulatory circuits in the secondary antibody response.

depends largely on circumstantial evidence. To understand both help and suppression, it is necessary to analyse the interrelationships and principal interactions among all the member cells in this complex and fascinating story. The authors will describe in this final section their personal view of the interactions involved in the suppression and regulatory circuits as represented in Fig. 71.1.

The authors propose that APC and antigen activate CTh1 and CTh2 under the influence of Ir genes expressed on APC (step 1 in Fig. 71.1). CTh1 and CTh2 give help to B cell subsets via cognate and non-cognate interactions. Whether or not different B cells are helped by different CTh has not been completely elucidated, and therefore only Th1–B cell interaction is shown in the figure. In addition, IgTh are first generated within the immune network system of the host, and are expanded by antigenic stimulation. Such IgTh should play a role in determining the quality of the antibody produced with respect to the expression of dominant idiotype, class distribution, maturation of antibody affinity, and allotypic deviation. IgTh may synergize with non-specific helper factors produced by CTh2 to convert the response into specific and meaningful form. Thus the first step in the regulation of the B cell response is the activation of the helper T cell lineage. The authors are aware of a number of problems yet to be resolved at this step, e.g. the nature and quantity of these Th subsets, the role of Ir and Is genes, MHC restriction, mediators of B cell activation, recognition of antigen and interacting cells by Th cells, etc.

The same antigen on APC should activate other regulatory pathways; the induction of CTs and CTa (step 2 in Fig. 71.1) which are true regulatory T cells for Th–B cell interactions. The first regulatory T cells are inducer type Tsi and Tai, which produce antigen-

specific suppressor and augmenting factors (TsiF and TaiF in Fig. 71.1). These factors are not the effector molecules, but act on the second T cell which are called transducer (Ttrans) or acceptor T cells to induce effector type Ts or Ta. The interaction between TsiF or TaiF and Ttrans have been shown to be restricted by MHC or Igh genes. Thus the transduction process is probably the contact point of carrier-specific and idiotype-driven regulation. This transduction process (step 3 in Fig. 71.1) could be either the direct activation of acceptor T cells to become effector T cells or the activation of a process where new effector T cells are generated from their own precursor pool. In any event, effector Ts and Ta (Tse and Tae in Fig. 71.1) are generated through the above complex transduction process. Tse and Tae may be either carrier specific (CTs and CTa) or Ig specific (IgTs and IgTa), depending on the transduction events. These effector type regulatory T cells produce the specific regulatory molecules that act directly on Th or, in certain cases, B cells (steps 4 and 5 in Fig. 71.1).

TseF or TaeF could be either MHC restricted, Ig restricted or only antigen specific in their action on Th, according to the transduction event. The relative activities of Tse and Tae (steps 4 and 5) should determine the ultimate activity of the cells in helping B cells. It is not known what determines these effector Ts and Ta activities. In the authors' experimental system, the contact of primed spleen cells with TsiF at the time of antigenic stimulation induced suppression, whereas one or two days after antigenic stimulation, the cells became resistant to TsiF and were susceptible preferentially to the effect of TaiF [17]. If the effects of Ts and Ta are distinct at their effector step (steps 4 and 5), the time of delivery of TseF and TaeF may have a key role to play: Th could easily be suppressed by TseF if they came into contact with TseF first. However, if Th were in contact with TaeF before TseF, they may become refractory to the effect of TseF. This latter situation is analogous to the effect of contrasuppression proposed by Gershon *et al.* [39], where contrasuppressor T cells rescue Th from suppression by Ts. Another published attempt is recommended to readers to help in the understanding of the different levels of suppression [40]. A discussion derived from the network concept, which suggests that the induction of help is due to de-repression of some Th precursors from predominant natural Ts, is also available [41].

These considerations are important for the further analyses of both suppressor and helper circuits, composed as they are of multiple interacting T cells producing the final regulatory suppressor effect. They are connected by antigen, MHC products and Ig-related structures to constitute an immune system with inherent regulatory principles. The 'middle age' of cellular immunology with over-simplified Th and Ts is now over, and the newly emerging technologies and concepts will help provide insights into this highly sophisticated regulatory system.

References

1 HERZENBERG L.A., BLACK S.J. & HERZENBERG L.A. (1980) Regulatory circuit and antibody responses. *Eur. J. Immunol.* **10**, 1.

2 CANTOR H. & GERSHON R.K. (1979) Immunological circuits: cellular composition. *Fedn Proc.* **38**, 2058.

3 GERSHON R.K. (1980) Immunoregulation *circa* 1980: Some commments on the state of the art. *J. Allergy clin. Immunol.* **66**, 18.

4 RAJEWSKY K. & ROTTRANDER E. (1967) Tolerance specificity and immune response to lactic dehydrogenase isozymes. *Cold Spring Harb. Symp. quant. Biol.* **32**, 547.

5 MITCHISON N.A. (1971) The carrier effect in the secondary response to hapten–protein conjugates. (II) Cellular cooperation. *Eur. J. Immunol.* **1**, 18.

6 TADA T., TAKEMORI T., OKUMURA K., NONAKA M. & TOKUHISA T. (1978) Two distinct types of helper T cells involved in the secondary antibody response: independent and synergistic effects of Ia$^-$ and Ia$^+$ helper T cells. *J. exp. Med.* **147**, 446.

7 MARRACK P.C. & KAPPLER J.W. (1975) Antigen-specific and nonspecific mediators of T cell/B cell cooperation. (I) Evidence for their production by different T cells. *J. Immunol.* **114**, 1116.

8 HERZENBERG L.A., OKUMURA K., CANTOR H., SATO V.L., SHEN F.W., BOYSE E. & HERZENBERG L.A. (1976) T-cell regulation of antibody response: demonstration of allotype-specific helper T cells and their specific removal by suppressor T cells. *J. exp. Med.* **144**, 330.

9 OKUMURA K., METZLER C.M., SU T., HERZENBERG L.A. & HERZENBERG L.A. (1976) Two stages of B-cell memory development with different T cell requirements. *J. exp. Med.* **144**, 345.

10 JERNEWAY C.A. JUN., RURGITA R.A., WEINBAUM F.I.,

ASOFSKY R. & WIGZELL H. (1975) Evidence for an immunoglobulin-dependent antigen-specific helper T cell. *Proc. natn. Acad. Sci. U.S.A.* **74**, 4582.

11 BOTTOMLY K. & MOSIER D.E. (1979) Mice whose B cells cannot produce the T15 idiotype also lack an antigen-specific helper T cell required for T15 expression. *J. exp. Med.* **150**, 1399.

12 WOODLAND R. & CANTOR H. (1978) Idiotype specific T helper cells are required to induce idiotype positive B memory cells to secrete antibody. *Eur. J. Immunol.* **8**, 600.

13 FRIDMAN W.H., RABOURDIN-COMBE C., NEAUPORT-SAUTES C. & GISLER R.H. (1981) Characterization and function of T cell Fcγ receptor. *Immunol. Revs.* **56**, 51.

14 ISHIZAKA K. (1983) IgE-binding factors from rat T lymphocytes. *Lymphokines*, **8**, 41.

15 SUEMURA M., SHIHO O., DEGUCHI H., YAMAMURA Y., BOTTCHER I. & KISHIMOTO T. (1981) Characterization and isolation of IgE class-specific suppressor factor (IgE-TsF). *J. Immunol.* **127**, 465.

16 KIYONO H., MCGHEE J.R., MOSTELLER L.M., ELDRIDGE J.H., KOOPMAN W.J., KEARNEY J.F. & MICHALEK S.M. (1982) Murine Peyer's patch T cell clones. Characterization of antigen-specific helper T cells for immunoglobulin A responses. *J. exp. Med.* **156**, 1115.

17 TOKUHISA T., TANIGUCHI M., OKUMURA K. & TADA T. (1978) An antigen-specific I region gene product that augments the antibody response. *J. Immunol.* **120**, 414.

18 MIYATANI S., HIRAMATSU K., NAKAJIMA P.B., OWEN F.L. & TADA T. (1983) Structural analysis of antigen-specific Ia-bearing regulatory T-cell factors: Gel electrophoretic analysis of the antigen-specific augmenting T-cell factor. *Proc. natn. Acad. Sci. U.S.A.* **80**, 6336.

19 ASANO Y. & HODES R.J. (1984) T cell regulation of B cell activation: MHC-restricted T augmenting cells enhance the B cell responses mediated by MHC-restricted cloned T helper cells. *J. Immunol.* **132**, 1151.

20 GERSHON R.K. (1974) T-cell control of antibody production. *Contemp. Top. Immunobiol.* **3**, 1.

21 TADA T. & OKUMURA K. (1979) The role of antigen-specific T cell factors in the immune response. *Adv. Immunol.* **28**, 1.

22 EARDLEY D.D., HUGENBERGER J., MCVAY-BOUDREAU L., SHEN F.W., GERSHON R.K. & CANTOR H. (1978) Immunoregulatory circuits among T-cell sets. (I) T-helper cells induct other T-cell sets to exert feedback inhibition. *J. exp. Med.* **147**, 1106.

23 TANIGUCHI M., SAITO T. & TADA T. (1979) Antigen-specific suppressor factor produced by a transplantable I-J bearing T cell hybridoma. *Nature*, **278**, 555.

24 YAMAUCHI K., CHAO N., MURPHY D.B. & GERSHON R.K. (1982) Molecular composition of an antigen-specific, Ly-1 T suppressor inducer factor: One molecule binds antigen and is I-J$^-$, does not bind antigen, and imparts Igh-variable region linked restriction. *J. exp. Med.* **155**, 655.

25 KRUPEN K., ARANEO B.A., KAPP J.A., STEIN S., WIEDER K.J. & WEBB D.R. (1982) Purification and characterization of a monoclonal T cell suppressor factor specific for poly(L-Glu^{60}-L-Ala^{30}-L-Tyr^{10}). *Proc. natn. Acad. Sci. U.S.A.* **79**, 1254.

26 FRESNO M., MCVAY-BOUDREAU L., NABEL G. & CANTOR

H. (1981) Antigen-specific T lymphocyte clones. (II) Purification and biochemical characterization of an antigen-specific suppressive protein synthesized by cloned T cells. *J. exp. Med.* **153,** 1260.

27 HERZENBERG L.A., CHAN E.L., RAVITCH M.M., RIBLET R.J. & HERZENBERG L.A. (1973) Active suppression of immunoglobulin allotype synthesis. (III) Identification of T cells as responsible for suppression by cells from spleen, thymus, lymph node and bone marrow. *J. exp. Med.* **137,** 1311.

28 EICHMANN K. (1975) Idiotype suppression. (II) Amplification of suppressor T cell with anti-idiotypic activity. *Eur. J. Immunol.* **5,** 511.

29 NISONOFF A., JU S.-T. & OWEN F.L. (1977) Studies of structure and immunosuppression of a cross-reactive idiotype in strain A mice. *Immunol. Revs.* **34,** 89.

30 TAKEMORI T. & RAJEWSKY K. (1984) Specificity, duration and mechanisms of idiotype suppression induced neonatal injection of monoclonal anti-idiotype antibody into mice. *Eur. J. Immunol.* **14,** 656.

31 OWEN F.L., FINNEGAN A., GATES E.R. & GOTTLIEB P.D. (1979) A mature T lymphocyte subpopulation marker closely linked to the Ig-1 allotype C_H locus. *Eur. J. Immunol.* **9,** 948.

32 KARASUYAMA H., KIM M., OKUMURA K. & TADA T. (1984) Heterogeneity of Igh-linked allotypic determinants expressed on functional T cell subsets as detected by monoclonal antibodies. *Eur. J. Immunol.* **14,** 413.

33 SUNDAY M.E., BENACERRAF B. & DORF M.E. (1981) Hapten-specific T cell responses to 4-hydroxy-3-nitrophenyl acetyl. (VIII) Suppressor cell pathways in cutaneous sensitivity response. *J. exp. Med.* **153,** 811.

34 DOHI Y. & NISONOFF A. (1979) Suppression of idiotype and generation of suppressor T cells with idiotype conjugated thymocytes. *J. exp. Med.* **150,** 909.

35 WEIDER K.J., ARANEO B.A., KAPP J.A. & WEBB D.R. (1982) Cell-free translation of a biologically active antigen-specific suppressor T cell factor. *Proc. natn. Acad. Sci. U.S.A.* **79,** 3599.

36 ABE R., KARASUYAMA H., YAGI J. & TADA T. (1984) Regulation of allotype-linked NP^b idiotype by an idiotype positive soluble factor derived from a T cell hybridoma—coupling of the circuit regulation to the network concept. *Int. Archs Allergy appl. Immunol.* **174,** 289.

37 SERCARZ E.E., YOWELL R.L., TURKIN D., MILLER A., ARANEO B.A. & ADORINI L. (1978) Different functional specificity repertoire for suppressor and helper T cells. *Immunol. Revs.* **39,** 108.

38 KOHNO Y. & BERZOFSKY J.A. (1982) Genetic control of the immune response to myoglobulin. (V) Antibody production *in vitro* is macrophage and T cell dependent and is under control of two determinant-specific Ir genes. *J. Immunol.* **128,** 2458.

39 GERSHON R.K., EARDLEY D.D., DURUM D.D., SHEN F.W., YAMAUCHI K., CANTOR H. & MURPHY D.B. (1981) Contrasuppression: A novel immunoregulatory activity. *J. exp. Med.* **153,** 1533.

40 GREEN D.R., CHUE B. & GERSHON R.K. (1983) Discrimination of 2 types of suppressor T cells by cell surface phenotype and by function: The ability to regulate the contrasuppressor circuit. *J. Mol. cell. Immunol.* **1,** 19.

41 EICHMANN K., FALK L., MELCHERS I. & SIMON M.M. (1980) Quantitative studies on T cell diversity. *J. exp. Med.* **152,** 477.

Chapter 72
Overview: Ir genes

B. BENACERRAF

Basis for specificity of MHC
restriction of T cells, 72.2

The major histocompatibility complex (MHC) has presented a considerable intellectual challenge to immunologists, as it is evident that the rejection of allografts does not have survival value and that this complex and costly system did not evolve for this trivial purpose. The development of this complex system of genes, which is found in many other vertebrate species besides mammals, must have other very important evolutionary significance and functions. The answer to this question was unexpected and was provided by developments in a completely different field from transplantation immunology, the discovery of immune response (Ir) genes and the demonstration that Ir genes code for transplantation antigens of the major histocompatibility complex [1–5]. The subsequent finding that Ir gene phenomenology is selectively concerned with the specific activation of T lymphocytes [6,7] stimulated studies of the specificity of T lymphocytes and of their regulatory interactions with other cells of the immune system, where MHC antigens play a critical role.

The following points have been established.

1 MHC antigens are concerned with our ability to distinguish self from non-self.

2 T lymphocytes develop receptors for self MHC antigens during differentiation; however, only mature T cells with specific receptors against self MHC of low affinity are allowed to migrate from the thymus [8].

3 T cells react to conventional foreign antigens only when presented on cell surfaces in conjunction with autologous MHC antigens [9,10].

4 MHC molecules, therefore, govern the necessary cell interactions concerned with antigen induced stimulation between the various cells of the immune system, T cells, B cells [11], and macrophages [9].

5 The extensive polymorphism of MHC antigens has the result that individuals differ in their ability to respond specifically to selected antigens and to develop immunological diseases [5,12].

6 Alloreactivity and our inability to transplant tissues is the price we pay for the benefits to the species of this complex recognition system [13,14].

The insight into the biological function of MHC molecules came from several experimental approaches. Initial studies in the author's [1] and McDevitt's [2] laboratories revealed that genes in the I region of the murine H-2 complex determine the ability of T lymphocytes to respond to a thymus dependent antigen. The author and McDevitt called these genes immune response genes or Ir genes [5]. Different individual and different inbred strains varied, therefore, in their ability to respond to an antigen under Ir gene control and were classified as responder and non-responder. Numerous studies in these and other laboratories established over the years that Ir genes do indeed code for the polypeptide chains of the class II MHC (Ia) molecules expressed for this purpose on the membrane of antigen-presenting cells and of B lymphocytes [15,16]. In an attempt to elucidate the function of Ir genes, several laboratories focussed their attention on the role of Ia molecules in specific immune responses. Rosenthal & Shevach, in Paul's laboratory at the National Institutes of Health, demonstrated that T lymphocytes only react to foreign antigens if they are presented by antigen-presenting cells together with autologous Ia antigens [17]. Moreover, the T cell clones in an F1 animal were shown to be restricted specifically to one or the other parental Ia molecule and the foreign antigen [18]. Accordingly anti-Ia antibody was able to block specifically the interaction of antigen presenting cells and antigen-specific T lymphocytes [19].

At the time when these findings were made the author, together with Katz, Hamaoka, & Dorf at Harvard, noted that the interaction between helper T cells and the B cells they regulate is equally restricted by Ia molecules [20]. The helper T cell is restricted to interact with a B cell bearing the same autologous Ia molecule as the macrophage that originally stimulated it with antigen. In addition, this restriction is clearly concerned with Ir gene function since a (responder × non-responder) T cell can provide help for a responder B cell and not for a non-responder B cell [21]. The author and his colleagues concluded that T helper lymphocytes are specific for both autologous Ia molecules and foreign antigens presented jointly, and that a T cell clone so selected in the course of immunization is restricted to interact with B lymphocytes bearing antigen in the same manner. The more recent experiments with cloned B cell and T cell lines have substantiated these conclusions for a category of B cells (Ly B5-) [22].

Following a different line of investigation in Australia, Zinkernagel & Doherty arrived independently at substantially identical conclusions with respect to class I MHC molecules and cytolytic T lymphocytes. They reported that cytolytic T lymphocytes (CTL) of mice specific for the lymphochoriomeningitis virus (LCMV) lyse LCMV-infected target cells bearing the same class I MHC antigen as the immunized host, but not LCMV-infected allogeneic cells bearing distinct type I MHC antigens. They concluded that CTLs are restricted to interact with foreign antigens only when presented in the context of autologous class I MHC antigens [10].

Thus different classes of T lymphocytes are restricted by different classes of MHC molecules in their ability to interact with foreign antigens.

Because of the extensive polymorphism of both class I and class II antigens, Ir gene phenomena have been described involving both class I [5] and class II [23] molecules.

It appears, therefore, that all T lymphocytes only recognize foreign antigens when perceived together with one or another class of MHC gene product, depending on the T cell subclass, and that this is a fundamental property of T cells.

Recent studies with human CTL cloned lines by Schlossman *et al.* have established that in man also different classes of T lymphocytes are specific for class I and for class II MHC antigens [24]; CTL specific for class I alloantigens bear the T8 surface antigen, whereas CTLs specific for human class II alloantigens (DR) bear T4 membrane glycoproteins. In addition, anti-T8 and anti-T4 antibody inhibit lysis of CTL specific for class I and class II antigens respectively, suggesting that, in man, T4 and T8 glycoproteins are directly concerned with the specificity of MHC restriction phenomena in this species.

Broadening further the phenomenon of MHC restriction of T lymphocytes, the author has recently established, with Greene, Dorf, and Sy in their laboratories, that suppressor T lymphocytes are restricted by another class of MHC molecule on antigen presenting cells, the product of the I–J subregion [24,25,26].

Basis for specificity of MHC restriction of T cells

The specificities of T cells for self MHC antigens in conjunction with foreign antigens determine restrictions in the ability of T cells to react with these foreign molecules, so that animals with certain MHC haplotypes are responders and others with other MHC haplotypes are non-responders to the same antigen. This fundamental behaviour, which is the basis of Ir gene phenomenology, has been noted for both class I and class II MHC antigens [5,23].

Two types of explanation have been proposed to account for the manner in which MHC molecules affect the specific pattern of immune reactivity of T lymphocytes.

1 Rosenthal [27] and the author [28] postulated that the specific interaction of Ia molecules with foreign antigens on the surface of antigen-presenting cells posed certain restrictions on the preferential orientation of these molecules and restricted their ability to bind to T cell specific receptors, thus introducing the concept of determinant selection on foreign antigens as a consequence of Ia molecule–antigen interactions. The major criticism directed against this hypothesis is the lack of heterogeneity in Ia molecules in any given individual. Two classes of Ia molecules exist in an individual mouse heterozygous at these loci; there can be, at most, eight distinct molecules in such an individual, taking advantage of interchain co-operation in the cis as well as in the trans configuration. This number of distinct Ia molecules would appear to be too small to account for the extent of Ir gene specific restrictions observed.

Yet evidence has been obtained compatible with a specific antigen–Ia molecule interaction at the level of the antigen presenting cell [29,30,31,32]. A unique prediction of the specific association model is that distinct antigens, which use the same interaction site, should compete for association with Ia molecules and subsequent presentation under limiting conditions [30]. In the course of studies characterizing a series of antigen-specific, Ia-restricted T cell hybridomas a specific competition was observed between structurally related copolymers under Ir gene control. Moreover, the competition at the level of the antigen-presenting cell has been localized and its specificity documented [30].

2 The other hypothesis postulates that the Ir gene defects are the result of clonal deletion at the level of the T cell, and that during differentiation, while T cells are rendered tolerant to self antigen in relation to autologous MHC antigens, certain foreign antigens plus self MHC molecules mimic some autologous molecule in the context of the same self MHC molecules. This results in the deletion of these T cell clones and in the inability to respond to these selected foreign antigens for animals of these precise MHC haplotypes [34,35]. This hypothesis is indeed very attractive but difficult to prove. Nevertheless, the author emphasizes that the two mechanisms proposed are not mutually exclusive and both may very well be operative.

References

1 LEVINE B.B., OJEDA A. & BENACERRAF B. (1963) Studies on artificial antigens. The genetic control of the immune response to hapten–poly-L-lysine conjugates in guinea pigs. *J. exp. Med.* **118**, 953.

2 McDEVITT H.O. & SELA M. (1965) Genetic control of the antibody response. (I) Demonstration of determinant specific differences in response to synthetic polypeptide antigens in two strains of inbred mice. *J. exp. Med.* **122**, 517.

3 McDEVITT H.O. & CHINITZ A. (1969) Genetic control of antibody response: relationship between immune response and histocompability (H-2) type. *Science*, **163**, 1207.

4 ELLMAN L., GREEN I., MARTIN W.J. & BENACERRAF B. (1970) Linkage between the PLL gene and the locus controlling the major histocompability antigens in strain 2 guinea pigs. *Proc. natn. Acad. Sci. U.S.A.* **66**, 322.

5 BENACERRAF B. & McDEVITT H.O. (1972) The histocompability linked immune response genes. *Science*, **175**, 273.

6 LEVINE B.B., OJEDA A. & BENACERRAF B. (1963) Basis for the antigenicity of hapten–poly-L-lysine conjugates in random-bred guinea pigs. *Nature*, **198**, 1215.

7 GREEN I., PAUL W.E. & BENACERRAF B. (1966) The behavior of hapten–poly-L-lysine conjugates as complete antigens in genetic responder and as haptens in non-responder guinea pigs. *J. exp. Med.* **123**, 859.

8 BEVAN M.J. (1977) In a radiation chimera, host H-2 antigens determine immune responsiveness of donor cytotoxic cells. *Nature*, **269**, 417.

9 SHEVACH E.M. & ROSENTHAL A.S. (1973) Function of macrophages in antigen recognition by guinea pig lymphocytes. (II) Role of macrophages in the regulation of genetic control of the immune response. *J. exp. Med.* **138**, 1213.

10 ZINKERNAGEL R.M. & DOHERTY P.C. (1975) H-2 compatibility requirement for T cell mediated lysis of target cells infected with choriomeningitis virus. Different cytotoxic cell specificities are associated with structures coded for in H-2K or H-2D. *J. exp. Med.* **141**, 1427.

11 KATZ D.H., HAMAOKA T. & BENACERRAF B. (1973) Cell interactions between histoincompatible T and B lymphocytes. (II) Failure of cooperative interactions between T and B lymphocytes from allogeneic donor strains in humoral response to hapten–protein conjugates. *J. exp. Med.* **137**, 1405.

12 GRIFFING W.L., MOORE S.B., LUTHER H.S., McKENNA C.H. & FATHMAN C.G. (1980) Association of antibodies to native DNA with HLA-DRw3. A possible major histocompatibility complex linked human immune response gene. *J. exp. Med.* **152**, 319.

13 FINBERG R., BURAKOFF S.J., CANTOR H. & BENACERRAF B. (1978) The biologic significance of alloreactivity. T cells stimulated by sendai virus coated syngeneic cells specifically lyse allogeneic target cells. *Proc. natn. Acad. Sci. U.S.A.* **75**, 5145.

14 BENACERRAF B. (1981) Role of MHC gene products in immune regulation. Nobel lecture. *Science*, **212**, 1229.

15 McDEVITT H.O., DEAK D.B., SHREFFLER D.C., KLEIN J., STIMPFLING J.H. & SNELL G.D. (1972) Genetic control of the immune response. Mapping of the Ir.1 locus. *J. exp. Med.* **135**, 1259.

16 BENACERRAF B. & GERMAIN R.N. (1978) The immune response genes of the major histocompatibility complex. *Immunol. Revs.* **38**, 70.

17 ROSENTHAL A.S. & SHEVACH E.M. (1973) Function of macrophages in antigen recognition by guinea pig lymphocytes. (I) Requirement for histocompatible macrophages and lymphocytes. *J. exp. Med.* **138**, 1194.

18 SHEVACH E.M., PAUL W.E. & GREEN I. (1972) Histocompatibility linked immune response gene function in the guinea pigs. Specific inhibition of antigen induced lymphocyte proliferation by alloantisera. *J. exp. Med.* **136**, 1207.

19 PAUL W.E., SHEVACH E.M., PICKERAL S., THOMAS D.W. & ROSENTHAL A.S. (1977) Independent populations of F1 guinea pig T lymphocytes respond to antigen-pulsed parental peritoneal cells. *J. exp. Med.* **145**, 618.

20 KATZ D.H., HAMAOKA T., DORF M.E., MAURER P.H. & BENACERRAF B. (1973) Cell interactions between histocompatible T and B lymphocytes. (III) Demonstration that the H-2 gene complex determines successful physiologic lymphocyte interactions. *Proc. natn. Acad. Sci. U.S.A.* **70**, 2624.

21 KATZ D.H., HAMAOKA T., DORF M.E., MAURER P.H. & BENACERRAF B. (1973) Cell interactions between histocompatible T and B lymphocytes. (IV) Involvement of the immune response (Ir) gene in the control of lymphocyte interactions in responses controlled by the gene. *J. exp. Med.* **138**, 734.

22 SINGER A., ASANO Y., SHIGETA M., HATHCOCK K.S., AHMED A., FATHMAN C.G. & HODES R.J. (1982) Distinct B cell subpopulations differ in their genetic requirements for activation by helper T cells. *Immunol. Revs.* **64**, 137.

23 FINBERG R. & BENACERRAF B. (1981) Induction, control and consequences of virus specific cytotoxic T cells. *Immunol. Revs.* **58**, 157.

24 MEUER S.C., SCHLOSSMAN S.F. & REINHERZ E.L. (1982) Clonal analysis of human cytotoxic T lymphocytes: T4+ and T8+ effector T cells recognize products of different major histocompatibility complex regions. *Proc. natn. Acad. Sci. U.S.A.* **79**, 4395.

25 TAKAOKI M., SY M.S., TOMINAGA A., LOWY A., TSURUFUJI M., FINBERG R., BENACERRAF B. & GREENE M.I. (1982) I-J restricted interactions in the generation of azobenzenearsonate specific suppressor T cells. *J. exp. Med.* **156**, 1325.

26 MINAMI M., HONJI N. & DORF M.E. (1982) Mechanism responsible for the induction of I-J restrictions on Ts3 suppressor cells. *J. exp. Med.* **156**, 1502.

27 ROSENTHAL A.S., BARCINSKI A.M. & BLAKE T.J. (1977)

Determinant selection is a macrophage dependent immune response gene function. *Nature*, **267**, 156.

28 BENACERRAF B. (1978) A hypothesis to relate the specificity of T-lymphocytes and the activity of I region specific Ir genes in macrophages and B lymphocytes. *J. Immunol.* **120**, 1809.

29 WERDELIN O. (1982) Chemically related antigens compete for presentation by accessory cells to T cell. *J. Immunol.* **129**, 1883.

30 ROCK K.L. & BENACERRAF B. (1983) Inhibition of antigen specific T lymphocyte activation by structurally related Ir gene controlled polymers: evidence of specific competition for accessory cell antigen presentation. *J. exp. Med.* **157**, 1618.

31 MATIS L.A., JONES P.P., MURPHY D.B., HEDRICK S.M., LERNER E.A., JANEWAY C.A. JUN., MCNICHOLAS J.M. & SCHWARTZ R.H. (1982) Immune response gene function correlates with the cell surface expression of an Ia antigen.

(II) Quantitative deficiency in Ae.Eα complex expression causes a corresponding defect in antigen-presenting cell function. *J. exp. Med.* **155**, 508.

32 MCNICHOLAS J., MURPHY D.B., MATIS L.A., SCHWARTZ R.M., LERNER E.A., JANEWAY C.A. JUN. & JONES P.P. (1982) Immune response gene function correlates with the expression of an Ia antigen. (I) Preferential association of certain Ae and Eα chains results in a quantitative deficiency in expression of an Ae.Eα complex. *J. exp. Med.* **155**, 490.

33 ISHII N., NAGY L.A. & KLEIN J. (1982) Restriction molecules involved in the interaction of T cells with allogeneic antigen-presenting cells. *J. exp. Med.* **156**, 622.

34 JERNE N.K. (1971) The somatic generation of immune recognition. *Eur. J. Immunol.* **1**, 1.

35 SCHWARTZ R.H. (1978) A clonal deletion model for Ir gene control of the immune response. *Scand. J. Immunol.* **7**, 3.

Chapter 73
Overview: Idiotypic regulation

K. RAJEWSKY

Antibodies with complementary binding sites, 73.1

The network hypothesis, 73.1

Experimental evidence for the components of a formal idiotypic network in the immune system, 73.2

Experimental evidence for idiotypic control, 73.2

Limitations of the network hypothesis, 73.3

Puzzles and questions, 73.3

Conclusion, 73.4

Antibodies with complementary binding sites

Nomenclature

The variable regions of antibody molecules, like any other macromolecular structure, carry antigenic determinants against which antibodies can be raised. These determinants are called idiotypic determinants or idiotopes and the corresponding antibodies are anti-idiotope antibodies. A set of idiotopes, be it expressed on a single antibody molecule or a family of antibodies, is called an idiotype and the corresponding set of anti-idiotopes, anti-idiotypic antibodies. One should keep in mind that the terms 'idiotope' and 'idiotype' on the one hand, and 'anti-idiotope' and 'anti-idiotype' on the other, are merely operational: one usually calls an antibody 'anti-idiotypic' if it was raised against a given antibody or set of antibodies (the 'idiotype'). However, since at the molecular level 'idiotype' and 'anti-idiotype' represent functionally equivalent molecules with complementary binding sites, one could also have raised the 'idiotype' by immunization with 'anti-idiotype', as has indeed been verified experimentally. In this case, one would have called the 'idiotype' 'anti-idiotype' and vice versa.

In order to avoid this problem, one often calls the antibody against which an anti-idiotype was raised, antibody 1 (ab1), and the anti-idiotype, ab2. Ab2 may fall into two classes, namely antibodies expressing a structure (idiotope) resembling the antigenic determinant against which ab1 was raised. These antibodies are called ab2β or the *internal image* of the immunizing antigenic determinant. The second class of ab2, ab2α, recognizes idiotopes on ab1 which are unrelated to the antigen binding site (paratope) of ab1. (Note that the terms 'idiotope' and 'paratope' are again no more than operational terms. 'Paratope' designates the classical hapten binding site of an antibody. Clearly, however, in idiotypic interactions of antibodies, paratopes recognize idiotopes as well as vice versa. Thus paratopes and idiotopes are indistinguishable in molecular terms and can be localized anywhere in the variable region of an antibody, although both will presumably be mostly associated with the hypervariable regions. Significantly, these latter sequences form both the grooves and the protusions of the variable (V) domains.)

As in the case of ab2, ab3 (antibodies raised against ab2) can be divided into two classes, namely ab3β (idiotypically resembling ab1) and ab3α (recognizing idiotopes on ab2 unrelated to the structure involved in the interaction of ab2 with ab1). The same rule holds for ab4, ab5, etc.

The network hypothesis

Since the discovery of T–B cell collaboration it has been clear that the cells of the immune system interact with each other in a functional way. The network hypothesis, formulated by Niels Jerne [1], sees the immune system as a system of interacting cells, the interactions being mediated by complementary receptors, be they cell surface bound or, like humoral antibodies, circulating in the serum. Idiotypic interactions are thus thought to be the language by which lymphocytes communicate. This language is imprinted into the immune system because of the diversity of antibody V region which leads to the expression of a large fraction of the universe of antigenic determinants within the population of V regions itself, i.e. within the immune system (see discussion of internal images above). The network hypothesis can be stated in various forms. For example, the immune system can be visualized as an equilibrium of idiotypic and anti-idiotypic receptors leading to a state of general suppression. The introduction of antigen disturbs this equilibrium and leads to a new equilibrium, characteristic of the state of immunity or tolerance. How is the original equilibrium reached? Here one might consider that as the receptor repertoire is generated from the germ line and diversified by somatic mutation, a state will be reached where the system is so diverse that each newly arising somatic mutant will already find its anti-idiotypic counterpart present and will thus be suppressed. Thus the network may both 'breed' somatic mutants and limit the extent to which they are allowed to contribute to the receptor repertoire. Every immune system may in this way establish its own, individual repertoire of binding sites in ontogeny. Alternatively, one might consider the naive immune system as a collection of functionally non-connected cells. Only when certain sets of clones are expanded through antigenic stimulation will idiotypic control be set in motion to regulate the immune response. Various mathematical models have been developed which describe such types of network regulation. Some of these models take into account both the interaction of the various cell types in the immune system (B cells, helper T and suppressor cells) and of free receptor molecules such as antibodies. All these components are considered to be part of a functional idiotypic network.

Experimental evidence for the components of a formal idiotypic network in the immune system

It has been established beyond doubt that idiotypes and anti-idiotypes co-exist in the immune system. Thus anti-idiotypic antibodies can be raised against apparently any antibody, even within inbred stains of mice. In addition, and definitely proving the point, anti-idiotypic antibodies arise spontaneously in the course of a variety of immune responses. It has also been shown that T cells can both express idiotypic determinants related to those on B cells and recognize B cell idiotypes in that they are able to specifically control idiotype expression by B cells (see also below). Thus, at least in a formal sense, an idiotypic network exists in the immune system and comprises both B and T cells.

There is also evidence for the existence of internal images of external antigens at the level of antibody variable regions. Most striking in this sense, perhaps, are experiments showing that fractions of anti-idiotypic antibodies against antibodies with specificity for certain hormones can bind to cellular receptors for those hormones and sometimes even mimic their physiological effects. In general, however, the bulk of anti-idiotypic antibodies do not seem to fall into the internal image category.

Experimental evidence for idiotypic control

There is a large body of evidence demonstrating that antibodies can control the expression of their complementary counterparts. When animals are immunized with an ab1, they will produce (anti-idiotypic) ab2. Such animals, when immunized with the antigen specific for ab1, will produce an immune response lacking the idiotypic determinants of ab1. However, when animals are primed with ab2 and subsequently immunized with the antigen specific for ab1, their immune response will consist predominantly of antibodies expressing idiotypic determinants of ab1, although in the response of a normal animal these determinants may be expressed only on a minor fraction of the total antibody population.

More convincing in the sense of a physiological role of humoral antibodies in idiotypic control are experiments in which antibodies with defined idiotypic or anti-idiotypic specificity are introduced into the immune system in free form and minute quantities. The application of nanogram quantities of anti-idiotype (even in the form of monoclonal, isogeneic antibody) to adult mice enhances the expression of the corresponding idiotype in subsequent immune responses, even when the latter are induced several months after anti-idiotype administration. In contrast, microgram amounts of anti-idiotype lead to long-term suppression of idiotype expression. Long-term suppression is also seen when anti-idiotypic antibody is administered to animals at birth (neonatal suppression). It has also been shown that the injection of microgram amounts of idiotypically defined antibodies can lead to the enhanced expression of *the same idiotype* in subsequent immune responses (idiotypic memory).

It is hard to escape the conclusion that reactions of this type occur physiologically in the immune system. For example, antibodies transmitted from the mother to the offspring should affect the antibody repertoire in the latter (maternal effect); experimental evidence for this phenomenon has been collected. Likewise, antibodies produced by an animal will affect the antibody repertoire in the same animal. Does this make sense in physiological terms? In the nanogram range (in which 'natural' antibodies may often occur), antibodies will expand the repertoire of cells expressing receptors with complementary binding sites. This mechanism could play an important role in the somatic generation of the antibody repertoire through network control (see also below). In the microgram range, antibodies inhibit the production of anti-antibodies. This is clearly a requirement of classical immunological tolerance and leads to the stabilization of the *expressed* repertoire. However, as pointed out below, idiotype suppression may be a mechanism of self-tolerance also to antigens other than antibody variable region.

As to the mechanisms by which antibodies exert their regulatory effects via idiotypic interactions, it seems clear that both enhancement and suppression involve both T and B cells, although the initial reaction may always be the interaction of the antibody with a complementary (idiotypic or anti-idiotypic) receptor on the B cell surface. There is good evidence that in the case of idiotype suppression by anti-idiotypic antibody, at least two different mechanisms operate, namely the elimination or blockade of newly arising B cells in the bone marrow (acute suppression) and the induction of regulatory T cells which prevent the expression of the target idiotype in the B cell population (chronic suppression). Whether anti-idiotypic B cells also play a role remains to be elucidated.

With respect to the nature of T cell control of idiotype expression by B cells, a variety of mechanisms are supported by experimental evidence. In the case of suppression, a cascade of interacting idiotypic and anti-idiotypic suppressor-inducer and suppressor-effector cells may be set in motion, their target being either an idiotype-specific helper T cell or the idiotype-bearing B cell itself. In the case of idiotype-specific help, anti-idiotypic helper cells may directly interact with B cells, or idiotypically related B and helper T cells may be bridged by anti-idiotypic antibody.

A recent analysis of idiotype suppression [3,6] has led to a model in which the binding of a ligand (anti-idiotypic antibody or antigen) to antigen receptors mediates the induction of regulatory (suppressive) T cells with specificity for the idiotype of the receptor. Indeed, recent experiments [9] show that chronic idiotype suppression can be induced not only by anti-idiotypic antibody but also by antigen. T cell mediated idiotype suppression may, therefore, be a general mechanism for the maintenance of self-tolerance.

Limitations of the network hypothesis

Idiotypic control of immune responses induced by external antigen

While idiotypic interactions may well play some role in the control of such responses, it also seems clear that antigen plays a dominant role in antibody selection. There are only a few exceptions to the general rule that idiotypes associated with a given antigen-specific immune response are confined to antigen-binding antibodies in the immune serum, although at the level of the total repertoire many of the corresponding idiotopes are also expressed in antibodies of unrelated antigen-binding specificity. This finding agrees with

the general observation that while anti-idiotypic antibodies in native (non-cross-linked) forms are powerful regulators of antigen-driven immune responses, they are poor inducers of antibody responses.

It is also clear that idiotype-specific T cells are not required for the induction of B cell responses, since cloned, antigen-specific helper T cells are able to induce normal B cell responses *in vitro* and *in vivo* in the absence of other types of T cells. This appears also true for primary *in vivo* responses [5]. Idiotypic control by T cells would thus be restricted to a modulation of the response itself and/or the pre-selection of the B cell repertoire and/or the activation of antigen-specific T cell help.

Genetic control of the idiotypic repertoire

Recent evidence indicates that in genetically identical animals the immune response is often much more homogeneous than one might have anticipated. In mice, a number of responses have been shown to be dominated by the products of a few germ line V, D and J genes and their somatically mutated progeny. These responses differ in different strains of mice because of polymorphism of the antibody structural genes. In line with these observations is evidence indicating that in a given strain at least part of its idiotope repertoire is regularly expressed and that, in a first approximation, the repertoire is incomplete because of polymorphism of the corresponding antibody structural genes. In F crosses between strains differing with respect to the expression of a given idiotope, idiotope expression is dominant but restricted to antibodies with the constant region of the idiotope-positive parent. It is unclear at present whether a functional idiotypic network exists to an appreciable extent at the level of the 'primary' repertoire of antibody V regions (i.e. the repertoire generated in the bone marrow by VDJ joining). The available structural information on anti-idiotypic antibodies argues rather against it [7]. At the antibody level, a functional network may connect the 'primary' repertoire and somatic antibody mutants and thus keep the latter in the system (see below), but clearly, at least in young mice, the repertoire of somatic mutants is insufficient to disturb the dominance of germ line encoded responses.

Puzzles and questions

1 How can we explain idiotype sharing between antibodies and T cell receptors? If anti-idiotypic antibodies contain internal images of the antigen against which the corresponding idiotypic antibody had been raised, then it is not surprising to find cross-reaction of the anti-idiotypes with T cells specific for the same antigen. However, experimental evidence indicates that, depending on the immunoglobulin heavy chain linkage group, a given strain will express or not express a cross-reactive idiotype at both the antibody and the T cell level. This result can be interpreted to mean that the genes encoding heavy chain variable regions are also expressed in T cell receptors. Evidence from molecular biology now argues strongly against this notion. This favours a second interpretation, namely that T cells adapt their receptor repertoire to that of B cells through idiotypic interactions in ontogeny. This would imply a functional network at the level of T–B interactions in a most fundamental sense, which leads us to the next question.

2 Do T cells play a role in the selection of the B cell repertoire? There is no question that T cells can do so in animals suppressed by anti-idiotype, and there is some evidence to suggest that similar situations are sometimes encountered in non-manipulated animals ('silent clones'). There is also controversial evidence indicating that in certain cases, idiotype dominance in normal animals depends upon the presence of idiotype-specific T cells, and that these T cells arise only in an environment in which idiotype-bearing B cells are present [8]. It has been speculated in this context that immunoglobulin idiotypes may function as restriction elements in T cell recognition of antigen, similar to the class I and II histocompatibility antigens. If T cells play a role in selecting the B cell repertoire, do they do so in the absence of external antigen and/or upon the induction of an antigen-driven immune response?

3 Does the induction of immune responses involve release from a general suppression brought about by network interactions? There is some evidence suggesting that the induction of both regulatory and effector T cells may require release from idiotypic suppression.

4 Is the idiotypic network involved in the somatic diversification of the antibody repertoire? The enhancement of idiotype expression by nanogram doses of anti-idiotype could reflect a general mechanism by which somatic mutants complementary to antibodies already produced by the system (e.g. those encoded by the germ line) are expanded and maintained in the system.

5 Do idiotypes and anti-idiotypes play a role in disease? This important question, which is in part connected with the internal image problem, is widely discussed and investigated in clinical immunology [4].

6 Can anti-idiotypic antibodies specific for idiotypes associated with antibodies of a given antigen binding specificity be used for the manipulation of immune responses of practical importance? Further investigations on internal images and idiotype polymorphism are needed in order to approach this problem further.

Conclusion

Extensive research on idiotypic control over the last years has convincingly shown that idiotypic determinants are recognized by both T and B lymphocytes and play a regulatory role in the sense of both enhancing and suppressing the expression of complementary binding sites. In this sense, idiotypes behave like external antigens except that their regulatory function is not obscured by the wide range of physico-chemical properties encountered at the level of the latter. The sensitivity of the immune system to idiotypic manipulations is most impressive. However, it still remains to be determined to what extent and at which level the idiotypic network determines the generation and expression of the receptor repertoire under physiological conditions. Further investigations on the role of the idiotypic network, in cell interactions in the T cell compartment and in the selection both of the T cell repertoire and of B cells bearing somatic mutants of antibody variable regions, appear to be of particular importance.

Most of the matters dealt with in this article have been recently reviewed [2–4]. References 5–8 refer to more recent work.

References

1 JERNE N.K. (1974) Towards a network theory of the immune system. *Ann. Immunol.* (Inst. Pasteur) **125C**, 373.
2 RAJEWSKY K. & TAKEMORI T. (1983) Genetics, expression, and function of idiotypes. *Ann. Rev. Immunol.* **1**, 569.
3 MÖLLER G. (ed.) (1984) Idiotypic networks. *Immunol. Rev.* **79**.
4 LAMBERT P.H. (ed.) (1983) Immunopathology of idiotypic inter-actions. *Springer Semin. Immunopath.* **6**, no. 1.
5 SMITH F.I., TESCH H. & RAJEWSKY K. (1984) Heterogenous and monoclonal helper T cells induce similar anti-(4-hydroxy-3-nitro-phenyl)acetyl (NP) antibody populations in the primary adoptive response. II. Lambda light chain dominance and idiotope expression. *Eur. J. Immunol.* **14**, 195.
6 TAKEMORI T. & RAJEWSKY K. (1984) Specificity, duration and mechanism of idiotype suppression induced by neonatal injection of monoclonal anti-idiotope antibodies into mice. *Eur. J. Immunol.* **14**, 656.
7 SABLITZKY F. & RAJEWSKY K. (1984) Molecular basis of an isogenic anti-idiotypic response. *EMBO J.* **3**, 3005.
8 MARTINEZ-A.C., PEREIRA P., BERNABE R., BANDEIRA A., LARSSON E-L., CAZENAVE P-A. & COUTINHO A. (1984) Internal complementarities in the immune system: regulation of the expression of helper T cell idiotypes. *Proc. natn. Acad. Sci. U.S.A.* **81**, 4520.
9 TOKUHISA T. & RAJEWSKY K. (1985) Antigen induced chronic idiotype suppression. Proc. natn. Acad. Sci. U.S.A. (in press).

Chapter 74
Overview: epitope-specific regulation

LEONORE A. HERZENBERG

The concept: integrated
regulatory circuits and
antibody production, 74.1
The findings: selective control of
IgG responses to individual
epitopes, 74.2
Selective isotype and allotype
regulation, 74.2

Bistable regulation, 74.2
The induction of epitope-specific
suppression, 74.3
Induction of suppression for
subsets of anti-epitope
antibodies, 74.3
Epitope-specific regulation and
other regulatory systems, 74.4

Epitope-specific regulation,
immunologic memory and
immune tolerance, 74.5
Methods and protocols: *in vivo
veritas*, 74.6
Characteristics of the
epitope-specific system
(summary), 74.6

The epitopes on a typical T-dependent antigen collectively stimulate production of a highly heterogeneous set of antibody molecules that vary with respect to constant region structure and combining-site specificity. Even the response to a single epitope in a single animal consists of several Ig heavy chain isotypes (e.g. IgM, IgG1, IgG2a) in association with a wide variety of idiotype and combining-site structures. Thus, as a rule, immunizations generate a vast number of different antibody molecules that can be subdivided along general lines (isotype, light chain type, combining-site specificity for individual epitopes, etc.) and classified into a myriad of small subsets when all of these properties are jointly taken into account.

Immunoregulatory studies have traditionally avoided addressing this extensive heterogeneity by adopting what might be termed 'isolationist' strategies, e.g. concentrating on the production of a particular isotype, allotype or idiotype in an antibody response; concentrating on genetically controlled responses to particular antigens or epitopes; concentrating on antibody responses to haptens on particular carriers (T dependent or T independent); and/or concentrating on carrier-specific mechanisms that exert an equal influence over the production of antibodies to all epitopes on an antigen.

These simplification strategies brought immunology through its formative years; however, at this point, more can be gained by treating individual regulatory mechanisms as components of an integrated system that selectively control the production of various kinds of antibodies. Once this concept is accepted, a wholly new perspective develops: previously unsuspected relationships among regulatory mechanisms begin to emerge; studies of one mechanism reveal key aspects of another; the inte-

grated operation of two mechanisms accounts for findings that neither mechanism alone could explain; and many of the bizarre phenomena associated with *in vivo* antibody responses become understandable in terms of the operations of a highly organized regulatory system.

The author's experience with the epitope-specific regulatory system illustrates this approach.

The concept: integrated regulatory circuits and antibody production

Several years ago, the author published some theoretical papers [1,2] suggesting that antibody responses are controlled by sets of integrated regulatory circuits, each centred around a 'core circuit' that regulates the expression of a small number of memory B cells committed to producing very similar antibody molecules (same isotype, same allotype, similar idiotype, similar combining site). As proposed, this core circuit can be induced either to support or suppress antibody production by its covey of B cells but cannot be induced to support antibody production by some and suppress production by others. Thus it constitutes the basic unit of specificity in the system.

In this model, several 'auxillary circuits' (carrier-specific, allotype-specific, etc.) are linked to each core circuit. These sense conditions in the immunological environment calling for the production (or non-production) of particular subsets of antibody molecules and then pressure the core circuit to act accordingly. The state (suppression or support) to which an individual core circuit will be induced is determined by the net pressure from all of its auxillary circuits.

The core circuit proposed here is configured such that it will tend to maintain itself in its initially induced state but will still be capable of shifting to the alternate state in response to a drastic change in the immunological environment. By and large, therefore, the operation of this circuit will perpetuate the response pattern determined by the conditions in the immunological environment when an epitope is first introduced. These characteristics, which define the core circuit as a bistable regulatory mechanism, introduce currently intriguing possibilities *vis à vis* the mechanisms responsible for immunologic memory and tolerance. It must be admitted, however, that the author was only dimly aware of these possibilities when she completed her work on the model and moved on to more concrete studies.

The findings: selective control of IgG responses to individual epitopes

Several years later, while investigating the selective regulation of memory B cell development and expression in allotype suppressed mice, the author made a series of observations that were difficult to reconcile with accepted dogma. These observations, however, were readily predictable from the bistable properties of the integrated circuits in the model she had proposed. Thus this model became a guide for real-life studies characterizing what we now call the 'epitope-specific' regulatory system.

Nearly all of the author's work in this area has been published and reviewed in detail quite recently [3–12]. In the interests of brevity, therefore, she presents a summary of her findings at the end of this article and a discussion here to highlight the major concepts developed in the course of these studies.

In essence, the author's initial studies with the epitope-specific system showed that primary immunization with a hapten–carrier conjugate induces equivalent IgG anti-hapten memory B cell populations in carrier primed mice and unprimed mice. Despite the presence of these memory cells, however, IgG anti-hapten antibody production fails markedly in the carrier primed mice. Thus, even when stimulated repeatedly with the hapten–carrier conjugate, these mice still tend to produce antibody responses to hapten that are substantially lower in magnitude and affinity than the primary IgG anti-hapten responses produced by control mice immunized initially with the hapten–carrier conjugate.

Subsequent studies showed that the 'carrier/hapten–carrier' immunization sequence induces a specific and persistent suppression for IgG antibody production to the 'new' epitope (hapten) belatedly introduced on the carrier molecule. Once induced, this suppression impairs antibody responses to the hapten presented on a variety of carrier molecules but does not interfere with antibody production to other epitopes on the carrier molecules. Therefore it is epitope-specific in the sense that it controls antibody production to individual epitopes on the carrier molecule.

In a more precise terminology, this mechanism should probably be described as combining-site specific since it selectively impairs production of a subset of anti-hapten antibodies that have relatively high combining affinities for the hapten. This specificity suggests a close similarity (or identity) between the mechanisms that mediate epitope-specific suppression and idiotype-specific suppression, i.e. both are capable of specifically regulating antibody production according to variable region structure. The specificity of the epitope-specific mechanism also approximates that defined for the core circuit in the model discussed above.

Selective isotype and allotype regulation

In general, IgG1 antibody responses are the most difficult to suppress initially, the most difficult to turn off once initiated and the first to escape suppression after repeated stimulation with hapten–carrier conjugates. IgG2a, IgG2b and IgG3 responses, in contrast, are more easily suppressed and more easily maintained under suppression. Each of the isotypes, however, is independently regulated since individual animals not infrequently produce one (or two) without the others. Furthermore, certain immunization and treatment protocols tend to selectively induce suppression for IgG1 responses (M. Waldor, K. Hayakawa, R.R. Hardy & L.A. Herzenberg, unpublished observations).

These findings suggest that the effector mechanism that mediates epitope-specific suppression is capable of recognizing and selectively controlling the expression on B cells committed to the production of antibodies that have different Ig heavy chain constant regions. Thus, in addition to being epitope specific (or combining-site specific), this effector mechanism might appropriately be described as Igh restricted.

Bistable regulation

Data from sequential immunization studies with carriers and hapten–carriers indicate that the mechanism that mediates epitope-specific regulation is bistable. Like the core circuits discussed earlier, it appears to have two mutually exclusive stable states (support and suppression), and generally tends to remain in its initially induced state. Thus suppression tends to be maintained despite repeated stimulation with hapten–carrier conjugates at dose levels sufficient to easily induce antibody production in non-suppressed animals; and support tends to be maintained despite immunization with the carrier/hapten–carrier sequence at dose levels sufficient to induce clear-cut suppression in non-immunized animals.

However, in keeping with the definition of a bistable system, both suppression and support can be eroded by strong stimulation towards the alternate state. Thus suppressed animals can initiate antibody production if given enough antigen in immunogenic form; and antibody-producing animals can terminate antibody production if exposed to a sufficiently strong suppression-induction stimulus.

The ability to maintain a stable state requires the ability to prevent the induction of the alternate state under conditions where it would normally have been induced. This means that support (once induced) prevents the induction of suppression and vice versa. As a practical matter, therefore, conditions that determine which state is induced first will, by and large, determine the state that will be maintained throughout subsequent immunizations. In other words, the conditions under which an animal initially encounters an epitope will define its immediate response and will strongly influence (but not absolutely determine) its future response to that epitope.

The induction of epitope-specific suppression

The induction of suppression for IgG anti-hapten antibody production in carrier/hapten–carrier immunized animals traces to the presence of functional carrier-specific suppressor T cells (CTs) in carrier primed animals. Direct isolation and transfer studies show that such CTs induce epitope-specific suppression for IgG antibody responses to haptens on the priming carrier (presumably by presenting hapten to the relevent cells in the epitope-specific suppression effector mechanism). Thus there is good reason to believe that CTs induced by carrier priming subsequently induce suppression for IgG anti-hapten antibody responses in carrier/hapten–carrier immunized animals.

The induction of this clear-cut suppression is possible because the hapten is introduced after CTs have matured to full function and before the animal has had the opportunity to induce stable anti-hapten antibody production. Introducing the hapten and establishing antibody production before CTs mature basically prevents suppression induction (or markedly reduces it). Thus, since functional CTs usually emerge a few days after animals are primed with a T-dependent antigen, there is reason to suspect that these well-known regulatory cells play a kind of scavenger role in animals producing normal primary responses to the antigen. That is, once mature, the CTs may serve to

induce suppression for antibody production to priming antigen epitopes that have not yet succeeded in inducing stable support for antibody production.

Scavenging of this sort could account for the selective antibody responses produced to epitopes on protein antigens. The tendency for individual animals to respond to different epitopes on a single protein (a phenomenon well known to serologists and immunogeneticists) has previously been explained in terms of the dominance of individual B cell clones in the memory pool; however, assigning responsibility for this selectivity to an epitope-specific system is equally consistent with the data.

Induction of suppression for subsets of anti-epitope antibodies

The epitope-specific regulatory system can be induced to selectively suppress or support the production of distinctive subsets of antibody molecules to a given epitope. As indicated above, the effector mechanism is Igh-restricted in the sense that it selectively regulates production of individual isotype and allotype anti-epitope responses. Furthermore, it can selectively suppress or selectively support individual idiotype-marked antibody responses (L.A. Herzenberg & T. Tokuhisa, unpublished observations).

This selectivity is characteristic of the partially suppressed anti-hapten responses found in carrier/hapten–carrier immunized animals that were poorly suppressed initially or are escaping from suppression following repeated hapten–carrier stimulations. In addition, it characterizes responses to epitopes on priming antigens in several kinds of immunodefective mice and probably defines the patterns of isotype and allotype representation typical of antibody responses to different kinds of antigens and immunization protocols.

The mechanisms responsible for the induction of these various selective suppressions have yet to be clearly defined; however, most of the cases that the author has investigated can be explained by the failure to generate stable support for a particular segment of the antibody response before CTs mature into full function and induce suppression for that response segment. That is, in general, suppression appears to be induced for a particular subset of the antibodies normally produced in response to a given antigen whenever conditions in the regulatory environment prevent the antigen from rapidly stimulating production of those antibodies (i.e. before CTs mature).

For example, if animals are immunized during a period when they are temporarily unable to produce allotype-marked antibodies, they develop a long-term suppression that is specific for allotype-marked antibodies to the epitopes on the priming antigen. Later, when they have recovered their overall ability to produce allotype-marked antibodies, they still retain the 'scars' of this earlier encounter in that they fail to produce allotype-marked antibodies to the priming antigen epitopes, even when these epitopes (haptens) are presented on a different carrier molecule. Thus a transient allotype suppression results in the induction of a restricted epitope-specific suppression that continues to impair production of the initially suppressed antibodies long after the initial suppression has dissipated.

Epitope-specific regulation and other regulatory systems

There is clearly a close functional relationship between carrier-specific and epitope-specific regulation. As already indicated, CTs induce the epitope-specific system to suppress antibody production. In addition, CTh (carrier-specific helper T cells) very likely induce the system to support antibody production. Thus the carrier-specific system can be viewed as the basic induction mechanism for epitope-specific regulation and the epitope-specific system as providing the basic effector mechanism for carrier-specific regulation.

Idiotype-specific regulation also fits easily into this construction. Idiotype-specific suppressor T cells suppress production of idiotype-bearing antibody molecules with particular variable region (combining-site) structures. Idiotype-specific helper T cells, in contrast, support production of such molecules. By definition, therefore, idiotype-specific systems can be viewed as individual regulatory modules that collectively comprise the effector mechanism of the epitope-specific system. In other words, epitope-specific suppression for anti-hapten antibody production appears to be a concerted idiotype-specific suppression induced to selectively impair production of anti-hapten antibodies.

The Igh (isotype/allotype) restrictions in epitope-specific regulation would appear to negate the direct involvement of idiotype-specific regulatory cells, since idiotype-specific regulation does not appear to be additionally specific for individual isotypes. However, judgement should be reserved on this point until idiotype-specific suppressor T cells are cloned and shown to regulate production of the idiotype on more than one isotype.

This overall hypothesis, too lengthy to defend fully here, also suggests that the induction of idiotype suppression may be a two-step process. That is, the injection of anti-idiotype antibodies, which temporarily compromises the ability to rapidly produce idiotype-bearing antibodies, may serve only to prepare the animal for suppression induction. The actual induction of suppression, in contrast, would occur when the compromised animal is immunized with an appropriate epitope (to which idiotype-bearing antibodies bind) and the suppression would be specific for those idiotype-bearing molecules that actually bind the inducing epitope.

According to this view, the immunization procedure used to determine whether suppression has been induced in an animal treated with anti-idiotype antibodies is responsible for inducing the stable idiotype-specific suppression that is observed. Furthermore, the fine specificity of this suppression is determined by the inducing antigen, i.e. the suppression induced will be specific for idiotype-bearing molecules that bind to the inducing epitope rather than for all idiotype-bearing molecules that can be produced. Thus our hypothesis accounts for the available facts: the induction of idiotype-specific suppression becomes a special case of the induction of epitope-specific suppression in which only a single module of the epitope-specific system is activated to suppress antibody production.

These ideas, which unite idiotype-specific, epitope-specific and carrier-specific regulation, also lay the groundwork for integrating other commonly studied regulatory systems into a comprehensive framework. Basically, all such systems can be viewed as operating through mechanisms that selectively influence the induction of stable support or suppression for antibody production to epitopes presented on priming antigens. That is, the specific regulation provided by these systems can be explained by their tendency to selectively impair the initiation of certain kinds of antibody production (and hence to favour the induction of epitope-specific suppression for those antibody responses).

Ir gene control mechanisms, also, need only prevent the rapid initiation of antibody production to epitopes on the target antigen. A short delay would be sufficient to allow CTs to mature to the point where they could induce long-term suppression for such antibody production to the epitopes on the antigen. Thus, as the author has shown, immunizing non-responder animals with a hapten coupled to the genetically controlled antigen results in the induction of epitope-specific suppression for antibody responses to the hapten (and presumably for antibody responses to the protein epitopes on the antigen as well). Similarly, as indicated earlier, immunizing allotype-suppressed animals induces stable, allotype-restricted, epitope-specific suppression that persists after the generalized allotype suppression disappears.

The epitope-specific system as a whole, therefore, emerges as a modular (idiotype-specific) regulatory system that provides a common channel through which many (all) of the known regulatory mechanisms operate to selectively control antibody production. The behaviour of the bistable modules in this system approximates the behaviour of the integrated regulatory circuits that the author proposed some time ago. Thus, in theory, the epitope-specific regulatory system provides a mechanism for taking into account all of the various pressures that favour and oppose the production of individual antibodies when defining the long-term response that an animal will tend to produce to a given set of epitopes.

Epitope-specific regulation, immunologic memory and immune tolerance

The epitope-specific system controls antibody production by controlling the expression of memory B cells. It does not appear to affect memory B cell development since suppressed (carrier/hapten–carrier immunized) animals that fail to mount even a primary level IgG anti-hapten antibody response *in situ* have substantial anti-hapten memory B cell populations. In fact, when compared in adoptive (co-transfer) assays, the memory populations in these mice are usually indistinguishable from the memory populations found in non-suppressed (hapten-carrier primed) animals that produce normal *in situ* primary and secondary anti-hapten antibody responses.

Normal anti-hapten memory B cell populations can also be found when epitope-specific suppression is induced in other ways. For example, in some (or perhaps all) responses under Ir gene control, suppression for anti-hapten antibody responses is induced when non-responder animals are challenged with a hapten coupled to the antigen to which they cannot respond. These animals produce minimal IgG anti-hapten responses, even when immunized subsequently with the hapten on a carrier to which they respond normally. Nevertheless, their anti-hapten memory B cell populations are equivalent to the anti-hapten memory populations in Ir congenic mice that respond strongly to the initial stimulation (K. Hayakawa & L.A. Herzenberg, unpublished observations).

Similar results are again obtained when allotype suppression is responsible for the induction of epitope-specific suppression. Thus the author's experience with a variety of regulatory systems indicates that suppressed animals generally have fully competent (albeit unexpressed) memory populations. The induction of B cell memory, therefore, is necessary but not sufficient for the production of *in situ* IgG secondary (anamnestic) antibody responses, i.e. epitope-specific suppression frequently prevents such responses and consequently obscures the presence of otherwise normal memory B cell populations.

Carrier-specific helper T cells (CTh) can be similarly 'hidden' by the induction of epitope-specific suppression, particularly when anti-hapten responses are suppressed and the response to the hapten is taken as an index of CTh activity. In general, suppressed animals have normal levels of CTh activity, detectable either in adoptive assays or *in situ* (as the ability to help IgG responses to epitopes that accompany the hapten on a carrier molecule). Thus epitope-specific suppression can mimic CTh development or depletion defects; however, CTh activity in suppressed animals is usually present at normal levels when measured appropriately.

These findings introduce a new perspective on the mechanisms responsible for immunologic memory and acquired immunologic tolerance. In essence, the author demonstrated the presence of equivalent CTh and memory B cell populations in animals that show diametrically opposed antibody response patterns (memory or tolerance) when challenged with a previously encountered antigen. These findings largely exclude CTh and memory B as populations responsible for maintaining these response differences (which are determined by the conditions surrounding the initial antigenic stimulation and maintained thereafter with considerable fidelity). Therefore they suggest that immunologic memory and at least some forms of tolerance represent learned responses that are remembered and mediated by a system(s) evolved to provide consistent control for antibody production to epitopes encountered under a variety of conditions.

The epitope-specific system has much to recommend it for this role. It is selectively inducible to support or suppress production of individual components of an antibody response. Furthermore, once induced, it acts as a guardian of the *status quo* in that it perpetuates initial antibody responses and discourages the entrance of new responses into the pool. Thus it provides a basic mechanism capable of memorizing regulatory decisions made when an epitope is first introduced and then controlling subsequent responses to the epitope accordingly.

The epitope-specific system, therefore, appears to be the repository for a new kind of immunologic memory that records a regulatory programme to be followed in the initial and subsequent responses to a given epitope. The author views this 'regulatory memory' as responsible for: (1) maintaining what is classically called immunologic memory (by 'remembering' to support the expression of large numbers of high affinity clones); (2) maintaining immunologic tolerance (by 'remembering' to suppress the expression of most of the clones capable of participating in the response); and (3) maintaining the individuality of antibody responses (by selectively supporting or suppressing the expression of different subsets of memory B cells in different animals). Thus both tolerance and classical memory (augmented antibody production) are seen as anamnestic responses that reflect regulatory memory programmes recorded with the epitope-specific system when the antigen was first introduced.

Methods and protocols: *in vivo veritas*

The author's work on this project largely represents a return to the kinds of sequential immunization studies that were in vogue years ago, about the time that hapten–carrier conjugates were first introduced as immunogens. These earlier studies were severely hampered by technical limitations and by the lack of direct knowledge about the cells and cell interactions of the immune system. Thus is is not surprising that they fell into disfavour when the introduction of cell culture and transfer methods opened a more direct access to the cells and mechanisms involved in antibody production.

The development of an accurate picture of how the immune system functions, however, clearly requires precise knowledge of how animals respond to different kinds of immunizations. Hypotheses that incorrectly predict the behaviour of the intact system must either be incomplete or wrong, no matter how rational they are or how consistent they may be with data from cellular studies. Thus, to evaluate current thought, we have either to rely on data from studies based on outdated methodologies and concepts or to commit ourselves to repeating parts of those studies with additional controls and response measurements so that the older data becomes interpretable in a modern context.

The use of this latter approach in re-examining previously known *in vivo* defects in antibody production revealed some of the key characteristics of the epitope-specific system. For example, to measure anti-hapten antibody responses, the author used newly developed radioimmune assays (RIA) that allowed her to determine the amount and affinity of the various allotype and isotype anti-hapten antibodies present in serum samples from individual mice [13]. These assays proved sensitive enough to accurately distinguish typical primary anti-hapten responses from lesser (suppressed) responses that are usually tenfold lower in affinity and fivefold lower in amount. Furthermore, they enable rapid and accurate measurements of primary and secondary IgG anti-carrier responses. Thus the author was able to determine whether a given anti-hapten response was suppressed and whether such suppression was accompanied by the suppression of antibody production to other

epitopes on the carrier on which the hapten was presented.

The author also used a variety of hapten–carrier cell transfer and culture methods in these studies in order to evaluate the status of memory B cells, CTh and CTs populations in animals immunized in different ways. The inclusion of anti-carrier antibody response measurements in the CTh and CTs experiments helped to resolve several (previously unrecognized) ambiguities that hampered interpretation of earlier data on carrier-specific regulatory mechanisms. Furthermore, the examination of memory B cell populations in non-responding animals brought new insights into the distinctions between those regulatory mechanisms that control memory B cell development and those that control memory B cell expression. All of the author's findings in these studies were consistent with earlier observations; however, the additional information she gathered led to the development of substantially new concepts of how memory B cells and regulatory T cells work.

These concepts led in turn to the framing of the overall epitope-specific regulation hypothesis presented here, which accounts for many of the characteristics of *in situ* antibody responses and offers plausible explanations for a number of the more bizarre 'phenomena' associated with such responses. The author is certain that this hypothesis will need corrections and additions as more data accrue; however, at the moment it meets the basic test for a description of the immune system, i.e. the predictions it makes accord well with *in situ* (as well as *in vitro* and adoptive) response patterns.

Characteristics of the epitope-specific system (summary)

Several recently published reviews [2–6] and papers [7–12] describe the epitope-specific system in detail. Briefly summarized, these show the following characteristics.

Specificity

Epitope-specific suppression is mediated by a mechanism that selectively controls the production of IgG antibodies to individual epitopes on complex antigens: this mechanism can be induced to suppress IgG anti-hapten responses to a hapten–carrier conjugate without interfering with primary or secondary antibody responses to the carrier protein epitopes; once induced to suppress antibody production to a hapten, it will suppress such antibody production regardless of the carrier on which the hapten is presented; it can be induced to suppress antibody production to epitopes on one of the proteins in a protein–protein conjugate without interfering with antibody production to epitopes on the other protein; and it can be (and generally is) induced to selectively suppress high affinity IgG anti-hapten antibody production without impairing production of low-affinity antibodies to the same hapten.

The suppression effector mechanism also appears to be Igh restricted in that it selectively regulates isotype and allotype representation in IgG antibody responses: it can be induced to suppress IgG2a, IgG2b and IgG3 anti-hapten antibody production without interfering with the production of IgG1 anti-hapten antibodies; it can be induced to suppress Igh-1b (IgG2a) allotype anti-DNP responses without interfering with Igh-1a anti-hapten responses; and it apparently maintains the isotype and allotype representation patterns characteristic of responses produced to epitopes on different kinds of carriers, e.g. proteins, erythrocytes.

Mechanism

The suppression effector mechanism blocks memory B cell expression (rather than development): normal anti-hapten memory B cell populations (demonstrable in adoptive assays) are present in severely suppressed animals; suppression for anti-hapten antibody production can be induced in animals currently producing a primary IgG anti-hapten response.

The effector mechanism does not interfere with carrier specific helper T cell (CTh) activity: CTh-supported primary and secondary antibody responses to other epitopes on carrier proteins proceed normally despite the suppression of antibody responses to haptens presented on the carrier.

The suppression is mediated by T cells: treatment with anti Thy-1 plus complement abrogates the ability to transfer a suppressed response with spleen cells from a suppressed animal.

The effector mechanism is bistable, i.e. it has two alternate regulatory states (suppression or support for antibody production) and tends to maintain itself in its initially induced state: by definition, the induction of suppression for anti-hapten antibody production specifically interferes with the subsequent stimulation of anti-hapten antibody production; similarly, the induction of anti-hapten antibody production specifically interferes with subsequent induction of suppression for anti-hapten antibody production; however, sufficient stimulation can induce a shift to the alternate state and thus either terminate an ongoing response or initiate a previously suppressed response.

Induction

Carrier priming results in the induction of epitope-specific suppression for antibody production to 'new' epitopes presented on the carrier molecule once carrier priming is complete: sequential immunizations with a carrier protein and a hapten conjugated to the immunizing carrier protein (carrier/hapten–carrier immunization) induce suppression for IgG anti-hapten antibody production; traditional carrier-specific suppressor T cells such as those that recognize keyhole limpet haemocyanin (KLH) are responsible for inducing this suppression (presumably by presenting the hapten in stimulatory fashion to an appropriate cell in suppression effector mechanism); thus the epitope-specific system is the effector mechanism that mediates carrier-specific suppression.

Regulatory defects such as Ir gene control, allotype suppression, and X-linked immunodeficiency frequently result in the induction of epitope-specific suppression: the induced suppression is specific for antibody responses that tend to fail initially because of the defect (presumably because the initiation of such antibody production is delayed beyond the time when CTs mature to full function); e.g. Ir gene controlled responses, specific suppression for anti-hapten antibody responses is induced by immunizing with the hapten on an antigen that cannot stimulate IgG antibody production in the immunized animal; the suppression persists indefinitely and maintains its initial specificity, regardless of whether the inducing defect disappears.

References

1 HERZENBERG L.A., BLACK S.J. & HERZENBERG L.A. (1980) Regulatory circuits and antibody responses. *Eur. J. Immunol.* **10**, 1.

2 HERZENBERG L.A., TOKUHISA T. & HAYAKAWA K. (1983) Epitope-specific regulation. *Ann. Rev. Immunol.* **1**, 609.

3 HERZENBERG L.A., TOKUHISA T., PARKS D.R. & HERZENBERG L.A. (1981) Hapten-specific regulation of heterogeneous antibody responses: Intersection of theory and practice. In *The Immune System*, (eds. Steinberg Ch. M. & Le Kovits I.). Karger, Basel.

4 HERZENBERG L.A., TOKUHISA T. & HERZENBERG L.A. (1981) Carrier-specific induction of hapten-specific suppression. *Immunology Today*, **2**, 40.

5 HERZENBERG L.A. (1983) Allotype suppression and epitope-specific regulation. *Immunology Today*, **4**, 113.

6 HERZENBERG L.A., HAYAKAWA K., HARDY R.R., TOKUHISA T., OI V.T. & HERZENBERG L.A. (1982) Molecular, cellular and systemic mechanisms for regulating IgCH expression. *Immunol. Revs.* **67**, 5.

7 HERZENBERG L.A., TOKUHISA T. & HERZENBERG L.A. (1980) Carrier-priming leads to hapten-specific suppression. *Nature*, **285**, 664.

8 HUBER B.T., TOKUHISA T. & HERZENBERG L.A. (1981) Primary and secondary *in situ* antibody response: Abnormal maturation pattern in mice carrying the XID gene. *Eur. J. Immunol.* **11,** 353.

9 HERZENBERG L.A. & TOKUHISA T. (1982) Epitope-specific regulation: I. Carrier-specific induction of suppression for IgG anti-hapten antibody responses. *J. exp. Med.* **155,** 1730.

10 HERZENBERG L.A., TOKUHISA T., PARKS D.R. & HERZENBERG L.A. (1982) Epitope-specific regulation: II. A bistable, Igh-restricted regulatory mechanism central to immunologic memory. *J. exp. Med.* **155,** 1741.

11 HERZENBERG L.A., TOKUHISA T. & HERZENBERG L.A. (1982) Epitope-specific regulation: III. Induction of allotype-restricted suppression for IgG antibody responses to individual epitopes on complex antigens. *Eur. J. Immunol.* **12,** 814.

12 HERZENBERG L.A., TOKUHISA T., HAYAKAWA K. & HERZENBERG L.A. (1982) Lack of immune response (IR) gene control for the induction of hapten-specific suppression by the TGAL antigen. *Nature,* **295,** 329.

13 HERZENBERG L.A., BLACK S.J., TOKUHISA T. & HERZENBERG L.A. (1980) Memory B cells at successive stages of differentiation: Affinity maturation and the role of IgD receptors. *J. exp. Med.* **151,** 1071.

Chapter 75
Overview: T cell clones

H. CANTOR

T cell sets—definition,
75.1
Regulation of immunity—
co-operating
cell sets, 75.2

T cell products, 75.3
Molecules synthesized
by inducer T cell
clones, 75.4

Definition of cells and
molecules that directly
mediate specific
immunologic suppression, 75.5
Summary, 75.6

T cell sets—definition

Early experiments were consistent with the idea that T cells represented a uniform population capable of a variety of immunologic functions, including activation or suppression of immune responses. According to this view, external conditions, such as the type or mode of antigenic stimulation, determined which T cell function was expressed. The alternative notion was that T cells consisted of specialized subpopulations, each equipped for a particular T cell function. This question resolved itself into the practical problem of finding out whether it was possible to subdivide the T cell population into different sets that, when confronted with antigen, were able to make only one or another of the possible T cell responses. The most effective technique for identifying and separating subpopulations of peripheral T cells came from studies of cell surface glycoproteins expressed on cells undergoing thymus-dependent differentiation using antibodies that specifically react with these surface glycoproteins. These antibodies bind to lymphocyte surface antigens expressed on thymocytes and lymphocytes, but not on cells of other tissues such as brain, kidney, liver or epidermal cells. Studies of these cells in mice and, more recently, man indicate that they are specified by genes expressed exclusively during thymocyte differentiation. For example, Ly1 glycoprotein, coded for by a gene on chromosome 19, and the Ly2 and Ly3 glycoproteins, both coded for by genes on chromosome 6, are expressed on thymocytes and on some peripheral T cells. These last two Ly gene products (Ly2 and Ly3) are tentatively treated together because the two genes are tightly linked and their two products have not yet exhibited any differences other than the fact that they are coded for by distinguishable loci. A second type of thymus-specific antigen, the TL glycoprotein, is also expressed on thymocytes but not peripheral T cells. In general, the approach to defining the antigenic markers on T cells involves a cytotoxicity assay similar to the complement-dependent haemolytic tests used to identify markers on red cells. More recently, antibodies bound to beads or dishes have been used to 'positively' select cells (see Chapter 55).

This revealed that the peripheral T cell pool contains at least three separate T cell sets, according to their unique surface molecular labels and functional potential. They are referred to as the precursor set, the inducer set, and the cytotoxic/suppressor set, and these account for 50%, 30%, and 10% respectively of the peripheral T cell pool. Thus, according to the criterion of selective expression of gene products on the cell surface and associated immunologic function, T cells are divisible into three groups of cells that each follow a different set of genetic instructions. Inducer cells ($Ly1^+2^-$) activate other cell types ('effector cells') to divide and/or differentiate. For example, they induce B cells to secrete antibody, and they stimulate monocytes, mast cells, and precursors of T-killer cells to participate in cell-mediated immune responses. In contrast, cells of the $Ly1^-2^+$ set are genetically programmed to kill or suppress other cells.

Judged both by their different functional potentials and by their cell surface phenotypes, inducer and cytotoxic/suppressor cells represent distinct and specialized cells. They could be two stages of a single line of differentiation, in which case one of them must give rise to the other. Alternatively, they may represent two branches of thymus-directed differentiation. The two T-cell sets were isolated according to their surface markers and used to re-populate the lymphoid tissues of syngeneic hosts that lacked all T cells. These recipients were observed for over six months. Mice given $Ly1^+2^-$ cells were equipped for inducer function but not killer function; and mice given $Ly1^-2^+$ cells were equipped for primary killer function but not for helper function. Thus even after prolonged residence in hosts in which all physiological controlling mechanisms should be set to favour expansion of alternate population, there was no appreciable generation of another cell set. These findings show that inducer T cells and cytotoxic/suppressive cells have already exercised differentiative options that prevent them from giving rise to one another. In other words, these two sets belong to different lines of cellular differentiation and are not sequential stages of a single progression.

Co-recognition by T cell sets

A fundamental property of T cells—specificity of the major histocompatibility gene products—can also be predicted from their surface markers. In mice, inducer cells recognize a set of MHC gene products called class II molecules, which are displayed mainly on B cells and macrophages. Class II molecules are expressed on the subset of macrophages ('antigen-presenting cells') which stimulate inducer cells to divide and synthesize inducer proteins. Inducer cells use these class II MHC products as 'self marking' molecules. They are activated following co-recognition of complexes formed class II molecules, and conventional antigens. This 'co-recognition' may actually represent binding of inducer cells to 'variants' of class II molecules which are mimicked by close association of class II molecules with antigens such as viral proteins. Class II molecules are also expressed on many targets of activated inducer cells. In the case of antibody induction, class II molecules displayed on B cells allow inducer cells that have been stimulated by co-recognition of a class II molecule and, say, a viral protein to locate B cells displaying the same class II-antigen complex. Some of these B cells also display the virus because they possess membrane Ig specific for the viral protein. These later cells are preferentially activated, and secrete antibodies specific for that viral protein.

Class II molecules are not recognized well by the second mature T cell set: Ly23 cells. Many of these cells are effector T cells that recognize antigen associated with class I MHC gene products, which are expressed on virtually all the cells of the body. Cytotoxic Ly2$^+$ cells thus can lyse virtually any somatic cell that displays an altered or variant class I surface molecule. Taken together, this information indicates that thymus-dependent differentiation gives rise to at least two separate sublines of mature T cells. One is programmed to induce or help other cell types and is activated by antigen associated with class II MHC products. The second is programmed for killer/suppressor activity and responds preferentially to class I MHC products. The net result is the formation of two screening systems. Selective altering of either by foreign or altered MHC region products activates immune reactions already programmed in either T cell set.

Antigen-reactive T cells (ARC)

The numerically largest population of T cells in mice bear the Ly123 phenotype and has been the least well defined. This is because many of these cells appear to represent a store of receptor-positive intermediary cells which lack a direct immunologic function but can develop into mature Ly1 and Ly23 cells. For example, cell lines generated from Ly123$^+$ cells by continuous stimulation *in vitro* by conventional or MHC antigens, or maintenance through addition of 'growth factors', give rise to Ly23 cells, which account for 90–100% of the cells' cytolytic or suppressive activity, or to Ly1 T-helper cells. This suggests that progressive loss of Ly1 or Ly23 from Ly123 precursors correlates with the acquisition of the mature cytolytic or inducer function.

Regulation of immunity—co-operating cell sets

Antigen-stimulated Ly1 cells, or proteins produced by these cells, induce antigen-reactive cells (ARC) bearing the Ly123 phenotype to become antigen specific Ly23 T-suppressive (Ts) cells. This interaction has been called feedback suppression because (a) the degree of suppressive activity exerted by a fixed number of Ly123 cells increases in direct proportion to the numbers of antigen-activated Ly1 cells, and (b) the major target of mature Ly23 Ts is the inducer cell responsible for activation of this pathway.

These experiments have shown that activated inducer cells stimulate B cells to secrete antibody and also induce Ts cells that, rather ungratefully, inactivate the very cells responsible for their generation. This results in reduced B cell stimulation and progressively less generation of Ts cells. Although the genetic and cellular mechanism of these interactions are not well understood, one clear conclusion is that, like the formation of antibody by B cells, the generation of suppression by Ly23 cells is not an autonomous function: both require induction by Ly1 cells.

The notion that feedback suppression is essential for well controlled immune responses and for the prevention of potentially harmful immune reactions has been tested. Mice which have been experimentally depleted of Ly123 and Ly23 T cell sets (suppressive/cytotoxic) developed substantial amounts of auto-antibodies for prolonged periods. In other words, in the absence of Ts and their precursors, auto-antibody production is a common outcome of environmental immunization. Furthermore, several inbred strains of mice that spontaneously develop auto-immune disease harbour specific defects in the ability to induce effective T-suppressor cells. The general principle that has emerged from these studies is that the genetic programme of each specialized T cell type combines information for unique cell surface glycoproteins or 'markers' and a particular immunologic function. This principle has been applied to the definition of homologous cell sets in man, again according to expression of unique surface markers. Studies of people with deficiencies or disproportions of T cell sets indicate a corresponding disorder of immunologic competence. Acute episodes of multiple sclerosis and rheumatoid arthritis in children are preceded by a loss of T-suppressor cells in both blood and the relevant tissue. For example, virtually all lymphocytes in the joint spaces of patients with rheumatoid arthritis are activated inducer cells; suppressor cells are virtually undetectable. Moreover, these inducer cells secrete peptides which activate mast cells and monocytes to destroy cartilage and bone. Although steroids and inhibitors of prostaglandin synthesis dampen these effects, such drugs are not effective in long-term control of what amounts to a chronic disregulation of inducer T cell activity.

This represents one example of inducer:acceptor cell-cell interaction. Activated inducer T cells or clones of these cells stimulate division and/or maturation of many other cell types, including B cells, suppressive and cytotoxic T lymphocytes, macrophages, and precursors of haematopoietic cells.

Clonal analysis of T cell clones: co-ordinate T cell programming

In a broader sense, the reliability of these markers for predicting the function and MHC specificity of a cell needs to be stringently tested for both practical and theoretical reasons. A direct approach to this problem could be to select T cells solely according to Ly phenotype, to derive clones from them, and to determine whether or not the function and antigen specificity of these clones could be predicted from their Ly phenotype.

In a large series of experiments T cells were stimulated by cells which express complete or nearly complete MHC differences. The T cells were separated solely on the basis of their Ly phenotype and were immediately put in cultures to derive large numbers of clones. Over thirty such clones were studied periodically over eighteen months. The clones that were initially selected for the $Ly1^+2^-$ phenotype ('Ly1 clones') were uniformly $Ly1^+2^-$ for over one year, while those selected for the $Ly1^-2^+$ phenotype ('Ly2 clones') retained this phenotype for the same period.

All Ly1 clones expressed inducer functions after stimulation. None caused detectable lysis even at high effector-to-target cell ratios. All $Ly2^+$ clone cells specifically lysed targets bearing appropriate class I antigens, and none had inducer function after stimulation. In sum, extensive testing of more than thirty clones over 16–18 months showed complete correlation of Ly phenotype with function; no evidence was obtained for a single clone which could mediate both helper and cytolytic activities. Moreover, correlation of Ly phenotype with MHC recognition was equally clear-cut. All Ly1 clones recognized class II MHC products; all Ly2 clones recognized class I region products.

This confirms at the clonal level initial observations of a remarkably consistent and predictive correlation between Ly markers, MHC specificity and function. *They show that expression of Ly antigens by a T cell is part of a co-ordinate genetic programme that also determines its function and MHC specificity.*

These results directly bear on analysis of human T cell sets based on the murine model. Over the past several years, a large number of antibodies have been developed which apparently distinguish among human inducer, cytolytic, and suppressor T cells. Some identify surface molecules that have been claimed to be 'evolutionary analogues' of the Ly1 and Ly2 gene products expressed in mice. However, this requires careful re-evaluation: there is no evidence that human T cells expressing surface antigens ($T4^+$) thought to be analogous to the inducer set in mice ($Ly1^+2^-$ cells) kill target cells bearing autologous HLA-D antigens. However, there is, in contrast to murine studies, good evidence that clones of '$T4^+$' cells lyse *foreign* $HLA-D^+$ cells. Human clones derived from T cells isolated solely according to expression of a particular surface antigen are necessary for this evaluation. In experiments analogous to those performed to test the predictive value of Ly1 and Ly2 in animals, each clone should be tested for stability of phenotype, immunologic function, and MHC specificity. This assessment is essential for further progress in understanding T cell regulation of the immune response in normal individuals and in patients with chronic disorders.

T cell products

The past ten years has witnessed major conceptual advances in immunology. However, less progress has been made in defining endogenous regulatory molecules produced by suppressor and inducer T cells. Such progress requires continuously growing, homogeneous cells that secrete large amounts of the regulatory molecule. For example, homogeneous tumours that secrete immunoglobulins ('myelomas') allowed definition of the structure of antibody molecules. Unfortunately, neoplastic T cells have not proved so useful. Many do not grow well in continuous culture and very few express immunologic function.

The central technical advance in this area has been the development of general methods to produce clones: all of the cells within a clone are derived from a single parent cell. Cloned cells can be frozen for storage and after thawing and regrowth, they continue to express the molecular labels and functional properties of antigen-specific inducer or suppressor cells. The cloning procedure does not require hybridization to tumour cells, although such hybridization may be useful under certain circumstances. Inducer and suppressor clones that have been separately developed continue to secrete proteins that either specifically induce or suppress immunity. Clones of Ts cells have already provided the first cellular source for identification and purification of a molecule that directly suppresses immunity to foreign substances. The aim of this effort is to define the structural and genetic basis of the different activities of endogenous immunoregulatory molecules.

Molecules synthesized by inducer T cell clones

Non-specific peptides secreted by inducer cells

After stimulation, inducer T cell clones stimulate division and/or maturation of many other cell types, including B cells, suppressive and cytotoxic T lymphocytes, macrophages, and precursors of haematopoietic cells. Clones of T-inducer cells activate one or another of these target cell populations by secretion of a family of peptides. Each peptide is specialized to trigger a particular target cell type.

One of these peptides has an apparent Mr of 30 000 according to Sephacryl chromatography and initially fits previous descriptions of factors that stimulate growth of cytotoxic and possibly suppressive T cells. However, further biochemical analysis of this molecule has shown that it is composed of two subunits having Mr of 16 kDa and 14 kDa. Mitogenic activity is carried by the 14 kDa chain, while the 16 kDa chain focusses the 14 kDa growth peptide onto T lymphocytes and not other target cells.

Inducer molecules that activate B cells to divide and secrete antibodies have also been examined. A polypeptide having an apparent relative molecular mass of 45 kDa and pI of 6.0 stimulates B cells to secrete Ig but not to divide. This 45 kDa protein is normally associated with the 14 kDa mitogenic peptide described above. The intact (45 kDa + 14 kDa) molecule selectively activates B cells both to divide and to

secrete Ig, and has no effect on other types of lymphocyte. These peptides, as well as other inducer molecules responsible for stimulation of haematopoietic cells, have been purified to homogeneity for sequencing and, ultimately, to define the genetic and structural basis of their biological activities.

Molecules that activate specific antibody responses

Current data support the view that inducer cells secrete a modified form of their surface receptor. The cell-bound receptor on inducer cells has the following properties: (1) it distinguishes almost completely between closely related determinants; (2) it recognizes a portion of the MHC-linked class II gene products (the HLA-D gene products in man); and (3) it does not recognize antigen conjugated to peptides which do not associate with the correct class II gene products. The specificity of secreted inducer proteins also displays these features. Thus they have the same capacity as the receptor for discrimination among closely related determinants and they recognize the same MHC class II molecule as does the receptor. Thus, secreted peptides that induce antibody formation by B cells have properties analogous to those displayed by the cell-bound receptor and most likely represent a modified form of this structure.

These findings indicate that at least some antibody responses to proteins may not depend directly on B cell–T cell interactions. Instead, a secreted form of the inducer T cell receptor may activate antibody secretion by antigen-specific, I-A identical B cells. The fine specificity of secreted inducer molecules ensures that B cell clones activated by these secreted molecules belong to the same pool as those triggered by the intact inducer cell.

It is important to note that in contrast to peptides synthesized and secreted by these inducer clones, it is difficult to show that inducer cells bind specifically to free antigen (although they may bind Ia-antigen complexes). The following observations are relevant: (1) the specificity of binding by secreted inducer cell molecules accounts precisely for the specificity of MHC-associated activation of the cloned inducer cells by antigen; (2) secreted inducer molecules that bind free antigen are composed of at least two chains as determined under reducing conditions on SDS-PAGE. Possibly the binding of secreted peptides to nominal antigen may depend upon contributions by two closely linked polypeptides chains. If so, linkage of these two polypeptides in the membrane of inducer cells may also be required for antigen specific binding. This notion implies that these antigen-binding chains are normally *not* associated in the lipid bilayer of inducer cell membranes: they are brought together only by simultaneous recognition of class II molecules and nominal antigen on the surface of APC.

Definition of cells and molecules that directly mediate specific immunologic suppression

Another application of T cell clones has come from studies of a T-suppressor clone that expresses surface receptors for glycophorin expressed on sheep erythrocytes. Analysis of this T cell clone has suggested that these cells share several major characteristics with antibody-forming B cells. Both display a similar number of surface receptors that bind to antigen in the absence of major histocompatibility complex (MHC) products. Both respond to signals from inducer T cells by secretion of antigen-binding proteins. The cells secrete a 70 kDa protein that binds to antigen and mediates suppression. Picogram amounts of purified antigen-binding proteins specifically inhibit an on-going immune response to the antigen.

One approach to the analysis of the structural basis of this activity comes from studies of degradation of the purified Ts molecule with proteolytic enzymes. Although the 70 kDa protein is sensitive to digestion by several different proteases, including pepsin and trypsin, papain yielded the most reproducible cleavage; this enzyme splits almost 100% of the 70 kDa antigen binding molecule into two subunits of Mr 45 kDa and 24 kDa. Both were resistant to further degradation and represented 70% to 85% of the fully digested 70 kDa product. Since this was a reproducible characteristic of the protein, the biological activity of the two cleavage products was defined. The 45 kDa subunit retained suppressive but not binding activity; the 24 kDa peptide lacked suppressive activity but retained specific binding to antigen.

A critical point is that *binding* of the intact 70 kDa protein to antigen also results in cleavage and production of the 45 kDa and 24 kDa subunits; these expressed the same biological activities as the two peptides obtained after enzymatic digestion of the parent molecule. The 45 kDa and 24 kDa subunits can be distinguished from one another serologically. An antibody made against myeloma proteins that recognizes V_H sequences of immunoglobulins reacts with the 70 kDa parent molecule and the 24 kDa subunits but not the 45 kDa subunit. A rabbit antibody that reacts with several other 70 kDa Ts molecules specific for different antigens binds to the 45 kDa but not the 24 kDa subunit of the Ts molecule.

Thus the combined activities of the separate 45 kDa and 24 kDa peptides account for the biological activity of the parent molecule and the two peptides probably represent two distinct domains of the Ts proteins. It is formally possible, albeit extremely unlikely, that the 24 kDa peptide is a breakdown product of the 45 kDa peptide. Nonetheless, definitive evidence that the 45 kDa and 24 kDa peptides represent independent domains of the 70 kDa parent molecule requires amino acid sequencing and analysis of the mRNA that codes for the 70 molecule.

Analogies between Ig and the Ts molecule

Papain digestion of Ig chains produces two fragments, Fc and Fab. The Ig chain fragment contained within the Fab fragment has an average Mr of 22 kDa, carries the antigen-binding site of the Ig chain, and contains sequences encoded by V_H genes. The Fc fragment has a mean Mr of 50 kDa, mediates the biological activity of the different classes of immunoglobulin and is encoded by C genes. Each C gene product displays characteristic 'isotypic' determinants which are serologically defined by antibodies. T-suppressor (Ts) molecules purified from cloned T cells also appear to consist of two functionally distinct domains as judged by papain digestion: a V region (24 kDa) that binds specifically to antigen but lacks suppressive activity and a C region (45 kDa) that does not bind antigen but suppresses antibody responses to a variety of antigens. As noted above, the 45 kDa protein of this molecule appears to share serologic determinants with partially purified Ts proteins which are specific for other antigens. Since these determinants are not detected on T-inducer proteins, they may represent isotypic determinants on T cell molecules that suppress immune responses.

Functional properties of the Ts molecule

Picogram amounts of purified 70 kDa Ts protein turn off the entire response to a complex cellular antigen even when administered after immunization to the antigen. The structural properties of this molecule suggest the following mechanism to account for its biological activity. Binding of the 70 kDa molecule to T-inducer cells that have bound to correct antigenic determinant is followed by increased sensitivity of the Ts molecule to a surface protease on target T-inducer cells and the consequent release of the 45 kDa subunit. This subunit suppresses all T-inducer cells specific for determinant on the same molecule that bears the epitope for which the Ts molecule is specific. The net effect of this reaction is suppression of an immune response to a complex foreign cell by a monoclonal Ts molecule specific for one site on that cell. An important feature of this mechanism is that it ensures efficient suppression of immunity to complex foreign cells or molecules by a relatively small number of Ts clones. An additional practical feature comes from the observation that T_H cells to randomly chosen proteins which have been covalently attached to the sheep erythrocyte are also suppressed. A possible therapeutic application would follow if T_H cells specific for an autologous protein involved in an auto-immune response are susceptible to suppression by the 70 kDa peptide and SRBC–protein conjugate.

Summary

Recent advances in lymphocyte culture technology allow production of large amounts of homogeneous T cells which secrete immunoregulatory peptides. This means that it is now possible to define and purify non-toxic peptides that either specifically turn off or turn on immune responses. For example, monoclonal peptides synthesized by inducer cells each activate a different target cell to divide or differentiate. One activates stem cells to differentiate into red cells and white cells, another stimulates B cells to secrete antibody, and another induces mast cells to divide and perhaps to differentiate. Perhaps the most informative point that has come from these studies is that each peptide that has been isolated from T cell clones exerts powerful regulatory effects on either the intensity or type of the immune response. The hope is that some of these immunoregulatory molecules or their analogues can be used as potent therapeutic agents for certain chronic diseases. Since purified inducer and suppressive peptides will be available in large amounts within the next several years, it will not be long before this strategy can be thoroughly evaluated.

Homogeneous T cell populations that mediate antigen-specific help or suppression represent highly attractive material for biochemical analysis. But there is an additional major point that can be made from close examination of immunologic activity of clones of T cells expressing defined function and specificity. Insights into the events that regulate the molecular cascade controlling blood clotting or complement activation has come from analysis of the contribution of each purified component to this biological reaction. This reductionist analysis has precisely defined the critical molecular events that amplify or suppress these two biological systems.

This approach may soon be applied to define the cascade of cell–cell interactions that regulate antibody and cellular immune responses. This strategy depends on 'building' or synthesizing the minimal cellular components required for an immune response, using well-characterized lymphocyte clones that belong to different regulatory T cell sets, supplemented by homogeneous populations of B cells and monocytes. What are the central genetic and molecular events to regulate this synthetic system? Do the interactions among this collection of cells obey the rules that have been derived from analysis of heterogeneous cell populations.

Further reading

1 CANTOR H. & BOYSE E.A. (1975) Functional subclasses of T lymphocytes bearing different Ly antigens. (I) The generation of functionally distinct T cell subclasses is a differentiative process independent of antigen. *J. exp. Med.* **141**, 1376.

2 CANTOR H. & BOYSE E.A. (1975) Functional subclasses of T lymphocytes bearing different Ly antigens. (II) Cooperation between subclasses of Ly^+ cells in the generation of killer activity. *J. exp. Med.* **141**, 1390.

3 CANTOR H., SHEN F.W. & BOYSE E.A. (1976) Separation of helper T cells from suppressor T cells expressing different Ly components. (II) Activation by antigen: After immunization, antigen-specific suppressor and helper activities are mediated by distinct T cell subclasses. *J. exp. Med.* **143**, 1391.

4 EARDLEY D.D., HUGENBERGER J., McVAY-BOUDREAU L., SHEN F.W., GERSHON R.K. & CANTOR H. (1978) Immunoregulatory circuits among T cell sets. (I) T-helper cells induce other T cells to exert feedback inhibition. *J. exp. Med.* **147**, 1106.

5 FATHMAN C.G. & FITCH F.W. (eds.) (1982) *Isolation and Utilization of T-cell Clones*. Academic Press, New York.

6 FRESNO M., McVAY-BOUDREAU L. & CANTOR H. (1981) Antigen specific T lymphocyte clones. (III) Papain splits purified T-suppressor molecules into two functional domains. *J. exp. Med.* **155**, 981.

7 GERSHON R.K. (1974) T-cell control of antibody response. *Contemp. Top. Mol. Immunol.* **3**, 1.

8 HUBER B., CANTOR H., SHEN F.W. & BOYSE E.A. (1978) Independent differentiative pathways of Ly1 and Ly23 subclasses of T cells. Experimental production of mice deprived of selected T-cell subclasses. *J. exp. Med.* **144**, 1128.

9 JANDINSKI J., CANTOR H., TADAKUMA T., PEAVY D.L. & PIERCE C.W. (1976) Separation of helper T cells from suppressor T cells expressing different Ly components. (I) Polyclonal activation: Suppressor and helper activities are inherent properties of distinct T cell subclasses. *J. exp. Med.* **143**, 1382.

10 KAPPLER J.W. & MARRACK P. (1978) The role of H-2 linked genes in helper T cell function. IV. Importance of T-cell genotype and host environment in I-region and Ir gene expression. *J. exp. Med.* **148**, 1510.

11 NABEL G., FRESNO M., CHESSMAN A. & CANTOR H. (1981) Use of cloned populations of mouse lymphocytes to analyse cellular differentiation. *Cell*, **23**, 19.

12 NAGY Z.A., KUSNIERCZYK P. & KLEIN J. (1981) Terminal differentiation of T cells specific for mutant H-2K antigens. Conversion of Lyt-1,2 cells into Lyt-2 but not Lyt-1 cells, *in vitro. Eur. J. Immunol.* **11**, 167.

13 PAUL W.E. & BENACERRAF B. (1977) Functional specificity of thymus-dependent lymphocytes. *Science*, **195**, 1293.

14 RAO A., ALLARD W.J., HOGAN P.G., ROSENSON R.S. & CANTOR H. (1983) Alloreactive T-cell clones. Ly pheno-

types predict both function and specificity for major histocompatibility complex in mice. *Immunogenetics*, **17**, 147.

15 REINHERZ E., KAMP P.F.C., GOLDSTEIN G. & SCHLOSSMAN S.F. (1979) Separation of functional subsets of human T-cells using monoclonal antibody. *Proc. natn. Acad. Sci. U.S.A.* **76**, 4061.

16 REINHERZ E.L., WEINER H.L., HAUSER S.L., COHEN J.A., DISTASO J.A. & SCHLOSSMAN S.F. (1980) Loss of suppressor T-cells in active multiple sclerosis. *New Engl. J. Med.* **303**, 125.

17 SCHREIER M.H., ISCOVE N.N., TEES R., AARDEN L. & VON BOEHMER H. (1980) Clones of killer and helper T cells: growth requirements, specificity and retention of function in long term culture. *Immunol. Rev.* **51**, 315.

18 SHEN F.W., MCDOUGAL J.S., BARD J. & CORT S.P. (1980) Developmental and communicative interactions of Ly123 and Ly1 cells sets. *J. exp. Med.* **151**, 566.

19 ZINKERNAGEL R.M., ALTHAGE A., WATERFIELD E., KINDRED B., WELSCH R.M., CALLAHAN G. & PINCETH P. (1980) Restriction specificities, alloreactivity, and allotolerance expressed by T cells from nude mice reconstituted with H-2-compatible or -incompatible thymus grafts. *J. exp. Med.* **151**, 376.

Chapter 76
Subtractive cDNA hybridization and the T-cell receptor genes

M. M. DAVIS

Isolation of T-cell receptor cDNA clones, 76.1

Method for subtractive cDNA hybridization, 76.2

T-cell receptor protein structure, 76.6

Additional hypervariable regions, 76.7

Gene structure, 76.8

Expression in T-cell subsets, 76.9

Expression during thymic differentiation, 76.9

Since the first indications that the immune system consisted of cellular (T-cell) as well as humoral (B-cell) components [1], immunologists have been trying to determine how T-cells recognize foreign entities. Because the quantities of receptor protein involved are so much smaller than is the case with immunoglobulins, this has proved to be a very difficult problem, with the first indications of success coming only in the last few years. In particular, this depended on the contributions of many workers, first in the establishment of functional lines and hybridomas of T cells [2], later in the use of anti-idiotypic antisera [3] and particularly monoclonals [4–11] to characterize an 80–90 kDa disulphide-linked heterodimer (α and β) on both helper and cytotoxic T cells. Particularly important to efforts at structural characterization has been the isolation of cDNA clones for the β [12–14] and later the α chains [15–17] of the receptor and the confirmation of the identities of those clones by partial amino acid sequences in the human [18,19] and mouse systems (C. Hannum, personal communication). Characterization of these clones has permitted the determination of the complete primary sequence of both α and β chains, as well as turning up an as yet unexplained third type of possible receptor molecule (γ) [20]. The isolation of these cDNA clones and the corresponding genomic clones makes likely the 'engineering' of the expression of large amounts of receptor protein at will in the near future. This will make possible the detailed biochemical characterization of receptor binding properties, something that is very difficult with the currently available quantities. In the longer term, this should lead to X-ray crystallographic studies of receptor structure. What follows is a detailed review of the subtractive cDNA methodology that the author and colleagues have used to isolate these genes, followed by a summary of their current knowledge of receptor gene structure and expression.

The subtractive cDNA approach is particularly relevant to the (many) other genes which one might hope to isolate from lymphoid and other specialized cell types.

Isolation of T-cell receptor cDNA clones

T-cell receptor cDNA clones have been isolated by subtractive hybridization [13,15,16,20], differential hybridization [12] and oligonucleotide probes based on partial amino acid sequence [17]. This last methodology is one of the most common ones in current usage and yet perhaps the most difficult to employ in this case because of the problems in generating enough purified protein for sequencing. Its application to systems where sufficient quantities of pure protein are available for sequencing has been reviewed elsewhere [21]. Subtractive hybridization and differential hybridization are similar in that they both employ randomly labelled cDNA probes for the initial screening and depend on differential expression of the RNA species of interest. The differential or 'plus-minus' screening approach suffers from a relative lack of sensitivity because of signal to noise problems (as reviewed in reference 22) but it has been successful in a number of cases [23–24], including the isolation of the human β chain gene [12]. In general, this procedure is adequate for species which are present at levels of 0.01% or higher in the mRNA population of interest. Subtractive hybridization, which utilizes hydroxyapatite to physically remove sequences that are shared between two populations (the cDNA:mRNA hybrids), has long been employed in various forms for comparing different mRNA populations [25–26] and was first used to isolate specific genes in the relatively abundant classes by Alt [27], Mather [28] and Timberlake and their respective colleagues [29]. Since the feasibility of either of the two procedures depends on there being as small a difference as possible between the mRNA populations employed, it is important to note measurements which show that B cells and T cells differ by only a small fraction of their gene expression [30; M.M. Davis, S.M. Hedrick and W.E. Paul, unpublished]. Specifically it was found that only $2\% \pm 0.5$ of the mass of the mRNA was B or T cell specific, representing approximately 200 different species. Even smaller differences (0.3%) distinguished T-cell hybridomas (*op. cit.*). By modifying existing procedures to isolate such small quantities in high yield (see next section) [30,31] and by the use of secondary and tertiary selections, the author and others have been able to isolate a number of important lymphocyte specific genes, notably cDNA clones encoding all three of the known T-cell receptor molecules (α, β and γ) [13,15,16,20], A_α [31], and the XLR gene family implicated in the xid mutation of the CBA/N mouse [32–33]. The subtraction procedure given in the methods section has also been used to isolate the lymphocyte cell surface markers Leu 2 and Leu 3 from positively transformed L cell lines (subtracted with normal L cell RNA) [34–36] and an IgE regulatory factor [37]. Because of the very small differences between mRNA populations in all of these cases, the species of interest are greatly enriched (50–1000-fold) in the cDNA probe and thus very rare messages are detectable (0.001% in some cases [22]). This means that even gene transcripts that are present in a few copies of mRNA per cell can be identified. This is particularly important to note since approximately 90% of the gene expression in lymphocytes and other cell types is in the rare abundance class [13,38]. Coupled with the use of subtracted probes in some cases has been the use of subtracted cDNA libraries, first introduced in references 31 and 39 and also utilized in references 13, 14, 16, 20, and 32. This involves only a slight modification of the basic procedure (see next section) and allows the concentration of a subtracted probe on to a relatively small number of filters (typically 10–20-fold fewer than with an unsubtracted library [31]). This can be important since the relative intensity of rare species hybridization will be directly proportional to the concentration of the probe. This is due to the fact that a rare species will not be concentrated enough under typical circumstances to hybridize completely to a colony or plaque on a filter (see discussion in the next section).

In addition to the basic subtraction strategies discussed above, secondary and tertiary selections are often employed. In the case of the T-cell receptor [31], these have taken the form of using membrane-bound polysomal RNA as the starting material, given the fact that these are cell-surface molecules and this results in a 3–10 × selection. A third selection, not so generally

applicable, was the criterion of rearrangement between T-cell and non-lymphoid DNAs. Another very T-cell receptor specific type of selection involved the preparation of a 'V-region' specific probe to isolate the murine α chain gene [15]. This involved the subtraction of randomly primed cDNA from a T cell of one specificity with mRNA from T cells of other specificities. This results in a necessarily very stringent selection and thus might be useful in systems where other types of recombining gene segments might be employed. Another type of secondary selection would involve specific units of the genome either as whole chromosomes [32], or cosmid clones [31] or (potentially) minichromosomes of various sorts. The use of L cells transformed for specific cell surface markers also results in a very specific selection [34–36]. Also useful is size selection of mRNA and message selected translation where a translation system has been established (as in reference 37). Another possibility is negative selection with one RNA, followed by positive selection with another, as employed by Mather *et al.* [28] to isolate a J chain cDNA clone (see next section).

Method for subtractive cDNA hybridization

Equipment

The only equipment necessary is a water-jacketed column and a circulating water bath which can maintain the column at either 60 °C or 97–100 °C. Haake or Lauda brand water baths or their equivalents are available from a number of distributors. Suitable water-jacketed columns are more difficult however, as the author has not found any company which makes a good one. However, nucleic acid hybridization people have traditionally had columns made by glass-blowers (any chemistry department shop) who cut the bottoms off reflux columns and replace them with a porous glass fret and a teflon valve. One such column of this type is shown in Fig. 76.1. It is also important to locate the apparatus near an air supply (preferably filtered) to allow a gentle air pressure on the column. An alternative to being able to boil off the material bound to the column is to use high concentrations of phosphate buffer (0.4 M). This results in lower yields of the double-stranded fraction and makes quantification difficult, but it allows the use of a constant 60 °C water bath and more makeshift water-jacketed columns (down to and including a Pasteur pipette plugged with glass wool embedded into a large stretch of tubing). The true yield of double-stranded material can be obtained from such columns by dissolving the hydroxyapatite in 50% nitric acid and counting an aliquot. This dilution of nitric acid is also useful for cleaning out the columns after use.

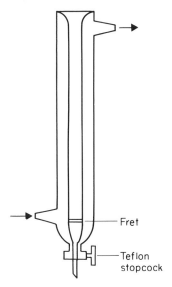

Fig. 76.1. Typical water-jacketed column made from a reflux column.

Materials

The authors have had good experience with Bio-Rad nucleic acid grade hydroxyapatite and deoxynucleotide triphosphates from P.L. Biochemicals. ^{32}PdCTP is from Amersham or New England Nuclear.

Procedure

cDNA synthesis

Hot cDNA (2×10^8 c.p.m./μg) is synthesized in the following manner after Chien *et al.* [40] in 50–200 μl volumes.

50 mM-Tris, pH 8.3
6 mM-MgCl$_2$, kept as a 10 × stock
60 mM-NaCl
1 mM-dATP ⎫
1 mM-dGTP ⎬ kept as 20 mM aliquots at -70 °C
1 mM-dTTP ⎪
30 μM-dCTP ⎭
3–12 μM-^{32}P dCTP (typically half of the final volume of 400–3000 Ci/mmol aqueous material)
100 μg/ml Actinomycin D (Sigma) (1 mg/ml stock aqueous material)
20 mM-Dithiothreitol (1 M stock)
20 μg/ml Oligo dT (1 mg/ml stock)
2–5 μg Poly (A)$^+$ RNA per 100 μl reaction (stored in 10 mM-Tris, pH 7.5, 1 mM-EDTA)
10 units avian reverse transcriptase per microgram of poly (A)$^+$ RNA

Incubate at 42 °C for 1–2 h. An alternative to oligo dT priming is random priming with nuclease digested calf thymus DNA [41]. This provides a more equal representation of mRNA (oligo dT priming tends to be 3′ biased—especially if there is any nuclease contamination).

Base hydrolysis

1 Remove RNA template by bringing the reaction mixture to 10 mM-EDTA, 0.1 M-NaOH and heating at 70 °C for 20 min.
2 Cool on ice and neutralize with 1 M-HCl.
3 Add sodium acetate (pH 7.0) to 0.2 M and SDS to 0.1% (for column).

Removal of incorporated nucleotides

1 Exclude cDNA on a 2 ml G-50 F Sephadex column in a Pasteur pipette plugged with silanized glass wool. Column buffer: 0.1 M-NaCl, 0.05 M-Tris, pH 7.5, 0.001 M-EDTA, 0.02% SDS.
2 Take successive 0.1 ml fractions into Eppendorf tubes. Yield should be 20–80% of input poly A RNA.
3 Combine excluded fractions (usually #7–12) into a silanized Eppendorf tube, concentrate to 0.4–0.5 ml with sec-butanol [42], add 50 μg tRNA as carrier, 2 vols. of ethanol, and precipitate on dry ice by allowing to freeze. Allow to thaw briefly and spin in an Eppendorf centrifuge for 15 min.
4 Remove ethanol supernatant with a slightly drawn Pasteur pipette and dry pellet on the edge of a fume hood with the window almost closed or apply a gentle vacuum briefly until just dry.

First subtractive hybridization (Fig. 76.2)

1 Resuspend pellet in 4–7 μl of poly (A)$^+$ RNA (1–2 mg/ml in 10 mM-Tris, pH 7.5, 1 mM-EDTA). (This usually produces a 5–10 excess of mRNA over cDNA and is sufficient. If total RNA is used, do not use more than 100–200 μg without a high salt RNAse treatment [26] or the column will be saturated and some double-stranded material may come out in the single-stranded fraction.)
2 Add 1 μl of 4 M-phosphate buffer (PB) (2 M-disodium and 2 M-monosodium phosphate, chelexed and Millipore filtered).
3 Add $\sim$0.1 μl 10% SDS (with a 5 μl glass capillary) $\sim$0.1 μl 0.5 M-EDTA and double-distilled filtered or autoclaved water to 8 μl. Seal into a 20 μl silanized glass capillary using a bunsen burner.
4 Heat in a boiling water bath for 30 s to disaggregate, and thereafter at 68 °C for 4–20 h, depending on desired C_0t value. In 0.5 M-PB at 68 °C (μg/ml of poly

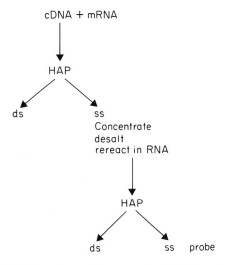

Fig. 76.2. Subtractive probe preparation. Multiple solution hybridizations and passages over hydroxyapatite result in probe suitable for library screening or in material that can be double-stranded and cloned directly.

(A)$^+$ RNA) (μg/ml poly (A)$^+$ RNA) $(0.07) = C_0t$s per hour. Most reactions terminate at C_0t values of 1500–3000. For analytical reactions, a given reaction mixture can be divided into 1 μl aliquots incubated in 5 μl capillary tubes to different times (up to 4 days).

Hydroxyapatite chromatography

1 Swell hydroxyapatite (HAP) in several volumes of buffer (0.12 M-PB, 0.1% SDS), decant once and apply to a water-jacketed column at 60 °C; the remainder can be stored for some months.

2 After approximately 1 ml (1 × 1 cm) has settled, equilibrate the column by washing through about 10 ml of the buffer. Use enough air pressure to provide a gentle but steady flow. Break ends of the capillary tube containing the reaction mixture using a triangular file and dilute into 1 ml of buffer.

3 Apply reaction mixture directly to the column avoiding the sides. Force material through with gentle air pressure as before, until buffer layer completely enters the column, collecting into disposable plastic tubes (but before dryness, when bubbles appear under the fret).

4 Repeat with successive 1 ml aliquots of buffer, washing the sides of the column in the process. Seven to eight aliquots should be sufficient and most of the single-stranded material will be in the first three fractions. Leaving the column valve open over an empty tube increase bath temperature to 97–98 °C (approximately 15 min). This will melt the double-stranded material and allow it to be eluted from the column. One to two minutes after reaching this temperature, turn the water bath down to 60 °C and elute the bound material with five successive 1 ml aliquots of buffer. Count aliquots of all fractions to determine the percentage of double-stranded cDNA. A good first reaction with closely related mRNA/cDNA populations should be 90–95% double stranded. If the number is lower, then the reaction is probably not going to completion. Columns can be cleaned with 50% nitric acid (which dissolves HAP) and rinsed with distilled water.

Concentration for re-reaction

Since phosphate buffer interferes with precipitations, it is necessary to first remove the phosphate ions by column chromatography. To allow the use of a small (Pasteur pipette) column, the material is concentrated with sec-butanol.

1 Combine the two or three best single-stranded fractions into a polypropylene tube and add an equal volume of secondary-butyl alcohol (Fisher). Invert several times, then remove the upper (butanol layer) when the phases separate. Sec-butanol removes water from an aqueous solution leaving charged salts and nucleic acids behind [42]. It will remove SDS as well (G. Galau, personal communication).

2 Repeat extraction until the aqueous layer has been concentrated to 0.25 ml.

3 Remove butanol by extracting once with an equal volume of chloroform and transfer to a silanized Eppendorf tube.

4 Remove chloroform by incubating at 37 °C for 15 min or aerating with nitrogen. This prevents the chloroform from extracting material from the column.

5 Add SDS to 0.1% and desalt by passage over a G-50 F Sephadex column as before.

6 Add carrier tRNA to the excluded fractions, transfer to a silanized Eppendorf tube, and ethanol precipitate as before. If there is difficulty achieving quantitative precipitation, add $MgCl_2$ to 10 mM. Resuspend and react as previously, although a smaller final volume (4–6 μl) and hybridization in a smaller (10 μl) capillary will conserve RNA. After the second hydroxyapatite passage (typically 20–60% double-stranded), the probe is ready to use to screen colonies or plaques. Although it has a significant amount of unreactable cDNA, this material is very small in size and does not seem to generate appreciable background.

Library screening with subtracted probes

Since rare species in a typical probe will be very dilute

(only 1% able to hybridize under most conditions), it is very important to keep it as concentrated as possible and to use every available rate accelerator. Therefore, after wetting and prehybridizing in the normal fashion, the author hybridizes a large (132 mm) nitrocellulose filter in a sealed bag with 1 ml of hybridization solution consisting of: 5 × SSPE [43], 5 × Denhardts [43], 100 μg/ml salmon sperm DNA, 10% dextran sulphate at 68 °C. This mixture produces a threefold better signal with single-stranded probes than the typical 50% formamide mixture with dextran sulphate [44] (M. Davis, unpublished observations). Care should be taken to remove most bubbles or to shift them away from the filter. Washing with 1–2 × SSPE 0.1% SDS at 55 °C is usually sufficient, although an additional wash at 0.2 × SSPE may be necessary.

Back reactions

For the purposes of quantification or use of specific probes to explore relationships between different subsets, it is often important to 'back react' a subtracted probe to its original template RNA. This allows one to remove most of the non-reactable cDNA (sometimes as much as 80% of the labelled material). This is accomplished by concentrating the probe as before (after the second subtraction) and hybridizing the original RNA to completion. After hydroxyapatite fractionation, the double-stranded material is eluted, alkaline hydrolysed to remove any RNA (as in the base hydrolysis), concentrated and desalted over G-50 F Sephadex, precipitated and resuspended in TE for further use.

Selected cDNA libraries

The same basic procedure is used to construct a cDNA subtracted library [31,39]. The only modifications are that only trace amounts of label are used in the cDNA synthesis and that the cold dCTP concentration is brought up to 1 mM. This typically increases the size of the single-stranded material and results in higher reactivities (94–96% in the first hybridization of a B*-T library [31]). One [31,39] or two [20] rounds of subtraction are feasible. At this point the cDNA is made double-stranded with DNA polymerase I or Klenau and can be cloned in a variety of ways.

Notes and recommendations

Yield losses

Because many steps are involved in subtraction strategies, it is critical to keep yields high. Even under the best of circumstances one can expect yields of 50–70%

per cycle of hybridization. The main problem is sticking of material (especially single-stranded nucleic acid) to glassware or plasticware. To minimize this it is necessary to use detergent (SDS) in solutions wherever feasible and to silanize all glassware and plasticware which comes in contact with the probe. Plastic tubes and pipettes are usually not a problem when SDS is present, but as this is not possible during the ethanol precipitations (due to the solubility of SDS in ethanol), Eppendorf tubes should be silanized when used for this purpose. Capillary pipettes for reactions, Pasteur pipettes for Sephadex columns and glass wool are routinely silanized with dichlorodimethylsilane by evaporation in a desiccator [43]. Other plasticware and the water-jacketed column should not be silanized.

Cytoplasmic versus total RNA

A large number of sequences are transcribed in nuclear RNA [38] versus those which appear in the cytoplasm (5–10 × more sequence complexity). Although not all of it is polyadenylated, enough is to add many more sequences to a preparation of total poly(A)+ RNA versus its cytoplasmic counterpart. Therefore, to avoid isolating transcripts which do not represent expressed genes, it is important to use cytoplasmic RNA as the starting material for a cDNA probe or library. The author uses one of the NP-40 lysis procedures which works well for B- and T-cell tumours [45], although different cell types can present various problems with respect to ease of lysis or abundance of endogenous nucleases. It may also be important to use cytoplasmic RNA in the subtraction, since in at least some systems, transcripts which are differentially expressed in the cytoplasm of different tissues are expressed equally well in the nucleus [46].

Analytical reactions

It is important to quantify a given subtractive reaction on an analytical scale in order to define the differences between any two RNA populations. Even in cases where this has already been done it can be a useful measure of how well the preparative reactions are going. Examples of how to do this for small differences are given in references 13 and 47. Knowing how many genes are different between two RNA populations is also important to planning a cloning strategy, whether secondary or tertiary selections are needed, etc. Needless to say, a good knowledge of nucleic acid hybridization theory and the basic chemistry is essential to doing this properly. In fact, the discovery by Wetmur & Davidson [48] that the renaturation of DNA followed simple chemical kinetics is one of the triumphs of physical chemistry over the behaviour of biologically important macromolecules. It is also worth noting that this work, together with the discovery of repetitive sequences by Britten & Kohne [49], rendered completely worthless an entire literature dealing with the phenomenology of hybridizations that had been accumulating up to that point.

Hybridization kinetic principles were extended to cDNA:mRNA hybridizations by Bishop [50] and further refined by Galau *et al*. [51]. Lewin's *Gene Expression II* (2nd edn.) [38] contains a comprehensive and authoritative review of the principles and literature dealing with this subject, and *Biochemistry*, by Wood *et al*, [52], contains very useful summaries and problem sets. It is of particular importance to note the effects of concentration, salt, temperature, size, complexity and G/C content on the rate of reaction and relative stability of a given duplex. Since these texts only deal with hybridizations in solution, it should be noted that those involving reactants fixed to solid substrates (i.e. filters) are generally about three times slower.

Reaction problems

If preparative reactions are falling substantially short (5% or more) of the analytical ones, there is usually something inhibiting the reaction. This is often excess salt which has come down in the precipitation and can be removed by additional precipitations or washing with 70% ethanol. Pay particular care to the physical appearance of the pellets after ethanol precipitation and brief drying (without catching too many β rays). They should be almost clear and barely visible scraps of material. Large, white pellets indicate the presence of salt. Large, grey pellets which dissolve poorly indicate that chloroform was present in the material put over the G-50 column and that part of the column was extracted into the effluent. If this is the case more care should be taken to be sure that all the chloroform is gone before loading the column (sniffing the tube is the best assay!). Another cause of low reactivity is a high proportion of short (< 300 nucleotide) cDNA. In this case one should try different lots of reverse transcriptase to find one which gives larger material (assuming the initial RNA is not degraded). Alkaline agarose gels are good for assessing cDNA size [43]. Problems have also been encountered with metal ions in the phosphate buffers which will cause strand scissions at high temperatures, but the simple chelex treatment step recommended in the protocol should take care of this.

Rescreening

Because of the generally small amount of probe and large numbers of positives in a typical screen it is best to rescreen in multiple arrays on the same plate. Alternatively, one could perform the initial screen at a very low density so that there is generally no need for rescreening. The usual practice of rescreening each positive on a single plate will spread a given probe very thin and may result in the loss of weak positives. As mentioned previously, this is where having a subtracted library makes life much easier, particularly if it is in a plasmid vector (which is easier to put in arrays on a plate than λ phage cDNA clones). Typically, the author will pick an area around a positive and streak this out on a plate: from this plate he will pick five to twenty individual colonies to put in an array. In this fashion, as many as fifty or more different positives can fit on to one large (150 mm) plate and a corresponding nitrocellulose (Millipore) filter. Once specific clones have been screened and rescreened positive, it is generally convenient to perform Northern (RNA) blot analysis [43,44] on each one to determine which are the same and which are different as well as to weed out any false positives (as in reference 13).

Repeated sequences

Repeated sequences in the 3′ untranslated region of mRNAs, while fairly common, does not seem to represent a problem in most subtraction reactions. That is, repeated sequences on mRNAs of one tissue generally are not present in mRNA of another tissue (M. Davis and W. Paul, unpublished observations). This is not true for nuclear RNA transcription [38]. Therefore if cDNA clones are being screened with poly(A)$^+$ cytoplasmic RNA derived probes there is usually no problem. Screening genomic clones is a much more sensitive proposition (since all repeats are, by definition, present many times in the genome) and in that case care should be allowed to fragment (by autoradiolysis [31] and/or random priming [41]) the cDNA to a small but still reactable size (500 nt average) and co-hybridize this with fragmented total genomic DNA along with the RNA used for subtraction. In this scheme [31], the genomic DNA only hybridizes to a repetitive C_0t while the RNA goes to completion, making both repetitive sequences and shared sequences double stranded and removable on hydroxyapatite. Fragmentation is also advisable if one suspects that different exons of the same gene are utilized in different populations.

T-cell receptor protein structure

Despite the different requirements for T-cell and B-cell recognition, the polypeptides encoded by the α and β chain genes (as well as the putative γ chain), are

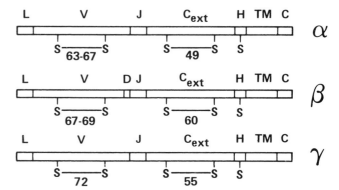

Fig. 76.3. Schematic of T-cell receptor protein structure. α, β and γ chains are compared. S indicates the presence of cysteine residues and presumptive sulphydryl bonds are shown. An additional cysteine residue in the middle of the β chain constant region is not depicted for the sake of simplicity.

remarkably immunoglobulin-like in their structure [12,14–17]. This is illustrated in Fig. 76.3, with the location of the intrachain sulphydryl bonds based on analogy to immunoglobulin. They all appear to have leader (L), variable (V), joining (J) and constant (C) region portions which are indistinguishable in size and location from those of immunoglobulin. Furthermore, the β chain molecules also have a diversity (D) elements [53–57] similar to those of the heavy chain genes [58, 59]. Evidence indicates that there is no D region associated with the γ chain or one which only provides Z nucleotides between V and J [100]. It may also be significant that the α chain V regions have a more light chain-like spacing between cysteines (63–67 a.a.) [15–17,79] whereas those of the β chain have a more heavy chain-like spacing (67–69 a.a.) [65]. This may reflect general constraints in how these peptides might have to fold around each other. By this criteria the γ chain spacing is more like that of the β chains (72 a.a.) and thus it might be an alternative for that peptide. One apparent difference from the structural requirements of immunoglobulins is that both J region elements of the α [79] and β chains [60] are similar to the heavy chain immunoglobulin Js in size (17–20 a.a.) rather than the shorter light chain J regions (13 a.a.). They are also shifted over one amino acid towards the N-terminus with respect to immunoglobulins. The constant regions also follow the immunoglobulin pattern, although there is only one globular domain, followed by a short, hinge-like region which appears to contain the extra cysteine involved in heterodimer formation, a transmembrane region and a short cytoplasmic anchor [12,14,60]. It has also been suggested that some parts of these regions act as connecting peptides [61]. It should be emphasized that all assignments of function to portions of the constant region are provisional pending definitive biochemical experiments. Both α and β chains are N-glycosylated, with each murine chain and the human α estimated to have at least three sites [14,65] and the human β to

have two [64]. This is supported by the amino acid sequence data which indicates 4–5 potential sites in the murine β chain [14,65] and two in the human [12]. The murine and human α chains each have four potential sites [15–17], two which are conserved in the constant region. The γ chain sequence has no apparent N-linked sites [20], although it (and the others) could have significant amounts of O-linked glycosylation.

This striking homology to immunoglobulin heavy and light chain genes indicates that both T cells and B cells utilize the same basic genetic strategies for antigenic recognition. It remains to be determined how antigen-MHC co-recognition is accomplished, especially with respect to the very strong evidence for the single receptor models [66–68]. Particularly important in this regard has been the work of Marrack *et al.*, showing that a monoclonal antibody which recognizes a particular T-cell receptor idiotype and precipitates a particular pair of α and β chains, correctly predicts the fine specificity of an independently derived T hydridoma [69]. That this does not necessarily mean a single receptor binding site is discussed in the next section.

Additional hypervariable regions

The identification of hypervariable and framework regions in immunoglobulin V residues by Kabat & Wu [70] provided the first clues regarding the antigen contact regions in antibody molecules, especially when their initial hypothesis was confirmed by X-ray crystallography [71,72]. By analogy to this initial work, we might hope to learn about T-cell receptor complementarity determining residues by a similar analysis of α and β chain V regions. The first such study by Patten *et al.* [65] examined seven V sequences and indicated that there were seven distinct regions of hypervariability. Three of these are analogous to those of immunoglobulins (CDR1, CDR2, CDR3) but the other four are in the framework portions of light and heavy chains. If these additional hypervariable regions are superimposed on an antibody three-dimensional structure, one is located deep within the globular domains, perhaps indicating a more open configuration, and the other three would be relatively close to each other on the outside of the Ig binding site [65]. It has been suggested that this cluster of additional hypervariable residues might form a second site of interaction for polymorphic determinants, possibly those of the MHC [65]. Support for the possibility that these additional hypervariable sites might be important in determining T-cell specificity was recently obtained by Sim & Augustin who found that several of the mutations which appear to alter the alloreactivity of a T-cell hybrid [73] are occurring in these regions (personal communication). While it should be emphasized that these analyses are still in the speculative stage, binding studies with purified receptor molecules and *in vitro* mutagenesis of transfected genes should be possible in the very near future.

One corollary to the abundance of hypervariable regions in the β chain has been the fact the V_βs are very dissimilar to each other, ranging from only 18 to 51% amino acid homology in one comparison [65], compared with 40–98% immunoglobulin homology [74]. This is also reflected in the fact that V_βs often hybridize to single bands on Southern analysis, whereas up to 60 bands are sometimes seen with Ig V region probes [75–77]. The explanation for this is may lie in the observation that hypervariable regions diverge more quickly than framework regions and that a greater proportion of sequence devoted to hypervariable residues necessitates a more rapid rate of divergence [78].

These analyses of the V_β sequences are particularly interesting considering the recent finding that many V_α genes occur in large cross-reactive gene families and that there appear to be fewer hypervariable regions and less overall variability [79]. Thus there may be important differences between α and β chain V regions which have no parallel in the antibody system. Once again, however, the functional significance of these findings are controversial [106] and a proper resolution of these questions must await more direct experiments, particularly structural studies.

Gene structure

The sequence organization of the β chain genes is illustrated in Fig. 76.4. The β chain gene is the best studied as of this writing and consists of at least twelve [65; and unpublished results] distinct V_β segments, five or more D elements [55,56,80], twelve potentially functional J regions localized in two separate clusters [60] and followed in each case by two very similar C regions. Exactly as in the case of immunoglobulin heavy chain genes [59], there is a D region element located just 5' to each J cluster [55,56]. In fact, all of the features of immunoglobulin gene organization are represented here, including the conserved seven and nine nucleotide sequences implicated in the variable region formation of immunoglobulins [53–57]. This underscores the common evolutionary origins of this gene complex. One departure from the immunoglobulin pattern is the fact that while the 12/23 rule [58,81] which seems to govern recombination is preserved in both systems, in the β chain it appears to allow direct V–J joining and possibly D–D joining as well [53–56], whereas in immunoglobulins it does not [58,81]. Less is currently known about the α chain locus, although there is a single constant region gene, and at least twenty-three J region elements [79, 103–105]. The J regions and the C region also seem to be spaced a considerable distance apart (T. Lindsten *et al.*, work in progress). The organization of the γ chain gene seems more like that of λ light chain [82], with multiple C regions widely spaced and preceded by a single J element [100]. All of the three T-cell receptor gene families are localized on different chromosomes in the mouse, as are the three immunoglobulin genes [83–85,102].

The C_β exons are organized somewhat like the heavy chain genes of immunoglobulin (Fig. 76.4), with the single immunoglobulin domain, the hinge region and the transmembrane region as separate exons [60,61]. The cytoplasmic anchor and the 3' untranslated region are fused into a fourth exon, reminiscent of the C_μ heavy chain gene [86]. The two β chain constant regions are almost identical, differing by only four amino acids in the mouse [60] and ten in the human

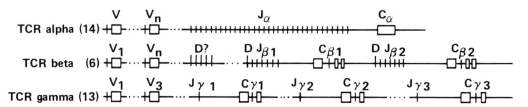

Fig. 76.4. T-cell receptor gene structure. Sequence organization of the α, β and γ chain genes. That of the α chain gene is generalised from references 103–105. Chromosomal localizations are indicated by parentheses.

case [87,88] (which has a very similar organization). This near identity and the fact that different helper phenotype cells can use either locus indicates that the two C_β regions are not functionally different. The duplication of the β chain locus is not a recent event however since the divergence of the 3′ untranslated regions in the mouse indicate that this occurred well before mammalian speciation [60].

Expression in T-cell subsets

In both human and murine systems all functional helper and cytotoxic T-cell lines and hybrids appear to use the same β chain constant and J region gene segments [20,53,89–91]. In at least one case the same V_β is used in both a class II restricted helper line and a class I directed alloreactive cytotoxic cell line [65; S. Hedrick *et al.*, personal communication]. Preliminary indications are that helper and cytotoxic cells will use the same α chain gene segments as well [15,16]. Thus, despite the different MHC class preferences of these cells, they appear to access the same repertoire of recognition structures (although presumably there will be some skewing in the choices that are made). The status of the suppressor T cells is less certain, clear evidence having been obtained that most functional murine suppressor hybridomas could not be using the β chain gene [91,101] and thus either have no antigen specificity or utilize a different locus. This contrasts with the reports of a number of groups working with human suppressor lines, all of which rearrange and express the β chain gene and in at least some cases, express α:β heterodimers on their surface [89,90]. This apparent contradiction is, at least in part, semantic since the assays used in the mouse and human systems are completely different and there is no indication that the same types of T cells are involved.

The case of the γ chain expression seems clearer, since while the overall expression in spleen and thymus is low (less than fifty times that of the β chain [15]) it has been found to be expressed in most functional cytotoxic T cells but not in many helper T cells [92]. Thus, it is the only currently known T-cell receptor-like molecule which differs between T-cell subsets. It does not appear to have much capacity for polymorphism both from the relatively small number of available gene segments and from the finding that a number of alloreactive cytotoxic T-cell lines all used the same V and J and differed only in the point of joining [92]. Although it can be argued that the anti-idiotype experiment of Marrack *et al.* [69] excludes the involvement of any chains other than α and β in determining specificity, this experiment does not rule out the possible use of only slightly polymorphic structures and in any case has not been done with

cytotoxic T cells. Although no role in T-cell recognition has yet been demonstrated for the γ chain, it is hard to imagine that an immunoglobulin-like, T-cell subset-specific gene family which is conserved in distantly related species (i.e. human; J. Seidman, personal communication) would not be important. To paraphrase Mae West (whose penchant for immunology has not been widely appreciated) 'There is no such thing as a bad gene', merely some that we know the function of and some that we do not. The existence of the γ chain gene also raises the possibility that an equivalent gene specific to helper cells might be isolated.

Expression during thymic differentiation

The precise time at which T-cell receptors first appear in ontogeny has been a matter of some controversy and yet is crucial in terms of understanding the different lineage relationships between subsets and when repertoire selections might be taking place. In this respect, the KJ16 monoclonal antibody of Haskins *et al.* [93,94] has been important in giving the first indications of the appearance of receptor on the surface of some cells early in thymic ontogeny. However, it is not yet clear exactly what this marker sees as only 20% of peripheral cells are stained [93,94]. There are now definitive indications that the thymus plays a role in inducing the expression of α and β chain genes and that expression occurs in a sequential fashion. As summarized in Fig. 76.5, it is now clear

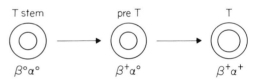

Fig. 76.5. Sequential expression of the T-cell receptor genes in thymic ontogeny. Evidence now indicates that both α and β chain genes are first expressed in the thymus and that β precedes α [95–98].

that at least some thymocytes do not express the β chain [93,94] (although most do) and that only after β chain rearrangement and expression does the α chain appear [95]. This was first suggested by the frequency measurements of Chien *et al.* [15] and recently confirmed by the work of Samelson, Lindsten *et al.* [95] and Raulet *et al.* [97]. We are thus able to define a true pre-T cell phenotype as being $\beta^+\alpha^0$ and that of an even earlier T cell as lacking both chains. Fetal thymocyte RNAs also show sequential expression of these loci with β appearing at day 15 and α at day 17 [97,98].

Acknowledgements

The author would like to thank his colleagues for the communication of experimental results prior to publication, the NIH and the Weingart Foundation for grant support, and K. Redman and S. Frankel for secretarial assistance in the preparation of this manuscript.

References

1   MILLER J.F.A.P. (1961) Immunological function of the thymus. *Lancet*, **i**, 748.
2   FATHMAN C.G. & FRELINGER J.G. (1983) T-lymphocyte clones. *Ann. Rev. Immunol.* **1**, 633.
3   INFANTE A.J., INFANTE P.D., GILLUS S. & FATHMAN C.G. (1982) Definition of T cell idiotypes using anti-idiotypic antisera produced by immunization with T cell clones. *J. exp. Med.* **155**, 1100.
4   ALLISON J.P., MACINTYRE B.W. & BLOCK D. (1982) Tumor specific antigen and murine T-lymphoma defined with monoclonal antibody. *J. Immunol.* **129**, 2293.
5   HASKINS K., KUBO R., WHITE J., PIGEON M., KAPPLER J. & MARRACK P. (1983) The major histocompatibility complex-restricted antigen receptor on T cells. I. Isolation with a monoclonal antibody. *J. exp. Med.* **157**, 1149.
6   MEUER S.C., FITZGERALD K.A., HUSSEY R.E., HODGDON J.C., SCHLOSSMAN S.F. & REINHERZ E.L. (1983) Clonotypic structures involved in antigen-specific human T cell function. Relationship to the T3 molecular complex. *J. exp. Med.* **157**, 705.
7   SAMELSON L.E., GERMAIN R.N. & SCHWARTZ R.H. (1983) Monoclonal antibodies against the antigen receptor on a cloned T-cell hybrid. *Proc. natn. Acad. Sci. U.S.A.* **80**, 6972.
8   KAYE J., PORCELLI S., TITE J., JONES B. & JANEWAY C.A. (1983) Both a monoclonal antibody and antisera specific for determinants unique to individual cloned helper T cell lines can substitute for antigen and antigen-presenting cells in the activation of T cells. *J. exp. Med.* **158**, 836.
9   ACUTO O., HUSSEY R.E., FITZGERALD K.A., PROTENTIS J.P., MEUER S.C., SCHLOSSMAN S.F. & REINHERZ E.L. (1983) The human T cell receptor: Appearance in ontogeny and biochemical relationship of α and β subunits on IL-2 dependent clones and T cell tumors. *Cell*, **34**, 717.
10 KAPPLER J., KUBO R., HASKINS K., HANNUM C., MARRACK P., PIGEON M., MCINTYRE B., ALLISON J. & TROWBRIDGE I. (1983) The major histocompatibility complex-restricted antigen receptor on T cells in mouse and man: Identification of constant and variable peptides. *Cell*, **35**, 295.
11 STAERZ U.D., PASTERNACK M.S., KLEIN J.R., BENEDETTO J.D. & BEVAN M.J. (1984) Monoclonal antibodies specific for a murine cytotoxic T-lymphocyte clone. *Proc. natn. Acad. Sci. U.S.A.* **81**, 1799.
12 YANAGI Y., YOSHIKAI Y., LEGGETT K., CLARK S.P., ALEKSANDER I. & MAK T.W. (1984) A human T cell-specific cDNA clone encodes a protein having extensive homology to immunoglobulin chains. *Nature*, **308**, 145.
13 HEDRICK S.M., COHEN D.I., NIELSEN E.A. & DAVIS M.M. (1984) The isolation of cDNA clones encoding T cell-specific membrane-associated proteins. *Nature*, **308**, 149.
14 HEDRICK S.M., NIELSEN E.A., KAVALER J., COHEN D.I. & DAVIS M.M. (1984) Sequence relationships between putative T-cell receptor polypeptides and immunoglobulins. *Nature*, **308**, 153.
15 CHIEN Y., BECKER D.M., LINDSTEN T., OKAMURA M., COHEN D.I. & DAVIS M.M. (1984) A third type of murine T cell receptor gene. *Nature*, **312**, 31.
16 SAITO H., KRANZ D.M., TAKAGAKI Y., HAYDAY A.C., EISEN H.N. & TONEGAWA S. (1984) A third rearranged and expressed gene in a clone of cytotoxic T lymphocytes. *Nature*, **312**, 36.
17 SIM G.K., YAGUE J., NELSON J., MARRACK P., PALMER E., AUGUSTIN A. & KAPPLER J. (1984) Primary structure of human T-cell receptor α-chain. *Nature*, **312**, 771.
18 ACUTO O., FABBI M., SMART J., POOLE C.B., PROTENTIS J., ROYER H.-D., SCHLOSSMAN S. & REINHERZ E.L. (1984) Purification and N-terminal amino acid sequence of the β subunit of a human T cell antigen receptor. *Proc. natn. Acad. Sci. U.S.A.* **81**, 3855.
19 HANNUM C.H., KAPPLER J.W., TROWBRIDGE I.S., MARRACK P. & FREED J.H. (1984) Immunoglobulin-like nature of the alpha-chain of a human T-cell antigen-MHC receptor. *Nature*, **312**, 65.
20 SAITO H., KRANZ D.M., TAKAGAKI Y., HAYDAY A.D., EISEN H.N. & TONEGAWA S. (1984) Complete primary structure of a heterodimeric T-cell receptor deduced from cDNA sequences. *Nature*, **309**, 757.
21 SUGGS S.V., HIROSE T., MIYAKE T., KAWASHIMA E.H., JOHNSON M.J., ITAKURA K. & WALLACE R.B. (1981) Use of synthetic oligodeoxyribonucleotides for the isolation of specific cloned DNA sequences. In *Developmental Biology Using Purified Genes*, (UCLA Symposia), Vol. 23, (ed. Brown D.D.), p. 683. Academic Press, New York.
22 DAVIS M.M., CHIEN Y., GASCOIGNE N.R.J. & HEDRICK S.M. (1984) A murine T cell receptor gene complex: isolation, structure and rearrangement. *Immunol. Revs.* **81**, 235.
23 DWORKIN M.B. & DAVID I.B. (1980) Use of a cloned library for the study of abundant poly(A)+ RNA during *Xenopus laevis* development. *Devl Biol.* **76**, 449.
24 GRAY P.W., LEUNG D.W., PENNICA D., YELVERTON E., NAJARIAN R., SIMONSEN C.C., DERYNCK R., SHERWOOD P.J., WALLACE D.M., BEYER S.L., LEVINSON A.D. & GOEDDEL D.V. (1982) Expression of human immune interferon cDNA in *E. coli* and monkey cells. *Nature*, **295**, 503.
25 HASTIE N.D. & BISHOP J.O. (1976) The expression of three abundance classes of mRNA in mouse tissues. *Cell*, **9**, 761.
26 GALAU G.A., KLEIN W.H., DAVIS M.M., WOLD B.J., BRITTEN R.J. & DAVIDSON E.H. (1976) Structural gene sets active in embryos and adult tissues of the sea urchin. *Cell*, **7**, 487.

27 ALT F.W., KELLEMS R.E., BERTINO J.R. & SCHIMKE R.T. (1978) Selection multiplication of dihydrofolate reductase genes in methotrexate-resistant variants of cultured murine cells. *J. Biol. Chem.* **253**, 1357.

28 MATHER E.L., ALT F.W., BOTHWELL A.L.M., BALTIMORE D. & KOSHLAND E. (1981) Expression of J chain RNA in cells lines representing different stages of B lymphocyte differentiation. *Cell*, **23**, 369.

29 ZIMMERMAN C.R., ORR W.C., LECLERC R.F., BARNARD E.C. & TIMBERLAKE W.E. (1980) Molecular cloning and selection of genes regulated in *Aspergillus* development. *Cell*, **21**, 709.

30 DAVIS M.M., COHEN D.I., NIELSEN E.A., DeFRANCO A.D. & PAUL W.E. (1982) The isolation of B and T cell specific genes. In *B and T cell Tumors*, (UCLA Symposia), Vol. 24, (ed. Vitetta E. & Fox C.F.), p. 215. Academic Press, New York.

31 DAVIS M.M., COHEN D.I., NIELSEN E.A., STEINMETZ M., PAUL W.E. & HOOD L. (1984) Cell-type-specific cDNA probes and the murine I region: The localization and orientation of A_{α}^{d}. *Proc. natn. Acad. Sci. U.S.A.* **81**, 2194.

32 COHEN D.I., HEDRICK S.M., NIELSEN E.A., D'EUSTACHIO P., RUDDLE F., STEINBERG A.D., PAUL W.E. & DAVIS M.M. (1985) Isolation of a cDNA clone corresponding to an X-linked gene family (*XLR*) closely linked to the murine immunodeficiency disorder, xid. *Nature*, **314**, 369.

33 COHEN D.I., STEINBERG A.D., PAUL W.E. & DAVIS M.M. (1985) Expression of an X-linked gene family (*XLR*) occurs in late stage B cells and is altered by the xid mutation. *Nature*, **314**, 372.

34 KAVATHAS P., SUKHATME V.P., HERZENBERG L.A. & PARNES J.R. (1984) Isolation of the gene coding for the human T lymphocyte differentiation antigen Leu-2 (T8) by gene transfer and cDNA subtraction. *Proc. natn. Acad. Sci. U.S.A.* **81**, 2460.

35 LITMAN D.R., THOMAS Y., MADDON P.J., CHESS L. & AXEL R. (1985) The isolation and sequence of the gene encoding T8: a molecule defining functional classes of T-lymphocytes. *Cell*, **40**, 237.

36 MADDON P.J., LITTMAN D.R., GODFREY M., MADDON D.E., CHESS L. & AXEL R. (1985) The isolation and nucleotide sequence of a cDNA clone encoding the T-cell surface protein T4: a new member of the immunoglobulin gene family. *Cell*, **42**, 93.

37 MARTENS C.L., HUFF T.F., JARDIEU P., TROUNSTINE M.L., COFFMAN R.L., ISHIZAKA K. & MOORE K.W. (1985) cDNA clones encoding IgE-binding factors from a rat-mouse hybridoma. *Proc. natn. Acad. Sci. U.S.A.* **82**, 2460.

38 LEWIN B. (1980) *Gene Expression II*, 2nd edn. Wiley (John) & Sons Ltd., New York.

39 SARGENT T. & DAWID I. (1983) Differential gene expression in the gastrula of *Xenopus laevis*. *Science*, **222**, 135.

40 CHIEN Y. & THOMPSON E.B. (1980) Genomic organization of rat prolactin and growth hormone genes. *Proc. natn. Acad. Sci. U.S.A.* **77**, 4583.

41 TAYLOR J.M., ILLMENSEE R. & SUMMERS J. (1976) Efficient transcription of RNA into DNA by Avian Sarcoma Virus polymerase. *Biochim. biophys. Acta*, **442**, 324.

42 STAFFORD D.W. & BIEBER D. (1975) Concentration of DNA solutions by extraction with 2-Butanol. *Biochim. biophys. Acta*, **378**, 18.

43 MANIATIS T., FRITSCH E.F. & SAMBROOK J. (1982) *Molecular cloning*. Cold Spring Harbor Laboratory.

44 WAHL G.M., STERN M. & STARK G.R. (1979) Efficient and rapid transfer of large DNA fragments from agarose gels to diazobenzyloxymethol-paper and rapid hybridization by using dextran sulphate. *Proc. natn. Acad. Sci. U.S.A.* **76**, 3683.

45 WALL R., LITTMAN S., TOTH K. & FEDEROFF N. (1977) A general method for the large scale isolation of polysomes and messenger RNA applied to MOPC 21 mouse myeloma tissue. *Analyt. Biochem.* **82**, 115.

46 WOLD B.J., KLEIN W.H., HOUGH-EVANS B.R., BRITTEN R.J. & DAVIDSON E.H. (1978) Sea urchin embryo sequences expressed in the nuclear RNA of adult tissues. *Cell*, **14**, 941.

47 GROUSE L.D., SCHRIER B.K., LETENDRE C.H., ZUBAIRI M.Y. & NELSON P.G. (1980) Neuroblastoma differentiation involves both the disappearance of old and the appearance of new poly(A)+ messenger RNA sequences in polyribosomes. *J. Biol. Chem.* **255**, 3871.

48 WETMUR J.G. & DAVIDSON N. (1968) Kinetics of renaturation of DNA. *J. Mol. Biol.* **31**, 349.

49 BRITTEN R.J. & KOHNE D.E. (1968) Repeated sequences in DNA. *Science*, **161**, 529.

50 BISHOP J.O., MORTON J.G., ROSBASH M. & RICHARDON M. (1974) Three abundance classes in HeLa cell messenger RNA. *Nature*, **250**, 199.

51 GALAU G.A., BRITTEN R.J. & DAVIDSON E.H. (1977) Studies on nucleic acid reassociation kinetics: rate of hybridization of excess RNA with DNA, compared with the rate of DNA renaturation. *Proc. natn. Acad. Sci. U.S.A.* **74**, 1020.

52 WOOD W.B., WILSON J.H., BENBOW R.M. & HOOD L.E. (1981) *Biochemistry*, 2nd edn., Benjamin/Cummings Publishing Co., Menlo Park.

53 CHIEN Y., GASCOIGNE N.R.J., KAVALER J., LEE N.E. & DAVIS M.M. (1984) Somatic recombination in a murine T cell receptor gene. *Nature*, **309**, 322.

54 SIU G., CLARK S.P., YOSHIKAI Y., MALISSEN M., YANAGI Y., STRAUSS E., MAK T.W. & HOOD L. (1984) The human T cell antigen receptor is encoded by variable, diversity, and joining gene segments that rearrange to generate a complete V gene. *Cell*, **37**, 393.

55 KAVALER J., DAVIS M.M. & CHIEN Y. (1984) Isolation of a T cell receptor Diversity (D) region element. *Nature*, **310**, 421.

56 SIU G., KRONENBERG M., STRAUSS E., HAARS R., MAK T.W. & HOOD L. (1984) The D_{β} gene segments of the murine T-cell antigen receptor: Structure, rearrangement and expression. *Nature*, **311**, 344.

57 CLARK S.P., YOSHIKAI Y., TAYLOR S., SIU G., HOOD L. & MAK T.W. (1984) Identification of a diversity segment of human T-cell receptor β-chain, and comparison with the analogous murine element. *Nature*, **311**, 387.

58 EARLY P., HUANG H., DAVIS M., CALAME K. & HOOD L.

(1980) An immunoglobulin heavy chain variable region gene is generated from three segments of DNA: V$_H$, D and J$_H$. *Cell*, **19**, 981.

59 SAKANO H., KUROSAWA Y., WEIGERT M. & TONEGAWA S. (1981) Identification and nucleotide sequence of a diversity DNA segment (D) of immunoglobulin heavy-chain genes. *Nature*, **290**, 562.

60 GASCOIGNE N.R.J., CHIEN Y., BECKER D.M., KAVALER J. & DAVIS M.M. (1984) Genomic organization and sequence of T cell receptor β-chain constant and joining region genes. *Nature*, **310**, 387.

61 MALISSEN M., MINARD K., MJOLSNESS S., KRONENBERG M., GOVERMAN J., HUNKAPILLER T., PRYSTOWSKY M.D., YOSHIKAI Y., FITCH F., MAK T.W. & HOOD L. (1984) Mouse T cell antigen receptor: Structure and organization of constant and joining gene segments encoding the β polypeptide. *Cell*, **37**, 1101.

62 MCINTYRE B.W. & ALLISON J.P. (1984) Biosynthesis and processing of murine T-cell antigen receptor. *Cell*, **38**, 654.

63 KAYE J. & JANEWAY C.A. (1984) Tunicamycin inhibits post-translational modification of the 31kd α and β subunit precursors of the murine T cell antigen/Ia receptor. *J. Immunol.* **133**, 2291.

64 TERHORST C. (1984) Cell surface structures involved in human T lymphocyte specific functions: analysis with monoclonal antibodies. In *Antibodies to Receptors: Probes for Receptor Structure and Function*, (ed. Greaves M.E.) Chapman and Hall, London.

65 PATTEN P., YOKOTA T., ROTHBARD J., CHIEN Y., ARAI K. & DAVIS M.M. (1984) Structure, expression and divergence of T cell receptor β-chain variable regions. *Nature*, **312**, 40.

66 KAPPLER J.W., SKIDMORE B., WHITE J. & MARRACK P. (1981) Antigen inducible, H-2 restricted, interleukin-2-producing T cell hybridomas. Lack of independent antigen and H-2 recognition. *J. exp. Med.* **153**, 1198.

67 HEBER-KATZ E., SCHWARTZ R.H., MATIS L.A., HANNUM C., FAIRWELL T., APPELLA E. & HANSBURG D. (1982) Contribution of antigen-presenting cell major histocompatibility complex gene products to the specificity of antigen-induced T cell activation. *J. exp. Med.* **155**, 1086.

68 HUNIG T.R. & BEVAN M.J. (1982) Antigen recognition by cloned cytotoxic T lymphocytes follows rules predicted by the altered self hypothesis. *J. exp. Med.* **155**, 111.

69 MARRACK P., SHIMONKEVITZ R., HANNUM C., HASKINS K. & KAPPLER J. (1983) The major histocompatibility complex restricted antigen receptor on T cells. IV. An anti-idiotypic antibody predicts both antigen and I-specificity. *J. exp. Med.* **158**, 1635.

70 WU T.T. & KABAT E.A. (1970) An analysis of the sequences of the variable regions of Bence Jones proteins and myeloma light chains and their implications for antibody complementarity. *J. exp. Med.* **132**, 211.

71 AMZEL L.M., POLJAK R.J., SAUL F., VARGA J.M. & RICHARDS F.F. (1974) The three dimensional structure of a combining region-ligand complex of immunoglobulin NEW at 3.5-A resolution. *Proc. natn. Acad. Sci. U.S.A.* **71**, 1427.

72 DAVIES D.R. & METZGER H. (1983) Structural basis of antibody function. *Ann. Rev. Immunol.* **1**, 87.

73 AUGUSTIN A.A. & SIM G.K. (1984) T-cell receptors generated via mutations are specific for various major histocompatibility antigens. *Cell*, **39**, 5.

74 KABAT E.A., WU T.T., BILOFSKY H., REID-MILLER M. & PERRY H. (1983) *Sequences of Immunological Interest*. U.S. Dept. of Health and Human Services, Washington DC.

75 SEIDMAN J.G., LEDER A., NAU M., NARMAN B. & LEDER P. (1978) Antibody diversity. *Science*, **202**, 11.

76 CORY S., TYLER B.M. & ADAMS J.M. (1981) V$_\kappa$ gene families in mice. *J. Mol. appl. Genet.* **1**, 103.

77 BRODEUR P.H. & RIBLET R. (1984) The immunoglobulin heavy chain variable region (Igh-V) locus in the mouse. I. 100 Igh-V genes comprise 7 families of homologous genes. *Eur. J. Immunol.* **14**, 922.

78 NEI M. (1983) Genetic polymorphism and the role of mutation in evolution. In *Evolution of Genes and Proteins*, (eds. Nei M. & Koehn M.), p. 165. Sinauer, Massachusetts.

79 BECKER D.M., PATTEN P., CHIEN Y., YOKOTA Y., WOLF R., ESHHAR Z., GIEDLIN M., ARAI K. & DAVIS M.M. (1985) V$_\alpha$ gene structure. *Nature*, **317**, 430.

80 CHIEN Y., KAVALER J. & DAVIS M.M. (1985) D and J region usage and the absence of somatic mutation in cDNA clones which utilize the same T cell receptor variable region gene. Manuscript in preparation.

81 TONEGAWA W. (1983) Somatic generation of antibody diversity. *Nature*, **302**, 575.

82 BLOMBERG B., TRAUNECKER A., EISEN H.N. & TONEGAWA W. (1981) Organization of four mouse λ light chain immunoglobulin genes. *Proc. natn. Acad. Sci. U.S.A.* **78**, 3765.

83 CACCIA N., KRONENBERG M., SAXE D., HAARS R., BRUNS G.A.P., GOVERMAN J., MALISSEN M., WILLARD H., YOSHIKAI Y., SIMON M., HOOD L. & MAK T.W. (1984) The T cell receptor β chain genes are located on chromosome 6 in mice and chromosome 7 in humans. *Cell*, **37**, 1091.

84 LEE N.E., D'EUSTACHIO P., PRAVTCHEVA D., RUDDLE F., HEDRICK S.M. & DAVIS M.M. (1984) One chain of the murine T cell receptor is encoded on chromosome six. *J. exp. Med.* **160**, 905.

85 COLLINS M.K.L., GOODFELLOW P.N., DUNNE M.J., SPURR N.K., SOLOMON E. & OWEN M.J. (1984) A human T-cell antigen receptor β chain gene maps to chromosome 7. *EMBO J.* **3**, 2347.

86 EARLY P., ROGERS J., DAVIS M., CALAME K., BOND M., WALL R. & HOOD L. (1980) Two mRNAs can be produced from a single immunoglobulin μ gene by alternative RNA processing pathways. *Cell*, **20**, 313.

87 YOSHIKAI Y., ANATONIOU D., CLARK S.P., YANAGI Y., SANGSTER R., VAN DEN ELSEN P., TERHORST C. & MAK T.W. (1984) Sequence and expression of transcripts of the human T-cell receptor β chain genes. *Nature*, **312**, 521.

88 JONES N., LEIDEN J., DIALYNAS D., FRASER J., CLABBY M., KISHIMOTO T., STROMINGER J.L., ANDREWS D., LANE W., & WOODY J. (1985) Partial primary structure of

the alpha and beta chains of human T cell receptors. *Science*, **227**, 311.

89 YOSHIKAI Y., YANAGI Y., SUCIU-FOCA N. & MAK T.W. (1984) Presence of T-cell receptor mRNA in functionally distinct T cells and elevation during intrathymic differentiation. *Nature*, **310**, 506.

90 ROYER H.D., BENSUSSAN A., ACUTO O. & REINHERZ E.L. (1984) Functional isotypes are not encoded by the constant region genes of the β subunit of the T cell receptor for antigen/MHC. *J. exp. Med.* **160**, 947.

91 HEDRICK S.M., GERMAIN R.N., BEVAN M.J., DORF M., FINK R., GASCOIGNE N.R.J., GREENE M., KAPP J., KAUFFMAN Y., MELCHERS F., PIERCE C., SORENSON C., TANIGUCHI M. & DAVIS M.M. (1985) Expression of the T cell receptor β chain in T lymphocyte subsets. *Proc. natn. Acad. Sci. U.S.A.* **82**,531.

92 KRANZ D.M. SAITO H., HELLER M., TAKAGAKI Y., HAAS W., EISEN H.N. & TONEGAWA S. (1985) Limited diversity of the rearranged T-cell and γ gene. *Nature*, **313**, 752.

93 HASKINS K., HANNUM C., WHITE J., ROEHM N., KUBO R., KAPPLER J. & MARRACK P. (1984) The major histocompatibility complex-restricted antigen receptor on T cells. VI. An antibody to a receptor allotype. *J. exp. Med.* **160**, 452.

94 ROEHM N., HERRON L., CAMBIER J., DiGUISTO D., HASKINS K., KAPPLER J. & MARRACK P. (1984) The major histocompatibility complex-restricted antigen receptor on T cells: Distribution on thymus and peripheral T cells. *Cell*, **38**, 577.

95 SAMELSON L., LINDSTEN T., FOWLKES B.J., VAN DEN ELSEN P., TERHORST C., DAVIS M.M., GERMAIN R.N. & SCHWARTZ R.H. (1985) The expression of genes of the T cell antigen receptor complex in precursor thymocytes. *Nature*, **315**, 765.

96 TROWBRIDGE I.S., LESLEY J., TROTTER J. & HYMAN R. (1985) Thymocyte subpopulation enriched for progenitors with an unrearranged T-cell receptor β-chain gene. *Nature*, **315**, 666.

97 RAULET D.H., GARMAN R.D., SAITO H. & TONEGAWA S. (1985) Developmental regulation of T-cell receptor gene expression. *Nature*, **314**, 103.

98 BORN W,. YAGÜE J., PALMER E., KAPPLER J. & MARRACK P. (1985) Rearrangement of T cell receptor β-chain genes during T-cell development. *Proc. natn. Acad. Sci. U.S.A.*, **82**, 2925.

99 KABAT E.A., WU T.T. & BILOFSKY H. (1978) Variable region genes for the immunoglobulin framework are assembled from small segments of DNA-A hypothesis. *Proc. natn. Acad. Sci. U.S.A.* **75**, 2429.

100 HAYDAY A.C., SAITO H., GILLIES S.D., KRANZ D.M., TANIGAWA G., EISEN H. & TONEGAWA S. (1985) Structure, organization and somatic rearrangement of T cell gamma genes. *Cell*, **40**, 259.

101 KRONENBERG M., GOVERMAN J., HAARS R., MALISSEN M., KRAIG E., PHILLIPS L., DELOVITCH T., SUCIU-FOCA & HOOD L. (1985) Rearrangement and transcription of the β-chain genes of the T-cell antigen receptor in different types of murine lympocytes. *Nature*, **313**, 647.

102 KRANZ D.M., SAITO H., DISTECHE C.M.,, SWISSHELM K., PRAVTCHEVA D., RUDDLE F.H., EISEN H. & TONEGAWA S. (1985) Chromosomal locations of the murine T-cell receptor alpha chain gene and the T-cell gamma gene. *Science*, **227**, 941.

103 HAYDAY A.C., DIAMOND D., TANIGAWA G., HEILIG J., FOLSOM U., SAITO H. & TONEGAWA S. (1985) Unusual features of the organization and diversity of T-cell receptor & chain genes. *Nature*, **316**, 828.

104 WINOTO A., MJOLSNESS S. & HOOD L. (1985) Genomic organization of the genes encoding the mouse T-cell receptor α chain. *Nature*, **316**, 832.

105 YOSHIKAI Y., CLARK S.P., TAYLOR S., SOHN U., WILSON B., MINDER M. & MAK T.W. (1985) Organization and sequences of the variable, joining and constant regions of the human T-cell receptor α chain. *Nature*, **316**, 837.

106 BARTH R., KIM B., LAN N., HUNKAPILLER T., SOBIECK N., WINOTO A., GERSTENFELD H., OKADA C., HANSBURG D., WEISSMAN I. & HOOD L. (1985) The murine T-cell receptor employs a limited repertoire of expressed $V_β$ gene segments. *Nature*, **316**, 517.

Chapter 77
Detection of suppressor cells and suppressor factors for delayed-type hypersensitivity responses

S. D. MILLER & M. K. JENKINS

Methods for induction and transfer of delayed hypersensitivity in mice, 77.3

Methods for induction of suppressor T cells and suppressor T cell factors, 77.7
Methods for assay of afferent suppression, 77.8

Methods for assay of efferent suppression, 77.10
Method for assay of suppressor T cell auxiliary cells, 77.11

T lymphocytes involved in delayed-type hypersensitivity (DTH) reactions have been shown to play a critical role in graft rejection, graft vs. host disease, auto-immunity, and immunity to intracellular parasites and tumours [1–5]. Elucidation of the mechanisms underlying induction and regulation of DTH reactions is critically important to our basic understanding of these disease processes. Therefore the study of antigen-specific, suppressor-T-cell-(Ts)-mediated immunologic control of DTH responses has been an area of intense investigation in recent years. This chapter will introduce methods for the induction and measurement of DTH reactions in mice to both contact sensitizers and protein antigens and for the induction and testing of antigen-specific Ts and their factors (TsF) on these DTH reactions.

DTH, as opposed to antibody-mediated hypersensitivities, is a T-cell-dependent reaction characterized by a delayed inflammatory reaction (peaking 24–48 h after injection) at the site of antigenic challenge. The classical DTH reaction is indurated in character as a result of the accumulation of mononuclear cells (T cells and macrophages) at the challenge site. DTH was first described in 1890 by Koch, who observed that challenge of infected, but not uninfected, guinea-pigs with tubercle bacilli resulted in an intense inflammatory reaction [6]. The cellular nature of the DTH reaction was first reported by Landsteiner & Chase in 1942 [7]. Experimental models of DTH usually employ sensitization of animals with protein antigens emulsified in Freund's complete adjuvant (FCA) with DTH reactivity lasting for months [1]. Contact sensitivity is a short-lived (5–7 days) form of DTH which is observed following epicutaneous exposure to chemically reactive compounds such as dinitrofluorobenzene (DNFB) and trinitrochlorobenzene (TNCB) [8–10] or the subcutaneous injection of hapten- or antigen-coupled syngeneic spleen cells [11–14].

DTH reactivity can be separated into afferent (induction phase) and efferent (elicitation phase) limbs (Fig. 77.1). The afferent limb is composed of a complex series of events following presentation of antigen to immunologically naive animals. This phase of the DTH response develops over a matter of days and is completed when the animal can mount a measurable elicitation reaction. Antigen or contact sensitizer is 'processed' and displayed on the surface of antigen-presenting cells (APC) which may be macrophages, Langerhans' cells, or dendritic cells [15,16] in association with self major histocompatibiiity complex (MHC) gene products [12,14,17]. Lymph node cells draining the site of immunization contain Lyt 1^+2^-, I-A$^+$ helper T (Th) cells specific for antigen in conjunction with MHC I-region gene products [14]. These Th produce mitogenic and differentiative factors [18] which stimulate Lyt 1^+2^-, I-A$^-$, I-region restricted precursor delayed-hypersensitivity T cells (pT$_{DH}$) to divide and differentiate into effector T$_{DH}$ cells [14,17,19]. Two other subsets of antigen-specific T cells in the draining nodes of sensitized mice have also been identified—an Lyt 1^+2^-, I-A$^+$ T cell which proliferates upon restimulation with antigen in vitro (Tprlf), and an Lyt 1^+2^-, I-J$^+$, cyclophosphamide-(CY)-sensitive Ts-auxilliary cell (Ts-aux), which is required for the activity of efferent-acting Ts [14,20,21] (see below). The characteristics of these cell types are shown in Table 77.1. The efferent limb of DTH is characterized by the classical histological changes resulting from the release of lymphokines (and sub-

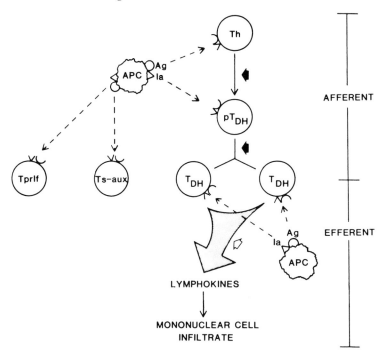

AFFERENT

EFFERENT

LYMPHOKINES

MONONUCLEAR CELL
INFILTRATE

Fig. 77.1. Scheme for the induction and regulation of DTH responses. The afferent limb of DTH is activated when antigen (Ag) is associated with Ia determinants on antigen-presenting cells (APC). This complex is recognized by antigen-specific helper T cells (Th) and precursor delayed-hypersensitivity T cells (pT$_{DH}$). pT$_{DH}$ cells proliferate and differentiate into effector T$_{DH}$ with the aid of Th. The Ag/Ia complex also stimulates induction of T cells, which proliferate upon re-exposure to antigen *in vitro* (Tprlf), and suppressor T cell-auxiliary cells (Ts-aux), which are required for expression of efferent-acting Ts activity. Following re-exposure to antigen, the efferent limb of DTH is activated by release of lymphokines from effector T$_{DH}$ cells leading to the classical mononuclear cell infiltrate characteristic of DTH reactions. Possible target sites of Ts regulation of the afferent (solid arrows) and efferent (open arrow) limbs are indicated.

Table 77.1. T cell subpopulations induced in sensitized mice

Characteristic	Th[a]	T$_{DH}$[b]	Tprlf[c]	Ts-aux[d]
Lyt determinants	1$^+$2$^-$	1$^+$2$^-$	1$^+$2$^-$	1$^+$2$^-$
Ia determinants	+	−	+	+
I–J determinants	−	−	−	+
Sensitivity to:				
cyclophosphamide	−	−	−	+
adult thymectomy	ND[e]	−	−	+
splenectomy	−	−	ND	−
Ts suppression	+	+	−	

[a] Helper T cell for DTH reactivity.
[b] T cell responsible for *in vivo* transfer of DTH.
[c] T cell responsible for *in vitro* antigen-driven proliferation.
[d] T cell required for the action of efferent-acting Ts.
[e] ND = not determined.

sequent attraction and activation of bystander mononuclear cells) from effector T$_{DH}$ cells following antigenic challenge, usually in a site distant from the initial sensitization. In guinea-pigs and man, DTH elicitation is usually performed by subcutaneous (s.c.) or intradermal injection of body skin. However, in the mouse, antigenic challenge is performed on the ears or

footpads [8,9]. This may be because these sites have adequate numbers of Langerhans' cells to act as APCs [15]. DTH is quantified with an engineer's micrometer by measuring incremental swelling (above pre-challenge thickness) in the ears or footpads due to mononuclear cell influx 24 h after antigenic challenge [8,9]. The ear swelling assay has generally proved to be more sensitive and reproducible than footpad swelling, or accumulation of ^{51}Cr-labelled syngeneic bone marrow cells or ^{125}I-UdR at the challenge site [22].

Experimental tolerance (unresponsiveness) in DTH systems dates back more than 50 years to the work of Sulzberger [23] who showed that intracardiac injection of free hapten led to reduced hapten-specific contact sensitivity. Later, Chase [24] showed that prolonged feeding of dinitrochlorobenzene to guinea-pigs induced antigen-specific unresponsiveness. The induction of tolerance depends on the route of antigen injection. Intravenous (i.v.) administration of free hapten or hapten-coupled syngeneic lymphoid cells favours tolerance induction, although epicutaneous or s.c. administration of these compounds favours the induction of DTH [11–14,25–29]. Tolerance induction via the i.v. route is directly proportional to the chemical reactivity of the contact allergen. Analogues of DNFB that are highly reactive in forming covalent bonds (e.g. DNFB itself) are more potent tolerogens than weakly reactive molecules (e.g. dinitrobenzene sulphonic acid—DNBS), and non-reactive molecules (e.g. DNP-lysine or DNP-mouse proteins) are not tolerogenic [30]. This implies that the effective tolerogen formed *in vivo* is the contactant coupled to some self component. Indeed, the authors [25] and others [11–14,26–29] have shown that the i.v. injection of hapten- or protein-coupled syngeneic spleen cells induces specific tolerance to both humoral and DTH responses.

Unresponsiveness induced by the i.v. administration of ligand-coupled syngeneic cells is due to two antigen-specific mechanisms—clonal inhibition and Ts activity [31]. Clonal inhibition is rapidly induced, long-lasting, CY-resistant, non-transferable and due to blockade of specific T cell clones. Ts activity is short-lived, Cy-sensitive, and transferable with T cells to naive recipients. Similarly, unresponsiveness induced by either oral [32,33] or i.v. [34,35] administration of free hapten or antigen is partly a result of the activity of Ts. A possible target for Ts regulation of DTH responses is the afferent limb, by inhibition of Th activity or by preventing activation and/or expansion of pre-T_{DH} cells. Alternatively, T_{DH} could be regulated at the efferent limb by preventing interaction of effector T_{DH} cells with APCs at the challenge site or preventing lymphokine release. Interestingly, Ts which regulate DTH activity have been shown to suppress either the generation of T_{DH} (afferent Ts), in which case they are effective only when given at the time of immunization, or the expression of T_{DH} activity (efferent suppression), when they are effective if administered at the time of challenge. Intravenous injection of trinitrobenzene sulphonic acid (TNBS) leads to the induction of Ts that inhibit the *expression* of TNP-specific DTH [34], although the i.v. injection of DNBS leads to the induction of Ts that inhibit the *induction* of DNP-specific DTH [35]. Study of Ts induction by the i.v. injection of ligand-modified syngeneic spleen cells in several antigenic systems has shown that Ts are not homogeneous in nature, rather Ts networks are induced [36–38]. This network is composed of at least three interacting subsets of cells (Ts-1, Ts-2, and Ts-3) and their corresponding soluble factors (TsF) which can be distinguished based on mode of activation, cellular phenotype, receptor specificity (idiotypic or anti-idiotypic), and functional targets (i.e. afferent or efferent limbs). The remainder of this chapter will describe methods for both the induction of DTH responses in mice and the assay of afferent- and efferent-acting Ts on DTH reactivity.

Methods for induction and transfer of delayed hypersensitivity in mice

Contact sensitivity

Contact sensitivity in mice is accomplished by sensitization of abdominal skin with a dilute solution of the contactant under study. Sensitization is followed 4–7 days later by applying a more dilute challenge solution of the contactant to the ear or footpad and measuring the increase in ear swelling 24 h thereafter [8,9]. Below, the authors detail the methods for induction and elicitation of contact sensitivity to both DNFB and TNCB. As these compounds are powerful sensitizers, they should be handled with gloves to avoid skin contact.

Procedure

Contactants

1 DNFB is obtained from Eastman Kodak Co., Rochester, NY, and TNCB from Matheson, Coleman and Bell, Cincinnati, OH. Stock solutions of DNFB (5% w/v) are prepared in 4:1 acetone:olive oil and can be stored in foil-wrapped (to prevent light inactivation), sealed 15 ml scintillation vials for up to one month.

2 For sensitization, the 5% stock solution is diluted 1:10 in acetone:olive oil, yielding a 0.5% working solution which can be stored for one week.

3 For challenge, the 5% stock solution is diluted 1:25 in acetone:olive oil yielding a 0.2% working challenge solution.

4 Seven per cent TNCB sensitizing solutions are always freshly prepared immediately prior to use in 4:1 acetone:olive oil.

5 One per cent (w/v) TNCB challenge solution is prepared in *pure* olive oil (to prevent high background swelling observed in mice challenged with TNCB diluted in acetone:olive oil) in a foil-wrapped, sealed scintillation vial containing a magnetic stirring bar.

6 Solubilization is achieved by rapid stirring for 24 h at room temperature. The challenge solution can be stored for 3–4 months.

Sensitization of mice

The abdominal hair of mice (preferably four or more mice per treatment group) is removed by shaving with an Oster Model A2 Small Animal Clippers (Milwaukee, WI) fitted with a Size 40 cutting head. It is important to remove as much hair as possible. For DNFB sensitization, 25 μl of the 0.5% working solution is applied to the shaved skin and evenly distributed with a glass rod on day 0 and again on day

1. For TNCB sensitization, 100 μl of freshly prepared 7% TNCB is applied in a similar manner *only* on day 0.

Elicitation and quantification of contact sensitivity

DNFB sensitivity is elicited on day 5 and TNCB sensitivity on day 6, relative to initial sensitization on day 0.

1   Mice to be challenged are lightly ether-anaesthetized until relaxation of the ears and tail are noted. A surgical dressing jar with a piece of window screen suspended about 2 cm from the bottom makes a convenient anaesthesia chamber. Mice are then grasped by the loose skin between the forepaws and held as shown in Fig. 77.2.

2   Basal ear thickness is measured with a spring-loaded Mitutoya Dial Thickness Gauge (Model No. 7326, range 0.001–0.050 in Schlessinger Tool Co, Brooklyn, NY). The 7326 gauge is only used for ear measurement due to its limited measurement range. The Mitutoya Model 7300 Dial Thickness Gauge is suitable for footpad measurements. Care must be taken to gently ease the gauge closed with the thumb without allowing the spring to compress the ear (this is especially important when measuring ears displaying large amounts of DTH). It is also important to place the pads of the gauge on only the outer two-thirds of the ear to avoid skin folds.

3   Normally the first measurement is discarded and then three subsequent readings are recorded and averaged.

4   The mouse is then re-anaesthetized (if necessary) and the challenge solution applied. Ten microlitres of 0.2% DNFB in acetone : olive oil is applied to the dorsal surface of the ear with an Eppendorf pipette and evenly distributing with a glass rod. TNCB challenge is accomplished by evenly distributing, with a glass rod, one drop of 1% TNCB in olive oil, from a 1 cm^3 disposable plastic syringe fitted with a disposable 25-gauge needle, to both the dorsal and ventral surfaces of the ear.

5   Twenty-four hours after challenge, the increase in ear thickness above baseline values is determined by re-measurement with the dial thickness gauge.

6   Again, the first measurement is discarded and three subsequent determinations are recorded and averaged.

7   The difference between the mean 24 h and mean pre-challenge readings is calculated and the results are expressed in units of 10^{-4} in.

8   Swelling obtained in sensitized mice must be compared to non-specific swelling seen in unsensitized mice challenged with the same contactant. This non-specific swelling varies with the challenge site (ear or footpad), strain of mouse, the contactant under study, and the vehicle in which the contactant is solubilized.

DTH to soluble protein antigens

Procedure

Immunizations

Protein antigen-specific DTH reactions are readily induced by subcutaneous injection of the protein emulsified in Freund's complete adjuvant (FCA) containing *Mycobacterium tuberculosis* H37Ra (Difco Laboratories, Detroit, MI).

1   Protein antigens dissolved in phosphate-buffered saline (PBS) are emulsified in an equal volume of FCA by repeated aspiration using a 1.0 ml glass syringe without a needle. Once emulsified the protein-FCA mixture will remain in the emulsified state for months, requiring only brief agitation before use.

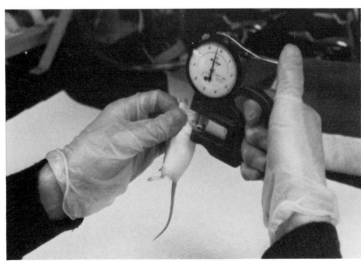

Fig. 77.2. Demonstration of ear measurement using engineer's micrometer.

2 Lightly anaesthetized mice are injected subcutaneously in the ventral surface of the tail base, between the caudal artery and vein, with 50 μl of antigen/FCA emulsion, using a 1.0 ml glass syringe fitted with a 27-gauge needle. The optimal immunizing dose varies with the antigen used, but generally falls in the 20–250 μg range.

3 Preliminary dose–response experiments are necessary to establish the optimal immunization conditions.

Elicitation and quantification of DTH

Between 7 and 21 days following immunization, pre-challenge ear measurements are recorded and DTH reactions elicited by intradermal injection of 10 μl of antigen (containing 1–10 μg of antigen) dissolved in PBS into the dorsal surface of the ear using a 100 μl Hamilton glass syringe fitted with a 30-gauge needle.

1 Lightly anaesthetized mice are suspended between the thumb and index finger of one hand, with the mouse's ear stretched over the index finger. The syringe is held in the other hand between the middle and index fingers (similar to holding a cigarette) with the thumb lightly resting on the end of the plunger. The needle is inserted into the dorsal dermal layer (bevelled side up) pointing toward the ear tip at about the midpoint (Fig. 77.3). Several cautions concerning ear injections should be noted. First, care should be taken to avoid damage to ear blood vessels as the resulting haematoma will lead to falsely high ear thickness readings. Second, ear injections are delicate and should be practised extensively before attempting a crucial experiment. Lastly, 30-gauge needles should be replaced after 8–10 injections as a considerable amount of needle dulling will occur. Proper injection will result in a small (8–10 mm) temporary bleb at the challenge site.

2 Twenty-four hours following ear challenge, the increase in ear thickness over pre-challenge measurements is determined.

3 Dose–response experiments should be performed to determine the optimal challenge dose, although 1–10 μg antigen per ear is generally sufficient to elicit a strong DTH reaction in primed mice.

DTH to ligand-coupled syngeneic spleen cells

Efficient DTH can also be induced by the s.c. injection of hapten- or protein antigen-modified syngeneic spleen cells [11–14,39]. Described below are the procedures for preparation, immunization and challenge of mice with DNP-, TNP-, and protein antigen-modified cells.

Procedure

Preparation of spleen cell suspensions

1 Mice are sacrificed by cervical dislocation, and their spleens are removed and dissected of fat and connective tissue.

2 Single cell suspensions are prepared by gently rubbing the spleens through 60-mesh stainless steel screens with the plunger of a 3 cm^3 disposable plastic syringe in a 100 cm Petri dish containing Mishell-Dutton balanced salt solution (BSS) [40]. The suspension is then aspirated through a 25-gauge needle, pelleted (250 **g**), and washed twice with BSS.

3 Erythrocytes are lysed by resuspending and immediately centrifuging the cell pellet in warm (37 °C) Tris-NH$_4$Cl (0.83% NH$_4$Cl, 0.017 M-Tris, pH 7.2). Following lysis, the spleen cells are washed in BSS and cell counts determined.

Preparation of hapten-modified spleen cells

1 Five millimolar DNFB solutions are prepared by dissolving 93 mg of DNFB in 0.5 ml of 70% ethanol followed by addition of 99.5 ml of 0.15 M-PBS, pH 7.2.

2 This mixture is stirred overnight in a foil-covered container.

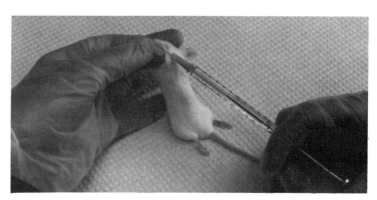

Fig. 77.3. Demonstration of intradermal ear injection.

3 Ten millimolar (2.93 mg/ml) trinitrobenzene sulphonic acid (TNBS, Sigma Chemical Co, St. Louis, MO) is prepared by a 1:16 dilution in BSS from a bicarbonate-neutralized (3 parts saline + 1 part 10% sodium bicarbonate) 50 mg/ml stock solution. For DNP-modification [25], washed, erythrocyte-free spleen cells are diluted to 5×10^6/ml in BSS. A total of 0.1 ml of a 5 mM-DNFB solution is added per millilitre of cells, yielding a final DNFB concentration of 0.5 mM.

4 The reaction is allowed to proceed for 30 min at room temperature, after which the coupled cells are washed twice in a twentyfold excess of BSS. Properly coupled cells will appear very pale yellow. For TNP-modification [14], washed, erythrocyte-free spleen cells are pelleted at 250 *g* and gently resuspended with a Pasteur pipette in 10 mM-TNBS at a concentration of 30×10^6/ml.

5 The cell suspension is incubated at 37 °C for 10 min, after which the cells are washed three times in a twentyfold excess of BSS. Properly coupled cells will appear bright orange.

6 Following hapten-modification, counts are performed and the cells diluted to the proper concentration in BSS and stored at 4 °C until use.

Preparation of protein-modified spleen cells

Coupling of protein antigens to spleen cells is accomplished with water-soluble 1-ethyl-3(3-dimethylaminopropyl) carbodiimide hydrochloride (ECDI) (Calbiochem-Behring Corp., La Jolla, CA), which promotes the formation of peptide bonds by an acid-catalysed condensation between free amino and carboxyl groups [13,39].

1 Washed, erythrocyte-free spleen cells (3.2×10^8) are pelleted in 17×100 mm tubes (Falcon No. 2057) and resuspended in 1.2 ml of the protein (5–10 mg/ml) to be coupled and 0.2 ml of ECDI (100 mg/ml). The ECDI should be dissolved *immediately* prior to use. Both the protein and the ECDI should be dissolved in saline or a buffer lacking amino, phosphate, or carboxyl groups which interfere with the coupling reaction. Reaction pHs of greater than 7 should be avoided because basic conditions will inhibit coupling. The reaction is carried out for 1 h at 0 °C, with intermittent stirring.

2 Cold BSS is added to the tube to terminate the reaction. The antigen-coupled cells are washed twice with BSS and kept on ice prior to use, to prevent internalization of the coupled ligand.

3 To confirm that coupling has taken place, 5 μl of an appropriate dilution of anti-protein antibody is added to 20 μl of the cell suspension (about 2×10^8 cells/ml)

on a glass slide. Rapid agglutination indicates that the protein is coupled to cell surface determinants.

Subcutaneous sensitization and elicitation of DTH

Ligand-coupled cells are potent inducers of DTH when injected s.c. [11–14,39].

1 Sensitization is accomplished by s.c. injection of ether-anaesthetized mice with a total of $3–5 \times 10^7$ coupled cells, in a total of 0.3 ml BSS, divided equally between each of three sites on the dorsal surface (the base of the neck, and the left and right rear flanks), using a 1.0 cm³ plastic syringe fitted with a 27-gauge needle. Subcutaneous injections are facilitated by lifting a fold of skin with the index finger and thumb and guiding the needle under the uplifted skin.

2 Five to seven days following sensitization, DTH reactions are elicited as described above for mice sensitized with contact sensitizers or protein/FCA.

3 Alternatively, DTH can be elicited by the intradermal injection of an appropriate number (5×10^5–10^6) of ligand-modified cells. (It is important to include injection of sham-coupled cells as a control due to increased non-specific swelling associated with cellular antigens.) In contrast to sensitization with antigen/FCA, sensitization with antigen-coupled cells results in strong cell-mediated responses, but no appreciable antibody production, and it is preferable when humoral effects are to be avoided.

Passive transfer of DTH to normal recipient mice

The hallmark of DTH is the ability to transfer the reaction with T lymphocytes. Procedures are now described for donor sensitization, preparation of lymph node cell suspensions, and cell transfer to, and challenge of, recipient animals.

Procedure

Sensitization of donor mice

The essential details for sensitization are described above. However, to increase the number of lymph node cells per donor, mice are sensitized at additional sites. For DNP-specific DTH, donors are sensitized with 0.5% DNFB—25 μl on the shaved abdomen and 5 μl on each ear and forepaw on day 0 and again on day 1. For TNP-specific DTH, mice are sensitized with 7% TNCB—100 μl on the shaved abdomen and 5 μl on each ear and forepaw only on day 0. For protein antigen-specific DTH, a protein/FCA emulsion is injected s.c. at the base of the tail (50 μl) and into the front and hind footpads (10 μl each).

Preparation of T_{DH} cells

Cells capable of transferring DTH reactivity are located mainly in the lymph nodes draining the sites of immunization; thus spleen is generally *not* used as a source of T_{DH} cells. Some investigators prefer to pre-treat with CY the donor mice (20–100 mg/kg) or the recipient mice (20 mg/kg), to enhance the degree of DTH transferred. However, this may interfere with certain Ts subpopulations in suppression experiments (see below). For transfer of DNP- and TNP-specific contact sensitivity, inguinal, axillary, brachial and cervical lymph nodes are collected on day 4. For transfer of protein antigen-specific DTH, inguinal, periaortic, axillary, brachial and popliteal lymph nodes are collected on day 5 or 6.

1 Single cell suspensions are prepared by gently rubbing the nodes through a 60-mesh stainless steel screen with the plunger of a 5 cm³ disposable plastic syringe in a 100 cm³ Petri dish containing BSS.
2 Resulting suspensions are aspirated through a 25-gauge needle, pelleted, and washed three times with BSS.
3 Viable cell counts are performed via trypan blue dye exclusion and the cells adjusted to a concentration of 5×10^7–10^8 cells/ml in BSS. The number of cells recovered per mouse varies with the immunization procedure, the antigen, and the mouse strain, but generally one can expect 5×10^7–10^8 cells per donor animal.

Transfer and elicitation of DTH

As DTH transfer is restricted by H-2 gene products [17], it is essential to use a recipient strain which is H-2 compatible with the T_{DH} donors. The appropriate number of sensitized lymph node cells are transferred to recipients in a volume of 0.5 ml or less via i.v. injection in the caudal vein using an appropriate mouse restraining device. Within 1 h of cell transfer, the recipients are challenged with the appropriate antigen (as described above) and increases in ear thickness is determined 24 h thereafter.

Methods for induction of suppressor T cells and suppressor T cell factors

Induction of suppressor T cells for DTH

As outlined in the introductory section, Ts active on either the afferent or efferent limbs of DTH responses can be induced by the i.v. injection of either reactive haptens [23,34,35,41] or ligand-modified syngeneic cells [25–29,38,39]. The mode of action of the Ts (afferent- or efferent-acting) induced by i.v. injection

of reactive haptens depends on: (1) the nature of the tolerogen (chemical form and chemical reactivity) [34,35]; and (2) the relative dose injected [42]. The mode of action of Ts induced by the i.v. injection of ligand-coupled cell tolerogens depends on: (1) the syngeneic or allogeneic origin of the cells [43–45]; (2) the epitope density of ligand on the cells [45; S.D. Miller, unpublished]; and (3) the receptor nature of the Ts (idiotypic or anti-idiotypic) [36–38].

Procedure

Ts induction with reactive haptens

1 Tolerance to DNFB is induced by the i.v. injection of 2,4-dinitrobenzenesulphonic acid sodium salt (DNBS—Eastman Kodak Co, Rochester, NY) [41]. A 30 mg/ml stock solution is prepared by dissolving the DNBS in distilled water and filtering through a 0.45 μm Millipore filter.
2 Mice are weighed individually and injected i.v. via the caudal vein with 0.025 ml DNBS per g of body weight (750 mg/kg).
3 Similarly, tolerance to TNCB is induced by the i.v. injection of TNBS [34]. A neutralized 50 mg/ml solution of TNBS is prepared as described previously and diluted 1:5 in normal saline, yielding a 10 mg/ml working solution.
4 Mice are weighed individually and injected i.v. via the caudal vein with 0.025 ml TNBS/g of body weight (250 mg/kg). Care should be taken, especially with TNBS, to use healthy mice of at least 18 g, as these compounds are toxic to sickly or underweight mice.
5 Ts can be demonstrated in the lymph nodes or spleens of such mice 5–7 days after tolerization.

Ts induction with ligand-coupled syngeneic cells

The number of cells required for efficient Ts induction should be determined for the antigen in use, but generally between 3×10^7 and 1×10^8 cells are required. Ligand-coupled cells are prepared as previously described and injected i.v. via the caudal vein in a volume of 0.5 ml or less of BSS. Ts can be obtained from spleen and/or lymph nodes 4–14 days following tolerization.

Preparation of suppressor T cell factors (TsF)

Essentially two methods have been used for the preparation of Ts factors in DTH systems. The first involves elaboration of TsF by *in vitro* culture of suspensions of lymphoid cells containing Ts [45,46]. The second involves the physical disruption, by sonication or freeze-thawing, of lymphoid cell suspensions containing Ts [48,49,54].

Procedure

Preparation of DNP- and TNP-specific TsF

TsF-containing supernates are prepared as described by Zembala & Asherson [46] following tolerization with reactive haptens (DNBS or TNBS) or with hapten-modified syngeneic spleen cells.

1   Mice are i.v. tolerized on day 0.

2   Five days later, the mice are sensitized on the shaved abdomen with 25 μl of 0.5% DNFB or 100 μl of 7% TNCB (see page 77.3) and with 5 μl, respectively, on the ears and forepaws.

3   Between 16 and 20 h later, superficial and mesenteric lymph nodes are removed and single cell suspensions prepared in BSS.

4   The cells are diluted to 10^7/ml in RPMI-1640 medium (Grand Island Biological Co., Grand Island, NY) containing 5% heat-inactivated fetal calf serum (FCS), 100 units of penicillin and 100 μg of streptomycin per ml. Ten millilitres of cells are cultured for 48 h in 100 × 20 mm sterile, disposable plastic tissue culture dishes for 48 h in a humidified atmosphere of 5% CO_2:95% air.

5   Supernatants are clarified by centrifugation at 450 g followed by a 10 000 g spin for 10 min, and are stored at −20 °C.

6   Control supernatants are prepared from mice that are not tolerized but that receive the epicutaneous hapten sensitization 16–20 h before culture.

7   Using this methodology, TsF can be obtained from cultures of lymph node, but not spleen cells. TsF activity can be obtained from the spleens of tolerant mice if they are not epicutaneously sensitized, and the tolerant cells are either physically disrupted or restimulated with hapten-coupled spleen cells in culture (J.W. Moorhead, personal communication). The authors have also recently prepared monoclonal T cell hybrids, by fusion of spleen cells from DNP-SP tolerant mice with the BW5147 thymoma line, which constitutively produce DNP-specific TsF [55].

Preparation of protein antigen-specific TsF

Intravenous injection of 5×10^7–10^8 protein antigen-coupled spleen cells results in specific unresponsiveness (tolerance) partly as a result of Ts activity [13,28,39,54].

1   Spleens and mesenteric, inguinal, and cervical lymph nodes from mice tolerized 7 days previously are

teased to single cell suspensions in BSS, and depleted of erythrocytes as described above.

2   The cells are counted, adjusted to 3×10^8 cells/ml in BSS and sonicated, on ice, with five 10 s, 4 A bursts using a Model S75 Branson Sonifier (Branson Instruments, Inc., Stamford, CT).

3   One or two drops of the sonicate should be examined under the microscope to ensure that complete cellular disruption has occurred. Protein denaturation can be minimized by avoiding foaming during the 10 s sonication steps and by keeping the sonicate on ice throughout the process.

4   Cellular debris is pelleted by centrifugation at 27 000 g and the supernatant sterilized through a 0.45 μm Millipore filter and stored frozen at −70 °C.

5   Sonicates should also be prepared from normal mice to control for non-specific suppressive effects. TsF can also be obtained by disrupting the tolerant cells by 3–4 cycles of freezing in an acetone/dry-ice bath, followed by rapid thawing in a 37 °C water bath. Supernates are clarified as described above.

Methods for assay of afferent suppression

Detailed below are methods for analysis of Ts and TsF that are used routinely in the authors' laboratory. The reader is referred to papers cited throughout this chapter for details of Ts analysis in other systems. As with all assays of specific Ts activity, antigen-specificity controls (the effects of a particular Ts population on responses to irrelevant antigens) should be routinely included. The reader should also be aware that some investigators achieve more consistent data when Ts are transferred to lightly irradiated (100–250 R) recipients. The reason behind this is not known, but it is thought to make available 'room' in recipient lymphoid organs for homing of the transferred cells [35].

Results must be subjected to appropriate statistical analysis. The authors routinely perform one-way analyses of variance and compare means of the treatment groups according to Scheffe's Multiple Comparison Test, as described by Steel & Torrie [50]. Mean differences are considered significant when $p < 0.05$.

Kinetic analysis

By definition, afferent-acting Ts or TsF are suppressive when injected early in the course of DTH sensitization and not suppressive when injected immediately prior to elicitation. Afferent-acting Ts displaying these characteristics have been identified in several experimental systems [33,35–39,44,45]. It is critical to test suppressive activity on both induction and elicitation of DTH as certain efferent-acting Ts also suppress the afferent limb of DTH due to the induction of an afferent-acting, second-order Ts-2 [38]. The afferent/efferent nature of a Ts population or soluble TsF in the DNFB DTH system is determined by passive transfer of 5×10^7–10^8 spleen and/or lymph node cells from tolerant donors or a suitable TsF preparation via i.v. injection to naive (or 250 R irradiated) syngeneic recipient mice before or at daily intervals after initiation of sensitization. Ts or TsF are transferred to recipients on days 0, 1, 2, 3, 4 or 5 relative to the start of sensitization on day 0 and challenge on day 5. Results of Ts recipient groups are compared to positive controls (mice receiving no Ts or cells from sham tolerized donors). Afferent-acting Ts from lymph nodes of mice tolerized 7 days before by the i.v. injection of DNBS are suppressive if transferred early during sensitization (days 0 or 1) and are not suppressive if transferred later (days 2–5).

Inhibition of lymph node cell proliferation

When mice are primed for DTH, the antigen stimulates T cells in lymph nodes draining the site of immunization to undergo DNA replication and cell proliferation. During DNFB contact sensitization, this proliferative response peaks 4–5 days after sensitization and declines rapidly thereafter [35]. As opposed to kinetic experiments, a more direct assay for an afferent-acting Ts or TsF is a test of their ability to inhibit the normal post-sensitization cell proliferation in the draining lymph nodes of recipient animals. Proliferation can be measured either *in vivo* or *in vitro*. Recipients of afferent-acting Ts (e.g. those induced by i.v. tolerization with DNBS) exhibit significantly reduced proliferative responses in either of these assays.

Procedure

In vivo assay for inhibition of lymph node cell proliferation

Incorporation of radio-labelled (^{125}I) 5-iodo-2′-deoxyuridine (IUdR) is used to measure lymph node cell proliferation *in vivo* [35,51].

1   Ts are i.v. transferred to naive recipient mice on day 0; these and positive controls (receiving no Ts) are DNFB sensitized on days 0 and 1, as described above.
2   On days 3, 4, 5, and 6 after sensitization, 4–6 mice per group, along with negative controls (4–6 unsensitized mice), are injected i.p. with 5×10^{-8} mol of fluorodeoxyuridine (FUdR—Sigma Chemical Co, St. Louis, MO) in 0.2 ml of sterile distilled water. Ten minutes later each animal receives 1 μCi of ^{125}IUdR

(Amersham-Searle Corp., Arlington Heights, IL) by the same route and in the same volume.
3   Five hours later, mice are sacrificed, and draining lymph nodes from individual mice are removed and placed in 1 ml of neutral buffered formalin in 10×75 mm disposable glass tubes. ^{125}IUdR incorporation is determined by counting in a gamma spectrometer.
4   Results are expressed as percentage uptake of input counts. This ranges between 0.15% and 0.50% for positive control mice assayed 4–5 days after sensitization.

In vitro assay for inhibition of lymph node cell proliferation

Proliferative activity of draining lymph nodes may also be assayed by measuring tritiated thymidine (^{3}H-TdR) incorporation *in vitro* [35,38,42,44].

1   Groups of positive control mice, Ts recipients, and negative controls are set up exactly as described for the *in vivo* assay.
2   On days 3, 4, 5, and 6 after sensitization, 4–6 mice per group are sacrificed, draining lymph nodes removed and single cell suspensions prepared in BSS.
3   To measure DNA synthesis, triplicate cultures of 10^6 cells/well are set up in 0.25 ml of RPMI-1640 medium containing 5% heat-inactivated FCS in 96-well, round-bottom tissue culture dishes (Costar Corp., Cambridge, MA).
4   The plate is incubated in a humidified atmosphere of 5% CO_2:95% air at 37 °C for 30 min and then pulsed with 1.0 μCi of ^{3}H-TdR (6.7 Ci/m Research Products International Corp., Mt. Prospect, IL) per well.
5   The cultures are incubated for an additional 5 h and trichloroacetic acid-precipitable radioactive material is collected with a semi-automated sample harvester (Brandel Model M24V, Rockville, MD) on to glass-fibre filter paper.
6   Radioactivity is counted in a liquid scintillation spectrometer and results are expressed as counts per minute (c.p.m.).

Induction and suppression of helper T cells for DTH reactions

The authors have recently developed a simple assay to measure the direct participation of Th cells in development of DTH reactions [14,54]. As Th would be a logical target for suppression by afferent-acting Ts (Fig. 79.1), this assay allows one to ask directly if Ts are suppressing either the development of Th or the delivery of help from Th. The authors have shown that the spleen and draining lymph nodes of mice optimally primed for DTH by the s.c. injection of ligand-coupled syngeneic spleen cells contain radioresistant, antigen-specific, H-2 I-region-restricted, Lyt 1^+2^-, I-A$^+$ T cells capable of enhancing the development of DTH responses in recipient animals primed s.c. with suboptimal doses of ligand-coupled syngeneic cells.

1 Spleen and/or lymph node cells, from mice primed s.c. with optimal doses $(3–5 \times 10^7)$ of ligand-coupled cells 5–14 days previously, are collected and single cell suspensions prepared in BSS.

2 Of these primed cells $5 \times 10^7–10^8$ are i.v. transferred to naive, syngeneic recipient mice, which are immediately s.c. primed with a suboptimal dose $(1–2 \times 10^6)$ of modified cells which by itself is not sufficient for DTH induction.

3 Suboptimally primed recipients of Th cells show significant levels of antigen-specific DTH, as opposed to recipients of Th cells alone or suboptimally primed mice not receiving Th cells.

4 The effect of Ts on Th cell development or expression is assessed by transferring Ts to donor mice prior to Th priming, or to recipient mice concomitant with Th transfer, respectively.

Methods for assay of efferent suppression

Kinetic analysis

By definition, efferent-acting Ts or TsF are suppressive when injected immediately before elicitation of DTH reactivity, but are not suppressive when transferred early in the course of sensitization. Efferent-acting Ts and TsF have been identified in several experimental systems [36–38,43,52]. The experimental set up for kinetic analysis of efferent-acting Ts and TsF in the DNFB DTH system is exactly as described earlier for afferent-acting Ts. The exception is that tolerance is noted if cells or factors are transferred immediately before challenge (days 4 or 5), but not when transferred before or shortly after sensitization (days 0–3). However, kinetic experiments should always be confirmed with more direct measurements of efferent suppression, as detailed below.

Inhibition of passive transfer of DTH

The DTH passive transfer assay is a direct correlate of the efferent limb of DTH as it measures the ability of effector T_{DH} cells to home to the site of antigen challenge and release lymphokines after encounter with antigen-MHC determinants. Efferent-acting Ts suppress elicitation of DTH responses by inhibiting this process at one or more points (Fig. 77.1). Thus a more direct and sensitive assay for efferent-acting Ts and TsF is to test their ability to suppress the passive transfer of DTH. Reproducible assays for inhibition

of efferent DTH by both Ts and TsF are detailed below.

Procedure

Inhibition of DTH passive transfer by suppressor T cells

This is a simple assay which involves determining the effect of co-transfer of a Ts population with effector T_{DH} cells on the magnitude of DTH responses elicited in normal recipient mice [34,43]. Spleen or lymph node cells from mice tolerized 7 days previously with syngeneic DNP-modified spleen cells (DNP-SP) contain Ts which specifically suppress passive transfer of DNP-specific DTH.

1 Single cell suspensions from DNP-SP tolerant mice and immune lymph node cells from DNFB sensitized donors are prepared and adjusted to 10^8 cells/ml as previously described.

2 Equal volumes of the two suspensions are mixed and 1.0 ml $(5 \times 10^7$ Ts $+ 5 \times 10^7$ $T_{DH})$ immediately injected i.v. into groups of 4–5 naive, syngeneic recipients.

3 The Ts recipients, positive controls (mice receiving only 5×10^7 T_{DH} cells), and negative controls (mice receiving no cells) are ear challenged with 0.2% DNFB within 1 h.

4 Increases in ear thickness are determined 24 h after challenge. Efferent-acting Ts will prevent the elicitation of DTH in the recipient animals.

Inhibition of DTH passive transfer by suppressor T cell factors

This assay involves pre-incubation of effector T_{DH} cells with a suppressor factor prior to passive transfer of DTH. Efferent-acting suppressive activity has been observed in TsF prepared from the lymph nodes of mice tolerized i.v. with the reactive haptens, DNBS, TNBS and azobenzenearsonate [46,47,52] (see above for preparation), and from a monoclonal DNP-specific, TsF-producing T cell hybrid derived from the fusion spleen cells of mice tolerized with syngeneic DNP-SP to the BW5147 thymoma line [55]. Effector T_{DH} cells are derived from immune lymph node cells of contact sensitized donors, as described previously (page 77.6).

1 T_{DH} cells $(5 \times 10^7–10^8$ cells/ml) are cultured with control or suppressor supernates in a 37 °C water bath for 1 h and then washed twice in BSS.

2 Viable cells $(4–5 \times 10^7)$ are then i.v. transferred to naive, syngeneic recipient mice.

3 Recipients are ear challenged within 1 h of transfer

and increases in ear thickness determined 24 h there-after.

4   Recipients of T_{DH} populations incubated in supernates containing active efferent-acting TsF will display significantly reduced DTH activity relative to T_{DH} incubated in control supernates.

Method for assay of suppressor T cell auxiliary cells

Recently, several investigators have described an I-J$^+$ T cell, termed Ts-auxiliary (Ts-aux) or Ts-3, which is required for the suppression of effector T_{DH} by efferent-acting Ts [20,21,53]. This cell was identified upon observing that DNP-specific, efferent-acting Ts could suppress the passive transfer of DTH mediated by immune lymph node cells obtained from normal, but not high dose CY-treated donors [20,21]. Suppression of effector T_{DH} from CY-treated donors (CY T_{DH}) could be restored if a small number of T cells from untreated, DNFB-sensitized donors, but not T cells from naive mice, were added prior to co-transfer. Thus the Ts-aux cell is induced by specific immunogenic, not tolerogenic, exposure to antigen and is required for the activity of efferent-acting Ts. Assay of Ts-aux activity involves the transfer of three separate cell populations to naive recipient mice. Single cell suspensions of spleen or lymph node cells from mice tolerized 7 days before with syngeneic DNP-SP, and suspensions of DNFB-immune lymph node cells from both normal and CY-treated (100–200 mg/kg i.v. 2 days before sensitization) are prepared and adjusted to 1.67×10^8 cells/ml. Co-transfer of 5×10^7 Ts and 5×10^7 normal T_{DH} to naive, syngeneic recipients results in suppression of passive transfer of DTH, as described previously (page 77.7). Co-transfer of 5×10^7 Ts and 5×10^7 CY T_{DH} does not result in suppression. However, transfer of 5×10^7 each of Ts, CY T_{DH}, and normal T_{DH} (the Ts-aux source) results in profound suppression of DTH passive transfer even though the number of effector T_{DH} cells is doubled.

Conclusions

Delayed-type hypersensitivity reactions comprise a fundamental component of the immune response to infectious agents and foreign grafts. Therefore elucidation of the mechanisms underlying induction, elicitation and regulation of DTH responses is critically important to our basic understanding of disease processes. The authors hope that the procedures outlined in this chapter will be useful in furthering the investigation of these questions.

References

1 CROWLE A.J. (1975) Delayed hypersensitivity in the mouse. *Adv. Immunol.* **20**, 197.

2 LOVELAND B.E., HOGARTH P.M., CEREDIG R.H. & MCKENZIE I.F.C. (1981) Cells mediating graft rejection in the mouse. (I) Lyt-1 cells mediate skin graft rejection. *J. exp. Med.* **153**, 1044.

3 PREHN R.T. & MAIN J.M. (1957) Immunity to methylcholanthrene-induced sarcomas. *J. Nat. Cancer Inst.* **18**, 769.

4 GREENE M.I. (1980) The genetic and cellular basis of regulation of the immune response to tumor antigens. *Contemp. Top. Immunobiol.* **11**, 81.

5 NAOR D. (1979) Suppressor cells: permitters and promoters of malignancy? *Adv. Cancer Res.* **29**, 45.

6 DAVID J.R. (1974) Delayed hypersensitivity. In *Progress in Immunology II, Biological Aspects II*, (eds. Bent L. & Holborow J.) p. 123. North–Holland Publishing Co., Amsterdam.

7 LANDSTEINER K. & CHASE M.W. (1942) Experiments on transfer of cutaneous sensitivity to simple chemical compounds. *Proc. Soc. exp. Biol. (NY)* **49**, 688.

8 ASHERSON G.L. & PTAK W. (1968) Contact and delayed hypersensitivity in the mouse. (I) Active sensitization and passive transfer. *Immunology*, **15**, 405.

9 PHANUPHAK P., MOORHEAD J.W. & CLAMAN H.N. (1974) Tolerance and contact sensitivity to DNFB in mice. (I) *In vivo* detection by ear swelling and correlation with *in vitro* cell stimulation. *J. Immunol.* **112**, 115.

10 CLAMAN H.N. & MOORHEAD J.W. (1976) Tolerance to contact hypersensitivity. *Contemp. Top. Immunobiol.* **5**, 211.

11 GREENE M.I., SUGIMOTO M. & BENACERRAF B. (1978) Mechanisms of regulation of cell-mediated immune responses. (I) Effect of the route of immunization with TNP-coupled syngeneic cells on the induction and suppression of contact sensitivity to picryl chloride. *J. Immunol.* **120**, 1604.

12 BACH B.A., SHERMAN L., BENACERRAF B. & GREENE M.I. (1978) Mechanisms of regulation of cell-mediated immunity. (II) Induction and suppression of delayed type hypersensitivity to azobenzenearsonate-coupled syngeneic spleen cells. *J. Immunol.* **121**, 1460.

13 MILLER S.D., WETZIG R.P. & CLAMAN H.N. (1979) The induction of cell-mediated immunity and tolerance with protein antigens coupled to syngeneic lymphoid cells. *J. exp. Med.* **149**, 758.

14 MILLER S.D. & BUTLER L.D. (1983) T cell responses induced by the parenteral injection of antigen-modified syngeneic cells. (I) Induction, characterization, and regulation of antigen-specific T helper cells involved in delayed-type hypersensitivity responses. *J. Immunol.* **131**, 77.

15 SILBERBERG-SINAKIN I., BAER R.L. & THORBECKE G.J. (1978) Langerhans cells. A review of their nature with emphasis on their immunologic functions. *Prog. Allergy* **24**, 268.

16 STEINMAN R.M., KAPLAN G., WITMER M.D. & COHN Z.A. (1979) Identification of a novel cell in peripheral lymphoid organs of mice. (V) Purification of spleen dendritic

cells, new surface markers, and maintenance *in vitro. J. exp. Med.* **149**, 1.

17 MILLER J.F.A.P., VADAS M.A., WHITELAW A. & GAMBLE J. (1976) Role of major histocompatibility complex gene products in delayed-type hypersensitivity. *Proc. natn. Acad. Sci. U.S.A.* **73**, 2486.

18 COHEN S., PICK E. & OPPENHEIM J.J. (1979) *Biology of the Lymphokines.* Academic Press, New York.

19 VADAS M.A., MILLER J.F.A.P., MCKENZIE I.F.C., CHISM S.E., SHEN F.W., BOYSE E.A., GAMBLE J.R. & WHITELAW A.M. (1976) Ly and Ia antigen phenotypes of T cells involved in delayed-type hypersensitivity and in suppression. *J. exp. Med.* **144**, 10.

20 SY M.S., MILLER S.D., MOORHEAD J.W. & CLAMAN H.N. (1979) Active suppression of DNFB-immune T cells requires an auxiliary T cell which is induced by antigen. *J. exp. Med.* **149**, 197.

21 MILLER S.D., BUTLER L.D. & CLAMAN H.N. (1982) The role of suppressor T cell networks in the regulation of DNFB contact sensitivity: Receptor–anti-receptor interactions in efferent suppression. *Ann. N.Y. Acad. Sci.* **392**, 122.

22 ROBINSON J.H. & NAYSMITH J.D. (1976) A comparison of four methods for measuring cutaneous delayed-type hypersensitivity reactions to protein antigens in the mouse. *Scand. J. Immunol.* **5**, 299.

23 SULZBERGER M.B. (1929) Hypersensitivity to arsphenamine in guinea pigs. *Archs Derm. Syph.* **20**, 699.

24 CHASE M.W. (1946) Inhibition of experimental drug allergy by prior feeding of the sensitizing agent. *Proc. Soc. exp. Biol. Med.* **61**, 257.

25 MILLER S.D. & CLAMAN H.N. (1976) The induction of hapten-specific T cell tolerance using hapten-modified lymphoid cells. (I) Characteristics of tolerance induction. *J. Immunol.* **117**, 1519.

26 BATTISTO J.R. & BLOOM B.R. (1966) Dual immunological unresponsiveness induced by cell membrane coupled hapten or antigen. *Nature,* **212**, 156.

27 DOHI Y. & NISONOFF A. (1979) Suppression of idiotype and generation of suppressor T cells with idiotype conjugated thymocytes. *J. exp. Med.* **150**, 909.

28 CHEUNG N.-K., SHERR D.H., HEGHINIAN K.M., BENACERRAF B. & DORF M.E. (1978) Immune suppression *in vivo* with antigen-modified syngeneic cells. (I) T cell-mediated suppression to the terpolymer (Glu,Lys,Phe)n. *J. exp. Med.* **148**, 1539.

29 FINBERG R., BURAKOFF S.J., BENACERRAF B. & GREENE M.I. (1979) The cytolytic T lymphocyte response to trinitrophenyl-modified syngeneic cells. (II) Evidence for antigen-specific suppressor T cells. *J. Immunol.* **123**, 1210.

30 CLAMAN H.N. (1976) Tolerance and contact sensitivity to DNFB in mice. (V) Induction of tolerance with DNP compounds and with free and membrane-associated DNFB. *J. Immunol.* **116**, 704.

31 MILLER S.D., SY M.S. & CLAMAN H.N. (1977) The induction of hapten-specific T cell tolerance using hapten-modified lymphoid cells. (II) Relative roles of suppressor T cells and clone inhibition in the tolerant state. *Eur. J. Immunol.* **7**, 165.

32 ASHERSON G.L., ZEMBALA M., PERERA M.A.C.C., MAYHEW B. & THOMAS W.R. (1977) Production of

immunity and unresponsiveness in the mouse by feeding contact sensitizing agents and the role of suppressor cells in the Peyer's patches, mesenteric lymph nodes and other lymphoid tissues. *Cell. Immunol.* **33**, 145.

33 MILLER S.D. & HANSON D.G. (1979) Inhibition of specific immune responses by feeding protein antigens. (IV) Evidence for tolerance and specific active suppression of cell-mediated immune responses to ovalbumin. *J. Immunol.* **123**, 2344.

34 ASHERSON G.L. & ZEMBALA M. (1974) Suppression of contact sensitivity by cells in the mouse. (I) Demonstration that suppressor cells act on the effector stage of contact sensitivity; and their induction following *in vitro* exposure to antigen. *Proc. R. Soc. Series B; Biological Sciences,* **187**, 329.

35 MOORHEAD J.W. (1976) Tolerance and contact sensitivity to DNFB in mice. (VI) Inhibition of afferent sensitivity by suppressor T cells in adoptive tolerance. *J. Immunol.* **117**, 802.

36 SY M.S., DIETZ M.H., GERMAIN R.N., BENACERRAF B. & GREENE M.I. (1980) Antigen and receptor driven regulatory mechanisms. (IV) Idiotype-bearing I-J$^+$ suppressor T cell factors induce second order suppressor T cells which express anti-idiotypic receptors. *J. exp. Med.* **151**, 1183.

37 WEINBERGER J.Z., GERMAIN R.N., BENACERRAF B. & DORF M.E. (1980) Hapten-specific T cell responses to 4-hydroxy-3-nitrophenyl acetyl. (V) Role of idiotypes in the suppressor pathway. *J. exp. Med.* **152**, 161.

38 MILLER S.D., BUTLER L.D. & CLAMAN H.N. (1982) Suppressor T cell circuits in contact sensitivity. (I) Two mechanistically distinct waves of suppressor T cells occur in mice tolerized with syngeneic DNP-modified lymphoid cells. *J. Immunol.* **129**, 461.

39 JENKINS M.K., LEI H.Y., WALTENBAUGH C. & MILLER S.D. (1984) Immunoregulatory pathways in adult responder mice. (I) Induction of GAT-specific tolerance and suppressor T cells for cellular and humoral responses. *Scand. J. Immunol.* **19**, 501.

40 MISHELL R.I. & DUTTON R.W. (1967) Immunization of dissociated spleen cell cultures from normal mice. *J. exp. Med.* **126**, 423.

41 PHANUPHAK P., MOORHEAD J.W. & CLAMAN H.N. (1974) Tolerance and contact sensitivity to DNFB in mice. (III) Transfer of tolerance with 'suppressor T cells'. *J. Immunol.* **113**, 1230.

42 THOMAS W.R., WATKINS M.C. & ASHERSON G.L. (1979) Suppressor cells for the afferent phase of contact sensitivity to picryl chloride: inhibition of DNA synthesis induced by T cells from mice injected with picryl sulfonic acid. *J. Immunol.* **122**, 2300.

43 MILLER S.D., SY M.S. & CLAMAN H.N. (1978) Suppressor cell mechanisms in contact sensitivity. (I) Efferent blockade by syninduced suppressor T cells. *J. Immunol.* **121**, 265.

44 MILLER S.D., SY M.S. & CLAMAN H.N. (1978) Suppressor cell mechanisms in contact sensitivity. (II) Afferent blockade by alloinduced suppressor T cells. *J. Immunol.* **121**, 274.

45 PIERRES A., BROMBERG J.S., SY M.S., BENACERRAF B. & GREENE M.I. (1980) Mechanisms of regulation of cell-

mediated immunity. (VI) Antigen density dependence of the induction of genetically restricted suppressor cells. *J. Immunol.* **124**, 343.

46 ZEMBALA M. & ASHERSON G.L. (1974) T cell suppression of contact sensitivity in the mouse. (II) The role of soluble suppressor factor and its interaction with macrophages. *Eur. J. Immunol.* **4**, 799.

47 MOORHEAD J.W. (1977) Soluble factors in tolerance and contact sensitivity to DNFB in mice. (I) Suppression of contact sensitivity by soluble suppressor factor released *in vitro* by lymph node cell populations containing specific suppressor cells. *J. Immunol.* **119**, 315.

48 TAKEMORI T. & TADA T. (1975) Properties of antigen-specific suppressive T-cell factor in the regulation of antibody responses of the mouse. (I) *In vivo* activity and immunochemical characterizations. *J. exp. Med.* **142**, 1241.

49 WALTENBAUGH C., THEZE J., KAPP J.A. & BENACERRAF B. (1977) Immunosuppressive factor(s) specific for L-glutamic acid^{50}-L-tyrosine^{50} (GT). (III) Generation of suppressor T cells by a suppressive extract derived from GT-primed lymphoid cells. *J. exp. Med.* **146**, 970.

50 STEEL R.G. & TORRIE J.H. (1960) *Principles and Procedures of Statistics.* McGraw-Hill Book Co., New York.

51 PRITCHARD H. & MICKLEM H.S. (1972) Immune responses in congenitally thymus-less mice. (I) Absence of response to oxazolone. *Clin. exp. Immunol.* **10**, 151.

52 DIETZ M.H., SY M.S., BENACERRAF B., NISONOFF A., GREENE M.I. & GERMAIN R.N. (1981) Antigen and receptor driven regulatory mechanisms. (VII) H-2-restricted anti-idiotypic suppressor factor from efferent suppressor T cells. *J. exp. Med.* **153**, 450.

53 SY M.S., NISONOFF A., GERMAIN R.N., BENACERRAF B. & GREENE M.I. (1981) Antigen and receptor driven regulatory mechanisms. (VIII) Suppression of idiotype-negative, *p*-azobenzenearsonate-specific T cells results from the interaction of an anti-idiotypic second order T suppressor cell with a cross-reactive idiotype-positive, *p*-azobenzenearsonate-primed T cell target. *J. exp. Med.* **153**, 1415.

54 JENKINS M.K., WALTENBAUGH C. & MILLER S.D. (1985) Immunoregulatory pathways in adult responder mice. (II) Regulation of DTH responses by GAT-specific suppressor factors present in GAT-tolerant adult responder mice. *J. Immunol.* **134**, 114.

55 MILLER S.D. (1984) Suppressor T cell circuits in contact sensitivity. (II) Induction and characterization of an efferent-acting, antigen-specific, H-2-restricted, monoclonal T cell hybrid-derived suppressor factor specific for DNFB contact hypersensitivity. *J. Immunol.* **133**, 3221.

Chapter 78
Detection of suppressor cells and suppressor factors for antibody responses

C. WALTENBAUGH & B. S. KIM

Common materials and methods,
    78.1
Methods for assay of non-specific
    suppressor cells and factors,
    78.4

Methods for assay of specific
    suppressor cells and factors,
    78.5
Media and buffers, 78.14

Modern cellular immunology began with the realization of two major compartments of the immune system responsible for humoral and cellular immune responses, i.e. B and T lymphocytes. Common to all B lymphocytes is the expression of surface-bound immunoglobulin. Upon suitable stimulation, B cells mature into antibody-secreting or plasma cells. As a population, B cells are fairly limited in function. T lymphocytes, on the other hand, display a far wider range of functional heterogeneity, serving in effector and regulatory roles. The majority of humoral immune responses require co-operation between T cells and B cells (T-dependent responses) and involve multiple cell interactions. Pioneer studies of regulation of humoral responses by Claman et al. [1] and Miller & Mitchell [2–5] showed T cells to help the immune response, i.e. helper T (Th) cells. Gershon & Kondo [6–8] first described another type of regulatory T cell, the suppressor T (Ts) cell, which diminishes the immune response. Cantor & Boyse [9,10] demonstrated that T cells that express Lyt-2,3 antigens were potent suppressors, whereas Th bear Lyt-1 antigens. Ts are either specific [6,7,11–14] or non-specific [15–17], suggesting heterogeneity of Ts populations, and Ts play a major role in regulating many cellular and humoral immune responses.

The large number of monospecific lymphocytes in the immune system and the wide variety of antigens recognized by this system present a problem in resolving the mechanism(s) of lymphocyte interaction. Lymphocytes must either come into intimate contact, or a lymphocyte-produced soluble mediator (factor) must carry an immunological signal between lymphocyte populations. Intimate contact requires that at least two cells must physically touch in order to interact. A circulating factor *in vivo* eliminates the necessity of cell–cell contact. Soluble factors have been described in several suppressor systems [18–22] and these T-cell derived suppressor factors (TsF) have a profound effect on the humoral immune response.

This chapter describes methods for the assessment of Ts in humoral immune responses. The wide variety of experimental systems and the extensive heterogeneity of Ts subpopulations require detailed descriptions of only a few representative experimental models. The authors have chosen to describe several experimental methods for induction of suppressor cells and their factors. The induction of allotype-, epitope-specific Ts, and contra-suppressor (Tcs) cells are treated in lesser detail as they are covered in other chapters of this volume.

Common materials and methods

Animals

Mice used in Ts studies ideally should be 2–4 months old at the time of assay. Only healthy mice should be used and it is particularly important that mice are not subjected to unnecessary stress before initiation of an experiment. If at all possible, investigators should maintain their own mouse breeding facilities and pay careful attention to proper animal husbandry procedures. As this is not often possible, the investigator must rely upon a steady supply of animals from an outside vendor. In our experience, animals subjected to the stress of shipping exhibit altered immune responsiveness for 2 weeks or more after shipment. It is best to allow 3–4 weeks for mice to become acclimatized to the new environment, microflora, and diet. The period of acclimatization improves the effectiveness of immune response assays. In the authors' facility, animals are fed standard laboratory mouse blocks and provided with acidified ($\sim$pH 5), chlorinated water (5 ml sodium hypochloride, Chlorox, per 20 l H_2O, to minimize bacterial growth in water) *ad libitum*.

Haemolytic plaque assay

The reader is referred to Chapter 64, by D.W. Dresser, which describes a wide range of different PFC techniques. In the present chapter, the authors describe a slide modification of the original Jerne haemolytic plaque assay in agar [23,24] and its application for the detection of PFC.

Equipment

Slide trays

Agarose, containing indicator cells and lymphocytes (see below), is poured (~2 mm thick) on to standard microscope slides (25 × 75 mm) and allowed to gel. To aid in subsequent handling, incubation, application of developing antisera, and complement, the slides are placed on Plexiglass trays. Chapter 64 details a slide tray constructed from Plexiglass. A similar tray is commercially available from Bellco Glass, Inc, Vineland, NJ (haemolytic plaque assay rack, stock number 7741-04000). Fig. 78.1 illustrates dimensions for a slide tray used in our laboratory, which has a greater slide holding capacity and slides and agarose are not as easily disturbed in handling as with other trays. The tray is easily constructed by cementing Lucite strips of indicated dimensions to a Lucite sheet.

Water bath and incubator

A water bath maintained at 45±1 °C keeps the agarose–indicator cell mixture soluble. A low-form (17.8 cm height) water bath (NAPCO, model #103) allows particularly easy access for the numerous pipetting operations required in the PFC assay. An incubator maintained at 41 °C is best suited for incubation of the plaque assay. Water-jacketed incubators (such as NAPCO models 2100 or 2200 or Forma Scientific model 3173) are less subject to transient temperature drops resulting from repeatedly opening the chamber door.

Microscope, illuminator and electronic plaque counter

A low-power (10–13×) dissecting type microscope is used for viewing plaques. The authors use American Optical Cycloptic (AO, model 58Fl, 13×) dissecting microscopes fitted with concave substage mirrors (AO part number 192) and AO model 653 illuminators. This microscope–illuminator combination allows the pseudo-darkfield viewing of zones of lysis (plaques). Plaques are counted with the aid of an electronic counter (Bel-Art, Pequannock, NJ, TechniLab Instru-

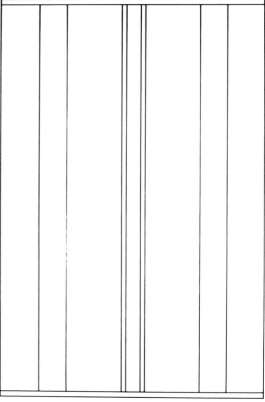

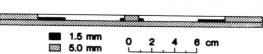

■ 1.5 mm
▨ 5.0 mm   0 2 4 6 cm

Fig. 78.1. Dimensions for slide holding tray for the haemolytic plaque assay. Tray has the capacity to hold forty-eight 25 × 75 mm microscope slides.

ments model 257). A needle probe is used together with a reference electrode to count across conductive surfaces such as agarose. By touching the plaques on the agarose with the needle probe, the counter advances.

Materials

Sheep erythrocytes (SRBC) vary in their susceptibility to lysis by mouse antibody and complement. The best approach is to screen several different lots of SRBC obtained from individual sheep for their applicability to the plaque assay. It is preferable to use erythrocytes from only one or two known animals, as this leads to greater consistency in PFC results. Two US sources (Colorado Serum Company, Boulder, CO and

GIBCO Diagnostics, Madison, WI) will supply investigators with bleeds from selected individual sheep on a standing order basis. SRBC listed by these suppliers as 'high titre' sheep erythrocytes, are more immunogenic in Mishell–Dutton type cultures [25,26] and are also more suitable for the plaque assay. SRBC are collected sterile as whole blood in Alsever's solution [27] and stored at 4 °C (for 4–6 months) until use.

The plaque assay relies upon the interaction of mouse immunoglobulin with antigens native to the SRBC surface or antigens chemically bound to the SRBC surface. Cells are resuspended and aseptically removed from Alsever's solution and washed by centrifugation (800 *g* for 10 min) in saline (0.15 M-NaCl). After the first wash, the white-cell rich buffy coat is removed from the surface of the red cell pellet by aspiration. The SRBC are resuspended in saline and washed at least two to three more times or until the supernatant is clear. The source of agarose used in the plaque assay is crucial. Agarose A37° (Induboise A37°, L'Industrie Biologique, Francaise, Paris, US supplier, Accurate Scientific, Hicksville, NY) is used by most laboratories. Seakern LE (FMC Corporation, Marine Colloids Div., Rockland, ME) is an alternative agarose source. To alleviate anti-complementary activity sometimes found in even these highly refined agaroses, 0.5 mg DEAE-Dextran (Pharmacia Fine Chemicals) is added per millilitre of final agarose solution. Freshly frozen guinea-pig serum is used as a source of complement. Although a number of suppliers offer this product, at least two US suppliers (Pel-Freez Biologicals, Rogers, AR, and Hazelton-Dutchland, Inc., Denver, PA) offer large quantities (100–500 ml) at reasonable prices.

Procedures

Haemolytic plaque assay

For a more detailed description of the haemolytic plaque assay see Chapter 64.

1 Six hundred milligrams agarose, 50 mg DEAE-Dextran and 100 ml Hank's balanced salt solution (HBSS) are boiled with stirring until the agarose dissolves.

2 Three hundred microlitres of agarose solution is pipetted into 10×75 mm glass tubes pre-warmed in the 45 °C water bath.

3 Fifty microlitres of 1% fetal bovine serum (FBS) in HBSS (v/v) are added to each tube which allows the indicator cells to distribute into an even lawn when the agarose is poured on to the microscope slide.

4 If required by the assay procedure, inhibitors are added to the appropriate tubes. Two drops (40–60 μl)

of the appropriate indicator cells (see below) are added from a Pasteur pipette.

5 Microscope slides (25×75 mm, frosted one end), previously coated with 0.1% agar dissolved in distilled water and air-dried (this procedure allows the agarose–indicator cell mixture to adhere to the slide), are placed upon a dry level surface (such as sheet of plate glass). The experimental groups and (optional) inhibitors are indicated on the frosted area of the microscope slide with a pencil mark.

6 The lymphocyte suspension to be assayed (0.1 ml) is pipetted into each tube; the agarose suspension is mixed by vortexing and the warm mixture is immediately poured on to agarose-painted microscope slides and allowed to gel (1–5 min). Slides are then inverted and placed face down in the recess of the slide tray, the tray is loosely covered with a plastic film (to retard evaporation) and placed in the 41 °C incubator for 1 h.

7 The trays are then removed from the incubator. The recessed trough is then flooded with guinea-pig complement diluted to suitable concentration (usually 1:20 to 1:25) with complement diluent (see 'Media and buffers', page 78.14, for preparation of diluent), and the tray is returned to the incubator for 1 h.

8 After this final incubation, complement is poured off and replaced with HBSS. PFC are counted under a low-power dissecting microscope with the aid of the electronic colony counter.

Notes

Mouse IgG is inefficient in fixing guinea-pig complement; therefore the above procedure will result in IgM plaques. If IgG PFC are to be counted, a developing or facilitation step must be added to the above procedure between the initial incubation period and the addition of guinea-pig complement. A suitable dilution (1:150 to 1:300) of rabbit anti-mouse Ig in HBSS is pipetted into the recess of the tray and the slide trays are returned (without the plastic film) to the incubator for a second 1 h incubation. The trays are removed from the incubator, and are tilted to pour the rabbit anti-mouse Ig solution to drain off. Complement is then added and the procedure is followed as detailed above.

Spleen cell cultures

Modifications of either the Mishell–Dutton [25,26] or the Marbrook [28] spleen cell culture systems are commonly used for Ts induction and assay. The Mishell–Dutton system probably finds the widest application in Ts experiments, although the carrier specific system of Tada *et al.* [29–31] is a notable exception. Mishell & Dutton [25,26] detail the salient requirements for primary immunization of lymphocyte suspension cultures.

1 Modified Mishell–Dutton culture medium is detailed at end of this chapter. Spleens are aseptically removed, teased, washed once by centrifugation in HBSS, and resuspended to 16×10^6 viable cells/ml in modified Mishell–Dutton medium containing fetal bovine serum (FBS) (see 'Media and buffers', page 78.14).

2 The cell suspension is distributed in 0.5 ml (8×10^6 cells) aliquots into 24-well, flat-bottom tissue culture plates (Linbro 76-033-05, Flow Laboratories, McLean, VA) and antigen and/or factors are added to the cultures.

3 Cultures are placed in a sealable incubator chamber (Modular Incubator Chamber, 61-530-00, Flow Laboratories). The incubator chamber is humidified, by placement of an open Petri dish containing distilled water, gassed with a mixture of 83% N_2, 10% CO_2, 7% O_2, and placed at 37 °C on a rocker platform (Bellco 7740–10010) at 7–12 oscillations per minute. Culture wells are fed daily by the addition of 50–60 μl (2 drops from a Pasteur pipette) of feeding mixture containing 50% nutritional cocktail (see below) and 50% FBS.

4 On the fourth or fifth day, cultures are harvested with a Pasteur pipette, cells washed three times in HBSS, and the cell pellet is resuspended to 1.0–2.5 ml in HBSS containing 1% FBS for the PFC assay.

The Marbrook system [28] allows a layer of cells on a dialysis membrane to be immersed in a reservoir of culture medium. Preparation and size of culture vessels and number of cells per chamber vary widely; the reader is referred to articles in this handbook, as well as elsewhere [27], for details. Major advantages of the Marbrook system are that the cultures do not require special medium, special gassing mixtures, or the repeated supply of additives. Its major drawback is time and expense required for the preparation of the culture chambers.

Radioimmunoassay

Radioimmunoassay (RIA) and enzyme-linked immunosorbent assay (ELISA) are alternatives to the haemolytic plaque assay for the measurement of specific antibody. These techniques are usually employed to measure serum antibody levels, as opposed to the measurement of antibody produced by single cells in the plaque assay. Various approaches to the RIA are described in detail in Chapter 26. The authors outline the application of RIA for detection of total specific antibody and/or idiotype (Id) detection. These same principles can be applied to using the ELISA assay; see Chapters 26 & 32 for detailed methodology.

A solid-phase RIA is one of the more convenient ways in which to determine the total specific antibody levels. Various concentrations of antigen (preferably purified) are immobilized on polystyrene tubes or polyvinyl chloride, 96-well microwell plates. A standard curve is generated to determine at which concentration of antigen known concentrations of specific antibodies react. The specific antibodies, reacted with the immobilized antigen subsequently measured after radiolabelled second antibodies (e.g. goat anti-mouse Ig to detect mouse specific antibodies), are allowed to bind. This standardized curve serves as reference for the determination of antibodies of unknown concentration. Alternatively, inhibition of the antigen–antibody reaction between immobilized known antibody and radiolabelled antigen by unknown samples are determined.

Detection of a level of specific allotype- and idiotype (Id)-bearing antibodies using RIA is somewhat restricted because both antigen and antibodies are both Igs generally derived from the same species. Determination of concentrations of specific allotype are detailed in Chapter 97 by Herzenberg. To determine the level of a given Id concentration, radiolabelled Id-bearing Ig and/or Fab fragments are used as probes [32,33]. Optimal concentration of anti-Id antibody ($\sim 70\%$ of maximal binding) for quantitative RIA is determined by titration over a wide range of antibody concentration (1:100–1:100 000) and a fixed concentration of radiolabelled Id (5000–100 000 c.p.m.). A standard inhibition curve is then established, based upon the inhibition of ^{125}I-Id–anti-Id reaction by known concentrations of purified Id. Inhibition by samples of unknown Id concentration are determined by comparison with the standard inhibition curve obtained with the purified Id standard. Generally, affinity purified myeloma proteins or monoclonal antibodies produced by hybridomas are used as a source of the radiolabelled probes.

Methods for assay of non-specific suppressor cells and factors

Con A-induced suppressor cells

Addition of concanavalin A (con A, derived from the jack bean, *Canavalia ensiformis*) to Mishell–Dutton spleen cell cultures either enhances or suppresses *in vitro* PFC responses to both T-dependent and T-independent antigens [16,17,34]. Submitogenic concentrations (0.001–0.01 μg/ml) of con A enhance the immune response, while optimal mitogenic ($\geqslant 1$–2 μg/ml) concentrations of con A added to mouse spleen cell cultures suppress *in vitro* primary and secondary immune responses. These phenomena result from the selective stimulation of Th or Ts, respectively. The Thy-1, Lyt-2$^+$,3$^+$, con A-induced Ts diminish PFC responses to classic T-dependent antigens such as SRBC and TNP-KLH (trinitrophenylated keyhole limpet haemocyanin) [16,34,35]. Con A Ts are demonstrable *in vivo* in animals treated with high dose of con A. Rich & Pierce [34] found that T cells from mice injected 24 h earlier with 150 μg con A suppress the PFC responses of normal spleen cells to SRBC *in vitro*.

Induction of con A-stimulated suppressor cells

Procedure

The method of Rich & Pierce [16,34] is described.
1   Twice crystallized con A (ICN Nutritional Biochemicals, Cleveland, OH, Stock number 10140) in a saturated NaCl solution is sterilized by membrane filtration (0.45 μm) and stored at room temperature.
2   Sterile dilutions are prepared in HBSS, stored at 4 °C and used within 1 week. Spleen cells of C57BL/6 mice (Jackson Laboratory, Bar Harbor, ME) are cultured under Mishell–Dutton conditions for 48 h either in the absence (control) or presence (Ts) of 750 ng to 1 μg con A/ml.
3   The cells are harvested, washed four times in HBSS at 150 *g* for 10 min, resuspended in fresh Mishell–Dutton medium (see 'Media and buffers', page 78.14), and graded numbers of viable cells are added to fresh Mishell–Dutton cultures containing 2×10^6 SRBC as antigen.
4   Cultures are harvested after 5 days and assayed for anti-SRBC PFC activity using the haemolytic plaque assay.

Notes

As few as 10^5 con A-activated spleen cells suppress either fresh or 48 h SRBC-stimulated cultures. The con A-induced Ts bear Thy-1, and Lyt-1$^-$,2$^+$ markers [36] and suppress the generation of both humoral (anti-SRBC) and cellular (cytotoxic T lymphocyte) immune responses [37] non-specifically.

Soluble immune response suppressor (SIRS)

Rich & Pierce [38] demonstrated that normal mouse spleen cell cultures, when activated by mitogenic concentrations of con A, produce a non-specific soluble immune response suppressor (SIRS) factor which suppresses both T-dependent and T-independent PFC responses.

Procedure

Culture supernatants containing SIRS are prepared as follows.
1   Five millilitre cultures containing 5×10^7 normal C57BL/6 spleen cells are incubated in 60 mm tissue culture dishes (Falcon Plastics 3002) for 48 h in Mishell–Dutton type cultures containing 2% FBS. Between 0.75 and 1.0 mg con A is added per ml at culture initiation.
2   SIRS-containing culture supernatants are collected by centrifugation at the end of this period.
3   Residual con A is removed by absorbing the supernatant fluids twice with Sephadex G-75 (Pharmacia Fine Chemicals) hydrated with Mishell–Dutton medium containing 2% FBS [38]. Approximately 30 ml packed, hydrated G-75 is used to absorb 70 ml culture supernatant for 1 h at 4 °C.
4   Supernatants are collected by centrifugation, membrane filter sterilized (0.45 μm) and stored at -20 °C until use.
5   The SIRS-containing supernatants maximally suppress ($>85\%$) the anti-SRBC PFC responses of Mishell–Dutton type cultures at 1:40 to 1:80 final concentration. Dilutions of $\leqslant 1:20$ are cytotoxic.

Methods for assay of specific suppressor cells and factors

Sheep erythrocytes (SRBC) suppressor cells and factors

Gershon & Kondo [6–8] first described the induction of antigen-specific Ts. They found that tolerance induction to a large dose of RBC in mice was T-cell dependent. Subsequent experiments by these investigators demonstrated that Ts were very efficient in inducing PFC unresponsiveness. Moreover, unresponsiveness was 'infectious', and could be transferred to naive syngeneic animals by tolerant splenic T cells (infectious tolerance). Eardley, Gershon and co-workers [39,40] defined the necessary conditions for the induction of Ts in Mishell–Dutton cultures.

Procedure

1   Normal, unprimed spleen cell suspensions are depleted of Ig$^+$ cells to yield a T cell enriched population [39].
2   One millilitre of 10^7 Lyt-2$^+$ T cells is then cultured with 25 μl 1% SRBC for in plastic tissue culture dishes (Falcon 3008).
3   After a 4 day culture period, the spleen cells are harvested, washed, counted, and treated with anti-Lyt-1 plus complement.
4   Graded numbers of these SRBC-specific Ts con-

taining cells suppress the ability of Mishell–Dutton normal spleen cell cultures to make PFC responses to normal immunogenic doses (10^6) of SRBC.

Procedure

An SRBC suppressor factor can be induced *in vitro* from SRBC tolerant splenic T cell cultures [39,40].
1   Ten million Ig$^+$-depleted spleen cells (T cells) are incubated with 2×10^6 SRBC in tissue culture plates under non-rocking conditions in 5% CO_2 at 37 °C in modified Mishell–Dutton media.
2   After 4 days of culture, the T cells are centrifuged (800 *g* for 15 min) over Lymphocyte-M (Cedarlane Laboratories, Hornby, Ontario, Canada) and the interface layer collected which contains viable mouse lymphocytes free from dead cells and SRBC.
3   The T cells are resuspended to 10^7 cells/ml in Mishell–Dutton medium and incubated for an additional 6 h at 37 °C.
4   The cultures are harvested, centrifuged, and the cell-free supernatant is added to Mishell–Dutton cultures at 1:10 final concentration, together with SRBC. Greater than 50% suppression of the primary *in vitro* anti-SRBC PFC response is seen.

Procedure

Yamauchi *et al.* [41] describe preparation of a SRBC-specific I-J$^+$ TsF produced by Lyt-1$^+$ Ts or Ts inducer factor (TsiF).
1   C57BL/6 or BALB/c mice are immunized twice i.p. with 0.2 ml 20% SRBC (v/v) in PBS at a 2 week interval.
2   The animals are sacrificed, spleens removed, and single-cell suspensions are prepared.
3   'Lyt-1$^+$ cells' are prepared by treatment of the whole spleen cell population with anti-Lyt-2 plus rabbit complement.
4   The Lyt-1-depleted cells are then cultured *in vitro* without antigen at 10^7 cells/ml in Mishell–Dutton medium.
5   The cultures are harvested after 48 h, supernatants collected following centrifugation (1000 *g* for 20 min), and sterilized by membrane filtration.
6   TsiF produced in this manner is added to primary Mishell-Dutton cultures at 1:10 final dilution. TsiF is composed of two chains: one is I-J$^+$ and V$_H$-restricted, while the other is I-J$^-$, binds antigen, and is antigen specific [41].

Carrier-specific (KLH) suppressor cells and factors

Tada *et al.* [11,19,29,31,42] described carrier-specific Ts and TsF. Antigen-specific Ts are induced with relatively high immunizing doses of keyhole limpet haemocyanin (KLH). The induced Ts suppress primary and secondary anti-hapten PFC responses both *in vivo* and *in vitro*. Carrier suppression is usually measured *in vitro* by the ability of Ts and TsF to diminish secondary anti-hapten responses of spleen cells. A hapten, such as the dinitrophenyl group (DNP), is coupled to the homologous carrier (KLH) as antigen in these cultures. Tada *et al.* [18,19] were the first to describe the production of an antigen-specific TsF. The factor was extracted by sonication and ultracentrifugation from thymocytes and spleen cells of mice immunized with high doses of KLH. The factor suppresses primary and secondary anti-DNP PFC responses.

Assay of KLH-specific responses

BALB/c, C57BL/6, or DBA/2 mice (from Jackson Laboratory), as well as other inbred strains, can be used. Preparation of KLH (Calbiochem, San Diego, CA) and DNP-KLH are described in Chapter 3. In general, KLH is dinitrophenylated according to the method of Eisen *et al.* [43] to make 700–800 DNP groups per KLH (assuming a 7 000 000 Da) molecule. Mice are primed with a single 200 μl i.p. injection of 100 μg DNP-KLH containing 10^9 killed *Bordetella pertussis* (alum-adsorbed vaccine may be obtained from Michigan Department of Public Health, Lansing, MI) organisms. Primary anti-DNP PFC responses are determined 4–8 days after primary immunization. Secondary anti-DNP PFC responses are induced *in vivo* by priming mice i.p. with 200 μl containing 100 μg DNP-KLH without adjuvant and boosting i.p. 4 weeks later with 100 μg DNP-KLH with(out) adjuvant. Anti-DNP PFC responses are determined 3 days after secondary immunization.

Procedure

For *in vitro* studies, mice are primed i.p. with a single injection of 200 μl saline suspension containing 100 μg DNP-KLH and 10^9 killed *Bordetella pertussis* organisms. Six weeks later, *in vitro* secondary PFC responses are induced in the Marbrook type [28] culture system.
1   Briefly, 10^7 DNP-KLH primed spleen cells in 1 ml minimum essential medium (MEM, Gibco, Grand Island, NY), supplemented with 10% FBS, are placed in the upper chamber of a Marbrook [28] vessel.
2   The cells are stimulated with 0.1 μg DNP-KLH/ml. Cultures are maintained in an atmosphere of 10% CO_2 in air for 5 days.
3   The cells are harvested at termination of culture and the number of anti-hapten PFC are determined in

the haemolytic plaque assay using TNP-SRBC as indicator cells.

TNP-SRBC can detect either anti-DNP or anti-TNP PFC responses and are prepared by modification of the method originally described by Rittenberg & Pratt [44].

Procedure

1 Dissolve 60 mg picryl sulphonic acid (P-5878, Sigma Chemical Corp., St. Louis, MO) in 21 ml PBS (phosphate-buffered saline) in a foil-wrapped 50 ml Erlenmeyer flask, include a small stirring bar to aid dissolution.
2 Add 3.0 ml packed (i.e. from centrifugation pellet) washed SRBC. Stir, allowing mixture to react for 10 min at room temperature.
3 The reacted cells are transferred to a 50 ml centrifuge tube and 35 ml PBS containing 22 mg glycyl-glycine (Sigma, G-1002) is added. The reactants may be scaled down to one-third the above procedure to couple 1.0 ml packed SRBC. Glycyl-glycine removes unreacted picryl sulphonic acid.
4 Centrifuge at 800 g for 10 min, remove yellow supernatant, and wash cells two or three times, or until the supernatant is clear.
5 Adjust the cells to ~10% in PBS (v/v) for use in PFC assay. TNP-SRBC are usable as indicator cells in the plaque assay for up to 2 weeks.

Induction of KLH-specific Ts

Procedure

1 KLH-primed Ts are derived from donor mice immunized with two i.p. 200 μl injections of 100 μg KLH without adjuvant at 2 week intervals.
2 Animals are sacrificed 2 weeks after the second injection, spleens and thymuses removed, and single-cell suspensions of these tissues prepared by mincing with forceps. Cellular clumps are removed by straining through a 200-mesh stainless steel screen (Small Parts, Inc, Miami, FL) and cells are washed three times in HBSS.
3 Carrier-primed cells (5×10^7), injected i.v., will transfer suppression to normal or KLH-primed syngeneic recipients.
4 Cell transfers are made 2–3 days after primary or simultaneous with secondary DNP-KLH challenge.
5 Splenic PFC responses are determined 3 days after secondary immunization. Alternatively, 10^6 carrier-primed spleen cells will suppress 10^7 DNP-KLH primed spleen cells *in vitro* when added at culture initiation.

Induction of KLH-specific suppressor factor

Procedure

1 Mice are immunized twice i.p. without adjuvant with 200 μl KLH at 2 week intervals.
2 Mice are sacrificed 2 weeks after second injection, their spleen and thymuses removed, tissues teased, washed twice in MEM (Eagle's minimum essential medium), and resuspended to 6×10^8 cells/ml. Cells are sonicated at 4 °C (UR-150 sonicator, Tomy Seiko Co. Ltd., Tokyo, Japan) followed by ultracentrifugation at 20 000 g for 1 h. Cell-free supernatants can be used immediately or stored at -80 °C until use.

TsF-producing T hybrids have been described that constitutively produce KLH-TsF [29] and can often be used instead of factor-containing lysates. KLH-specific TsF activity is usually measured *in vitro*. Extract equivalent to 1×10^7 carrier-primed cells is added to 10^7 cells on day 2 of Marbrook cultured DNP-KLH-primed spleen cells. DNP-specific PFC are enumerated in the haemolytic plaque assay 5 days after culture initiation. The KLH-TsF bears I-J determinants [42] and causes 50–80% suppression of the secondary anti-DNP PFC response.

Copolymer-specific (GAT/GT) suppressor cells and factors

Genes located in the I-region of the murine major histocompatibility complex (H-2) regulate specific immune responses to a number of antigens [45]. The most extensive studies of specific immune suppression in copolymer systems have used the synthetic copolymers of L-amino acids poly($\text{Glu}^{60}\text{Ala}^{30}\text{Tyr}^{10}$) (GAT) and poly($\text{Glu}^{50}\text{Tyr}^{50}$) (GT). The genetic basis of Ts induction to GAT and GT, the heterogeneity of Ts subpopulations, and the relative ease of induction and assay of specific Ts and TsF both *in vivo* and *in vitro* have been responsible for the extensive use of these copolymers. H-2^{a,b,d,k} strains respond to GAT both *in vivo* and *in vitro*; H-2^{p,q,s} haplotype strains are unresponsive [46–51]. GAT injection stimulates the development of Ts and TsF in non-responder haplotype mice [12,13,20,52]. Non-responders make anti-GAT PFC responses to the immunogenic form of GAT, GAT–MBSA (GAT coupled to methylated bovine serum albumin), indicating that these mice do not have genetically defective B cells. In contrast to GAT, most inbred strains of mice are non-responders to GT [14,48,53,54]. GT injection of H-2^{d,k,s} mice results in the development of GT-specific Ts and GT–TsF which suppress primary GT–MBSA PFC responses [14]. H-2^{a,b} mice are both non-responders and non-suppressors to GT [53]. H-2^b mice produce GT–TsF following

GT injection, although they cannot be suppressed by this factor [55,56]. In contrast, H-2^a mice are genetically incapable of producing GT–TsF following GT injection, although they develop specific second order Ts (Ts2) upon exposure to the appropriate GT–TsF [21,56]. Gene complementation between H-2^a and H-2^b non-suppressor parental strains circumvents parental genetic defects and leads to GT-suppressor F1 mice, which produce both GT-specific Ts and TsF [56].

Assay of GAT/GT responses

Non-responders make anti-GAT or anti-GT humoral responses following immunization with GAT– or GT–MBSA. Copolymers are commercially available from Sigma Chemical Corporation, St. Louis, MO; Vega Biochemicals, Tucson, AZ; or Miles Laboratories, Elkhart, IN. These poly-L-amino acids should be > 25 000 Da and be prepared by base-initiated polymerization of *N*-carboxyanhydrides; see Chapter 1.

Procedure

1 Copolymer stock solutions (10 mg/ml) are prepared by dissolving 250 mg copolymer in 5 ml 5% Na$_2$CO$_3$ (w/v in H$_2$O), with 20 ml saline added (final pH 9–11) for a final volume of 25 ml. The stock solutions are membrane filter sterilized (0.45 μm) and can be stored indefinitely at 4 °C.
2 MBSA-coupled forms of the copolymers are readily prepared. MBSA is available commercially from Sigma (A-1009) or can be easily synthesized by the method of Seuoka & Chang [57,58]. A membrane-filtered sterile stock solution of MBSA (5 mg dry weight/ml H$_2$O) is required. Copolymer–MBSA compounds are prepared by the dropwise addition of 8.0 ml of sterile 1 mg/ml (in PBS) copolymer solution into 5.6 ml sterile MBSA stock solution. The sterile components are reacted within a tissue culture hood in a sterile beaker with spin bar. The mixture is stirred (10–40 rev./min) for 20 min to allow maximum flocculation. Precipitates are washed four or five times at 800 *g* for 3 min in sterile plastic centrifuge tubes. A 50% coupling efficiency is usual. A 1.0 mg/ml stock solution is prepared by resuspending the precipitate to 4.0 ml with PBS.
3 Anti-copolymer responses can be induced either *in vivo* or *in vitro*. Mice are immunized i.p. with a single 100 μl PBS suspension containing 10 μg (10 μl stock solution) copolymer–MBSA together with Maalox (10 μl, aluminium–magnesium hydroxide gel: W.F. Roher, Ft. Washington, PA) and *Bordetella pertussis* (50 μl containing 2 × 10^9 killed organisms: Michigan Department of Public Health, Lansing, MI) as adjuvant. Ten micrograms (10 μl) sterile copolymer–MBSA suspension per culture well is an optimal immunogenic dose. Anti-GAT or anti-GT humoral immune responses are usually measured in the haemolytic plaque assay on day 7 (*in vivo*) or day 5 (*in vitro*) after immunization.

Copolymer-specific PFC responses are determined by an inhibition assay. GAT–SRBC are used as indicator cells for anti-GAT, anti-GT, or anti-poly-(Glu^{60}Ala^{40}) (GA) PFC responses. GAT is coupled to SRBC using chromium chloride (CrCl$_3$.6H$_2$O: Baker Chemical Corp, 1-1588). The original CrCl$_3$ technique [59] has been modified to couple GAT to SRBC [60].

Procedure

1 A solution of 10 mg/ml (w/v) CrCl$_3$ is prepared immediately before coupling. SRBC are washed in saline (do not use PBS!), as described above.
2 One millilitre of packed, washed SRBC and 1.0 ml of GAT stock solution are pipetted into a 50 ml centrifuge tube.
3 To this mixture is added 0.2 ml fresh CrCl$_3$ solution, and the reactants are gently mixed for 1 min. The quantity of CrCl$_3$ solution to be added must be determined empirically, depending upon the lot of GAT being used, and can vary from 0.1 to 1.0 ml.
4 The reaction is stopped by adding PBS, and the cells are washed three or four times in PBS by centrifugation. Adjust the cells to ~ 10% (v/v) for use in the PFC assay. GAT–SRBC should be prepared fresh on the day of plaque assay.
5 Four glass tubes containing agarose are set up in the 45 °C water bath (see above) for each experimental group. All tubes contain 0.3 ml agarose, 50 μl 1% FBS in HBSS, and GAT–SRBC as indicator cells.
6 Fifty microlitres of a 1:20 to 1:40 dilution (in HBSS) of the GAT stock solution is added as inhibitor to two of the four glass tubes.
7 Lymphocyte suspension (0.1 ml) is added to each well and the agarose–lymphocyte–indicator cell mixture is poured on to microscope slides. PFC are developed with rabbit anti-mouse Ig, complement is then added, and the PFC are counted.
8 The number of copolymer-specific PFC are determined by subtracting the number of PFC detected in the presence of inhibitor from the number of PFC detected with GAT–SRBC in the absence of inhibitor. Data are expressed as PFC per spleen or culture.

Induction of GAT/GT suppressor cells

GAT–Ts or GT–Ts are induced in H-2^{p,q,s} or H-2^{d,k,s} non-responder haplotype mice, respectively. Ts are induced *in vivo* by a single injection of GAT or GT in Maalox.

Procedure

1   A 100 μl suspension containing 1 μl GAT stock solution (10 mg/ml), 10 μl Maalox, and 89 μl saline is injected i.p. into GAT-suppressor haplotype mice. GT-suppressor haplotype mice receive a 100 μl injection, i.p., containing 10 μl GT stock solution (10 mg/ml), 10 μl Maalox, and 80 μl saline. GAT–Ts or GT-Ts can also be induced by incubating 10 μg sterile GAT or GT with $1-10 \times 10^6$ suppressor haplotype spleen cells under Mishell–Dutton type culture conditions. Splenic Thy-1, Lyt-2$^+$, I-J$^+$ Ts appear within 3 days [13,14].

2   These copolymer-specific Ts suppress the autologous GAT– or GT–MBSA PFC responses or can be transferred to a syngeneic animal or Mishell–Dutton culture. Ts can also be generated by copolymer-specific suppressor factors; see below.

3   Adult GAT-responder mice can be induced to produce GAT-Ts by the i.v. injection of GAT-coupled syngeneic spleen cells. Normal, untreated GAT responder mice are sacrificed, their spleens removed, and single-cell, erythrocyte-free lymphocyte (using Tris-NH$_4$Cl) suspensions are prepared. Washed spleen cells (4×10^8) are suspended in 1.5 ml GAT stock solution. To this mixture is added 250 μl (100 mg/ml saline) water-soluble carbodiimide HCl (Calbiochem-Behring, catalogue number 341006) and the suspension is incubated at 4 °C.

4   After 1 h incubation, cells are washed three times in HBSS. Injection of 10^7-10^8 GAT-coupled spleen cells i.v. induces the generation of GAT-specific Ts 3–5 days later.

Induction of GAT/GT suppressor factors

Procedure

1   Suppressor haplotype mice are injected i.p. in a mixture of copolymer and Maalox, as detailed in the paragraph above.

2   Three days later, the mice are sacrificed and their spleens and thymuses removed; tissues are teased into single-cell suspensions, washed twice in HBSS, and resuspended to a final concentration of 6×10^8 cells/ml in HBSS.

3   Cells are sonicated (Sonifier Cell Disruptor model W-104E, equipped with microtip, Branson Ultrasonics, Plainview, NY) by applying 50 W for 3 min, or until no intact cells are visible in the microscope.

4   The lysate is centrifuged (40 000 *g* for 45 min), and the resulting supernatant is collected and stored at -80 °C until use.

TsF-producing T hybrids have been described that constitutively produce GAT–TsF or GT–TsF [61,62] and often can be interchanged with factor-containing lysates. The TsF-containing lysates suppress GAT–MBSA or GT–MBSA responses *in vivo* or *in vitro*. Immune responses are suppressed *in vivo* by the i.v. injection of a 0.5 ml dilution (1 : 2 to 1 : 8) TsF-containing lysate. The GAT–MBSA or GT–MBSA (with adjuvant) responses of such immunized mice are suppressed immediately and for a period of several weeks thereafter. TsF-containing lysates are membrane filter sterilized and added at 1 : 200 to 1 : 3200 final concentration to Mishell–Dutton cultures containing the appropriate copolymer–MBSA suspension. Copolymer specific TsF used *in vitro* or *in vivo* at the indicated concentrations causes the generation of specific Ts within 3–5 days in the absence of copolymer–MBSA complexes. Mechanisms of these interactions are detailed elsewhere [21,63].

Idiotype-specific suppressor cells

Antigenic determinants reflecting conformation of antibody-combining sites are referred to as idiotypes (Id) [64,65]. The recent finding that B and T cells bear either cross-reactive Id or complementary anti-Id receptors [66,67] implies that Id functions both as a specific receptor for antigen and as a signal for Id–anti-Id interactions in immunologic activation and suppression. In fact, production of antibodies bearing Id or cross-reactive Id (CRI) can be specifically suppressed or elevated by injection with anti-Id antibody depending upon the Id system and the concentration as well as the isotype of the anti-Id antibody [65,67,68].

Representative experimental systems for suppression of Id-bearing antibody production include anti-phosphorylcholine (PC), anti-*p*-azophenylarsonate (Ar), anti-streptococcal A carbohydrate (A-CHO), and anti-4-hydroxy-3-nitrophenylacetyl (NP) systems (Table 78.1). For suppression of the major CRI of anti-Ar or anti-A-CHO antibodies, xenogeneic anti-Id antibodies are used following absorption with normal Ig. In addition, multiple antigenic stimulation was given after injections with anti-Id antibody [69,70]. In contrast, for suppression of the major Id of anti-PC and anti-NP antibodies, allogeneic anti-Id antibodies are used. Moreover, no deliberate antigenic stimulation is given for the latter system [66,68,71,72]. The Id suppression is generally compensated for by an increased production of antigen-specific antibodies lacking the suppressed Id [67,70]. However, suppression of

Table 78.1. Experimental schemes for the induction of idiotype suppression *in vivo*

	Antibody systems			
	Anti-Ar	Anti-A-CHO	Anti-PC	Anti-NP
Idiotypes	CRI	A5A	T15	NP[b] (B1–8)
% Antibody	20–70	60–70	>90	10–100
Recipient mice and age	A/J	A/J	BALB/c	C57BL/6
	8 weeks	6–8 weeks	1–3 days	10 weeks
Anti-Id source	Rabbit	Guinea-pig	A mice and hybridoma	Hybridoma
Antigen pre-treatment	2×	6×	None	None
Antigen	Ar-KLH	Group A streptococci	R36A/R36a pneumococci	NP-Fowl Ig
Total specific antibody	Normal	Normal	<10%	Normal
Ts specificity	Anti-CRI	Anti-A5A	Anti-T15	Anti-NP[b]
References	[32,70,73]	[67,69]	[66,71,72]	[68,74]

the major Id (T15Id) of anti-PC antibody renders the host completely tolerant to PC, with no apparent compensation for the suppressed Id [66,71,72]. The lack of compensation may be attributed to the exceptionally high degree of the T15Id dominance (>90%).

Id-suppressed animals demonstrate the lack of the suppressed Id-bearing B cells and the presence of Ts specific for the Id. The sequence of events leading to the generation of anti-idiotypic Ts in response to anti-Id antibody is presently undefined. Anti-Id antibody may induce Id-bearing antigen-specific Ts which subsequently generate Id-specific Ts [73]. However, concrete evidence that anti-Id antibody induces the Id-bearing antigen-specific Ts population has yet to be demonstrated, although such antibody elicits Th bearing the corresponding Id [66]. Therefore it is conceivable that anti-Id antibody stimulates corresponding Id-bearing Th which, in turn, induce anti-idiotypic Ts [74].

Assay of anti-PC-Id responses

In many experimental protocols, bacteria vaccine is used as an immunizing antigen to raise Id responses. For example, *Streptococcus pneumonia* strain R36a/R36A is used for the anti-PC response and group A streptococci; strain J17A4 is used to induce anti-A-CHO responses [66,67]. In addition, chemical conjugates of hapten to immunogenic carrier are also used, e.g. PC-KLH for anti-PC, Ar-KLH for anti-Ar, and NP-Fowl Ig for anti-NP responses (see also Table 78.1). The procedures for chemical coupling of hapten to carrier molecules are detailed in Chapter 3.

As an example, the PC system will be described in detail.

Procedure

1   Immunization of 8–10 week old BALB/c mice or their spleen cell cultures ($1.0–1.5 \times 10^7$ cells/ml) with rough strain pneumococci (*Streptococcus pneumoniae* R36a) results in a vigorous anti-PC response in 4 days. Between 1 and 10×10^8 formalin-killed R36a cells are injected i.v. in 0.2 ml saline for *in vivo* immunization, or $1–5 \times 10^6$ organisms in 30 μl culture medium are added to 1 ml Mishell–Dutton type cultures for *in vitro* immunizations. Viable seed cultures of both rough strain (R36a, #27336) and smooth strain (R36A, #11733) pneumococcus can be obtained from the American Type Culture Collection, Rocksville, MD. In order to prepare pneumococcal vaccine, seed bacteria are first grown in a small volume (50–100 ml) of sterile Columbia Broth or Brain Heart Infusion medium (Difco Laboratories, Detroit, MI; or BBL, Div. Beckton-Dickinson, Cockeysville, MD) at 37 °C for 1–2 days. Bacteria in exponential growth are then inoculated into 2000 ml of the same medium in a 4 l Erlenmeyer flask. After an 18–36 h incubation at 37 °C, the bacteria are centrifuged at 8000 *g* for 30 min and the pellet is resuspended in 200 ml saline containing 0.5% formalin for 1–2 h. The formalin-treated bacteria are washed three times with sterile saline and then adjusted to a 10% solution (v/v) for storage at 4–7 °C.

2   Specific antibody response is determined either by RIA as outlined above or by enumerating PFC. In order to prepare target SRBC, pneumococcal C-polysaccharide (PnC), extracted from R36A/R36a, is often used [66,71,72].

3   The C-polysaccharide is extracted according to the method of Liu & Gotschlich [75]. In a typical prep-

aration, R36a are exponentially grown in 4 l medium. After the bacteria are washed three times with saline, they are resuspended in 100 ml of a 0.1% sodium deoxycholate (Sigma, D-6750) in PBS solution. The suspended pellet is brought to pH 7.0 with 1 M NaOH, and is incubated at room temperature for 15 min. Two millilitres 2 M acetic acid are added to the mixture and the vessel containing this mixture is placed in a boiling water bath for 15–20 min to extract the C-polysaccharide. The heated mixture is centrifuged at 8000 g for 20 min and the resulting supernatant is mixed with 400 ml of 95% ethanol. The alcohol mixture is then placed overnight at −20 °C. For further purification, the precipitate in the chilled mixture is collected by centrifugation at 10 000–12 000 g for 20 min and resuspended in 30 ml distilled H_2O. The extract is then exhaustively dialysed against H_2O and lyophilized. The lyophilized PnC preparation is resuspended in saline to a 1 mg/ml (w/v) final concentration. Further removal of insoluble precipitates by centrifugation and digestion of DNA with DNase may be necessary, depending upon the preparation.

4   To coat SRBC with PnC, SRBC are washed three times with saline and the SRBC pellet is adjusted to 50% with saline (v/v). One hundred and fifty microlitres of freshly prepared CrCl$_3$ (1 mg/ml in saline) are added dropwise to 1.0 ml SRBC suspension. After a 10 min incubation at room temperature, 1.0 ml of a pre-titrated concentration of PnC (0.1–0.7 mg/ml) is slowly added. The mixture is incubated for 1 h at room temperature, and then stored in PBS as a 5% suspension for up to 3 weeks. The coating efficiency can be checked by either a spot haemolytic assay on a PnC–SRBC–agar slide (see 'Haemolytic plaque assay', page 78.3) using culture supernatants of IgM anti-PC producing hybridoma lines [72] or by haemagglutination with diluted (1:100–1:10 000) ascites fluid of the TEPC–15 plasmacytoma. PFC producing IgM anti-PC antibodies display clear, uniformly sized plaques. IgG and IgA plaques can be assayed after treatment with rabbit anti-mouse IgG or anti-IgA antisera, as detailed above.

Alternatively, *p*-diazonium phenylphosphorylcholine (DPPC) solution can be used to couple PC directly on to SRBC [76]. Commercially prepared DPPC is not yet available. However, DPPC can be prepared by reducing the amine of *p*-nitrophenylphosphorylcholine (Calibiochem-Behring Co., La Jolla, CA) and then diazotizing it with NaNO$_2$, as described by Chesebro & Metzger [77].

Id production is determined either by inhibition of ^{125}I-Id and anti-Id antibody reaction or by inhibition of plaque formation by PFC in the presence of anti-Id antibody. Both methods are frequently used, but the PFC assay is simple and convenient as long as one can prepare sensitive antigen-coated indicator cells. Fifty microlitres of a 1:20–1:100 dilution of anti-Id antiserum is used to inhibit anti-PC PFC similar to the method outlined above for copolymer systems. Anti-Id can be added either directly to the agarose–lymphocyte–indicator cell mixture or a further dilution of the anti-Id solution can be made (dilution is determined empirically) and poured into the slide tray recess before adding complement. The numbers of PFC developed in the presence and absence of anti-Id are compared to calculate the percentage of PC-specific PFC. Hapten specificity of PFC can be assessed by inhibiting anti-PC plaque formation of PnC-SRBC by the addition of 50 μl of 10 mM phosphorylcholine chloride (Sigma, P-0378) solution to the agarose–indicator cell mixture. Generally, >90% plaques induced by injection with R36a is PC-specific [78].

Induction of anti-Id suppressor cells

Conventionally, anti-Id Ts are induced in mice by injection with anti-Id antibody (Table 78.1). Injection(s) of antigen following the anti-Id antibody treatment generally enhances the level of anti-idiotypic Ts [69,70]. As illustrated in Table 78.1, age, genetic background and antigenic stimulation appear to play important roles in the generation of Id-specific Ts. In the PC system, injection of anti-Id (10–50 μl/animal) into neonates is necessary to induce such Ts; older animals are harder to suppress [71]. No subsequent antigen injection is required in the PC Id-suppression system. However, antigen may play an important role in the generation of PC-Ts, as PC is a cellular constituent of many gut microflora which may serve to continuously stimulate the immune system [79]. In addition, the Id assay involves co-culturing Ts (10^4–10^7 cells) with normal spleen cells (1–1.5 × 10^7 cells/culture) for 4 days in the presence of antigen. Therefore this brief *in vitro* exposure to antigen may be sufficient to activate the Ts population [72].

Recently, Id-specific Ts have been induced *in vivo* by injection of normal syngeneic recipients with either antigen-specific Ts or their products (TsF), (GAT- and GT-Ts and TsF) [62,80,81], Id-coupled syngeneic spleen cells [82] or Id-bearing myeloma or hybridoma proteins [83,84]. Similarly, Ts can be generated *in vitro* within 2–3 days by incubating normal spleen cells with antigen-specific Ts or TsF [21], antigen-Id complexes [85], or antigen plus anti-Id antibody [86]. Id-specific Ts appear to recognize Id-bearing Th (for T-dependent antigens) and/or B cells (T-independent antigens) and bear Lyt-2 and I-J antigenic markers [72,74,87].

As originally shown with antigen-specific Ts, the presence of anti-Id Ts was initially demonstrated by adoptive transfer [69,70]. Briefly, 2–3 × 10^7 spleen cells from Id-suppressed mice are injected into lightly (200 R) irradiated syngeneic recipients. At various times after transfer, the recipients are treated with the specific antigen before anti-Id Ts activity is measured. Different immunization schedules are used depending upon the Id system. For anti-A-CHO, recipients are immunized with six i.v. injections of antigen within 10 days, 6 weeks after the initial cell transfer [69]. However, in the anti-Ar system, the cell recipients are injected with Ar-KLH in complete Freund's adjuvant on days 2 and 9 after cell transfer [70]. The levels of specific antibody and Id production in sera are determined 5–12 days after the last antigen injection.

As *in vitro* culture techniques become better defined and manageable, more experiments are performed *in vitro*. In the PC system, graded numbers of spleen cells from neonatally anti-T15Id suppressed mice are cultured with normal spleen cells (1:1–1:4 ratios) for 4 days in the presence of R36a. Since volume and cell density significantly affect the anti-PC response *in vitro*, constant volume (1.0 ml) and cell density (not more than 2×10^7 cells/culture) are maintained by adding syngeneic, irradiated (3000 R), normal spleen cells as fillers [72]. For example, cultures containing 1×10^7 normal spleen cells and 1×10^7 spleen cells from Id-suppressed mice are incubated for 4 days in the presence of R36a. As a cell density and volume control, 1×10^7 irradiated normal spleen cells are added instead of Id-suppressed spleen cells. The Id specificity is determined by the inhibition of plaque formation using anti-Id antibody (see above). In addition to the stimulation of cultures with PC antigen, a minimum of one unrelated antigen is used to stimulate cultures to determine the specificity of the suppression. When various serological reagents (e.g. anti-Thy-1 and C) are used to characterize the Ts population, the cell number should be readjusted by making up the balance of lost (killed) cells with irradiated normal spleen cells.

Allotype-specific suppressor cells

Prenatal and/or neonatal exposure of rabbits [88] or mice [89,90] to anti-allotype antibodies chronically suppresses the production of that allotype in animals genetically predisposed to produce that allotype. Fetal exposure of $(Igh^a \times Igh^b)F_1$ animals to antibody specific for the IgG_{2a} allotype of Igh^a are suppressed in the production of the a but not the b allelic form of the IgG_{2a}. Some animals display a transient remission from suppression, although this episode is followed by a chronic suppression. Diminished allotype expression results from the presence of allotype-specific Ts whose target is an allotype-specific Th [91]. Allotype Ts bear Lyt-1^-,2^+ antigens and genetic markers of the H-2 I-J

subregion [92]. A similar form of chronic allotype suppression can be demonstrated by adoptive transfer of thymocytes from Igh^b immunized, Igh^a-producing BALB/c mice into irradiated Igh^b-producing C.B17 congenic mice [93].

Procedure

1 In order to induce chronic allotype suppression, BALB/c (Igh^a) females are immunized against IgG1b by injection of 10 μg IgG1b (in complete Freund's adjuvant) reactive to BALB/c H-2 antigen. After 2 weekly i.p. booster injections in a volume of 20 μl in saline, the high anti-IgG1b antibody titre is maintained by monthly injection.

2 These immunized BALB/c females are then mated with normal SJL (Igh^b) males to obtain (BALB/c × SJL)F1 offspring. About half the progeny do not produce IgG1b up to 6 months of age.

3 The production of IgG1b is estimated by either RIA using a ^{125}I-IgG1b probe (see Chapter 32 by Herzenberg) or IgG1b PFC responses to conventional antigens such as DNP–KLH or SRBC [89,90].

4 Allotype-specific Ts can be detected by a short-term adoptive transfer system using sublethally irradiated (600 R) BALB/c mice. Spleen cells (1×10^7) from allotype-suppressed mice previously primed with antigen (e.g. SRBC) are transferred i.v. into BALB/c recipients irradiated 18 h previously at the same time as immunization.

5 Seven days after the adoptive transfer and immunization, specific donor allotype-producing PFC are enumerated [91].

6 Alternatively, such allotype-specific Ts activity is demonstrated *in vitro* [94]. Spleen cells (3×10^6) from antigen-primed (4×10^8 SRBC, 2–5 months previously) (BALB/c × SJL)F1 non-suppressed mice are co-cultured for 1 week with 1×10^6 spleen cells from suppressed mice in the presence of SRBC.

Epitope-specific suppressor cells

Herzenberg *et al.* [95–97] (see Chapter 74 of this handbook) have recently described a phenomenon that they term epitope-specific suppression. Carrier priming has the paradoxical effect of limiting anti-hapten responses when the same animal is boosted one or more times with a hapten conjugated to the homologous carrier [95]. A strong suppression of the IgG antibody response to the hapten results. Suppressor T cells do not eliminate carrier-specific Th, and the anti-carrier response is unimpaired, suggesting that carrier-specific cells (Ts or Th?) induce hapten-specific Ts [96]. The epitope-specific system suggests an immunoregulatory pathway distinct from carrier- or idiotype-specific Ts. Although the epitope-specific suppression has been described for haptens [95,97] the same phenomena are applicable to other antigenic systems. BALB/c mice receiving a single i.p. injection of 10 μg GAT as GAT–MBSA in Maalox and *B. pertussis* as adjuvant make a good anti-GAT- and MBSA-specific PFC response, Table 78.2. Injection of these mice with GAT→GAT–MBSA does not significantly diminish the anti-GAT PFC response, but causes nearly 60% suppression of the anti-MBSA PFC response. Conversely, injection of BALB/c mice with MBSA, followed 7 days later with GAT–MBSA, suppresses nearly 80% of the anti-GAT PFC response, while the anti-MBSA PFC response is unaffected, Table 78.2. These data demonstrate that the phenomenon of 'epitope-specific' suppression is applicable to larger molecules containing more than a single epitope. For a detailed review of this subject, the reader is referred to Chapter 74 of this handbook.

Table 78.2. Evidence for MBSA, GAT–MBSA epitope-specific suppression in BALB/c

Treatment[a]		Antigen-specific PFC per spleen[b]	
Day 0	Day 7	GAT	MBSA
—	GAT/MP	$13\,400 \pm 5100$	NT[c]
—	GAT–MBSA/MP	$12\,900 \pm 1400$	$26\,600 \pm 1200$
GAT/MP	GAT–MBSA/MP	9600 ± 2600	$11\,100 \pm 1300$
MBSA/MP	GAT–MBSA/MP	2800 ± 2200	$28\,200 \pm 500$

[a] BALB/c mice (4 per group) were primed with 10 μg GAT or 10 μg MBSA in Maalox and 10^9 *B. pertussis* organisms as adjuvant. Seven days later (day 7), the mice received 10 μg GAT/MP or 10 μg GAT as GAT–MBSA/MP. M = Maalox, P = pertussis.
[b] Antigen-specific plaque forming cells per spleen were determined seven days after last injection (day 14). Underlining indicates significant (p = 0.01) suppression of the PFC response.
[c] Not tested.

Contrasuppressor cells

Gershon *et al.* [98,99] recently described a novel immunoregulatory system. The cells mediating this unique form of immunoregulation are Lyt-2+, I-J+ T cells bearing a high density of Thy-1 antigen were termed 'contrasuppressors' (Tcs). Contrasuppression augments immune responses by interfering with Ts function. The phenotype of the Tcs distinguishes it from Th. The I-J determinant on the Tcs is distinct

from I-J determinants found on Ts [100]. Tcs are found in normal unprimed Lyt-2 T cell populations and were originally as few as 2×10^5 unprimed T cells were found to inhibit suppression caused by 3×10^4 Lyt-2, SRBC-primed Ts. Contrasuppression can also be demonstrated in copolymer systems. Injection of GT non-suppressor C57BL/6 (B6) mice results in a strong (approximately 14 000 PFC $\times$/spleen) *in vivo* anti-GT PFC response, Table 78.3. Injection of these mice with an I-J^k-bearing monoclonal GT–TsF 3 days before GT–MBSA immunization has no inhibitory effect. If, however, B6 mice are treated with monoclonal anti-I-J^b antibody (WF9.1.4), which eliminates Tcs in B6 mice [100], then monoclonal GT–TsF suppresses >50% of the GT–MBSA PFC response. Injection with a monoclonal anti-I-J^b antibody (WF9.40.5) which does not affect Tcs function [100] does not allow suppression of B6 GT–MBSA PFC responses by GT–TsF, Table 78.3. The monoclonal anti-I-J^b antibodies are not reactive with I-J^k determinants found on the monoclonal GT–TsF [62]. These data indicate that Tcs may play a role in the regulation of immune responses in Ir gene-controlled copolymer systems, and may suggest a possible explanation for the occurrence of non-suppressor, non-responder (e.g. B6) mice.

Table 78.3. Elimination of contrasuppression allows suppression of non-responder C57BL/6 mice

Anti-I-J[b] treatment[a]	Factor treatment[b]	Antigen[c]	% Control GT–MBSA PFC per spleen[d]
Day 0	Day 5	Day 8	Day 15
		GT–MBSA	100
	I-J^k GT–TsF	GT–MBSA	113
WF9.1.4	I-J^k GT–TsF	GT–MBSA	45
WF9.40.5	I-J^k GT–TsF	GT–MBSA	114

[a] Five hundred microlitres monoclonal anti-I-J^b-containing ascites diluted 1:10 in HBSS were injected i.v. WF9.1.4 and WF9.40.5 indicate different anti-I-J^b-secreting hybridoma clones derived from the same fusion [62].
[b] Five hundred microlitres monoclonal GT–TsF$_1$ (WF11.3A.1)-containing culture supernatant diluted 1:10 in HBSS were injected i.v. The I-J^k, monoclonal GT–TsF$_1$ was derived from the fusion of GT-primed B10.BR (H-2^k) spleen cells with the BW5147 thymoma [62].
[c] Ten micrograms GT, as GT–MBSA emulsified in complete Freund's adjuvant in a total volume of 0.2 ml, was injected i.p.
[d] PFC responses were determined 7 days after GT–MBSA immunization.

Media and buffers

Hank's balanced salt solution (HBSS)

HBSS is prepared either from commercial powdered tissue culture medium (GIBCO 450–1200) or from individual salts. Stock solution is maintained as a 5× sterile stock solution and does not contain sodium bicarbonate. The working solution does not require 5% CO_2 in air.

1 Preparation from commercial powder. Add contents of a 50 l package to 10 l of tissue-culture-grade distilled water. When all powder is dissolved proceed to step 3.

2 Preparation from individual chemicals. Dissolve in order:

KCl, 20.00 g
KH_2PO_4, 3.00 g
NaCl, 400.00 g
Na_2HPO_4, 2.40 g
Glucose, 50.00 g
$MgSO_4 \cdot 7H_2O$, 9.99 g
$CaCl_2$, 7.00 g
Phenol red, 0.50 g
Distilled H_2O to 10.0 l.

When all chemicals are dissolved, proceed to step 3.

3 Adjust 5× stock solution to pH 6.70–6.72 with NaOH, which upon dilution with tissue-culture-grade distilled H_2O will yield a pH 7.2 1× working solution. Use a membrane filter (0.22 μm to sterilize 5× stock solution. Store at 4 °C.

4 To make a 1× working solution admix 1 part 5× HBSS to 4 parts distilled H_2O.

Complement diluent

This is a 1× working solution and can be stored at 4 °C for several months.

NaCl, 34.00 g
$CaCl_2$, 0.073 g
$MgCl_2 \cdot 6H_2O$, 0.407 g
Na_2HPO_4, 3.060 g
KH_2PO_4, 0.696 g
Distilled H_2O to 4.0 l

Adjust to pH 7.2 ± 0.1 with HCl or NaOH.

Phosphate-buffered saline (PBS)

A 10× stock solution can be kept at room temperature for many months without contaminant microbial growth.

Na_2HPO_4, 153.30 g
$NaH_2PO_4 \cdot H_2O$, 57.96 g

NaCl, 1227.24 g
Distilled H_2O to 15.0 l

Adjust 10× stock solution to pH 6.5 ± 0.1, which upon dilution with tissue-culture-grade distilled H_2O will yield a pH 7.2 ± 0.1 1× working solution. Working solution (1×) 0.01 M-PO_4 + 0.14 M-NaCl = 0.15 M.

Mishell–Dutton culture medium

Most media components are obtainable from Whittaker M.A. Bioproducts (MAB), Baltimore, MD; catalogue numbers are in parentheses below. All solutions are sterile.

MEM, Eagle (MAB 12-126), 100.0 ml
MEM non-essential amino acids (100×, MAB 13-606), 1.0 ml
L-Glutamine (200 mM, MAB 17-605), 1.0 ml
Sodium pyruvate (100 mM, MAB 13-115), 1.0 ml
Penicillin-streptomycin (5000 U/5000 mg, MAB 17-603), 1.0 ml
FBS (selected for Mishell–Dutton cultures; see text), 10.0 ml
$NaHCO_3$ (7.5% solution in H_2O), 4.0 ml
2-Mercaptoethanol (1 M, Sigma M-6250), 5.0 μl

Mishell–Dutton nutritional cocktail

HBSS without $NaHCO_3$ (1×; see above), 25.0 ml
Dextrose (500 mg/ml), 0.5 ml
MEM essential amino acids (50×, MAB 13-606), 1.0 ml
MEM non-essential amino acids (100×, MAB 13-606), 0.5 ml
L-Glutamine (200 mM, MAB 17-605), 0.5 ml
$NaHCO_3$ (7.5% solution in H_2O), 2.0 ml

Mishell–Dutton feeding mixture

Mix equal parts FBS and Mishell–Dutton nutritional cocktail. Feed cultures 2 drops per well from a Pasteur pipette (~50 μl) daily.

References

1 CLAMAN H., CHAPERON E. & TRIPLETT R. (1966) Thymus-marrow cell combinations. Synergism in antibody production. *Proc. Soc. exp. Biol. Med.* **122,** 1167.
2 MILLER J. (1961) Immunological function of the thymus. *Lancet,* **ii,** 748.
3 MILLER J. (1962) Effect of neonatal thymectomy on the immunological responsiveness of the mouse. *Proc. R. Soc.* Series B, **156,** 415.
4 MITCHELL G.F. & MILLER J.F.A.P. (1968) Cell to cell interaction in the immune response. (II) The source of

hemolysin-forming cells in irradiated mice given bone marrow and thymus or thoracic duct lymphocytes. *J. exp. Med.* **128**, 821.

5 MILLER J.F.A.P. & MITCHELL G.F. (1968) Cell to cell interaction in the immune response. (I) Hemolysin-forming cells in neonatally thymectomized mice reconstituted with thymus or thoracic duct lymphocytes. *J. exp. Med.* **128**, 801.

6 GERSHON R. & KONDO K. (1971) Antigenic competition between heterologous erythrocytes. (I) Thymic dependency. *J. Immunol.* **106**, 1524.

7 GERSHON R. & KONDO K. (1972) Degeneracy of the immune response to sheep red cells. Thymic dependency. *Immunology*, **23**, 335.

8 GERSHON R. & KONDO K. (1972) Degeneracy of the immune response to sheep red cells. *Immunology*, **23**, 321.

9 CANTOR H. & BOYSE E. (1975) Functional subclasses of T lymphocytes bearing different Ly antigens. (I) The generation of functionally distinct T-cell subclasses is a differentiative process independent of antigen. *J. exp. Med.* **141**, 1376.

10 CANTOR H. & BOYSE E. (1975) Functional subclasses of T lymphocytes bearing different Ly antigens. (II) Co-operation between subclasses of Ly^+ cells in the generation of killer activity. *J. exp. Med.* **141**, 1390.

11 TADA T. & TAKEMORI T. (1974) Selective roles of thymus-derived lymphocytes in the antibody response. (I) Differential suppressive effect of carrier primed T cells on hapten-specific IgM and IgG antibody responses. *J. exp. Med.* **140**, 239.

12 KAPP J., PIERCE C. & BENACERRAF B. (1974) Genetic control of immune responses *in vitro*. (III) Tolerogenic properties of the terpolymer L-glutamic acid[60]-L-alanine[30]-L-tyrosine[10] (GAT) for spleen cells from non-responder (H-2[S] and H-2[q]) mice. *J. exp. Med.* **140**, 172.

13 KAPP J., PIERCE C. & BENACERRAF B. (1974) Genetic control of immune responses *in vitro*. (V) Stimulation of suppressor T cells in nonresponder mice by the terpolymer L-glutamic acid[60]-L-alanine[30]-L-tyrosine[10] (GAT). *J. exp. Med.* **140**, 648.

14 DEBRE P., KAPP J. & BENACERRAF B. (1975) Genetic control of specific immune suppression. (I) Experimental conditions for the stimulation of suppressor cells by the copolymer L-glutamic acid[50]-L-tyrosine[50] (GT) in nonresponder BALB/c mice. *J. exp. Med.* **142**, 1436.

15 PIERCE C. & KAPP J. (1976) Regulation of immune responses by suppressor T cells. In *Contemporary Topics in Immunobiology*, Vol. 5, (ed. Wiegle W.O.), p. 91. Plenum, New York.

16 RICH R. & PIERCE C. (1973) Biological expressions of lymphocyte activation. (II) Generation of a population of thymus-derived suppressor lymphocytes. *J. exp. Med.* **137**, 649.

17 DUTTON R. (1972) Inhibitory and stimulatory effects of concanavalin A on the response of mouse spleen cells suspensions to antigen. (I) Characterization of the inhibitory cell activity. *J. exp. Med.* **136**, 1445.

18 TAKEMORI T. & TADA T. (1975) Properties of the antigen-specific suppressive T-cell factor in the regulation of antibody response of the mouse. (I) *In vitro* activity and immunochemical characterizations. *J. exp. Med.* **142**, 1241.

19 TANIGUCHI M., HAYAKAWA K. & TADA T. (1976) Properties of the antigen-specific suppressive T cell factor in the regulation of antibody response of the mouse. (II) *In vitro* activity and evidence for the I region gene product. *J. Immunol.* **116**, 542.

20 KAPP J., PIERCE C., DE LA CROIX F. & BENACERRAF B. (1976) Immunosuppressive factor(s) extracted from lymphoid cells of nonresponder mice primed with L-glutamic acid[60]-L-alanine[30]-L-tyrosine[10] (GAT). (I) Activity and antigenic specificity. *J. Immunol.* **116**, 305.

21 WALTENBAUGH C., THEZE J., KAPP J. & BENACERRAF B. (1977) Immunosuppressive factor(s) specific for L-glutamic acid[50]-L-tyrosine[50] (GT). (III) Generation of suppressor T cells by a suppressive extract derived from GT-primed lymphoid cells. *J. exp. Med.* **146**, 970.

22 WALTENBAUGH C., THEZE J., DORF M. & BENACERRAF B. (1977) Immunosuppressive factor(s) specific for L-glutamic acid[50]-L-tyrosine[50] (GT). (I) Production, characterization, and lack of H-2 restriction for activity in recipient strain. *J. Immunol.* **118**, 2073.

23 JERNE N., NORDIN A. & HENRY C. (1963) The agar plaque technique for recognizing antibody-producing cells. In *Cell Bound Antibodies*, (eds. Amos B. & Koprowski H.), p. 109. Wistar Inst. Press.

24 JERNE N., HENRY C., NORDIN A., FUJI H., KOROSS A. & LEFKOVITS I. (1974) Plaque forming cells: methodology and theory. *Transplant. Rev.* **18**, 130.

25 MISHELL R. & DUTTON R. (1967) Immunization of dissociated spleen cell cultures from normal mice. *J. exp. Med.* **126**, 423.

26 DUTTON R. & MISHELL R. (1967) Cell populations and cell proliferation in the *in vitro* response of normal mouse spleen to heterologous erythrocytes. *J. exp. Med.* **126**, 443.

27 MISHELL B.B. & SHIIGI S.M. (1980) *Selected methods in cellular immunology*. W.H. Freeman and Co., San Francisco.

28 MARBROOK J. (1967) Primary immune response in cultures of spleen cells. *Lancet*, **ii**, 1279.

29 TADA T., TANIGUCHI M., OKUMURA K., HAYAKAWA K., HIRAMATSU K. & SUZUKI G. (1981) Ia antigens on T-cell factors produced by hybridomas. In *Immunobiology of the Major Histocompatibility Complex*, p. 69. Karger, Basel.

30 TANIGUCHI M., TADA T. & TOKUHISA T. (1976) Properties of the antigen-specific suppressive T-cell factor in the regulation of antibody response of the mouse. (III) Dual gene control of the T-cell-mediated suppression of the antibody response. *J. exp. Med.* **144**, 20.

31 TOKUHISA T., TANIGUCHI M., OKUMURA K. & TADA T. (1978) An antigen-specific I region gene product that augments the antibody response. *J. Immunol.* **120**, 414.

32 HART D.A., WANG A.-L., PAWLAK L.L. & NISONOFF A. (1972) Suppression of idiotypic specificities in adult mice by administration of antiidiotypic antibody. *J. exp. Med.* **135**, 1293.

33 KIM B.S. & BENEWICZ B.J. (1980) The lack of compensatory increases of cells producing anti-phosphorylcholine antibodies bearing other idiotypes in TEPC–15 idiotype-

suppressed inbred and outbred mice. *Eur. J. Immunol.* **10**, 171.

34 RICH R. & PIERCE C. (1973) Biological expressions of lymphocyte activation. (I) Effects of phytomitogens on antibody synthesis *in vitro. J. exp. Med.* **137**, 205.

35 JACOBS D. (1975) Effects of Concanavalin A on the *in vitro* responses of mouse spleen cells to T-dependent and T-independent antigens. *J. Immunol.* **114**, 365.

36 JANDINSKI J., CANTOR H., TADAKUMA T., PEAVY D. & PIERCE C. (1976) Separation of helper T cells from suppressor T cells expressing different Ly components. (I) Polyclonal activation: suppressor and helper activities are inherent properties of distinct T-cell subclasses. *J. exp. Med.* **143**, 1382.

37 PEAVY D. & PIERCE C. (1974) Cell-mediated immune responses *in vitro.* (I) Suppression of the generation of cytotoxic lymphocytes by Concanavalin A and Concanavalin A-activated spleen cells. *J. exp. Med.* **140**, 356.

38 RICH R. & PIERCE C. (1974) Biological expression of lymphocyte activation. (III) Suppression of plaque-forming cell responses *in vitro* by supernatant fluids from Concanavalin A-activated spleen cell cultures. *J. Immunol.* **112**, 1360.

39 EARDLEY D.D. & GERSHON R.K. (1976) Induction of specific suppressor T cells *in vitro. J. Immunol.* **117**, 313.

40 EARDLEY D.D., SHEN F.W., CONE R.E. & GERSHON R.K. (1979) Antigen-binding T cells: dose response and kinetics studies on the development of different subsets. *J. Immunol.* **122**, 140.

41 YAMAUCHI K., CHAO N., MURPHY D.B. & GERSHON R.K. (1982) Molecular composition of an antigen-specific, Ly-1 suppressor inducer factor. One molecule binds antigen and is I-J$^-$; another is I-J$^+$, does not bind antigen, and imparts an Igh-variable region-linked restriction. *J. exp. Med.* **155**, 655.

42 TADA T., TANIGUCHI M. & DAVID C. (1976) Properties of the antigen-specific suppressive T-cell factor in the regulation of antibody response of the mouse. (IV) Special subregion assignment of the gene(s) that codes for the suppressive T-cell factor in the *H-2* histocompatibility complex. *J. exp. Med.* **144**, 713.

43 EISEN H.N., BELMAN S. & CARSTEN M.E. (1953) The reaction of 2,4-dinitrobenzenesulfonic acid with free amino group proteins. *J. Am. Chem. Soc.* **75**, 4583.

44 RITTENBERG M. & PRATT K. (1969) Antitrinitrophenyl (TNP) plaque assay. Primary response of Balb/c mice to soluble and particulate immunogen. *Proc. Soc. exp. Biol. Med.* **132**, 575.

45 BENACERRAF B. & MCDEVITT H. (1972) Histocompatibility-linked immune response genes. *Science*, **175**, 273.

46 PINCHUCK P. & MAURER P. (1965) Antigenicity of polypeptides (poly alpha amino acids). (XV) Studies on the immunogenicity of synthetic polypeptides in mice. *J. exp. Med.* **122**, 665.

47 MARTIN W., MAURER P. & BENACERRAF B. (1971) Genetic control of immune responsiveness to a glutamic acid, alanine, tyrosine copolymer in mice. (I) Linkage of responsiveness to H-2 genotype. *J. Immunol.* **107**, 715.

48 MAURER P. (1964) Use of synthetic polymers of amino acids to study the basis of antigenicity. *Prog. Allergy*, **8**, 1.

49 PINCHUCK P. & MAURER P. (1965) Antigenicity of polypeptides (poly amino acids). (XVI) Genetic control of immunogenicity of synthetic polypeptides in mice. *J. exp. Med.* **122**, 673.

50 PIERCE C. & KAPP J. (1977) L-Glutamic acid^{60}-L-alanine^{40}-L-tyrosine^{10} (GAT): a probe for regulatory mechanisms in antibody responses. In *Immunobiology of Proteins and Peptides I*, (eds. Atassi M.Z. & Stavitsky A.B.), p. 419. Plenum Press, New York.

51 KAPP J., PIERCE C. & BENACERRAF B. (1973) Genetic control of immune responses *in vitro.* (I) Development of primary and secondary plaque-forming cell responses to the random terpolymer L-glutamic acid^{60}-L-alanine^{30}-L-tyrosine^{10} (GAT) by mouse spleen cells *in vitro. J. exp. Med.* **138**, 1107.

52 GERSHON R., MAURER P. & MERRYMAN C. (1973) A cellular basis for genetically controlled immunologic unresponsiveness in mice: tolerance induction in T-cells. *Proc. natn. Acad. Sci. U.S.A.* **70**, 250.

53 DEBRE P., KAPP J., DORF M. & BENACERRAF B. (1975) Genetic control of specific immune suppression. (II) H-2-linked dominant genetic control of immune suppression by the random copolymer L-glutamic acid^{50}-L-tyrosine^{50} (GT). *J. exp. Med.* **142**, 1447.

54 LEI H.-Y., MELVOLD R., MILLER S. & WALTENBAUGH C. (1982) Gain/loss of poly(Glu^{50}Tyr^{50})/poly(Glu^{60}-Ala^{30}Tyr^{10}) responsiveness in the *bm12* mutant strain. *J. exp. Med.* **156**, 596.

55 GERMAIN R., WALTENBAUGH C. & BENACERRAF B. (1980) Antigen-specific T cell-mediated suppression. (V) H-2-linked genetic control of distinct antigen-specific defects in the production and activity of L-glutamic acid^{50}-L-tyrosine^{50} suppressor factor. *J. exp. Med.* **151**, 1245.

56 LEI H.-Y., DORF M. & WALTENBAUGH C. (1982) Regulation of immune responses by I-J gene products. (II) Presence of both I-J^b and I-J^k suppressor factors in (nonsuppressor × nonsuppressor) F$_1$ mice. *J. exp. Med.* **155**, 955.

57 SUEOKA N. & CHENG T.-Y. (1962) Fractionation of Nucleic acids with the methylated albumin column. *J. Mol. Biol.* **4**, 161.

58 WILLIAMS C.A. & CHASE M.W. (1967) *Methods in Immunology and Immunochemistry. Vol. I. Preparation of Antigens and Antibodies.* Academic Press, New York.

59 GOLD E.R. & FUDENBERG H.H. (1967) Chromic chloride: a coupling reagent for passive hemagglutination reactions. *J. Immunol.* **99**, 859.

60 NATHAN C., MURRAY H. & COHN Z. (1980) The macrophage as an effector cell. *New Engl. J. Med.* **303**, 622.

61 KAPP, J.A., ARANEO B.A. & CLEVINGER B.L. (1980) Suppression of antibody and T cell proliferative responses to L-glutamic acid^{60}-L-alanine^{30}-L-tyrosine^{10} by a specific monoclonal T cell factor. *J. exp. Med.* **152**, 235.

62 WALTENBAUGH C. (1981) Regulation of immune responses by I-J gene products. (I) Production and characterization of anti-I-J monoclonal antibodies. *J. exp. Med.* **154**, 1570.

63 GERMAIN R. & BENACERRAF B. (1981) A single major

pathway of T-lymphocyte interactions in antigen-specific immune suppression. *Scand. J. Immunol.* **13**, 1.

64 OUDIN J. & MICHEL M. (1963) A new form of allotypy of rabbit gammaglobulins apparently correlated with antibody function and specificity. *C.r. hebd. Séanc. Acad. Sci.* **257**, 805.

65 KUNKEL H.G., MANNIK M. & WILLIAMS R.C. (1963) Individual antigenic specificities of isolated antibodies. *Science*, **140**, 1218.

66 COSENZA H., JULIUS M.H. & AUGUSTIN A.A. (1977) Idiotypes as variable region markers: analogies between receptors on phosphorylcholine-specific T and B lymphocytes. *Immunol. Revs.* **34**, 3.

67 EICHMANN K. (1978) Expression and function of idiotypes on lymphocytes. *Adv. Immunol.* **26**, 195.

68 KELSO G., RETH M. & RAJEWSKY K. (1980) Control of idiotype expression by monoclonal anti-idiotype antibodies. *Immunol. Revs.* **52**, 75.

69 EICHMANN K. (1975) Idiotype suppression. (II) Amplification of a suppressor T cell with anti-idiotypic activity. *Eur. J. Immunol.* **5**, 511.

70 NISONOFF A. & BANGASSER S.A. (1975) Immunological suppression of idiotypic specificities. *Transplant. Rev.* **27**, 100–134.

71 STRAYER D.S., COSENZA H., LEE W., ROWLEY D.A. & KÖHLER H. (1974) Neonatal tolerance induced by antibody against antigen-specific receptor. *Science*, **186**, 640.

72 KIM B.S. & GREENBERG J.A. (1981) Mechanisms of idiotype suppression. (IV) Functional neutralization in mixtures of idiotype-specific suppressor and hapten-specific suppressor T cells. *J. exp. Med.* **154**, 809.

73 HIRAI Y. & NISONOFF A. (1980) Selective suppression of the major idiotypic component of an anti-hapten response by soluble T cell-derived factors with idiotypic or anti-idiotypic receptors. *J. exp. Med.* **151**, 1213.

74 MINAMI M., AOKI I., HONJI N., WALTENBAUGH C. & DORF M. (1983) The role of I-J and Igh determinants on T1-derived suppressor factor in controlling restriction specificity. *J. exp. Med.* **158**, 1428.

75 LIU T. & GOTSCHLICH E.C. (1968) The chemical composition of pneumococcal C-polysaccharide. *J. Biol. Chem.* **238**, 1928.

76 CLAFLIN J.L., LIEBERMAN R. & DAVIE J.M. (1974) Clonal nature of the immune response to phosphorylcholine. (I) Specificity, class, and idiotype of phosphorylcholine-binding receptors on lymphoid cells. *J. exp. Med.* **139**, 58.

77 CHESEBRO B. & METZGER H. (1972) Affinity labeling of a phosphorylcholine binding mouse myeloma protein. *Biochemistry*, **11**, 766.

78 COZENZA H. & KÖHLER H. (1972) Specific suppression of the antibody response by antibodies to receptors. *Proc. natn. Acad. Sci. U.S.A.* **69**, 2701.

79 POTTER M. (1971) Antigen-binding myeloma proteins in mice. *Ann. N.Y. Acad. Sci.* **190**, 306.

80 SY M.-S., DIETZ M.H., GERMAIN R.N., BENACERRAF B. & GREENE M.I. (1980) Antigen- and receptor-driven regulatory mechanisms. (IV) Idiotype-bearing I-J+ suppressor T cell factors induce second-order suppressor T

cells which express anti-idiotypic receptors. *J. exp. Med.* **151**, 1183.

81 WEINBERGER J., GERMAIN R.N., BENACERRAF B. & DORF M.E. (1980) Hapten-specific T cell responses to 4-hydroxy-3-nitro-phenyl acetyl. (V) Role of idiotypes in the suppressor pathway. *J. exp. Med.* **152**, 161.

82 SY M.-S., BACH B.A., BROWN A., NISONOFF A., BENACERRAF B. & GREENE M.I. (1979) Antigen- and receptor-driven regulatory mechanisms. (II) Induction of suppressor T cells with idiotype-coupled syngeneic spleen cells. *J. exp. Med.* **150**, 1229.

83 ROHRER J.W. & LYNCH R.G. (1978) Antigen-specific regulation of myeloma cell differentiation *in vivo* by carrier-specific T cell factors and macrophages. *J. Immunol.* **121**, 1066.

84 ABBAS A.K., BURAKOFF S.J., GEFTER M.L. & GREENE M.I. (1980) T lymphocyte-mediated suppression of myeloma function *in vitro*. (III) Regulation of antibody production in hybrid myeloma cells by T lymphocytes. *J. exp. Med.* **152**, 969.

85 CAULFIELD M.J., LUCE K.J., PROFFITT M.R. & CERNY J. (1983) Induction of idiotype-specific suppressor T cells with antigen/antibody complexes. *J. exp. Med.* **157**, 1713.

86 KIM B.S. (1979) Mechanisms of idiotype suppression. (I) *In vitro* generation of idiotype-specific suppressor T cells by anti-idiotype antibodies and specific antigen. *J. exp. Med.* **149**, 1371.

87 GREENE M.I., SY M.-S., NISONOFF A. & BENACERRAF B. (1980) The genetic and cellular basis of antigen and receptor stimulated regulation. *Mol. Immunol.* **17**, 857.

88 DRAY S. (1979) Immunoglobulin allotype suppression in rabbits. *Ann. Immunol.* (Paris), **130**, 481.

89 JACOBSON E.B. & HERZENBERG I.A. (1972) Active suppression of immunoglobulin synthesis. (I) Chronic suppression after perinatal exposure to maternal antibody to paternal allotype in (SJL × BALB/c)F1 mice. *J. exp. Med.* **135**, 1151.

90 JACOBSON E.B., HERZENBERG L.A., RIBLET R. & HERZENBERG L.A. (1972) Active suppression of immunoglobulin synthesis. (II) Transfer of suppressing factor with spleen cells. *J. exp. Med.* **135**, 1163.

91 HERZENBERG L.A., OKUMURA K., CANTOR H., SATO V.L., SHEN F.-W., BOYSE E.A. & HERZENBERG L.A. (1976) T-cell regulation of antibody responses: demonstration of allotype-specific helper T cells and their specific removal by suppressor T cells. *J. exp. Med.* **144**, 330.

92 MURPHY D., HERZENBERG L., OKUMURA K., HERZENBERG L. & McDEVITT H. (1976) A new I subregion (I-J) marked by a locus (Ia-4) controlling surface determinants on suppressor T lymphocytes. *J. exp. Med.* **144**, 699.

93 BOSMA M.J. & BOSMA G.C. (1976) Chronic suppression of immunoglobulin allotype. *Nature*, **259**, 313.

94 JACOBSON E.B. (1963) *In vitro* studies of allotype suppression in mice. *Eur. J. Immunol.* **3**, 619.

95 HERZENBERG L.A., TOKUHISA T. & HERZENBERG L.A. (1980) Carrier-priming leads to hapten-specific suppression. *Nature*, **285**, 664.

96 HERZENBERG L.A. (1983) Allotype suppression and epitope-specific regulation. *Immunol. Today*, **4**, 113.

97 HERZENBERG L.A. & TOKUHISA T. (1982) Epitope-specific regulation. (I) Carrier-specific induction of suppression for IgG anti-hapten antibody responses. *J. exp. Med.* **155**, 1730.

98 GERSHON R.K., EARDLEY D.D., DURUM S., GREEN D.R., SHEN F.-W., YAMAUCHI K., CANTOR H. & MURPHY D.B. (1981) Contrasuppression. A novel immunoregulatory activity. *J. exp. Med.* **153**, 1533.

99 YAMAUCHI K., GREEN D.R., EARDLEY D.D., MURPHY D.B. & GERSHON R.K. (1981) Immunoregulatory circuits that modulate responsiveness to suppressor cell signals. Failure of B10 mice to respond to suppressor factors can be overcome by quenching the contrasuppressor circuit. *J. exp. Med.* **153**, 1547.

100 GREEN D.R., CHUE B. & GERSHON R.K. (1983) Discrimination of 2 types of suppressor T cells by cell surface phenotype and function: the ability to regulate the contrasuppressor circuit. *J. Mol. cell. Immunol.* **1**, 19.

Chapter 79
Contrasuppressor T cells: a practical guide to the identification of contrasuppressive effects in immunoregulatory systems

D. R. GREEN

The basic immunoregulatory T cell circuit in mice, 79.1
Nature of observations, 79.1

Approaches to the discrimination of contrasuppression, 79.2

Conclusion: contrasuppression in immunoregulation, 79.7

Contrasuppression is an immunoregulatory T cell activity which functions to interfere with suppressor cell signals. Contrasuppressor activity has been observed in cultures of *in vitro* educated suppressor cells [1], in regulatory T cell factors [2], in the spleens of hyperimmune mice [3], and in the Peyer's patch of the gut associated lymphoid tissue [4]. It has been implicated in contact sensitivity [5] and in the immune response to malaria [6]. Contrasuppressor effector cells have been generated by culturing spleen cells from neonatal animals [7], auto-immune animals [8], and old animals [6]. Finally, they can be generated in cultures of normal adult spleen cells if these have been treated with a reagent (F7D5) which removes a subset of splenic T cells [9]. Several potential examples of contrasuppression exist in man. All of this will be discussed in more detail.

The purpose of this review is not so much to consider all that is known about contrasuppression, but rather to act as a guide to the methodology which may be used to elucidate the role played by this activity in any given system. Examples are used throughout in an attempt to illustrate the practicality of each method.

The basic immunoregulatory T cell circuit in mice

The contrasuppressor T cell circuit was elucidated by many of the methods to be discussed in the following sections. The basic approach employed was that of identifying unique profiles of antigenic surface markers and correlating these with a unique function. The use of this strategy in the study of regulatory circuits has been reviewed in detail [10].

The contrasuppressor circuit is shown schematically in Fig. 79.1. The contrasuppressor inducer cell is an I-J$^+$, Ly-2 T cell [1]. It acts via a cell-free factor [2]

through a contrasuppressor transducer cell, which is an I-J$^+$, Ly-1,2 T cell [1,2]. Without the transducer cell neither the inducer cell nor its factor have an effect.

The contrasuppressor effector cell, once generated, can function without the transducer cell. The effector cell is an I-J$^+$, Ly-1 T cell which adheres to the *Vicia villosa* lectin. This cell renders helper T cells resistant to suppressor cell signals [3,7].

There is no evidence that contrasuppressor cells inactivate suppressor cells. In fact, it is postulated that in the presence of contrasuppression, suppressor cells produce increased quantities of suppressor factors [3]. The contrasuppressive effect appears to occur at the target of the suppressor cell signal, interfering with suppression and rendering the target resistant to subsequent suppressive signals [3,7].

With this basic circuit in mind, it is possible to begin the consideration of how to identify contrasuppressive effects.

Nature of observations

The basic function of the contrasuppressor circuit is to interfere with suppressor cell signals. Any system involving the loss of suppressor cell activity is ripe for investigation of contrasuppressive effects. Similarly, the uncovering of 'covert' suppression [11] by the removal of other cells suggests a potential contrasuppressive phenomenon. A simple test is to ask whether suppression or its absence is the dominant activity.

When spleen cells from adult mice are cultured for several days, potent suppressor cells appear. Spleen cells from one-week-old mice treated in an identical manner do not produce such suppression [12]. It was found that addition of these non-suppressive pre-cultured neonatal cells to primary anti-SRBC cultures containing suppressor cells or factors caused the

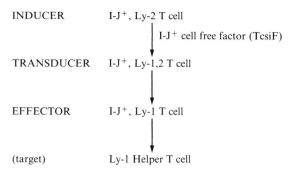

INDUCER   I-J$^+$, Ly-2 T cell

                  I-J$^+$ cell free factor (TcsiF)

TRANSDUCER   I-J$^+$, Ly-1,2 T cell

EFFECTOR   I-J$^+$, Ly-1 T cell

(target)   Ly-1 Helper T cell

Fig. 79.1. The contrasuppressor circuit.

suppression to be ignored, i.e. the absence of suppressive activity in the pre-cultured neonatal spleen cells was dominant [7]. This phenomenon has been examined by several methods discussed below and shown to be a prime example of contrasuppression.

Other examples of the basic function (interference with suppression) have not been examined in as much detail. Ly-2 suppressor T cells specific for the SIII pneumococcal polysaccharide were isolated from tolerized animals by the removal of an Ly-1$^+$ cell which interfered with the suppressive activity [13]. In the rat, density fractionation of spleen cells revealed a fraction rich in suppressor cells for the concanavalin A mitogenic response [14]. Reconstitution of the cell populations caused this suppression to disappear. In man, 'covert' suppressor activity was observed in the peripheral blood lymphocytes of patients with Crohn's disease [11]. No suppressor cell activity could be demonstrated unless T cells were purified through affinity columns. Whether, indeed, contrasuppressor cells were removed during the purification to reveal active suppressor cells is an open question.

In another system removal of human T cell subsets allowed the production of suppressor factors at antigen doses that do not ordinarily (apparently) induce such factors [15]. Loss of suppressor T cell function has been observed in patients with systemic lupus erythematosis [16] and 'auto-immune' chronic active hepatitis (CAH) [17], and in the synovial T cells of patients with rheumatoid arthritis [18]. Defective suppressor cell function in CAH was reversed by a short *in vitro* pulse of corticosteroid [19]. It is possible that this treatment removed a contrasuppressor cell which masked suppression. In every case, more approaches are needed to determine whether these phenomena are an effect of contrasuppressive activity. These approaches will now be considered.

Approaches to the discrimination of contrasuppression

By cell surface phenotype

When a cell such as a lymphocyte differentiates, presumably by the activation of a discrete family of genes, a profile of molecular entities encoded by some of these genes may appear on the cell surface. Thus the surface phenotype of a cell is associated with its specialized function in the organism. Using specific reagents directed at such surface markers, unique profiles of cell surface molecules can be correlated with distinct functional populations (such as contrasuppressor T cells). There is no requirement in such an approach for knowledge of what each surface label is actually doing there, only that it is present on one type of cell and not on another. On the other hand, such knowledge may be extremely valuable in understanding the mechanism of a cellular activity.

There are several surface markers which have been associated with elements of the contrasuppressor circuit (discussed above). Two of these, I-J and the receptor for *Vicia villosa* lectin, are especially valuable in the discrimination of contrasuppressor cells.

I-J

Antisera that discriminate between lymphoid cells from B10.A(3R) and B10.A(5R) animals (defining the I-J subregion) are extremely useful in the identification of immunoregulatory T cells [20]. As already discussed, all of the T cells involved in the contrasuppressor circuit have been shown to be I-J$^+$, i.e. their activity can be removed with anti-I-J antibody plus complement.

Not all anti-I-J reagents react with contrasuppressor cells, however. A number of monoclonal anti-I-J reagents were found to react with suppressor cells while having no effect upon cells of the contrasuppressor circuit [21]. On the other hand, some anti-I-J reagents have been found to react preferentially with contrasuppressor cells [22].

Applicable systems

To analyse a regulatory population in terms of surface phenotype (such as reactivity with anti-I-J or *V. villosa* lectin) it is important that the population be available for *in vitro* manipulation. It is possible, however, that *in vivo* manipulation may be accomplished by injection of anti-I-J antibodies reactive with contrasuppressor cells (C. Waltenbaugh, personal communication). Most remarkably, recent evidence suggests that both antisera and monoclonal antibodies specific for I-J react with *human* contrasuppressor T cells but not with human suppressor cells [41]. Thus, I-J is a useful marker in studies of both murine and human regulation by contrasuppressor cells.

Reagents

Anti-I-J antiserum or antibody.
Rabbit serum (screened for complement activity and low background cytotoxicity; Pelfreeze, Rogers, AR, permits aliquot screening).
Balanced salt solution (with Ca^{2+} and Mg^{2+}).

Procedure

1 Suspend lymphocytes at a concentration of 1×10^7 cells per ml of appropriately diluted antibody (approximately 1:5 for conventional allosera; higher for monoclonal antibodies).
2 Incubate at room temperature for 30 min.
3 Wash cells.
4 Resuspend at 1×10^7 cells per ml of diluted rabbit complement.
5 Incubate at 37 °C for 30 min.
6 Wash cells.
7 Evaluate for activity in assay.

Notes and recommendations

This analysis requires important controls. Anti-I-J treated cells should be compared for function with cells treated with complement only. In addition, anti-I-J antisera should be absorbed for 1 h on ice with one of two populations of spleen cells before treatment. One population should match the antiserum specificity at I-J; the other should not. This procedure will determine whether the reactivity detectable in the serum is, in fact, related to I-J (e.g. absorption of anti-I-J^b serum on B10.A(3R) spleen cells (I-J^b) removed the ability of the serum to destroy I-J^b contrasuppressor effector cells whereas the same serum absorbed on B10.A(5R) cells (I-J^k) retained its anti-contrasuppressor cell activity [7]).

These antibodies are extremely valuable in the discrimination of contrasuppressor cell activity from that of conventional T helper cells (which are I-J$^-$) [7]. Reports of I-J$^+$ 'helper' T cells [23,24] suggest that either (a) helper T cells bearing I-J encoded determinants exist and therefore more characteristics than this are required for identification of contrasuppressor cells, or (b) in each case a contrasuppressor cell (which is I-J$^+$) was actually being described. The second possibility is an important consideration in light of observations that Ly-1 T helper cells may often be protected from suppressive influences by contrasup-

pressor cells. Removal of the contrasuppressor cell can, therefore, lead to a loss of activity, making it appear that the helper cell itself was I-J$^+$ (J. Rohrer & J. Kemp, manuscript in preparation). This is further discussed under 'Adoptive transfer', on page 79.5.

Vicia villosa *lectin*

Certain T cell subsets have been found to bind to the *Vicia villosa* lectin. Such cells can be eluted from the lectin with the sugar *N*-acetyl-D-galactosamine. In this way, adherent contrasuppressor effector cells can be separated from non-adherent helper cells [7]. This particular means of identification is likely to be effective in discrimination of contrasuppressor cells in man.

The method described herein is adapted from one developed by Dr A. Kimura.

Applicable systems

(Same as above.)

Reagents

Vicia villosa lectin (E-Y Laboratories, San Mateo, CA).
Citrate Buffer (pH 5.5).
N-Acetyl-D-galactosamine (Sigma).

Materials

Plastic Petri dishes (Fisher) (100 mm are convenient).

Procedure

1 Dissolve lectin at 2 mg/ml in citrate buffer (as little as 0.5 mg/ml may be used, but the higher concentration is more effective). This solution may be stored at 4 °C for several months and may be reused several times for coating plates.
2 Apply enough solution (3–5 ml) to cover bottom of each Petri dish.
3 Incubate at room temperature for 1 h.
4 Recover lectin for reuse.
5 Wash plates 3 times with buffered saline. Final wash should contain 2% calf serum and be allowed to incubate at room temperature for at least 15 min.
6 Up to 10 ml of $5–7 \times 10^6$ cells/ml can be applied to each plate.
7 Incubate for 45 min at 37 °C.
8 Gently remove non-adherent cells by washing several times. Do not pipette vigorously, otherwise adherent cells may be dislodged as well.
9 Elute adherent cells by adding 5 ml *N*-acetyl-D-

galactosamine (2 mg/ml in buffered saline), incubating for 10 min at 37 °C, then washing.

Notes

Using this technique, contrasuppressor effector cells were separated from the spleens of mice hyperimmunized with sheep red blood cells (SRBC) (unpublished observation), from cultures of neonatal spleen cells [7,25], and from animals immunized for contact sensitivity [5] (see section on 'Adoptive transfer', page 79.5). It should be noted that some suppressor T cells may be adherent to this lectin as well (unpublished observations), perhaps making it an unsuitable general approach to unmasking covert suppression.

By function

Circuit disruption

In several cases it has been possible to employ knowledge of the circuit shown in Fig. 79.1 in order to demonstrate contrasuppressive effects. In such cases suppression was revealed upon removal of the contrasuppressor inducer cell (or factor) co-existing with the suppressor effector cell (or factor). Similarly suppression could be revealed by removal of the contrasuppressor transducer cell from the assay population. This is shown schematically in Fig. 79.2.

Removal of the contrasuppressor inducer cell from the suppressor cell population can be achieved by treatment with anti-I-J reagents plus complement in those cases in which the suppressor effector cell is $I\text{-}J^-$ [1]. This was also found to be effective in removal of a contrasuppressor inducer factor (using a column of anti-I-J antibody bound to sepharose) from a suppressor factor specific for SRBC [2]. In this case it was also found that the contrasuppressor inducer factor could be removed by absorption with horse red blood cells which would not absorb the suppressor factor. In each case, removal of the contrasuppressor inducer cell or factor revealed potent suppressor effector activity. Removal of the contrasuppressor transducer cell can

be readily achieved by treatment of the assay population with anti-Ly-2 antibody plus complement. When this was done, the remaining cells were then readily suppressed, regardless of the presence of contrasuppressor inducer cells.

Applicable systems

Demonstration of contrasuppression by circuit disruption requires: (a) a population of putative regulatory cells or factors thought to contain elements of suppressor and contrasuppressor cell circuits; (b) an assay in which addition of regulatory cell populations is known to have identifiable effects.

Reagents

Antibodies or antisera reactive with regulatory subsets. Examples are anti-I-J (see above), anti-Ly-1 and anti-Ly-2 (e.g. New England Nuclear), and, in human systems, anti-T4 and anti-T8 (Ortho diagnostics).

Rationale

If suppressive influences in the regulatory population (as well as immune elements necessary for positive responses in the assay culture) survive any treatment that destroys a vital element of the masking contrasuppressive effect; then, following such treatment, addition of the regulatory population to the assay will result in suppression (where none could be observed without treatment).

Notes and recommendations

The procedure obviously depends entirely upon the nature of both the regulatory cells and the assay population. Therefore an example from previous studies will be given to illustrate the concept.

A practical example of this procedure was observed in the addition of naive Peyer's patch T cells to spleen cells in an *in vitro* response to SRBC [4]. Peyer's patch Ly-2 T cells from most mouse strains show no effects

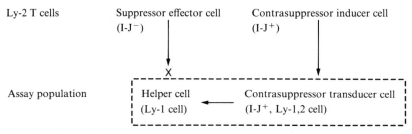

Fig. 79.2. Circuit disruption. Removal of either the contrasuppressor inducer or transducer cell reveals suppressor cell activity in the Ly-2 T cell population.

when added to normal spleen cells. When Ly-2 T cells from Peyer's patches were treated with anti-I-J plus complement, however, they became potently suppressive. This suppressor cell was observed to be an I-J$^-$, Ly-2 T cell. Suppression could also be revealed by adding Peyer's patch Ly-2 T cells to spleen cells that had been treated with anti-Ly-2 plus complement. Thus an I-J$^+$, Ly-2 cell in the Peyer's patch interacted with an Ly-2$^+$ (probably Ly-1,2) cell in the spleen culture to obscure the suppression produced by the Peyer's patch Ly-2 suppressor cell. Only after disruption of the contrasuppressor circuit could these effects be observed. For an example employing a human regulatory T cell system see Lehner [15,41].

Adoptive transfer

In most cases immune memory can be transferred by intravenous injection of immune cells into a recipient only if that recipient is irradiated [26], or treated with a low dose of cyclophosphamide (Cy) [27]. Some types of immunity, however, can be readily transferred into untreated recipients. One example is contact sensitivity.

Applicable systems

Any system in which immunity can be adoptively transferred by systemic introduction of immune cells into untreated naive recipients may be analysed in this way.

Reagents

Anti-I-J antibodies and/or *V. villosa* lectin (see above). Cyclophosphamide (Cytoxan, Mead Johnson).

Rationale

Adoptive transfer of immunity into the suppressive environment of an untreated, naive recipient might require the presence of contrasuppressor cells in the immune inoculum from the donor. Removal of such a contrasuppressive population would then yield immune cells which transfer immunity into recipients pre-treated to remove suppressor cells (by cyclophosphamide) but not into normal recipients. Re-addition of the contrasuppressor cells (which display no immunity in adoptive transfer alone) restores the response in untreated recipients.

Procedure

1 Recipients are untreated, or treated 24 h earlier with approximately 50 mg/kg Cy injected i.p.

2 Immune cells are treated with anti-I-J or separated on *V. villosa* lectin coated dishes (see above).
3 Treated immune populations are injected into normal and treated recipients. (Cell numbers are determined beforehand using untreated immune cells into normal recipients.)
4 Assess immunity as appropriate for system.

Notes and recommendations

X-ray irradiation (250 R) can theoretically be substituted for Cy pre-treatment.

Suitable controls for this analysis require injection of both treated and untreated cell populations into normal and Cy pre-treated animals.

Two sets of experiments have illustrated the activity of contrasuppressor cells in the adoptive transfer of contact sensitivity [5]. These are shown schematically in Table 79.1. Immune cells were transferred into normal and Cy treated recipients. One day later ears were painted with the sensitizing agent (picryl chloride) and the ear swelling response at 24 h was ascertained. Fractionation of the immune cells on *Vicia villosa* lectin coated plates revealed that two populations were active (Experiment I). The *V. villosa* non-adherent cells could transfer immunity only into

Table 79.1. Adoptive transfer of contact sensitivity

Immune T cells	Recipient	Immunity
Experiment I		
Unfractionated	Normal	+ +
Unfractionated	Cy	+ +
V. villosa adherent	Normal	−
V. villosa adherent	Cy	−
V. villosa non-adherent	Normal	−
V. villosa non-adherent	Cy	+ +
Reconstituted (adherent + non-adherent)	Normal	+ +
Reconstituted (adherent + non-adherent)	Cy	+ +
Experiment II		
Ly-1 T	Normal	+ +
Ly-1 T	Cy	+ +
I-J$^-$, Ly-1 T	Normal	−
I-J$^-$, Ly-1 T	Cy	+ +

Immune T cells were treated as shown and transferred by intravenous injection into normal or cyclophosphamide (Cy) treated recipients. Ly-1 T cells (Experiment II) were prepared by treatment of T cells with anti-Ly-2 + C'. Ears were painted immediately following transfer and immunity was assessed by ear swelling 24–40 h later [5].

Cy treated recipients. The *V. villosa* adherent population, while incapable of transferring immunity, served to protect the immunity of the non-adherent population when transferred into normal recipients.

Similarly (Experiment II), removal of an I-J$^+$, Ly-1 cell had no effect upon transfer of immunity into Cy treated recipients, but expression of this immunity was prevented in normal recipients. Thus a population of cells with no immune reactivity themselves functioned to protect an immune population from a cyclophosphamide sensitive inhibitory activity. These protective cells were observed to be I-J$^+$ and *V. villosa* lectin adherent, two markers associated with contrasuppression.

Intermediate culture

The intermediate culture system was developed to examine whether effects of regulatory cell interactions persist after the regulatory cells have been removed. Using this system it was determined that: (1) suppressor T cells can render helper T cells inactive such that they will not induce B cells even after removal of the suppressor cells [28]; (2) contrasuppressor effector cells can interfere with this interaction and leave the helper cells active; and (3) such 'contrasuppressed' helper T cells remain relatively resistant to suppressor T cell signals even after removal of the contrasuppressor cells [3,7]. In this system T cells were co-cultured for 48 h, following which the helper cells were isolated by the use of specific antisera against the other subsets. The helper cells were then added to B cells under conditions for a primary *in vitro* SRBC response. This system proved somewhat awkward in its requirement for multiple controls for each antiserum treatment. Therefore another system was developed that did not require such treatments.

Applicable systems

Three separate cell populations are required: suppressor cells, suppressor cell targets (e.g. helper T cells), and the putative contrasuppressor cells. Following intermediate culture, the target population must be assayed for activity; for example, regulated helper cells added to B cells under conditions for an *in vitro* immune response can be used to determine the activity of the regulated population. Addition of fresh suppressor cells to the assay can be used to evaluate the sensitivity of the regulated population to inhibitory signals.

Materials

Periscopic double Marbrook chambers (Bellco, Vineland, NJ).

Unipore membranes (approx. 0.1–0.4 μm) (Biorad).

Procedure

1   Assemble double Marbrook chambers with membranes and autoclave.
2   Prepare cell populations (suppressor, contrasuppressor, and targets) as available to system.
3   Regulatory cells are placed in the upper chamber, target cells in the lower. Add tissue culture medium until above membrane in upper chamber (25–30 ml).
4   Culture for 48 h at 37 °C in 5% CO_2–95% air.
5   Recover target population from lower chamber.
6   Add target population to assay cultures (plus or minus suppressor cells) to determine level of activity and sensitivity to subsequent suppressor cell signals.

Notes and recommendations

This technique is useful if the contrasuppressor cells represent an effector cell population. Inducer cells, however, might require a transducer cell population in order to have an effect. This population could be missing, or else the interaction between subsets might require longer than the allotted 48 h.

A contrasuppressor effector cell present in the spleens of hyperimmunized animals was elucidated in this way [3]. Naive Ly-1 T cells were used as a source of helper cells and placed in the lower chamber. Pre-cultured suppressor T cells plus or minus splenic T cells from SRBC hyperimmune animals (haemagglutination titres greater than ten doubling dilutions) were placed in the upper chamber, separated from the helper cells by a 0.4 μm, cell impermeable membrane. After 48 h the helper cells from the lower chamber were recovered and added to B cells (+/− suppressor T cells) in assay cultures (*in vitro* primary anti-SRBC responses). Helper cells that were co-cultured with suppressor cells were inactivated (failed to stimulate normal levels of plaque forming cells), while those co-cultured with suppressor cells plus hyperimmune T cells were not only active but subsequently resistant to suppression [3, and unpublished observation]. By using the intermediate culture system it was therefore possible to assess the contrasuppressive activity of hyperimmune T cells without the effects of the potent suppressor-resistant helper cells also present in the spleens.

Culture activation

Under various conditions, cells cultured in the absence of antigen for 5–6 days produce potent contrasuppressor effector cells. This technique was useful in the detection of contrasuppressive potential in the spleens of neonatal animals (5–14 days old) [7], old animals (> 20 months old) [6], and in experimentally induced auto-immune animals [8]. Contrasuppressor effector cells were also produced by culture of normal adult spleen cells that had been treated with low concentrations of a monoclonal anti-T cell antibody, F7D5 (available from Olac, Oxon, England). F7D5 at low concentrations removes a subset of splenic T cells which appear to inhibit the generation of contrasuppressor cells in this system [9].

Applicable systems

Potent suppressor T cells can be produced by culture of normal adult splenic T cells in the absence of antigen for several days. Failure to generate suppressor cells might reflect activation of contrasuppressor cells in the cultures. This phenomenon may in turn reflect the immunoregulatory status of the spleen cell donors. To evaluate, any immune response susceptible to regulation may be employed.

Materials

75 cm^2 tissue culture flasks (Costar).

Procedure

1 Prepare a suspension of the cell population to be activated.
2 Bring cell concentration to 5×10^6 cells/ml in tissue culture medium.
3 Up to 30 ml of suspension may be cultured in each flask.
4 Culture horizontally for 5–6 days at 37 °C in 5% CO_2–95% air.
5 Recover and wash cultured cells.
6 Assay by addition to assay cultures (plus or minus suppressor cells).

Notes and recommendations

The contrasuppressor effector cells generated in the cultures have in all cases been shown to be I-J$^+$ and to interfere with suppressor cell function *in vitro*. In the case of the cultured neonatal cells the contrasuppressive activity was demonstrated in intermediate culture as well [7, and unpublished observations].

Conclusion: contrasuppression in immunoregulation

In this discussion an attempt has been made to describe the approaches which may be used to identify contrasuppression in immunoregulatory phenomena. Although many of the procedures are simple, their

application has demonstrated the involvement of contrasuppression in many systems. Three physiologic roles for contrasuppression have been proposed: (1) in recovery from suppression, (2) in anatomically localized immune responses, and (3) in the generation of suppression-resistant states. Although many of the phenomena have been discussed throughout this review, they are again briefly mentioned in this context.

The recovery from suppression might simply involve the loss of active suppressor cells. In those cases where it has been studied, however, the event seems to be an active one, i.e. involving contrasuppression. Potent contrasuppressor cell activity can be demonstrated in animals that have recovered from immunosuppressive non-fatal malaria infections [6] and burn-trauma-induced suppression [38]. Contrasuppressor cell activity can be generated in the cells of neonatal mice during the immunosuppressed state which follows birth [7] and may be necessary for proper immune maturation to responsiveness [6].

Localization of an immune response to an anatomical site can be achieved by the localization of contrasuppressor cells in systemically suppressed animals. One example might be the immune response of gut associated lymphoid tissue (GALT). Antigen that enters the gut tends to produce potent suppressor cell activity [29] and systemic tolerance with concomitant gut immunity [30]. This might be explained if contrasuppressor cells in the GALT sheltered the local environment from the effects of circulating suppressor factors and thereby allowed a local response. The finding that Peyer's patches contain contrasuppressor inducer cells supports this idea [4]. Other anatomical sites which may be similarly sheltered to produce immunity are the bone marrow [31] and the skin [5].

Finally, contrasuppression may be involved in the generation of states that are resistant to the effects of suppressor T cells. Potent suppressor factors can be collected from the secretions of hyperimmunized T cells [32] and isolated from the serum of such animals [33]. Nevertheless, hyperimmune animals appear to be resistant to the effects of these factors as they continue to produce active immune responses. Contrasuppressor cells have been identified in the spleens of these animals [3]. Helper cells isolated from hyperimmune animals remain resistant to suppression even after removal of contrasuppressor cells, an observation consistent with the action of contrasuppressor cells in other experimental situations [3,7]. It is therefore likely that contrasuppression plays an important part in the generation of the hyperimmune state.

A similar situation is seen in some forms of auto-immunity. In such cases, auto-immunity proceeds in the face of general systemic suppression.

Examples are the MRL murine model of systemic lupus erythematosis [34] and auto-immunity associated with old age [35] and malaria [36]. In all cases contrasuppression has been implicated in some way, and it remains to be seen whether a cause and effect relationship can be established.

The author has recently induced antigen-specific contrasuppressor cells and factors that produce a resistance to suppression of contact sensitivity to simple haptens. This was accomplished by the administration of haptenated immunoglobulin [39, 40] and by the use of antigen–antibody complexes (submitted for publication). These recent findings open new avenues for the characterization of this regulatory phenomenon.

Contrasuppression may well have other physiologic functions. It is the author's hope that this review may help in the determination of these additional roles. With its activity associated with adoptive transfer, hyperimmunity, auto-immunity, resistance to parasitic infection and more, contrasuppression stands out as an important immunoregulatory activity. Rapid advances that are occurring in cellular immunology ensure that a fuller understanding of contrasuppression and its prospects cannot be far off.

Acknowledgement

DRG is supported by a grant from the UNDP/World Bank/WHO special program for research in tropical disease and by the Department of Surgery, Yale University. Author's current address: Department of Immunology, University of Alberta, Canada.

References

1   GERSHON R.K., EARDLEY D.D., DURUM S., GREEN D.R., SHEN F.W., YAMAUCHI K., CANTOR H. & MURPHY D.B. (1981) Contrasuppression: a novel immunoregulatory activity. *J. exp. Med.* **153,** 1533.

2   YAMAUCHI K., GREEN D.R., EARDLEY D.D., MURPHY D.B. & GERSHON R.K. (1981) Immunoregulatory circuits that modulate responsiveness to suppressor cell signals: the failure of B10 mice to respond to suppressor factors can be overcome by quenching the contrasuppressor circuit. *J. exp. Med.* **153,** 1547.

3   GREEN D.R. & GERSHON R.K. (1982) Hyperimmunity and the decision to be intolerant. *Ann. N.Y. Acad. Sci.* **392,** 318.

4   GREEN D.R., GOLD J., ST. MARTIN S., GERSHON R. & GERSHON R.K. (1982) Microenvironmental immunoregulation: the possible role of contrasuppressor cells in maintaining immune responses in gut associated lymphoid tissue. *Proc. natn. Acad. Sci. U.S.A.* **79,** 889.

5   IVERSON G.M., PTAK W., GREEN D.R. & GERSHON R.K. (1983) The role of contrasuppression in the adoptive transfer of immunity. *J. exp. Med.* **158,** 982.

6   GREEN D.R. (1981) *Contrasuppression: an immunoregulatory T cell activity.* Ph.D. Thesis. Yale University, New Haven, CT.

7   GREEN D.R., EARDLEY D.D., KIMURA A., MURPHY D.B., YAMAUCHI K. & GERSHON R.K. (1981) Immunoregulatory circuits which modulate responsiveness to suppressor cell signals: characterization of an effector cell in the contrasuppressor circuit. *Eur. J. Immunol.* **11,** 973.

8   SMITH H.R., GREEN D.R., RAVECHE E.S., SMATHERS P.A., GERSHON R.K. & STEINBERG A.D. (1982) Studies of the induction of anti-DNA in normal mice. *J. Immunol.* **129,** 2332.

9   GREEN D.R., CHUE B. & GERSHON R.K. (1985) Discrimination of 2 types of suppressor cells by function (ability to regulate contrasuppression) as well as by cell surface phenotype. *J. cell. Mol. Immunol.* **1,** 19.

10   GREEN D.R., FLOOD P.J. & GERSHON R.K. (1983) Immunoregulatory T cell pathways. *Ann. Rev. Immunol.* **1,** 439.

11   ELSON C.O., GRAEFF A.S., JAMES S.P. & STROBER W. (1981) Covert suppressor T cells in Crohn's disease. *Gastroenterology,* **80,** 1513.

12   ROLLWAGEN F.W. & STUTMAN O. (1979) Ontogeny of culture generated suppressor cells. *J. exp. Med.* **150,** 1359.

13   BRALEY-MULLEN H. (1980) Direct demonstration of splenic suppressor T cells in mice tolerant to type III pneumococcal polysaccharide: two-step requirement for development of detectable suppressor cells. *J. Immunol.* **125,** 1849.

14   BELL E.T. & BELL J.E. (1982) Regulation of the immune response in the rat: evidence for the existence of contrasuppressor cells. *Cell. Immunol.* **71,** 388.

15   LEHNER T. (1982) The relationship between human helper and suppressor factors to a streptococcal protein antigen. *J. Immunol.* **129,** 1936.

16   FAUCI A.S., STEINBERG A.D., HAYNES B.F. & WHALEN G. (1978) Immunoregulatory aberrations in system lupus erythematosis. *J. Immunol.* **121,** 1473.

17   ALEXANDER G.J.M., NOURIA K., HEGARTY J.E., EDDLESTON A.L.W.F. & WILLIAMS R. (1982) Relationship of T cell subsets of suppressor cell function in chronic liver disease. *Gut,* **23,** A461.

18   KEYSTONE E.C., GLADMAN D.D., BUCHANAN R., CANE D. & POPLONSKI L. (1980) Impaired antigen-specific suppressor cell activity in patients with rheumatoid arthritis. *Arthrit. Rheum.* **23,** 1246.

19   NOURI-ARIA K.T., HEGARTY J.E., ALEXANDER G.J.M., EDDLESTON A.L.W.F. & WILLIAMS R. (1982) Effect of corticosteroids on suppressor cell activity in 'autoimmune' and viral active hepatitis. *New Engl J. Med.* **307,** 388.

20   MURPHY D.B. (1978) The I-J subregion of the murine H-2 gene complex. *Springer Semin. Immunopath.* **1,** 111.

21   GOLDE W.T., GREEN D.R., WALTENBAUGH C.R. & GERSHON R.K. (1982) Different I-J specificities define different T-cell regulatory pathways. *Fedn Proc.* **41,** 190.

22   YAMAUCHI K., TANIGUCHI M., GREEN D.R. & GERSHON R.K. (1982) The use of a monoclonal anti-I-J antibody to distinguish cells in the feedback suppression circuit from those in the contrasuppressor circuit. *Immunogenetics,* **16,** 551.

23   TADA T., TAKEMORI T., OKUMURA K., NONAKA M. &

TOKUHISA T. (1978) Two distinct types of helper T cells involved in the secondary antibody response. *J. exp. Med.* **147**, 446.

24 JAYARAMAN S., SWIERKOSZ J.E. & BELLONE C.J. (1982) T cell replacing factor substitutes for an I-J$^+$, idiotype specific T helper cell. *J. exp. Med.* **155**, 641.

25 PTAK W., GREEN D.R., DURUM S.K., KIMURA A., MURPHY D.B. & GERSHON R.K. (1981) Immunoregulatory circuits that modulate responsiveness to suppressor cell signals: contrasuppressor cells can convert an *in vivo* tolerogenic signal into an immunogenic one. *Eur. J. Immunol.* **11**, 980.

26 CELADA F. (1966) Quantitative studies for the adoptive immunological memory in mice. (I) An age dependent barrier to syngeneic transplantation. *J. exp. Med.* **124**, 7.

27 EARDLEY D.D. & GERSHON R.K. (1975) Feedback induction of suppressor T-cell activity. *J. exp. Med.* **142**, 524.

28 GREEN D.R., GERSHON R.K. & EARDLEY D.D. (1981) Functional deletion of different Ly-1 T cell inducer subset activities by Ly-2 suppressor T lymphocytes. *Proc. natn. Acad. Sci. U.S.A.* **78**, 3819.

29 MATTINGLY J.A. & WAKSMAN B.H. (1978) Immunologic suppression after oral administration of antigen. (I) Specific suppressor cells found in rat Peyer's patches after oral administration of sheep erythrocytes and their systemic migration. *J. Immunol.* **121**, 1878.

30 CHALLACOMBE S.J. & TOMASI T.B. (1980) Systemic tolerance and secretory immunity after oral immunization. *J. exp. Med.* **152**, 1459.

31 MICHAELSON J.D. (1982) *The characterization and functional analysis of immunoregulatory cells in murine bone marrow.* Thesis. Yale Univ. Sch. Med., New Haven, CT.

32 YAMAUCHI K., MURPHY D.B., CANTOR H. & GERSHON R.K. (1981) Analysis of an antigen specific H-2 restricted, cell free product(s) made by 'I-J$^-$' Ly-2 cells (Ly-2 TsF) that suppresses Ly-2 depleted spleen cell activity. *Eur. J. Immunol.* **11**, 905.

33 IVERSON G.M., EARDLEY D.D., JANEWAY C.A. & GERSHON R.K. (1983) The use of anti-idiotype immunosorbents to isolate circulating antigen specific T cell derived molecules from hyperimmune sera. *Proc. natn. Acad. Sci. U.S.A.* **80**, 544.

34 GERSHON R.K., HOROWITZ M., KEMP J.D. & MURPHY D.B. (1978) The cellular site of immunoregulatory breakdown in the 1pr mouse. In *Genetic Control of Autoimmune Disease*, (eds. Rose N.R., Bigazzi R.E. & Warner N.L.). Elsevier/North-Holland, New York.

35 MAKINODAN T. & KAY M.B. (1980) Age influence on the immune system. *Adv. Immunol.* **29**, 287.

36 POELS L.G. & VAN NIEKERK C.C. (1977) *Plasmodium bergheii*: Immunosuppression and hyperimmunoglobulinemia. *Expl Parasitol.* **42**, 235.

37 BRALEY-MULLEN, H. (1984) Regulation of the antibody response to type III pneumococcal polysaccharide by contrasuppressor T cells. *J. exp. Med.* **160**, 42.

38 KUPPER T.S. & GREEN D.R. (1984) Immunoregulation after thermal injury: Sequential appearance of I-J$^+$, Ly-1$^+$, 2$^-$ T suppressor-inducer cells and Ly-1$^-$,2$^+$ T suppressor-effector cells following thermal trauma in mice. *J. Immunol.* **133**, 3047.

39 PTAK W., BERETA M., MARCINKIEWICZ J., GERSHON R.K. & GREEN D.R. (1984) Production of antigen-specific contrasuppressor cells and factor and their use in augmentation of cell mediated immunity. *J. Immunol.* **133**, 623.

40 PTAK W., BERETA M., PTAK M., GERSHON R.K. & GREEN D.R. (1984) Regulatory T cell interactions with an antigen-specific T contrasuppressor factor in contact sensitivity: Eradication of the tolerant state. *J. Immunol.* **133**, 1124.

41 LEHNER T., BRINES R., JONES T. & AVERY J. (1984) Detection of cross-reacting murine I-J like determinants on a human subject of T8$^+$ antigen binding, presenting, and contrasuppressor cells. *Clin. exp. Immunol.* **58**, 410.

Chapter 80
Antigen-specific suppressor molecules produced by T cells

M. TANIGUCHI & T. TOKUHISA

Methods for the preparation of antigen-specific suppressor T cell factors, 80.1

Methods for the preparation of antibodies reactive to the antigen-specific suppressor T cell factor, 80.3

Assay systems for the detection of the suppressor factor, 80.3

Methods for the preparation and detection of mRNAs coding for suppressor molecules, 80.5

Methods for the reconstitution of suppressor activity with mRNA translation products and isolated free chains, 80.8

It has been well established that an antigen-specific suppression of immune response is mediated by soluble factors derived from suppressor T cells [reviewed in 1]. This strongly suggests that direct cell-to-cell contact is not necessary in the regulatory T cell interactions. Therefore characterizations of functional and molecular features of soluble suppressor factors are important for understanding the mechanisms of T cell interactions in the regulation of immune responses. Recently developed new technology to establish constitutive T cell lines, such as T cell hybridomas and TCGF (T cell growth factor)-dependent T cell clones, permit us to characterize T cell mediated functions at biochemical and molecular levels. In fact, it is obvious that these methods provide important strategy for determining the functional and molecular structure of T cell factors, which are devices for T cells to recognize antigens and to collaborate with other subsets of T cells. The purpose of this chapter is to describe in detail the methods for characterization of suppressor molecules that regulate immune responses in an antigen-specific fashion. Several suppressor factors with different immunological properties have been described [2–20], but the authors will mainly confine themselves to a discussion of the antigen-specific suppressor T cell factor composed of two polypeptide (heavy and light) chains.

Methods for the preparation of antigen-specific suppressor T cell factors

Conventional suppressor factor extracted from thymus or spleen cells

Procedure

The method for obtaining an antigen-specific suppres-sor T cell factor is originally described by Tada et al. [2].

1 Mice were intraperitoneally immunized twice with 100–200 μg of antigen (i.e. keyhole limpet haemo-cyanin: KLH, sheep red blood cell: SRBC, or ovalbu-min: OVA, etc.) at a 2-week interval.

2 Ten days after the second immunization, lymphoid cell suspensions from spleen or thymus were prepared at a concentration of $1–4 \times 10^8$ cells per ml in 0.01 M sodium phosphate buffered saline (PBS), pH 7.2, containing 0.2 mM-phenylmethylsulphonylfluoride (PMSF: Sigma, St. Louis, Mo.) and then subjected to sonication for 2 min in ice with a sonicator (Tommy UR-150P, Tommy Seiko Co. Ltd., Tokyo, Japan), or to freezing and thawing ten times in dry ice with acetone.

3 The cell-free supernates were obtained by ultracentrifugation at 40 000 g for 1 h, and were used as the conventional extracted suppressor T cell factor.

Monoclonal suppressor factor obtained from T cell hybridomas

T cell hybridomas were made by fusion of a thymoma cell line, (i.e. BW5147), which lacks the enzyme hypoxanthine guanine phosphoribosyl transferase (HGPRT$^-$), with suppressor T cells specific for antigen (i.e. KLH) [17,18]. In order to effectively obtain antigen-specific suppressor T cell hybridomas, the KLH-specific suppressor T cells were enriched by allowing Ig-negative spleen cells from KLH primed mice to bind to KLH-coated Petri dishes [21] or to KLH-conjugated Sepharose column [22] before cell fusion.

Procedure

The procedure for enriching antigen-specific suppressor T cells is presented in schematic form in Fig. 80.1.
1 Anti-mouse Ig coated culture-grade Petri dishes (Falcon #3002) were prepared by incubation of dishes with 3 ml of purified rabbit antibodies (100–1000 μg/ml) overnight at 4 °C. Dishes were extensively washed with 0.01 M-PBS, pH 7.2, and twice with RPMI-1640 before use. 2.5 ml of spleen cell suspensions (1×10^7 cells per ml) from mice primed with a high dose of antigen was incubated for 1 h on ice in culture-grade Petri dishes coated with affinity purified rabbit anti-mouse immunoglobulins (Ig) to remove Ig-bearing B cells. Incubation with radioactively labelled γ-globulin showed that under these conditions, 15–25 μg protein was bound and <0.1 μg was released during the subsequent removal of adherent spleen cells.
2 After incubation, the plates were swirled, and the non-adherent cells were recovered for further separation. Usually 20–30% of the initial cell population was recovered at this stage and shown to contain more than 95% of Ig-negative spleen cells.
3 Of this cell population 2.5 ml (5×10^6 cells per ml) was further incubated at room temperature for 1 h in

Petri dishes pre-coated with 3 ml of KLH solution (100 μg/ml) for 4 h at room temperature.
4 The non-adherent cells were then removed by swirling and the plates were put on ice for 30 min.
5 The antigen-binding cells were released by flushing cold medium with a syringe wearing a 27-G needle. By this procedure, about 0.1–0.5% of original spleen cells were recovered, but the suppressor activity was enriched about 100-fold.
6 The enriched suppressor T cells were hybridized with thymoma cells (BW5147) (cell ratio = 1:1) in the presence of polyethylene glycol (Mr 1500: BDH Chem. Ltd., Poole, UK).
7 After cell hybridization, the cell mixture was plated with a feeder layer (1×10^6 cells per well) in 96-well microculture plates (Falcon #3042) in 0.1 ml of RPMI-1640 enriched with 20% fetal calf serum (FCS) per well.
8 Progressive chemical selection was carried out for two weeks. One hundred microlitres of HAT medium (20% FCS-RPMI-1640 containing 1×10^{-4} M-hypoxanthine, 4×10^{-7} M-aminopterin, 1.6×10^{-5} M-thymidine) was added on day 1 and half the medium (0.1 ml) was replaced with fresh HAT medium every two days.
9 Cells grown in HAT medium were harvested and reacted with antibodies against the antigen-specific suppressor factor (see Chapters 77 and 78), followed by staining with fluorescein-conjugated rabbit anti-mouse Ig.
10 The stained cells were separated by a fluorescence activated cell sorter (FACS-IV, Becton-Dickinson & Co., Sunnyvale, Calif.) and cloned with limiting dilution.
11 Hybrid cells with antigen-specific suppressor activity were further selected by functional assays. Suppressor T cell hybridomas easily lose their antigen-specific activity. It is, therefore, necessary to reclone functionally active cells. In this respect, hybridomas with antigen-specific suppressor activity are successfully selected by fluorescence-staining with monoclonal antibodies reactive to the factor on FACS.

Extracted suppressor factor derived from hybridoma cells

Procedure

Cell-free extracts were obtained by ultracentrifugation, at 40 000 **g** for 1 h, of the frozen and thawed materials of the suppressor T hybridoma cells (1×10^7 cells/ml in 0.01 M-PBS containing 0.2 mM-PMSF), as described above.

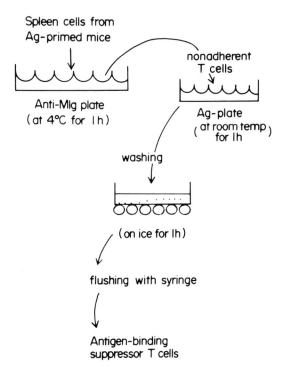

Fig. 80.1. Outline of the technique for enriching antigen-specific suppressor T cells.

Secreted suppressor factor derived from hybridoma cells

Procedure

The secreted form of the suppressor factor can be obtained in ascites of hybridoma-bearing syngeneic F_1 or nude mice that have been intraperitoneally transplanted with $5-10 \times 10^7$ hybrid cells. This procedure usually allows us to obtain strong suppressor activity in a small amount of ascitic fluid (i.e. sometimes the $1:10^{-3}$ diluted ascites still have the activity).

Methods for the preparation of antibodies reactive to the antigen-specific suppressor T cell factor

Several types of antibodies reactive to suppressor T cells and antigen-specific suppressor T cell factors have so far been described [9–15,23–26,32–36]. In this section, the authors present the alloantibodies specifically reactive to the antigen-specific suppressor factor.

Owen *et al.* have originally reported that some BALB/c (Ig^a, $H-2^d$) alloantisera prepared against Ig congenic CAL-20 (Ig^d, $H-2^d$) splenic T cells that had been stimulated with concanavalin A contain antibodies reactive with the determinants exclusively expressed on suppressor T cells [27,28]. It has also been reported that conventional and monoclonal alloantibodies made by BALB/c (Ig^a,$H-2^d$) anti-CB-20 (Ig^b, $H-2^d$) recognize constant region determinants on the antigen-specific suppressor T cell factors of Ig^b mice [29–31]. The immunization procedures are essentially the same as those reported by Owen *et al.* [27]. Weekly injections at least fifteen times of 10^7 concanavalin A stimulated splenic T cells treated with mitomycin C are generally sufficient to obtain specific alloantibodies. However, antisera prepared in this manner contain antibodies reactive with a variety of cell surface products. It is therefore better to establish specific monoclonal antibodies by somatic cell hybridization technique.

The specific monoclonal antibodies are easily screened by functional assays (see next section) [31].

Procedure

The culture supernates from hybridomas made by the fusion of HGPRT negative mutant myeloma cells (i.e. P3U1, NS-1) and spleen cells (i.e. BALB/c:Ig^a) hyperimmunized with splenic T cells from Ig allotype congenic mice (CB-20:Ig^b) are added to the culture of spleen cells (i.e. C57BL/6:Ig^b) and the suppressor factor (i.e. C57BL/6:Ig^b) with identical Ig allotypes to those of the immunizing donors (i.e. CB-20). If hybridoma supernates contain the antibody reactive to the factor, the factor-mediated suppression of the *in vitro* antibody responses is greatly abrogated by the specific antibody. Control experiments should be included with the assay using spleen cells and suppressor factors from mice with different Ig allotypes from the antibody specificity expected.

Another type of alloantibody reactive to the factor has been reported by several investigators using different systems [9–15,32–36]. The conventional and monoclonal antibodies are raised in the special combinations of B10.A(3R) ($H-2^{i3}$) and B10.A(5R) ($H-2^{i5}$), or B10.HTT ($H-2^{t3}$) and B10.S(9R) ($H-2^{t4}$). The immunizing procedures for raising the alloantibodies are essentially the same as those described above. For screening of the monoclonal antibodies reactive to the factor, the assay system has to use responding primed spleen cells and the suppressor factor of mice (i.e. C57BL/6:$H-2^b$) with the same $H-2$ haplotypes as the specificity of the antibody (i.e. B10.A(5R) anti-B10.A(3R)) expected. Serological and genetic studies have demonstrated that the difference between B10.A(3R) and B10.A(5R), or B10.HTT and B10.S(9R), in the I region of the $H-2$ complex is only the I-J subregion [32]. Moreover, the conventional and monoclonal alloantibodies raised in the combinations mentioned above specifically reacted with suppressor T cells and their factors. However, recent molecular genetic studies on the I-J subregion genes reported by Steinmetz *et al.* have demonstrated the possibilities that the I-J subregion is not encoded in the I region between the I-A and I-E subregions [37]. Therefore the genes coding for the products on suppressor T cells or factors defined by the antibodies have not been precisely mapped. In any case, it is clear that suppressor T cells and their factors carry the determinants detected by alloantibodies made in combinations of B10.A(3R) and B10.A(5R), or B10.HTT and B10.S(9R).

Assay systems for detection of the suppressor factor

It has so far been very hard to demonstrate the suppressor factor by biochemical means, probably because of the difficulty in collecting sufficient materials from suppressor T cells. However, it is easy to detect functional activities with minute amounts of the conventional or monoclonal suppressor factor. Therefore the most popular analyses of the immunochemical properties of an antigen-specific suppressor molecule are functional assays.

Functional assay

Procedure

The modified Mishell–Dutton culture system [38] was utilized to investigate the effects of suppressor factors on the *in vitro* secondary antibody responses.

1 Mice were primed with an i.p. injection of 100 μg of antigen (i.e. 2,4-dinitrophenylated KLH: DNP-KLH) together with 10^9 *Bordetella pertussis* vaccine (Chiba Serum Institute, Chiba, Japan) as an adjuvant.

2 Four weeks after the immunization, 4×10^6/ml primed spleen cells were cultured with 0.1 μg/ml of immunizing antigen (i.e. DNP-KLH) in RPMI-1640 enriched with 10% heat-inactivated FCS and 2×10^{-5} M-2-mercaptoethanol in 1 ml Mishell–Dutton plates (Falcon #3008) in quadruplicate or in 0.2 ml microculture plates (Falcon #3042) in six wells per group. The culture was maintained at 37 °C in an atmosphere of 10% CO_2 in air for 5 days. The cell-free extracts (100 μl in 1 ml plate or 10 μl in 0.2 ml plate at a dose comparable to 1×10^7/ml of primed-thymocyte or primed-spleen cells, or to 3×10^5/ml of hybridoma cells) or the secreted materials in ascitic fluid at a final dilution of 1:1 to $1:10^{-3}$ were added at the beginning of the culture.

3 After a 5-day culture, numbers of antigen (DNP)-specific plaque-forming cells (PFC) were assayed in a Cunningham chamber by using sheep erythrocytes coupled with DNP-heterologous carrier (i.e. DNP$_{31}$-bovine serum albumin) [39,40].

Absorption and elution of the factor using immunoadsorbent columns

Procedure

As the antigen-specific suppressor factor causes decreased numbers of PFC responses in an antigen-specific manner when added to the *in vitro* or *in vivo* antibody responses, it is easy to investigate suppressor activity of the materials before or after absorption with immunoadsorbent columns.

1 Immunoadsorbent columns were prepared as described by Axen *et al.* [41] with the use of Sepharose CL-4B beads (Pharmacia Fine Chemical, Uppsala, Sweden) covalently conjugated with antigen or antibodies.

2 Either 200 μl of the 1:2 diluted ascites or 200 μl of hybridoma-extracts (1×10^7 cells per ml) was applied to 1 ml of immunoadsorbent columns (1 ml plastic syringe) equilibrated with RPMI-1640 containing 20 mM-N-2-hydroxyethylpiperazine-N-2-ethanesulphonic acid (HEPES: Nakarai Chem. Ltd., Kyoto, Japan) and was incubated for 1 h at 4 °C.

3 After 1 h incubation, the column was washed with 5 ml of chilled RPMI-1640.

4 The absorbed materials were eluted with 2 ml of 0.175 M-glycine-HCl buffer, pH 3.2. Then 2.0 ml of eluate was collected in tubes with 0.3 ml of 0.5 M sodium bicarbonate, dialysed against 0.01 M-PBS, pH 7.2, and concentrated up to the final volume of 200 μl

with Sephadex powder. These procedures should be carried out at 4 °C. The materials were added to the *in vitro* culture system in order to investigate suppressor activity.

Notes and recommendations

From the results obtained by absorption studies, several important properties of the antigen-specific suppressor T cell factor have been demonstrated [42].

1 The KLH-specific suppressor factor (KLH-TsF) obtained from KLH-primed thymocytes or KLH-specific suppressor T cell hybridomas possesses the ability to bind to the relevant antigen KLH column, but not to the irrelevant antigen (i.e. OVA or *Ascaris suum* extracts, etc.), suggesting that the factor carries specific antigen-binding affinity like immunoglobulins. Neither constant region determinants nor the Fab portion of immunoglobulins were, however, demonstrated on the factor [15].

2 The factor was found to be composed of two distinct polypeptide chains. One is the heavy chain (Mr 45 000) with antigen-binding moiety and constant determinants (Ct) unique to suppressor T cells and their factors. The T cell constant region determinants were demonstrated by conventional and monoclonal antibodies made by the Ig allotype congenic pair of mice (BALB/c anti-CB-20), because the monoclonal BALB/c (Ig^a) anti-CB-20 (Ig^b) antibody absorbed conventional KLH-TsF derived from Ig^b mice, such as C57BL/6, CB-20, CWB and BAB-14 mice, but not those from mice with other Igh allotypes, i.e. BALB/c (Ig^a), C3H (Ig^j) or C3H.SW (Ig^j) etc. [29–31]. The other is the light chain (Mr 28 000) with the determinant detected by conventional or monoclonal antibodies raised in B10.A(5R) and B10.A(3R) combinations [33,35].

3 The heavy or the light chain per se could not express any functional activity. However, the mixture of the two molecules reconstitutes the active suppressor factor [43,44]. It is thus apparent that both heavy and light chains of the factor are required for the functional expression of the factor.

4 The heavy and light chains of the factor seem to be independently synthesized in the cytoplasm and are covalently associated with disulphide bonds when they are secreted [44].

Solid-phase radioimmune assay: plate binding assay

At least two monoclonal antibodies recognizing different epitopes on the antigen-specific suppressor factor are necessary for this assay. The authors recently established two monoclonal alloantibodies reactive to the constant region allotypic determinants on the suppressor factor [31]. These two antibodies (Ab1 and Ab2) recognize distinct epitopes on the same suppressor molecule.

Procedure

1 Wells in a 96-well microtitre plate (Dynatech, Alexandria, Va.) were incubated with 70 μl/well of Ab1 solution (1 mg/ml), in 0.01 M-PBS, pH 7.2, at room temperature for 1 h to coat the Ab1 on to the plate, followed by washing with 0.01 M-PBS, pH 7.2, containing 0.5% bovine serum albumin (BSA). The plate was further reacted with 0.01 M-PBS, pH 7.2, enriched with 20% FCS to block the residual reactive sites on the plate.
2 After extensive washing by flicking, the plate was reacted with 50 μl of the antigen-specific extracted suppressor factor (equivalent to $2–8 \times 10^8$ cells per ml) on ice for 1 h, and the unbound materials were removed by flicking. The procedures were repeated five times.
3 The wells were subsequently washed three times with 200 μl of 0.01 M-PBS containing 0.5% BSA, followed by reacting with 50 μl of ^{125}I-labelled Ab2 (800 000 c.p.m. per well) for 1 h at 4 °C. The plate was washed at least five times and counted for 3 min by a gamma counter. The experiments should be done in triplicate.

Notes and recommendations

Data showing a typical plot (linear) of the solid-phase radioimmune assay by using monoclonal BALB/c (Ig^a) anti-CB-20 (Ig^b) for the detection of the suppressor factor in the thymocyte extracts from C57BL/6 (Ig^b) are presented in Fig. 80.2. For control, the same amounts of BALB/c (Ig^a) thymocyte extracts were used. As the BALB/c anti-CB-20 recognizes allotypic determinant (Ct^b) on the constant region of the factor, the assay system measures the relative amounts of Ct^b-bearing molecules of the factor. Moreover, the suppressor activity of the materials obtained by this method is shown to correlate with the amounts of suppressor molecules detected.

Methods for the preparation and detection of mRNAs coding for suppressor molecules

Because hybridoma cells or cloned T cell lines consist of homogeneous cell populations, it is useful in obtaining mRNAs encoding molecules with specific T cell functions. In this section, the authors describe methods for preparing mRNAs and detecting minute amounts of products of mRNAs translated in *Xenopus laevis* oocytes.

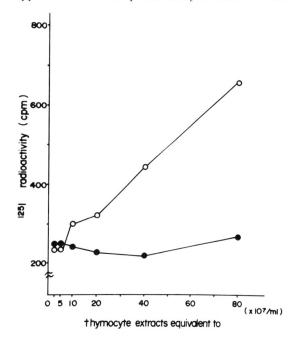

Fig. 80.2. Binding of the factor to the plate coated with specific monoclonal antibodies, BALB/c (Ig^a) anti-CB-20 (Ig^b). Thymocyte extracts derived from BALB/c (Ig^a) (●) or C57BL/6 (Ig^b) (○) bound to the plates were detected by radioimmune assay.

Preparation of mRNAs

Isolation with phenol-metacresol

Procedure

1 The well washed hybridoma cells (10^9) were suspended in 10 ml of 0.1 M-Tris-HCl, pH 9.0, containing 0.25 M-sucrose, 0.1 M-NaCl and 5 u/ml RNase inhibitor or rat liver as described [45].
2 The cells were homogenized with a Potter homogenizer (Wheaton #200) and the homogenized materials were centrifuged at 10 000 *g* for 20 min.
3 The supernates were collected and added with an equal volume of phenol:metacresol (9:1) containing 0.1% 8-hydroxyquinolin. The mixture was vigorously shaken for 10 min and centrifuged at 10 000 *g* for 20 min.
4 After centrifugation, the mixture was separated into two phases (an upper layer: aqueous phase; and a lower layer: phenol phase). As RNAs were dissolved in the aqueous phase, the upper layer was collected and again mixed with an equal volume of phenol:metacresol solution. This procedure was repeated several times until the proteins were completely removed. The

interphase between the aqueous and phenol phases should contain proteins. If the proteins were removed completely by this procedure, the interphase became clear.

5 The aqueous phase after complete removal of proteins was mixed with $\frac{1}{10}$ vol. of 3 M sodium acetate buffer, pH 5.5, and 2 vols. of ethanol, and left to stand for 10 h at $-20\,^{\circ}$C to precipitate RNAs.

6 The total RNAs were pelleted by centrifugation at 2000–3000 g for 20 min at 4 $^{\circ}$C. The pellets were gently rinsed with 10 ml of 80% ethanol.

7 The supernates were discarded, and the pellets were dried and then dissolved in 10 ml of distilled water. By this method, about 10 mg of RNAs was usually obtained from 10^9 cells.

Isolation with guanidine/cesium chloride

Procedure

This method was originally described by Chirgwin *et al.* [46].

1 The washed pellets of 10^9 hybridoma cells were resuspended in 10 ml of guanidine thiocyanate solution (GTC solution: 4.2 M guanidine thiocyanate, pH 7.0, containing 5 mM sodium citrate, 0.1 M-2-mercaptoethanol and 0.1% antiform A).

2 The cell suspensions were homogenized with a Potter homogenizer. They were centrifuged at 500 g for 5 min, and the small bubbles on the top layer were removed by aspiration.

3 The homogenized materials were overlayed on 5.7 M-CsCl$_2$, 0.1 M-EDTA, pH 7.0, (CsCl$_2$ solution) (volume ratios of materials/CsCl$_2$ solution = 2:1) in a polyallomer tube (1.3 × 13 cm, 13 PA tube, Hitachi Koki Co. Ltd., Tokyo, Japan) and centrifuged at 170 000 g for 15 h at 15 $^{\circ}$C by a swing rotor (RPS-40T, Hitachi Koki, Co. Ltd., Tokyo, Japan). During centrifugation, only RNAs form pellets on the bottom of the tube, while most DNAs and proteins float on the CsCl$_2$ solution.

4 After centrifugation, the solution containing DNAs and proteins was removed by aspiration. The walls of the centrifuge tubes were gently washed three times with 1 ml of GTC solution. The pellets were then rinsed with 2 ml of cold 80% ethanol, dried and resuspended in 3 ml of distilled water, followed by precipitation of the RNAs with ethanol, as described in the previous section. After ethanol precipitation, the RNAs were resuspended in 5–10 ml of distilled water. By this procedure, 5–8 mg of RNAs was generally obtained from 10^9 cells. Moreover, the RNAs isolated with guanidine/cesium chloride were usually intact when compared with other methods.

Purification of polyadenylated RNA

Procedure

Several techniques have been developed to separate poly(A) positive RNA from non-adenylated RNAs. The method described here is chromatography on oligo(dT)-cellulose [47].

1 The RNA solution (10 ml of 1 mg/ml), which had been adjusted at a final concentration of 10 mM-Tris-HCl, pH 7.4, 0.1 mM-EDTA, 0.5 M-KCl, was applied to the column (1.5 × 5 cm) composed of 5 ml of oligo(dT)-cellulose Type 7 (PL Biochemicals Inc., Milwaukee, Wisconsin) equilibrated with Tris-HCl buffer containing 0.5 M-KCl (10 mM-Tris-HCl, pH 7.4, 0.1 mM-EDTA, 0.5 M-KCl).

2 The column was thoroughly washed with 100–150 ml of Tris-HCl buffer with 0.5 M-KCl solution. Only poly (A) positive RNAs (mRNA) were retained by the oligo(dT)-cellulose column, and r-RNAs and t-RNAs passed through the column.

3 mRNAs were then eluted with 15 ml of Tris-HCl buffer under monitoring by 260 nm with a UV monitor (Model UA-500, ISCO, Nebraska).

4 The purified mRNAs were again applied to the second oligo(dT)-cellulose column.

5 The column was washed with 50 ml of Tris-HCl buffer with 0.5 M-KCl followed by washing with Tris-HCl buffer with 0.2 M-KCl.

6 The mRNAs were then eluted with Tris-HCl buffer, pelleted with ethanol-precipitation, and dissolved in distilled water (5 mg/ml). The procedures are carried out at room temperature. Generally, mRNAs thus obtained are 1–2% of the total RNA.

Sucrose density gradient centrifugation

Procedure

1 The mRNA solution was heated at 75 $^{\circ}$C for 10 min and subsequently cooled in ice before use.

2 Heated 200–500 μg (5 mg/ml) mRNA was overlayed on to 12.8 ml of 5–22% linear sucrose gradient in a polyallomer centrifge tube (Hitachi 13 PA tube). This was ultracentrifuged at 170 000 g for 16 h at 15 $^{\circ}$C by a Hitachi SCP70H with a RPS-40T swing rotor.

3 After centrifugation, samples were fractionated with a density gradient fractionator (Model 640, ISCO, Nebraska).

4 mRNA in each fraction was precipitated with ethanol and suspended in distilled water at a concentration of 0.5 mg/ml.

Translation of mRNA injected into **Xenopus laevis** oocytes

Procedure

The methods to translate mRNA in *Xenopus laevis* oocyte have been described by Gurdon *et al.* [48].

1   Between 30 and 50 nl of the mRNA dissolved in distilled water was injected into fully grown oocytes from healthy, adult female *Xenopus* using a fine micropipette under an inverted light microscope.

2   Immediately after the injection, ten oocytes injected with the same fraction of mRNA were incubated at 19–21 °C for 36 h in 100 μl of a sterile Barth's medium (88 mM-NaCl, 1 mM-KCl, 0.33 mM-Ca(NO$_3$)$_2$, 0.41 mM-CaCl$_2$ 0.82 mM-MgSO$_4$, 2.4 mM-NaHCO$_3$, 10 mM-HEPES, pH 7.4, containing 10 mg/ml penicillin and 10 mg/ml streptomycin sulphate).

3   The translation products were prepared by centrifugation of homogenates of oocytes injected with mRNAs at 100 000 *g* for 1 h. After centrifugation, there will be two distinct phases: an upper phase, which contains the translation products, and a lower phase of yolk and pigment granules of oocytes. Therefore the upper phase was collected, added with 0.2 mM-PMSF, and stored at −80 °C until use.

Notes and recommendations

The mRNAs injected into oocytes are much more efficiently translated than those in the reticulocyte or wheatgerm system when translation products are detected by the cytotoxic inhibition assays as described below (see next section). In fact, the mRNA directing the heavy chain of the suppressor factor is translated about ten times more efficiently in *Xenopus* oocytes than in a reticulocyte lysate, and about fifty times more efficiently in *Xenopus* than in wheatgerm.

Detection of translation products of mRNAs coding for the suppressor T cell factor

Translation products of the fractionated mRNA were tested for their ability to inhibit the cytotoxic activity of the monoclonal antibody against the antigen-specific suppressor factor [49]. The cytotoxic inhibition assay is very sensitive and easily detects minute amounts of the suppressor factor in the translation products of mRNA. However, it is necessary to use the monoclonal antibody and monoclonal target cell lines, such as T cell hybridomas or TCGF-dependent cell lines.

Procedure

1   Target cells (10^4) and 10 μl of the diluted monoclonal antibody that gave the endpoint of maximum cytotoxic activity, were mixed with 10 μl of the translation products of the mRNA or the oocyte extract as an inhibitor. The mixture was incubated for 30 min on ice in a V-bottom 96-well microplate (Dynatech, Alexandria, Va).

2   The cells were pelleted and resuspended in 20 μl of rabbit complement, followed by further incubation for 30 min at 37 °C. Dead and viable cells were counted under a light microscope by dye exclusion. The percentage cytotoxicity and percentage inhibition of the cytotoxicity were calculated.

Functional detection of the suppressor activity in the translation products of mRNAs

The *in vitro* spleen cell culture can be used for the detection of the suppressor activity in the translation products of the fractionated mRNA. As it is apparent from functional assays using extracted or secreted suppressor T cell factors that both heavy and light chains of the factor are necessary for the expression of the antigen-specific suppressor function [43,44], the translation products of two fractionated mRNAs were mixed in appropriate combinations and added to the *in vitro* antibody response to test their suppressor activity. A higher concentration of oocyte extracts per se sometimes causes non-specific inhibition of the *in vitro* antibody responses. It is thus necessary to titrate the suppressor activity of the mRNA translation products in comparison with the dose effects of the uninjected oocyte extracts on the antibody formation. In fact, Fig. 80.3 demonstrates the effects of oocyte extracts on the *in vitro* secondary anti-DNP IgG

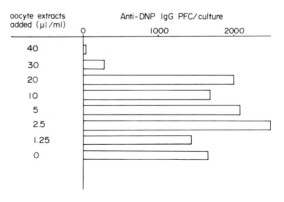

Fig. 80.3. Effects of oocyte extracts on the *in vitro* secondary antibody (PFC) responses.

antibody PFC responses. The addition of more than 30 μl/ml of oocyte extracts into the *in vitro* culture system inhibited PFC responses, while no significant effect was observed by the addition of 1.25–20 μl/ml of oocyte extracts obtained from ten oocytes cultured for 36 h in 100 μl of Barth's medium.

Data showing typical results obtained by using translation products of fractionated mRNAs from KLH-specific suppressor T cell hybridoma are presented in Fig. 80.4. The mixture of translation products of the 11S and 13S mRNAs or the 11S and 18.5S mRNAs reconstitutes KLH-specific suppressor function, while the double volume of each mRNA translation product did not show any effects on the PFC responses [49].

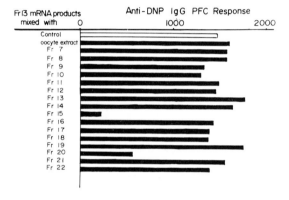

Fig. 80.4. Reconstitution of suppressor activity with the mixture of translation products of mRNAs in fraction 13 (11S mRNA) and fraction 15 (13S mRNA) or fraction 20 (18.5S mRNA). mRNAs from KLH-specific suppressor T cell hybridomas were fractionated by sucrose density gradient centrifugation; 1.25 μl of each fractionated mRNA product was mixed and added to the culture.

Methods for the reconstitution of suppressor activity with mRNA translation products and isolated free chains

The mixture of the translated heavy and light chains (13S and 11S mRNA products) successfully reconstitutes the active form of suppressor factor that mediates the antigen-specific and genetically restricted suppressor activity. The use of mRNA translates of the factor permits the investigation of the biological roles of the heavy and light chains of suppressor factor because they provide the homogeneous active materials of heavy or light chains. The extracted materials from primed thymocytes contain three forms of suppressor T cell factor: free heavy chains, free light chains and the non-covalently associated form of these two, and they seem to be in a state of equilibrium.

Therefore, it is possible to isolate free heavy and light chains from the extracted suppressor factor and to reconstitute suppressor factor with mRNA translates.

Preparation of free heavy and light chains of the suppressor factor

Procedure

The methods for the preparation of the free heavy and light chains are carried out under the same conditions as described in the section under 'Absorption and elution of the factor using immunoadsorbent columns'.

1 For the preparation of the antigen-binding heavy chains with distinct specificities, i.e. KLH or OVA, 100 μl of the KLH- or OVA-primed thymocyte extracts (equivalent to 1.5×10^7 cells) was applied to the first column composed of 1 ml of anti-I-J-coupled Sepharose beads. The effluent contains only the free heavy chain while the free light chain and the associated form are retained on the anti-I-J column. Thus, it is possible to use the effluent as a source of the free light chains of the factor.

2 The effluent was further incubated with the second KLH or OVA column in order to isolate the free heavy chain. The absorbed materials were eluted with 0.175 M-glycine HCl buffer, pH 3.2, and used as the antigen-binding heavy chain because the free heavy chain itself possesses the ability to bind to the native antigen.

3 Similar procedures can be used to prepare the I-J positive light chain. The antigen-primed thymocyte extracts from H-2^b or H-2^k mice were reacted with the first antigen column under the same conditions described above. Again, it is possible to use the effluent as a source of the free light chains.

4 The effluent was successively applied to the second anti-I-J^b or anti-I-J^k column.

5 The acid eluate from the anti-I-J column was immediately neutralized and dialysed against PBS, pH 7.2. This contains the I-J positive light chains.

Reconstitution of the isolated heavy or light chains and the mRNA translation products

One hundred microlitres of the isolated heavy chain with KLH- or OVA-binding activity (obtained from the extracted factor equivalent to 1.5×10^7 cells) was mixed with 1.25 μl of the 11S mRNA translate of the I-J positive light chain. The mixture was added to the 1 ml culture of spleen cells 4 weeks previously primed with 100 μg DNP-KLH or DNP-OVA and *B. pertussis* vaccine as described above. It is essential that the H-2 haplotype between the factor and responding spleen cells is identical.

Notes and recommendations

The data on the shuffling experiments [50] using the mRNA translates and the isolated chains, revealed the functional roles of the heavy and light chains of the suppressor factor:

1 The antigen-binding heavy chain determines the antigen specificity of the factor. The mixture of the translated light chain and the isolated KLH-binding heavy chain suppressed only the responses against DNP-KLH but not those to DNP-OVA, whereas the mixture in combination with the isolated OVA-binding heavy chain mediated the suppressor function in the responses to DNP-OVA but not to DNP-KLH.

2 The light chain determines the genetic specificity of the suppressor factor. The mixture of the $I-J^k$ positive light chain obtained from C3H and the translate of 13S mRNA from C57BL/6 derived KLH-specific suppressor T cell hybridoma suppressed the response of C3H but not C57BL/6 mice. However, C57BL/6 but not C3H response was preferentially suppressed when the same translated heavy chain was mixed with the $I-J^b$ positive isolated light chain from C57BL/6.

3 There is no genetic preferential combination between heavy and light chains in the reconstitution of the functional suppressor molecule.

Acknowledgements

The authors wish to thank the entire staff of their laboratory, especially Dr Masamoto Kanno, Dr Masatoshi Tagawa and Mr Toshihiro Itoh for the preparation and testing of mRNA and their translation products, and Miss Hisano Nakajima for her generous help in preparation of this manuscript.

References

1 TADA T. & OKUMURA K. (1979) The role of antigen-specific T cell factors in the immune response. *Adv. Immunol.* **28**, 1.

2 TADA T., OKUMURA K. & TANIGUCHI M. (1973) Regulation of homocytotropic antibody formation in the rat. (VIII) An antigen-specific T cell factor that regulates anti-hapten homocytotropic antibody response. *J. Immunol.* **111**, 952.

3 KONTIAINEN S. & FELDMANN M. (1978) Suppressor-cell induction *in vitro*. (IV) Target of antigen-specific suppressor factor and its genetic relationships. *J. exp. Med.* **147**, 110.

4 ZEMBRA M. & ASHERSON G.L. (1974) T cell suppression of contact sensitivity in the mouse. (II) The role of soluble factor and its interaction with macrophages. *Eur. J. Immunol.* **4**, 799.

5 GREENE M.I., FUJIMOTO S. & SEHON A.H. (1977) Regulation of the immune response to tumor antigen. (III) Characterization of thymic suppressor(s) produced by the tumor bearing host. *J. Immunol.* **119**, 757.

6 TAKEI F., LEVY H.G. & KILBURN D.G. (1978) Characterization of a soluble factor that specifically suppresses the *in vitro* generation of cells cytotoxic for syngeneic tumor cells in mice. *J. Immunol.* **120**, 1218.

7 THEZE J., WALTENBAUGH C., GERMAIN R.N. & BENACERRAF B. (1977) Immunosuppressive factor(s) specific for L-glutamic acid^{60}-L-tyrosine^{50}. *In vitro* activity and immunochemical properties. *Eur. J. Immunol.* **7**, 705.

8 FRESNO M., McVAY-BOUDREAU L., NABEL G. & CANTOR H. (1981) Antigen-specific T cell clones. (II) Purification and biological characterization of an antigen-specific suppressive protein synthesized by cloned T-cells. *J. exp. Med.* **153**, 1260.

9 TANIGUCHI M. & MILLER J.F.A.P. (1978) Specific suppression of the immune response by a factor obtained from spleen cells of mice tolerant to human γ-globulin. *J. Immunol.* **120**, 21.

10 THEZE J., KAPP J. & BENACERRAF B. (1977) Immunosuppressive factor(s) extracted from lymphoid cells of nonresponder mice primed with L-glutamic acid^{60}-L-alanine^{30}-L-tyrosine^{10} (GAT). (III) Immunochemical properties of the GAT-specific suppressive factor. *J. exp. Med.* **145**, 839.

11 GREENE M.I., PIERCE C.A., DORF M.E. & BENACERRAF B. (1977) The I-J subregion codes for determinants on suppressor factor(s) which limit the contact sensitivity response to picryl chloride. *J. exp. Med.* **146**, 293.

12 MOOREHEAD J.W. (1977) Soluble factors in tolerant and contact sensitivity to 2,4-dinitrofluobenzene in mice. (I) Suppression of contact sensitivity by soluble suppressor factor released *in vitro* by lymph node cell populations containing specific suppressor cells. *J. Immunol.* **119**, 315.

13 YAMAUCHI K., MURPHY D., CANTOR H. & GERSHQN R.K. (1981) Analysis of antigen-specific, Ig-restricted cell-free material made by I-J$^+$ Ly-1$^+$ cells (Ly-1 TsF) that induces Ly-2$^+$ cells to express suppressor activity. *Eur. J. Immunol.* **11**, 905.

14 SY M.S., DIETZ M.H., GERMAIN R.N., BENACERRAF B. & GREENE M.I. (1980) Antigen- and receptor-driven regulatory mechanisms. (IV) Idiotype-bearing I-J$^+$ suppressor T cell factors induce second-order suppressor T cells which express anti-idiotypic receptors. *J. exp. Med.* **151**, 1183.

15 TANIGUCHI M., HAYAKAWA K. & TADA T. (1976) Properties of antigen-specific suppressive T-cell factor in the regulation of antibody response of the mouse. (II) *In vitro* activity and evidence for the I region gene product. *J. Immunol.* **116**, 542.

16 KONTIAINEN S., SIMPSON E., BORER E., BEVERLEY P.C., HERZENBERG L.A., FITZPATRICK W.C., VOGT P., TORANO A., McKENZIE I.F.C. & FELDMANN M. (1978) T cell lines producing antigen-specific suppressor factor. *Nature*, **274**, 477.

17 TANIGUCHI M. & MILLER J.F.A.P. (1978) Specific suppressive factors produced by hybridomas derived from

the fusion of enriched suppressor T cells and a T lymphoma cell line. *J. exp. Med.* **148**, 373.

18 TANIGUCHI M., SAITO T. & TADA T. (1979) Antigen-specific suppressive factor produced by a transplantable I-J bearing T cell hybridoma. *Nature*, **278**, 555.

19 MINAMI M., OKUDA K., FURUSAWA S., BENACERRAF B. & DORF M.E. (1981) Analysis of T cell hybridomas. (I) Characterization of H-2 and Igh-restricted monoclonal suppressor factors. *J. exp. Med.* **154**, 1390.

20 WATANABE T., KIMOTO M., MARUYAMA T., KISHIMOTO T. & YAMAMURA Y. (1978) Regulation of antibody response in different immunoglobulin classes. (V) Establishment of T hybrid cell line secreting IgE class-specific suppressor factor. *J. Immunol.* **121**, 2113.

21 TANIGUCHI M. & MILLER J.F.A.P. (1977) Enrichment of specific suppressor T cells and characterization of their surface markers. *J. exp. Med.* **146**, 1450.

22 OKUMURA K., TAKEMORI T., TOKUHISA T. & TADA T. (1977) Specific enrichment of the suppressor T cell bearing I-J determinants: parallel functional and serological characterizations. *J. exp. Med.* **146**, 1234.

23 BACH B.M., GREENE M.I., BENACERRAF B. & NISSONOFF A. (1979) Mechanisms of regulation of cell mediated immunity. (IV) Asobenzenearsonate (ABA) specific suppressor factor(s) bear cross-reactive idiotype (CRI) determinants the expression of which is linked to the heavy chain allotype linkage group of genes *J. exp. Med.* **149**, 1084.

24 TADA T., HAYAKAWA K., OKUMURA K. & TANIGUCHI M. (1980) Coexistence of variable region of immunoglobulin heavy chain and I-region gene products on antigen-specific suppressor T cells and suppressor T cell factor. A minimal model of functional antigen receptor of T cells. *Mol. Immunol.* **17**, 867.

25 KONTIAINEN S. & FELDMANN M. (1979) Structural characteristics of antigen-specific suppressor factors: definition of 'constant' and 'variable' region determinants. *Thymus*, **1**, 59.

26 GERMAIN R.N., JU S., KIPPS J., BENACERRAF B. & DORF M.E. (1979) Shared idiotypic determinants on antibodies and T-cell-derived suppressor factor specific for the random terpolymer L-glutamic acid[60]-L-alanine[30]-L-tyrosine[10]. *J. exp. Med.* **149**, 613.

27 OWEN F.L., FINNEGAR A., GATES E.R. & GOTTLIEB P.O. (1979) A mature T lymphocyte subpopulation marker closely linked to the Igh-1 allotype CH locus. *Eur. J. Immunol.* **9**, 948.

28 OWEN F.L. (1980) A mature T lymphocyte marker closely linked to Igh-1 that is expressed on the precursor for the suppressor T cell regulating a primary response to SRBC. *J. Immunol.* **124**, 1411.

29 TOKUHISA T. & TANIGUCHI M. (1982) Two distinct allotypic determinants on the antigen-specific suppressor and enhancing T cell factors that are encoded by genes linked to the immunoglobulin heavy chain locus. *J. exp. Med.* **155**, 126.

30 TOKUHISA T. & TANIGUCHI M. (1982) Constant region determinants on the antigen-binding chain of the suppressor T cell factor. *Nature*, **298**, 174.

31 TOKUHISA T., KOMATSU Y., UCHIDA Y. & TANIGUCHI M. (1982) Monoclonal alloantibodies specific for the con-

stant region of the T cell antigen-receptors. *J. exp. Med.* **156**, 888.

32 MURPHY D.B., HERZENBERG L.A., OKUMURA K., HERZENBERG L.A. & McDEVITT H.O. (1976) A new I subregion (I-J) marked by a locus (Ia-4) controlling surface determinants on suppressor T lymphocytes. *J. exp. Med.* **144**, 699.

33 TADA T., TANIGUCHI M. & DAVID C.S. (1976) Properties of antigen-specific suppressive T-cell factor in the regulation of antibody response of the mouse. (IV) Special subregion assignment of the gene(s) codes for the suppressive T-cell factor in the H-2 histocompatibility complex. *J. exp. Med.* **144**, 713.

34 THEZE J., WALTENBAUGH C., DORF M.E. & BENACERRAF B. (1977) Immunosuppressive factor(s) specific for L-glutamic acid[50]-L-tyrosine[50] (GT). (II) Presence of I-J determinants on the GT-suppressive factor. *J. exp. Med.* **146**, 287.

35 KANNO M., KOBAYASHI S., TOKUHISA T., TAKEI I., SHINOHARA N. & TANIGUCHI M. (1981) Monoclonal antibodies that recognize the product controlled by a gene in the I-J subregion of the mouse H-2 complex. *J. exp. Med.* **154**, 1290.

36 WALTENBAUGH C. (1981) Regulation of immune response by I-J gene products. (I) Production and characterization of anti-I-J monoclonal antibodies. *J. exp. Med.* **154**, 1570.

37 STEINMETZ M., MINARD K., HOVATH S., McNICHOLAS J., FRELINGER J., WAKE C., LONG E., MACH B. & HOOD L. (1982) A molecular map of the immune response region from the major histocompatibility complex of the mouse. *Nature*, **300**, 35.

38 MISHELL R.I. & DUTTON R.W. (1967) Immunization of dissociated spleen cell cultures from normal mice. *J. exp. Med.* **126**, 423.

39 EISEN H.N., BELMAN S. & CARSTEN M.E. (1953) The reaction of 2,4-dinitrobenzenesulfonic acid with free amino group of proteins. *J. Am. chem. Soc.* **75**, 4583.

40 CUNNINGHAM A.J. & SZENBERG A. (1968) Further improvements in the plaque technique for detecting single antibody-forming cells. *Immunology*, **14**, 599.

41 AXEN R., PORATH J. & ERNBACK S. (1967) Chemical coupling of peptides and proteins to polysaccharides by means of cyanogen halides. *Nature*, **214**, 1302.

42 TANIGUCHI M., SAITO T., TAKEI I., KANNO M., TOKUHISA T. & TOMIOKA H. (1982) Suppressor T-cell hybridomas and their soluble products. In *Lymphokines*, Vol. 5, (ed. Feldmann M. & Schreier M.H.), p. 77. Academic Press, New York.

43 TANIGUCHI M., TAKEI I. & TADA T. (1980) Functional and molecular organization of an antigen-specific suppressor factor derived from a T cell hybridoma. *Nature*, **283**, 227.

44 TANIGUCHI M., SAITO T., TAKEI I. & TOKUHISA T. (1981) Presence of interchain disulfide bonds between two gene products that compose the secreted form of an antigen-specific suppressor factor. *J. exp. Med.* **153**, 1672.

45 HONJO T., SHIMIZU A., TSUDA M., NATORI S., KATAOKA T., DOHMOTO C. & MANO Y. (1977) Accumulation of immunoglobulin messenger ribonucleic acid in immunized mouse spleen. *Biochemistry*, **16**, 5764.

46 CHIRGWIN J.M., PREZYBYLA A.E., MacDONALD R.J. & RUTTER W.J. (1979) Isolation of biochemically active

ribonucleic acid from sources enriched in ribonuclease. *Biochemistry*, **18**, 5294.

47 AVIV H. & LEDER P. (1972) Purification of biologically active globulin messenger RNA by chromatography on oligothymidylic acid-cellulose. *Proc. natn. Acad. Sci. U.S.A.* **69**, 1408.

48 GURDON J.B., LANE C.D., WOODLAND H.R. & MARAIX G. (1971) Use of frog eggs in oocytes for the study of mRNA and its translation in living cells. *Nature*, **233**, 177.

49 TANIGUCHI M., TOKUHISA T., KANNO M., YAOITA Y., SHIMIZU A. & HONJO T. (1982) Reconstitution of antigen-specific suppressor activity with translation products of mRNA. *Nature*, **298**, 172.

50 TANIGUCHI M., TOKUHISA T., ITOH T. & KANNO M. (1984) Functional roles of two polypeptide chains that compose an antigen-specific suppressor T cell factor. *J. exp. Med.* **159**, 1096.

Chapter 81
Immunosuppressive agents

D. J. G. WHITE & J. F. L. SHAW

Immunosuppressive agents, 81.1
History of immunosuppression in
 transplantation, 81.1
Review of techniques for

assessing immunosuppressive
 activity, 81.2
Experimental immunosuppressive
 procedures, 81.3

Monoclonal antibodies as
 immunosuppressive agents,
 81.10
Cyclosporin A, 81.10

Immunosuppressive agents

There are a large number of diseases in which lesions are produced as a consequence of inappropriate activity (or inactivity) by various components of the immune system. These can be categorized under the three general headings: immunodeficiencies, autoimmunity and allograft responses. It is primarily the latter two conditions that may require treatment with immunosuppressive agents. During the last decade our ability to dissect and analyse various components of the immune system has increased and with it our understanding of these inappropriate responses. Our capacity to intervene successfully to prevent or, more appropriately, halt such responses remains very limited.

There has long been a dichotomy between the search for 'immunosuppressive agents' that are primarily directed at preventing graft rejection and non-steroidal anti-inflammatories that are primarily directed at treatment of autoimmune conditions. One of the differences between these two conditions is that in transplantation the advent of the immune response may be predicted. The site and aetiology of the stimulating antigens is known and the clinician can institute an appropriate immunosuppressive action in advance of the anticipated adverse immunological responses to the transplant. It should also be appreciated that the allograft reaction is an artificial response which in some respects is greater than that elicited by non-major histocompatibility complex antigens. In autoimmune conditions the clinician is faced with treating an established immune response in which the effector cell population has already been generated and whose aetiology is for the most part poorly understood. Those seeking to treat patients suffering from autoimmune conditions are also faced with the dilemma that while these conditions may cause considerable discomfort and often reduce the individual's lifespan, rarely are such diseases immediately life-threatening. Thus while one may be justified in making heroic efforts involving the risk of lethal infections to prevent the rejection of say a heart transplant, such efforts would not be justifiable in the treatment of rheumatoid arthritis. It is inevitable, therefore, that as experience with immunosuppression is obtained in organ transplantation, the successful regimens are adapted for use in the treatment of autoimmunity as their safety and efficiency are established. Although this chapter describes the current status of experimental immunosuppressive agents for use in transplantation, their possible relevance to other conditions should not be ignored.

History of immunosuppression in transplantation

The stimulus which induced research workers to try to suppress the immune system was provided largely by the desire of surgeons to treat by transplantation terminal single organ failure diseases, particularly of the kidney. A series of elegant, innovative experiments performed by Medawar et al. demonstrated that rejection is an immune process [1]. Furthermore, these workers found that it was possible to manipulate the immune system so that it would accept foreign grafts [2]. The successful grafting of a kidney between identical twins showed that organ transplantation was a potentially beneficial therapy for kidney failure if rejection could be overcome [3].

The principles involved in the development of antigen-specific non-responsiveness are described in detail elsewhere in this volume (Chapter 80). While such donor-specific immunosuppression must ultimately be the goal for those seeking to control allograft rejection, the clinician faced with the urgency of treating fatal disease has turned to the less subtle but currently available approach of non-specific immunosuppression.

Initial attempts at non-specific depression of the immune system were with the use of whole body irradiation. This approach met with some success in that it was found possible to irradicate the immune system with irradiation and thus permit the acceptance of a subsequent transplant. Unfortunately recipients of such treatment rapidly succumbed to uncontrolled and uncontrollable infection. It became clear that more selective means of regulating the immune system were required so that the individual could be left with enough immune function to prevent trivial infections becoming fatal while providing sufficient immunosuppression to prevent graft rejection.

The demonstration by Schwartz & Damashek [4] of the induction of immunological tolerance to proteins in rabbits treated with 6-mercaptopurine led Calne [5] to demonstrate that this agent would prevent kidney graft rejection in dogs. 6-Mercaptopurine proved to be too toxic for clinical use. However, azathioprine (Fig. 81.1), an analogue of 6-mercaptopurine, was shown by Calne to be less toxic and as immunosuppressive as unmodified 6-mercaptopurine [6]. It was the introduction of this drug and its subsequent combination by Starzl with high dose steroids that established transplantation as a practical therapy for kidney failure [7]. This double-drug approach has formed the basis for immunosuppressive therapy from that time until the present day. With these two agents results from the treatment of renal failure by kidney grafting improved steadily during the 1960s both in terms of patient and graft survival. By the early 1970s, just over half the kidneys transplanted could be expected to retain life-supporting function for more than one year.

During the 1970s, knowledge of the processes involved in immune responses increased substantially. Major advances were made in understanding the HLA system, although the contribution of tissue typing to improvement in cadaveric graft survival remains disappointing. On the immunosuppressive front anti-lymphocyte serum (or its derivatives anti-lymphocyte globulin and anti-thymocyte globulin), was introduced into clinical use and proved to be a potent immunosuppressive, although its successful use has been restricted to a few centres. However, by the end of the decade results in kidney transplantation were,

despite considerable amounts of time, money and effort invested in research, only marginally improved over those achieved at its beginning. It is to be hoped that the recent advances that have been made in the development of immunosuppressive agents mean that the next decade will see more substantial advances.

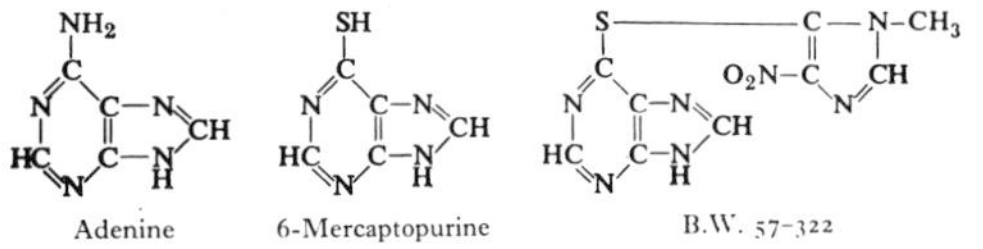

Review of techniques for assessing immunosuppressive activity

Almost any assay of immune responsiveness, the majority of which are described in other sections of this handbook, can be suitably adapted to measure the effect of potentially immunosuppressive agents. The procedural detail will therefore not be given here. Of those *in vitro* assays which can measure immune responses in man the mixed lymphocyte* culture and cell mediated lympholysis have proved to be of greatest value in screening for potential immunosuppressive agents for use in transplantation [8,9]. However, agents which are immunosuppressive *in vitro* often prove to be of little value *in vivo*. Thus one is forced to evaluate these agents in animal models of transplantation. Most immunologists tend to consider that the height of their surgical skills would probably not stretch further than performing skin grafts [10]. While it is true that organ transplantation in large animals requires specialized premises and trained expertise in the techniques of vascular surgery, recent developments in microvascular surgery have meant that some organ grafts in small animals can now be performed with a minimum of surgical education. One of the most commonly used organ grafts for testing immunosuppressive agents is the heterotopic heart transplant in the rat. The original technique for performing this procedure was described by Ono & Lindsey [11] and in essence required the anastomosis of the great vessels of the heart to the rat aorta and vena cava below the liver. This involved opening the peritoneal cavity with the possible risk of peritonitis and performing arterial and venous anastomoses on relatively small vessels. These anastomoses, particularly when performed by the unskilled individual, tended either to thrombose or to leak, causing death of the recipient by haemorrhage. The development of the cuffing procedure for joining vessels, first described by Heron and modified by Dunn and later by Kamada, has made this procedure much easier [12–14]. The heart can now be placed in the neck rather than the abdomen and the vessels joined without the use of sutures. This procedure (Fig. 81.2) reduces the risk of

Fig. 81.1. Azathioprine and its relationship to 6-mercaptopurine and purine.

---

* The correct procedure for these assays is of importance for the valid interpretation of any data obtained by their use. The problems with the assay are reviewed in ref. 8.

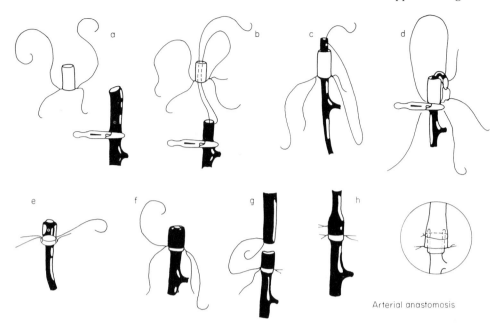

Arterial anastomosis

Fig. 81.2. A polythene prosthesis about 3 mm long is prepared from tubing of about 2.0 mm external diameter. Two 7/0 silk sutures are tied at opposite sides of one end of the prosthesis (a). One of these is used to pull the recipient artery through the prosthesis as in b and c. This suture is tied with one double throw and pulls the end of the artery forward (d). The second suture is then passed through the opposite edge of the artery and tied with one double throw. Front and back walls of the vessel now lie in front of the cuff (e). The cuff is then held with a pair of straight forceps and the knots are allowed to slip just enough to allow the front wall of the artery to be everted over the back of the cuff. Both knots are then tied and the artery is ready for anastomosis (f). The suture needles are passed through the opposite corners of the donor artery, and the vessel is pulled down behind the cuff (g). The first throws of the knots are held in forceps and the anterior wall of the donor vessel is slowly stretched over the cuff. The knots are tied (h). A circumferential 7/0 silk ligature completes the anastomosis. No bleeding occurs from this anastomosis. (Reproduced by kind permission of D.C. Dunn [13].)

thrombosis and haemorrhage and means that six heart grafts a day can be easily performed. Placing the heart graft in the neck makes it easy to ascertain function. The graft can be exposed and removed without threat to the animal's life and, if desired, a second heart can be placed using the contralateral vessels [15].

Experimental immunosuppressive procedures

Total lymphoid irradiation (TLI)

The problems of overcoming the side-effects induced by irradiation and the success of pharmacological immunosuppression meant that the interest in ionizing irradiation as a means of preventing graft rejection, which had flourished in the 1950s, waned [16]. However, over the intervening years our understanding of the fundamental biological mechanisms underlying the effects of ionizing irradiations on cells has improved considerably. Ionizing irradiation produces its lethal effect upon cells usually by the production of a

lesion in DNA, which causes the cell to die during attempted mitotic division. Many of these radiation-induced lesions can be repaired by the action of enzymes in advance of any attempted division. However, there is a population of highly radiosensitive cells, including the small resting lymphocyte, which die as a result of radiation damage during interphase. The mechanism by which this cell death is induced is not clearly understood. Thus, when irradiation doses are fractionated over several days, repair processes occur in most cells between successive exposures. In the radiosensitive cell population, however, no such repair occurs and an almost linear dose–response curve can be achieved with this fractionated treatment.

As a result of this peculiar radiosensitivity of the small lymphocyte, the treatment by fractionated radiation therapy of Hodgkin's disease has proved a highly effective treatment for an otherwise fatal condition. Detailed studies have revealed that a dose of approximately 4000 rads given as a fractionated treatment is capable of irradicating the disease from an involved lymph node. However, because of the meta-static nature of this condition, it is necessary to treat all the involved lymph nodes and this necessity has led to an expansion in the size of the field irradiated. This expansion has resulted in the use of the 'mantle field', which encompasses the submental, submandibular, cervical, supraclavicular, infraclavicular and axillary lymph nodes bilaterally, as well as the mediastinal and hilar nodes, while the lung and heart remain shielded. In order to include a group of patients who have subdiaphragmatic involvement, the radiation field can be further extended by the use of the inverted Y field, which permits irradiation of the spleen and the abdominal and pelvic retroperitoneal nodes. It has been found that most patients could tolerate the very high doses of irradiation remarkably well and such total lymphoid irradiation made it possible to offer a permanent cure for at least 70% of all patients with this once invariably fatal disease.

There has been little clinical evidence to suggest that patients treated with TLI for Hodgkin's disease have any impairment of their immune function. There has been no evidence of any discernible long-term increase in the frequency of infections in this patient population. However, it was found that these patients had a substantial deficiency in their T cell functions. This was manifested as a T lymphocytopenia and a B lymphocytosis, depression of responsiveness both in mixed lymphocyte reaction and to PHA mitogenesis and a loss of delayed type hypersensitivity responses to rechallenge with skin sensitive agents [17]. It was these observations that led Slavin & Strober to consider the use of TLI as an immunosuppressive agent in transplantation. Their initial experiments were performed using skin grafts between H2 incompatible strains of mice [18]. These workers demonstrated that Balb C mice given 200 rads per day five times a week to a total of 3400 rads of irradiation, rejected skin grafts from C57BL/K mice placed one day after the end of the treatment for a median of 49.1 days, compared with 10.7 days for controls. They also showed that a single injection of bone marrow cells produced stable chimaeras in similarly TLI-treated recipients. Skin grafts of donor origin placed on these chimaeras then survived indefinitely in seven out of eight such recipients. These authors extended their studies to the rat given either a skin graft, for which established chimaerism was needed to achieve indefinite survival, or a heart graft, where established chimaerism was not required to produce indefinite survival [19].

It is perhaps not surprising that a total cumulative dose of more than 3000 rads should prove to be immunosuppressive. However, the remarkable observation that it proved possible to establish chimaeras by transfer of fully allogeneic bone-marrow cells without any indication of graft-versus-host disease was of great potential clinical significance. Since graft-versus-host disease is fundamentally a property of the transferred donor cells, which of course have not received any irradiation, this observation would suggest that some fundamental modification of the immune system has taken place. Slavin *et al.* suggested that the TLI treatment alters the structure of the reticuloendothelial and lymphoid tissues [20]. These changes then bring about the tolerance of residual host lymphocytes to transplantation antigens from the graft and inhibit the proper maturation of the cells derived from the transplanted bone marrow.

Because of the logistic complexities and financial commitment necessary to maintain a state of TLI readiness in a clinical environment, the end product in terms of graft and patient well-being needs to be greater than a marginal improvement on results achieved with established immunosuppressive techniques. The potential attraction of TLI therapy in clinical use would thus seem to be its apparent ability to permit the safe establishment of chimaerism and hence specific graft tolerance. This possibility was given extra credence by the report from the Stanford group that they were successfully able to induce chimaerism, as assessed by blood grouping and sex karyotyping, between unrelated mongrel dogs preconditioned with TLI [21]. However, when these workers subsequently came to test the acceptance of specific heterotopic heart grafts in these dogs, all the animals tested rejected the graft [22].

These observations are in contrast to those of Raaf *et al.* who found induction of chimaerism in dogs using TLI extremely difficult, requiring very high doses of irradiation and associated with a high rate of mortality and morbidity [23]. However, successful chimaerism in their hands resulted in indefinite survival of the specific test graft (a kidney). One possible explanation for these divergent results is that the Stanford group were not establishing true chimaerism and Raaf *et al.* have pointed to the extreme technical difficulty involved in performing the confirmatory tests in dogs, which are needed to support any statement concerning the establishment of chimaerism. Another possibility is that a variation in the irradiation regimes or fields used by the two different groups was allowing the establishment of split tolerance by the Stanford group but full chimaerism in New York.

Contradictory results have also been published by Rynasiewicz *et al.* [24] who used the same rat heart model as Slavin *et al.* [19] and, although Rynasiewicz was able to produce a retardation in the rejection time of the heterotopic heart grafts in these rats, he was unable to get indefinite survival, as had been reported by Slavin & Strober. Furthermore, when Rynasiewicz used TLI and allogeneic bone marrow transplantation to precondition the rats, either no graft prolongation occurred (at 1.2×10^7 bone marrow cells) or the recipients died of chronic graft-versus-host disease ($1-3 \times 10^8$ bone marrow cells per rat).

Despite these disappointing results with bone marrow transplantation, all groups who have worked with TLI have shown that it is immunosuppressive and both Raaf and Rynasiewicz have shown that its effects could be greatly enhanced by the addition of small amounts of other immunosuppressive agents [23,24]. Myburgh *et al.* have undertaken over the past few years a major study into the use of TLI in primates. They have demonstrated that a single dose of TLI was ineffective in inducing graft prolongation but that multiple dose therapy produced prolonged graft survival, in particular a priming regime of 2200 rads over a period of 3 months followed by monthly boosts of 200 rads until transplantation proved highly effective. Using this protocol long-term survival of kidney grafts in baboons could be achieved either with or without concurrent bone marrow transplantation [25].

Only two substantial series of clinical transplants immunosuppressed with TLI have so far been reported [26,27,91]. A total of twenty-two high-risk patients were treated with TLI prior to transplantation of a kidney graft. A twenty-third patient died during the conditioning phase and was never transplanted. Results from this trial showed that of the twenty-two patients transplanted sixteen (72%) are alive and well with functioning grafts at between 5 and 36 months post-transplant. One graft was lost from rejection and four deaths account for the remaining graft losses. These results compare very favourably with a comparable historical conventionally immunosuppressed group. However, the price paid in terms of side-effects resulting from the TLI preconditioning was high, with seventeen patients having complications as a result of the TLI conditioning which required interruption of the dosing schedule.

Immune monitoring of patients receiving TLI showed a dose-dependent depression of circulating T cell numbers with maximal depression being achieved after 2000 rads. There was also a loss of responsiveness to allogeneic and mitogenic stimulation which was not solely as a result of depletion of T cells since comparable numbers of T cells were assessed irrespective of the overall counts. This implies that the remaining T cells are functionally disturbed by the TLI. Preliminary studies suggest that this may be due to a greater depletion of helper cells leaving a higher proportion of suppressor cytotoxic cells.

Najarian's clinical studies [26] have also demonstrated that, unlike patients treated for Hodgkin's disease, most of those receiving TLI prior to renal transplantation recover from its immunosuppressive effects. Similar immunological recovery has been reported by Trentham *et al.* who used TLI to treat refractory rheumatoid arthritis [28]. In Najarian's study all those patients whose immune systems recovered had demonstrable graft rejection. This poses two problems, which are currently unresolved. The first is that these patients require pharmacological immunosuppression in addition to the TLI and there is a relationship between the dose of TLI delivered and post-operative immunosuppressive protocol used. The second problem is that the length of time between completion of irradiation and transplantation is important. Those patients for whom it is difficult to find a suitable cross-matched cytotoxic negative transplant may require a substantial number of 'topping up' irradiation treatments. The correct protocol, immunological value and side-effects of this treatment have yet to be clearly defined. It is likely, however, that a maintenance irradiation schedule provides the potential to add substantially to the cumulative pre-transplant irradiation dose and this may well incur an increase in the side effects of TLI.

Thoracic duct drainage

The rationale for using thoracic duct drainage as an immunosuppressive agent was provided by a series of experiments from Gowans *et al.* made as a result of the observation that lymphocytes recirculate from the blood into lymph [29]. Rats challenged with tetanus toxoid or sheep erythrocytes, after thoracic duct drainage had been maintained for 5 days, failed to produce antibodies to such challenges [30]. McGregor & Gowans [31] went on to demonstrate that lymphocyte depletion by chronic drainage from a thoracic duct fistula prolonged the survival of skin grafted between members of an outbred rat colony with many of the grafts surviving permanently. Untreated rats from this colony rejected such skin grafts in 14 days. Woodruff & Anderson [32] were able to demonstrate that there was a substantial synergistic effect between thoracic duct drainage and anti-lymphocyte serum and, on the basis of these initial animal studies, thoracic duct drainage was introduced into the clinic as an adjunct to immunosuppressive therapy for renal transplantation. The first attempts at the clinical use of thoracic duct drainage were made by Newton [33] and Franksson [34]. The technique requires the insertion of a catheter into the thoracic duct, which is normally approached by an incision in the left subclavian region. The construction of this cannula is of some importance, most success being achieved with the double lumen type catheter permitting the infusion of heparinized saline through one lumen while lymph is collected from the other. Machleder & Paulus [35] advocate the use of a tapering double-lumen catheter made from soft-grade silicone rubber reinforced by coiled wire incorporated into the wall to keep the tube from kinking as a result of subsequent neck movements. The outflowing lymph is collected, centrifuged to remove the white cells and cell-free lymph can then be reinfused into the patient on a daily basis. Klintmalm *et al.* [36] have shown that this re-infusion may not be necessary if adequate volumes of electrolyte solutions are given intravenously instead.

A critical aspect of thoracic duct drainage as an immunosuppressive agent is the timing, with both the duration of the procedure and its initiation in relation to implantation of the graft being important. Machleder & Paulus [35] in their study on the immunological consequences of thoracic duct drainage stress the difference between short-term (i.e. 1–2 weeks) lymphocyte diversion, which they show to have minimal effects on the immune system, and long-term (1–3 months) lymphocyte depletion, which they demonstrate had profound immunosuppressive consequences. It is unfortunate that most of the animal studies on thoracic duct drainage fall into the former category and therefore these results are difficult to interpret.

The most persuasive evidence that thoracic duct drainage is of value for immunosuppressing human allografts comes from the study of Levine *et al.* [37]. These workers placed skin grafts from unrelated donors on to six patients receiving thoracic duct drainage for the treatment of rheumatoid arthritis. These grafts were placed either shortly before or just after the termination of prolonged (1–3 months) thoracic duct drainage treatment and survived for between 16 and 550 days (mean 124 ± 86 days, median 30 days) compared with control values taken from the literature of between 8 and 11 days. Furthermore one of these patients developed donor-specific tolerance to his skin graft as demonstrated by the acceptance of a second graft from the original donor but the prompt rejection of a third party graft (in 11 days). To the best of the authors' knowledge this is the only documentation of donor-specific skin graft acceptance induced by immunological manipulation (as opposed to bone marrow grafting and chimaerism) to have been achieved in man. The effect of the total lymphoid irradiation on the rheumatoid arthritis was limited in that the condition recurred at some time after the cessation of the ductal drainage. A detailed study of thoracic duct drainage in kidney transplantation by Klintmalm *et al.* [36] confirms the immunosuppressive potency of this technique for allografts and also emphasizes the importance of prolonged drainage in excess of 28 days to achieve the necessary immunosuppressive potency.

Serial assay of absolute lymphocyte counts has demonstrated a progressive absolute lymphopenia in both the blood and lymph of patients receiving thoracic duct drainage treatment. The proportion of B lymphocytes increases in lymph with a reciprocal decrease in T lymphocytes, although this change is not consistent unless drainage is continued to the 14th week. Bone marrow biopsies before and after drainage show no alteration in lymphocyte concentration or morphology. Serial assays of immunoglobulin concentrations show a substantial decline in the IgG concentration from an average of 1450 to 980 mg/dl during the first week of drainage with little subsequent change. IgA declines by 40% over a period of 6 weeks. No changes in IgM levels have been noted. The drop in IgG occurs far more rapidly than would have been anticipated from the B cell depletion alone and much faster than changes in other immunoglobulin levels. It has been suggested that this might be due to a shift in T cell subpopulations resulting in a switch off of immunoglobulin production [35]. Thoracic duct drainage has been shown to inhibit delayed hypersensitivity type reactions as assessed by serial intradermal skin tests with these tests becoming negative between the 30th and the 35th day after starting drainage. Thoracic duct drainage also impairs humoral immunity as assessed by the ability of patients to respond to secondary challenge to typhoid H antigen at the conclusion of their thoracic duct drainage. However, challenge of such patients with KLH demonstrated similar amounts of antibody production as is achieved in the normal control population.

Infection, particularly as a result of the presence of the catheter or the continuous reinfusion of cell-free lymph, has proved to be a hazard encountered by most groups using thoracic duct drainage although the routine prophylactic use of antibiotics has controlled this problem in the series reported in the literature. Occasional opportunistic infections have also been reported by some groups. Perhaps the most significant impediment to the continued use of thoracic duct drainage as a means of immunosuppression is the necessity for continual close hospital supervision of the patient over a period of several months. Unless this can be overcome by some major advance in the current technique [95], thoracic duct drainage will not become a practical economically acceptable immunosuppressive therapy.

Arachidonic acid metabolites and their inhibition as immunosuppressive agents

Cells metabolize arachidonic acid to prostaglandins, thromboxanes, prostacyclins and leucotrienes [38]. Many of these substances appear to be involved in the control of cellular activity, often via changes in cyclic AMP availability. These substances may also function as locally active hormones enabling cells to communicate with each other. Their rapid production from cell membrane phospholipids by preformed enzymes and their rapid degradation to inactive metabolites make them ideally suited for this purpose. It has been shown that arachidonic acid metabolites are involved in a wide range of physiological processes. Some of them are produced by cells of the immune system and these have been shown to be involved in regulation of cellular, humoral and inflammatory components of the immune system.

There is evidence that prostaglandins of the E group have immunosuppressive activity [39,40]. Prostaglandin E1 has also been shown to prolong the survival of hampster to rat heart xenografts from a median of 73.5 h in controls to 94 h in animals treated with PGE1 [41]. Mundy *et al.* [42] have demonstrated that PGI2 infusion inhibited hyperacute rejection of renal allografts in specifically pre-sensitized dogs and in cat to dog renal xenografts. It has also been shown that both PGE2 and PGF2 reduce antibody mediated damage to rat hearts and a combination of PGE1 and procarbazine led to prolonged survival of mouse skin allografts [43,44].

The authors have studied the effect of modifying the normal physiological balance of arachidonic acid metabolites (Fig. 81.3) on the rejection of rat heterotopic hearts transplanted between the DA and PVG strains. Treatment was, where practical, given by eight hourly subcutaneous injections. In the case of PGI2

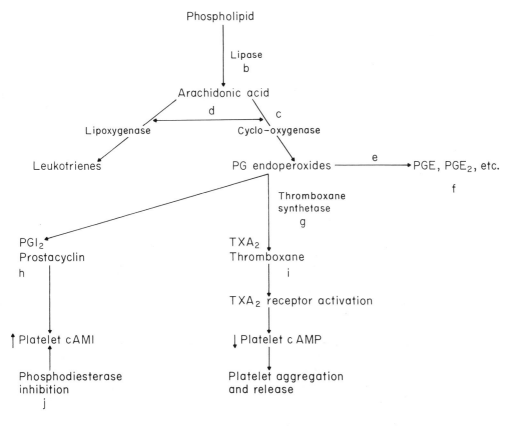

Fig. 81.3. Schematic representation of arachidonic acid metabolites and the site of action of drugs tested. (a) Control of precursor supply; (b) inhibited by steroids; (c) inhibited by aspirin; (d) inhibited by BW 755C (Wellcome); (e) inhibited by Surgam (Roussel); (f) inhibited by specific antibodies; (g) inhibited by UK-38,485 (Pfizer); (h) addition of exogenous PGI2 (Upjohn); (i) EIP (Upjohn) Inhibition; (j) phosphodiesterase inhibition by dipyridamole (Boehringer-Ingelheim).

which has a very short half-life at physiological temperature and pH, it was necessary to develop a system for continuous infusions lasting many days to be given into the inferior vena cava of a mobile rat. This was done with the use of a lightweight flexible stainless steel coil running from the base of the rat's tail to a cooled infusion box. A cannula was passed from the cool box to the inferior vena cava via the right femoral vein inside this coil so that it was protected from being bitten or broken by the rat. The authors showed that there was no suppression of the immune response from using this technique due to any adrenal related stress, as has been described for closely confined rats. Using this system there was no loss of PGI2 activity during storage and delivery, as assessed by the ability to inhibit ADP-induced aggregation of human platelet rich plasma in a Born aggregometer [31].

The authors have tested the following drugs for their immunosuppressive potency.

1 Intralipid 20% (KabiVitrum Ltd.): to increase supply of essential fatty acids.

2 Naudicelle (Bio Oil Research Ltd.) (oil of evening primrose) 500 mg/kg/day: supply of precursor essential fatty acids.

3 Hydrocortisone succinate (1.2 mg/kg/day): phospholipase inhibition.

4 BW 755C (Wellcome Research Laboratories) 100 mg/kg/day: lipoxygenase inhibition.

5 Aspirin (Aspro Clear) 200 mg/kg/day: cyclo-oxygenase inhibitor.

6 Timegadine (Leo Pharmaceutical Products Ltd.) 200 mg/kg/day: lipoxygenase and cyclo-oxygenase inhibition.

7 Tiaprofenic acid (Surgam) (Roussell Laboratories Ltd.) 200 mg/kg/day: strong inhibition of the synthesis of PGE2 and PGF2α; reduced inhibitory effect on PGI2.

8 UK-38,485 (Pfizer Ltd.) 200 mg/kg/day: thromboxane synthetase inhibitor.

9 9,11-Epoxyiminoprosta-5,13-dienoic acid (Upjohn Co. Ltd.) 1 mg/kg/day: selective thromboxane A2 receptor antagonist.

10 Dipyridamole (Boehringer Ingelheim Ltd.) 75 mg/kg/day: a phosphodiesterase inhibitor.

11 AHP 719 SCI (Boehringer Ingelheim Ltd.) 25 mg/kg/day: phosphodiesterase inhibitor.

12 Prostaglandin E1 (Upjohn Ltd.) 10 μg/kg/day: delivered by osmotically powered infusion pumps implanted into the peritoneal cavity.

13 Ketanserin (Janssen Pharmaceuticals) 40 mg/kg/day: 5-HT2-receptor blocking agent.

14 Sodium salicylate (B.D.H. Chemicals Ltd.) 200 mg/kg/day: weak cyclo-oxygenase inhibitor.

15 Prostacyclin I2 (Wellcome Research Labora-tories) 250 ng/kg/min by continuous intravenous infusion in glycine buffer at pH 9.8.

16 Anti-PGE1 antibodies (a gift from Drs Mertin and Stackpole) 0.2 ml/day.

The graft survival times achieved by the various treatment schedules are shown in Table 81.1. Of all the drugs used only aspirin, sodium salicylate and prostacyclin infusion prolonged graft survival significantly, while timegadine and antibodies to prostaglandin E1 reduced graft survival times. Since neither BW 755C nor timegadine were beneficial in prolonging graft survival, it would seem unlikely that the leucotrienes are important in graft rejection in this particular model. Surgam caused death in all the five rats studied between days 4 and 6 and this drug clearly warrants further studies at lower dose ranges. Neither EIP nor UK-38,485 affected graft rejection and this would suggest that thromboxane A2 does not play a primary role in the control of allograft rejection. Similarly, phosphodiesterase inhibitors were without effect. In contrast to the results of Favalli *et al.* and Strom *et al.* [45,46], the authors failed to show in these experiments that PGE1 infusion could prolong graft survival. However, this observation does not exclude the possibility that this prostaglandin is a natural inhibitor of immune mechanisms. PGE1 is rapidly inactivated by passage through the lungs and only a low dose was used in these studies. Further studies await the availability of a more stable analogue of this prostaglandin, and it may well be of significance that the removal of prostaglandin E1 with antibodies hastened graft rejection. Prostacyclin and aspirin both prolonged graft survival whether given from day 1 or from day 5 when rejection was already well established. At the doses of drug used (which were the maximum doses tolerated by PVG rats) aspirin was more effective than PGI2 and occasionally led to very prolonged graft survival. When PGI2 was infused from day 1 it was less effective in prolonging graft survival than when infused from day 5, although this difference was not statistically significant. A possible explanation for this is the loss of sensitivity of adenyl cyclase to PGI2 stimulation after prolonged infusion of PGI2 [47,48]. It seems probable in view of the results obtained by interfering with thromboxane A2 production and thromboxane A2 receptor blockade, that prostacyclin I2 and aspirin prolong graft survival by mechanisms other than the reduction of platelet accumulation and graft ischaemia, perhaps by directly reducing the severity of the immune attack.

There is now evidence that cell mediated immunity *in vitro* can be suppressed by PGI2 [49]. If cyclo-oxygenase products such as PGE1 and PGE2 are natural inhibitors of the immune response, then inhibition of cyclo-oxygenase by timegadine or their removal with

Table 81.1. Results of testing potential immunosuppressive agents (see text) on rat heart graft rejection

Drug used	Graft survival (days)	Mean	Difference vs. Control (Wilcoxon) (n.s. = not significant)
None: saline 0.2 ml/day	6, 7, 7, 7, 7, 7, 7, 8, 8, 8, 8, 9.	7.4	—
Intralipid 20% 5 ml/day	†, †, 7, 7, 7.	7.0	n.s.
Naudicelle 500 mg/kg/day	6, 6, 6, 7, 8.	6.4	n.s.
Hydrocortisone 1.2 mg/kg/day	7, 7, 8, 8, 11.	8.6	$P < 0.05$
BW 755C 100 mg/kg/day	6, 7, 8, 8, 8.	7.6	n.s.
Aspirin 200 mg/kg/day	8, 8, 9, 9, 10, 10, 11, 11, 11, 14, 63, > 6/12.	> 14.9	$P < 0.01$
Timegadine 200 mg/kg/day	6, 6, 6, 6, 7.	6.3	$P < 0.05$
Surgam 200 mg/kg/day	†, †, †, †, †.	—	—
UK-38, 485 200 mg/kg/day	7, 7, 8, 8, 8.	7.7	n.s.
EIP 1 mg/kg/day	6, 7, 7, 7, 8.	7.0	n.s.
Dipyridamole 75 mg/kg/day	7, 8, 8, 8, 8.	7.9	n.s.
AH-P 719 SC1 25 mg/kg/day	7, 7, 8, 8, 8.	7.7	n.s.
PGE_1 10 μg/kg/day	7, 8, 8, 8, 9.	8.0	n.s.
Ketanserin 40 mg/kg/day	7, 7, 7, 8, 8.	7.3	n.s.
PGI_2 continuous infusion μg/min/from day 1	8, 8, 8, 9, 9, 9, 10.	8.7	$P < 0.05$
PGI_2 continuous infusion from day 5	8, 9, 9, 9, 9, 9, 9, 9, 9, 11, 13.	9.4	$P < 0.01$
Anti-PGE_1 antiserum (0.2 ml per day)	5, 6, 6, 6, 6, 6, 7.	6.0	$P < 0.05$
Sodium salicylate 200 mg/day	11, 11, 13, 28, 48, 60, > 100, > 100, > 100, > 100, > 100, > 100.	> 64.2	$P < 0.001$

antibodies would accelerate rejection, as indeed the authors found to be the case in these studies. However, sodium salicylate, which is a weak cyclo-oxygenase inhibitor, was found to be a very powerful suppressor of graft rejection and this may well be due to a direct effect of the salicylate moiety upon the immune system and be entirely independent of prostaglandin inhibition. Thus aspirin could be expected to exhibit opposing activities; its induction of cyclo-oxygenase inhibition by acetylation would accelerate graft rejection while the presence of the salicylate moiety would induce delayed graft rejection. This would imply that the major immunological modulatory effect of aspirin is via mechanisms other than those associated with the metabolites of arachidonic acid, e.g. by acting as a free oxygen radical scavenger.

Monoclonal antibodies as immunosuppressive agents

Elsewhere in this volume (Chapter 78) the various mechanisms by which intervention with antibodies might control specific immune responses are outlined. The advent of monoclonal antibodies has made the production of suitable reagents a practical possibility. As yet, no clinically applicable antigen-specific immunosuppressive protocol has been devised, although such manipulations have been performed in experimental systems. Intervention with monoclonal antibodies, along the lines pioneered by users of heterologous anti-lymphocyte sera or anti-thymocyte sera, are now being attempted in a number of centres. The principle of this approach is to use the monoclonal to remove or inactivate a relevant cell population, thus depriving the immune system of a necessary component. The attractive feature of such an approach is that by careful selection of the monoclonal, a very discrete population of cells can be attacked, eliminating only a small part of the individual's immune repertoire. As yet our understanding of the functions fulfilled by the various cellular populations that comprise the immune system is not sufficient to predict with any certainty the outcome of such interventions. Thus at present most studies have been directed towards eliminating the total T cell population with pan T reagents. It is to be hoped that these studies will eventually lead to control mechanisms involving more restricted subpopulations.

The major drawback of this scheme, however, is the inherent immunogenicity of rodent immunoglobulin, which is currently used for such interventions. For example, OKT3, a pan T reagent, has been used by Cosimi's group in association with conventional immunosuppressive agents to treat acute rejection crises in renal allograft recipients [50]. Such treatment resulted in the rapid disappearance of OKT3 reactive cells from the peripheral blood and prompt reversal of the rejection crisis. These encouraging results, however, have to be treated with some caution since it has become clear that the initial potency of the OKT3 reagent diminishes with time as a result of the recipient mounting an immune response against mouse immunoglobulin despite that recipient's depressed state [51]. A recent randomized trial by Chatenoud *et al.* used OKT3 as the sole immunosuppressive agent [52]. These workers found that despite continued treatment with the monoclonal antibody, T cells that had disappeared 1 h after giving the first dose would reappear into the circulation 2 to 3 days later. Furthermore these T cells, which would normally have expressed the OKT3 antigen, had become OKT3-negative, although they continued to express other surface markers characteristic of T cells (OKT4 or OKT8). Cultured *in vitro* in the absence of OKT3, these cells were found to re-express the OKT3 antigen. A randomized controlled trial of OKT-3 has demonstrated the efficiency of this agent in reversing rejection episodes [92]. Thus the OKT3 monoclonal was modulating the target antigen rather than eliminating the relevant cell population. Clearly it should be possible to overcome this problem by using suitable fragments of the OKT3 antibody and experiments to test this are currently in progress. However, the problem of immune responses to mouse immunoglobulin inactivating the reagent would seem to require the development of suitable human-derived monoclonals for its solution.

Cyclosporin A

The discovery of cyclosporin A is one of the most exciting advances to have occurred in the development of immunosuppressive agents in recent years. This compound is a metabolite isolated from cultures of the fungal species *Tolyplocadium inflatum*. It is a neutral, extremely hydrophobic cyclical polypeptide comprising 11 amino-acids (Fig. 81.4). One of these amino-acids (the open-ring 9-carbon structure) is unique to the cyclosporins [53]. Because of its extremely hydrophobic nature the drug has to be dissolved in oil for its administration. The drug was first isolated in the Sandoz Laboratories in Basle as part of a search for biologically produced anti-fungal agents. Although the compound proved to have only mild anti-fungal activity, it was discovered by Borel to influence the immune system [54–56].

In summary, what Borel showed was as follows.
1 Cyclosporin A exerts an immunosuppressive action on both humoral and cell mediated immunity.
2 It fails to suppress the antibody response to lipopolysaccharides in nude mice.
3 It depresses chronic but not acute inflammatory reactions.
4 It inhibits lymphocyte proliferation.
5 It affects mitogenic triggering but not mitosis.
6 It has no influence on preformed cytotoxic cells.
7 It is not lymphocytotoxic or myelocytotoxic.

It was also demonstrated [57] that the drug had no effect on the myeloid compartment of the immune system and these authors also confirmed the observation of Borel that the drug preferentially affected the activated but not the resting T cell at an early stage in the cell activating process.

One of the problems in the *in vivo* use of cyclosporin A was to devise a procedure for administering a water-insoluble compound to animals. Borel's original *in vivo* experiments were performed giving the drug orally mixed with tragacanth. In the initial

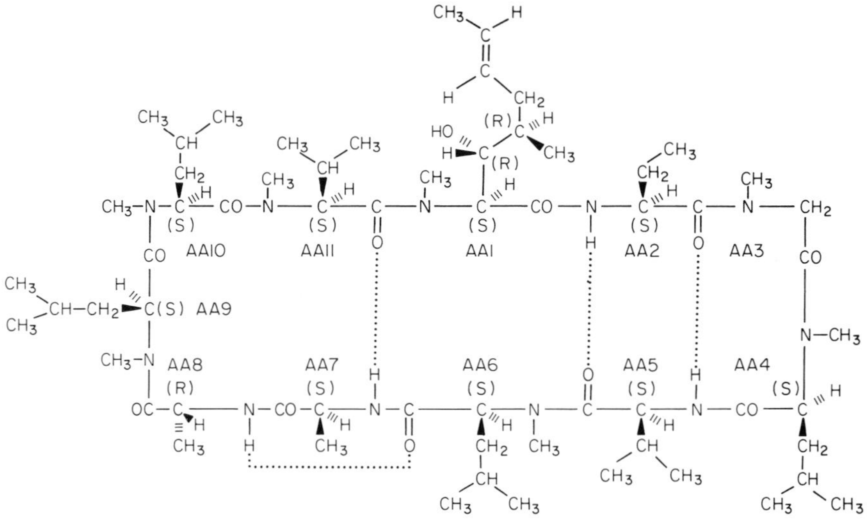

Fig. 81.4. Structure of cyclosporin A.

experiments of Kostakis *et al.* [58], in which the drug was tested for its immunosuppressive potency in suppressing the rejection of rat heart transplants, it was given by intramuscular injection dissolved in absolute alcohol, using the same dose (250 mg/kg/day) as that used by Borel in his mice studies [54]. However, these workers quickly discovered that at this dose toxic effects occurred as a result of both the alcohol and high doses of the drug. This problem was resolved by injecting the agent intramuscularly dissolved in olive oil at (up to) 50 mg/ml at a greatly reduced dose (in this form the LD50 in a rat is between 50 and 100 mg/kg/day, depending on the rat strain). It was found that at a dose of 20 mg/kg administered on days 0, 2, 4 and 6, post-transplant, very prolonged graft survival could be achieved (42 days versus 9 days in controls) [59]. If the animal was treated with the cyclosporin A for longer than this then the graft survived for the lifetime of the rat [60]. The immunosuppressive potency of cyclosporin A for the prevention of allograft rejection was confirmed by testing it in mongrel dogs given kidney grafts after bilateral nephrectomy [61] and in pigs transplanted with tissue-typed incompatible orthotopic heart grafts [62]. In both species the drug proved an extremely potent suppressor of graft rejection (Tables 81.2 and 81.3).

Since that time the potency of cyclosporin A to prevent graft rejection in animals has been proved in many different species using a large variety of organs and tissues as test transplants (Table 81.4). Of particular interest clinically is the possibility of grafting intestines or lungs or the adnexa (ovaries and fallopian tubes), though this last possibility may pose complex ethical problems. Reitz *et al.* have already established a successful clinical heart and lung transplant programme using cyclosporin A immunosuppression [63].

Cyclosporin A was first introduced into clinical practice in 1978 as an immunosuppressive agent to inhibit rejection of organ and bone marrow allografts [64,65]. Since that time its superiority as an immuno-

Table 81.2. Survival of bilaterally nephrectomized mongrel dogs with renal allografts

Treatment	Number	Survival in days	Median survival
Azathioprine 5 mg/kg/day	10	48, 38, 35, 30, 28, 27, 25, 19, 17, 9.	27.5
CyA 50 mg/kg/day	17	> 275, > 198, 147, 68, 62, 52, 35, 33, 28, 21, 20, 19, 17, 13, 11, 11, 10.	31
CyA 25 mg/kg/day	8	> 220, > 113, > 79, 152, 61, 22, 22, 14.	67

Table 81.3. Comparison of survival in days of pigs with orthoptic heart transplants receiving a variety of immunosuppressive regimens

Immunosuppression*	Survival (days)	Median survival (days)
Mismatched: Nil	5, 6, 6	6
Identical siblings: Nil	74, 132, 191	132
Mismatched: azathioprine (5) + methylprednisolone (5)	4, 5, 6, 6, 16, 51	6
Mismatched: azathioprine (5) + carrageenan + promethazine	3, 4, 6, 6, 14	6
Mismatched: Asta 036.5122 (5)	4†, 4, 5, 6, 8, 20	5.5
Mismatched: cyclosporin A (15) on days 0, 2, 4	19, 21, 22, 33, 33	22
Mismatched: cyclosporin A (25)	22, 43, 72, 223, >280, >301, >306, >322	>251

* Doses (shown in parentheses) are in mg/kg/day.
† With azathioprine (10).

Table 81.4. Transplant models in which cyclosporin A has proved to be a potent immunosuppressive agent

Cyclosporin A has been shown to be a potent suppressor of rejection in:	
Rat	Kidney, heart, pancreas, liver, skin, bone marrow
Dog	Kidney, pancreas, skin, bone marrow, intestine, lung
Pig	Heart
Rabbit	Skin, cornea, kidney, bone marrow, adnexa
Monkey	Kidney, heart, heart-and-lung
Man	Kidney, liver, pancreas, bone marrow, heart, heart-and-lung
Impotent	
Rat	Islet cell transplants
Dog	DLA identical bone marrow

suppressive agent for these indications has been demonstrated by a number of different centres comparing it with a range of different control protocols (Fig. 81.5). Use of cyclosporin A immunosuppression has proved particularly beneficial in human cardiac transplantation [66]. The details of the different clinical approaches to the use of this drug and its side-effects have been recently reviewed [67,68].

The process by which cyclosporin A exerts its immunosuppressive action is still very much a matter of debate. For example, it is not clear to what extent cyclosporin A has selectivity of action within the lymphoid compartment in so far as it affects T cells but spares B cell activity. The observation of Borel that cyclosporin A had no effect on the production of antibodies to lipopolysaccharides in nude mice would support the contention that the drug's activity is restricted to the T cell compartment. This view is further supported by the observation that cyclosporin A fails to inhibit the *in vitro* proliferation of B cells at doses which cause inhibition of T cell activity [69,80]. In contrast to this there are reports that cyclosporin A affects B and T cell transformation to the same extent when B cells are triggered by either pokeweed mitogen or *Staphylococcus aureus*. However, the problem with such experiments is that the B cell activation resulting from the exposure to these mitogens may not be entirely T cell independent and that the cyclosporin A inhibition observed could still be a result of inhibition of T cell activity.

The clearest studies on the effect of cyclosporin A on the B cell compartment have been performed by Kunkel & Klaus [71] who have demonstrated that in the mouse there are two groups of T-independent antigens which equate with two different subsets of B cells. One group will elicit normal or supranormal antibody responses in mice fully immunosuppressed with cyclosporin A, while antibody to the second group (which includes lipopolysaccharides) is totally suppressed by the cyclosporin A.

Cyclosporin A does not inhibit human NK cells directly. However, it does affect the performance of these cells indirectly by interfering with the T-dependent production of interferon-γ, a positive modulator of NK cells. It has been suggested [72] that cyclosporin A acts by being specifically cytotoxic for the proliferating cell. However, monitoring of total T cell counts (by use of the monoclonal OKT3) in transplant recipients immunosuppressed with cyclosporin A, failed to show any post-transplant changes. Furthermore, subpopulation studies using the monoclonal antisera OKT4 (helper T) and OKT8 (suppressor cytotoxic) subpopulations are unchanged by immunosuppression with cyclosporin A, although some reports have suggested that a change in the 4/8 ratio takes place post-transplant [73,74].

Both dose- and time-dependent inhibition by cyclosporin A of mitogen-induced and mixed lymphocyte responses of T cells have been demonstrated in a variety of different species, including man. This inhibitory effect can be reversed by thorough washing of the cells, followed by overnight culture in cyclosporin-A-free medium and then restimulation of the cell population, which will then respond in a normal 'first set' fashion. However, the proliferative effect of phorbol myristic acid on thymus cells is unaffected by cyclo-

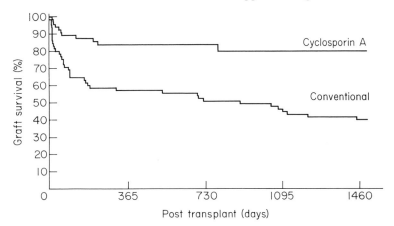

Fig. 81.5. Comparison of kidney graft survival between cyclosporin A and conventional immunosuppression.

sporin A. The generation of effector cytotoxic lymphocytes, as a result of a mixed lymphocyte reaction, is prevented by cyclosporin A but once generated their cytotoxic activity is not inhibited by the drug [54]. Animals given cyclosporin A at doses which produce prolonged survival of organ allografts show a marked reduction in the size and cellularity of the thymic medulla, splenic marginal zones, and splenic periarterial sheath, all compartments thought to contain cells of the T cell lineage helper activity [75].

Thus most of the data on the mode of action of cyclosporin A suggests an inhibitory effect on the T helper cell subpopulation. Cyclosporin A effectively suppresses primary T-dependent antibody responses in rodents. It has been shown that secondary antibody responses are far less susceptible to suppression by the drug than are primary responses [71,76]. Klaus's review [77] using a hapten carrier conjugate test system in the mouse has shown that this difference reflects a difference in the susceptibility between the unprimed and the primed T helper cell to cyclosporin A. These workers have also suggested that cyclosporin A does not directly influence the priming of the helper T cell to the T-dependent antigen but inhibits the effector function of that helper T cell when primed in the presence of cyclosporin A. If, however, priming takes place in the absence of cyclosporin A, the effector function which would otherwise have been inhibited by the drug, becomes cyclosporin A resistant. As Klaus points out, the significance of these observations for our understanding of the mode of action of cyclosporin A is considerable. It seems clear from these studies that cyclosporin A works by inhibiting not the antigenic priming of T cells but some event which takes place subsequent to that priming [93].

Another possible explanation for the action of cyclosporin A is that it acts preferentially on enhancing the suppressor T cell subpopulation. Tutschka &

Santos [78] have suggested that cyclosporin A administered *in vivo* facilitates the induction of alloantigen-specific suppressor cells, which appear rapidly in the spleen cells of rat bone marrow chimaeras. They found that *in vitro* addition of cyclosporin A inhibited the induction of cytotoxic effector but not T suppressor cells [79]. Since the suppressor activity of cyclosporin-A-treated cultures was never greater than in untreated controls, it appears most likely that cyclosporin A spares and preserves but does not induce suppressor cell activation. In support of this hypothesis Leapman *et al.* [80] found that *in vitro* addition of cyclosporin A did not affect the generation or function of con-A-induced human T suppressor lymphocytes. Further support comes from the evidence that cyclosporin-A-treated renal allograft recipients display a depressed number of inducer helper cells with maintenance of normal numbers of suppressor cytotoxic subpopulations and an unchanged total T cell count, suggesting that cyclosporin A administration distorts the relative number of immunoregulatory T lymphocytes [74].

These data suggest most strongly that cyclosporin A exerts a specific activity on T lymphocytes. The most likely mechanism by which this specific activity is achieved is through the existence of specific surface ligands or receptors. Studies on the surface binding of labelled cyclosporin A have yielded conflicting results. Using radioactive iodinated cyclosporin A (which is not biologically active) no increased binding to lymphocyte surfaces could be demonstrated [81]. However, using tritium-labelled dihydrocyclosporin C as the tracer molecule that is biologically active, a specific binding pattern was observed [82]. In a murine test system these workers found that cortisone-sensitive thymus cells bound more cyclosporin C than peripheral T lymphocytes, which in turn bound more than B lymphocytes. No preferential binding to macrophages was observed on a cell-for-cell basis. These workers concluded that it only required a few of the high affinity sites to be occupied for immunosuppression to occur.

In a study using tritiated cyclosporin A, Kahan *et al.* [83] found that helper T cells displayed a marked avidity for binding the drug unlike a T suppressor cell line and a B cell line, both of which showed slow, prolonged, less avid uptake without a detectable saturation point. In addition it was impossible to displace the cyclosporin A bound to suppressor and B cells with the active structural analogue cyclosporin D, whereas this was possible in the helper T cell population. However, these studies utilize neoplastic T cells and the exact correlation between this and binding studies in the human awaits clarification.

There are at present two different hypotheses on the subcellular mechanism of action of cyclosporin A.

1 *Inhibition of activation.* The experiments of Larsson [84] have suggested that cyclosporin A acts by inhibiting expression of the receptor for interleukin-2. Palacios & Moller [85] have confirmed these observations and reported failure to detect the expression of Ia on the surface of activated T cells inhibited with cyclosporin A. Recently Britton & Palacios [86] have reported that T cells exposed by cyclosporin A no longer bind OKT3 monoclonal antibody. This suggests that both these reagents are reacting with the same cell surface receptor or very closely associated receptors and there is some evidence to suggest that this receptor is the structure involved in antigen recognition by T cells [87]. If this interpretation is correct it clearly has major implications for our understanding of the mechanisms available for controlling the immune system.

2 *Inhibition of second signal.* It has been suggested [88] that cyclosporin A does not affect the activation of T cells but works by exerting a selective inhibitory effect on the secretion and/or production of interleukin-2 (IL-2). In addition, it reduces the number of potentially active IL-2-secreting T cells by inhibiting the release of IL-1. This inhibition is not due to an effect on the IL-1-secreting macrophage but rather to a deficiency in either expression or function of a T cell population which induces the macrophage to secrete the IL-1. Experimentally it has been possible to partially overcome the inhibitory effects of cyclosporin A by the addition of exogenous IL-2 but not by the addition of IL-1, which made only a marginal difference. This view is supported by Kronke's observations [94].

A detailed analysis by Fidelius *et al.* [89] of the response of T cell clones to cyclosporin has done much to clarify the subcellular mechanism of action of the drug. Using IL-2-dependent T cell clones these authors showed that the IL-2 driven proliferative response was unaffected by cyclosporin A whereas the specific antigen driven proliferation of these clones could be completely abolished by the drug. These authors suggest that their data shows cyclosporin A to act by inhibiting the antigenic signal for cell division.

The recent total synthesis of cyclosporin A [53] has made it much more likely that this agent is going to be the first of a new generation of immunosuppressive drugs, which will enable us to control the various aspects of the immune system involved in a whole range of undesirable pathogenic processes in a much safer and more specific fashion.

A recent report on the Second Dusseldorf Workshop on autoimmunity [90] reviews the use of cyclosporin A or cyano-aziridines (as well as monoclonal antibodies to T-cell or Ia antigens) and concludes that the prospects for T-lymphocyte directed methods for immunosuppression and modulation look very promising.

References

1 GIBSON T. & MEDAWAR P.B. (1943) The fate of skin homografts in man. *J. Anat.* **77,** 299.

2 BILLINGHAM R.E., BRENT L. & MEDAWAR P.B. (1956) The antigenic stimulus in transplantation immunity. *Nature,* **178,** 514.

3 HUME D.M., MERRILL J.P. & MILLER, B.F. (1952) Homologous transplantation of human kidneys. *J. clin. Invest.* **31,** 640.

4 SCHWARTZ R. & DAMASHEK W. (1959) Drug-induced immunological tolerance. *Nature,* **183,** 1682.

5 CALNE R.Y. (1960) The rejection of renal homografts. Inhibition in dogs by 6-Mercaptopurine. *Lancet,* **i,** 417.

6 CALNE R.Y. (1961) Inhibition of the rejection of renal homografts in dogs by purine analogues. *Transplant. Bull.* **28,** 65.

7 STARZL T.E., MARCHIORO R.L. & WADDELL W.R. (1963) The reversal of rejection in human renal homografts with subsequent development of homograft tolerance. *Surgery Gynec. Obstet.* **117,** 385.

8 KNIGHT S.L. & BURMAN S. (1981) Control of mixed lymphocyte reactions by cellular concentration. Studies in 20 µl hanging droplet cultures. *Transplant. Proc.* **13,** 1637.

9 GOULMY E., BRADLEY B.A., LANSBERGEN Q. & VAN ROOD J.J. (1978) The importance of H–Y incompatibility in human organ transplantation. *Transplantation,* **25,** 315.

10 BARKER C.F. & BILLINGHAM R.E. (1973) Skeletal muscle as a privileged site for orthotopic skin allografts. *J. exp. Med.* **138,** 289.

11 ONO K. & LINDSEY E.S. (1969) Improved technique of heart transplantation in rats. *J. thorac. cardiovasc. Surg.* **57,** 225.

12 HERON I. (1971) A technique for accessory cervical heart transplantation in rabbits and rats. *Acta path. microbiol. scand.* **79,** 366.

13 DUNN D.C. (1976) Orthotopic renal transplantation in the rabbit. *Transplantation*, **22**, 427.

14 KAMADA N. & CALNE R.Y. (1983) A surgical experience with 530 liver transplants in the rat. *Surgery*, **93**, 64.

15 KASAHARA K., WHITE D.J.G. & CALNE R.Y. (1982) Antigen dependence of Cyclosporin A induced allograft acceptance. *Transplantation*, **34**, 216.

16 HAMBURGER J., VAYSSE J., CROSNIER J., AUVERT J., LALANNE C.M. & HOPPER J. (1962) Renal homotransplantation in man after radiation of the recipient. *Am. J. Med.* **32**, 854.

17 FUKS Z., STROBER S. & BABROVE A.M. (1976) Long term effects of radiation on T and B lymphocytes in peripheral blood of patients with Hodgkin's disease. *J. clin. Invest.* **58**, 803.

18 SLAVIN S., STROBER S., FUKS Z. & KAPLAN H.S. (1976) Long term survival of skin allografts in mice treated with fractionated total lymphoid irradiation. *Science*, **193**, 1252.

19 SLAVIN S., REITZ B., BIEBER C.P., KAPLAN, H.S. & STROBER S. (1978) Transplantation tolerance in adult rats using total lymphoid irradiation. Permanent survival of skin, heart and marrow allografts. *J. exp. Med.* **147**, 963.

20 SLAVIN S., KAPLAN H.S. & STROBER S. (1978) Transplantation of allogeneic bone marrow without graft versus host disease using total lymphoid irradiation. *J. exp. Med.* **147**, 700.

21 SLAVIN S., GOTTLIEB M., STROBER S., BIEBER C., HOPPE R., KAPLAN H.S. & GRUMET F.C. (1979) Transplantation of bone marrow in outbred dogs without graft-versus-host disease using total lymphoid irradiation. *Transplantation*, **27**, 139.

22 KORETZ S.H., GOTTLIEB M.S., STROBER S., PENNOCK J., BIEBER C.P., HOPPE R.T., REITZ B.A. & KAPLAN H.S. (1981) Organ transplantation in mongrel dogs using total lymphoid irradiation. *Transplant. Proc.* **13**, 443.

23 RAAF J., BRYAN C., MONDEN M., BRAY A., KIM J.H., CHU F., CHAGANTI R.S.K., SHANK B., CAHAN A. & FORTNER J.G. (1981) Bone marrow and renal transplantation in canine recipients prepared by total lymphoid irradiation. *Transplant. Proc.* **13**, 429.

24 RYNASIEWICZ J.J., SUTHERLAND D.E.R., KAWAHARA K., KIM T. & NAJARIAN J.S. (1981) Total lymphoid irradiation in rat heart allografts. Dose, fractionation and combination with Cyclosporin A. *Transplant. Proc.* **13**, 452.

25 MYBURGH J.A., SMIT J.A. & BROWDE S. (1981) Transplantation tolerance in the primate following total lymphoid irradiation and bone marrow injection. *Transplant. Proc.* **13**, 434.

26 NAJARIAN J.S., SUTHERLAND D.E.R., FERGUSON R.M., SIMMONS R.L., KERSEY J., MAUER S.M., SLAVIN S. & KIM T.H. (1981) Total lymphoid irradiation and kidney transplantation. A clinical experience. *Transplant. Proc.* **13**, 417.

27 NAJARIAN J.S., FERGUSON R.M., SUTHERLAND D.E.R., SLAVIN S., KIM T., KERSEY J. & SIMMONS R.L. (1982) Fractionated total lymphoid irradiation as preparative immunosuppression in high risk renal transplantation. *Ann. Surg.* **196**, 442.

28 TRENTHAM D.E., BELLI J.A., ANDERSON R.J., BUCKLEY J.A., GOETZL E.J., DAVID J.R. & AUSTEN K.F. (1981) Clinical and immunologic effects of fractionated total lymphoid irradiation in refractory rheumatoid arthritis. *New Engl. J. Med.* **305**, 976.

29 GOWANS J.L. (1959) The recirculation of lymphocytes from blood to lymph in the rat. *J. Physiol.* **146**, 54.

30 GOWANS J.L., McGREGOR D.D., COWEN A. & FORD W. (1962) Initiation of immune responses by small lymphocytes. *Nature*, **196**, 651.

31 McGREGOR D.D. & GOWANS J.L. (1964) Survival of homografts of skin in rats depleted of lymphocytes by chronic drainage from the thoracic duct. *Lancet*, **i**, 629.

32 WOODRUFF M.F.A. & ANDERSON N.F. (1963) Effect of lymphocyte depletion by thoracic duct fistula and ALS on the survival of skin homografts in rats. *Nature*, **200**, 702.

33 NEWTON W.T. (1965) The biological basis of tissue transplantation. *Surg. Clins N. Am.* **45**, 393.

34 FRANKSSON C. (1964) Survival of homografts of skin in rats depleted of lymphocytes by chronic drainage from the thoracic duct. *Lancet*, **i**, 1331.

35 MACHLEDER H.I. & PAULUS H. (1978) Clinical and immunological alterations observed in patients undergoing long-term thoracic duct drainage. *Surgery*, **84**, 157.

36 KLINTMALM G., IWATSUKI S., KANO T., IWAKI Y., TERASAKI P.I., SCHROTER G., KOEP L., WEIL R. & STARZL T.E. (1981) Determinants of effectiveness of thoracic duct drainage for primary cadaver kidney transplantation. *Transplant. Proc.* **13**, 537.

37 LEVINE S., HSU S., SPARKES R.S., PAULUS H.E. & MACHLEDER H.I. (1975) Skin homograft survival in humans after lymphocyte depletion by prolonged thoracic duct drainage. *Archs Surg., Lond.* **110**, 736.

38 STENSON W.F. & PARKER C.W. (1980) Prostaglandins, macrophages and immunity. *J. Immunol.* **125**, 1.

39 GOODWIN J.S. & WEBB D.R. (1980) Regulation of the immune response by prostaglandins. *Clin. Immunol. Path.* **15**, 108.

40 PELUS L.M. & STRAUSSER H.R. (1977) Prostaglandins and the immune response. *Life Sciences*, **20**, 903.

41 KAKITA A., BLANCHARD J. & FORTNER J.G. (1975) Effectiveness of prostaglandin E1 and procarbazine hydrochloride in prolonging the survival of vascularized cardiac hampster-to-rat xenografts. *Transplantation*, **20**, 439.

42 MUNDY A.R., BEWICK M., MONCADA S. & VANE J.R. (1980) Short term suppression of hyperacute renal allograft rejection in presensitized dogs with prostacyclin. *Prostaglandins*, **19**, 595.

43 PAUSESCU E., LAKY D. & POPESCU M.V. (1981) *In vivo* and *in vitro* morphological studies on myocardial protection induced by PGE2 and PGF2 against immune aggression. *Eur. surg. Res.* **13**, 1.

44 QUAGLIATA F., LAWRENCE V.J.W. & PHILLIPS-QUAGLIATA J.M. (1973) Prostaglandin E1 as a regulator of lymphocyte function. *Cell. Immunol.* **6**, 457.

45 FAVALLI C., MASTINO A., JEZZI T., RINALDI C., GARACI E. & JAFFE B.M. (1982) Influence of PGE on immune response in normal and immunosuppressed mice. *Proceedings of V International Conference on Prostaglandins*, p. 638.

46 STROM T.B., CARPENTER C.D., CRAGOE E.J., NORRIS S.,

DEOLIN R. & PERPER R.J. (1977) Suppression of *in vivo* and *in vitro* alloimmunity by prostaglandins. *Transplant. Proc.* **9**, 1075.

47 GOODWIN J.S., BANKHURST A.D. & MESSNER R.P. (1977) Suppression of human T cell mitogenesis by prostaglandin. *J. exp. Med.* **146**, 1719.

48 WEBB D.R. & NOWOWIEJSKI I. (1981) Control of suppressor cell activation via endogenous prostaglandin synthesis. The role of T cells and macrophages. *Cell. Immunol.* **63**, 321.

49 LEUNG K.H. & MIHICH E. (1980) Prostaglandin modulation of development of cell-mediated immunity in culture. *Nature*, **288**, 597.

50 COSIMI A.B., COLVIN R.B., BURTON R.C. *et al.* (1981) Use of monoclonal antibodies to T-cell subsets for immunological monitoring and treatment in recipients of renal allografts. *New Engl. J. Med.* **305**, 308.

51 JAFFES G., COLVIN R.B., COSIMI A.B., GIORGI J.V., FULLER J.C., LILLEHEI C. & RUSSELL P.S. (1983) The human immune response to murine OKT3 monoclonal antibody. *Transplant. Proc.* **15**, 646.

52 CHATENOUD L., BAUDRIHAYE M.F., CHKOFF N., KREIS H. & BACH J.F. Immunologic follow-up of renal allograft recipients treated prophylactically by OKT3 alone. *Transplant. Proc.* **15**, 643.

53 WENGER R. (1982) Chemistry of Cyclosporin. In *Cyclosporin A*, (ed. White D.J.G.), p. 19. Elsevier Biomedical Press.

54 BOREL J.F. (1976) Comparative study of *in vitro* and *in vivo* drug effects on cell mediated cytotoxicity. *Immunology*, **31**, 631.

55 BOREL J.F., FEURER C., MAGNEE C. & STAHELIN H. (1977) Effects of the new anti-lymphocytic peptide Cyclosporin A in animals. *Immunology*, **32**, 1017.

56 BOREL J.F. (1982) The history of Cyclosporin A and its significance. In *Cyclosporin A*, Chapter 2, (ed. White D.J.G), p. 5. Elsevier Biomedical Press.

57 WHITE D.J.G., PLUMB A.M., PAWELEC G. & BRONS G. (1979) Cyclosporin A: an immunosuppressive agent preferentially active against proliferating T-cells. *Transplantation*, **27**, 55.

58 KOSTAKIS A.J., WHITE D.J.G. & CALNE R.Y. (1977) Toxic effects in the use of Cyclosporin A in alcoholic solution as an immunosuppressant of rat heart allografts. *IRCS Med. Sci.* **5**, 243.

59 KOSTAKIS A.J., WHITE D.J.G. & CALNE R.Y. (1977) Prolongation of rat heart allograft survival by Cyclosporin A. *IRCS Med. Sci.* **5**, 280.

60 WHITE D.J.G., ROLLES K. & OTTAWA T. (1980) CyA induced long-term survival of fully incompatible skin and heart grafts in rats. *Transplant. Proc.* **12**, 261.

61 CALNE R.Y. & WHITE D.J.G. (1977) Cyclosporin A—a powerful immunosuppressant in dogs with renal allografts. *IRCS Med. Sci.* **5**, 595.

62 CALNE R.Y., WHITE D.J.G., ROLLES K., SMITH D.P. & HERBERTSON B.M. (1978) Prolonged survival of pig orthotopic heart grafts treated with Cyclosporin A. *Lancet*, **i**, 1183.

63 REITZ B.A., WALLWORK J.L., HUNT S.A., PENNOCK J.L., OYER P.E., STINSON E.B. & SHUMWAY N.E. (1982) Cyclosporin A for combined heart-lung transplantation.

In *Cyclosporin A*, Chapter 42, (ed. White D.J.G.), p. 473. Elsevier Biomedical Press.

64 CALNE R.Y., WHITE D.J., THIRUS, EVANS D.B., MCMASTER P., DUNN D.C., CRADDOCK G.N., PENTLOW B.D. & ROLLES K. (1978) Cyclosporin A in patients receiving renal allografts from cadaver donors. *Lancet*, **ii**, 1323.

65 POWLES R.L., BARRELL A.J. & CLINK H. (1978) Cyclosporin A for the treatment of graft versus host disease in man. *Lancet*, **ii**, 1327.

66 OYER P.E., STINSON E.B., REITZ B.A. *et al.* (1982) Preliminary results with Cyclosporin A in clinical cardiac transplantstion. In *Cyclosporin A*, Chapter 41, (ed. White D.J.G.), p. 461. Elsevier Biomedical Press.

67 CALNE R.Y. (1980) Immunosuppression for organ grafting. Observations on Cyclosporin A. *Immunol. Revs.* **46**, 113.

68 WHITE D.J.G. & CALNE R.Y. (1982) The use of Cyclosporin A immunosuppression in organ grafting. *Immunol. Revs.* **65**, 115.

69 BIRD A.G., MCLACHLAN S.M. & BRITTON S. (1980) Cyclosporin A promotes spontaneous outgrowth *in vitro* of E-B virus induced V cell lines. *Nature*, **289**, 300.

70 WHITE D.J.G., CALNE R.Y. & PLUMB A. (1979) Mode of action of Cyclosporin A: a new immunosuppressive agent. *Transplant. Proc.* **11**, 855.

71 KUNKEL A. & KLAUS G.G.B. (1980) Selective effects of Cyclosporin A on functional B cell subsets in the mouse. *J. Immunol.* **125**, 2526.

72 GREEN C.J. & ALLISON A.C. (1978) Extensive prolongation of rabbit kidney allograft survival after short-term Cyclosporin A treatment. *Lancet*, **i**, 1182.

73 MORRIS P.J. (1983) Renal Transplantation–1982. *Transplant. Proc.* **15**, 1033..

74 KAHAN B.D., KERMAN R.H., AGOSTINO G., FRIEDMAN A. & LEGRUE S.J. (1982) The action of Cyclosporin A on human lymphocytes. In *Cyclosporin A*, (ed. White D.J.G.), p. 281. Elsevier Biomedical Press.

75 BALDWIN W.M., HUTCHINSON I.F., MEIJER C.J.L.M. & TILNEY N.L. (1981) Marked decrease in medullary and splenic T lymphocytes after Cyclosporin A treatment. *Transplantation*, **31**, 117.

76 LINDSEY N.J., HARRIS K.R., NORMAN H.B., SMITH J.L., LEE H.A. & SLAPAK M. (1980) The effect of Cyclosporin A on the primary and secondary immune response in the rabbit. *Transplant. Proc.* **12**, 252.

77 KLAUS G.B. (1981) Cyclosporin A: its influence on T and B cells. *Immunology Today*, **2**, 83.

78 TUTSCHKA P.J., HESS A.D., BESCHORNER W.E. & SANTOS A.D. (1981) Suppressor Cells in transplantation tolerance. *Transplantation*, **32**, 203.

79 HESS A.D., TUTSCHKA P.J. & SANTOS G.W. (1982) The effect of Cyclosporin A on T-lymphocyte subpopulations. In *Cyclosporin A*, Chapter 19, (ed. White D.J.G.), p. 209. Elsevier Biomedical Press.

80 LEAPMAN S.B., FILO R.S., SMITH E.J. & SMITH P.G. (1980) Effects of Cyclosporin A on the generation of primed lymphocytes *in vitro. Transplant. Proc.* **13**, 405.

81 LEONI P., GARCIA R.C. & ALLISON A.C. (1978) Effects of Cyclosporin A on human lymphocytes in culture. *J. Clin. Lab. Immunol.* **1**, 67.

82 RYFFEL B., DONATSCH P., COTZ U. & TSCHOPP M. (1980)

Cyclosporin receptor on mouse lymphocytes. *Immunology*, **41**, 913.

83 KAHAN B.D., VAN BUREN C.T., LIN S.N., RIED M. & LE GRUE S.J. (1982) Pharmacokinetics of Cyclosporin A in renal allograft recipients. In *Cyclosporin A*, (ed. White D.J.G.), p. 413. Elsevier Biomedical Press.

84 LARSSON E.L. (1980) Cyclosporin A and Dexamethasone suppress T cell responses by selectively acting at distant sites of the triggering process. *J. Immunol.* **124**, 2828.

85 PALACIOS R. & MOLLER G. (1981) Cyclosporin A blocks receptors for HLA-DR antigens on T cells. *Nature*, **290**, 792.

86 BRITTON S. & PALACIOS R. (1982) Cyclosporin A—usefulness, risks and mechanism of action. *Immunol. Revs.* **65**, 70.

87 CHANG R., KUNG P. & GINGRES S. (1981) Does OKT3 monoclonal antibody react with an antigen recognition structure on human T cells? *Proc. natn. Acad. Sci. U.S.A.* **78**, 1805.

88 BUNJES D., HARDT C., SOLBACH W., DEUSCH K., ROLL-INGHOFF M. & WAGNER H. (1982) Studies on the mechanism of action of Cyclosporin A in the murine and human T cell response *in vitro*. In *Cyclosporin A*, Chapter 22, (ed. White D.J.G.), p. 261. Elsevier Biomedical Press.

89 FIDELIUS R.K., FERGUSON R.M., WIDMER B.M., WEE S.L., BACH F.H. & OROSZ C.G. (1982) Effect of Cyclo-sporin A on murine and human T helper cell clones. *Transplantation*, **34**, 308.

90 KOLB H. & TOYKA K.V. (1984) New concepts in immunotherapy. *Immunology Today*, **5**, 307.

91 CORTESINI R., MOLAJON R.E., MONARI C., FAMULARI A., BERLOCO P., CAPUA A., MORINUCCI G. & ALFANI D. (1985) Total lymphoid irradiation in clinical transplantation: experience in 30 high-risk patients. *Transplant. Proc.* **17**, 1291.

92 ORTHO MULTICENTER TRANSPLANT (1985) Study Group. A randomized clinical trial of OKT-3. Monoclonal antibody for acute rejection of cadaveric renal transplants. *New Engl. J. Med.* **313**, 337.

93 WHITE D.J.G., MCNAUGHTON D. & WATSON J.V. (1985) A cellular analysis of *in vitro* and *in vitro* activation of lymphocytes in the presence of Cyclosporin A. *Transplant. Proc.* **18**, 595.

94 KRONKE M., LEONARD W.S., DEPPER J.M., ARYA S.K., WONG-STAAL F., GALLO R.C., WALDMANN T.A. & GREEN W.C. (1984) Cyclosporin A inhibits T cell growth factor gene expression at the level of a RNA transcription. *Proc. natn. Acad. Sci. U.S.A.* **81**. 3209.

95 WILLIAMSON E.B.M. & SELLS R.A. (1985) The chilo-oesophageal fistula: successful internal drainage of the thoracic duct without fluid replacement. Transplant. Proc. (in press).

Chapter 82
Studies of autoimmune disease

ELIZABETH S. RAVECHE & A. D. STEINBERG

Introduction to murine models of
  lupus, 82.1
Serological studies, 82.1
Studies of kidney inflammation,
  82.6
Studies of B cell hyperactivity,
  82.6

Studies of abnormal
  immunoregulation, 82.8
Genetic tools useful in
  autoimmune disease, 82.13
Techniques for the development
  of autoimmunity, 82.15

Techniques for cytogenetic
  analysis of autoimmune NZB
  cells, 82.16
Molecular genetic analysis, 82.16
Conclusion, 82.18

Introduction to murine models of lupus

There are a large number of spontaneously occurring autoimmune diseases of humans. For many of these, animal models have been developed. These include animals immunized with various self-antigens such as thyroid (to induce thyroiditis) and myelin basic protein (to induce demyelinating diseases). In addition, spontaneously occurring abnormalities in certain animals resemble certain human diseases. Thus certain mice have features of human systemic lupus erythematosus (NZB, BXSB, MRL-*lpr/lpr*) [1]. Spontaneously occurring thyroiditis has been studied in the buffalo rat [2] and the obese strain chicken [3]. Recently a chicken model of fibrosing diseases has been described [4].

In view of the large number of autoimmune diseases, it it impossible to outline all of the laboratory procedures useful for investigating them. Each requires its own analysis. The abnormalities in different disorders are different and require separate assays. In general, there are assays for clinical abnormalities, and for pathogenic defects. Ultimately one would like to understand the genetic basis for disease, the gene products that are abnormal, how such abnormalities lead to the phenotypic expression of the disorder, and the pathogenetic mechanisms that follow. Where environmental factors are important, one wishes to understand the interactions between the environmental factors and the host, including the genetic basis for susceptibility (Fig. 82.1).

In this chapter, the authors will confine their consideration to murine lupus as an example of an auto-immune model of a human disease. The murine models of lupus vary in their clinical and serological abnormalities (Table 82.1). As a result, each mouse strain or cross requires somewhat different serological

and clinical measures or different time frames for study. All have polyclonal B cell activation at the height of illness with hypergammaglobulinaemia; however, the pace and isotype expression vary.

Serological studies

Technique for measurement of antibodies reactive with DNA

Murine lupus, like human lupus, is characterized by antinuclear antibodies. These are often measured by immunofluorescence using various substrates such as liver cells, leucocytes, or *Crithidia lucilia*. Many investigators wish to know the antibody activity directed toward individual nuclear components. Antibodies reactive with histones, RNA (tRNA, ssRNA, dsRNA, small nuclear RNAs), DNA (ssDNA, native DNA, synthetic dsDNA, Z DNA), DNA–histones, and nuclear non-histone proteins may be measured separately (Fig. 82.2). The most commonly used assays are radio-immunoassays and the ELISA (enzyme-linked immunosorbant assay). The latter offers the advantage of allowing the identification of isotype and avoids the requirement for radioactive ligand and a liquid scintillation counter (Fig. 82.3).

ELISA technique

Equipment

Micro-ELISA auto reader (Dynatech Instruments, Santa Monica, CA).

Procedure

The technique has been published [5].
1 To 96-well Immulon microtitre plates (Dynatech,

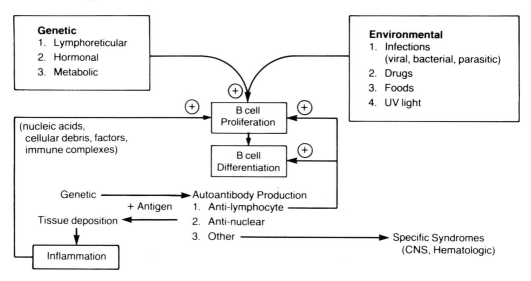

Fig. 82.1. Factors involved in the initiation and perpetuation of SLE. Techniques employed in analysis of the factors involved in SLE will be the subject of the following sections.

Alexandria, VA), 100 μl of 10 μg/ml methylated bovine γ-globulin (MBGG) was added at room temperature for 3 h.

2 The plates were thoroughly washed and calf thymus DNA (either nDNA or heat-denatured ssDNA obtained by heating nDNA to 100 °C and rapidly chilling in ice water with stirring) was added at 5 μg/ml in a total volume of 100 μl.

3 The plates were incubated for 3 days at 4 °C, after which they were thoroughly washed and 'blocked' with 100 μl of 2% bovine serum albumin (BSA) in phosphate-buffered saline (PBS) containing 0.05% Tween 20 detergent.

4 Ten microlitres of test sera were added to the wells at room temperature for 75 min.

5 After a thorough washing of the plates, peroxidase-conjugated anti-mouse IgG or IgM (Kirkegaard-Perry Laboratories, Alexandria, VA) was then added; after a 75 min incubation, the enzyme substrates were added (o-phenylenediamine 1/20 and H_2O_2 1/100 by volume to the buffer) and the optical density read at completion (40 min; 405 nm).

6 Background binding by normal mouse serum was minimal and was subtracted from the results; known positives gave a substantial response. Human anti-ssDNA and -nDNA from patients with systemic lupus erythematosus were used as controls for the species specificity of the anti-Ig reagents. Their binding was equivalent to that of the blank. A positive control is a pool of serum from old female (NZB × NZW)F$_1$ mice.

Notes and recommendations

The time for incubation with DNA can be reduced. It is desirable to read the optical density at 20, 30, and 40 min. Plates should be kept in the dark for step 5. This assay can be modified for the measurement of antibodies with many different specificities.

Farr assay

The ELISA assay measures low and high affinity antibodies. In contrast, the Farr assay preferentially measures high affinity antibody.

Procedure [44]

A commercial source of labelled *E. coli* DNA (e.g. New England Nuclear, Boston, MA) was used with an activity of 2500 d.p.m./10 μl. Before the DNA was used in an assay, it was made single-stranded by heating in a water bath for 10 min at 100 °C and then immersed in an ice bath with constant stirring. The DNA was diluted with borate buffer (1 part DNA and 4 parts buffer) and 50 μl added to 10 × 75 mm test tubes. Then 40 μl of borate buffer and 10 μl of sera (which had previously been heated for 30 min at 56 °C) were added. (In some cases 25 μl of borate buffer and 25 μl of sera were employed). The tubes were shaken, covered with parafilm and incubated at 37 °C for 30 min and then placed at 4 °C overnight. One hundred microlitres of 70% $(NH_4)_2SO_4$ were added in the cold (giving a final concentration of 35%) and the tubes

Table 82.1. Abnormalities in murine lupus erythematosus

Feature	Strain			
	NZB	(NZB × NZW)F$_1$	MRL-MP/lpr/lpr*	BXSB
Genetic	At least six autosomal genes	Multiple genes, some from NZW	Multiple background genes, lpr = major accelerator	Multiple background genes; Y chromosome gene = major accelerator
Major histocompatibility	d/d	d/z	k/k	b/b
Sex	Little effect; recessive gene for androgen insensitivity	Marked effect; androgens protect, oestrogens worsen	Androgens protect	Marked acceleration in males not hormonal
Immunoglobulins	Increased IgM	Increased IgM and IgG	Increased IgG1 and IgG2a	Increased IgG1 and IgG2b
Lymphoid organs	Lymphoid hyperplasia	Lymphoid hyperplasia	Marked increase in T cells	Moderate increase in B cells
Effect of *xid*	Prevents disease	Prevents disease	Retards disease	Prevents disease
Disease manifestations	Anti-T-cell antibodies; Coombs-positive haemolytic anaemia; splenic hyperdiploidy	Anti-DNA; lupus erythematosus cells membranoproliferative glomerulonephritis; Sjögren's syndrome	Marked lymphadenopathy; anti-DNA; anti-Sm; arthritis and anti-Ig; membranoproliferative glomerulonephritis; vasculitis	Immune complex glomerulonephritis; degenerative coronary artery disease; fewer serologic abnormalities than others; moderate adenopathy
Median survival (months)	Female 15 Male 17	Female 10 Male 16	Female 5–7 Male 7–8	Female 15 Male 7

* The *lpr/lpr* genotype has been bred into other genetic backgrounds. There is anti-DNA production and premature death in all; however, severe renal disease is not common unless the background is autoimmune-prone [49].

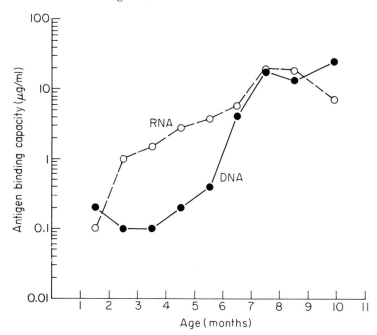

Fig. 82.2. Age-dependent formation of anti-RNA and anti-DNA antibodies in (NZB × NZW)F₁ female mice.

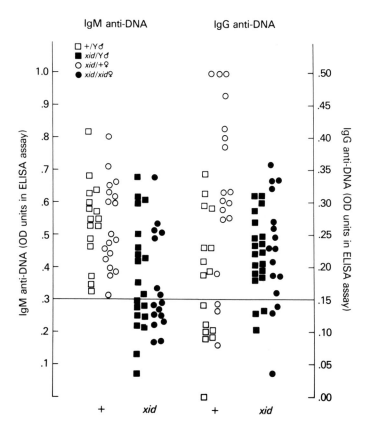

Fig. 82.3. Representative results obtained by the ELISA technique for determination of class specific anti-DNA antibodies in MRL-*lpr/lpr* mice with and without the *xid* gene defect. Each point represents the results of an individual animal.

were incubated in an ice bath for 1 h. The tubes were then centrifuged at 1000 *g* for 20 min and 100 μl of supernatant removed and placed in counting vials. Ten millilitres of ultrafluor (National Diagnostic, Somerville, NJ) counting solution were added and the tubes were counted for 10 min (Nuclear Chicago Scintillation Counter). The amount of total radioactivity present was obtained by placing a sample of the DNA in separate counting vials. Several known positive and negative controls were used. Background counts were subtracted from each sample. The same assay can be used for native DNA, RNA, etc.

Calculations

The procedure is based on the solubility of unbound ^{14}C-DNA in ammonium sulphate while antibody bound ^{14}C-DNA complexes are precipitated by ammonium sulphate. The percentage binding is calculated by the formula:

Percentage bound =
$$\frac{\text{input d.p.m.} - 2\,(\text{d.p.m. in 100 } \mu\text{l of sample supernatant})}{\text{input d.p.m.}}$$

Technique for measurement of naturally occurring thymocytotoxic auto-antibodies (NTA)

Anti-T cell auto-antibodies have been found in NZB mice and are associated with an age-dependent loss of T cells in these mice [6]. These antibodies impair cellular responses and cause a loss of suppressor T cells [7].

Procedure [8]

1 Target thymocytes from C57BL/6 mice were chromium labelled by incubation with 30 μCi of ^{51}Cr per 10^7 cells for 30 min at 37 °C in RPMI 1640 medium.
2 Labelled thymocytes (5×10^4) were added to 50 μl of serially diluted test serum and incubated for 30 min at room temperature followed by 30 min at 4 °C.
3 Cells were centrifuged, washed twice in medium, and incubated with 50 μl of a 1:5 dilution of rabbit complement (previously absorbed with mouse thymocytes) for 30 min at 37 °C.
4 The suspension was then centrifuged, and 50 μl of supernate removed and counted in a gamma spectrometer.
5 The positive control was a pool of NZB sera with known NTA activity; the negative control consisted of sera from 1-year-old female DBA/2 mice. Maximum ^{51}Cr release was obtained by freeze-thawing three times. Cytotoxicity of complement (C) alone was also determined. Percentage cytotoxicity was calculated as

$$\frac{(\text{c.p.m. test serum} - \text{c.p.m. C})}{(\text{c.p.m. freeze-thaw} - \text{c.p.m. C})} \times 100$$

All sera were assayed in duplicate with good reproducibility. The cytotoxic titre was the last dilution giving 50% ^{51}Cr release. A positive titre in this assay is 1:4.

Notes and recommendations

The source of complement is the major problem with this assay. Complement should be screened for non-specific killing and ability to lyse nearly all of the appropriate target. Low-tox complement (Accurate Chemical and Scientific Corp., Westbury, NY) should be screened as well if it is to be employed in the assay.

Technique for measuring anti-erythrocyte auto-antibodies

Haemolytic anaemia due to the loss of red blood cells caused by anti-erythrocyte auto-antibodies is present in ageing autoimmune NZB mice [1].

Procedure: direct Coombs' assay of anti-erythrocyte auto-antibodies

1 Blood from each mouse was collected in preservative-free heparin and centrifuged at 322 *g* for 10 min. The erythrocytes were washed three times with phosphate-buffered saline, pH 7.2, and resuspended at a final concentration of 1%.
2 Polyvalent sheep anti-mouse-Ig serum was heated at 56 °C for 30 min and adsorbed with a 1/4 volume of packed mouse erythrocytes overnight at 4 °C.
3 The direct Coombs' assay was performed by adding to microtitre wells 50 μl of a 1% erythrocyte suspension and 50 μl of serial twofold dilutions of the adsorbed sheep anti-mouse Ig starting at 1:10 dilution.
4 The wells were then examined for agglutination after an incubation of 1 h at 37 °C. A positive result was assigned to erythrocyte samples that showed agglutination of an anti-Ig dilution of 1:4 (1:40 final dilution). Known positives, blood from old NZB mice, and negative controls, usually blood from young BALB/C mice, were run with each assay.

Notes and recommendations

The dilution of anti-Ig should be chosen on the basis of preliminary experiments so as to conserve reagents. With a very high-titred reagent, old NZB red blood cells can have titres > 40 wells. The authors usually calibrate the test so that a decent positive is > 9 wells and call all > 12 wells positives just > 12 without going to a separate plate.

Studies of kidney inflammation

Proteinuria

Renal inflammation can be measured by testing voided urine for proteinuria. A mouse is picked up and usually it will urinate. Gentle massaging of the lower abdomen may facilitate urination. The voided urine can be caught on a small piece of parafilm and tested with chemically treated paper (Albustix, Miles Laboratories, Eklhart, IN). The accompanying colour code gives an estimation of the urine protein concentration. Proteinuria of 3+ or 4+ is very abnormal (300–2000 mg/dl). In females, 2+ is abnormal. Since males often have proteinuria unrelated to renal disease, 2+ is not a reliable measure for males.

Histological studies of kidneys

Renal inflammation is also assessed by sacrificing the animal and examining the kidneys histologically. Thin sections, 4 μm, allow evaluation. Thick sections prevent easy assessment. Routine staining with hae-matoxylin and eosin is usually sufficient; however, PAS stains are helpful. Glomeruli can be graded individually and a score for each mouse provided [9].

Renal functional deterioration is accompanied by a rise in serum nitrogen waste products. Serum urea or urea nitrogen may be measured to assess renal function.

Studies of B cell hyperactivity

B cell hyperactivity is a common feature of murine models of autoimmunity. The abnormalities could arise from abnormalities in stem cell production of B lymphocytes, an intrinsic abnormality of B cells, or an abnormality resulting from abnormal T cell regulation of B cells (Fig. 82.4).

IgM secretion in short-term cultures

In several autoimmune strains there is a marked spontaneous hypersection of IgM by splenic B cells in short-term cultures.

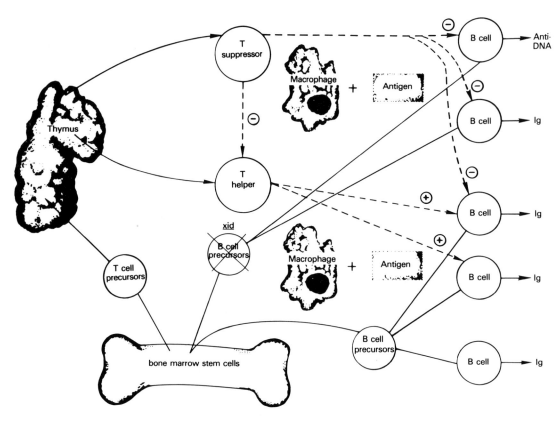

Fig. 82.4. Immunoregulatory abnormalities in autoimmunity which may result in B cell hyperactivity.

Procedure [10]

1 Spleen cells from mice, killed by cervical dislocation, were prepared by gentle teasing and the cells were washed in balanced salt solution. The standard tissue culture medium consisted of RPMI 1640 supplemented with 10% fetal calf serum, 200 mM-glutamine, 0.15 mM-HEPES, non-essential amino acids, sodium pyruvate, 5×10^{-5} M-2-mercaptoethanol, 100 U/ml penicillin, and 100 μg/ml streptomycin.

2 Cells (2×10^6 in 250 μl) were cultured in Costar 3596 plates in a humidified 5% CO_2–95% air incubator at 37 °C for 24 h.

3 Culture supernatants were then assayed for immunoglobulin levels. A solid-phase enzyme-linked immunoabsorbent assay (ELISA) was developed for assay of supernatant immunoglobulin.

4 U-bottom polystyrene plates (Immulon I, Dynatech Laboratories, Alexandria, VA) were incubated with 5 μg/ml of goat anti-mouse IgG (or IgM) in phosphate-buffered saline, pH 7.2, overnight at 4 °C. After extensive washing with PBS/0.05% Tween 20 and distilled water, the plates were blocked with 2.0% BSA.

5 The test supernatants diluted 1:200 in PBS/0.05% Tween 20, were added to the coated plates and incubated for 60 min at room temperature.

6 The plates were washed with PBS/Tween 20 and then distilled water. A previously titred peroxidase-conjugated goat anti-mouse IgG (Kirkergaard and Perry Laboratories, Gaithersburg, MD) (or peroxidase-conjugated goat anti-mouse IgM) was diluted in PBS containing 2.0% BSA and then added to each well in a volume of 0.1 ml.

7 The plates were again incubated for 60 min at room temperature and then washed as before.

8 A substrate solution of previously titred hydrogen peroxide and *o*-phenylenediamine was freshly prepared and added to each well (see anti-DNA above).

9 After incubation in the dark for 15 min, the absorbance of each well at 450 nm was measured with an automated reader (Titertek Multiscan, Flow Laboratories, McLean, VA).

10 Known positive and negative controls were included in each assay.

Notes and recommendations

The cultures can be extended to 4 and/or 6 days which generates additional information.

Anti-μ activation of B cell cultures

In vitro analysis of the response of autoimmune B cells to polyclonal B cell activators points to different B cell defects in different autoimmune strains [11].

Procedure

B cells can be obtained from a variety of techniques and then cultured with anti-IgM.

High-dose anti-μ

1 Cell suspensions were treated with monoclonal anti-thy-1.2 (New England Nuclear, Boston, MA) and complement (C: guinea-pig serum, Flow Labs, McLean, VA) to obtain T-depleted spleen cells.

2 Cells were washed and layered on top of a discontinuous gradient composed of 70%, 60% and 50% Percoll (Pharmacia Fine Chemicals, Piscataway, NJ).

3 The gradient was centrifuged at 2300 *g* for 12 min at 5 °C.

4 The cells at each interface were collected from above with a Pasteur pipette. Low-density fractions were above 50% Percoll (1.062 sp. gr.); intermediate density (1.062–1.074), between 50 and 60% Percoll; dense (1.074–1.086), between 60 and 70% Percoll.

5 Cells obtained after Percoll density separation were cultured according to the method previously described [12]. Briefly, cells were cultured in serum-free medium Iscove's/F-12. Cells (3×10^6) were cultured in 1 ml of medium in 16 mm diameter (24 wells/plate), flat-bottomed tissue culture wells (3524, Costar, Cambridge, MA).

6 Cultured cells were stimulated with affinity-purified goat anti-μ antibody (50 μg/ml) or with LPS (50 μg/ml) (Difco, Detroit, MI) in the presence of colcemid (25 ng/ml) (GIBCO, Grand Island, NY) added after the first 24 h.

7 After 48 h the cultures were harvested and analysed for individual cellular DNA content by staining with propidium iodide (see pp. 82.8–82.9).

The percentage of cells responding is the number of cells in the S+, G_2+M phases of the cell cycle. For determining the uptake of ^{3}H-thymidine, cells were cultured at 2×10^5 cells/well in flat-bottomed 96-well microtitre plates (3596; Costar).

Applications

Following *in vitro* stimulation with high-dose anti-μ, cells from old autoimmune NZB and MRL-*lpr/lpr* mice failed to proliferate. In contrast, cells from young autoimmune mice proliferated in response to high-dose anti-μ.

Stimulation with low-dose anti-μ and B-cell growth factor (BCGF)

Purified B cells (>95% Ig by flow cytometric analysis) from autoimmune mice can be cultured with anti-μ according to a method previously described [13].

1   Briefly, mice are T-depleted *in vivo* by injection of 0.04 ml of rabbit anti-mouse thymocyte serum (MA Bioproducts, Walkersville, MD) 2 days prior to sacrifice. The spleen is removed and a single cell suspension of spleen cells is treated with anti-thy 1.2 and complement.

2   Macrophages are depleted by adherence to plastic Petri dishes at 37 °C for 1 h in 10% FCS.

3   B cells are further purified by passage through a Sephadex G10 column and finally B cells are positively selected by panning on anti-Ig-coated plastic Petri dishes.

4   Proliferative responses of these highly purified B cells may be obtained in a co-stimulating assay. Briefly, a low number of cells (5×10^4/well) cultured in RPMI 1640 medium supplemented with 10% FCS L-glutamine (200 mM), 100 U/ml penicillin, streptomycin (50 μg/ml), and 2-mercaptoethanol (5×10^{-5} M) were stimulated with a low concentration of goat anti-IgM antibodies (5 μg/ml), various concentrations of partially purified BCGF (B-cell growth factor) obtained from supernatant of phorbol myristate acetate (PMA)-stimulated EL-4 cells, or both.

By this method, the signals which lead to activation and proliferation of B cells may be studied both in normal and pathological situations. The authors have compared the proliferative responses of autoimmune mice (2–3-month-old female NZB) with age- and sex-matched controls. Whereas normal mice showed a maximum ^{3}H-thymidine incorporation only when both goat anti-μ and BCGF were added to the culture, NZB mice manifested similar responses to BCGF alone, and BCGF$^+$ anti-μ. These results suggest that B cells from autoimmune animals are already 'in vivo' activated, with the activation signal delivered by anti-μ being unnecessary [14]. As more pure cytokines become available, assays without anti-μ will be especially useful.

Assay for spleen immunoglobulin-secreting cells

Polyclonal B cell activation can be manifested by a non-specific increase in numbers of Ig-secreting cells (IgSC). To study total IgSC a reverse plaque forming cell assay can be employed with anti-mouse-Ig-coupled sheep red blood cells as targets and class-specific anti-mouse reagents as developers [15].

Studies of abnormal immunoregulation

Abnormal autologous mixed lymphocyte reaction

The autologous mixed lymphocyte reaction (AMLR) is the proliferation that results when T cells are co-cultured with autologous or syngeneic non-T cells.

The AMLR may be an *in vitro* manifestation of *in vivo* T cell regulation of other lymphocytes. It may serve as the major 'immunostat' *in vivo*. The AMLR is abnormal in autoimmune states. In young autoimmune mice, the AMLR is intact, but it is greatly reduced in older mice with autoimmune disease. The AMLR defect in older autoimmune mice appears to reside in the responder T cells [16].

Procedure

1   Preparation of responder cells: lymph node T cells were obtained by passage over a nylon wool column. The nylon non-adherent cell population contained less than 1% surface Ig-bearing cells by direct immunofluorescence and less than 1% macrophages by the criterion of latex ingestion. This population was used as a source of responder T lymphocytes.

2   Preparation of stimulator cells: the peritoneal cavities of unimmunized mice were lavaged with 15 ml of Hanks' balanced salt solution (HBSS) and the cells obtained used as stimulator cells. This population consisted of 50–70% macrophages by latex ingestion, 15–20% T cells using fluorescein-labelled anti-brain antibody, and 10–15% B lymphocytes by surface staining for Ig. Whole spleen was also used as a source of stimulator cells in some experiments. All stimulator cells received 2500 rad with a cesium source before use in culture.

3   Culture conditions and assay of DNA synthesis: T lymphocytes were mixed with irradiated stimulator cells in medium RPMI 1640 containing 4% polyethylene glycol (PEG) (Mr 6000; Sigma Chemical Co., St. Louis, MO), L-glutamine (300 μg/ml), penicillin-streptomycin, 2-mercaptoethanol (5×10^{-5} M), sodium pyruvate, and 0.5% fresh syngeneic normal mouse serum obtained from young mice. A constant number of responder cells, 4×10^5, was cultured with varying numbers of stimulator cells in a total volume of 0.2 ml in round-bottomed microtitre plates for 5 days at 37 °C in 5% CO$_2$; 18–24 h before harvesting, 1 μCi of tritiated thymidine (^{3}H-TdR, sp. ac. 6.7 Ci/mM, New England Nuclear Corp., Boston, MA) was added to each well, and the amount of radioactive uptake was measured. The amount of ^{3}H-TdR incorporated into DNA was used as a measure of the magnitude of the AMLR.

Method for cell cycle analysis of lymphocyte activation

The proportion of cells that are in the S and G$_2$ phases of the cell cycle is an indication of the percentage of proliferating cells. This measure is more precise than ^{3}H-TdR incorporation into cellular DNA.

Procedure

1 Remove tissue to be studied, such as lymph node, bone or spleen. In the case of the lymph node and spleen, mince in cold HBSS.
2 Bone-marrow cells are flushed from femurs and tibias with a 25-gauge needle attached to a 3 ml syringe containing cold HBSS.
3 Single cell suspensions are counted and centrifuged.
4 The pellet is resuspend to $3-5 \times 10^6$ cells/ml in a hypotonic solution of propidium iodide (propidium iodide 5 mg/100 ml in 0.1% sodium citrate). The hypotonic solution causes cell lysis but leaves nuclei intact.
5 The stained cells are excited at 488 nm with a flow cytometer. The amount of fluorescence emitted is proportional to the DNA content of individual nuclei. Cell cycle analysis was performed by computer-assisted data analysis, and the percentage of cells in G_0/G_1, S, and G_2+M phases of the cell cycle determined. If no cell cycle program is available, simple integration techniques for the area under the G_0/G_1 peak can be employed. Analysis of the number of mitotic cells by phase-contrast microscopy before staining with propidium iodide and after staining and cytometric study indicated that under the conditions employed, mitotic nuclei remained intact.

Method for determining RNA content of individual cells

As cells become activated, the cells progress through the cell cycle. An early event is cellular enlargement and an increase in RNA content as the cells leave G_0 and enter G_1 phase of the cycle.

Equipment

Fluorescence activated cell sorter or analyzer.

Materials

Pyronin Y: technique for single parameter analysis of RNA content of individual cells.
Acridine orange: technique for dual-parameter simultaneous analysis of DNA and RNA content of individual cells.

Procedure 1

Pyronin Y (PY) technique [17]. Single cell suspensions are obtained and cells are fixed in 70% ETOH. After 1 day of fixation, cells are washed and stained with a solution containing 0.01 mg/ml PY (Polysciences Inc.,

Warrington, PA) and analysed on a fluorescence activated cell sorter.

Procedure 2

Published techniques for staining with acridine orange are employed [18]. Young autoimmune NZB mice that do not have increased numbers of proliferating cells in the spleen have cells with increased RNA content.

Notes and recommendations

To determine the amount of RNA content in G_0, leucocytes from normal murine peripheral blood can be used as a standard.

Enumeration of subsets of T and B lymphocytes by flow cytometric techniques

Autoimmune mice have been found to have abnormal percentages of lymphocytes. As they age, the percentage of sIg cells decreases, as does the percentage of T cells. A variety of antibodies recognizing subsets of T and B cells, as well as antibodies which distinguish differentiation pathways of T and B cells, are available. These antibodies, coupled with flow cytometric analysis, have been very useful in augmenting our understanding of autoimmunity.

Using two-colour flow cytometry, a subset of B cells, Lyl^+, IgM^+, has been identified [19]. The Lyl B cells are increased in NZB mice and may account for the B cells that are spontaneously hyperactive in NZB mice [19a].

Abnormal generation of primary cytotoxic T lymphocytes

NZB spleen cells appear to have abnormal responses to minor antigenic determinants in primary cultures. NZB ($H-2^d$) spleen cells can generate, *in vitro*, a vigorous primary response against non-NZB $H-2^d$ spleen cells. Normal strains of mice respond to such determinants vigorously only in a secondary culture after priming. In addition, NZB cytotoxic T lymphocytes, in response to allogeneic stimulation, appeared earlier than the response of non-autoimmune $H-2^d$ strain cells to allogeneic stimulation. The accelerated generation of cytotoxic lymphocytes in NZB cultures could result from abnormal immunoregulation with an excess of helper function or previous priming *in vivo* with cross-reacting antigens. To assay this, cells from $H-2^d$ donor strains were stimulated *in vitro* with spleen cells from C57BL/6 mice ($H-2^b$) and assayed with EL-4 ($H-2^b$) tumour targets in a 4 h chromium release assay [20].

Procedure

1   Single spleen-cell suspensions were prepared in HBSS from non-primed mice.

2   C57BL/6 spleen cells, to be used as *in vitro* stimulator cells, were exposed to 1500 rad of gamma irradiation.

3   Cells were cultured in modified Eagle's minimum essential medium (MEM) with 10% heat-inactivated, mycoplasma-screened fetal calf serum (FCS) (Grand Island Biological Co., Grand Island, NY), in 16 mm, flat-bottomed culture wells (Costar, Data Packaging, Cambridge, MA). Six hundred and twenty-four replicate wells that contained 1×10^7 responder cells and 1×10^6 irradiated stimulator cells were cultured in a final vol of 1.5 ml.

4   Cultures were incubated for the specified number of days in a humidified atmosphere of 10% CO_2, 7% O_2, and 83% N_2 at 37 °C.

5   These effector cells were washed and resuspended in MEM with 10% FCS to the desired concentration of viable cells, and mixed with equal volumes (0.1 ml) of ^{51}Cr-labelled target cells (see below) in serological tubes.

6   Effector and target cells were incubated for 4 h at 37 °C in a humidified atmosphere with 5% CO_2; radioactivity released into the supernate was measured in a gamma spectrometer (model 8000; Beckman Instruments, Inc., Spinco Div., Palto Alto, CA).

Each determination was assayed in duplicate. Spontaneous ^{51}Cr release was determined by incubating 0.1 ml of target cells with 0.1 ml of MEM with 10% FCS. Maximum release was determined by three cycles of freezing and thawing similar cultures. Spontaneous release was determined for each time-point in an assay. Data from 4 h fixed-endpoint experiments are expressed as percentage specific lysis and were calculated by the formula:

Percentage specific lysis =

$$\frac{100 \times (\text{experimental release} - \text{spontaneous release})}{(\text{maximum release} - \text{spontaneous release})}$$

EL-4 tumour cells were used as targets and 2×10^7 tumour cells were incubated with 100 μCi of ^{51}Cr ($Na_2[^{51}CrO_4]$) in 1 ml of HBSS with 10% FCS for 30 min at 37 °C, and washed twice with HBSS before use in assay above.

Tolerance defects

Several murine models of autoimmunity have been found to lack the ability to become tolerant to heterologous serum proteins. Studies of the defect in tolerance induction may provide insight into the pathogenesis of the loss of self-tolerance which gives rise to autoimmunity [21] (Fig. 82.5).

Procedure

Tolerization and immunization with bovine γ-globulin (BGG)

1   Purified BGG (Cohn fraction II, Mann Research Laboratories, New York, NY) (40 mg/ml) in phosphate-buffered saline (PBS), pH 7.2, was spun in a Beckman L2-65 ultracentrifuge using a fixed-angle rotor (Type 65) at 105 000 ***g*** for 2 h.

2   The top one-third of the ultracentrifuged preparation was carefully removed, and 10 mg of deaggregated BGG was immediately injected intraperitoneally (i.p.) into each animal.

3   These mice and untreated controls were challenged

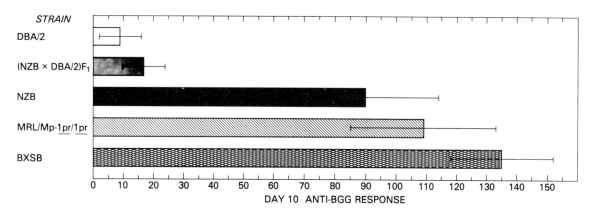

Fig. 82.5. Anti-BGG response 10 days following a tolerizing dose of ultracentrifuged BGG. Autoimmune mice were not tolerant when challenged with BGG in Freund's adjuvant. All mice were 2–3-month-old females except for the BXSB strain in which males were employed.

i.p. 10–14 days later with 0.5 mg BGG emulsified with complete Freund's adjuvant (CFA; H37Ra, Difco Co., Detroit, MI).

4 Mice were bled 10 and 30 days after challenge by retro-orbital puncture under light ether anaesthesia. The blood was allowed to clot at room temperature for about 2 h. The sera were removed, centrifuged to remove cellular debris, and stored at $-20\,°C$ until tested.

Assay of antibodies to BGG

A solid-phase immunoradiometric assay was used.

1 One hundred microlitres of a 10 μg/ml solution of DEAE-Sephacel purified BGG in PBS were allowed to incubate overnight at 4 °C in each well of a flexible round-bottomed microtitre plate (Cooke Co., Alexandria, VA).

2 The wells were rinsed with cold PBS (4 °C), and then 100 μl of 0.1% rabbit serum albumin (RSA; Miles Laboratories, Inc., Kankakee, IL) in PBS were added to each well. This was incubated for 30 min at 37 °C and then for 1 h at 4 °C. The wells were again washed with cold PBS.

3 Fifty microlitres of 1:50 dilutions of serum samples were added to the wells.

4 Each sample was run in duplicate. Each plate also contained 1:50 duplicate dilutions of standard pooled sera from BALB/c mice hyperimmunized with BGG, and pooled normal mouse sera. Incubation of all these specimens was again 30 min at 37 °C and 1 h at 4 °C. After extensive washing with cold PBS, 50 μl of 0.05%

Tween 20 in PBS, containing 20 ng of ^{3}H-labelled, affinity-purified rabbit anti-mouse Ig, were added to each well for 30 min at 37 °C and 1 h at 4 °C. After a final rinse, the wells were individually cut out and counted for 1 min in a liquid scintillation counter. The amount of labelled anti-mouse Ig bound per millilitre of sample was calculated according to the following formula:

$$\mu g\ ^3\text{H-labelled anti-Ig bound/ml} = \frac{(\text{c.p.m.} - \text{background}) \times \text{dilution factor}}{\text{specific activity of } ^3\text{H-labelled anti-Ig}}$$

An ELISA assay (as described above for anti-DNA) can also be used [5].

Technique for measuring IL-2 production

Murine models of autoimmunity have profound defects in mitogen-induced *interleukin-2* (IL-2) production and proliferation [22]. Studies of IL-2 production may help elucidate sequences involved in the activation of T cells (Fig. 82.6).

Procedure

1 Single cell suspensions of spleen cells were cultured at 5×10^6 cells/ml in 1 ml RPMI 1640 supplemented with 20 mM-HEPES, 2 mM-L-glutamine, 100 U penicillin, 50 μg streptomycin and 5% heat-inactivated FCS in a humidified atmosphere containing 5% CO_2, 5 μg con A (Pharmacia, Piscataway, NJ).

2 Five nanograms of phorbol myristate acetate

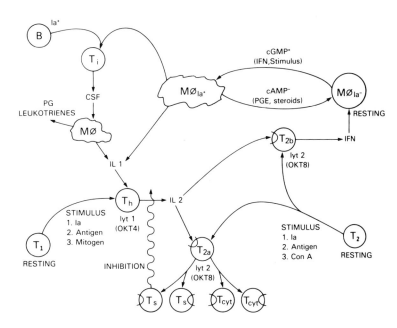

Fig. 82.6. Role of soluble factors in the activation of T cells.

(PMA) or 5 μg con A plus 5 ng of PMA were added to 16-well Costar plates for various times.

3 The wells were harvested, centrifuged at 600 g for 10 min, passed through a 0.45 μm filter (Millipore Corp., Bedford, MA) and stored at $-20\,°C$ until use.

4 To measure the IL-2 produced, supernatants were tested for their ability to maintain the growth of the IL-2-dependent CT6 cells [23].

Applications

Autoimmune mice produce subnormal amounts of IL-2 when cultured in the presence of Con A. This defect was repaired by the addition of PMA. It appears that autoimmune-prone mice are capable of producing IL-2 provided that the comitogen is present [24], or that the cells are pre-cultured for several days prior to stimulation with con A [45].

Techniques for detection of immune interferon

Immune interferon (IFN) is a lymphokine that is produced in response to mitogenic lectins and specific antigens [25] and is thought to participate in a variety of immunoregulating events. This is the lymphokine most responsible for immune regulatory abnormalities in lupus. It is spontaneously produced in large amounts by mice with lupus [26].

Procedure

1 Interferon is measured either in serum or in supernatants of stimulated lymphocytes. For the latter, 5 μg of con A or medium alone were added in 20 μl aliquots to 1 ml of 5×10^4 spleen cells in 24-well plates (Costar, Cambridge, MA) and cultured for variable periods of time.

2 Individual wells were harvested, centrifuged at 600 g for 10 min, passed through a 0.45 μm filter (Millipore Corp., Bedford, MA) and stored at $-20\,°C$ until assayed for IFN activity.

3 Supernatants or sera (fresh) were assayed for IFN by the reduction of plaque formation of vesicular stomatitis virus on mouse L cells. Briefly, 5×10^4 murine L cells, in 100 μl of RPMI 1640 with 1% FCS, were dispensed in flat-bottomed microculture plates. Serial dilutions of the test sample were then added in 50 μl aliquots to triplicate cultures, and the plates were incubated at 37 °C for 25 h. The cultures were then drained, and the monolayers in each well were inoculated with 50 plaque-forming units of vesicular stomatitis virus for 90 min. The wells were then drained and overlayered with 50 μl of a methyl cellulose solution for 24 h at 37 °C. The viral plaques were subsequently visualized by staining with a neutral red solution. The

IFN titre, expressed as units per millilitre, is the reciprocal of the logarithm of the dilution of the test sample, which produces a 50% reduction of the plaque-forming cell response of control cultures (calculated by linear regression).

Notes and recommendations

IFN found in the serum of MRL-*lpr/lpr* and MRL-*lpr/lpr·xid* mice was detected most easily in fresh serum. Frozen serum gave reduced and more variable results [46]. In contrast, IFN generated by *in vitro* stimulation was stable upon freezing and storing.

Methods for studying stem cell abnormalities in autoimmune disease

Several studies have suggested that the auto-immune disease which spontaneously occurs in several murine lupus models may have a primary defect in stem cell response to differentiation signals. Analysis of stem cell activity may be performed by several techniques.

Colony formation—CFU (colony forming units)

Endogenous CFU: these represent the expansion and differentiation of endogenous pluripotent stem cells into cells of the myeloid and lymphoid series. Auto-immune NZB mice, both young and old, have increased numbers of CFUs when compared to normal strains of mice [27,28] (Fig. 82.7).

Procedure

Mice are irradiated with 650 rad and spleens removed 6–10 days later. The time selected as the endpoint following sub-lethal irradiation should be the same for each datum in a given experiment, but can be chosen to maximize the information. In a situation where large numbers of colonies are produced, by day 8 the colonies will have overgrown the spleen and counting of individual colonies becomes hampered. Such animals are best studied on day 6 or 7. On the chosen day, mice are killed and the spleens are fixed in 5–10 ml of the following solution: 70% ETOH, 20 parts; 30% formaldehyde, 1 part; glacial acetic acid, 1 part. The colonies are enumerated with the aid of a dissecting microscope.

Exogenous CFU. In this case analysis of the ability of injected cells to form CFUs in the spleens of irradiated animals is assessed. By this technique it is possible to study stem cell activity in several organs.

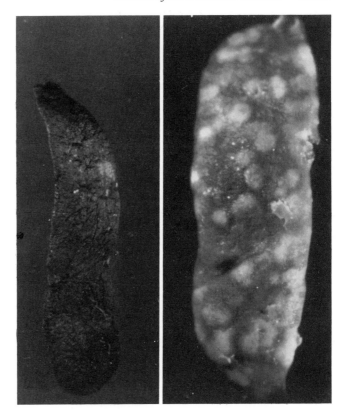

Fig. 82.7. Endogenous spleen colony formation in 2–3-month-old female mice following irradiation with 650 rad. The left fixed spleen is from a DBA/2 female and the right spleen is from a NZB female.

Procedure

Recipient animals are irradiated with 950 rad and injected with a source of stem cells (bone marrow, spleen, etc.). Non-autoimmune mice are readily repopulated with bone marrow or spleen as sources of pluripotent stem cell. Spleens of repopulated animals are removed and processed as above.

Bone marrow B cell colonies

Various monoclonals directed against markers of B-cell maturation are now available. With the use of these markers to deplete mature B cells from the bone marrow it is possible to study the maturation of B cells. At a young age, NZB marrow contains large numbers of sIg$^-$ B cell precursors that can respond to mitogens in semi-solid agar cultures without preculture [29,30]. Briefly, the procedure involves removing cells from the bone marrow and depleting sIg$^+$ cells by adherence to anti-Ig-coated plastic Petri dishes. Adherent cells are removed by passing cell suspensions through Sephadex G-10 columns. Depletion of 14.8$^+$ cells is accomplished by panning. Semi-solid agar cultures are established with (LPS) (25 μg/plate) as a potentiator of colony formation.

Genetic tools useful in autoimmune disease

An understanding of the types of inheritance patterns which are operative in murine autoimmunity has become a valuable tool for dissecting the regulation of autoimmune disease. (Exceptions are matings with non-autoimmune mice produce F$_1$ progeny which may produce auto-antibodies but generally do not die from autoimmune disease. (The exceptions are matings with NZW or SWR mice.) The genetic make-up of the non-NZB parent influences the expression of autoimmunity and suggests that a number of genes determine the expression of autoimmunity.

Development of recombinant inbred lines

The analysis of F$_2$ mice allows study of gene assortment and segregation of traits. This can be extended to studies of large numbers of identical F$_2$ mice by creating recombinant inbred lines. These lines serve an important function because often one wishes to study many traits in the F$_2$ and it may not be possible to do all of the studies on one mouse (one mouse cannot be killed at several different ages, one study may prevent another or interfere with it, etc.) This problem is, to some extent, overcome by taking the F$_2$ mice and brother–sister mating; after many generations, most of the loci become homozygous and different lines will have different sets of genes from a given parental strain. Each line is characterized with regard to different traits. After each line is analysed, the various lines are compared. This technique gives an estimate of the number of genes required for a given trait [31] as well as linkages among traits [48]. Ultimately gene mapping and molecular genetic studies can be done.

Breeding congenic and recombinant inbred autoimmune mice

In order to analyse the effect of a single gene on the autoimmune syndrome, it is useful to have congenic mice which differ by only that gene. Although this ideal is never achieved in practice, it is possible to prepare mice that differ by only a very small number of genes. An example is the introduction of the *xid* gene (on the X chromosome of CBA/N mice) into NZB, NZW, BXSB, and MRL-*lpr/lpr* mice. The authors will use the NZB mouse an an example. NZB females are mated with CBA/N males. The F$_1$ offspring are *xid/+*, i.e. one X chromosome has the *xid* gene and one has the wild type (+). These F$_1$ females are mated with NZB males. The male offspring which have only one X are either *xid* or + in a 1:1 ratio. The *xid*/Y males are selected for further mating. This is done by testing the response to TNP–Ficoll (immunize with TNP–Ficoll, 10 μg in saline i.p. and bleed 5 days later and test for antibodies by haemagglutination with TNP–RBC) or serum IgM levels (by radial immunodiffusion or ELISA). An absent response to TNP–Ficoll and a low serum IgM level allow the selection of the *xid*/Y male. For simplicity, one can designate that male as 75% NZB with the *xid* gene. It is mated with NZB females to produce *xid/+* female offspring which are approximately 87.5% NZB. These are mated with NZB males and the male offspring are 93.75% NZB; half are *xid*/Y and half are +/Y. The *xid* males are selected for continued mating. Thus, in every other mating, the selected *xid*/Y male is used to mate with NZB females and in alternate matings the *xid/+* females are used to mate with NZB males. The procedure is continued until the mice are highly inbred. At some point, one can start to brother–sister mate mice in order to generate an NZB.*xid* line. This is done by mating an *xid/+* female with her *xid*/Y son so as to produce *xid/xid* and *xid/+* females. These are tested for the *xid/xid* genotype with TNP–Ficoll or serum IgM levels and the *xid/xid* females are mated with *xid*/Y males to maintain the line. How far should the breeding be maintained before such inbreeding is done? At least twenty back-crosses are necessary and forty would be

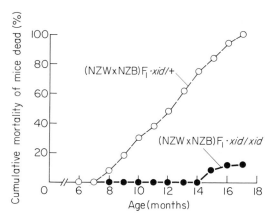

Fig. 82.8. Survival of female (NZW × NZB)F$_1$ females with and without the *xid* defect (*xid/xid*).

better. The ideal would be always to outbreed to NZB mice to avoid genetic drift from the parent strain.

In addition to *xid*, other genes can be bred on to the NZB background. In addition, NZB mice can be prepared with other Ig allotypes or different H-2 types (Fig. 82.8).

Influence of sex on the expression of inherited autoimmune traits

In the murine models of autoimmunity, females develop autoimmune features earlier than males with the exception of the BXSB strain where males develop an accelerated disease which does not have a hormonal basis. In order to determine patterns of inheritance of auto-immune traits, the effects of sex hormones must be considered [32].

Procedures

Animals to be studied can be surgically castrated pre-pubertally and hormone manipulations performed. In female mice, the ovaries can be removed through two bilateral flank incisions. In males, both testes can be removed through a single scrotal incision. The *vas deferens* is tied, and each testis and epididymis removed.

For hormonal manipulation, silastic capsules containing hormones can be implanted subcutaneously high in the back. The silastic capsules (Dow Dorning Corp., MI) 0.155 mm in diameter and 5 mm long contain either 2.5 mg 5-α-dihydrotestosterone or 2.0 mg 17-β-oestradiol (Sigma Chem. Co., Mo). Before capsules are implanted, they are soaked in phosphate-buffered saline for 24 h to allow for equilibration. Serum testosterone and oestrogen levels, as measured by a radioimmunoassay, were normal.

Techniques for the development of autoimmunity

B cells capable of making auto-antibodies are present in normals (both mice and humans). The development of an autoimmune response must, therefore, under normal circumstances, be under some regulatory control. Studies aimed at determining procedures which result in the development of autoimmunity are helpful in determining what regulatory controls are operative in the normal situation.

Induction of autoimmunity with polyclonal B cell activators

Polyclonal B cell activation appears to be fundamental to the development of autoimmunity. Polyclonal B cell activators are capable of inducing auto-antibodies in non-autoimmune mice [33,34] and can also accelerate disease in autoimmune-prone mice [35].

Procedure

To polyclonally stimulate mice *in vivo*, mice can be injected i.p. three times weekly with LPS (Difco Lab, Detroit, MI). In order to eliminate endotoxin shock from high doses the LPS is given increasing doses according to the following schedule: 25 μg per mouse three times weekly for 1 week, 50 μg per mouse three times a week for the duration of the experiment. Poly rI rC (P.L. Biochemicals Inc., WI) can also be used and is given i.p. at 10–100 μg three times weekly [36].

Induction of autoimmunity with bone marrow transfers

Numerous studies have shown that NZB bone marrow has the potential to transfer autoimmune disease to irradiated non-autoimmune mice. The use of the irradiated host allows for reconstitution with sub-populations of autoimmune marrow. With reconstitution experiments, it is possible to determine the proliferative and differentiative capacity of auto-immune stem cells. In addition, irradiated hosts can be repopulated with combinations of normal and auto-immune bone marrow. With the use of allele-specific surface markers, such as Lyb 2.1 (Fig. 82.9) or strain-dependent expression of surface antigens, such as ThB, the origin of the various cells in the repopulated recipient can be determined.

Dietary regulation of autoimmunity

Studies have shown that caloric restrictions sufficient to reduce animal weight by 30% reduce many features of murine autoimmunity [37]. Other variations in diet may have important modulatory effects on the expression of autoimmunity.

Procedure for dietary enrichment with the polyunsaturated fatty acid eicosapentaenoic acid (EPA) [38]

Diets

The basic diet consisted of a fat-free powder (ICN Nutritional Biochemicals, Cleveland, OH), which contains, by weight, 21% casein, 15.6% cellulose, 58.5% sucrose, and 4% balanced salt mixture, plus essential vitamins. This was mixed three parts to one by weight with refined whole menhaden oil (Zapata Haynie Company, Reedville, VA), a source rich in EPA.

Notes and recommendations

Since reduced food intake and decreased weight can ameliorate the autoimmune syndrome in mice, it is

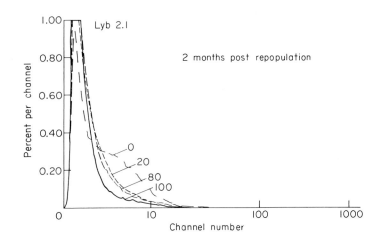

Fig. 82.9. Flow cytometric profiles obtained after staining radiation chimeras with allele-specific Lyb 2.1 which recognizes a subset of DBA/2 B cells but not NZB. The chimeras were repopulated with combinations of NZB and/or DBA/2 marrow: 0, 0% NZB + 100% DBA/2; 20, 20% NZB + 30% DBA/2; 80, 80% NZB + 20% DBA/2; 100, 100% NZB + 0% DBA/2.

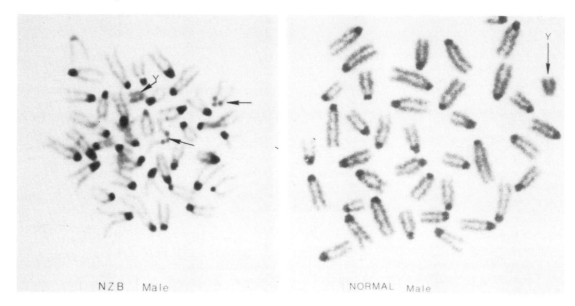

Fig. 82.10. Mitotic spleen cells from 2–3-month-old NZB or DBA/2 mice. NZB cells in addition to the Y chromosome have a marker pair of chromosomes which lack terminal C bands (indicated by arrows).

necessary to make sure that all groups have compatible weights until terminal illness develops.

Techniques for cytogenetic analysis of autoimmune NZB cells

C-banding of marker chromosomes

All mitotic cells of NZB mice possess a marker chromosome pair with abnormal centromeric-banding (C-banding) [39]. This permits the identification of NZB cells in situations where non-NZB cells are also present (Fig. 82.10).

Procedure

1 Single cell suspensions are obtained. Cells are washed in HBSS, centrifuged for 5 min at 200 g and resuspended in 0.075 M-KCl. The cells were swollen in the KCl for 30 min, centrifuged, and resuspended in 3:1 methanol:glacial acetic acid fixative.
2 After 10 min of fixation, the cells were centrifuged and resuspended in fixative, and slides were made and set aside.
3 After 2–3 days, the slides were incubated in 0.2 M-HCl at room temperature for 1 h, rinsed with deionized water, and incubated in $Ba(OH)_2$ (20–30 ml of 0.3 M-$Ba(OH)_2$ (Sigma) in 100 ml of deionized water) for 90 s at room temperature and then in an SSC solution (0.03 M-sodium citrate and 0.3 M-NaCl) at 60 °C for 1 h.

4 The slides were then rinsed and stained in a freshly prepared 4% Giemsa solution for 1 min.
5 In order to obtain both darkly staining C-banding regions and lightly staining G-banding regions, a modification of the normal C-banding technique was employed: 1-day-old slides were incubated with 0.10–0.15 M-HCl and treated with a weaker $Ba(OH)_2$ solution (10–15 ml of 0.3 M-$Ba(OH)_2$ in 100 ml of deionized water).

Analysis of hyperdiploid cells

As they age NZB mice develop cells in their spleen with extra chromosomes. This was found to be an inherited trait and present in association with other manifestations of immunological hyper-reactivity [39]. Hyperdiploid cells can be analysed cytogenetically, as described above (Fig. 82.11), or observed by flow cytometric techniques (Fig. 82.12).

Molecular genetic analysis

Oncogenes are the genetic elements in acute transforming retroviruses that are associated with the ability of these viruses to neoplastically transform cells. DNA sequences (c-*onc* genes) homologous to viral oncogenes (v-*onc* genes) have been conserved through evolution and can be found in most mammalian cells. Their ubiquitous presence and homology to the transforming genes in viruses suggest that they must play fundamental roles in normal cell growth or

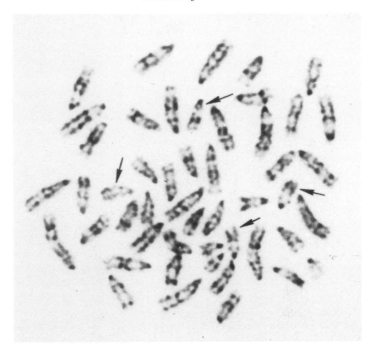

Fig. 82.11. Mitotic hyperdiploid spleen cell from 1-year-old female NZB. Normal spleen cells have 40 chromosomes, whereas this NZB had a modal number of 52 chromosomes. Arrows indicate chromosome #17. This cell had two extra copies of chromosome #17.

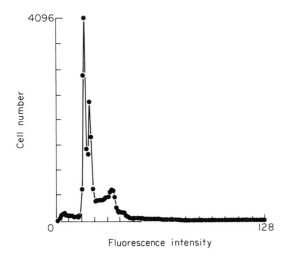

Fig. 82.12. Flow cytometric profile of the DNA content of spleen cells from a hyperdiploid NZB mouse. The first peak represents the normal G_1 cells and the second peak represents the hyperdiploid G_1 cells.

metabolism. One reasonable role that one or more oncogenes may play in non-transformed cells is the stimulation or regulation of cellular proliferation. Expression of varying levels of RNA transcribed from many *onc* genes can be detected in normal cells. An increased amount of *myc* RNA has been observed following *in vitro* activation of lymphocytes [40]. Thus it seems reasonable to test whether the abnormal proliferation of cells in autoimmune mice might be associated with increased expression of one or more cellular oncogenes. Several oncogenes were used to probe poly (A) RNA from spleens and lymph nodes of autoimmune and control mice.

Procedure

1 In each experiment, spleens from twenty normal or ten autoimmune mice of a single strain or cross were removed and gently teased into single cell suspensions in cold Hanks balanced salt solution buffered with 10 mM-HEPES, pH 7.4.

2 In some experiments, lymph nodes, thymuses or spleen are directly studied. In others, B cells or T cells were isolated. For B cell isolation macrophages were depleted by allowing them to adhere to plastic Petri dishes at 37 °C; T cells were depleted by treatment with anti-thy 1 and complement; the remaining cells, highly enriched in B cells, were used immediately for RNA isolation.

3 RNA isolation, blotting and hybridization: the guanidine thiocyanate method of Chirgwin *et al.* [41] was used to rupture cells and denature ribonuclease simultaneously. The RNA was separated from DNA and proteins by the cesium chloride centrifugation technique of Glisin *et al.* [42]. For final purification, the RNA was extracted once in chloroform/phenol and once in chloroform. The poly (A)$^+$ RNA fraction was obtained by passing the total purified RNA twice over an oligo(dT)-cellulose column and elution with low-salt buffer.

4 Ten micrograms of poly (A)$^+$ RNA was denatured in 14 mM-methylmercury hydroxide and subjected to electrophoresis in 1.5% agarose/5 mM-methylmercury hydroxide gels.

5 The RNA was blotted on to *o*-diazophenyl thioether paper, prehybridized and hybridized with 1–3 × 10^6 c.p.m./ml of different DNA probes that had been labelled with ^{32}P by nick translation to a specific activity of 1.4–2.0 × 10^8 c.p.m./μg. Ethidium bromide staining of the gel before and after confirmed that nearly equal amounts of RNA were blotted to the paper.

6 After washing under stringent conditions the hybridized blots were exposed to Kodak AR-2 film at −70 °C in the presence of an intensifying screen.

7 The autoradiographs were scanned with a GS 300 scanning densitometer (Hoefer Scientific Inst., San Francisco, CA).

8 The RNA blots were later stripped in 100% formamide at 65 °C for 2–6 h to remove traces of radioactive hybridized probe.

9 The blots were then pre-hybridized and hybridized with other probes to ensure that approximately equal amounts of poly (A)$^+$ RNA were present on the blots [43].

DNA probes

The c-*myc* probe was 5.5. kilobase (kb) Bam HI fragment containing mouse c-*myc* gene segments that had been isolated from a mouse plasmacytoma S107 bacteriophage library and subcloned into pBR322. The v *myb* probe was a 1.3 kb Kpn I-Xba I fragment isolated from cloned avian myeloblastosis virus and subcloned in pBR322. The v *abl* probe was a 1.2 kb Bgl II fragment isolated from cloned A-MuLV and subcloned using Eco RI linkers into pBR322.

Synthesis of cDNA and hybridization enrichment

1 Complementary DNA (cDNA) was synthesized in a final reaction volume of 0.2 ml containing 5 μg poly (A)$^+$ RNA, 2 μg of oligo-(dT), 60 U reverse transcriptase (Life Sciences Inc., St. Petersburg, FL), 1 mmol each of dATP, dGTP, dTTP and ^{32}P dCTP (Amersham Corp., Arlington Heights, IL, 10 mCi/ml; 3000 Ci/mmol) plus cold dCTP at a concentration of 75 μM, 5 μM-dithiothreitol, 20 μg actinomycin D, 6 mM-MgCl, 90 mM-KCl and 50 mM-Tris (pH 8.1 at 42 °C).

2 After incubation at 42 °C for 2 h and base

hydrolysis of the mRNA in 0.1 M-NaOH at 70 °C for 20 min, the cDNA was separated from the reaction mixture components on a column of Sephadex G-50 fine in a Pasteur pipette and ethanol precipitated with 50 μg of carrier tRNA.

3 A 20-fold excess of poly (A)$^+$ RNA was mixed with the ^{32}P cDNA in an ultracentrifuge tube, precipitated in ethanol and pelleted together. The pellet was resuspended in 5 μl of water, 1.5 μl of 2.0 M-phosphate buffer, 0.1 μl of 20% SDS, and 0.1 μl of 0.1 M-EDTA.

4 The 7 μl reaction volume was hybridized by heating in a sealed 20 μl capillary tube to 98 °C for 30 s, then 68 °C for 20 h.

5 Hybridization was followed by hydroxyapatite chromatography at 60 °C to allow isolation of the unhybridized single-stranded cDNA, followed by elution of double-stranded cDNA-poly (A)$^+$ RNA at 98 °C.

6 The single-stranded cDNA was hybridized to RNA blots at a final specific activity of 1–3 × 10^6 c.p.m./ml of hybridization solution as previously described [44] except that 1 mg yeast t-RNA, 100 μg poly-A, 100 μg poly-C, and 50 μg sheared *E. coli* DNA were added during pre-hybridization and hybridization. Hybridization was carried out at 45 °C for 8 h.

7 The blots were stringently washed twice in 2 × SSC for 30 min at 37 °C, then twice in 0.1 × SSD for 30 min at 65 °C.

In vitro *translation of mRNA*

In vitro translation was performed using micrococcal nuclease-treated rabbit reticulocyte lysates (New England Nuclear, Boston, MA). The reactions were carried out in a volume of 50 μl containing 1 μg mRNA, 1 mM-dithiothreitol, 19 amino acids at 0.05 mM each, ^{35}S-methionine (50 μCi) and the reticulocyte lysate system (optimized for translating B cell mRNA) with incubation for 90 min, at 36 °C. An aliquot was removed for counting of trichloroacetic acid insoluble counts and equal amounts of radioactive protein were subjected to electrophoresis on a 10% polyacrylamide gel. The gels were dried and exposed to X-ray film.

Conclusion

In summary, the above techniques are not unique to investigations in murine autoimmunity but, rather, modifications of existing techniques with special applications to autoimmune analysis.

References

1 STEINBERG A.D., HUSTON D.P., TAUROG J.D., COWDERY J.S. & RAVECHE E.S. (1981) The cellular and genetic basis of murine lupus. *Immunol. Revs.* **55,** 121.

2 NOBLE B., YOSHIDA T., ROSE N.R. & BIGAZZI P.E. (1976) Thyroid antibodies in spontaneous autoimmune thyroiditis in the Buffalo rat. *J. Immunol.* **117**, 1447.

3 PONTES DE CARVALHO L.C., WICK G. & ROITT I.M. (1981) Requirement of T cells for the development of spontaneous autoimmune thyroiditis in obese strain (OS) chickens. *J. Immunol.* **126**, 750.

4 GERSHWIN M.E., ABPLANALP H., CASTLES J.J., IKEDA R., VAN DER WATER J., EKLUND J. & HAYNES D. (1981) Characterization of a spontaneous disease of White Leghorn chickens resembling progressive systemic sclerosis (scleroderma). *J. exp. Med.* **153**, 1640.

5 STEINBERG E.B., SANTORO T.S., CHUSED T.M., SMATHERS P.A. & STEINBERG A.D. (1983) Studies of congenic MRL/lpr/lpr.xid mice. *J. Immunol.* **131**, 2789.

6 SHIRAI T. & MELLORS R.C. (1972) Natural cytotoxic autoantibody against thymocytes in NZB mice. *Clin. exp. Immunol.* **12**, 133.

7 HUSTON D.P., RAVECHE E.S. & STEINBERG A.D. (1980) Preferential lysis of undifferentiated thymocytes by NTA from NZB mice. *J. Immunol.* **124**, 1635.

8 RAVECHE E.S., STEINBERG A.D., KLASSEN L.W. & TJIO J.H. (1978) Genetic studies in NZB mice. (I) Spontaneous autoantibody production. *J. exp. Med.* **147**, 1487.

9 GELFAND M.C., SCHUR P.H., ASOFSKY R. & STEINBERG A.D. (1976) Therapeutic studies on NZB/W mice IV. Effect of combination drug therapy on immune complex deposition. *Arthrit. Rheum.* **19**, 43–47.

10 SMITH H.R., RAVECHE E.S., YAFFEE L., CHUSED T. & STEINBERG A.D. (1985) Analysis of autoantibody production by a subset of B cells. *Cell Immunol.* **92**, 190.

11 RAVECHE E.S., STEINBERG A.D., DeFRANCO A.L. & TJIO J.H. (1982) Cell cycle analysis of lymphocyte activation in normal and autoimmune strains of mice. *J. Immunol.* **129**, 1219.

12 DeFRANCO A.L., RAVECHE E.S., ASOFSKY R. & PAUL W.E. (1982) Frequency of B lymphocytes responsive to anti-immunoglobulin. *J. exp. Med.* **155**, 1523.

13 HOWARD M., FARRAR J., MILLIKER M., JOHNSON B., TAKATSU K., MAMAOKA T. & PAUL W.E. (1982) Identification of T cell-derived B cell growth factor distinct from interleukin 2. *J. exp. Med.* **155**, 914.

14 GUTIERREZ C., RAVECHE E.S., HOWARD M. & STEINBERG A.D. Features of proliferative responses to B cell growth factor in autoimmune mice. (Submitted.)

15 MOLINARA C.A. & DRAY S. (1974) Antibody-coated erythrocytes as a manifold probe for antigen. *Nature*, **248**, 515.

16 GLIMCHER L.H., STEINBERG A.D., HOUSE S.B. & GREEN I. (1980) The autologous mixed lymphocyte reaction in strains of mice with autoimmune disease. *J. Immunol.* **125**, 1832.

17 POLLACK A., PRUDHOMME D., GREENSTEIN D., IRVIN G.L., CLAFIN A.J. & BLOCK N.C. (1982) Flow cytometric analysis of RNA content in different cell populations using pyronin Y and methyl green. *Cytometry*, **3**, 28.

18 DARZYNKIEWICZ Z., ANDREEFF M., TRAGANOS F., SHARPLESS T. & MELAMED M.R. (1978) Discrimination of cycling and non-cycling lymphocytes by BUdR-suppressed acridine orange in a flow cytometric system. *Expl Cell Res.* **115**, 31.

19a HAYAKAWA K., HARDY R.B., PARKS D.R. & HERZENBERG L.A. (1983) The Ly 1 B cell subpopulation in normal, immunodefective and autoimmune mice. *J. exp. Med.* **157**, 202.

19 MONOHAR V.L., BROWN E.M., LEISERSON W.M. & CHUSED T.M. (1982) Expression of Ly 1 by a subset of B lymphocytes. *J. Immunol.* **129**, 532.

20 HUSTON D.P. & STEINBERG A.D. (1980) NZB cytotoxic lymphocyte responses. *J. exp. Med.* **152**, 748.

21 LASKIN C.A., TAUROG J.D., SMATHERS P.A. & STEINBERG A.D. (1981) Studies of defective tolerance in murine lupus. *J. Immunol.* **127**, 1743.

22 WOLFSY D., MURPHY E.D., ROTHS J.B., DAUPHINEE M.J., KIPPER S.B. & TALAL N. (1981) Deficient interleukin 2 activity in MRL/M and C57BL/6J mice bearing the lpr gene. *J. exp. Med.* **154**, 1671.

23 WATSON I., GILLIS S., MARBROOK J., MOCHIZUKI D. & SMITH K. (1979) Biochemical and biological characterization of lymphocyte regulatory molecules I. Purification of a class of murine lymphokines. *J. exp. Med.* **150**, 849.

24 SANTORO T.J., LUGER T.A., RAVECHE E.S., SMOLEN J.S., OPPENHEIM J.J. & STEINBERG A.D. (1983) In vitro correction of the interleukin 2 defect of autoimmune mice. *Eur. J. Immunol.* **13**, 601.

25 SONNENFIELD G.A., MANDEL A.D. & MERIGAN T.C. (1979) In vitro production and cellular origin of murine type II interferon. *Immunology*, **36**, 883.

26 SANTORO T.J., BENJAMIN W.R., OPPENHEIM J.J. & STEINBERG A.D. (1983) The cellular basis for immune interferon production in autoimmune MRL/lpr mice. *J. Immunol.* **131**, 265.

27 MORTON J.I. & SIEGEL B.V. (1978) Transplantation of autoimmune potential (III) Immunological hyper-responsiveness and elevated endogenous colony formation in lethally irradiated recipients of NZB bone marrow cells. *Immunology*, **34**, 863.

28 RAVECHE E.S., CHUSED T.M., STEINBERG A.D., LASKIN C.A., EDISON L.J. & TJIO J.H. (1985) Comparison of response to stem cell differentiation signals between normal and autoimmune mouse strains. *J. Immunol.* **134**, 865.

29 KINCADE P.W., LEE G., FERNANDES G., MOORE M.A.S., WILLIAMS N. & GOOD R.A. (1979) Abnormalities in clonable B lymphocytes and myeloid progenitors in autoimmune NZB mice. *PNAS*, **76**, 3464.

30 JOYONOUCHI H., KINCADE P.W., GOOD R.A. & FERNANDES G. (1981) Reciprocal transfer of abnormalities in clonable B lymphocytes and myeloid progenitors between NZB and DBA/2 mice. *J. Immunol.* **127**, 1232.

31 RAVECHE E.S., NOVOTNY E.A., HANSEN C.T., TJIO J.H. & STEINBERG A.D. (1981) Genetic studies in NZB mice V. Recombinant inbred lines demonstrate that separate genes control autoimmune phenotype. *J. exp. Med.* **153**, 221–234.

32 RAVECHE E.S., TJIO J.H., BOGEL W. & STEINBERG A.D. (1979) Studies of the effects of sex hormones on autosomal and X-linked genetic control of induced and spontaneous antibody production. *Arthrit. Rheum.* **22**, 1177.

33 FOURNIE G.J., LAMBERT P.H. & MIESCHER P.A. (1974) Release of DNA in circulating blood and induction of

anti-DNA antibodies after injection of bacterial lipopoly-saccharides. *J. exp. Med.* **140**, 1189.

34 IZUI S., KOBAYAKAWA T., LOUIS J. & LAMBERT P.H. (1979) Induction of thymocytotoxic autoantibodies after injection of bacterial lipopolysaccharide in mice. *Eur. J. Immunol.* **9**, 338.

35 STEINBERG A.D., BARON S.H. & TALAL N. (1969) The pathogenesis of autoimmunity in NZB mice. (I) Induction of anti-nucleic acid antibodies by polyinosinic-poly-cytidylic acid. *PNAS*, **63**, 1102.

36 SMITH H.R., GREEN D.R., SMATHERS P.A., GERSHON R.K., RAVECHE E.S. & STEINBERG A.D. (1983) Induction of autoimmunity in normal mice by thymectomy and administration of polyclonal B cell activators: association with contrasuppressor function. *Clin. exp. Immunol.* **51**, 579–586.

37 FERNANDES G., YUNIS E.J. & GOOD R.A. (1976) Influence of diet on survival of mice. *PNAS*, **73**, 1279–1283.

38 PRICKETT J.D., ROBINSON D.R. & STEINBERG A.D. (1981) Dietary enrichment with the polyunsaturated fatty acid eicosapentaenoic acid prevents proteinuria and prolongs survival in NZB × NZW F mice. *J. clin. Invest.* **68**, 556.

39 RAVECHE E.S., TJIO J.H. & STEINBERG A.D. (1979) Genetic studies in NZB mice. II. Hyperdiploidy in the spleens of NZB mice and their hybrids. *Cytogenet. Cell Genet.* **23**, 182.

40 KELLY K., COCHRAN B.H., STILES C.D. & LEDER P. (1983) Cell-specific regulation of the c *myc* gene by lymphocyte mitogens and platelet-derived growth factor. *Cell*, **35**, 603.

41 CHIRGWIN J.M., PRZYBYLA A.E., MACDONALD R.J. & RUTTER W.J. (1979) Isolation of biologically active ribonucleic acid from sources enriched in ribonuclease. *Biochemistry*, **18**, 5294.

42 COX R.A. (1968) The use of guanidinium chloride in the isolation of nucleic acids. *Meth. Enzym.* **128**, 120.

43 MOUNTZ J.D., STEINBERG A.D., KLINMAN D.R., SMITH H.R. & MUSHINSKI J. (1984) Autoimmunity and increased *c-myb* transcription. *Science*, **226**, 1087.

44 PARKER L.M. & STEINBERG A.D. (1983) The antibody response to polyinosinic-polycytidylic acid. *J. Immunol.* **110**, 742.

45 ROSENBERG Y.J., STEINBERG A.D. & SANTORO T.J. (1984) T cells from autoimmune 'IL-2 defective' MRL-*lpr/lpr* mice continue to grow *in vitro* and produce IL-2 constitutively. *J. Immunol.* **133**, 2545.

46 STEINBERG E.B., SANTORO T.J., CHUSED T.M., SMATHERS P.A. & STEINBERG A.D. (1983) Studies of congenic MRL-*lpr/lpr·xid* mice. *J. Immunol.* **131**, 278.

47 DAVIDSON W.F., ROTHS J.B., HOLMES K.L., RUDIKOFF E. & MORSE H.C. (1984) Dissociation of severe lupus-like disease from polyclonal B cell activation and IL-2 deficiency in CBH-*lpr/lpr* mice. *J. Immunol.* **133**, 1048.

48 MILLER M.L., RAVECHE E.S., LASKIN C.A., KLINMAN D.M. & STEINBERG A.D. (1984) Genetic studies in NZB mice. VI. Association of autoimmune traits in recombinant inbred lines. *J. Immunol.* **133**, 1325.

49 IZUI S., KELLY V.E., MASUDA K., YOSHIDA H., ROTHS J.B. & MURPHY E.D. (1984) Induction of various auto-antibodies by mutant gene lpr in several strains of mice. *J. Immunol.* **133**, 227–233.

Chapter 83
Primary immunodeficiencies: definitions and diagnosis

F. S. ROSEN

Definitions of
  immunodeficiencies, 83.1

Diagnosis of B-cell
  immunodeficiencies, 83.3

Diagnosis of T-cell
  immunodeficiencies, 83.4

The purpose of this chapter is to describe the primary immunodeficiency diseases in man and the approach to their diagnosis. The details of methods for evaluation of human immunodeficiency disease are described elsewhere in this book. The minimal definition of each one is given and is followed by a section devoted to the laboratory methods presently available to aid in the diagnosis of these syndromes.

Definitions of immunodeficiencies

X-linked agammaglobulinaemia (XLA)

Boys with XLA usually have undetectable levels of serum immunoglobulin A (IgA) and IgM from birth onward [2]. The IgG that traverses the placenta is lost by the age of 6–9 months and is not replaced, so that the serum of affected boys contains < 100 mg% of IgG. Mature B cells are absent from the blood, bone marrow, spleen and lymph nodes, but the bone marrow contains normal numbers of pre-B cells [3]. These pre-B cells can be transformed with Epstein–Barr virus [4]. They continue to synthesize $C\mu$ chains, but the μ chain messenger RNA is defective in that the V, D and J genes are not expressed [5]. By and large, obligate female heterozygotous carriers of the trait cannot be detected.

X-linked hypogammaglobulinaemia with growth hormone deficiency

One kindred has been described with the findings like those of XLA. The affected males also had short stature, retarded bone age, small phallus and delayed puberty. Growth hormone was deficient and could not be elicited with arginine or insulin stimulation [6].

Autosomal recessive agammaglobulinaemia

Sporadic and rare cases of agammaglobulinaemia have been reported in females that cannot be distinguished from XLA.

Immunoglobulin deficiency with increased IgM (and IgD) (hyper-IgM immunodeficiency; dysgammaglobulinaemia)

Patients with a deficiency of IgG, IgA and IgE who have high normal or elevated levels of IgM fall into this category. Usually IgD levels are also high in serum. B cells bearing surface μ or $\mu + \delta$ are present in the blood together with large plasmacytoid cells that are spontaneously secreting IgM [8]. These patients almost invariably have IgM autoantibodies to the formed elements of the blood, platelets, leucocytes, erythrocytes and T cells.

IgA deficiency

As many as 1 in 700 people lack serum IgA and most of these individuals are asymptomatic [9,10]. The blood of IgA-deficient individuals contains $\mu + \alpha$ surface-bearing B cells that cannot be induced to become mature IgA-secreting cells.

Selective deficiency of other immunoglobulin isotypes

No clinical consequences have been reported from selective deficiencies of IgD and IgE, but rare cases of selective IgM deficiency have been associated with severe recurrent sepsis [11]. Selective deficiency of IgG subclasses have been reported in patients with recurrent, pyogenic infections. Deficiency of IgG1 or IgG2 or both appears to be of clinical significance, whereas deficiency of IgG3 or IgG4 might not [12,13].

κ-Chain deficiency

In only one kindred has a complete absence of κ chains been described so that the proposita had only Igs of λ type and none of κ type in serum and supernatants of pokeweed-stimulated lymphocytes *in vitro* [14].

Antibody deficiency with normal γ-globulin levels or hypergammaglobulinaemia

An immunodeficiency had been described in which there is a failure of specific responses to a battery of antigens despite normal serum levels of immunoglobulins [15]. The pathogenesis of this defect has not been well studied.

Immunodeficiency with thymoma

A small but significant number of patients with thymoma have panhypogammaglobulinaemia. Such patients lack pre-B cells in their bone marrow and consequently have no B lymphocytes in peripheral blood or tissues [16].

Transient hypogammaglobulinaemia of infancy

Normally, serum levels of immunoglobulins begin to rise in infants in the fifth month of life. In some infants the IgG levels remain extremely low for 30–36 months and then rapidly rise to normal levels. During this phase of IgG deficiency the T-helper subset is diminished in absolute numbers in the blood, but B cells are present in normal numbers [17].

Common variable immunodeficiency

This term includes a variety of B-cell defects that do not appear to be inherited. The acquisition of agammaglobulinaemia may occur at any age. Most patients with this syndrome have nearly normal numbers of predominantly $\mu+\delta+$B cells [18] but a smaller number of these patients have no B cells [19]. Another group of patients has been described with $\mu+\gamma+$ or $\gamma+$ B cells that synthesize but do not secrete immunoglobulin [19,20]. One group of patients has normal or increased numbers of $\mu+\delta+\gamma+$, or $\mu+\delta+\alpha+$ B cells that do not terminally differentiate [18]. Common variable immunodeficiency may also result from a deficiency of T-helper cells [21] or from an excess of activated T-suppressor cells (Ia^+) [22]. Patients with autoantibodies to T or B cells have been described and this state may also cause common variable immunodeficiency [23,24].

Transcobalamin II deficiency

The genetic deficiency of the principal B12 serum transport protein causes early onset of severe megaloblastic anaemia and agammaglobulinaemia. B cell numbers are normal but apparently will not terminally differentiate in the absence of vitamin B12. Administration of B12 rapidly reverses the anaemia and agammaglobulinaemia [25].

Severe combined immunodeficiency (SCID)

SCID is a group of inherited disorders in which there is a profound deficiency of T lymphocytes. SCID may be inherited as an autosomal or X-linked recessive phenomenon [1]. There is profound lymphopaenia in the blood and tissues but the pathognomonic sign of the disease resides in the abnormalities of the thymus gland, which is fetal in appearance and composed of nests of endothelial cells that have failed to become lymphoid and lack Hassall's corpuscles [1].

Severe combined immunodeficiency with adneosine deaminase (ADA) deficiency

One form of SCID results from the genetically determined deficiency of ADA [26]. ADA deficiency is found in approximately half the SCID patients with the autosomal recessive form of the syndrome [27]. ADA is a ubiquitous enzyme in mammalian cells [28], yet its deficiency affects only the lymphoid system. This unique effect has been attributed to abnormal accumulation of deoxy-ATP in T lymphoid stem cells that are poisoned by this metabolite which inhibits ribonucleotide reductase [29]. Some rare mutant forms of the enzyme do not cause immunodeficiency [30]. An excellent review of the biochemical perturbations in ADA deficiency describes the metabolic alterations associated with ADA deficiency and their consequences [29].

Purine nucleoside phosphorylase (PNP) deficiency

PNP deficiency results in a severe T cell defect. There are normal numbers of B cells, and immunoglobulin levels in the serum are normal, but cell-mediated immune function is grossly impaired [31]. Deoxy-GTP has been incriminated as the principal metabolic toxin that accumulates in PNP deficiency [32]. Carson has reviewed the reasons for the greater T cell toxicity of deoxy-ATP compared to deoxy-GTP in ADA and PNP deficiencies [33].

Immunodeficiency with unusual response to Epstein–Barr virus (EBV)

A number of boys in several kindred have died from EBV infections with fatal mononucleosis, bone-marrow aplasia or B-cell lymphoma [34]. Some of these boys developed agammaglobulinaemia following EBV infection. Although the syndrome appears to be inherited as an X-linked recessive phenomenon, sporadic cases have been reported in females. Prior to EBV infection, these children appear to be completely normal; however, an acute EBV infection results in depletion of T lymphocytes from peripheral blood and the appearance of large numbers of NK cells [35].

Wiskott–Aldrich syndrome

This syndrome is inherited in an X-linked recessive pattern. Affected boys have eczema, thrombocytopaenia, and progressively profound T-cell depletion with increasing age. Most patients die in the first decade of life from haemorrhage or overwhelming infection. The T lymphocytes have a defect in one of the major constitutive glycoproteins of the T-cell membrane, gpL 115 [36].

Ataxia telangiectasia

This disease is inherited in an autosomal recessive pattern. Patients become ataxic in the second year of life and develop telangiectasia in the sixth year of life. The serum α_1-fetoprotein is invariably elevated [37]. Seventy per cent of the patients have IgA deficiency and T-cell function and cell-mediated immunity are grossly impaired [38]. Ataxia telangiectasia cells are extremely sensitive to ionizing radiation and there is defective repair of DNA following irradiation. At least five complementation groups have been discerned by heterokaryon analysis [39].

Third and fourth pouch syndrome (DiGeorge's syndrome)

A congenital malformation can result from *in utero* injury early in gestation to derivatives of the third and fourth pharyngeal arch derivatives. As a consequence there is parathyroid and thymic aplasia or profound hypoplasia [40]. A constellation of cardiac malformations accompanies these defects and is the usual cause of death in these infants. The degree of T-cell deficiency in affected babies is very variable but B cells are normal.

Acquired immunodeficiency syndrome (AIDS)

In the past three years a profound form of cell-mediated immunodeficiency has been described in certain population groups at risk. These include homosexually active males, intravenous drug addicts, recipients of blood or certain blood products, and the spouses or offspring of the aforementioned. AIDS has also been diagnosed in Caribbean and Central African populations. The diagnosis rests on the occurrence of relentless, opportunistic infections and of bizarre malignancies in patients who have no other predisposing reason to be immunodeficient. AIDS is further characterized by a profound deficiency of the helper subset (T4 or Leu3) of T lymphocytes and the presence in peripheral blood of increased numbers of activated B cells. Recently, a human lymphocytotropic retrovirus (HTLV III or LAV) has been identified as the pathogenic agent that causes AIDS [41].

Diagnosis of B-cell immunodeficiencies

Most, if not all, of the methods described in this section can be found in detail elsewhere in this volume. Patients with primary immunodeficiency tend to fall into two easily definable groups. The first group are those patients with a predominant B cell defect. In these patients the clinical history is replete with recurrent pyogenic infections principally *Haemophilus influenzae* and *Streptococcus pneumoniae*. A number of patients will also have difficulty with *Pseudomonas aeruginosa*, *Streptococcus pyogenes* and other pyogenic bacteria. There is also a tendency amongst people with B-cell deficiencies to develop *Giardia lamblia* infection. Whenever symptoms of non-tropical sprue or persistent diarrhoea and weight loss are present *G. lamblia* should always be suspected as the causative organism in patients with B-cell deficiencies. Another unusual susceptibility that occurs, particularly in boys with X-linked agammaglobulinaemia, is a persistent inability to terminate infection with ECHO virus. These infections result in a progressive fatal neuromuscular disease. Recently, it has been possible to control these ECHO infections with high doses of intravenous γ-globulin containing high titres of antibody to the relevant ECHO virus.

Determination of immunoglobulins (see Chapter 126)

The most obvious manifestation of B-cell immunodeficiencies is depression of the serum immunoglobulins. There are a number of methods involving radial immunodiffusion or nephalometry to quantify the five Ig classes in the serum. It is also very valuable to be able to quantify the IgG subclasses. As previously mentioned, the subtle deficiencies of IgG1 or IgG2 or both can cause B-cell immunodeficiency disease. In patients with primary B-cell immunodeficiencies it is also important to determine a failure of specific antibody formation. Since there is universal immunization with diphtheria and tetanus toxoid, a measurement of antibodies to these two antigens is useful because all infants respond normally to these antigens. It also is useful to measure antibody titres to polysaccharide antigens, and this is most easily done by measuring titres of isohaemagglutinins in the blood. Infants do not normally make isohaemagglutinins until as late as 18 months of age, so that these measurements may not be of value in the very young. Another polysaccharide antigen that is widely measured is polyribose phosphate (PRP). The antibody to this capsular polysaccharide of *H. influenzae* type B is universally distributed in the adult population. It is predominantly an antibody of the IgG2 subclass and its measurement is a convenient measure of IgG2 subclass responses.

Enumeration of B lymphocytes (see Chapter 126)

Human blood contains 11% B lymphocytes. They are readily enumerated by examining lymphoid cells in the blood for cell surface immunoglobulin. These cells are absent in individuals with X-linked agammaglobulinaemia. In patients with common variable immunodeficiency, the distribution of these cells is abnormal, as outlined above. In patients with X-linked agammaglobulinaemia pre-B cells can be found in the bone marrow by staining with specific anti-Cμ antisera, and they are found in normal numbers in the bone marrow of boys with this disease. As previously mentioned, they are absent from the bone marrow in patients with immunodeficiency with thymoma.

The transformation of B lymphocytes with Epstein–Barr virus has been very useful because the transformed cells perpetuate the phenotypic abnormality in long-term culture. Thus the various B cell immunodeficiencies can be studied in *in vitro* cultures of these cells.

Miscellaneous testing

As mentioned above, one form of immunodeficiency results from the genetic deficiency of transcobalamin II. This form of immunodeficiency is always accompanied by megaloblastic anaemia and, when this is found, vitamin B12 assays should be performed. It is worth mentioning that as much as 50% of adults with common variable immunodeficiency develop megaloblastic anaemia and pernicious anaemia due to loss of intrinsic factor. Thus the measurement of vitamin

B12 in the serum of adults with agammaglobulinaemia is also a useful procedure. It has also been mentioned that growth hormone may be deficient in another form of X-linked agammaglobulinaemia, and this hormone can readily be measured by radioimmunoassay. The diagnosis of agammaglobulinaemia can sometimes be ascertained by X-ray because lateral view of the nasopharynx reveals an absence of adenoid and tonsillar tissue. The resultant widening of the upper airway is an invariable radiologic sign of X-linked agammaglobulinaemia.

Diagnosis of T-cell immunodeficiencies

In contrast to patients with B-cell immunodeficiencies who are subject to recurrent infection with pyogenic bacteria, patients with T-cell deficiencies tend to sustain recurrent and frequently fatal infections from opportunistic organisms. Opportunistic pathogens are those microorganisms that cause self-limited disease in a normal host. In individuals who are T-cell deficient, these pathogens cause fatal or near-fatal infections. Principal opportunistic infections that are observed in the T-cell deficient are caused by the large DNA viruses: varicella, herpes and cytomegalovirus. Other opportunistic infections observed in the T-cell deficient individual include those due to *Pneumocystis carinii*, adenovirus, measles virus, BCG, enteric Gram-negative bacilli and other ordinarily innocuous or nearly innocuous organisms found as part of the normal flora of the skin and mucous membranes.

Enumeration of T lymphocytes (see Chapter 126)

T lymphocytes in the peripheral blood can be readily enumerated by their capacity to rosette with sheep erythrocytes or by specific antisera now available to T-cell surface antigens. Furthermore, T-cell subsets can be enumerated with specific monoclonal antibodies to the helper or inducer subset or to the suppressor/cytotoxic subset. These subsets of cells are deranged in certain patients with common variable immunodeficiency and are, of course, important in the diagnosis of AIDS.

Mitogen responses (see Chapters 66 and 126)

It is always important to test the functional capacity of T cells obtained from these patients. This can best be performed with non-specific mitogens, such as phytohaemagglutinin, pokeweed or concanavalin A. These tests have largely replaced skin tests for cell-mediated immunity. Nonetheless, there is an advantage in using *Candida* antigen or streptokinase or other antigens to which there are universal cell-mediated responses in the intact host. T cells will also respond to specific antigens *in vitro* by increased thymidine incorporation or other measures of cell division.

Enzyme measurements

The measurements of erythrocyte adenosine deaminase, and nucleoside phosphorylase are useful assays to assess patients suspected of severe combined immunodeficiency. As described above, one or another of these two enzymes may be absent in about half the patients with the autosomal recessive form of severe combined immunodeficiency.

T-cell typing (see Chapters 59 and 126)

Mixed lymphocyte cultures and HLA typing are important markers of T-cell competence, particularly in patients with severe combined immunodeficiency in which the HLA markers are absent from the surface of the cells and the cells will not give positive MLC response. This so-called 'bare lymphocyte syndrome' is discerned in a number of children with severe combined immunodeficiency. Antibodies to T lymphocytes may also cause immunodeficiency. Autoantibodies to subsets of T lymphocytes, as well as pan T-cell cytoxic antibodies have been detected in the serum of patients with immunodeficiency. The production of interleukin-1 (IL-1) and interleukin-2 (IL-2) in mixed lymphocyte cultures and mitogen-stimulated cultures are also important functional measurements of T lymphocytes *in vitro*. Patients with IL-1 T-cell receptor defects have been described. The failure of IL-2 production is a common observation in patients with a generalized T-cell defect.

Miscellaneous

Measurement of α_1-fetoprotein is important in the diagnosis of ataxia telangiectasia. The measurement of serum calcium and phosphorus is important in ascertaining the diagnosis of the third and fourth pharyngeal pouch syndrome. Children with this syndrome almost invariably have neonatal tetany and the T-cell defect should be suspected in that setting. It is characteristic of the Wiskott–Aldrich syndrome that the volume of the platelets and the T cells is half-normal. This can be readily ascertained in a Coulter counter.

The tests for the establishment of the B- and T-cell immunodeficiencies are readily performed and easily available. The tests described are designed to conform to the definitions of the immunodeficiencies as outlined by the Immunodeficiency Working Party of the World Health Organization. Further details of their report are given in ref. 42.

References

1 ROSEN F.S., COOPER M.D. & WEDGWOOD R.J.P. (1984) The primary immunodeficiencies. (I) *New Engl. J. Med.* **311**, 235; (II) *New Engl. J. Med.* **311**, 300.

2 WEDGWOOD R.J. (1978) X-linked agammaglobulinemia. *CRC Handbook Series in Clin. Lab. Sci.* **1**(1), 41.

3 PEARL E.R., VOGLER L.B., OKOS A.J., CRIST W.M., LAWTON III & COOPER M.D. (1978) B lymphocyte precursors in human bone marrow: an analysis of normal individuals and patients with antibody-deficient states. *J. Immunol.* **120**, 1169.

4 FU S.M., HURLEY J.N., McCUNE J.M., KUNKEL H.G. & GOOD R.A. (1980) Pre-B cells and other possible precursor lymphoid cell lines derived from patients with X-linked agammaglobulinemia. *J. exp. Med.* **152**, 1519.

5 SCHWABER J., MOLGAARD H., ORKIN S.H., GOULD H.J. & ROSEN F.S. (1983) Early pre-B cells from normal and X-linked agammaglobulinemia produce $C\mu$ without an attached V_H region. *Nature*, **304**, 355.

6 FLEISHER I.A., WHITE R.M., BRODER S. *et al.* (1980) X-linked hypogammaglobulinemia and isolated growth hormone deficiency. *New Engl. J. Med.* **302**, 1429.

7 HOFFMAN T., WINCHESTER R., SCHULKIND M., FRIAS J.L., AYOUB E.M. & GOOD, R.A. (1977) Hypogammaglobulinemia with normal T cell function in female siblings. *Clin. Immunol. Immunopath.* **7**, 364.

8 GEHA R.S., HYSLOP N., ALAMI S., FARAH F., SCHNEEBERGER E.E. & ROSEN F.S. (1979) Hyper-immunoglobulin M immunodeficiency (dysgammaglobulinemia): presence of immunoglobulin M-secreting plasmacytoid cells in peripheral blood and failure of immunoglobulin M–immunoglobulin G switch in B-cell differentiation. *J. clin. Invest.* **84**, 385.

9 ROPARS C., MULLER A., PAINT N., BEIGE D. & AVENARD G. (1982) Large scale detection of IgA deficient blood donors. *J. immunol. Meth.* **54**, 183.

10 CONLEY M.E. & COOPER M.D. (1981) Immature IgA B cells in IgA-deficient patients. *New Engl. J. Med.* **305**, 495.

11 FAULK W.P., KIYASU W.S., COOPER M.D. & FUDENBERG H.H. (1971) Deficiency of IgM. *Pediatrics*, **47**, 399.

12 OXELIUS V.-A. (1974) Chronic infection in a family with hereditary deficiency of IgG2 and IgG4. *Clin. exp. Immunol.* **17**, 19.

13 SCHUR P.H., BOREL H., GELFAND E.W., ALPER C.A. & ROSEN F.S. (1970) Selective gamma-G globulin deficiencies in patients with recurrent pyogenic infections. *New Engl. J. Med.* **283**, 631.

14 ZEGERS B.J.M., MAERTZDORF W.J., VAN LOGHEM E., MUL N.A.J., STOOP J.W., VAN DER LAAG J., VOSSEN J.J. & BALLIEUX R.E. (1976) Kappa-chain deficiency: An immunoglobulin disorder. *New Engl. J. Med.* **294**, 1026.

15 BLECHER T.E., SOOTHILL J.F., VOYCE M.A. & WALKER W.H.C. (1968) Antibody deficiency syndrome: a case with normal immunoglobulin levels. *Clin. exp. Immunol.* **3**, 47.

16 ROGERS B.H.G., MANALIGOD J.R. & BLAZEK W.V. (1968)

Thymoma associated with pancytopenia and hypogammaglobulinemia: report of a case and review of the literature. *Am. J. Med.* **44**, 154.

17 SIEGEL R.L., ISSEKUTZ T., SCHWABER J., ROSEN F.S. & GEHA R.S. (1981) Deficiency of T helper cells in transient hypogammaglobulinemia of infancy. *New Engl. J. Med.* **305**, 1307.

18 PREUD'HOMME J.L., GRISCELLI C. & SELIGMANN M. (1973) Immunoglobulins on the surface of lymphocytes in fifty patients with primary immunodeficiency diseases. *Clin. Immunol. Immunopath.* **1**, 241.

19 GEHA R.S., SCHNEEBERGER E., MERLER E. & ROSEN F.S. (1974) Heterogeneity of 'acquired' or common variable agammaglobulinemia. *New Engl. J. Med.* **291**, 1.

20 SCHWABER J. & ROSEN F.S. (1979) Somatic cell hybrids of mouse myeloma cells and B lymphocytes from a patient with agammaglobulinemia: failure to secrete human immunoglobulin. *J. Immunol.* **122**, 1849.

21 REINHERZ E.L., COOPER M.D., SCHLOSSMAN S.F. & ROSEN F.S. (1981) Abnormalities of T cell maturation and regulation in human beings with immunodeficiency disorders. *J. clin. Invest.* **69**, 699.

22 REINHERZ E.L., RUBINSTEIN A.J., GEHA R.S., STRELKAUSKAS A.J., ROSEN F.S. & SCHLOSSMAN S.F. (1979) Abnormalities of immunoregulatory T cells in disorders of immune function. *New Engl. J. Med.* **301**, 1018.

23 GELFAND E.W., BOREL H., BERKEL A.I. & ROSEN F.S. (1972) Auto-immunosuppression: recurrent infections associated with immunologic unresponsiveness in the presence of an auto-antibody to IgG. *Clin. Immunol. Immunopath.* **1**, 155.

24 TURSZ R., PREUD'HOMME J.L., LABAUME S., MATUCHANSKY C. & SELIGMANN M. (1977) Autoantibodies to B lymphocytes in a patient with hypogammaglobulinemic characterization and pathogenic role. *J. clin. Invest.* **60**, 405.

25 HITZIG W.H., DOHMANN U., PLUSS H.J. & VISCHER D. (1974) Hereditary transcobalamin II deficiency: clinical findings in a new family. *J. Pediat.* **85**, 622.

26 GIBLETT E.R., ANDERSON J.E., COHEN F., POLLARA B. & MEUWISSEN H.J. (1972) Adenosine-deaminase deficiency in two patients with severely impaired cellular immunity. *Lancet*, **ii**, 1067.

27 HIRSCHHORN R., VAWTER G.F., KIRKPATRICK J.A. & ROSEN F.S. (1979) Adenosine deaminase deficiency: frequency and comparative pathology in autosomally recessive severe combined immunodeficiency. *Clin. Immunol. Immunopath.* **14**, 107.

28 SPENCER N., HOPKINSON D.A. & HARRIS H. (1968) Adenosine deaminase polymorphism in man. *Ann. Haman Genet.* **32**, 9.

29 THOMPSON L.F. & SEEGMILLER J.E. (1980) Adenosine deaminase deficiency and severe combined immunodeficiency disease. *Adv. Enzym.* **51**, 167.

30 HIRSCHHORN R., ROEGNER V., JENKINS T., SEAMAN C., PIOMELLI S. & BORKOWSKY W. (1979) Erythrocyte adenosine deaminase deficiency without immunodeficiency: evidence for an unstable mutant enzyme. *J. clin. Invest.* **64**, 1130.

31 GIBLETT E.R., AMMANN A.J., WARA D.W., SANDMAN R. & DIAMOND L.K. (1975) Nucleoside-phosphorylase deficiency in a child with severely defective T-cell immunity and normal B-cell immunity. *Lancet*, **i**, 1010.

32 GELFAND E.W., DOSCH H.-M., BIGGAR W.D. & FOX I.H. (1978) Partial purine nucleoside phosphorylase deficiency: studies of lymphocyte function. *J. clin. Invest.* **61**, 1071.

33 CARSON D.A., WASSON D.B., LAKOW E. & KAMATANI N. (1982) Possible metabolic basis for the different immunodeficiency states associated with genetic deficiencies of adenosine deaminase and purine nucleoside phosphorylase. *Proc. natn. Acad. Sci. U.S.A.* **79**, 3848.

34 PURTILO D.T., DEFLORIO D., HUTT L.M. *et al.* (1977) Variable phenotypic expression of an X-linked recessive lymphoproliferative syndrome. *New Engl. J. Med.* **297**, 1077.

35 SULLIVAN J.L., BYRON K.S., BREWSTER F.E., BAKER S.M. & OCHS H.D. (1983) X-linked lymphoproliferative syndrome: natural history of the immunodeficiency. *J. clin. Invest.* **71**, 1765.

36 REMOLD-O'DONNELL E., KENNEY D.M., PARKMAN R., CAIRNS L., SAVAGE B. & ROSEN F.S. (1984) Characterization of a human lymphocyte surface sialoglycoprotein that is defective in Wiskott–Aldrich syndrome. *J. exp. Med.* **159**, 1705.

37 WALDMANN T.A. & McINTIRE K.R. (1972) Serum-alpha-fetoprotein levels in patients with ataxia-telangiectasia. *Lancet*, **ii**, 1112.

38 WALDMANN T.A., BRODER S., GOLDMAN C.K., FROST K., KORSMEYER S.J. & MEDICI M.A. (1983) Disorders of B cells and helper T cells in the pathogenesis of the immunoglobulin deficiency of patients with ataxia telangiectasia. *J. clin. Invest.* **71**, 282.

39 PATERSON M.C. & SMITH P.J. (1979) Ataxia-telangiectasia: an inherited human disorder involving hypersensitivity to ionizing radiation and related DNA-damaging chemicals. *Ann. Rev. Genet.* **13**, 291.

40 LISCHNER H.W. & PUNNETT H.H. (1967) Lymphocytes in congenital absence of the thymus. *Nature*, **214**, 580.

41 SELIGMANN M., CHESS L., FAHEY J.L., FAUCI A.S., LACHMANN P., L'AGE-STEHR J., NGU J., PINCHING A.J., ROSEN F.S., SPIRA T.J. & WYBRAN J. (1984) AIDS: an immunologic reevaluation. Report of a joint IUIS/WHO Working Group. *New Engl. J. Med.* **311**, 1286.

42 ROSEN F.S., WEDGWOOD R.J., AIUTI F., COOPER M.D., GOOD R.A., HANSON L.A., HITZIG W.H., MATSUMOTO S., SELIGMANN M., SOOTHILL J.F. & WALDMANN T.A. (1983) Primary immunodeficiency diseases. Report prepared for the WHO by a Scientific Group on Immunodeficiency. *Clin. Immunol. Immunopath.* **28**, 450.

Chapter 84
Studying immune regulation with protein and peptide antigens

N. SHASTRI† & E. E. SERCARZ*

Ia specificity, 84.1
Determinant focussing, 84.2
Agretypy, 84.3

Dissociation of suppressor
   determinants from helper
   determinants, 84.3
Hierarchy, 84.5

T cell steering, 84.5
Idiotypy, 84.6
Compartmentalization, 84.7
Conclusions, 84.7

Almost twenty years ago, the authors' laboratory initiated the detailed study of the immune response to two well-characterized protein molecules, chicken egg-white lysozyme and *E. coli* β-galactosidase. Recently the authors have been absorbed in studying the cellular recognition of these antigens and the interactions of regulatory T cells and their target cell 'regulees' (such as T helper cell (Th) targets for T suppressor cells (Ts) and B cell targets for Th) in these systems.

Many of the parameters describing immune response gene control were first discovered using what were thought to be simple antigens, random polypeptides with known proportions of two or three components (e.g. glutamic acid and alanine; or glutamic acid, lysine and phenylalanine). In fact, it was soon realized that such antigens of compositional simplicity had immense complexity of sequence as well as unknown three dimensional structure. This is also the case for polymers of the type (T,G)-A-L, with mixed tyrosyl-glutamic acid end groups on polyalanyl sidechains protruding from polylysine backbones. Batch-to-batch variations add a further dimension of complexity.

The distinct advantages of the well-characterized monomeric protein antigens such as lysozymes, insulins, myoglobins, and cytochromes lie in their exact similarity and the known position of each amino acid residue. In the cases mentioned, nature has provided a large number of structurally similar congeners, each with several amino acid substitutions which can be used as probes for exploring the nature of T cell epitopes, macrophage presentation sites, and B cell

recognition. Now, with the ease of preparing polypeptides by solid-phase synthesis, it is possible to create additional variants of peptides known from earlier experiments with the native antigens to be important for the lymphocyte subpopulation in question. This is particularly true for T cells which appear to be able to respond to peptides with 8–10 amino acid residues.

There are certain obvious differences in studying regulation with monomeric protein antigens or their peptides *vis-à-vis* hapten or random polypeptide systems. For example, a single epitope will exist only once on the antigenic molecule and therefore, if the Th cell recognizes this epitope, antigen bridging rules between Th and B cells dictate that the latter would be recognizing a different epitope. However, in the case of hapten-carrier systems, hapten-specific Th cells can interact with hapten-specific B cells via carrier bridging.

The authors have formulated a set of rules that emerge from their previous studies in the aforementioned protein antigen systems, and that they hope will prove useful to neophytes initiating the exploration of their systems. Where pertinent, additions from the work of other investigators are included. The format employed is that of stating a 'principle' (italicized), which indeed is often merely an interpretation, and following it with one or several examples, and possibly some caveats.

Ia specificity

A determinant on a protein antigen that will elicit a T-helper response in one strain may not do so in another

An analysis of determinants recognized by antigen-specific T-helper cells must consider that Th cell recognition of antigens is fundamentally distinct from

† Recipient of a Leukemia Society of America Postdoctoral Fellowship.
* This work was supported by USPHS AI 11183, USPHS CA 24442, and ACS IM-263A.

that of antibody. Antibodies can bind free antigen either in solution or when the antibody molecule is present as the antigen receptor on the B cell surface. T-helper cells, in contrast, respond to antigen only in the context of Ia molecules encoded by the I region of the major histocompatibility complex or H-2 in the mouse. The function of providing the antigen-Ia context is carried out on the cell surface of antigen presenting cells (APC) which could be macrophages or B cells [1,2].

A characteristic feature of Th cell antigen recognition is the cross-reactivity between native and denatured forms of the antigen [3]. This is presumably a reflection of the process of antigen degradation which precedes antigen recognition. Analysis of the elicited specificity of Th cells relies on this property. Populations or clones of Th cells can be distinguished on the basis of responses to chemically derived fragments of the antigen in question. In addition, availability of closely related molecules such as species variants of many naturally occurring proteins can be used to identify significant residues involved in antigen recognition.

The antigen-specific repertoire of T cells, assayed by proliferation (incorporation of tritiated thymidine) and helper cell assays (described in Chapter 71), to several protein antigens has been found to vary as a function of the H-2 haplotype. It is clear that congenic pairs of mice differing only at the H-2 locus can show dramatic differences in the regions of a protein antigen chosen for responsiveness. In the lysozyme system, hen egg-white lysozyme (HEL)-primed lymph node cells from each of three congenic strains of mice show a characteristic specificity profile (Table 84.1) [4,5,6]. B10 respond to determinants only within the L2H (amino acids 13–105) region, while B10.D2 mice predominantly respond to determinants within L3H (amino acids 106–129), but also can respond to L2H. B10.A mice show an opposite pattern, responding preferentially to L2H and show poor recognition of the L3H peptide.

Similar haplotype-related specificity differences have been observed with T cell responses to sperm whale myoglobin where congenic mouse strains differ in their ability to respond to cyanogen bromide cleavage fragments 1–55 and 132–153 [7]. Specificity of response to A or B chains of insulins is also a function of MHC haplotype in both mice [8] and guinea-pigs [9]. Although T lymphocyte response to pigeon or moth cytochrome *c* in responder strains seems to be restricted to the carboxy-terminal cyanogen bromide cleavage fragment, fine specificity distinctions have been observed in the clonal repertoire of different strains [10,11].

Determinant focussing

Very few portions of a protein antigen are employed by the T cell system in any one haplotype

Perhaps an explanation of the MHC haplotype associated specificity of the Th response is that in any one given haplotype, there appears to be a dominance of response to certain determinants over others. One end of the spectrum is provided by the example of B10 responsiveness to HEL (Table 84.1). B10 mice respond

Table 84.1. MHC haplotype related differences in HEL-specific T cell repertoire

Strain	Response of HEL-primed lymph node T cells		
	HEL	L2H[b]	L3H[c]
B10	+[a]	+	−
B10.A	+ +	+ +	±
B10.D2	+ +	+	+ +

[a] Peripheral lymph nodes do respond to HEL, as detailed on page 84.7.
[b] L2H = cyanogen bromide cleavage fragment 2, amino acids 13–105 derived from reduced and carboxymethylated HEL.
[c] L3H = cyanogen bromide cleavage fragment 3, amino acids 106–129.

exclusively to determinants within the L2H region, completely ignoring determinants within L3H. Immunization with L3H likewise elicits no response. Still more striking was the clonal analysis of T cell lines derived from B10 mice primed to L2H [12;]. Like the lymph nodes from which they were derived, all clones were found to react to only the major trypsin derived fragment T-11 (amino acids 74–96). B10 mice seem to ignore other potential determinants within L2H, although immunization with HEL gave rise to a majority of non-T-11 responsive clones [47]. The B10.A response to the L2H peptide has a different dominant focus, including amino acids 13–17. (See 'Hierarchy' section below for further discussion.)

Restrictions of responsiveness to limited regions of protein antigens have been documented for insulin and cytochrome *c* [9,10,11]. These have been attributed to limited differences between the immunogen and the self analogue of mouse. However, such an explanation is not tenable for bird lysozymes where immense differences exist between the immunogen and the self mammalian lysozymes. Human lysozyme, for example, is known to differ at more than 50 amino acid residues from HEL such that except for residues involved in the active site, almost every surface amino acid is distinct.

The authors interpret the dominance of some determinants over others as a hierarchy which is set up during the course of the response. The underlying mechanisms are as yet obscure but may relate to suppression directed primarily towards certain regions of the molecule and/or to relative efficacy of antigen presentation (see below, pages 84.3–84.5).

Agretypy

A minimal peptide which can induce T cell activity requires both an agretope and an epitope

To explain the T cell specificity for both nominal antigen and Ia molecules, the hypothesis has been advanced that requires the antigen to physically associate with Ia molecules [13,14]. This process is considered a necessary condition for Th cell stimulation. Several results in independent antigen systems have strongly suggested that the determinant and the Ia molecule can each be visualized as consisting of two independent sites.

Heber-Katz, Hansburg & Schwartz [15] have proposed a convenient nomenclature for these sites. The T cell receptor recognizes the *epitope* on the antigen and a *histotope* on the Ia molecule. The antigen and Ia restricting element are brought in close proximity by interaction of an *agretope* on the antigen and a *desetope* on the Ia molecule. Thus a peptide antigen capable of T cell stimulation must possess both an agretope and an epitope for interaction with the Ia molecule and the T cell receptor. Such a concept leads to a useful definition of a T cell 'determinant' on a nominal antigen as comprised of epitope plus agretope. Potential reactivity thus depends on an appropriate desetope–agretope interaction at one site, followed by recognition by ambient T cells of epitypic subsites on the antigen as well as additional subsites such as the histotope on the Ia molecule. Alternatively, recognition could require simultaneous interactions of each member of the ternary complex.

The concept is based on the findings of parallel sets of non-cross-reactive T cells restricted in antigen recognition to the same Ia molecule and the same site on the cytochrome molecule (the agretope). For example, the T cell response of B10.A mice to the pigeon cytochrome *c* C-terminal cyanogen bromide cleavage fragment of two non-cross-reactive (native and acetimidated) molecules, shows a characteristic hierarchy of reactivity to species variant cytochrome molecules [16]. Moreover, mice immunized with the acetimidate derivatives show the same hierarchy pro-file using the derivatized species variant cytochromes, despite the lack of cross-reaction of these T cells with the native forms. Thus it is postulated that the agretypic site is preserved in both native and derivatized immunogens and was utilized for presentation of antigen to non-cross-reactive T cells. Similar parallel sets have also been described for responses to lysozyme [6] and myoglobin [17] in certain strains of mice.

More recently, studies with cytochrome *c* synthetic peptides with minimal substitutions have provided convincing evidence for separable T recognition and MHC interaction sites on an antigen fragment [18,19]. The epitypic site could be specified owing to the localization of the acetimidyl derivative on a particular lysine. Substitution of a glutamine at this position affected the specificity of the T lymphocyte population stimulated. Alterations at the nearby C-terminal residues (agretope) affected only the magnitude of the response without effect on the T cell specificity. Furthermore, a current report by Rock & Benacerraf [20] showed that shared structural features, which could be agretopes on a non-cross-reactive antigen, can inhibit presentation of the desired antigen to a reactive T cell clone, a finding which supports earlier experiments of Werdelin [21].

Dissociation of suppressor determinants from helper determinants

Suppressor-cell and helper-cell inducing determinants are generally non-overlapping. A non-immunogenic molecule can sometimes be dissociated to reveal both Th and Ts activity

One of the difficult problems in cellular immunology is deciding how many regulatory cells are present in a particular situation. Along with the evolution in thinking about the maturation of the B cell response came the information that T-helper cells were involved, and then T-suppressor cells; now it is clear that T-augmenting/contra-suppressor cells as well as an army of cells within the suppressive circuitry play a role in the eventual outcome of T–B collaboration [22,23,24]. Therefore it is naive to assume that a cell type is absent until it is explicitly excluded.

Two recent examples may suffice to illustrate immunologically the old adage that 'you can't tell a book by its cover'. In discussions about immune response gene control, it is often stated that an animal is a non-responder, with the implicit consideration that one reason may be the failure to present the antigen, and another, a gap in the T-cell repertoire. The coexistence of latent responsiveness and latent suppression is considered only a distant third possibility [25].

A second and correlative example occurs in discussions about immune tolerance where it is assumed that the failure to demonstrate suppression upon mixing a tolerant cell population with a normal, immunized target population reflects an absence of T-suppressor cells. In fact, Ts cells may be present but there may be a lack of T-suppressor inducer cells or, on the contrary, there may also be a contra-suppressive cell which prevents the activity of the Ts by interaction with the Th [24].

In either event, one possible approach to the demonstration of suppression is the uncovering of latent T cell activity to a molecule from which a suppressor cell inducing determinant (SD) has been removed. Not only does this provide some suggestive evidence for an SD, but also indicates that all the information is present for the presentation of at least one epitope on the protein to Tp/Th and as a corollary indicates that at least some T cells of this specificity exist in the repertoire.

Hen egg-white lysozyme

In accounting for T cell responses to epitopes on such foreign protein antigens as chicken lysozyme, a broad repertoire of reactivity might have been expected. Thus initially it might have been predicted that suppressive and helper T cell subpopulations would have each recognized the same heterogeneous set of determinants on HEL. It was therefore of some interest to discover that only a single determinant on HEL addressed the Ts population of certain mouse strains. HEL is non-immunogenic for the $H-2^b$ mouse after a typical immunizing intraperitoneal dose of 100 ng to 10 μg of HEL in CFA, a dose and route which induces strong reactivity in a congenic B10.A mouse [26]. Crucial to the identity of the SD for $H-2^b$ mice was a phenylalanine at amino acid residue 3. Lysozymes with tyrosine at this position did not induce suppression [27]. Utilizing the principle of amputation or removal of suppressor determinants, the large cyanogen bromide peptide, amino acids 13–105 (= L2H), was able to induce a normal proliferative T cell response in this strain [28]. It would therefore be predicted that the amputated dodecapeptide 1–12, or the N-terminal–C-terminal peptide from HEL, termed N–C (= 1–17 : cys 6–cys 127 : 120–129) would be able to induce T-suppressor cells that could prevent the revealed responsiveness to an epitope within L2H. Such was the case, but the suppression only occurred in the presence of a molecule containing both the SD and a helper determinant (HD) which could serve to bridge the T cells [28, 29, and unpublished].

Confirmation that a single SD exists on HEL for the $H-2^b$ strain also came via another approach. Removal of simply the three N-terminal amino acids from HEL would be predicted to relieve suppression. Removal was accomplished with *Aeromonas* aminopeptidase to produce des-lys-val-phe-HEL. This molecule induced a T-proliferative response in the non-responder rather than suppression, presumably because a unique SD had been deleted from the molecule [30].

In seeking peptides of HEL that might stimulate T cell proliferation or help, N–C and L3H have consistently failed to do so. In summary, the SD and HD for $H-2^b$ mice exist in non-overlapping portions of the HEL molecule.

As can be appreciated from the principle of hierarchy (page 84.5) subsidiary SDs may exist on the molecule and could conceivably play a role during, for example, attempted tolerance induction to some internal peptide of lysozyme.

β-Galactosidase (GZ)

Suppressor-inducing determinants on native protein molecules have also been demonstrated on the large *E. coli* β-galactosidase tetramer (Mr = 465 000). Priming with cyanogen bromide peptide 2 from GZ (CB-2 = amino acids 3–92) suppressed anti-GZ antibody formation or the appearance of anti-FITC plaque forming cells to GZ-FITC in *in vitro* studies [31 and unpublished]. It was likewise shown that CB-2 could induce Th cells in the popliteal node of CBA/J ($H-2^k$) mice [32]. Therefore it was conceivable that the Ts and Th inducing determinants were identical. In order to test this possibility, tryptic peptides from CB-2 were assessed for their regulatory activity. It was found that the fourth tryptic peptide from the N terminus (amino acids 27–37) could induce Ts which suppressed the *in vitro* anti-FITC response to GZ-FITC. Likewise, tryptic peptide 6, (amino acids 44–52) induced Th which increased the *in vitro* anti-FITC response to GZ-FITC as much as GZ-induced Th [31 and unpublished]. In this example also, the SD and HD are non-overlapping.

One possible explanation for this non-overlapping arrangement of HD and SD in particular haplotypes has been presented elsewhere [33]. In short, not only are there H-agretopes with affinity for sites on I-A and I-E molecules used to present antigen to class II-restricted Th cells but it is postulated that there are special S-agretopes whose interaction with MHC desetopes is based on chemically disparate forces. (For example, S-desetopes may only interact with a set of hydrophilic amino acid residues.) Presumably the MHC molecules bearing the restricting elements for suppressor cell activation would be different and might even appear on unique APC. It is evident that the same peptide might conceivably elicit a response from both Ts and Th, but in principle this should arise because there are both an H-agretope and an S-agretope within the peptide.

In summary, a protein or peptide may not elicit a proliferative or helper response despite the fact that latent epitopes exist within it capable of being recognized by the T cell system. This most often is owing to the coexistence of Ts and Th-inducing epitopes on the same molecule. The latent T cell reactivity both in the suppressor and helper compartments can be revealed by dissociating the molecule to separate these epitopes.

Hierarchy

In some cases, a strain may be able to respond to a particular determinant, but it will not be obvious when the native molecule is given. A hierarchy of choice exists, in which certain determinants are favoured over others when several can theoretically be utilized

The total response potential of a strain may sometimes not be evident when mice are immunized with the whole molecule. As discussed above (page 84.2), a given haplotype shows a dominant response to limited regions of the whole molecule. The region(s) not responded to can, however, in some cases be shown to be reasonably immunogenic if given alone. For example, immunization of B10.A mice with L3H leads to a strong HEL cross-reactive response [4]. This potential to respond to L3H is not evident, however, when B10.A mice are immunized with native HEL (Table 84.1). B10 mice do not respond even when immunized with L3H [5]. Thus a hierarchy of responsiveness to available determinants is established when animals are immunized with HEL. The response potential to poorly responded determinants can be realized in B10.A or B10.D2 but not in B10 by the simple expedient of immunizing with a peptide containing a single determinant. The situation in B10 mice can be considered an example of an 'absolute hierarchy'.

A somewhat similar situation has been documented in the response of BALB/c mice to insulins [34]. Immunization with porcine insulin leads to response directed to a determinant cross-reactive with bovine and ovine insulins. However, if the mice are immunized with bovine or ovine insulin, the only response obtained is that to the A chain and is not cross-reactive with porcine insulin. Thus presence of the dominant A chain determinant on bovine or ovine insulin obscures the potential to respond to the determinant cross-reactive with porcine insulin.

Finally, in the case of β-galactosidase, it appears that a very limited repertoire of Th cells is activated by the native immunogen, and the HD which gains preference is *different* from either of the 2 HDs which

could be demonstrated by peptide priming of Th [31,45]. The 'native GZ' HD expresses its dominance over these peptide-induced HDs in that the latter seem to not be expressed.

The reasons underlying this phenomenon could potentially lie in either a high precursor frequency of T cells specific for the dominant determinant or to relative differences in the efficacy of presentation of certain determinants over others (see page 84.2). Alternatively the dominance of certain determinants may be a result of suppressor mechanisms which effectively shut off certain specificities (see page 84.3).

T cell steering

The specificity of a particular effector cell will circumscribe the specificity of its target effector cell

The principle of antigen-bridging, that Th will recognize a different epitope from the B cells with which they collaborate, was first enunciated by N.A. Mitchison in his seminal contributions to cell co-operation theory [35].

The following questions may be asked. If an antigen specific Th cell recognizes a single epitope on an antigen, will help be provided for B cells specific for any other epitope on an antigen, or just certain epitopes? Are close or distant epitopes favoured? What are the limitations in the reactivities of effector Ts for their Th targets: are all Th on the same molecule susceptible? Although the use of T cell clones should finally permit the appropriate study of these issues, questions of this sort have engaged the authors' laboratory for many years.

HEL system

It is clear that AgTh specific for epitopes on the peptic LOOP peptide (amino acids 57–107) in B10.A mice will provide help for N–C-specific antibody formation when native HEL is used for challenge (Cecka, unpublished). Experiments are in progress to ask whether N–C-specific and L3-specific T cell clones can also provide such help.

In the interaction between antigen-specific Ts and Th, it must be realized that there is already a highly circumscribed specificity for antigen in any T cell subpopulation, as pointed out above (pages 84.2–84.5). Thus AgTs specific for the N terminus of HEL can interfere with the 'complete' responsiveness of the H-2^b animal at the T-proliferative and B cell levels; it is possible that the total Th/Tp repertoire may be directed against a single site on HEL. It may be that were a Th site to exist close to a Ts site, such Th would be 'protected' [36] or resistant to the suppression by the neighbouring Ts.

β-Galactosidase system

We are again confronted with a combination of circumscribed intercellular interactions as well as MHC-restricted opportunities for activation.

Since only CB-2 and CB-10 (amino acids 378–418) induced Th cells while only CB-2 and CB-3 (amino acids 93–187) could induce Ts cells, the authors explored the interaction of these various activated T cell populations with each other in the response to GZ-FITC. The peptide primed T cell populations were compared to populations primed with native GZ. The following interesting pattern of regulatory interaction was observed [45]: (1) GZ-induced Th were suppressed by Ts induced by CB-2 and CB-3 although CB-2-induced Th were not suppressible by CB-3-induced Ts. This result not only implies that the GZ and CB-2 induced Th are different, but also that the interactions between Th and Ts are highly ordered, involving T cells with carefully matched specificities. (2) CB-10-induced Th seemed to be totally unaffected by the suppression exerted by any Ts cell, including those induced by GZ. It could be deduced from the results in (a) that CB-10-induced Th do not appear regularly upon priming with GZ.

Another interesting set of proscriptions appeared in the comparison between cyanogen bromide peptides that could induce T cell proliferation and those that could induce T cell help [32]. Eight of the ten other cyanogen bromide peptides tested were able to induce T cell proliferation but not T cell help for the anti-FITC response. Thus the special requirements needed for inducing help are not agretypic in nature but seem to depend on the proximity of the FITC haptens to the Th sites on the GZ molecule [45,46]. (One of the six FITC per monomer is probably conjugated at the N-terminal residue, close to the Th-inducing determinant within CB-2.)

Even on a large protein antigen such as GZ, Ts and Th-inducing determinants are not widespread. An interesting conclusion is that this may not be owing exclusively to repertoire but rather, in addition, to the relative position of these determinants to B cell-reactive epitopes [45]. The interaction between Ts and Th cells seems to involve small fragments of antigen, presumably produced during antigen processing. The stringency concerning the targets which can be used by particular Ts probably reflects the requirement for the suppressor determinant to adjoin the helper determinant at a particular distance on a relevant interaction fragment. (It should be noted that the entire HEL molecule is just slightly larger than one of the GZ cyanogen bromide peptides such as CB-2.) It is to be expected that within the next few years, studies with T cell clones will clarify the special rules circumscribing

cellular interactions utilizing different antigenic determinants on a native protein.

Idiotypy

The idiotypic network exerts a powerful influence on the nature of the eventual response, both with regard to specificity and affinity

In many systems in which a predominant idiotype (IdX) exists among the antibodies produced, it is thought that a regulatory idiotope recognized by a Th or Ts cell is the instrument of selection. This regulatory idiotope need not reside within the antibody active site. Another possibility is that anti-IdX antibody molecules interact directly with IdX bearing cells to modulate their behaviour.

Examples from the lysozyme system will illustrate these notions. The primary antibody response has a minority representation of IdX^+ anti-HEL. However, antibodies arising in the secondary response are almost entirely IdX^+ [37]. This has been attributed to the positive selective influence of IdX-recognizing T-helper cells [38], although this has not been directly shown. Monoclonal antibodies, prepared from fusions with secondary response antibody forming cells can be specific for non-overlapping epitopes on the HEL surface, as established by competition studies [39]. What is relevant to the current discussion is that (1) all of the antibodies bearing the IdX have specificity for the same face of the HEL molecule, and (2) all antibodies must be capable of binding to HEL itself. For example, among anti-HUL (human lysozyme) antibodies, only the HEL–HUL cross-reactive molecules are IdX^+, and this generalization is also true for more closely related lysozymes. Thus there *is* a relationship to specificity that is undeniable but the requirements that are inclusive or exclusive for fitting under the IdX^+ umbrella are not yet obvious [39].

In many systems there are 'private' idiotypes which are characteristic of antibody molecules that share active site residues. When certain specificities of antibody are dominant in a response, it is reasonable then to wonder whether an idiotypic influence may be indirectly responsible. For example, during the primary anti-lysozyme response, from 30–60% of the cells are making antibodies that require the presence of the three N-terminal amino acids ('TIP-specific'). Evidence now being accumulated using anti-idiotypic serum directed against a monoclonal antibody with this TIP-specificity indicates that there is probably a shared TIP-related idiotope on all of the primary anti-TIP producers. One can entertain the suspicion that a TIP-Id-recognizing T-helper cell is involved and the authors are exploring this possibility.

Finally, the authors also have evidence that pre-treatment of mice with anti-IdX antibody molecules primes B cells bearing IdX, provided that HEL immunization soon follows [40]. Interestingly, in this situation, very high affinity anti-HEL appears early in the response suggesting a relationship of affinity to predominant idiotypy. This has not been characteristic of many systems, but it is mentioned here to reiterate the idea that idiotypic forces may strongly influence the outcome of a response.

Compartmentalization

Since immune responses often represent a balance between regulatory cells, some lymphoid compartments may display a response while others remain non-responsive in the same individual

In the H-2^b mouse such a non-homogeneous situation arises in comparison of the popliteal lymph node (P-LN) and the spleen in their response to HEL given as an emulsion in complete Freund's adjuvant. The spleen has the characteristic non-response phenotype after intraperitoneal injection of the antigen which can be attributed to the potent suppressor system induced by this antigen. However, following footpad injection, the P-LN provide an excellent source of HEL-specific proliferative and helper T cells as well as a somewhat delayed plaque forming cell response [41].

Analysis of the situation provided a reason for this anomaly [41,42]. The 9–10 day HEL-primed P-LN lacks the Lyt 1$^-$,2$^+$ IdX-bearing T suppressor cell (Ts) although there are active Lyt-1$^+$, 2$^-$, I-J$^+$ T-suppressor inducer (Tsi) cells. Later on, by the 21st day following priming, the Ts become demonstrable in the P-LN while the Tsi activity disappears: Tsi must be added extrinsically to obtain suppression. Presumably, these early Tsi are irreversibly suppressed by the late-developing or late-arriving Ts. In other experimentally manipulated situations, where a suppressor cell source is deprived of Tsi in one way or another (e.g. by anti-I-J treatment), it could be shown that the existence of active Tsi is a *sine qua non* for suppression [43].

An interesting corollary also revealed in the experiments was the existence of all the machinery to induce an antibody response in the 'non-responsive' H-2^b mouse: HEL-presenting cells, an appropriate receptor-bearing T cell population, as well as an available B cell repertoire. A second lesson is that in seeking Ts cells, one must be careful to ask whether all 'accessory' and inducing cells are present.

Conclusions

The preceding sections discuss some of the 'rules' discerned from studies of immune responsiveness to well-defined protein antigens. It is evident that many of the discovered principles, especially those related to distinctions among determinants addressing distinct cellular subpopulations could only be worked out with proteins of known sequence and structure. It should be emphasized that the rules presented here were derived from experience within a limited number of protein antigen systems and are representative of our current working hypotheses more than established fact.

Current goals of regulatory immunology are centred around exact descriptions of the recognition and restrictions of interacting cellular subpopulations. It is already clear that both responsiveness and lack of it are outcomes of a complex interactive system. Subpopulations with distinct functions have been described among all of the three major (T,B and accessory) classes of cells involved. The authors suggest that the communication among lymphocytes has evolved to be highly unambiguous. If each cell is circumscribed to the recognition of specific partners, this would necessitate the use of combined recognition of various structures: idiotopes, epitopes, MHC restriction elements, and even lymphocyte differentiation antigens. Future studies in immune regulation should include formulations of the precise rules of recognition that will permit integration of the current fragmental information. The authors are convinced that protein and peptide antigens with their clearly definable structure will certainly occupy a central position in future descriptions of cellular regulatory interactions.

References

1 ROSENTHAL A.S. & SHEVACH E.M. (1973) Function of macrophages in antigen recognition by guinea pig T lymphocytes. *J. exp. Med.* **138**, 1194.

2 CHESNUT R.W. & GREY H.M. (1981) Studies on the capacity of B cells to serve as antigen-presenting cells. *J. Immunol.* **126**, 1075.

3 CHESNUT R.W., ENDRES R.O. & GREY H.M. (1980) Antigen recognition by T and B cells: recognition of cross-reactivity between native and denatured forms of globular antigens. *Clin. Immunol. Immunopath.* **15**, 397.

4 MAIZELS R.M., CLARKE J.A., HARVEY M.A., MILLER A. & SERCARZ E.E. (1980) Epitope specificity of the T cell proliferative response to lysozyme: proliferative T cells react predominantly to different determinants from those recognized by B cells. *Eur. J. Immunol.* **10**, 509.

5 MAIZELS R.M., CLARKE J.A., HARVEY M.A., MILLER A. & SERCARZ E.E. (1980) Ir-gene control of T cell proliferative responses: two distinct expressions of the genetically unresponsive state. *Eur. J. Immunol.* **20**, 516.

6 KATZ M.E., MAIZELS R.M., WICKER L., MILLER A. & SERCARZ E.E. (1982) Immunological focussing by the mouse MHC: mouse strains confronted with distantly related lysozymes confine their attention to a very few epitopes. *Eur. J. Immunol.* **12,** 535.

7 BERZOFSKY J.A., RICHMAN L.K. & KILLION D.J. (1979) Distinct H-2 linked Ir genes control both antibody and T cell responses to different determinants on the same antigen, myoglobin. *Proc. natn. Acad. Sci. U.S.A.* **76,** 4046.

8 ROSENWASSER L.J., BARCINSKI M.A., SCHWARTZ R.H. & ROSENTHAL A.S. (1979) Immune response gene control of determinant selection. (II) Genetic control of the murine T lymphocyte proliferative response to insulin. *J. Immunol.* **123,** 471.

9 ROSENTHAL A.S., THOMAS J.W., SCHROER J. & BLAKE J.T. (1980) The role of macrophages in genetic control of the immune response. *Fourth International Congress of Immunology. Progress in Immunology IV,* (eds. Fougereau M. & Dausset J.), p. 458. Academic Press, New York.

10 ULTEE M.E., MARGOLIASH E., KIPKOWSKI A., FLOURET G., SOLINGER A.M., LEBWOHL D., MATIS L.A., CHEN C. & SCHWARTZ R.H. (1980) The T lymphocyte response to cytochrome c-II. Molecular characterization of a pigeon cytochrome c determinant recognized by proliferating T lymphocytes of the B10.A mouse. *Mol. Immunol.* **17,** 809.

11 HEDRICK S.M., MATIS L.A., HECHT T.T., SAMELSON L.E., LONGO D.L., HEBER-KATZ E. & SCHWARTZ R.H. (1982) The fine specificity of antigen and Ia determinant recognition by T cell hybridoma clones specific for pigeon cytochrome c. *Cell,* **30,** 141.

12 MANCA F., CLARKE J., SHASTRI N., MILLER A. & SERCARZ E.E. (1984) A limited region within hen eggwhite lysozyme serves as the focus for a diversity of T cell clones. *J. Immunol.* **133,** 2075.

13 BENACERRAF B. (1978) A hypothesis to relate the specificity of T lymphocytes and the activity of I region-specific Ir genes in macrophages against B lymphocytes. *J. Immunol.* **120,** 1809.

14 ZINKERNAGEL R.M. & DOHERTY P.L. (1977) Major transplantation antigens, virus and specificity of surveillance T-cell. The altered self hypothesis. *Contemp. Top. Immunobiol.* **7,** 179.

15 HEBER-KATZ E., HANSBURG D. & SCHWARTZ R.H. (1983) The Ia molecule of the antigen-presenting cell plays a critical role in immune response gene regulation of T cell activation. *J. Mol. cell Immunol.* **1,** 3.

16 HANSBURG D., HANNUM C., INMAN J.K., APPELLA E., MARGOLIASH E. & SCHWARTZ R.H. (1981) Parallel cross-reactivity patterns of 2 sets of antigenically distinct cytochrome c peptides: possible evidence for a presentational model of Ir gene function. *J. Immunol.* **127,** 1844.

17 BERKOWER I., BUCKENMEYER G.K., GURD F.R.N. & BERZOFSKY J.A. (1982) A possible immunodominant epitope recognized by murine T lymphocytes immune to different myoglobins. *Proc. natn. Acad. Sci. U.S.A.* **79,** 4723.

18 HANSBURG D., FAIRWELL T., PINCUS M., SCHWARTZ R.H. & APELLA E. (1983) The T lymphocyte response to cytochrome c. (IV) Distinguishable sites on a peptide antigen which affect antigenic strength and memory. *J. Immunol.* **131,** 319.

19 HANSBURG D., HEBER-KATZ E., FAIRWELL T. & APELLA E. (1983) Major histocompatibility complex-controlled, antigen-presenting cell-expressed specificity of T cell antigen recognition *J. exp. Med.* **158,** 25.

20 ROCK K.L. & BENACERRAF B. (1983) Inhibition of antigen specific T lymphocyte activation by structural related Ir gene-controlled polymers. Evidence of specific competition for accessory cell antigen presentation. *J. exp. Med.* **157,** 1618.

21 WERDELIN O. (1982) Chemically related antigens compete for presentation by accessory cells to T cells. *J. Immunol.* **129,** 1883.

22 TADA T. (1983) I region determinants expressed on different subsets of T-cells: their role in immune circuits. In *Immunogenetics,* (ed. Benacerraf B.). Masson, Paris.

23 GERMAIN R.N. & BENACERRAF B. (1981) A single major pathway of T-lymphocyte interactions in antigen-specific immune suppression. *Scand. J. Immunol.* **13,** 1.

24 GREEN D.R., FLOOD P.M. & GERSHON R.K. (1983) Immunoregulatory T cell pathways. *Ann. Revs. Immunol.* **1,** 439.

25 SCHWARTZ R.H. (1982) Functional properties of I region gene products and theories of immune response (Ir) gene function. In *Ia Antigens and their Analogues in Man and Other Animals,* (eds. Ferrone S. & David C.). CRC Press, Boca Raton, Florida.

26 HILL S.W. & SERCARZ E.E. (1975) Fine specificity of the H-2 linked immune response gene for the gallinaceous lysozymes. *Eur. J. Immunol.* **5,** 317.

27 ADORINI L., MILLER A. & SERCARZ E.E. (1979) The fine specificity of regulatory cells. (I) Hen-egg-white lysozyme-induced suppressor T cells in a genetically non-responder mouse strain do not recognize a closely related immunogenic lysozyme. *J. Immunol.* **122,** 871.

28 YOWELL R.L., ARANEO B.A., MILLER A. & SERCARZ E.E. (1979) Amputation of a suppressor determinant on lysozyme reveals underlying T cell reactivity to other determinants. *Nature,* **279,** 70.

29 ADORINI L., HARVEY M.A., MILLER A. & SERCARZ E.E. (1979) The fine specificity of regulatory T cells. (II) Suppressor and helper T cells are induced by different regions of hen egg-white lysozyme (HEL) in a genetically non-responder mouse strain. *J. exp. Med.* **150,** 293.

30 WICKER L., KATZ M., KRZYCH U., MILLER A. & SERCARZ E.E. (1981) Focussing in the immune response to a protein antigen. In *14th Leukocyte Culture Conference,* (eds. Kirchner H. & Resch K.), p. 99. Elsevier/North-Holland Biomedical Press.

31 KRZYCH U., FOWLER A.V. & SERCARZ E.E. (1983) Antigen structures used by regulatory T cells in the interaction among T suppressor, T helper and B cells. In *Protein Conformation as an Immunological Signal,* (eds. Celada F., Schumaker V. & Sercarz E.E.), p. 395. Plenum Press, London.

32 KRZYCH U., FOWLER A.V., MILLER A. & SERCARZ E.E. (1982) Repertoires of T cells directed against a large protein antigen, beta-galactosidase. (I) Helper cells have a more restricted specificity repertoire than proliferative cells. *J. Immunol.* **128,** 1529.

33 GOODMAN J.W. & SERCARZ E.E. (1983) The complexity of structures involved in T-cell activation. *Ann. Revs. Immunol.* **1**, 465.

34 COHEN I.R. & TALMON J. (1980) H-2 genetic control of the response of T lymphocytes to insulins. Priming of non-responder mice by forbidden variants of specific antigenic determinants. *Eur. J. Immunol.* **10**, 284.

35 MITCHISON N.A. (1971) The carrier effect in the secondary response to hapten protein conjugates II Cellular cooperation. *Eur. J. Immunol.* **1**, 18.

36 SERCARZ E.E. (1980) The concept of 'protected' help in Ir gene control. In *Strategies of Immune Regulation*, (eds. Sercarz E.E. & Cunningham A.J.), p. 359. Academic Press, New York.

37 METZGER D.W., FURMAN A., MILLER A. & SERCARZ E.E. (1981) Idiotypic repertoire of anti-hen egg white lysozyme antibodies probed with hybridomas. Selection after immunization of an IdX marker common to antibodies of distinct epitope specificity. *J. exp. Med.* **154**, 701.

38 ADORINI L., HARVEY M. & SERCARZ E.E. (1979) The fine specificity of regulatory T cells. (IV) Idiotypic complementarity and antigen-bridging interactions in the anti-lysozyme response. *Eur. J. Immunol.* **9**, 906.

39 MILLER A., CH'NG L.-K., BENJAMIN C., SERCARZ E., BRODEUR P. & RIBLET R. (1983) Detailed analysis of the public idiotype of anti-hen egg-white lysozyme antibodies in the idiotype network. In *Immune Networks* (eds. Bona C. & Kohler H.), *Ann. N.Y. Acad. Sci.* **418**, 140.

40 SERCARZ E.E. & BENJAMIN C.D. (1984) Manipulating an idiotypic system with asymmetric circuitry: antiidiotypic antibodies versus idiotype-recognizing T cells. In *Idiotypy*, (eds. Köhler H., Urbain J. & Cazenave P.-A.), p. 101. Academic Press, New York.

41 YOWELL R.L., ARANEO B.A. & SERCARZ E.E. (1979) Ir-gene defects may reflect a regulatory imbalance. (I) Helper T cell activity revealed in a strain whose lack of response is controlled by suppression. *J. Immunol.* **123**, 961.

42 ARANEO B.A., YOWELL R.L., & SERCARZ E.E. (1985) Recognition and display of the predominant idiotype among members of the regulatory circuitry controlling the anti-lysozyme immune response. *J. Immunol.* **134**, 1073

43 GREEN D.R., GERSHON R.K. & EARDLEY D.D. (1981) Functional deletion of different Ly-1 T cell inducer subset activities by Ly-2 suppressor T lymphocytes. *Proc. natn. Acad. Sci. U.S.A.* **78**, 3819.

44 WICKER L.S., KATZ M., SERCARZ E.E. & MILLER A. (1984) Immunodominant protein epitopes. I. Induction of suppression to hen eggwhite lysozyme is obliterated by removal of the first three N-terminal amino acids. *Eur. J. Immunol.* **14**, 442.

45 KRYZCH U., FOWLER A.V. & SERCARZ E.E. (1985) Repertoire of T cells directed against a large protein antigen, beta-galactosidase. II. Only certain T helper or T suppressor cells are relevant in particular regulatory interactions. *J. exp. Med.* **162**, 332.

46 MANCA F., KUNKL A,. FENOGLIO D., FOWLER A., SERCARZ E.E. & CELADA F. (1985) Constraints in T-B cooperation related to epitope topology on *E. coli* beta-galactosidase. I. The fine specificity of T cells dictates the fine specificity of antibodies directed to conformation-dependent determinants. *Eur. J. Immunol.* **15**, 345.

47 SHASTRI N., MILLER A. & SERCARZ E.E. (1984) The expressed T cell repertoire is hierarchical: The precise of focus of lysozyme-specific T cell clones is dependent upon the structure of the immunogen. *J. Mol. cell. Immunol.* **1**, 369.

Index

Abelson lymphoma 45.1
Absorption analysis for Ia alloantigen detection 48.10
Accessory cells 49.2
Acetate buffer 52.7
Acid hydrolase 47.3
Acquired immunodeficiency syndrome (AIDS) 83.3
Actin-binding proteins 41.5
Active oxygen species, biochemical methods 50.4
Active oxygen species, cytochemical studies 50.8
  monitoring 50.4
  release 50.1
Adherence, cell separation methods 58.8
Adjuvant, *B. pertussis* 67.3
Adneosine deaminase (ADA) deficiency with SCID 83.2
Adoptive host irradiation dosage 67.6
Adoptive transfer, contrasuppression in 79.5
Adoptive transfer, Ir 67.1
Affinity columns for cells 55.6
  method 55.7
Affinity purified reagents 44.9
Affinity separation in dishes (panning) 55.7
  method 55.8
Agammaglobulinaemia, autosomal recessive 83.1
  X-linked (XIA) 83.1
Agarose 55.5
Agarose leukocyte assay 51.4
  method 51.8
Agarose, in plaque assay 78.2
Agglutinin, peanut 55.9
  wheat germ 55.6
Agretope 84.3
Agretypy 84.3
AIDS 83.3
Albumin, bovine plasma (BPA) 49.3
Alkaline phosphatase immunoassay substrate 58.13
Alkaline phosphodiesterase I, assay 52.4
Alkoxy radicals 50.5
Allelic exclusion 56.1
Alloantibody, Ts lymphocyte factor preparation 80.3
Alloantigen, genetic background

effects 61.5
Ia, detection methods 48.10
lymphocyte cell surface 61.1
as marker 57.17
mouse, analysis
  functional 61.5
  genetic 61.4
  tissue distribution 61.5
classification 61.1
detection methods 61.4
  reagents 61.4
  test procedures 61.4
  fluorescence-activated cell sorter (FACS) 61.4
  identification 61.1
  monoclonal reagents 61.4
Qa series 61.1
TL series 61.1
Alloenzymes 56.7
Alloreactive clones 69.2
Alloreactivity 72.1
  measurement *in vitro* 66.6
Allorecognition 53.2
Allotype, determinant bearing (Ct^b) molecules 80.5
  regulation 74.2
  suppression 74.4
Allotype-specific suppressor cells 78.12
Allotype-Ts lymphocyte 78.1
Alpha-chain gene 53.3
Alum precipitation in mouse immunization 64.3
Amino acid, TIP-specific 84.6
Amino acid sequence of V_H gene 90.1
2-Aminoethylisothiouronium bromide 55.9
S-2-Aminoethylisothiouronium bromide hydrobromide 58.2
Analmias, mouse linkage map 104.12
Angiogenesis factor 47.4
Angiotensin-converting enzyme 47.2
Animal, marked 56.1
Animal techniques, mouse, genetic marker preparation 56.3
  inoculation, footpad 68.9
  intraperitoneal 45.1
Anti-albumin antibody, serological assay 67.7
Anti-γ-azophenylarsonate (Ar) 78.9
Anti-gamma-globulin antibody, serological assay 67.7
Anti-hapten antibody, serological

assay 67.7
Anti-Ia antibody, blocking function 72.1
Antibody, affinity prepared 64.19
  anti-albumin serological assay 67.7
  anti-DNP PFC response induction 78.6
  anti-gamma globulin serological assay 67.7
  anti-hapten serological assay 67.7
  anti-prostaglandin E1 81.8
  anti-receptor 48.2
  auto-, to erythrocytes 82.5
  auto-, production 75.2
  combining site 73.1
  deficiency 83.2
  DNA reactive 82.1
  direct binding 48.10
  erythrocyte rosetting 49.4
  expressed repertoire 73.2
  idiotype bearing suppression 78.9
  in idiotypic control 73.2
  indirect binding 48.10
  maternal effect 73.2
  monoclonal specificity 84.6
  production by regulatory circuits 74.1
  reactive to Ts lymphocyte factor 80.3
  response mechanism 75.5
  rosette test 58.4
  specific secretion assays 65.6
  subsets from epitope 74.3
  to T lymphocyte antigen 55.3
  in vitro lymphocyte 57.4
  specificity, in mouse V_H genes 90.5
Antibody-coated erythrocytes (EA) 49.3
Antibody-forming cell precursor (AFCP) 67.1
Antibody-mediated modulation 55.4
Anti-enzyme plaques 64.13
Antigen, activation by T lymphocytes 69.1
  allogeneic MHC 68.1
  assay methods 78.4
  avidin-biotin-complex (ABC) assay 43.9
  binding by lymphocytes 75.4
  bone-marrow-derived lymphocyte (MBLA) 67.1
  concentration calculation 43.6
  conformation copy 68.1

Antigen (*cont.*)
  cross-reactivity 68.1
  cytotoxic responses 68.2
  direct labelling 55.1
  DR (human) 45.8
  epitope-specific suppression 78.12
  erythrocyte (Ea) 61.1
  histocompatibility 62.4
  Ia 48.9
    on cell lines 45.8
  immune response idiotypic control 73.3
  immunoglobulin production induction 66.10
  incubation times 43.7
  indirect labelling 55.2
  lymphocyte (Ly) 61.1
  lymphocyte cooperation mediation 67.1
  of lymphoid cells 75.1
  macrophage-restricted 45.8
  major histocompatibility complex 68.1, 72.1
  male specific minor H, H-Y 68.3
  minor histocompatibility (H) 68.1.2
  minor transplantation 68.9
  mixed 64.9
  mouse tissue techniques 43.4
  non-erythrocyte 64.12
  plasma cell (P ca) 61.1
  presentation to B lymphocytes 48.5
  processing 68.2
  radiolabelled preparations 67.7
  reactive cells 57.1
  recognition 68.1
  skin (Sk) 61.1
  soluble cloning methods 69.5
  soluble protein, delayed type hypersensitivity 77.4
  solubilization 43.7
  T lymphocyte recognition 84.2
    specific 84.2
    suppressor factors 80.1
  thymocyte (Thy) 61.1
  transplantation 72.1
Antigen binding capacity (ABC) 67.6
Antigen-binding cells 55.13
  from spleen 80.2
Antigen binding site 73.1
Antigen-bridging 84.5
Antigen presenting cells 48.1, 68.1, 71.1
    in delayed type hypersensitivity 77.1
Antigen-reactive T cells (ARC) 75.2
Antigen sensitized T lymphocytes 69.8
Antigen specific helper hybrid identification 69.10
Antigen-specific suppressor T cell factor, preparation 80.1
Antigen specificity, T lymphocyte 53.2
Antigen–antibody complexes, macro-

phage line stimulation 45.6
Antigen–antibody interaction, specificity 55.5
Antigenic determinants, for idiotope 73.1
  internal image 73.1
  for *in vivo* adoptive immune response 67.1
Antigenic markers, cell surface 57.15
Anti-4-hydroxy-3-nitrophenylacetyl (NP) 78.9
Anti-idiotypic Ts lymphocyte induction 78.11
Anti-IgM 70.5
Anti-immunoglobulin sera 64.18
  absorption of antisera 64.20
  development and inhibition of plaques 64.20
  production 64.18
    antigen affinity columns 64.19
    to fragments (Fc, Fab) 64.19
    myeloma transplantation 64.18
    purification 64.19
Anti-lymphocytic antibody (ALS), production 67.4
Anti-lymphocytic globulin 81.2
Anti-phosphorylcholine (PC) 78.9
Anti-prostaglandin E1 antibodies 81.8
Antiserum, to mouse alloantigen 61.4
Anti-streptococcal A Carbohydrate (A-CHO) 78.9
Anti-thymocyte globulin 81.2
Anti-thymocyte serum (ATS) 67.4
Apoliprotein E 47.3, 14
Arachidonate, bioactive derivatives 47.6
Arachidonic acid 81.7
  continous infusion in rat 81.8
Arginase 47.3
ARS 90.1
Arsanyl 55.6
Aspirin, as immunosuppressive 81.8
Assay incubation time 68.7
Assay plate preparation 64.3
Assay well use 68.6
Ataxia telangiectasia 83.3
Auto-antibody production 75.2
Auto-immune inherited traits, influence of sex 82, 14
Auto-immune inbred mouse breeding 82.14
Auto-immune disease 82.1
  abnormal immunoregulation studies 82.8
  B lymphocyte hyperactivity studies 82.6
  development techniques 82.15
  genetic tools 82.13
  molecular genetic analysis 82.16
  serological studies 82.1
  stem cell abnormality studies 82.12
  tolerance defects 82.10

Auto-immunity, dietary regulation 82.15
  DTH reactions in 77.1
Autokilling by culture 68.13
Autologous mixed lymphocyte reaction (AMLR), abnormal 82.8
Autoradiography of enzymes 56.7
  for immunoglobulin-secreting cells 64.9
  of lymphocyte 57.8
  mouse tissue 43.6
Auxiliary circuits, antibody 74.1
Avidin-biotin-complex (ABC) antigen assay 43.9
p-Azophenylarsonate (ARS) 90.1
Azathioprine 81.2

BGDF, lymphocyte activator 70.3
  types
    Human I 70.3
    Human II 70.3
    Interleukin I 70.3
    Mouse-I 70.1
    Mouse-II 70.2
Beta-chain gene 53.3
B lymphocyte 62.2
  activation by BGDF 70.3
  activation of auto-immunity 82.15
  activators 63.1
    density cultures 63.1
      human 63.8
      method (mouse) 63.3
      purified, PBA response 63.4
      response measurement 63.5
        Ig secretion 63.6
        proliferation after subculture 63.6
  antigen presentation 48.5
  bone marrow colonies 82.13
  clones 75.4
  continuous cultivation lines 70.8
  culture activation 82.7
  cyclosporin A effect 81.12
  differentiation 57.17
  dinitrophenol-specific response 65.3
  effector function evaluation 46.6
  enumeration 83.4
  flow cytometry subset enumeration 82.9
  fluorescence 57.12
  Fc receptors 48.2
  growth factors (BCGF) 59.1, 70.1
  helper function assay 66.12
  heterogeneity 53.4
  homogeneous 75.6
  hyperactivity studies 82.6
  IgG coated 41.3
  immunodeficiency diagnosis 83.3
  intracytoplasmic staining 63.7
  long-term lines 70.7
  memory cells 53.4, 58.12, 74.1, 6
  migration 57.15

B lymphocyte (*cont.*)
  mitotic index   63.6
  phosphorylcholine-specific response
    65.3
  plaque assays   63.7
  recirculation   57.1
  saturation density   63.6
  separation from T cell   54.1
  suppressor functions assay   66.12
  surface immunoglobulin   53.1
  surface immunoglobulin assay   66.4
  uridine labelling   57.9
B-lymphocyte stimulating factor (BSF)
    71.2
BCG, in macrophage isolation   43.1
Bacteria, *Bordetella pertussis*   78.6
  Corynebacterium parvum   48.9
  Escherichia coli   48.9
  IgG-coated   41.1
  Klebsiella aerogenes   48.9
  macrophage interactions   45.8
  Neisseria gonorrhoeae   48.9
  phagocytosis assay   46.7
    culture   46.6
    intracellular killing   46.7
    pre-opsonization   46.7
  Salmonella typhimurium   48.9
  Staphylococcus albus   48.9
  Streptococcus pneumoniae   78.10
Balanced salt solution (BSS)   45.1
  for immune response assay   67.8
Basophil, Fc receptors   48.2
Benzoate decarboxylation   50.6
Benzoquinone conjugation   64.13
Berg's reagent, preparation and
    assay   52.6
Beta-carotene   50.7
Bilirubin   50.7
Biochemical markers   56.7
Bistable regulation   74.2
Blast cell, transformation   66.5
Blood, leucocytes, human   58.1
Blood, mononuclear cells from   66.1
Blood, natural killer cells from   60.2
Blood flow to lymphatic organs   57.1
  lymphocyte traffic   57.1
Bone marrow, allogeneic cell
    transfer   81.4
  auto-immunity induction   82.15
  B lymphocytes from   53.6
  B cell colonies   82.13
  chimaeras from   56.2
  lymphocyte traffic   57.5
  lymphocytes from   67.1
  for monocellular culture   45.2
  natural killer cells from   60.1
  phagocytes from   46.1
  separation of mononuclear cells
    66.2
Bone-marrow-derived lymphocyte
    antigen (MBLA)   67.1
Bone marrow graft, cyclosporin A
    81.11
Borate buffer for immune response

    assay   67.8
Bovine γ-Globulin (BGG), tolerization
    and immunization with
    82.10
  antibody assay   82.11
Bovine plasma albumin (BPA)   49.3
Bovine serum albumin (BSA)   54.7
  as immunogen   67.2
  methylated (MBSA)   78.7
Brucella, in macrophage activation
    48.11
Burnet, Sir F.M.   62.2

C gene   75.5
C receptor   45.8
  on macrophage lines   45.8
Calbiochem   47.15
Calcium ionophore A23187   50.3
Candida albicans for chemotaxis
    assay   51.11
Carbohydrate antigen, conjugation
    64.14
Carrier effect   67.1
Carrier-specific augmenting T cell
    (CTa)   71.3
Carrier-specific helper T cell
    (CTR)   71.1, 74.4
Carrier-specific (KLH) suppressor
    cells   78.6
Carrier-specific regulation   74.4
Carrier-specific and Ig-specific path-
    way interaction   74.4
Carrier-specific suppressor T cells
    (CTs)   71.3, 74.3
Casein, macrophage stimulator   48.11
Catalase   50.5
Cell, adherence separation   58.8
  binding of ligands   43.3
  chemotactic ratio   51.3
  dendritic (DC)   49.1
  effector   65.1
  gradient separation   58.9
  intact, for fibrinolysis assay   47.18
  ionising irradiation effects   81.3
  Langerhans   53.4
  natural killer   53.3, 60.1
  panning   53.1
  for phagocytosis tests   46.6
  proliferation system   44.1
  respiratory burst   50.3
  rosetting   53.1
  stem   53.5
    differentiation   75.6
Cell adherence to plastic   60.3
Cell affinity columns   55.6
Cell cooperation, anti-MBLA anti-
    serum in   67.1
  antigen-bridging   84.5
  antigen-mediated   67.1
  limited dilution analysis   65.1
Cell fixation   43.3
Cell fractionation techniques   52.3
Cell-free extracts of suppressor fac-
    tor   80.2

Cell-free fraction of macrophages
    47.19
Cell fusion techniques for macrophage
    cell lines   45.2
Cell lineages   53.5
Cell-mediated immunity   75.2
  sensitization *in vivo*   68.3
  in vitro suppression   81.8
Cell motility   41.5
Cell nylon wool column adherence
    60.3
Cell populations, genetic markers
    56.1
  interacting   68.2
  resolution   44.13
Cell protein assay, Lowry method
    43.12
Cell separation, design and analysis
    54.1
  by monoclonal antibody panning
    58.6
  variance   54.2
Cell streaming limit   54.5
Cell surface, alloantigens in
    mouse   61.1
  anti-receptor antibodies   48.2
  antigens, EA14236   48.7
    EA1423α   48.7
    Ly-5 (T200)   57.18
    OKT 11a   55.9
    Thy-1   57.17
  identification   53.1
Cell surface antigenic markers   57.15
Cell surface glycoproteins   53.2 75.1
  in MHC specificity   72.2
Cell surface markers   68.1
  hybridization confirmation   69.9
Cell surface phenotype   68.1, 79.2
Cell suspensions method   67.6
  preparation   64.17
  temperature   68.4
Cell tracing, intrinsic markers   57.17
Cell transfer method   67.5, 6
  for Ts protective response   68.3
Cerium based techniques   50.10
  perhydroxide   50.10
Cerous ions   50.10
Cerous salts   50·10
Cesium chloride   80.6
Cetrimiol counting solution   44.16
Chemiluminescence   50.1, 4
Chemokinesis   51.2
Chemotactic peptides   50.3
  in inflammatory response   48.9
Chemotactic ratio   51.3
Chemotaxis   51.3
Chicken gamma globulin as im-
    munogen   67.2
Chimaera, artificial   56.2
  of lymphocyte   81.4
  naturally occurring   56.2
  secondary   56.2
Chlamydia psittaci, macrophage cyto-
    toxicity to   45.8

Chromatography, gas 50.5
 hydroxyapatite 76.4
Chromic chloride, aged 58.13
 conjugation 64.12
 for rosetting 55.10
Chromium chloride coupling 78.8
Chromium-(^{51}Cr) label release
 assay 60.5, 68.5
Chromium-(^{51}Cr)-label target cell preparation 66.11
Chromium (^{51}Cr) labelled lymphocyte
 method 57.5
Chromosome, C-banding 82.16
 loss in T cell hybrids 69.10
 markers 56.2
 spreading 56.3
 staining 56.3
  giemsa 56.4
  orcein 56.4
 translocation 56.2
 X- 56.1
Chromosome analysis, bias avoi-
 dance 56.5
 for hybridization confirmation 69.9
 sources of error 56.4
Chronic active hepatitis (CAH) 79.2
Chronic granulomatous disease (CGD)
 50.9
Cinematography, time-lapse 51.11
Clark oxygen electrode 50.4
Clonal inhibition 77.3
Clonal selection theory 62.2
Cloning by limiting dilution 68.12
Coeliac disease, antigen frequency
 102.6
  D/DR associations 102.6
  inheritance 102.9
Cognate interaction, B cells 71.1
Collagen, for cell locomotion 51.13
Collagenase 47.1
Colony-forming cells, in spleen
 (CFU-S) 53.5
Colony forming units (CFU), in auto-
 immune disease 82.12
Colony-stimulating activities (CSA)
 45.6
Colony stimulating factor (CSF)
 44.1, 5, 45.6, 59.1
Competition assay for mouse tissue
 antigen 43.6
Complement, components 47.3
 purified 48.6
 (CR) 48.5
 cytotoxicity tests 48.10
 diluent preparation 78.14
 lymphocyte immunoselection 55.3
 macrophage synthesis 45.5
 in phagocytosis 41.1
 receptors 41.1
  detection on monolayers 48.7
  detection in suspension 48.7
  function regulation 41.6
  identification by erythrocytes
   48.1

rosettes (EAC) 55.10
Complement-mediated cytotoxicity
 55.3, 58.7
 assay 48.11
Concanavalin A 50.3, 58.10, 63.1, 8,
 14
 blast cultures 68.5
 mitogenic response 79.2
 in suppressor cell induction 78.4
Conditioned medium (CM) for
 clones 69.1
Conditioned medium preparation
 (LCM) 44.5
Conjugate cytotoxic assay 60.5
Constant region, determinants on Ts
 lymphocyte factor 80.3
 contrasuppression 71.6, 79.1
 adoptive transfer 79.5
 in immunoregulation 79.7
Contrasuppressive cell 84.3
Contrasuppressor cells 78.13
Contrasuppressor circuit 79.2
 disruption 79.4
Contrasuppressor inducer cell remo-
 val 79.4
Contrasuppressor T lymphocyte
 (Tcs) 78.1, 79.1
Coombs' assay of anti-erythrocyte
 auto-antibodies 82.5
Core circuit, antibody 74.1
Corticosteroids, macrophage matu-
 ration 45.7
Cosmid libraries for cloning MHC
 genes 68.3
Cosmid transfection 68.13
Coulter cell counter 54.4
Coupling reagent, benzoquinone
 64.13
 chromic chloride 64.12
 p-diazonium phenylphosphorylcho-
  line (DPPC) 78.11
 ECD 1 64.12
Crohn's disease, suppressor cell acti-
 vity 79.2
Cuffing procedure in microvascular
 surgery 81.2
Culture of lymphocyte 54.4, 75.6
Culture of T lymphocytes 63.9
 screening by inverted microscope
  63.4
Cunningham biological assay 64.7
Cunningham monolayer technique
 64.6
Cyclosporin A 81.10
 B lymphocyte effect 81.12
 graft rejection prevention 81.11
 in vivo use 81.10
 hypotheses on action mechanism
  81.14
 mode of action 81.13
 synthesis 81.14
 T lymphocyte response inhibition 81.13
Cyclosporin C, tritium labelled dihyd-

ro- 81.14
Cyclosporin D 81.14
Cytochalasins 41.5
Cytogenetic analysis of auto-immune
 mouse cells 82.16
Cytological markers 56.2
Cytolytic T lymphocyte (CTL) 63.13
 mouse 72.2
Cytoplasmic structural markers 56.7
Cytoplast 41.5
Cytoskeletal proteins 41.5
Cytotoxic activity developed per cul-
 ture 68.7
Cytotoxic assay, ^{125}IVαR test 57.10
Cytotoxic effectors, functional acti-
 vity 68.10
Cytotoxic inhibition assay for mRNA
 products 80.7
Cytotoxic responses to non-MHC
 antigens 68.2
Cytotoxic/suppressor set of T lympho-
 cyte 75.1
Cytotoxic T lymphocyte (CTL) 63.10
 response analysis 68.1
Cytotoxicity, complement-mediated
 55.3, 58.7
 non-specific killing 68.8
 positive selection 55.13
 target cells for 57.7
 towards tumour targets 45.9
Cytotoxicity assay *in vitro* 68.9
 methods 68.8

DEAE-dextran in plaque assay 78.3
Defibrinated blood for leucocytes 58.2
Degradation assays 43.12
Dendritic cells (DC) 49.1
 as accessory or stimulating cells
  49.2
 enumeration 49.7
 enrichment techniques 49.7
 features 49.1
 identification 49.1
 isolation techniques 49.3
 labelling 49.1
 as lymphocyte response stimulators 49.2
 preparation from human
  blood 49.6
 preparation from mouse 49.3
 preparation from rat 49.6
 purification 49.2
  cytolytic method 49.7
  physical method 49.7
Densitometer scanning 56.10
Density gradient centrifugation 55.10
 for natural killer cells 40.3
Density lymphocyte sedimentation
 54.5
Deoxycholate 50.3
Desetope 84.3
Determinant, hierarchy 84.5
Determinant focusing 84.2

Developing serum, correction factor titration 64.4
DEX3 90.1
Dexamethasone 47.8
Dexter mouse cultures 45.2
Dextran, cross-linked 55.5
α1, 3-Dextran 90.1
3, 3'-Diaminobenzidine (DAB) 50.9
Diazobicyclooctane 50.7
Diazonium salt of sulphanilic acid (DASA) 52.1
  assay 52.6
  resorcinol assay 52.6
o-Dibenzoylbenzene 50.7
C15-Dibenzoylethylene 50.7
DiGeorge's syndrome 83.3
Digitizer tablet 51.14
Digitonin 50.3
Dimeric C3b, binding 48.7
5,5-Dimethyl-1-pyroline-N-oxide (DMPO) 50.6
Dimethylsulfoxide methane assay test 50.5
Dimethyl sulphoxide (DMSO) for cloned cell storage 69.4
Dinitro fluorobenzene (DNFB) delayed type hypersensitivity 77.1
Dinitrophenol-specific responses in B lymphocytes 65.3
Dinitrophenyl (DNP), antibody to (in assay) 78.6
  in monoclonal antibody studies 64.15
2,4-Dinitrophenyl as immunogen 67.2
2,5-Diphenylfuran 50.7
1,3-Diphenylisobenzofuran 50.7
Dipyridamole 81.8
Direct plaque-forming cells (PFC) 64.1
DNA, antibody reaction measurement 82.1
  for cloning HC genes 68.3
  of defined cell populations 53.2
  markers 56.6
  in molecular genetic analysis 82.16
  sequences 53.3
  synthesis in lymphocyte 57.9
  in RNA hybrids 76.1
cDNA, clone isolation 76.1
  reaction problems 76.6
  rescreening 76.6
  subtracted library 76.5
  subtractive hybridization 76.1
  subtractive hybridization method 76.2
  synthesis 76.3
Double-drug therapy 81.2
Dulbecco's phosphate-buffered saline (PBS) 58.13, 60.9
  preparation 64.22
Dysgammaglobulinaemia 83.1

Ecto-enzymes 52.1
  mouse macrophage identification 52.1
Effector cells, limiting dilution analysis 65.1
Egg albumin as immunogen 67.2
Ehrlich, Paul 62.1
Eicosapentaenoic acid (EPA), dietary enrichment 82.15
Elastase 47.2
Elastin, lysis assay 47.21
  lysis enhancement with SDS 47.23
  substrate preparation 47.21
Electron microscopy, phagocytosis assessment 46.3
Electron spin resonance spectroscopy 50.7
Electrophoresis, for immunoselection of cell 55.13
  polyacrylamide gel 47.8, 53.1
  SDS-polyacrylamide gradient gel 47.10
Electrophoretic markers 56.7
Elicitation of macrophages 50.3
  or neutrophils 50.3
  condition 50.3
ELISA, DNA reactive with antibody technique 82.1
  for immunoglobulin synthesis 58.11
  virus antibody assay 58.11
End-point assay 51.5
Endotoxin 47.19
Enzyme, autoradiographic preparation 56.7
Enzyme markers 56.5
Eosinophil 50.3
  Fc receptors 48.2
Epitope, control of IgG responses 74.2
Epitope-specific regulation 74.1
  antibody subsets 74.3
Epitope-specific suppressor cells 78.12
Epitope-specific Ts lymphocyte 78.1
α, 11 Epoxyiminoprosta-5, 13-dienoic acid 81.8
Epstein–Barr virus, with immunodeficiency 83.3
  transformed lymphoblastoid lines 69.6
Equilibrium 73.1
E-rosette technique 55.8
Erythrocyte, antibody-coated (EA) 49.3
  antibody rosetting 49.4
  antigen (Ea) 61.1
  complement receptor identification 48.1
  dendritic cell preparation from 49.3
  dinitrophenyl as hapten 64.15
  Fc receptor detection 48.1
  in Fc receptor test 58.3

haemagglutination assays 65.6
  in haemolytic assays, chromic chloride method 64.12
  in haemolytic assays, ECDI method 64.12
  immune response assay 67.8
  IgG-coated 41.3
  as immunogen 67.4
  lysis using water 60.3
  preparation for rosetting 55.9
  removal before culture 68.5
  rosette-formation 55.9, 58.2, 60.4
Erythroprotein 47.6
Ethanol 50.7
4-Ethoxymethylene-2-phenyloxazolone as immunogen 67.2
Ethylene production by hydroxyl radicals 50.5

FACS (see Fluorescence-activated cell sorter)
Factor 1 (inactivator) 48.7
Factor increasing monocytopoiesis (FIM) 42.3
Farr assay 67.6
  for DNA antibody reaction measurement 82.2
Fatty acids 50.3
Ferricytochrome C 50.4
Fetal bovine serum 45.3
Fetal calf serum (FCS) 63.1
  T cell response determination 63.11
α-Fetoprotein, in diagnosis of ataxia telangiectasia 83.5
Feulgen–Rossbeck stain 56.6
Fibrin 47.22
Fibrin gel, for cell locomotion 51.13
Fibrin lysis zones 47.14
Fibrin plates, preparation 47.16
Fibrinogen, iodination 47.15
  proteolysis 47.2
  purification 47.15
Fibrinolysis, assay 47.18
Fibroblast, pinocytosis activity 42.2
Fibronectin 45.10, 47.4, 14
  in phagocytosis 41.1
Fibronectin receptors 41.7
Ficoll 44.17
Ficoll–Hypaque solution, preparation 44.17
  for cell separation 58.13
Filler cells for T lymphocyte clones 69.2
Filter assay 51.7
  automated 51.7
Flow cytofluorometry for lymphocytes 57.12
Flow cytometer, use of 44.11
Flow cytometry, T and B lymphocyte subset enumeration 82.9
Fluorescein (FITC) 55.6

Fluorescein conjugation to lympho-
    cyte 57.12
    preparation 57.13
Flurorescein diacetate 58.13
Fluorescein, *in situ* labelling 57.16
Fluorescence-activated cell sorter
    53.1, 54.1, 57.17
    cellular reactivity analysis 53.2
    for human leucocytes 58.5
    in lymphocyte separation 55.1
    for mouse alloantigens 61.4
Fluorescence detector with linear
    amplifier 44.13
    with logarithmic amplifier 44.13
Fluoride 50.3
Fluorimetry, antibody detection 48.2
Fluorochrome, for M.A labelling
    44.14
Fluorodeoxyuridine (FUα R) 57.11
Fluorograph gels 47.11
Formaldehyde from hydroxyl radi-
    cal 50.5
Formazan reaction product 50.8
Fragments, antiserum to 64.18
    MHC interaction sites 84.3
    T lymphocyte binding sites 84.3
    Ts and Th lymphocyte interac-
        tion 84.6
Fab, immunoglobulin activity 75.5
F(ab′)2, in indirect radioimmune bind-
    ing assay 43.5
    of rodent monoclonal antibodies
    44.7
Fc, immunoglobulin activity 75.5
    immunoglobulins binding to macro-
        phage 43.4
    macrophage binding 45.5
    rosetting 58.4
Fc receptor 41.3, 45.8, 53.1
    detection 58.3
        by erythrocyte 48.1
        methods 48.2
            in monolayers 48.3
            in suspension 48.2
    determination of number 48.4
    for IgG's 45.10
    macrophage 48.2
    on macrophage lines 45.8
    in mononuclear phagocytes 42.2
    mouse 48.2
    positive T cells 71.3
    rosettes 55.10
    types 41.6
Frozen section assay (Woodruff) of
    lymphocyte HEV binding
    57.19

GAT *see* Glucosamine, alanine, tyra-
    mine
Beta-galactosidase (GZ) 84.4
Gamma camera for spleen and lymph
    nodes 57.7
Gas chromatography 50.5
Gelatin-coated plate for cell sepa-

ration 55.13
Gelatin, Hanks' 64.22
    HEPES Eagles 64.22
Gelsolin 41.5
Gene, α-chain 53.3
    β-chain 53.3
    H-2 Ir, in graft rejection 68.3
    idiotypic repertoire control 73.3
    mapping technique 104.4
    structure 76.8
    transfer experiments 68.8
    VH sequence homology plot 90.1
Gene conversion 53.2
Genetic disparity in cytotoxicity 68.1
Genetic markers, alloantigen 61.1
    for cell populations 56.1
    criteria 56.1
    natural 56.2
    use in combination 56, 14
Genomic DNA for cloning MHC
    genes 68.3
Germinal center lymphocytes 57.15
Gey's solution 58.13
Giemsa staining 56.4
Glucocorticoid 47.2
Glucosamine, alanine, tyramine
    (GAT), Ts induction 78.7
    GAT/GT, response assay 78.8
        response induction 78.7
    GAT/GT, suppressor cell induc-
        tion 78.8
        suppressor factor, induc-
            tion 78.9
    GAT-MBSA,   epitope-specific
        sup pression 78.13
        Ts induction 78.7
    GAT-Ts 78.8
    GAT-TsF 78.9
Glucosamine, tyramine (GT), in Ts
    induction 78.7
Glucose 6-phosphate dehydrogenase
    (G6PDH)   electrophoresis
    56.12
Glucose phosphate isomerase (GPI-1),
    electrophoresis 56.13
Glycogen, macrophage stimulator
    48.11
Glycolipid assays for immunoglobulin-
    secreting cells 64.14
Glycoprotein, cell surface, T lympho-
    cyte isolation 75.1
    T zoo 55.4
    TL 75.1
Goat anti-rat Ig 44.9
Gradient cell separation method 58.9
Graft, skin 81.2
    rejection 81.1
        prevention with cyclosporin
            A 81.11
        DTH reactions in D 77.1
        mediation 68.3
        thoracic duct drainage in 81.6
Graft-versus-host reaction 77.1, 81.4
Granulocyte, human, phagocytosis

by 46, 10, 11
    intracellular killing by 46.12
    lymphokine growth factor 59.1
Granulomatous disease, chronic,
    phagocytosis in 46.2
Growth/differentiation factors 68.10
Growth hormone deficiency 83.1
Guanidine 80.6
Guinea pig, Fc receptors for
    IgG1 48.2
    IgG2 48.2
Gut associated lymphoid tissue
    (GALT) 79.7

Haemagglutination assay for specific
    antibody secretion 65.6
Haemolysis, localized in gel 64.1
Haemolytic complement, mouse link-
    age map 104.10
Haemolytic plaque assay 64.2, 67.7,
    78.2
Hank's balanced salt solution (HBSS),
    in plaque assay 78.3
    preparation 78.14
Hanks' gelatin (HG), preparation
    64.22
Hapten, as carrier determinant 67.3
    induction 74.7
    mechanism 74.7
    specificity 74.6
    epitope-specific suppression, induc-
        tion 74.3
    carrier-effect response 67.1
    conjugation to protein 67.3
    2,4-dinitrophenyl 64.15
    IgG antibody production 74.2
    immune response to 68.9
    in mixed lymphocyte cultures 68.2
    radiolabelled 67.7
Hapten-protein ratios 67.3
Hapten-specific   contact   sensiti-
        vity 77.2
Heart and lung transplant pro-
    gramme 81.11
Heart graft in pigs 81.11
Heavy chain, mouse sequence classifi-
    cation 90.1
    mouse VH gene antibody spec-
        ificity 90.5
    suppressor factor preparation 80.8
HEL system 84.5
Helper circuit 71.5
Helper determinant (HD) 84.4
    dissociation from suppressor deter-
        minant 84.3
Helper T cells *see* Th lymphocyte
Hen egg-white lysozyme *see* HEL
Heparinized   blood   for   leuco-
        cytes 58.2
Hepatitis, chronic immune (CAA),
    auto-immune 79.2
HEPES concentration for mouse cul-
    tures 68.5

HEPES Eagle's gelatin (HEG), preparation 64.22

Heterotopic heart transplant in rat 81.2

High endothelial venules (HEV) 57.18

Histidine 50.7

Histochemical markers 56.13

Histochemistry, phagocyte ectoenzymes 52.2

Histocompatibility antigens, complex loci 104.5

Histotope 84.3

Hodgkin's disease, radiation therapy 81.3

T cell deficiency 81.4

Homology plot of V_H gene sequences 90.1

Hormone, effects on auto-immune traits 82.14

Human alveolar macrophages 50.8

Human BCGF-I 70.3

Human BCGF-II 70.3

Human blood, dendritic cell preparation from 49.6

enrichment 49.7

mononuclear cells from 66.1

Human immune system 66.1

Human leucocyte subpopulations 58.1

Human lymphocyte function 66.1

Human serum albumin as immunogen 67.2

Human T lymphocyte cloning 69.6

Human T-T hybridoma production 69.8

fusion procedure 69.9

hybridization confirmation 69.9

Human tumours 45.2

Hydrocortisone succinate 81.8

Hydrogen peroxide 50.1

detection 50.9

release 50.5

Hydroxyapatite chromatography 76.4

Hydroxyl radical 50.1

chemical assays 50.2, 6

formation 50.5

inhibitors 50.7

measurements 50.5

4-Hydroxy-3-nitrophenacetyl as immunogen 67.2

4-Hydroxy-3-nitrophenyl acetyl 90.2

Hypersensitivity, delayed type cells (TDH) 68.3

after exposure to chemical compounds 77.1

method for induction and transfer in mouse 77.3

passive transfer 77.6

passive transfer assay 77.10

reactivity phases 77.1

syngeneic spleen cell method 77.5

Ts lymphocyte induction methods 77.7

Hypervariable regions 76.7

Hypochlorous acid (HOC1) 50.8

Hypogammaglobulinaemia, neonatal 83.2

Hypogammaglobulinaemia, X-linked 83.1

Ia antigens on cell lines 45.8

detection method 48.10

on macrophages 48.9

Ia specificity 84.1

Ia-antigen complex 75.4

Iα X 84.6

I-J determinant, on T lymphocyte contra-suppressor cell 78.13, 79.2

on T lymphocyte suppressor cell 78.13

IgA, deficiency 83.1

transport receptor 53.2

IgD 53.4

tracing by monoclonal antibody 57.17

IgE, erythrocyte phagocytosis 45.8

monocyte receptors 48.2

receptors on macrophage lines 45.8

IgG, antibody production to hapten 74.2

anti-carrier response assay 74.6

decline after thoracic duct drainage 81.6

deficiency 83.1

erythrocyte lysis 45.8

erythrocyte phagocytosis 45.8

fraction 55.7

ingestion by mononuclear phagocytes 42.2

mouse isotypes 45.8

in opsonization 46.1

proteolysis 47.2

receptors 41.1

response control by epitope 74.2

subclass formation by PBA 63.7

tumour target kill 45.8

IgG1, guinea pig receptors 48.2

monocyte receptors 48.2

IgG2, guinea pig receptors 48.2

preparation 48.2

IgG2a, mouse Fc receptors 48.2

IgG2b, mouse Fc receptors 48.2

IgG3, monocyte receptors 48.2

IgG4, monocyte receptors 48.2

IgM 53.4

anti in sensitizing B cells 70.5

culture secretion 82.6

kinetics in lymphocyte activation response 63.7

monocyte receptors 48.2

tracing by monoclonal antibody 57.17

transport receptor 53.2

Igh allotype markers 56.1

Igh locus 53.3

Idiotype 73.1

antibody role in control 73.2

enhancement 73.2

immune response control by antigen 73.3

recognition by T and B lymphocytes 73.4

regulation 73.1

repertoire 73.2

suppression 73.2

Idiotype determinants 73.1

Idiotype-specific suppressor cells 78.9

Idiotype-specific Ts *in vivo* induction 78.11

Idiotypic repertoire, genetic control 73.3

Idiotypy, specificity 84.6

Immotile cilia syndrome 51.2

Immune circuit 71.1

Immune complex, in macrophage activation 48.11

Immune interferon (IFN), detection 82.12

Immune regulation 84.1

Immune response, adoptive *in vivo* assay 67.1

adoptive transfer 67.1

assay methods 67.6

compartmentalization 84.7

genes, control 84.1

idiotypic control by antigen 73.3

soluble suppressor (SIRS) 78.5

suppression by Ts 75.5

Ts assessment in 78.1

to transplantation 81.1

Immune system network hypothesis 73.1

Immune tolerance 74.5

Immunoadhesion 55.5

Immunoadsorbent *see also* Enzyme-linked immunosorbent assay (ELISA)

for antigen-specific suppressor factor 80.4

in immunoglobulin assay 66.7

insoluble, preparation 64.20

Immunoblotting, Western 47.14

Immunocytochemical assay, for mouse tissue antigen 43.9

reagents 43.9

staining 43.10

Immunodeficiency, common variable 83.2

definitions 83.1

human diseases 83.1

severe combined (SCID) 83.2

X-chromosome linked 56.14

Immunofluorescence, assays for mouse tissue antigens 43.8

cell preparations, human leucocytes 58.5

FACS analysis 43.8

for Ia alloantigen detection 48.10

Immunogen, materials 67.2
    BSA 67.2
    CGG 67.2
    DNP 67.2
    HSA 67.2
    KLH 67.2
    MGG 67.2
    NIP 67.2
    OA 67.2
    OX 67.2
    preparation method 67.2
Immunoglobulin, antigen-induced pro-
    duction assay 66.10
    assay by ELISA 66.7
    B lymphocyte assay 66.4
    B lymphocyte surface 53.1
    binding of aggregated 48.3
    classes 64.1
    in culture supernatants 63.6
    deficiency with increased IgM 83.1
    determination 83.3
    gene rearrangements 53.2, 62.4
    genetic basis for formation 69.1
    goat anti-rat 44.9
    macrophage elastase from 47.22
    mouse variable region sequences
        90.1
    in PBA activation 63.6
    production evaluation *in vitro* 66.6
    production suppression 66.11
    PWM-induced production assay
        66.9
    secretion assay 66.9, 82.8
    selected isotype deficiency 83.1
    specific helper T cells (IgTh) 71.2
    subclass response to epitope 74.1
    synthesis by pokeweed mitogen
        58.10
    T-suppressor analogy 75.5
Immunoglobulin,-secreting cells 64.1
    affinity prepared antibodies 64.19
    autoradiography 64.6, 9
    Cunningham method 64.6
    Jerne plaque assay 64.2
    localized haemolysis in gel (LHG)
        64.1
    micromanipulation 64.7
    mixed antigens 64.9
    monolayer (Cunningham) technique
        64.6
    petri-dish (Jerne plaque) assay 64.2
    preparation of assay plates 64.3
    procedure 64.3
Immunoglobulin-specific Ts lympho-
    cyte 71.4
Immunogravitation 55.8
Immunolocalization 47.9
Immunological markers 56.13
Immunological memory 74.5
Immunology, history 62.1
Immunomagnetic methods for cell
    separation 55.12
Immunoperoxidase, antibody detec-
    tion 48.2

staining 57.16
    for Ia alloantigen detection
        48.10
Immunoprecipitation 47.13
Immunosuppression, agents 81.1
    arachidonic acid 81.7
    assessment techniques 81.2
    experimental procedures 81.3
    mediators 75.5
    monoclonal antibodies as agents
        81.10
    non-specific 81.2
    in transplantation 81.1
Immunotoxicity 55.3
Indirect binding assays (IBA) 43.4
Indirect plaque-forming cells (PFC)
    64.1
Indium-III lymphocyte labelling
    method 57.7
Inducer set of T lymphocyte 75.1
    peptide secretion 75.4
Inducer T cell 71.1
Inflammatory reaction, monocytes
    on 42.3
Inflammatory response, chemotactic
    peptides in 48.9
    lectin-like receptors in 48.9
Influenza virus, antibody response
    58.11
Intracellular recognition 53.2
Interferon 45.10, 47.4, 53.4, 59.1
    cyclosporin A effect 81.13
    immune (IFN), detection 82.12
    as NK regulator 60.1
    poly I: C induced 45.6
Interleukin 53.4, 59.1
    as NK regulator 60.7
    production 59.4
Interleukin 1 45.6, 47.4, 70.3
    release inhibition by cyclosporin
        A 81.14
Interleukin-2 68.1, 69.1
    biological activity 68.10
    human, for cloning human T lym-
        phocytes 69.6
        for supernatant production 69.7
    microassay method 69.3
    production inhibition by cyclosporin
        A 81.14
    production measurement 82.11
    receptor inhibition by cyclosporin
        A 81.14
    for T lymphocyte culture 69.1
    test for presence 68.11
International lymphokine workshop
    69.1
Intestines, grafting 81.11
Intracellular organisms, T lymphocyte
    defence 68.3
Intralipid 20% 81.8
Iodination, fibrinogen 47.15
    of ligands 43.11
    proteins 67.7
Iγ Code, T lymphocyte activation

72.1
Iγ genes 72.1
    transplantation antigen coding
        72.1
Iron, to remove phagocytes 55.12
Iron-dextran polymers 55.12
Irradiation, of cells 81.3
    inverted Y field 81.4
    mantle field 81.4
    of mouse 67.6
    total lymphoid, in clinical trans-
        plants 81.3
        in dogs 81.4
        immune monitoring 81.3
        in primates 81.3
    whole body 81.2
Isoelectrically focussed (IEF) over-
    lay 64.11
Isotype, regulation 74.2
IUDR-labelled target cell elimina-
    tion 60.6
^{125}IUd R, lymphocyte labelling
    method 57.10

Jerne, N.K. 62.2
Jerne plaque assay 64.2
Jurkat line of human T leukaemia
    69.9

K-chain deficiency 83.2
Ketanserin 81.8
2-Keto-4-thiomethylbutyric acid 50.5
Keyhole limpet haemocyanin (KLH)
    74.7
    as immunogen 67.2
    for suppressor factor preparation
        80.1
    specific, induction of Ts 78.7
    specific responses, assay 78.6
    specific suppressor factor (KLH-TsF)
        80.4
    specific, TsF induction 78.7
    trinitrophenylated-(TNP-
        KLH) 78.5
Kidney grafting, between twins 81.1
    rejection treatment by OKT3
        81.10
        thoracic duct drainage in 81.5
    inflammation studies 82.6
Klinokinesis 51.2
Küpffer cell *see also* Macro-
    phage 46.1
    in mice 42.2

Lactate dehydrogenase (LDH) 52.1
Lactoferrin 46.2, 48.1
Lactoperoxidase (LPO), in phagocy-
    tosis 41.3
LAF *see* Lymphocyte activating factor
Langerhans' cells 53.4
    in delayed type hypersensiti-
        vity 77.1
Laser, dye 44.14
Latex particles 50.1

Lazy leucocyte syndrome 41.5
Lectin, in chromatography 55.6
  T cell induction 63.8
    response analysis 63.11
    "step 1" and "step 2" activities 63.11
  Vicia Villosa assay 79.3
Lectin-like receptors 48.9
  detection methods 48.9
  in inflammatory response 48.9
Leishmania tropica, macrophage cytotoxicity to 45.8
Leucine aminopeptidase, assay 52.5
Leucine-^{14}C, lymphocyte labelling method 57.8
Leucine-^{3}H lymphocyte labelling method 57.8
Leucophoresis 57.3
Leukocyte, chemotaxis 51.1
  chambers 51.5
    demonstration 51.14
    visual assay 51.5
  common antigen 55.4
  contact guidance 51.3
  counting methods 51.7
  fluorescence activated cell sorting 58.5
  human, complement receptor 1 48.5
    complement receptor 2 48.5
    complement receptor 3 48.5
  indirect immunofluorescence 58.5
  isolation from blood 64.18
  of T lymphocytes from 69.9
  'leading front' migration measurement 51.7
  locomotion 51.1
    assay 51.4
    random 51.1
  oxygen excitation techniques 50.1
  phagocytic 41.6, 50.1
  in phagocytosis assay 46.6
  soluble stimuli 50.3
  subpopulations 58.1
  subset, function assays 58.9
    techniques 58.1
  time-lapse cinematography 51.11
Leukaemia lines, surface antigens 45.8
Leukotrienes 81.7
Library screening with subtracted probes 76.4
Ligand, attachment to carrier particles 48.1
  particulate 48.1
  physical nature 48.1
  soluble 48.1
Light chain, suppressor factor preparation 80.8
Lignocain hydrochloride 55.8
Limiting dilution analysis 65.1, 68.9
  assay systems 65.2
  limiting cell functions 65.3
  cloning 68.12
  of primed responder cells 69.4

for human T cell cloning 69.7
for T lymphocyte clones 69.2
Limiting effector cell, functional analysis 65.3
Linked recognition of cells 71.1
Lipopolysaccharide (LPS), for cell activation 63.1
  cytolytic activity 45.5
  cytotoxicity 45.8
Lipoprotein lipase 47.3
Listeria, in macrophage activation 48.11
Liver, lymphocyte traffic 57.5
Localized haemolysis, in gel (LHG) 64.1
  assay on slides 64.4
  cytotoxicity 64.12
Lowry protein assay 43.12
Luminol, phagocytic oxidation 50.4
Lungs, grafting 81.11
  lymphocyte traffic 57.5
Lupus erythematosus, mouse models 82.1
  Ts lymphocyte loss 79.2
Lymph node, blood flow to 57.2
  high endothelial venules in
  inhibition assay methods 77.9
  lymphocyte leaving rate 57.2
  lymphocyte traffic 57.2
  mononuclear cells from 66.3
  T cell localization 57.2
Lymphochoriomeningitis virus, (LCMV) 72.2
Lymphocyte activating factor (LAF)
  cytotoxic T cell induction 45.6
  production and assay 63.10
Lymphocyte, activity separation profile 55.2
  activators 63.1
  antigen (Ly) 61.1
  antigen receptors 67.1, 75.4
  assays
    cell density 63.1
    non-specific killer 63.10
    proliferation 63.10
  biology 62.1
  blast transformation, methods *in vitro* 66.5
    PWM or TT 66.6
    to T lymphocyte mitogens 66.6
  cell cycle analysis of activation 82.8
  cell surface alloantigens 61.1
  cell tracing 57.2
  chimaera 81.4
  chromium (^{51}Cr) labelled method 57.5
  communication 84.7
  counting 54.4
    culture for activation 75.6
  Ficoll-Hypaque 54.9
  depletion by thoracic duct fistula 81.6
  detection threshold 55.1
  differentiation 79.2

DNA synthesis 57.9
enrichment separation profile 55.2
fluorescence microscopy 57.12
fractionation of sub-populations 54.1, 55.1
  antibody coated column 55.7
  by electrophoresis 55.13
  by immunomagnetic methods 55.12
  by physical adherence 55.5
  by density 54.8
  electrophoresis 54.9
  by physical adherence 54.7
  by sedimentation 54.5
function evaluation *in vitro* 66.1
germinal center 57.15
growth and differentiation factors 62.4
HEV binding, frozen section assay 57.19
  quantification 57.20
  interaction *in vitro* assay 57.18
immunosuppressive antisera to 81.2
indium-III labelling method 57.7
influx measurement by rubidium-86 57.12
injected 57.16
interaction history 62.2
in vitro antibodies 57.4
in vitro enzymes 57.4
in vitro lectins 57.4
^{125}IU labelling method 57.10, 11
labelling 57.5
large granular (LGL) 60.1
leucine-^{14}C labelling method 57.8
leucine-^{3}H labelling method 57.8
life span 57.10
maturation 57.18
migration 57.1
overview 53.1
peripheral blood sampling 68.5
phenotyping 57.15
radioactive labelling 57.10, 63.10
  DNA precursors *in vivo* 57.10
  for DNA synthesis *in vivo* 57.10
  detection of labelled cells 57.11
    autoradiography 57.11
    organ counting 57.12
recirculating pool 57.1
rejection 57.4
responder cell 68.1
rosetting 55.8
size analysis 54.4
specific genes 76.2
stimulator cells 68.1
subsets 62.4
surface marker identification 66.3
suspensions, azide 55.2
suspension preparation 54.4
U-^{14}C-thymidine- labelling method 57.9
6-^{3}H-thymidine- labelling method 57.9
tracing by radioactive labelling

Lymphocyte (*cont.*)
  57.5
  traffic 57.1
    examination in bone-marrow
    57.5
      in liver 57.5
      in lungs 57.5
      in lymph nodes 57.5
      in Peyer's patches 57.5
    tracer sample principle 57.3
    uridine-5³-H labelling method 57.8
    uridine-¹⁴C(U) labelling method
    57.8
  vascular endothelium 57.1
  virgin 62.4
Lymphocyte activation 63.1
  culture 63.3
  method 63.3
  preparation of cultures 63.3
  preparation of suspensions 63.3
  response measurements 63.5
    Ig secretion 63.7
  subculture IgM kinetics 63.7
Lymphocyte-produced soluble media-
    tor (FACTOR) 78.1
Lymphoid cells, cyclosporin A
    action 81.12
  Fc receptor 48.2
  human population method 66.1
Lymphoid tissue, in antibody produc-
    tion 62.1
  antigen presenting 53.4
  cell harvesting 64.17
  peripheral 53.6
Lymphokine, cell biology 59.1
  comparison of assay systems 59.4
  culture from unfractionated cells
    59.2
  cytolytic activity 45.5
  cytotoxicity 45.8
  growth factors 59.1
  induction assays 59.5
  production from cloned T lympho-
    cytes 59.3
  production methods 59.2
  production, from T lymphocyte
    tumours 59.3
    from T lymphoma 69.1
  proliferative assays 59.5
  purification 59.6
  recombinant DNA production
    methods 59.6
  titration curves 59.6
  unit of activity definition 59.6
Lymphokine activated cells 50.3, 63.1
Lymphokine-mediated events 47.6
Lymphoma 57.19
  Abelson 45.1
Lymphoneogenesis 62.4
Lymphoproliferation assay method
    58.9
Lymphoreticular tumours for target
    cells 68.6
Lymphotoxin 59.1

Lysosomal enzymes, macrophage pro-
    duction 45.7
Lysozyme 46.2, 47.1
  determinant 84.4
  immune response 84.1
  from macrophage cell lines 45.5
  specificity 84.5
Lysozyme plate assay 47.24
Lytic activity per culture 68.7

Macrophage 46.1, 47.1
  acid hydrolases 47.3
  activated 47.1, 6, 48.11, 50.3, 52.3
  activation with intracellular path-
    ogens 48.11
  adherent cell removal 44.6
  alpha₂-Macroglobulin 47.3, 14
  as antigen presenting cell (APC)
    48.1, 9, 53.4
  cell culture 47.18
  cell-free fractions 47.19
  cell lines 45.1
    culture method 45.3
    cytolytic activity 45.3
    defects 45.9
    Fc-mediated effects 45.8
    harvesting 45.3
    Ia and macrophage-restricted
      antigen expression 45.9
    immature 45.6
    mature 45.5
    microbial parasites 45.7
    mouse 45.4, 6
    mycoplasma contamin-
      ation 45.4
    parasite–host interaction 45.8
    repositories 45.3
    secretions 45.5
    stability 45.4
    tumours 45.1
    viral transformation 45.2
  cell lysates 47.18
  cell suspension preparation 44.5
  in chronic inflammatory condi-
    tions 48.5
  coagulation factors 47.3
  conditioned medium collection
    47.18
  differentiation state responses 41.8
  elastase 47.2
    assay 47.21
  elicited 50.3
  environmental regulation 48.10
  factor B 47.3
  factor D 47.3
  fibrinolysis enhancement 47.20
  fibrinolytic activity 47.7
  Fc binding to immunoglobulin
    43.4
  Fc receptors 48.2
  growth factor 44.1
  human alveolar 50.8
  Ia antigens 48.9
  inflammatory 47.6

  inhibition factor (MIF) 59.1
  in vitro studies 42.2
  in intracellular killing test 46.8
  isolation, from lung 48.13
    mouse 45.2, 63.9, 68.6
    from peritoneum 48.12
    from tissue 48.14
  labelling method 47.9
  labelling with monoclonal antibodies
    (MAbs) 44.6
  lymphokine activated 50.3
  lymphokine growth factor 59.1
  lysosomal enzyme release 48.5
  lysozyme assay 47.24
  markers 47.6
  membrane receptors 48.1
  mouse 43.1
    adherent populations 43.12
    origin and function 48.11
    oxidative metabolism 50.3
    particle ingestion 41.3, 46.1
    in phagocytosis assay 46.7
    plasminogen activators 47.2
    procoagulant activity 47.3
    proteinases 47.1
      classification 47.3
    receptor signal generation 41.8
    resident 47.6, 48.11, 50.3
    secretion regulation 47.7
    secretory activity 41.7
    secretory products 47.1
    sources 47.18
      preparation and induction 48.12
    spreading rate 41.8
    stimulating agents 48.11
    surface receptors 41.10
    synthesis and secretion patterns
      47.12
    tissue 43.1
Macrophage lineage, human, imma-
    ture 45.7
  mouse, immature 45.6
Macrophage-restricted antigens 45.8
Major histocompatibility complex,
    antigens 62.4, 68.1
  function 72.1
  stimulation of immune sys-
    tem 72.1
  class I genetic organization 68.3
  co-recognition 75.2
  genetic mapping in mouse 53.2
  haplotype specificity 84.2
  I-A products 48.9
  Ir coding 72.1
  interaction sites 84.3
  in mouse genetic response 78.7
  precursor restriction to Th lympho-
    cyte 65.3
  restricted cytotoxic responses 68.2
  restricted function 65.3
  restricted virus specific cytotoxic
    cells 68.3
  restriction specificities 65.4
  role 62.3

Major histocomp. complex (*cont.*)
  significance 72.1
  and tissue transplantation 72.1
Major histocompatibility locus 53.2
Mancini radial immunodiffusion technique 64.21
Mannitol 50.7
Mannosyl, fucosyl receptor (MFR) 43.1
  assay method 43.11
    ligand iodination 43.11
  properties 43.3
Marker, non-antigenic 57.18
Marker chromosomes, C-banding 82.16
Mast cell, IgE receptor 48.2
  lymphokine growth factor 59.1
Mediator production assay 66.13
Medium, lymphocyte-conditioned 47.20
  for lymphocyte culture 78.3
  minimum essential (MEM) 82.10
Membrane, patching 44.14
Membrane receptors, macrophage 48.1
6-Mercaptopurine 81.2
Mercury-sulphur bridge, chemically cleavable 55.6
Methane production from dimethylsulfoxide assay test 50.5
Methionine 50.7
Methylated bovine serum albumin (MBSA) 78.7
Metrizoate–Ficoll separation 55.11
MHC *see* Major histocompatibility complex
Microcytotoxicity assay 69.9
Micromanipulation 64.7
  for T lymphocyte clones 69.2
Micropore filter assay 51.4
  method 51.5
Microvascular surgery 81.2
  cuffing procedure 81.2
Migration inhibition factor 47.7
Mineral oil, macrophage stimulator 48.11
Minor histocompatibility (H) antigens 68.1, 2
  immune response to 68.9
Mishell–Dutton medium 78.3
  preparation 78.14
Mishell–Dutton culture system 80.3
Mitogens 47.4
  of lymphocyte 59.3, 63.8, 66.6
  receptors 70.1
  responses to T cells 83.4
Mixed antigens 64.9
Mixed lymphocyte culture (MLC) 68.1, 69.5
  anti-hapten responses 68.2
  cytotoxic T cell ^{51}Cr assay 68.5
  cytotoxicity assay *in vitro* 68.9
    assessment of results 68.10

memory 68.2
minor histocompatibility antigens 68.2
preparation 68.6
primary 69.3
secondary 69.3
synergy 68.2
for T lymphocyte cytotoxic response *in vitro* 68.3
Mixed lymphocyte reaction, abnormal autologous 82.8
Molecular genetics 53.2
Molecular genetic analysis 82.16
  DNA probes 82.18
  cDNA synthesis 82.18
  mRNA *in vitro* translation 82.18
Monoblast, cell cycle 42.2
Monoclonal antibody, assay 80.3
  bound cell percentage 44.15
  fluorochrome labelling 44.14
  FcR Fc receptor 58.3
  functional assays 69.9
  functional human T-T production 69.8
  as immunosuppressive agent 81.10
  for labelling murine macrophages 44.6
    determining viability 44.7
    fixation of cells 44.7
    recommendations 44.7
    second reagents 44.7
  limiting dilution analysis 65.1
  for lymphokine purification 59.7
  in macrophage receptor function 41.9
  to mononuclear phagocytes 42.1
  to mouse macrophage 43.1
  to mouse alloantigen 61.4
  panning for cell separation 58.6
  secreted suppressor factor 80.3
  specificity 84.6
  suppressor factor from 80.2
  from T lymphocyte 69.1
  T lymphocyte assay 66.4
  T-T mouse production method 69.10
  techniques 53.1
Monoclonal suppressor factor 80.1
Monocyte, Fc receptors 48.2
  human intracellular killing 46.16
    in phagocytosis assay 46.6
  inflammatory reaction 42.3
  isolation from peripheral blood 48.14
  mouse kinetic studies 42.2
  PMA receptor 50.3
  production regulation 42.3
Monocyte production inhibitor (MPI) 42.4
Mononuclear phagocyte 42.1, 44.1, 46.1
  cell differentiation mechanism 44.1
  cell line 42.1
  characterization 42.1

clonal heterogeneity 44.1
counting methods 44.4
culture methods 44.5
enzyme markers 42.1
functional heterogeneity 44.1
monoclonal antibody reaction 42.1
mouse 43.1
preparation medium 44.16
protein radiolabelling method 47.9
receptors 42.1
solutions 44.16
system (MPS) 42.4
see also Monocyte *and* Macrophage
α Morpholinopropane sulphonic acid (α MOPS) 44.2
  preparation 44.16
Mouse antibodies to T lymphocyte antigens 55.3
BCGF-I 70.1
  assay 70.4
  properties 70.5
    purification method 70.6
  sources 70.5
  units 70.5
BCGF-II 70.2
cell surface alloantigens 61.1
contact sensitivity induction 77.3
delayed hypersensitivity method 77.3
  passive transfer 77.6
  sensitization 77.6
dendritic cells 49.1
  preparation 49.3, 5
Dexter cultures 45.2
Fc receptor 48.2
gamma globulin as immunogen 67.2
genetic marker preparation 56.3
glycoprotein T200 55.4
hyperdiploid cell analysis 82.16
  immunization method 67.3
inbred auto-immune 82.14
irradiation 67.6
lupus models 82.1
macrophage 43.1
  cell lines 45.4, 6
  enzymes 45.6
MHC general mapping 53.2
natural killer cells 60.2
recombinant inbred 61.5, 82.13
T-T hybrid production 69.10
tissue degradation assays 43.12
  single cell assays 43.12
V_H sequences classification 90.1
Multiple cell harvester 63.10
Murine sarcoma virus (MSV) 68.3
Mycobacterium, in macrophage activation 48.11
Mycology, DTH reactions 77.1
Mycoplasma contamination of cell lines 45.4
Myelin, basic protein 47.2
Myeloma, mouse transplantable 64.18

Myeloma protein mixture 44.17
Myeloperoxidase deficiency in phago-
        cytes 46.2
Myosin in phagocytosis 41.5

Natural killer (NK) cells 50.3, 53.3,
        60.1, 81.12
    adherence 60.3
    biological substance regulation of
        lysis 60.7
    definition 60.1
    density 60.3
    growth *in vitro* 60.8
    handling 60.1
    in vitro assays 60.4, 5
    morphology 60.7
    specificity 60.7
    subfractionation 60.3
    surface markers 60.4
    suspension preparation 60.2
    target cell elimination 60.6
Naudicelle 81.8
Neonatal hypogammaglobulinaemia
    83.2
Neonatal suppression of idio-
        type 73.2
Network hypothesis 73.1
    limitations 73.3
Neuraminidase 55.9
Neutrophil, Fc receptors 48.2
    locomotion 51.1
    oxygen consumption 50.3
Nitroblue tetrazolium (NBT) 46.5
    reduction 50.8
    test 50.9
Nitrogen, liquid for macrophage cell
        line storage 45.3
NK cells *see* Natural killer cells
Noncognate interactions of lympho-
        cytes 71.5
Non-erythrocyte antigens 64.12
Non-specific immunosuppression
    81.2
Nonspecific killer assay 63.10
Northern blot analysis 76.6
Nucleated target cells 64.16
5′-Nucleotidase as activation
        marker 52.2
    as ecto-enzyme 52.1
    assay method 52.3
Nylon wool column, cell adher-
        ence 60.3
    immunoselective method 55.5
    in lymphocyte separation 55.1

OKT3 for rejection treatment 81.10
OKT 4/OKT 8 ratio post-transplant
        change 81.13
Oligonucleotide probes 76.1
Oncogene 62.5, 82.16
Oncogenic viruses 68.3
Orcein staining 56.4
Orientation assay 51.4
    method 51.9

Orthokinesis 51.2
Oxygen, consumption 50.4
    leukocyte stimulation 50.1
    reactive metabolites 47.6
    singlet 50.1

PBS *see* Phosphate-buffered saline
PGK, blood analysis 56.12
Panning 55.7
Paraformaldehyde, buffered 44.16
Paraquat 50.11
Pasteur, Louis 62.1
Peanut agglutinin 55.9
Percoll cell fractionation 58.13
Periodate, lysine and paraformalde-
        hyde (PLP) fixative 43.11
Peripheral blood leukocytes (PBL)
        64.18
Peripheral blood lymphocytes
        (PBL) 69.6
Peripheral blood mononuclear (PBM)
        cells, separation 58.1, 66.2
Peripheral blood mononuclear leuco-
        cytes 69.9
Peritoneal cells from mouse 68.8
Peroxidase, as catalyst 50.5
    horseradish 50.5
    macrophage production 45.7
    secretion by macrophage lines 45.6
Peroxidase enzyme immunoassay sub-
        stance 58.15
Peroxidase-H_2O_2-halide systems 50.7
Peroxy radicals 50.5
Peyer's patch, dendritic cell pre-
        paration 49.5
    high endothelial venules (HEV)
        57.18
    lymphocyte traffic 57.5
    T lymphocytes 79.1, 4
    localization 57.18
PHA *see* Phytohaemagglutinin
Phagocyte analyses 44.10
    flow cytometry 44.11
    microscopic method 44.11
    attachment to 41.1
    autofluorescence 44.14
    chemical assays 50.2
    cytochemical assays 50.2
    ecto-enzymes 52.1
        assay 52.3
        histochemical techniques 52.2
    erythrophagocytosis, complement-
        coated red cells 42.3
    isolation, from blood 46.3
        from mouse 44.2
            alveoli 44.3
            bone marrow 44.2
            mouse peritoneum 46.6
            peripheral blood 44.8
            peritoneal exudate 44.3
    microbicidal system 46.3
        methods 46.3, 5
    myeloperoxidase deficiency 46.2
    particle engulfment 41.1

plasma membrane enzymes 52.2
polymorphonuclear 46.1
receptor function 41.1
respirometric studies 50.4
Phagocytic index 46.9
Phagocytic leukocytes 50.1
    oxidative metabolism 50.1, 8
    cytochemical techniques 50.2
Phagocytosis, antibody-dependent
        45.5
    assessment 46.3
    C-mediated 45.10
    EA 45.10
    complement 41.1
    for fibrinolysis 47.20
    homeostatic function 41.1
    immune 42.2, 45.5, 46.1
    inhibition 41.5
    in vitro methods 46.1
        bacteria 46.4
        calculations 46.9
        isolation of cells 46.3
        materials 46.5
            media and sera 46.5
            tubes 46.6
        particle isolation 46.2
        viability of cells 46.6
    killing index 46.9
    of latex or zymosan beads 45.5
    in leucocyte metabolism 50.1
    metabolic processes 41.5
    micro-method determination 46.8
    morphological assessment 46.7
    opsonization 46.1
    phosphorylation specificity 41.8
    plasma membrane receptors 41.10
    rate determination 46.4, 5
    receptor problems 41.9
    receptor-mediated ion flux 41.16
    test 46.9
        kinetics 46.10
        zipper mechanism 41.3, 46.2
Phagocytosis-promoting receptors
        41.2, 3
Phagolysosome, latex-contain-
        ing 41.5
Phagosome, formation 46.2
Phenol-metacresol 86.5
Phenotype analysis 79.2
Phenylmethylsulfonylfluoride
        (PMSF) 80.1
Phorbol myristate acetate (PMA)
        50.3, 59.3
    cell stimulation 69.2
    cytolytic activity 45.5
    cytotoxicity 45.6
    for IL-2 measurement 82.11
    macrophage line stimulation 45.6
    for mouse BCGF-I 70.5
    proliferative effect 81.13
Phosphate-buffered saline 44.16
    preparation 78.14
Phosphoglycerate kinase (PGK-1)
        56.7, 57.18

Phosphoryl choline, *in vitro* techniques 78.12
  idiotype response assay 78.10
Phosphorylcholine-specific responses in B lymphocytes 65.3
Photography, for immunoglobulin-secreting cells 64.9
Phytohaemagglutinin 58.10, 59.3, 63.1, 14
Pig, heart graft 81.11
Pinocytosis 45.10
Plaque assay, haemolytic 64.2
  reversed 64.16
Plaque definition 64.1
  inhibition 64.9
  pseudo- 64.17
  zones of inhibited phage 64.16
Plaque forming cells (PFC) 65.2
  assay method 66.7
  direct 64.1
  indirect 64.1
Plasma cell antigen 61.1
  investigation 62.1
Plasma membrane, enzymes 52.1
  markers 43.1
  macrophage changes 43.3
  phagocyte 52.2
Plasminogen activator 45.10, 47.1
  assay 47.14
  electrophoresis 47.20
  purification 47.17
Platelet, Fc receptors 48.2
PMA *see* Phorbol myristate acetate
Pneumococcal C-polysaccharide (PnC) extraction method 78.10
Pneumococcal vaccine preparation 78.10
Poisson distribution 68.10
Pokeweed mitogen (PWM) 58.10
  immunoglobulin synthesis by 58.10
Polyacrylamide 55.5
Polyacrylamide gel electrophoresis 47.8, 53.1
Polyanions, in macrophage activation 48.11
Polyclonal activators (PA) 63.1
Polyclonal B cell activator (PBA) 63.1
Polyclonal T cell activators 63.8
Polyethylene glycol for cell fusion 69.8
Poly Gluco, ALA 30, TYR 10 90.1
Polymethylmethacrylate 55.5
  beads 55.6
Polyribose phosphate 83.4
C-Polysaccharide, sheep erythrocytes coated in 78.11
Polystyrene 55.5
Polyvinyl pyrrolidone (PVP) 54.9
Precursor, *in vitro* isolation and expansion 65.4
Precursor set of T lymphocyte 75.1
Primed responder cells (PRC) 69.3
  limit dilution cloning 69.4

soft agar cloning 69.4
Procoagulant activity 45.10
Pronase 44.16
Properdin 47.3
Propidium iodide 44.7
Prostacyclins 81.7, 81.8
Prostaglandins 81.7
  E group 45.6, 81.7, 81.8
Protease peptone broth, macrophage stimulator 48.11
Protein, iodinated 67.7
  in lymphocyte activation 63.8
Proteinase 47.1
Alpha,-proteinase inhibitor, proteolysis 47.2
Proteinuria 82.6
Proteolytic enzymes 52.2
Prothymocyte 53.5
Protozoology, macrophage interactions 45.8
Pseudoplaques 64.17
Purine, metabolites 47.6
Purine nucleoside phosphorylase deficiency 83.2
Pyronin Y (PY) technique 82.9

R3 for complement 48.6
RNA, cytotoxic inhibition assays 80.7
  functional assays 80.7
  preparation 80.5
  purification 80.6
  sucrose density gradient centrifugation 80.6
  translation 47.8
    into oocytes 80.7
  translation product 80.7
  detection 80.7
  heavy or light chain reconstitution 80.8
Rabbit antibody in PCA 33.6
Radiation toxicity 57.7
Radioactive labelling of lymphocyte 57.10, 63,10
Radioimmunoassay, anti-hapten antibody responses 74.6
  autoradiography 43.6
  indirect binding assay 43.5
  intact cell procedure 43.5
  mouse antigen methods 43.4
  plate assay with immobilized cells 43.5
  soluble antigen procedure 43.6
  tube assay 43.6
  serum antibody measurement 78.4
  solid phase antibody 80.4
Radiolabelling of antigens 67.7
Rat, antibodies to T lymphocyte antigens 55.3
  dendritic cell preparation 49.6
  kappa allotype congenic 57.17
Rat techniques 81.2, 7
Receptors, phagocytosis-promoting 41.2, 3

Recloning 68.13
Recombinant DNA 62.3
  for cell lines 68.13
  methods, for lymphokine production 59.6
Recombinant inbred strains, mouse 104.4
Regression analysis 68.7
Regulatory circuits and antibody production 74.1
Regulatory idiotope 84.6
Regulatory memory 74.5
Replica analysis 64.8
Resorcinol assay of DASA 52.6
Respiratory burst of leucocytes 50.3
Reversed plaque assay 64.16
  universal method 64.17
Rheumatoid arthritis, Ts cell loss 79.2
  total lymphoid irradiation 81.5
Rheumatoid factor (RF) plaques 64.14
RIA *see* Radioimmunoassay
RNA, analytical reactant 76.5
  content determination 82.9
  cytoplasmic versus total 76.5
  in vitro translation 82.18
  mRNA population comparison 76.1
  repeated sequences 76.6
  subset, back reactions 76.5
Rosette aggregation 55.12
  assays 48.2
    method 48.2
    for Ia antigens 48.10
  direct formation method 58.5
  formation by lymphocyte 55.8
    method 55.10
    for T cell assay 66.3
  test, for antibodies 58.4
    for human leucocytes 58.2
  separation 55.10
RPMI-1640 60.9
Rubber policeman 55.8
Rubidium-86, to measure lymphocyte influx 57.12

Saturation indirect binding assay 43.4
Scopoletin 50.5
  and horseradish peroxidase 50.5
Sedimentation separation 54.5
Sensitization of skin 77.3
Sephadex 55.5
Sepharose 55.5
Serum, AB chelated with EDTA 48.7
  acid-treated 47.17
  anti-immunoglobulin 64.18
  anti-thymocyte 67.4
  antibody assay 67.7
  complement from 48.6
  developing 64.4
  fetal bovine 45.3
  opsonic activity 46.11

Severe combined immunodeficiency (SCID) 83.2
enzyme measurements 83.5
Sheep erythrocyte, 2-aminoethylisothiouronium-treated 66.11
for plaque assay 78.2
C-polysaccharide coated 78.11
factor 78.6
lymphatics 57.2
gamma camera imaging 57.8
rosetting 66.3
staphylococcal protein A-coated 66.7
suppressor cells 78.5
for suppressor factor preparation 80.1
Silent clones 73.4
Singlet oxygen 50.1
chemical assays 50.2
detection
formation 50.7
quenchers 50.7
Skin antigen 61.1
Skin grafts 81.2
Slice technique for cell assay 64.10
Sodium azide 44.17
Sodium dodecyl sulphate, elastinolysis enhancement 47.23
Sodium phosphate buffer 52.7
Sodium pyrophosphate 44.16
Sodium salicylate 81.8
Soft agar cloning of primed responder cells 69.4
Solid-phase radioimmune assay: plate binding assay 80.4
Soluble immune response suppressor 78.5
Soluble suppressor factors 80.1
Somatic mutation 80.1
Somatic variation 80.4
Sorensen's glycine II buffer, preparation 52.7
Specific lysis calculation 68.7
Specificity of antigen-antibody interaction 55.5
Spectroscopic measurement of assay 68.8
Spleen, antibody production 62.1
antibody-producing cells from 64.17
cell cultures 78.3
immunoglobulin-secreting cell assay 82.8
lymph node cell from 67.4
lymphocytes from 63.9, 68.4, 8
lymphocyte traffic 57.4, 5
mononuclear cells from 66.3
mouse hyperdiploid cell analysis 82.16
natural killer cells from 60.2
T lymphocyte suppressor factor 80.1
Staphylococcal protein A coated SRBC 66.7
plaque assay 63.7

Stem cells 53.5
abnormality studies 82.12
Steroids, high dose 81.2
Subtractive hybridization 76.1
Sucrose density gradient 80.6
Sudan black stain 56.7
Supernatant culture production method 69.2
containing human IL-2 69.7
Superoxide 50.1
dismutase (SOD) 50.4
release measurement 50.4
Superoxide anion, macrophage line secretion 45.6
Suppressor cell inducing determinant 84.4
Suppressor circuit 71.5
Suppressor determinant, dissociation from helper determinant 84.3
Suppressor factor, extraction from monoclonal antibody 80.2
secreted form 80.3
Surface active agents, for leucocyte metabolism 50.1
Surface antigen, in leukaemia cell lines 45.8
Systemic lupus erythematosus *see* Lupus erythematosus

T leukaemia cell lines 69.6
Jurkat line 69.9
T lymphocyte 62.2
acceptor 71.5
activation by antigen 69.1
pathways 68.2
activators 63.8
assays 63.10
methods 63.9
antigen-reactive 75.2
antigen receptors 53.2
antigen recognition 72.2
antigen sensitized 69.8
antigen-specific clones 70.7
mouse 69.6
repertoire 84.2
suppressor factor production 80.1
antigen specificity 53.2
antigenic markers 75.1
carrier-specific augmenting (CTa) 71.3
cell isolation and activation 69.9
cell separation 68.2
cell sets 75.1
co-recognition 75.2
cell surface glycoproteins 53.2
phenotypes 68.6
cloning 68.2
method 68.12
differentiation 68.10
frequency 68.12
function evaluation 66.10

limiting dilution analyses 68.9
precursor frequency 68.10, 12
protective response against viruses 68.3
responses, anti viral 68.2
cloned 69.1
clones 53.1, 68.1
analysis 75.3
antigen specificity 68.2
cell surface phenotype 68.3
definition 75.1
functional characteristics 68.2
generation and uses 68.2
growth and maintenance 69.1
homogeneous populations 68.3
human 69.6
immunologic activity 75.6
interleukin-2 dependent 68.2
receptor composition 68.3
target cell killing 68.2
specificity 68.2
in vitro 53.3
constant (C) regions 76.7
determinants 80.4
contrasuppressor 71.6, 78.1, 79.1
contrasuppressor effector cell culture 79.6
co-ordinate programming 75.3
^{51}Cr release assay 68.5
culture for activation 63.9
cytolytic 63.13
clones 69.1
cytotoxic 63.10, 68.1
abnormal generation 82.9
clones 68.13
differentiation 68.1
effectors 68.1
function assay 66.11
generation 68.13
in vitro 68.3
MHC restricted 68.1
response 68.2
analysis 68.1
to histocompatibility antigens 68.3
to MHC antigens 68.3
to minor histocompatibility antigens 68.3
separation of subpopulations 68.9
and assay *in vivo* 68.8
target cell specificity 68.1
transfectant analyses 68.13
delayed inflammatory reaction 77.1
delayed type hypersensitivity 68.3
depression after irradiation 81.4
determinant definition 84.3
effector 71.5, 75.2
assay 68.3
biological role 68.3
cell migration 68.3
enumeration 83.4
E-rosette technique 55.8

T lymphocyte (*cont.*

flow cytometry subset enumeration 82.9
fluorescence 57.12
Fc receptors 48.2
receptor-positive 71.3
freezing and storage of clone 69.4
genetic programme 75.3
glycoprotein 75.1
growth with conditioned medium 69.1
growth factors (TCGF) 63.8, 68.2
analysis "step 1" 63.11
analysis "step 2" 63.11
blast preparation 63.9
differentiation factors 68.2
interleukin-2 68.2
with limiting dilution of pTc 68.2
production and assay 63.9
quantitation 63.13
see also Interleukin-2
help evaluation 66.11
homogeneous 75.6
human cell lines 69.1
human, limiting dilution cloning method 69.7
hybridoma production 59.4
idiotype-specific 73.4
immune response 84.1
immunodeficiency diagnosis 83.4
immunoregulatory 79.1
inducer 71.1
clone, synthesis 75.5
interactions 68.2
intermediate culture system 79.6
irradiation deficiency 81.4
joining regions 76.7
leader regions 76.7
lectin-induced response analysis 63.8
limiting dilution analysis 65.1
lymphokine growth factors 59.1
lymphokine production 59.3
MHC effect, immune reactivity 72.2
MHC specificity in human 72.2
media and buffers 78.14
memory cells 58.12
migration 57.15
mitogen responses 83.4
mitogens from blast transformation 66.6
monoclonal antibodies 80.1
assay 66.4
production 69.1
monoclonal suppressor factor 80.1
mouse, cell lines 69.1
cloning methods with soluble antigen 69.5
cytolytic alloreactive cloning method 69.4
non-cytolytic, alloreactive, cloning methods 69.3
non-responder 72.1
Peyer's patch 79.1, 4

plating 68.6
poisson distribution 65.1
precursor effectors, limiting dilution 68.2
precursor frequency 68.2
probability distributions 65.1
products 75.3
proliferative response 68.2
receptors 62.3
against self MHC 72.1
constant region 53.3
genes 76.1
gene expression in thymic ontogeny 76.10
protein structure 76.6
subtraction strategies 76.2
recirculation 57.1
recognition site 84.3
regulatory 74.6
circuit 71.1
interaction 72.1
replacing factor (TRF) 70.2, 71.2
responder 72.1
response failure 84.4
response inhibition by cyclosporin A 81.13
restriction phenomenon 102.6
roles 78.1
rosette formation 66.3
separation from B cell 54.1
specificity 72.1, 76.8, 84.5
stable lines 68.2
steering 84.5
subpopulations in sensitized mice 77.11
subsets 53.4
expression 76.9
suppressor factor 78.1
surface Ia inhibition cyclosporin A 81.14
transducer 71.5
typing 83.5
uridine labelling 57.9
variable (V) regions 76.7
Tcs lymphocyte 79.1
I-J subregion 79.2
Tdh lymphocyte, preparation 77.7
Th lymphocyte 71.1
allotype-specific 71.2
antigen recognition 84.2
cell surface markers 68.1
phenotype 68.1
for DTH reaction preparation 77.9
epitope recognition 84.5
family 71.1
carrier-specific augmenting T cell (CTa)
carrier-specific helper T cell (Cth) 71.1
CTL 1 71.1
CTL 2 71.2
Ig specific helper T cells (IgTL) 71.2
frequency analysis 65.2

frequency assessment 68.11
function 65.4
hapten-specific 84.1
responses 65.6
heterogeneity 65.3
immunoglobulin specific 71.2
interaction 84.6
limiting dilution analysis 68.9, 11
activity assay 68.12
specificity 84.5
suppression 75.5
Ts lymphocyte 71.1
afferent suppression assays 77.8
kinetic analysis 77.8
lymph node inhibition 77.9
allotype- 78.1
allotype-specific 78.12
soluble factor 71.3
assay 77.11
assessment in immune response 78.1
carrier-specific 74.3
assay 78.6
clone 75.5
con A-induced 78.4
contrasuppression 78.13, 79.1
I-J determinant 78.13, 79.2
covert 79.1
cyclosporin A subpopulation effects 81.13
in delayed type hypersensitivity 77.1
delayed type hypersensitivity activity 77.3
detection 77.1
determinants 80.3
effector 71.3
efferent suppression assays
DTH passive transfer inhibition 77.10
kinetic analysis 77.10
epitope-specific 78.1, 78.12
families 71.3
carrier-specific suppressor T cells (CTs) 71.3
Ig-special Ts (IgTs) 71.4
functional properties 75.5
GAT/GT in immune suppression 78.7
GAT/GT induction 78.8
I-J$^+$ subregion 78.6
genes 80.3
idiotype-specific 74.4
induction 78.11
immunoglobulin analogy 75.5
Ig-specific 71.4
inducer 71.3
factor 78.6
induction 78.1
methods 77.7
interaction 84.6
KLH-specific induction 78.7
mouse studies 78.1
proteolytic cleavage 75.5

Ts lymphocyte (*cont.*)
recovery from 79.7
regulation 75.2
regulatory interactions 80.1
pathways 71.4
sheep erythrocyte 78.5
specificity 84.5
TsF lymphocyte antibody preparation to 80.3
assays
functional assay 80.3
immunoadsorbent columns 80.4
solid phase radioimmune assay 80.4
constant region determinants 80.3
heavy chain preparation 80.8
light chain preparation 80.8
preparation 77.7
in mRNA 80.7
reconstitution methods 80.8
sheep erythrocyte 78.5
for lymphokine production 69.1
Target cell addition 68.6
for cytotoxicity 57.7
H-2 matched 68.8
for lymphokine bioassay 59.4
nucleated 64.16
preparation 68.5, 13
sources 68.5
Thioglycollate, macrophage stimulator 48.11
preparation 44.16
3-Thiomethylpropionaldehyde (methional) 50.5
Thiourea 50.7
Third and fourth pouch syndrome 83.3
Thoracic duct, cannulation 57.3
for rubidium-36 lymphocyte influor 57.12
lymphocytes (TDL) 57.4
drainage 81.5
clinical use 81.5
in immunosuppression 81.5
in kidney transplantation 81.6
Thromboxanes 81.7
THY-1 loss variants 55.4
U-^{14}C-Thymidine-, lymphocyte labelling method 57.9
6-^{3}H-Thymidine, lymphocyte labelling method 57.9
radiation toxicity 57.9
Thymocyte (*see also* T lymphocyte)
antigens 75.1
Thymocyte, antigen (Thy) 61.1
immunosuppressive antisera to 81.2
subsets 57.15
Thymocytotoxic auto-antibody (NTA), measurement 82.5
Thymus, antibody-producing cells

from 64.18
differentiation of T cell genes 76.9
lymphocyte from 67.1, 75.2
suppressor factor 80.1
T lymphocytes from 53.5
suppressor factor 80.1
Thymus dependent antigen 72.1
Thymus hormone 62.4
Thymus lymphocytes, phenotypic analysis 57.17
Thyroiditis 82.1
Tiaprofenic acid (Surgam) 81.8
Time-lapse cinematography 51.11
Timegadine 81.8
TIP specific amino acids 84.6
Tissue, antigen, microscopic and photography 43.10
perfusion fixation 43.9
bone marrow 53.6
culture lines for NK cells 60.8
genetic marker preparation 56.3
mosaicism 56.1
mouse, cell preparations 43.10
section preparation 43.10
thymus 53.5
Tissue macrophages, mouse 43.1
Tissue transplantation, MHC 72.1
Tissue typing 81.2
Tolerance, in delayed type hypersensitivity 77.2
Toluidine blue stain 56.7
Tonsil, mononuclear cell from 66.3
Total lymphoid Irradiation (TLI) *see* Irradiation, total lymphoid
Toxic factor, soluble 45.9
Toxoplasma, in macrophage activation 48.11
Toxoplasma gondii, macrophage cytotoxicity to 45.8
Tracer sample principle 57.3
Transcobalamin II deficiency 83.2
Transduction 71.4, 5
Transfectant analysis with cytotoxic T cells 68.13
Transfection 68.8
Transformants 68.13
Transmembrane signalling 41.6
Transplantation, immunosuppression in 81.1
Travenol 60.9
Trichinella, in macrophage activation 48.11
Trichloroacetic acid precipitation 47.10
Trinitrobenzene sulphonic acid (TNBS) 77.3
Trinitrochlorobenzene (TNCB), in delayed-type hypersensitivity 77.1
Trinitrophenyl SRBC, indicator cells

78.7
Trinitrophenylated-keyhole limpet hemocyanin (TNP-KL) 78.5
TRIS-HCI buffer, preparation 52.7
Triton X-100 52.7
Trypan blue solution 60.9
Trypanosome, in macrophage activation 48.11
Tryptophan 50.7
Tumour, human 45.2
macrophage culture 45.1
restriction 68.3

Uridine-5-^{3}H, lymphocyte labelling method 57.8
Uridine-^{14}C(U), lymphocyte labelling method 57.8

Vaccine, preparation from pneumococcus 78.10
Variable region, mouse heavy chain sequences 90.1
Varicella zoster virus, antibody response 58.11
Vascular endothelium, and lymphocytes 57.1
Versene 58.13
Videotape, visual assay 51.11
film analysis 51.13
Viral transformation of macrophage cell lines 45.2
Virus, Epstein–Barr, with immunodeficiency 83.3
macrophage interactions 45.8
response against 68.3
specific kill 68.9
T lymphocyte effector responses 68.2

Western immunoblotting 47.14
Wheat germ agglutinin 55.6
WHO immunodeficiency working party 83.5
Wiskott–Aldrich syndrome 83.3

X-chromosome, inactivation 56.1
linked immunodeficiency 56.14
X-linked, agammaglobulinaemia (XIA) 83.1
hypogammaglobulinaemia 83.1
XLR gene family 76.2

Y chromosome, identification 56.3
Yeast cell walls, preparation 48.6

Zones of inhibited phage plaques (ZIPP) 64.16
Zymosan 50.1
macrophage line stimulation 45.6